DISCARD

THE ENGLISH AUGUSTANS

★

THE LIFE OF REASON

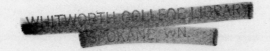

THE
LIFE OF REASON

HOBBES, LOCKE, BOLINGBROKE

BY

D. G. JAMES

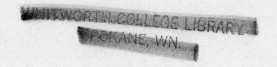

LONGMANS, GREEN AND CO
LONDON · NEW YORK · TORONTO

LONGMANS, GREEN AND CO LTD
6 & 7 CLIFFORD STREET LONDON W 1
ALSO AT MELBOURNE AND CAPE TOWN
LONGMANS, GREEN AND CO INC
55 FIFTH AVENUE NEW YORK 3
LONGMANS, GREEN AND CO
215 VICTORIA STREET TORONTO 1
ORIENT LONGMANS LTD
BOMBAY CALCUTTA MADRAS

First Published 1949

PRINTED BY
SPOTTISWOODE, BALLANTYNE AND CO. LTD
LONDON AND COLCHESTER

To
PHILIP R. MORRIS
THIS VOLUME IS
DEDICATED

Contents

ACKNOWLEDGEMENT

We are indebted to the author, the Rev. Father M. C. D'Arcy,
S.J., and Messrs Sheed and Ward Ltd. for permission to use
a passage from *The Nature of Belief*.

Introduction

THE title of this essay needs some explanation; and I shall try to give the reader some impression of what he may look for, if he troubles to read over the pages that follow.

I give the name of 'Augustans' to the leaders of thought and letters in that period of our history which we are accustomed to call indifferently the Age of Reason or the Age of Neo-classicism; and this period I take roughly as extending from 1650 to 1780. These are indeed rough limits: I give 1650 so as to show that I include the *Leviathan* at one end as a monument of Augustanism and, at the other, I give 1780 to cover (or very nearly) the appearance of Johnson's *Lives of the Poets*. In using the word Augustan as widely as this, I am indeed extending it beyond the limits employed by Mr. Saintsbury in his well-known book; but if we are going to use the word at all, it is hard to see how we can exclude so influential a maker of the age as Hobbes. He, more than any other great writer of the seventeenth and eighteenth centuries, preached the power and scope of human reason; and besides, his influence on Dryden was emphatic and acknowledged.

Yet, in this essay, I have written of only three great Augustans: Hobbes, Locke and Bolingbroke; and of these I have not written studies of their writings in all their aspects. Thus, all three were eminent political theorists; but the reader will find nothing here, or very little, of their ethical and political doctrines. Instead, I have tried to elicit the tone and spirit of those of their writings which treat of human knowledge, imagination and religious feeling; and even here, I cannot claim to have made anything approaching complete studies of their doctrines. What I have done is to speak of their writings with an eye to the consequences they were bound to have on the art of literature and on religion, but chiefly on the former; if the latter appears to the reader to loom sometimes large, it is only because I believe that in the last resort art and religion lie, in certain respects, very near to each other.

I have written in this volume about Hobbes, Locke and Bolingbroke, because I have thought that by speaking of these three I should be able to recreate something of the intellectual idiom in which the literary men of the first half of the period were reared, the intellectual attitudes and beliefs which lay behind and influenced Dryden, Pope, Swift, Addison, and which were to affect belief and feeling up to the end of Augustan times. To read the work of these three philosophers is perhaps the best introduction to the study of the state of affairs with which the literary men of the age had to come to terms and in which they must do the best they could.

I do not mean, of course, that Hobbes, Locke and Bolingbroke were, so to speak, all of a piece, and that their successive philosophies represent merely a continuing development of certain master-ideas. On the contrary, Locke was animated by a passionate antagonism to the leading intentions and motives of Hobbes's writings, even if he disdained open polemic with his doctrines; and Bolingbroke, acknowledging Locke for his master, twisted and changed his master's teaching nearly out of recognition. The term 'reason,' as we employ it in 'the Age of Reason,' is no fixed counter which remains legal tender as we progress through the Augustan years. We shall see this clearly enough. The unity of what I have written comes as much from reaction and perverse developments in those years as from continuous growth and flowering of enduring thoughts.

I had hoped in this essay to speak of Dryden, Congreve and Pope in order, by the study of their writings, to exhibit the ways in which the literary men dealt with the practical problems supplied to them by the philosophers. But I found that this would require a book at least as long as this one; and I shall hope to carry out such a study at another time. Indeed, the story might then be continued to treat of that middle generation, Berkeley (who may, for a number of reasons, appear in this group), Butler, Thomson, Gray and Collins, who in varying degrees and in different ways tried to break out of what was then becoming difficult for them; and then, at the end of the journey, of Hume and Johnson: Hume, in whom the age of reason performed its final demolition of any unified human experience, indeed made mock of all experience; and Johnson, afraid of life and death, clinging, in the surrounding darkness, to common-sense and to a simple and deeply moving Christian piety. These two compose the ends to which the Augustan story comes; but for us now, at the stage where we are in this volume, this is a long way off.

It is illuminating to keep the poets in mind as we read the philosophers, and the philosophers as we read the poets. This is not to say that we should read poetry for the philosophy in it or the philosophy for the poetry in it. And yet there is sense in saying that in any age the philosophers and the poets are alike involved in a single philosophical labour. The Augustan age is especially interesting in this respect, partly because the poets of the first half of the period wrote a good deal of what may be called philosophical poetry and partly because they read or listened to the philosophers with deep attention, if sometimes with uncomprehending ears. And on the other side, the philosophers were most frequently literary; they had, for much the bigger part, style; they were writers; and some of them, indeed the majority of them, take their place amongst the most splendid composers in the English tongue; of our three, Hobbes and Bolingbroke were masters of English prose.

But to say nothing of this, there is, in all truth, a philosophical labour common to philosophers and artists. But if there is, in some sense, a common philosophical labour, the problem with which all are concerned is not, as we would expect, equally clear to both. The philosophers formulate the problem; it is their job to do so with the greatest possible clearness; they state it and then wrestle with it. But the poets must largely suffer and endure it, without expressing it; or rather, they exhibit the problems in their practice; the problem shows itself in the forms their art takes; their poetry, in its varying forms, may be seen as symptoms of a distress and unease which they do not clearly apprehend and bring into sharp philosophical light; and because they are artists and so far not philosophers, they fight with an enemy they at best see only obscurely. Poetry, after all, as a great poet once said, is not so fine a thing as philosophy; it must move in a certain inevitable obscurity; and to leave the obscurity to try to solve the problem which ultimately agitates and distresses it, it must pass into philosophy. Pass into, indeed, but not necessarily be lost in, philosophy. The *Divine Comedy* stands for a warning against rash theory. Still, what was possible for Dante has been possible for no other poet; certainly it was not possible for Shakespeare; still less was it possible for a poet of the Augustan age. But it will be better to speak of these large matters at the end, instead of at the beginning, of our story.

Finally, it is only fair to the reader to tell him that I have tried, in the course of my narration, to suggest a view of human knowledge which may, I hope, be judged to do more justice to our experience in perception, art and religion than the Augustan philosophers of whom I speak were able or disposed to do. The doctrine I have put forward will at least, I trust, have the merit of throwing certain aspects of Augustan teaching into sharp relief, even if it be judged to be itself mistaken; it may at least play a rôle in narration, even if it is thought to fail as a construction. It consists in saying of human knowledge that it is essentially symbolical; and I shall argue that the chief lack in the Augustan mind is that it was not aware of symbolism in the sense in which I understand and try to expound it here. In doing this, I shall perhaps be able not only to bring out certain striking features of Augustan philosophy; I shall also be preparing the way for study of certain striking features of Augustan poetry.

I am conscious that to lead argument into a historical essay is a dangerous and risky business; and my readers may well judge that I have failed to justify my attempt to do so. But the historian of ideas owes it to his readers not to withhold judgement on the ideas he speaks of, however respectful of those ideas he may, and no doubt ought to, be. Merely to narrate the ideas of the past is certainly no work of supererogation; on the contrary, it is necessary, exacting and important. But one has to make up one's mind about them; and provided one tries to do so without rash pre-conception and prejudices, no harm can perhaps come of trying to make narrative serve the purpose of argument, and argument the purposes of narrative.

Besides, in writing about Hobbes, Locke and Bolingbroke, I could hardly fail to be aware of the relevance of what they were and what they said to our own times. This relevance will also be plain to the reader and I need not enlarge on it. But in writing about our great 'Age of Reason', I have wished to suggest a view of the life of reason more catholic than that which prevailed then and which finally produced Hume. And in our own time, it is natural to feel some dismay at the prevalent willingness of philosophers to concentrate on conceptual truth and then on the so-called analysis of propositions to the exclusion of the plain facts of perception, of art, of history, and of religion. There is, I believe, no more surprising thing, in this bewildering age, than the spectacle of philosophers who seem to be concerned only with thought in its narrowest sense; what is not surprising is that philosophical thought then turns out to be, in their hands, something of little human importance. I should be, I hope, the last man to wish to underestimate the value and importance of the intelligence; but so to lose sight of the wider life of reason, which is manifested in sense-perception, art, history and religion as well as in proposition and logical inference, is simply to play into the hands of irrationality. In saying this, I fear that I may appear disrespectful to some of my seniors, whose learning and mental powers are much greater than my own; but it has now, I should have thought, become fairly obvious that the outcome of much of the philosophy of our time is a harsh positivism which ignores clear facts of our experience and which commands reason to be silent on matters of palmary importance to human life. To say this is not, I am convinced, to say something which smacks of anti-intellectualism; and in what follows I have tried to outline a view of the life of reason as something growing from humble beginnings in perception into art, science and religion through an interplay of forces all of which manifest a rational principle. Tensions there may be between these forces; but they are family tensions only; they must be accepted as necessary features of the life of reason in its fullness and variety; and each of them has its part to play in bringing the mind to where alone it can find satisfaction.

I wish to express my gratitude to my friend Dr. Stephan Körner, who has read through the typescript and has made many valuable criticisms and suggestions. He himself works in a different philosophical tradition from that in which I have tried to write; and I have all the more appreciated the care and forbearance he has given to what I have tried to do. What errors remain are entirely my own.

I am again in the debt of my sister, Mrs. Frank Blackmore, for her excellent typing of my MS. My debt to my wife is so huge and circumambient a thing, that to thank her for helping me with the index seems little short of silly.

January, 1949.

CHAPTER ONE ... *The Proud Mind*

I SHALL plunge at once into narrative and begin by speaking of
Hobbes. It is, indeed, impossible to speak, in all strictness, of a
beginning of English Augustanism, as it is impossible to speak of
the absolute beginning of anything else. But it is in the writings of
Hobbes that English Augustan Æsthetic has its first philosophical
statement. It was to prove a potent statement. For Dryden read the
Sage of Malmesbury with care and respect; he refers to him in his
critical writings and acknowledges his debts to him in poetical theory;
and Aubrey has recorded Dryden's saying that he used his doctrines
in his plays. Certainly in Dryden's critical writings the alliance between Augustan philosophy and Augustan critical orthodoxy becomes
close enough.

I

Now at a later stage I shall try to recreate some of Hobbes's philosophical thinking. But first, it is necessary to observe certain facts in his
life story. The facts, in their bareness, are the grand preface to our long
narrative. They need only to be set out to become a part of the verit-
able history of Augustanism, and cannot fail to acquire in the mind of
the reader the depth and expressiveness of symbol.

To begin with, Hobbes's life stretches from 1588 to 1678. It is unlikely that any other pair of dates, marking the birth and death of any
great Englishman, can strike the imagination with such force; so many
years and experience of so many profound changes have been given to
few men of genius. If our minds travel back we may indeed recall the
long life of Isocrates, which began before the Peloponnesian War and
ended with (though not, perhaps, as Milton believed, on account
of) Chaeronea. Certainly the comparison, if we think of length of
years and the witness of many and mighty political changes, is enough
to hold the mind; but the likeness, if we think of the burden of their
writing and thought, quickly gives way to contrast. Isocrates was and
remains a notable figure in the history of humanist education and consistently upheld letters against philosophy; Hobbes deserted the cause
of humanism for a philosophy mastered, from its inception in his mind,
by mathematical abstractions; and certainly he acquired, as we may say

1

without prejudice, some of the views of some of the sophists whom
Plato combated and of whom Isocrates disapproved.

In the second place, there is some truth in saying that Hobbes was
nearly fifty before he became a philosopher. We must be careful not to
exaggerate; but it is at least true to say that it was in 1637 that his way
became finally clear to him and his perception of the world and of
human experience sharp and assured. Of his stay in Paris at the end of
the 1634–37 tour he says,

> Hic ego Mersennum novi, communico et illi
> De rerum motu quae meditatus eram.
> Is probat et multis commendat; tempore ab illo
> Inter philosophos et numerabar ego.[1]

Certainly the year 1637 is crucial in the life of Hobbes. To be
acknowledged by Mersenne, the friend and confidant of Descartes, and
the very meeting-place and changing-house of the new ideas, was
enough. But the year is important for other reasons. A year or so
earlier he had met Galileo, old, blind and a prisoner, and never lost his
reverence for him; Galileo he says 'was the first that opened to us the
gate of natural philosophy universal, which is the knowledge of the
nature of *motion*.' (E. 1. p. viii). But if Hobbes stood in reverence of
Galileo, he stood in no great awe of Descartes, whose *Discourse on
Method* was published in the very year of 1637; and against the *Meditations* Hobbes was to send some lively and assured objections in 1640.
In 1636 Corneille's *Le Cid* had been performed, and the French classical
drama, despite all that was urged against Corneille's play, was begun.
In the following year there was to appear in Italy a young English poet
who was to contemplate there the writing of an epic, but who was also
to listen to Galileo. It is impressive enough to reflect that 1637 saw
both Hobbes straightly upon his path, and the publication of the *Discourse*; it is perhaps still more impressive to reflect that within a few
years both Hobbes and Milton discussed natural philosophy with
Galileo. Galileo confirmed Hobbes in a resolve to make life and the
world extraordinarily simple and clear by the application of geometry;
and as Hobbes went on, to his own complete satisfaction, to do so, his
personality acquired indeed something of the neatness and assurance of
a proposition out of Euclid. But the neatness and adroitness of

---

[1] L. 1. p. xc.
    Quotations from Hobbes's writings will be made from Sir William Molesworth's edition,
London, 1839–45, except where otherwise stated. The references will be preceded by 'L'
or 'E', indicating the Latin and English works respectively.

Hobbes's mind certainly had no share in Milton's. The Tuscan artist no doubt helped to give to Milton a certain easy sense of the magnitude of the new universe, and thereby facilitated Satan's way across Chaos; but for the rest, what Milton felt of the new possibilities of science only added to the difficulties of a mind already sombre, complicated and uncertain of its way. The thought of the new powers which these men perceived science would afford was sedative for Hobbes; for Milton it was an added stimulant in a mind naturally more addicted to power than to the clemency and blandness of Christianity.

But my immediate purpose is not to look forward from this crucial year, but to look backwards into the earlier life of Hobbes. Hobbes had been lucky in his education. He had been taught Classics, Aubrey tells us,[1] by 'Mr. Robert Latimer, a young man of about 19 or 20, newly come from the University, who then kept a private schoole in Westport'; and Aubrey adds that 'this Mr. Latimer was a good Graecian, and the first that came into our parts hereabout since the Reformation.' Before Hobbes went to Magdalen Hall, at the age of fourteen, he had 'turned Euripidis *Medea* out of Greeke into Latin Iambiques, which he presented to his master.' Thus the new New Learning came into Wiltshire, and by good luck it was transmitted to young Hobbes.

Hobbes has left us two accounts of his life, both in Latin, one in prose, the other in elegiacs. In the prose autobiography he says of his Oxford days only that he was there for five years *operam impendens studio logicae physicae Aristotelicae* (L. 1. p. xiii). But his Muse tells us more. He was placed in the lowest logic class, he says, and listened carefully to his beardless lecturer on the Syllogism. Clearly the logic left him unmoved. The forms of the Syllogism *tarde disco, disco tamen, abjicioque* (L. 1. p. lxxxvii); and Aubrey says that 'he did not care much for logick, yet he learned it, and thought himself a good disputant.'[2] Nor did Aristotle's theory of perception move him to curiosity. Later, of course, he was to say some hard things about 'sensible species'; yet we might have expected that one who was to show such lively interest in the theory of perception would have been moved by them to reflection; but his time for thinking was not yet. It is clear that all the philosophy he was taught at Oxford meant nothing to him; all the doctrines he learnt, and there were many, went, he says, over his head. The truth is that his mind was elsewhere, in the reading of maps, in following Drake in imagination round the world, in thinking of the wonders of

[1] John Aubrey, *Brief Lives*, ed. Andrew Clark, Oxford, 1898, vol. i. pp. 328–29.
[2] *Ibid.*, p. 329.

unknown lands;[1] he was more a man of imagination than of thought; and was to remain so for some twenty years.

In 1609, the year after Hobbes left Oxford, Kepler published the first of the laws of motion, and Galileo was already far in his career of discovery. But if scholastic theory had not touched Hobbes into life, he also knew nothing of the new physics. Indeed, without interest in either philosophy or physics he stood, in the early years of his tutorship in the Cavendish family, to which he went soon after leaving Oxford, in danger of losing even his classics. It is natural to believe that it would have been easy for him at this time to sink into idleness and flaccidity of mind. Of very humble origin, he had become a tutor in a noble family, and might have rested content. But again Hobbes was lucky. The Earl of Devonshire sent him with young Cavendish to the Continent. He had been made a scholar by Latimer, fresh from the University, who brought to Malmesbury what had begun in Italy in the fourteenth century. But the impulse of Latimer's teaching had died; and Hobbes, sent abroad, now suffered, under the impact of Italy herself, a rebirth of love for the classics. No doubt it is unfair to give credit only to good luck. Hobbes deserved his good fortune. He was, he says in the prose autobiography, speaking of the time of his first tutorship, *temperans, sedulus, hilaris* (L. i. p. xiii). Certainly he was, and was to remain so. And if he had good fortune in being sent to Italy, he owed it to himself that he was sedulous. He came back from Italy, made himself a scholar accomplished in Greek and a fine composer in Latin and English.

He was to remain with the Cavendishes for twenty years—till 1628; and until this year he was a Renaissance scholar, immersed in classical antiquity, having thrown aside philosophy and logic. Two things at least he did and had to show for his labours. First, excellence in writing Latin, not, he tells us, floridly, but having *vim verborum cogitatis congruentem* (L. i. p. xiv); second, his translation of the greatest writer of history in the ancient world and perhaps of all time. Of his Thucydides and of his humanist period I shall speak later. But I wish now to mention his celebrated friendship with Francis Bacon which falls within this period, probably between the years 1620 and 1625. This will lead me on, as the reader will understand, to make some observations about the history of Hobbes's mind during the years from 1628 to 1637, when he was in process of becoming a philosopher. I shall then return to speak of his humanist phase.

[1] Aubrey. *loc. cit.*, vol. i. p. 329 and L. i. p. lxxxvii.

In the first half or so of the twenties 'the Lord Chancellour Bacon loved to converse with him'. 'His lordship', Aubrey goes on to say, 'was a very contemplative person, and was wont to contemplate in his delicious walks at Gorambery ' (p. 331). It was Bacon's habit to have someone attending on him 'with inke and paper ready to sett downe presently his thoughts. His lordship would often say that he better liked Mr. Hobbes's taking his thoughts, then any of the other, because he understood what he wrote . . .' There follows at once, in Aubrey's papers: 'It is to be remembered that about these times Mr. T. H. was much addicted to musique, and practiced on the base-violl'; and this scrap of information, coming thus in Aubrey's notes, comes like an inspired observation on Hobbes's indifference, if we are to judge by his own writings, to the thoughts of Bacon, which he yet transcribed so competently and so greatly to the satisfaction of the lord of Gorhambury. We may be surprised that the doctrines of sensible and intelligible species did not rouse Hobbes to philosophy; it is astonishing that Bacon thus appears neither then to have stirred him to thought nor later, in recollection, to have left an unmistakable mark upon his reflections. It is difficult to exaggerate the importance of this. Philosophy was not to begin in Hobbes's mind until about 1630, when he was some forty years of age; and it was neither the maker of the old nor the new Organon that was to set him on fire. For this, two things were necessary; one of them was to be indeed an 'Organon', one which Aristotle was too much of a biologist to have valued and about which Bacon knew little and cared as much. The other was the passionately felt need to philosophize, the urgent requirements of life. Later in the twenties the Organon was put, as it were, into his hands; and by that time the need and urgency were becoming strong in his mind.

The new instrument was geometry. 'He was 40 yeares old', says Aubrey, 'before he looked on geometry; which happened accidentally. Being in a gentleman's library . . . Euclid's Elements lay open, and 'twas the 47 El. libri I. He read the proposition. "By G—", sayd he, "this is impossible!" So he reads the demonstration of it, which referred him back to such a proposition, which proposition he read. That referred him back to another; which he also read. Et sic deinceps, that at last he was demonstratively convinced of that trueth. This made him in love with geometry' (p. 332). He was forty when he fell in love, and his love was to bring him a lot of trouble; but certainly he never fell out of love. It was some time between 1629 and 1631 that this incident occurred, when Hobbes was tutor to the son of Sir Gervase Clifton and had gone abroad with him. But by this time the constitutional struggle was well begun. Eliot was leading the Commons. A few years earlier Charles I's Parliament had impeached Buckingham; Eliot had been imprisoned; and writs of Habeas Corpus had been refused when the King's taxation was defied. In 1628 the Commons presented the Petition of Right, Buckingham was assassinated at Portsmouth, Wentworth went over to the King and Laud was promoted to be Bishop of London. In 1629 Finch was held down in the Chair while resolutions were passed declaring an enemy of the realm anyone urging innovation in religion or advising taxation without the approval of Parliament; and Parliament, dissolved, was not to meet again until 1640. The constitutional issues were thus, when Hobbes 'looked' as he tells us, 'on geometry', clearly enough defined. It was this that created the need for philosophy.

Now it was not until 1640 that, in *The Elements of Law*, Hobbes set forth his political doctrines; and we have nothing written by him at the time of his discovery of geometry which tells us of his feelings about the constitutional crisis. But it can hardly be imagined that Hobbes had been indifferent to the events of 1627 to 1629 and to what Charles's assumption of personal rule in 1629 signified. When Hobbes came back in 1637 from his third tour, his philosophical ideas and intentions, I have said, were formed. Body, Man and Society comprises all philosophy, he tells us in the verse life, in that part where he speaks of his return to England in 1637; and he intends three books, one on each of these departments of philosophy. His views on politics, like his views on body and on human nature, are formed in all essentials; and it is hard to believe that they did not spring from strong feelings roused in him, from the outset of the constitutional struggle, by the politics of England.

If this is so, we may say that in the years from 1628 (in which he temporarily left the service of the Cavendishes for that of Sir Gervase Clifton) to 1630 (or thereabouts, for we have not precise information) Hobbes both falls in love with geometric method and learns to hate the intransigence and disobedience of Parliament to the monarch. The instrument and the need to use it came closely together in Hobbes's life; and geometry, perhaps, will arrest the political struggle and ensure the obedience of the Commons. It was a bold mind which saw in geometry a means of solving political problems and of substituting for the violence of civil war a mathematical peace. The reader will understand that I am not at this stage concerned with the substance of Hobbes's thinking, but only with its origin and its sources of power. What neither Aristotle through the medium of a yet mediaeval Oxford, nor the very presence and converse of Francis Bacon could do, was done by an alliance of geometry with a bitter constitutional quarrel in which the authority of the monarch was at stake. There was a need and a problem, yearly more urgent and more pressing; not remote, but threatening the lives of all British subjects; and suddenly the means and the method for their treatment are in Hobbes's hands.

The problem, I have said, threatened the lives of all British subjects; and of these Hobbes was one. His own safety was at stake; and in fairness to him the Ethic he was to make did not allow for more than a calculating altruism. His philosophy is at least honest and consistent; and consistency requires that we should see his books as inspired in no small degree by his desire for personal safety and security. It is here, and it is hard to imagine Hobbes denying it, that we find much of the origin and source of his thought. It would have been more agreeable perhaps to trace the beginnings of his philosophy to Aristotle or to Bacon; it is ignominious perhaps to trace it only to Hobbes himself and his fearful nature. But we speak only in the spirit of Hobbes himself, and, apart from the evidence of his thought, he never tried to hide his timidity. Fear was his twin, he said. It was commonly held that he was afraid 'to lye alone at night in his chamber'; this, says Aubrey, was untrue; but he had often heard Hobbes say 'that he was not afrayd of sprights, but afraid of being knockt on the head for five or ten pounds, which rogues might thinke he had in his chamber'—the slander was not so slanderous, after all. (He had another reason for locking up at night. 'He had alwayes bookes of prick-song lyeing on his table:—e.g. of H. Lawes' etc. *Songs*—which at night, when he was abed, and the dores made fast, and was sure nobody heard him, he sang aloud (not that he had a very good voice) but for his health's sake: he did beleeve it did his lunges good, and conduced much to prolong his life') (p. 352). In 1640, with the Long Parliament installed and looking like remaining so, Hobbes, fearing that his *Elements of Law*, which had been circulating in manuscript, would get him into trouble, left discreetly for France. His fear was out of all proportion to the danger; but 'doubting how they would use him' Hobbes 'went over to France, the first of all that fled, and there continued eleven years, to his damage some thousands of pounds deep' (E. 4. p. 414). 'The first of all that fled', he says of himself. For once we suspect that Hobbes is here cherishing an illusion; and to our suspicion we add a mild curiosity to know how he calculated his 'damage'. But in 1651 he makes an escape in the opposite direction,

back to England. The conclusion of *Leviathan* had got him into difficulties with Charles's courtiers in Paris; he thought of Ambassadors
come abroad for the Parliament who had been stabbed to death by
Royalists, and again decides for safety—or what he judged to be greater
safety than he could have in France—and goes to England. The verses
in which he writes of his journey are touched with self-pity; in fairness
to him he did not try to build himself up into a hero:

> In patriam redeo tutelae non bene certus,
>   Sed nullo potui tutior esse loco;
> Frigus erat, nix alta, senex ego, ventus acerbus;
>   Vexat equus sternax et salebrosa via.   (L. i. p. xciii.)

He was not indeed cast for a heroic rôle; and he was to argue that the
monarch must certainly suffer at least one mitigation of his prodigious
authority: he might not compel any subject to serve in war.

And yet it would be absurd to represent Hobbes as a creature of fear.
Equally, it would be absurd to represent him as a man of brooding
melancholy. Physical fear he certainly had, and a love of security and
safety. But, as I have said, it required a bold mind to apply geometry
to politics; and the reader will recall his description of himself as
temperans, *sedulus* and *hilaris*. Dilthey has said of Hobbes that 'from the
depths of his personality, formed in travel, in courts and in watching
the tangles of politics, came his profound melancholy, his suspicions,
fearful diffidence of life, and his passionate desire for a peaceful and
assured condition'.[1] This is not true, or at best only partially. For nowhere does Hobbes give us an impression of melancholy and suspicion,
watchful as he was for his own safety and capable of making long-term
plans to ensure it. It is much safer to follow Hobbes himself than
Dilthey; for Hobbes's head was cool enough to see even himself with
few illusions, and he gives us no grounds for romanticizing him into a
sombre misanthrope. 'Being naturally of a cheerfull and pleasant
humour, he affected not at all austerity and gravity and to looke
severe', says Aubrey; and Aubrey further tells us that 'he had a good
eie, and that of a hazell colour, which was full of life and spirit, even to
the last. When he was earnest in discourse, there shone (as it were) a
bright live-coale within it. He had two kinds of looks:—when he
laugh't, was witty, and in a merry humour, one could scarce see his
eies; by and by, when he was serious and positive, he open'd his eies
round (i.e. his eie-lids)' (pp. 348–9). This is not a portrait of misan-
thropical melancholy.

[1] Dilthey, *Gesammelte Schriften*, vol. ii. p. 246.

The truth is that Hobbes was both physically timid and strikingly sanguine. Aubrey says that 'he was sanguineo—melancholicus'. But melancholy he was not except in a lively apprehensiveness for personal safety as well as for orderliness and peacefulness of life. Sanguine he certainly was, of a 'fresh, ruddie complexion', and having those properties of mind the word connotes, of courage, hope and confidence. It seems a curious mixture; but there is no doubt of its existence in Hobbes. After all, there were not twins but triplets: Hobbes, Fear and Sanguinity. For if his physical timidity made the contemplation of civil strife an impulse to reflection, there was also that in him that gave his mind a prodigious and dashing courage in devising and publishing a doctrine of an unheard-of heterodoxy whereby to ensure a quiet life for himself and everybody else. His assurance and courage in his philosophical thinking are clear; he never abated his confidence in mathematical method, and courageously carried it to its most logical conclusion in devising a thorough materialism and, for all theoretical (not practical) purposes, a thorough atheism; and he showed as much assurance in publishing these outrageous doctrines as in devising them. If it was fear that made him first to think, it was hope and confidence and courage that moved him to apply the instrument of mathematical method, so firmly and well, to the whole of experience.

The reader will recall that I have been led to speak of the years from 1628 to 1637 in Hobbes's life and of the circumstances of his becoming a philosopher, from observing that Bacon of all men, whom he knew well in the early twenties, did not rouse him to wish to be a philosopher. It was his fear, occasioned by political strife, and his sanguinity, called out by his lucky discovery of geometry, that roused him to be a philosopher ; and this was probably in the last year of the decade. It was not long before he was putting his philosophical thoughts on paper. It was probably as early as 1630 that he composed his first philosophical essay, selections from which Tönnies published in 1889. Here we are in a halfway house between what he learned at Oxford and what was to be his settled doctrine in physics, epistemology and ethics. At last he is thinking hard about sensible species; but motion is clearly becoming the mastering idea. From this time forwards his mind is in a ferment.

> Ast ego perpetuo naturam cogito rerum,
>   Seu rate, seu curru, sive ferebar equo.
> Et mihi visa quidem est toto res unica mundo
>   Vera, licet multis falsificata modis. (L. 1. p. lxxxix.)

In 1631 he comes back from abroad where he had been with the son of Sir Gervase Clifton. In the same year he returns to the Cavendishes, to educate the son of his former and late pupil; in 1634 he goes with him abroad, on the tour in which he was to meet Galileo, become the friend of Mersenne, and be counted amongst the philosophers.

Now when we consider in what way and by what occasion Hobbes became a philosopher, and reflect that the impact of English politics on his mind seems to have been greater than that of Francis Bacon, we find confirmation for our impression that Hobbes's prose is passionate enough. Certainly his philosophical thought will be as mathematical as he can make it. But it will be mathematical at the instance of strong feeling and of the most urgently desired practical effects; and from this passionate thought, as Mr. Pogson Smith observed, will come his *style*. For Hobbes's style is no accident; it is the image of a mind whose intelligence is not the servant of a free and disinterested curiosity, but of a total personality. Aubrey tells us that 'he did not care to give, neither was he adroit at, a present answer to a serious quaere: he has as lieve they should have expected an extemporary solution to an arithmeticall probleme, for he turned and winded and compounded in philosophy, politiques, etc., as if he had been at analyticall [mathematicall?] worke' (p. 340); and again, that '(though he was ready and happy in repartying in *drollery*) he did not care to give a present answer *to a question*' (p. 356). This signifies, we may think, the engagement of all of him in intellectual work ; he needed to marshal his whole personality before he could think well; philosophy was not an affair of quick wits but of directing and orientating his total mind. Thus, it was not his beardless praelector nor the greatest thinker of England who stirred his intellect into ceaseless life; more potent, we can believe, was the thought of Mr. Speaker Finch, held down in the Chair of the Commons. We are not far astray if we say that about 1629, under the combined impact of politics and geometry, of power and mathematics, Hobbes's intellect took fire. 'In his youth', Aubrey tells us, 'he was unhealthy and of an ill complexion (yellowish). His lord, who was a waster, sent him up and downe to borrow money, and to gett gentlemen to be bound for him, being ashamed to speake him selfe; he took colds, being wett in his feet (then there were no hackney coaches to stand in the streetes), and trod both his shoes aside the same way. Notwithstanding he was well beloved; they lov'd his company for his pleasant facetiousness and good-nature' (p. 347). It is a pathetic picture of the dependent humanist scholar. But Aubrey says: 'From forty, or better, he grew healthier, and then he had a fresh, ruddy complexion'. Hobbes was forty in 1628. The humanist becomes the rationalist but by no means unimpassioned philosopher. Coming back from Italy in 1610 he made himself a fine classical scholar, read prodigiously and translated Thucydides; but in later years 'he had very few books. I never sawe (said Sir William Petty) above halfe a dozen about him in his chamber . . .'; and Aubrey adds: 'his contemplation was much more then his reading. He was wont to say that if he had read as much as other men, he should have knowne no more then other men' (p. 349).

I turn now to the philosophy of reason and imagination which the mathematical philosopher was to give us. We shall come back later to the sickly, wet-footed, ill-complexioned humanist scholar.

II

I shall now try to reconstruct some of Hobbes's philosophical thinking. Hobbes, I have said, was a curious mixture of the timid and the sanguine; there moves through all his thinking the desire to establish secure power; he was sanguine that this could be done, and that great occasions for fear could thereby be removed. 'The end of knowledge is power; and the use of theories (which among geometricians, serve for the finding out of properties) is for the construction of problems; and, lastly the scope of all speculation is the performing of some action, or thing to be done.' So he writes in the opening of the *De Corpore* (E. 1. p. 7), which was completed in 1655, some four years after his melancholy return to England. Natural philosophy gives us architecture and navigation and 'instruments for all uses'; but moral and civil philosophy save us from 'all such calamities as may be avoided by human industry', and which 'arise from war, but chiefly [we might have expected him to say it] from civil war'; and the 'cause of civil war is, that men know not the causes of war nor peace, there being but few in the world that have learned those duties which unite and keep men in peace, that is to say, that have learned the rules of civil life sufficiently. Now, the knowledge of these rules is moral philosophy' (E. 1. p. 8). The chief end of philosophy is to secure that civil war becomes impossible and the power and authority of the state absolute. Philosophy will control nature by understanding it; it will also control man by understanding *him*. Philosophy *is* power. Power therefore is in the mind, or nowhere, and 'every man brought

Philosophy, that is, Natural Reason, into the world with him' (E. 1.
p. 1). 'Philosophy . . . the child of the world and your own mind', he
says in the *Epistle to the Reader*, which opens the English version of the
De Corpore, 'is within yourself; perhaps not fashioned yet, but like the
world its father, as it was in the beginning, a thing confused . . . Imitate
the creation: if you will be a philosopher in good earnest, let your
reason[1] move upon the deep of your own cogitations and experience;
those things that lie in confusion must be set asunder, distinguished,
and every one stamped with its own name set in order.' He himself,
in his own thinking, will follow the very order of creation. In the
beginning he will set up the light of reason; and in it a new heaven and
a new earth and a new man, subject to command, will arise. Reason
will make the world, and reason therefore will control it. And it will
not be Hobbes's private world, but the world of all men, in widest
commonalty spread. 'Have not all men one kind of soul, and the same
faculties of mind?' (E. 1. p. 8). Nothing less than the making of a
universe could serve for a theme for Milton's masterpiece. Nothing
less, we shall see, than the thought of making of a universe animated
Hobbes's thinking.

Hobbes defines philosophy in this way, in the first chapter of the
De Corpore: 'Philosophy is such knowledge of effects or appearances, as
we acquire by true ratiocination from the knowledge we have first of
their causes or generation: And again, of such causes or generations as
may be from knowing first their effects' (E. 1. p. 3). In Latin (and it is
the Latin alone that is strictly Hobbes's) it runs: 'Philosophia est
Effectuum sive Phaenomenwn ex conceptis eorum Causis seu Genera-
tionibus, et rursus Generationum quae esse possunt, ex cognitis
effectibus per rectam ratiocinationem acquisita cognitio' (L. 1. p. 2).
Much, we know, and Hobbes certainly knew, depends upon definitions;
and the whole of Hobbes's philosophy is implicit in this definition. In
section 8 of the same chapter he says: 'The *subject* of Philosophy, or the
matter it treats of, is every body of which we can conceive any generation (*corpus omne cuius generatio aliqua concipi . . . potest*)'. Philosophical knowledge, a very different thing from the knowledge we have
in 'sense and memory of things', is got by *ratiocination* whereby we
comprehend the causes or generations of things; that is to say, we have
philosophical knowledge only when we understand a thing's coming-

---

[1] The reader will understand that the word 'reason' as ordinarily employed by the
Augustan thinkers means 'ratiocination'. This is a narrow employment of a word which
should, as I suggested earlier, be used to mean something wider than conceptual knowledge. But we have, it seems, no alternative but to accept this two-fold usage.

to-be. Now at first sight this may seem harmless enough. But at later sight we see not only that it is not harmless (because theology is thus ruled out of the philosophical domain, for God did not come-to-be), but also because Hobbes requires of philosophy (which comprises both what we now understand by science and what we now understand by philosophy) that it understand, as we may be said to understand a theorem in Euclid, everything which has a place in the world. This he believes to be a not impossible task. On the contrary, if philosophy is not this, it is nothing. And it can come to this understanding because it can conceive the beginnings and coming-to-be of things. 'And this is the science of causes, or as they call it, of the διότι. All other science, which is called the ὅτι, is either perception by sense, or the imagination, or memory remaining after such perception' (E. 1. p. 66).

Now this is high rationalism. But before I go further, I remark two other features of this definition. First, I remark that his definition of philosophy, given in Chapter 1 of the *De Corpore*, is repeated in the first section of Chapter 6. But it is repeated with differences. 'Philosophy', the second statement runs, 'is the knowledge we acquire, by true ratiocination, of appearances, or apparent effects, from the knowledge we have of some possible production or generation of the same; and of such production, as has been or may be, from the knowledge we have of the effects' (E. 1. p. 65). The reader will observe that he speaks here 'of some *possible* production or generation'. Now either definition will serve Hobbes equally well. For what is in his mind is that if ratiocination can explain certain effects by its knowledge of an intelligible cause, it is indifferent whether in fact that cause is the real cause. God *may* have brought about certain effects by the use of another, and no doubt equally intelligible, cause; but it is enough for mortal ratiocination to know what might intelligibly have caused them, what may be *conceived* as a cause which would, inevitably, have *these* results. Thus Hobbes is less concerned to discover the methods of God in creation than to satisfy the rational requirements of the human mind; and whether in fact we know the real cause or another but equally intelligible cause, is immaterial to the results for human happiness. It is less reality than intelligibility that Hobbes looks for. This leads me to my second observation, which is concerned with the same matter.

The reader will notice a difference between the concluding clauses of the definitions. I italicize the relevant parts. In the first we have: 'And again, of such causes or generations *as may be* from knowing first their effects'. In the second we have: 'And of such production, *as has been or may be*, from the knowledge we have of the effects'. Now in the latter part of the definition Hobbes is speaking of that method of obtaining philosophical knowledge whereby instead of proceeding from cause to effect we proceed from effect to cause. Here, instead of knowing a cause from which we deduce certain effects, we observe certain effects and cast about to conceive a cause. But in this event, too, it is of little importance that we finally alight on the real cause; it is enough that we conceive an intelligible cause. Philosophical knowledge is of such production *as has been or may be*, he says; and presumably we have no means of knowing the 'has been' from the 'may be'; it is enough that our reason be satisfied.

Now of these two processes, moving forward from cause to effect and going backward from effect to cause, Hobbes clearly gives first place to the former. He explains in the sixth chapter of the *De Corpore* that it is possible for men to 'search after science either simply or indefinitely; that is, to know as much as they can, without propounding to themselves any limited question; or they enquire into the cause of some determined appearance . . . as what is the cause of *light*, of *heat*, of *gravity* . . . or the like'. Yet neither method required, in Hobbes's view, the use of experiment; and both therefore must seem to us strange and useless proceedings. Kant, a century later, was better able to understand what was involved in the scientific investigations and discoveries of Galileo and Torricelli than their contemporary Hobbes. Kant says that in the time of these scientists, 'a light broke upon all students of nature.' But the light of which Kant speaks did not, in fact, break upon Hobbes, who was nevertheless an ardent 'student of nature'. 'For Reason', said Kant, in a statement classical in all but its prose, 'must go to Nature to be taught by her. And in one hand Reason must have its principles, for only when appearances conform thereto can they (i.e. the principles) have validity as law; but in the other hand Reason must carry experiment, contrived also in accordance with these principles. But Reason will yet go to Nature not as a scholar who only recites what his teacher wishes, but as a judge having authority who compels witnesses to answer the questions he puts to them.'[1] But the idea of a fertile union of principles and experiment was lost on Hobbes. His contempt for the 'gentlemen of Gresham College' is well known; and 'not every one that brings from beyond the seas a new gin, or other jaunty device, is therefore a philosopher. For if you reckon that way,

<hr>

[1] *Kritik der Reinen Vernunft*, Hartenstein, Leipzig, 1867, vol. iii. p. 16.

not only apothecaries and gardeners, but many other sorts of workmen, will put in for and get the prize' (E. 4. p. 437). 'As for mean and common experiments', he says elsewhere, 'I think them a great deal better witness of nature, than those that are forced by fire, and known but to very few' (E. 7. p. 117).

Now if we undertake search for science *simpliciter*, we shall proceed, Hobbes tells us, by analysis, which he calls the method of attaining to the universal knowledge (notions) of things; by abstraction we will work back to know the 'causes of universal things, or of such accidents as are common to all bodies, that is, to all matter' (E. 1. p. 68). By this process we find three universal notions; there is motion, which is the universal cause, there is space in which motion occurs, and there is body. We may leave out, in our analytical search, all else but these; and what has been left out (and there are many things left out) may be deduced from these. All is body, motion and space ; and those things which seem not to be expressible in terms of them are yet, in fact, to be explained wholly by them.

It is a surprising method, and the results are as surprising as the method. For one thing, another rationalist philosopher, Descartes, sitting before his stove in 1619 and trying to find out, in an uncertain world, something of which he could be sure, decided that it was quite certain, and a clear and distinct idea, that he existed. The whole physical world, motion, matter, his own body, space, might be illusion, but he must at least exist before he could be so deceived. But what was *he*? The answer is 'a substance the whole essence or nature of which is to think'; and Descartes was quite clear that 'for its existence there is no need of any place, nor does it depend on any material thing'.[1] Thus, the rationalist philosopher of France and the rationalist philosopher of England came, by the employment of reason, to widely different conclusions; and we may surmise that reason is not perhaps what Descartes and Hobbes believed it to be, or that they are putting 'reason' to purposes it was never designed to serve. But however that may be, we must not let the philosophers make our heads spin, but consent for the present to agree with Hobbes, for the sake of further understanding what is in his mind, that if we are disposed to disagree with him, it is because we have had 'our natural discourse corrupted with former opinions received from our master', or because we 'do not at all bend our mind to the enquiring out of truth'.

One of these three universal notions indeed, namely, body, occupies

[1] *Philosophical Works of Descartes*, tr. Haldane and Ross, Cambridge, 1931, vol. i. p. 101.

a dubious and unhappy place in Hobbes's philosophy. Unlike Descartes he declined to identify body and space, which he might well have done; (and he was to say of body that it was 'a mere name', and that in it no form nor any other accident but quantity are at all considered' (E. 1. p. 118)); perhaps it was a piece of Aristotelianism with which he might have dispensed. Let us be content then with the notions of space and motion. Nor is there any reason why we should not be content; for with these we can make, or remake, the world. Now the reader will recall Hobbes's definition of philosophy; it is 'such knowledge of effects or appearances as we acquire by true ratiocination from the knowledge we have of their causes or generation . . .' Let us then consider, What in space and by motion may be 'generated'? The answer is, *figure*. 'He that conceived *motion* aright, cannot but know that *motion is the privation of one place, and the acquisition of another*'; and 'it remains, that we enquire what motion begets such and such effects; as, what motion makes a straight line, and what a circular . . . and so forwards, till we see what the effects of simple motion are; and then, in like manner, we are to observe what proceeds from the addition, multiplication, subtraction and division, of these motions, and what effects, what figures, and what properties, they produce; from which kind of contemplation spring that part of philosophy which is called geometry' (E. 1. pp. 70–71). That is to say, we can conceive the beginning and coming-to-be of geometrical figure. Indeed with space and motion we *make* geometrical figure; geometry is our creation, and the figures of geometricians do not exist in nature. Geometry therefore is pure philosophy, knowledge of effects or appearances acquired from the knowledge we have of their causes or generation. Our reason is moving upon the deep, and out of the vague and unfashioned are now appearing form and figure.

Now if, 'bending our minds to the enquiring out of truth', we are still disposed to listen to Hobbes, we may yet so far unbend our minds as to observe that after all he is speaking only of abstractions, and that he is still far from the real world which is the world of all of us. And we may further observe that it will not do to imply that geometry is in any sense our creation, seeing that space is presumably given to us and with it the ordering and relations of figures in it. But then, to our astonishment, Hobbes replies to our objection by saying that we must not imagine that space is real; it is, he says, a *phantasm* of our mind. Now this is certainly something for which we were unprepared; and we must pause to understand further.

'Space', says Hobbes, 'is the phantasm of a thing existing without the mind simply (*phantasma rei existentis, quatenus existentis*)' (E. 1. p. 94). For, he says, suppose the whole world of things destroyed, any man left over from the universal destruction would yet be conscious of space and time. But the space (and time) thus apprehended could only be a phantasm, seeing that all else had been destroyed. Space therefore is imaginary and merely phantasmal. This is a strange argument; for not only does the argument from a universal destruction seem quite unconvincing, but, we ask, if space is phantasmal, what of motion and body? (Besides, we shall see that he holds that what we see in sense is a '*seeming*, or fancy': the 'qualities called *Sensible*, are in the object that causeth them, but so many several motions of the matter, by which it presseth our organs diversly'; and therefore their 'apparence to us is Fancy, the same waking, that dreaming'.[1] So that what we see in sense is but 'phantasmal'). Space, body, motion, we had thought were the things alone really real. Yet are they now to be dissolved into mere imaginings of the *mind*? But in fact Hobbes said this only of space; motion and body, he held consistently, are real and not fictions of the mind.

Certainly Hobbes is in deep waters, and is all but collapsing into a subjectivism; and it is clear that he avoids doing so only by taking up positions which it is very easy to attack. He is treating of matters which will be endlessly debated for centuries to come; but he seems more often than not to be unaware of the frightful philosophical possibilities which stand everywhere about his path; and his sanguinity, his dash and his adroitness do not desert him. But I am not concerned to point out objections to Hobbes. No doubt he is, in certain respects, easy enough game. I want only to elicit the motives and direction of his mind. Yet it is obvious that Hobbes's whole philosophy is here trembling on the very brink of ruin. But because he was a clever man, and could not be wholly unaware of the dangers he was running, we can only assume that he had a strong motive in making space into a phantasm of the mind. And indeed, the motive is not far to seek. For in the next chapter it is made plain to us. Let us continue our intellectual experiment wherein we destroyed the universe and retained our consciousness of space ; and let us now begin to re-make the universe. Let us suppose a table called into existence. It would be a portion of *body*, and not at all

---

[1] *Leviathan*, Clarendon Press, 1929, p. 12. All quotations from *Leviathan* will be made from this edition. This edition is reprinted from the edition of 1651. *Leviathan* in Molesworth's edition is modernized.

dependent for its existence on our mind. *But it has to be fitted into our imaginary space;* and says Hobbes, 'body is called *subject* because it is laid and placed under imaginary space (*sub spatio imaginario substerni et supponi videtur*) so that not by the senses but only by the reason is anything understood to be there (*ut non sensibus sed ratione tantum aliquid ibi esse intelligatur*).'[1] Therefore the definition of body is: body is that which, not being dependent on our thought, is coincident or co-extended with some part of space.' Body then, which is a wholly external thing, enters into, is 'submitted' to, space, which is mental, and yet Hobbes holds that bodies have extension in their own right and in a *real* space. 'The extension of a body, is the same thing with the magnitude of it, as that which some call *real space*. But this *magnitude* does not depend upon our cogitations, as imaginary space does; for this is an effect of our imagination, but *magnitude* is the cause of it; this is an accident of the mind, that of a body existing out of the mind' (E. 1. p. 105). And as space is a phantasm relative to extension, time is a phantasm relative to motion. Hobbes's motive is clear. Space is an accident of the mind; the innumerable figures of geometry we *make* in this accident, and their generation is thus known to us; therefore we have truly philosophical knowledge of them. But happily, what is not an accident of the mind, namely, body in its extension (*quod appellari solet, propter extensionem quidem,* corpus) is subject to this accident; and therefore, considered as extension or quantity, body too is open to our philosophical investigation. And thus it comes about that the mind in search of science *simpliciter*, by deduction from the definitions of space and motion, is able wholly to understand, as it is able to understand a geometrical theorem, the structure of the universe; it can arrive at a 'science of causes of the διότι'. The knowledge we thus come by may be indeed only hypothetical; but it will serve.

> 'Tis onely God can know
> Whether the fair idea thou dost show
> Agree entirely with his own or no,
> This I dare boldly tell,
> 'Tis so like truth, 'twill serve our turn as well.

sang Cowley in his Pindaric Ode *To Mr. Hobbes*. We can re-construct, so to speak, the universe, by reasoning; thus re-making it is also the coming to philosophical knowledge of it; given space and time, to which magnitude and motion are subject, we can understand how the universe

---

[1] L. 1. p. 91. I give here a translation more accurate, I think, than that of the English Translation (E. 1. p. 102).

is made; it may not be the universe as God made it; it will be the universe as we have made it; and that is enough.

Thus from space and motion and body reason can re-construct the world, and not only the material world but also the world of life and mind—the world, as he calls it, of internal and invisible motion. For the method of analysis carried us back to space, motion and body; and all change whatsoever is motion (of which body is the mysterious vehicle) in space. The materialism is thorough and absolute. The qualities of light and heat are motions; seeing and feeling are motions; and 'that which thinks is something corporeal; for, as it appears, the subjects of all activities can be conceived only after a corporeal fashion'.[1] We may advance steadily from the philosophy of geometry to the philosophy of mechanics; thence to physics to treat of heat, light and sound and the processes whereby they are apprehended; thence to moral philosophy, and on to civil philosophy; and motion in space is everywhere the universal cause. 'And because all appearance of things to sense is determined, and made to be of such and such quality and quantity by compounded motions, every one of which has a certain degree of velocity, and a certain and determined way; therefore, in the first place we are to search out the ways of motion simply (in which geometry consists); next the ways of such generated motions as are manifest; and, lastly, the ways of internal and invisible motions (which is the enquiry of natural philosophy). And therefore, they that study natural philosophy, study in vain, except they begin at geometry; and such writers or disputers thereof, as are ignorant of geometry, do but make their readers and hearers lose their time' (E. 1. p. 73).

III

I have spoken of reason, in Hobbes's view, re-making the world. But can we in fact see it as necessarily *only re-making* it? Does it not perhaps make it? For we *make* geometrical figure, Hobbes tells us, from space and motion. But if space is only a phantasm, an accident of the mind, are not all things in it? Motion, Hobbes insists, is real. But, I have asked, can space be phantasmal and motion *real*? And of body, we have no *idea*, only ratiocinative knowledge. And if so, may not the whole universe be a creation of the mind, one mighty theorem, which we ourselves have constructed? For the structure of the universe as it will finally lie open to the eye of reason may be entirely of our own

[1] *Objections to Descartes, Works of Descartes,* tr. Haldane and Ross, vol. ii. p. 62.

making; it is indifferent to Hobbes whether it be so or not; for he explicitly declares, as we have seen, that 'philosophy is the knowledge we
acquire, by true ratiocination, of appearances or apparent effects, from
the knowledge we have of some *possible production or generation* of the
same; and of such production, *as has been or may be*, from the knowledge
we have of the effects'; the structure of the world 'disclosed' to reasoning may well be one made by reasoning; Hobbes is not in a position to
deny, and makes it clear that he does not wish to deny, that the intelligible universe is a human construction. Is not then humanity a God?
If we have philosophical knowledge of geometry because we *make*
figure, may we not also have philosophical understanding of the world
only because we make it also? The thought is dazzling; and our minds
go back to Hobbes's *Epistle to the Reader* which precedes the *De
Corpore*: 'Philosophy, therefore, the child of the world and your own
mind, is within yourself; perhaps not fashioned yet, but like the world
its father, as it was in the beginning, a thing confused . . . Let your
reason move upon the deep of your own cogitations and experience;
those things that lie in confusion must be set asunder, distinguished,
and every one stamped with its own name set in order; that is to say,
your method must resemble that of the creation.' And when we consider his philosophy, do we not see him near to ascribing to the mind
the actual creation of the universe? And might not perhaps, as another
rationalist was to suggest, perceptions be really only thoughts obscurely
thought, perceptions which could be dissolved by thought into theorem
and concept?

For this seventeenth-century mind was very complicated. On the
one side, he wanted power; and philosophical thought, demonstrable
knowledge, was the supreme power; by it alone could society be made
and kept stable. Therefore the mind was exalted to be the source of
power. But on the one hand only corporeal process is intelligible and
penetrable, as it were, by the light of reason. Therefore Hobbes's
materialism no less than his rationalism springs from his desire to set
no limits to the power of reason; his materialism and his rationalism
are inextricably intertwined; one without the other is of no use to him.
But it was a difficult alliance. His rationalism comes near to carrying
him over into an abyss of subjectivism; and of his materialism, had he
been less addicted to power and of a freer and more open mind, he
might have said what he exclaimed on reading Euclid for the first
time.

But we are more concerned to understand Hobbes than to criticize him; and at the risk of repetition, I re-emphasize the motive which animates this philosophy—it is the sense of the *creative power of reason* issuing into power. At one end it creates geometry; it erects an intelligibly ordered universe; it then creates a new man in a new Society. And it can create them only because it can know their generation and thereby understand them utterly. Only that which we can make can we understand; and only that which we both make and understand can we control and order.

And yet, in the interest of this rationalism and of the promise of power it gives, Hobbes was also a materialist. I said a moment ago that he might well feel tempted to consider all perceptions to be but obscure concepts. In fact, what he said was that 'whatsoever . . . we conceive has been perceived first by sense' (E. 3. p. 17). For reason indeed to master the world, the world must be wholly material; and then reason must itself be material. Hobbes wished to have it both ways. His entire philosophy is an attempt to run together two philosophical extremes, a rationalism and a materialism, which he labours cleverly and assiduously and in vain to put on the friendliest terms; in trying to do this, he makes man both into a God and into mere movements of matter; he makes truth man-made and eternal; he makes moral values relative and absolute; and man himself both a savage and a contriver of Leviathan. His philosophy is set fast in a violent contradiction which he will not see; he sees as a system what in fact is split from top to bottom.

IV

I can best illustrate the contradiction in which Hobbes's philosophy is set by speaking of his doctrine of names.

His doctrine of names has an agreeable simplicity which masks a typical adroitness. Like much of Hobbes's writing, it has great force and the appearance of coming from an unclouded and disinterested intelligence which seeks only clarity and ordering. But in fact it is a subtle and daring *tour de force* which at once satisfies (or rather, appeared to Hobbes to satisfy) the two great and diametrically opposed movements of his philosophical thinking. To read Hobbes with attention is to see beneath the objective and authoritative manner a play of conflicting philosophical impulse and aim; beneath the calm surface there is agitation and labour; and we have the feel of Hobbes's mind only when, having this agitation in clear view, we see with what adroitness and skill he seeks to hide its existence from himself no less than from us. He does not of course hide it successfully from us; it was quite impossible that he should. But his deception was at least accomplished; his philosophical manner had a fine air of assurance; and he never comes near to losing his confidence. But if his philosophy has something of the finished performance of a man of the world who plays out the game with assurance, it is perhaps only because, like the man of the world, it had to keep up a fair pace and not stop too long to think; and if his philosophizing with all its clear confidence and authority is also strangely crude, it is only because his anxiety for power both committed him to, and prevented him from discerning, an inevitable clash of doctrine. For his philosophical intention was at once to show that reason is creative and that it is an accident of body. How to his own complete satisfaction he resolved this conflict in his doctrine of names, it is interesting to observe.

His resolution consists, simply, in saying that reason and reasoning is a matter of words, or speech; reason is speech, and speech reason. And if this is so, two consequences appear to follow. First, that reason is sensualized, brought down firmly into the world of sense and particulars. Second, that as speech is man-made, the entire structure of truth is reared by the human intelligence. It is a prodigious, cunning and daring doctrine; and it is as prodigious in its two-fold convenience for Hobbes's purposes as it is prodigious in its falsity. But what we are especially concerned to point out is that Hobbes is not, and cannot be, loyal to his doctrine; *he carries it off*, appearing to hold it; but he also constantly says things which make it clear that he does not. For if thought is speech, it is certain that we do not think and are not therefore rational; and if truth is indeed man-made, it is not really truth. On the one side he wishes to reduce reason to motion and then makes it an affair of sounds; but if so, it is nonsense to say that we are rational. On the other side, he wishes to make us the creators of truth; but if he does so, he in effect denies that there is such a thing as truth to be had and known. In this impossible position, he must resort to exposition which *trims* with all the subtlety he can muster, whereby he may deceive himself and us. He deceives himself because he wants to be deceived; he was an eminently passionate nature. Yet he can hardly deceive us.

But let us see how he proceeds. 'But the most noble and profitable invention of all other, was that of SPEECH, consisting of *Names* or *Appellations*, and their Connexion; whereby men register their Thoughts; recall them when they are past; and also declare them one to another for mutuall utility and conversation; without which, there had been amongst men, neither Common-wealth, nor Society, nor Contract, nor Peace, no more than amongst Lyons, Bears and Wolves' (*Lev.*, p. 24) and in *De Corpore* he says that 'for the acquiring of philosophy, some sensible moniments are necessary, by which our past thoughts may be not only reduced, but also registered every one in its own order. These moniments I call MARKS, namely, sensible things taken at pleasure, that, by the sense of them, such thoughts may be recalled to our mind as are like those thoughts for which we took them' (E. 1. pp. 13–14). Then, he says, when these marks are also employed to communicate our thoughts to others, they are also *signs*; and 'words so connected as that they become signs of our thoughts, are called SPEECH, of which every part is a *name*' (E. 1. p. 15).

Now it is to be noticed that he does not here identify thought with speech. We may, he implies, have thoughts before we have speech; words register and recall thoughts, he says; he does not say they are identical with them. Still, he certainly means to say that thought without speech would be a negligible confusion; it is by means of speech that we, as it were, *hold* our thoughts and then order them; so that we are lifted above what would otherwise be little more than a flux of mere experience.

But there was that in Hobbes which urged him to go father than this. The impetus of his materialism drove him towards *identifying* thought and speech; and we are not surprised when, in Chapter 4 of *Leviathan*, we read this: 'When a man, upon the hearing of any Speech, hath those thoughts which the words of that Speech, and their connexion, were ordained and constituted to signifie; Then he is said to understand it: *Understanding* being *nothing else, but conception caused by* Speech [the italics are mine] (*Lev.*, p. 31). And therefore if speech be peculiar to man, as for ought I know it is, then is Understanding peculiar to him also.' Here, conception *follows* speech; there are now no thoughts to be recalled or registered; the thoughts are *caused* by speech. I said that we are not surprised to come upon this in Hobbes's exposition; it is what we should have expected. For as a materialist, he would naturally wish to reduce thought to sense; but this he could hardly do, because he knew that when he thought of 'man' he did not entertain a composite image which was not of any one man, and that there can be no 'universal' image (E. 4. p. 22); and he was therefore all the more willing to make the word 'man' the very thought of man. Therefore Hobbes comes near to an extreme nominalism, which makes the thought a word; and it is very easy to expound him as saying so; indeed he gives authority for our saying so when he declares that understanding 'is caused by speech.'

And yet, the fact is that, while having the air of believing this, Hobbes does not believe it, or at most believes it with a half of his mind which he does not suffer to know what the other half is doing. For if he really believed it, what sense was there in saying that one of the 'special uses of speech' was 'to Register, what by cogitation, wee find to be the cause of any thing, present or past? (*Lev.*, p. 25). Or again that 'a *man* denotes any one of a multitude of men . . . *by reason of their similitude*'? (E. 1. p. 18, my italics). It is obvious that Hobbes's philosophical method was to suggest rather than to declare, and to slip over from one doctrine to another with as little fuss as possible; he exerts a philosophical trimming which looks for the advantages of a number of contradictory doctrines. The fact appears to be that Hobbes dare not be a nominalist nor a conceptualist; he must keep moving back and fore between the two doctrines with all the adroitness he can muster. He has to be both a materialist and a rationalist.

But there is another aspect of his doctrine of language which exhibits the same sleight of mind. The moniments, which he calls marks, are, he said in what I quoted a moment ago, taken *at pleasure* that our thoughts may be recalled to our mind. He says again, a little later: 'A NAME is a word taken at pleasure to serve for a mark, which may raise in our mind a thought like to some thought we had before, and which being pronounced to others, may be to them a sign of what thought the speaker had, or had not before his mind' (E. 1. p. 16). Now it is certain from this that Hobbes intends that any general name does not denote any thing or reality; it is a device for calling up a thought in our mind or for letting someone know that a certain thought is in our mind. Now if we ask, what is meant by a 'thought'? Hobbes, as we have seen, will give no consistent answer: he will not say, simply, the word itself or an image, or a concept. But we leave this now, and observe the development of his doctrine of names. A name, he has said, is not of any part of reality, but a mark for calling up a thought in our minds; it is, strictly, a device and not a name. Therefore, as we might expect, Hobbes goes on to say that a name is given arbitrarily: any word will do to call up a thought in my mind, provided I continue to use the same word for this purpose. Then he says: 'it is true (for example) that *man is a living creature*, but it is for this reason, that it pleased men to impose both those names on the same thing' (E. 1. p. 36). Let us now overlook that he here speaks of 'imposing names on things', which seems to be inconsistent with what he has said above; and let us take him as saying that quite arbitrarily men have used 'man' and 'living creature' to call up the same thought in their minds. This being so, when we say 'man is a living creature' we are really only saying that we use 'man' and 'living creature' for the same purpose. In other words, the 'truth' of the proposition turns out to be an affair of how we use language. In this way necessary knowledge is really linguistic; we do not, in Hobbes's whole scheme of deductive science, get beyond our arbitrary use of sounds. We do not, in 'necessary' knowledge, get beyond names to reality; we are really making elaborate patterns of knowledge which are not of reality, but airy systems of relations between names, which are *not* the names of things or of realities. What we call rational knowledge, in which philosophy consists, is of our own making, or rather comes from our employment of arbitrary marks; and the entire deductive system of knowledge, from which Hobbes expects such immense practical results and hitherto unimagined power, turns out to be an affair of arbitrary linguistics.

Now this is quite incredible. And Hobbes himself only contrives to give an air of believing it. Once again, there was a half of him which did not believe it. But before justifying this last observation, let us ask, why did Hobbes, if only with a half of his mind, want to believe it? The answer is clear: because in this way reason is resolved into something non-rational and springs from the arbitrary and utterly irrational. This certainly appears to be perverse; but Hobbes was a materialist, and reason must be resolved into motion. Reason is in the last resort something which springs from the arbitrary employment of certain sounds which are really motion.

But there is another reason, equally potent in Hobbes's mind. It is that reason is man's creation. It is true that it is man's arbitrary creation; but that it was arbitrary makes it, in its way, still more impressive; philosophy, and the world as it is apprehended by philosophy, is created by the arbitrary fiat of the human mind, which then takes on a God-like stature. Philosophical truth is not something discovered by man; it is truth because it was created by man. Beyond this, mortal pride cannot go; it is the zenith of the pride of the Renaissance. On the one hand, Hobbes reduces reason to motion; and then words are wholly arbitrary signs of thoughts. But on the other hand, he also wished to make reason and a rational universe a creation of man's mind; for if man *makes* truth, he can command the universe and no part of it will escape him. His knowledge will be absolute; for it will be knowledge he has made.

And yet Hobbes cannot be content with all this. And he cannot be content with it because, according to this doctrine, the mind cannot apprehend *truth*. The contradiction in which Hobbes is caught here, which however he will not see for a contradiction because of the passion and intellectual greed of his mind, is in the sentence: 'it is true (for example) that *Man is a living creature*, but it is for this reason, that it pleased men to impose both those names on the same thing'. But if all rational knowledge is deduced from definitions wholly arbitrary, we cannot end up with truth for the good reason that we have not begun from it; if universal propositions which are really only about the way we use words are the source of our thinking, our thinking neither begins nor ends with knowledge or reality; there is no bridge here between names and the world; we are confined to a game which is conducted in at best a spirit of caprice and fancy. But Hobbes will not have it that this is so; it is *true*, he says, that man is a living creature; and by saying so he breaks right out of the prison of names. Or again, he goes on to say that we impose 'those names *on the same thing*', thereby going beyond his doctrine of the name as a mark used for recalling a thought. Or again, he says: 'wherefore, in every proposition three things are to be considered, *viz.*, the two names, which are the *subject*, and the *predicate*, and their *copulation*; both which names raise in our mind the thought of one and the same thing; but the copulation makes us think of the *Cause for which those names were imposed on that thing*' (E. 1. p. 31, my italics). But to say this is indeed to give away the game; if there *is* such a cause, the doctrine of caprice and arbitrariness has been yielded up; or rather would have been yielded up, had Hobbes been bent less on power than on truth. Or again he says: 'And therefore those propositions only are *necessary*, which are of sempiternal truth, that is, true at all times. From hence also it is manifest, that truth adheres not to things, but to speech only, for some truths are eternal ; for it will be eternally true, *if man, then living creature*; but that any *man*, or *living-creature*, should exist eternally, is not necessary' (E. 1. p. 38). But if necessary propositions arise from arbitrary naming, what purpose is there in speaking of eternal truth? And if truth adheres to speech only, how can it be eternal? Hobbes's bland persistence in self-deception never deserts him. There was too much at stake for him to stop quietly to think with genuine detachment about his doctrines. The more we read Hobbes the less we think of his doctrines in an intellectual point of view; but also, the more fascinated we become by *him*, in a human point of view. He enthrals us the more as a figure in human history in proportion as we observe the contradictions in his thought which he passionately overlooks.

Of the leading motives in Hobbes's thinking I have said enough. I remark only in passing, before going on to speak of what he has to say about perception, that he treats morality as he treats rational knowledge. Truth, he will have us believe, is of our making and yet is sempiternal; similarly, morality is of our making and yet has absolute claims on us. 'But whatsoever is the object of any mans Appetite or Desire; that is it, which he for his part calleth *Good* : And the object of his Hate, and Aversion, *Evill*; And of his Contempt, *Vile* and *Inconsiderable*. For these words of Good, Evill, and Contemptible, are ever used with relation to the person that useth them: There being nothing simply and absolutely so; nor any common Rule of Good and Evill, to be taken from the nature of the objects themselves . . .' (*Lev.*, p. 41). Good and evil are therefore strictly relative terms; and man is actuated, without freedom, by egotistic passion. And yet it is this creature, whose will can be no more than strength of animal appetite, who is the creator of Leviathan whereby his pride, through the power of reason, is tamed. Thought is ultimately motion; it yet resolves the chaos of experience into intelligible order and constructs a rational universe. Passion is the law of man's nature; it yet contrives a rational society of law. The morality by which man lives springs from the arbitrariness of appetite, as eternal truth springs from the arbitrariness of naming.

V

Now when Hobbes goes over to ethics and to the theory of perception, he cannot exhibit our passions or our knowledge of sense-qualities as mere movements of physical particles. No doubt he believes that that is what, in the last resort, they are; but he certainly cannot deduce them from mathematical propositions. What he does instead is to represent, when he can, the passions and what happens in perception in terms of imagery derived from the physical world; he can only suggest vague analogies with happenings in the material universe. We shall find illustrations of this in what follows.

My purpose now is to transfer attention from his doctrine of creative reason to consequences it has for the doctrine of the imagination. It has been held by many, at widely different times, that the rôle

of reason is to discover, that of the imagination to create. But Hobbes,
whose ambition for reason is so unlimited, is unlikely to suffer any
counterclaim from the imagination. I turn now to his doctrine of perception and fancy.

All sensible qualities, he says, 'are in the object that causeth them, but
so many several motions of the matter, by which it presseth our organs
diversly. Neither in us that are pressed, are they any thing else, but
divers motions; (for motion produceth nothing but motion)' (*Lev.*,
p. 12). Now it is not easy to understand how a patch of red, whether
objective, or, as Hobbes believes, subjective, is nothing but motion;
but we must take it that Hobbes found no difficulty in this. Also, we
can hardly forbear to think that if the so-called secondary qualities are
to be dealt with in this way, the so-called primary must suffer the same
fate. But here, as everywhere in his philosophizing, Hobbes is walking
a knife-edge. We can only acknowledge that he walks it with verve and
aplomb; for he coolly remarks: 'And though at some certain distance,
the reall, the very object seem invested with the fancy it begets in us;
Yet still the object is one thing, the image or fancy is another. So that
Sense in all cases, is nothing els but original fancy, caused (as I have
said) by the pressure, that is, by the motion, of external things upon
our Eyes, Eares, and other organs thereunto ordained.'

But if 'sense is originall fancy', and if 'there is no conception in a
mans mind, which hath not at first, totally or by parts, been begotten
upon the organs of *Sense*' (*Lev.*, p. 11), what shall we say of the imagination? Hobbes's celebrated answer is that it 'is nothing but *decaying
sense*'. 'And as wee see in the water, though the wind cease, the waves
give not over rowling for a long time after; so also it happeneth in that
motion, which is made in the internall parts of a man, when he Sees,
Dreams, etc. For after the object is removed or the eye shut, wee still
retain an image of the thing seen, though more obscure than when we
see it' (*Lev.*, p. 13). This is imagination or fancy; and like sense or
original fancy it is an effect set up by body in body. It is a curious doctrine. For in it sense is fanciful, and what is fanciful only sense. Sense-
perception is given powers of creation (however Hobbes may deny it
and call sense only motion) which transform a universe of dull quantities into a universe of surpassing beauty; but the imagination can only
repeat, and obscurely and tamely, what sense provides. Imagination
therefore is only memory. 'This *decaying sense*, when wee would express
the thing itself, (I mean *fancy* it selfe), wee call *Imagination*, as I said before: But when we would express the *decay*, and signifie that the Sense

is fading, old and past, it is called *Memory*. So that *Imagination* and *Memory*, are but one thing, which for divers considerations hath divers names' (*Lev.*, p. 14).

Memory proper then, is imagination; and the succession of images in the memory, being but motions within us, are 'reliques of those made in the Sense; And those motions that immediately succeeded one another in the sense, continue also together after sense . . . [so] that in the Imagining of anything, there is no certainty what we shall Imagine next; Onely this is certain, it shall be something that succeeded the same before at some time or another' (*Lev.*, p. 19). And I need not observe that whatever this may be said to explain, it does not explain, precisely, *memory*. Then he goes on to speak of complicated trains of thought, of 'Mentall Discourse' as he calls it. He tells us there are two kinds of discourse, the one unguided, the other regulated. I shall quote the entire paragraph in which he expounds his idea of unguided discourse, if only because the beauty of its prose is quite extraordinarily striking; it shows the *wholeness* of Hobbes in his philosophizing, the impregnation of the language of thought with passion, a rationalist thinker having the finest susceptibilities to language, a perfection of exposition along with the indetectable subtleties of the artist. 'This Trayne of Thoughts, or Mentall Discourse, is of two sorts. The first is *Unguided, without Designe*, and inconstant; wherein there is no Passionate Thought, to govern and direct those that follow, to it self, as the end and scope of some desire, or other passion: In which case the thoughts are said to wander, and seem impertinent to one another, as in a Dream. Such are Commonly the thoughts of men, that are not onely without company, but also without care of any thing; though even then their Thoughts are as busie as at other times, but without harmony; as the sound which a Lute out of tune would yeeld to any man; or in tune, to one that could not play. And yet in this wild ranging of the mind, a man may oft-times perceive the way of it, and the dependance of one thought upon another. For in a Discourse of our present civill War, what could seem more impertinent, than to ask (as one did) what was the value of a Roman Penny? Yet the Cohaerence to me was manifest enough. For the Thought of the warre, introduced the Thought of the delivering up the King to his Enemies; The Thought of that, brought in the Thought of the delivering up of Christ; and that again the Thought of the 30 pence, which was the price of that treason: and thence easily followed that malicious question; and all this in a moment of time; for Thought is quick' (*Lev.*, pp. 19–20).

Of this we can only say that a paragraph, devoted to the thought of unguided discourse 'wherein there is no Passionate Thought', could hardly have come to a more surprising end.

But Hobbes's fast progress along his narrow, hedged-in path is un-arrested; and he goes on in his next paragraph to speak blandly of 'discourse *regulated* by some desire, and designe'. Of such there are two kinds: 'one, when of an effect imagined, wee seek the causes, or means that produce it; and this is common to Man and Beast. The other is, when imagining any thing whatsoever, wee seek all the possible effects, that can by it be produced . . .' This he says is 'nothing but *Seeking*, or the faculty of Invention' (p. 20). But at this sub-rational level of knowledge we have not only sagacity, which we share, along with sense and memory, with the animals; there is also prudence, which again we share with the animals. 'Prudence is a *Præsumtion* of the *Future*, contracted from the *Experience* of time *Past*'; by it we may anticipate and expect on the grounds of experience in the past.

Now it is to be emphasized that sense, imagination, memory, sagacity, prudence, all belong to us as animals. They occur at the level of 'experience' merely, where the mind trafficks only in particulars. And at the end of the third chapter in *Leviathan*, from which I have been quoting, he says: 'There is no other act of mans mind, that I can remember, naturally planted in him, so, as to need no other thing, to the exercise of it, but to be born a man, and live with the use of his five Senses. Those other Faculties, of which I shall speak by and by, and which seem proper to man onely, are acquired, and encreased by study and industry; and of most men learned by instruction, and discipline; and proceed all from the invention of Words, and Speech . . .' (p. 22). Now if so, we begin with a sharp dichotomy between sense and thought, particular and universal.

Now it is true that he goes on at once to say that 'by the help of Speech, and Method, the same Facultyes may be improved to such a height, as to distinguish men from all other creatures'. They 'may be improved', he says; for, as we saw earlier, by 'marks' we may hold firmly in our minds what sense and memory provide; what sense provides is 'apt to slip out of our memory'; and speech comes as an enormous facilitation of 'remembrance'. Thus it comes about that speech acts, at the level of 'experience' to extend further these animal powers. These powers remain, by nature, what the animals also have; but they become more efficient by the employment of the tools we call words. Here then speech is to be regarded not as that which lifts us into being rational creatures (though it certainly does that also); it but makes us more efficient animals; and it is as improved animals that we sense, remember, are sagacious and prudent.

It is clear then that Hobbes sustains a sharp dichotomy between sense and reason. 'Experience concludeth nothing universally' (E. 4. p. 18); but philosophy, whereby we apprehend universal truth, and construct a deductive system of causes and effects, comes of the employment of names in the way we spoke of in the preceding section. That Hobbes is now nominalist and now certainly not nominalist in his treatment of language as an instrument of reason is not here relevant; what is here relevant is that he distinguishes between the use of language by experience for the knowledge of the particular, and the use of language by philosophy, for the knowledge of the universal. We may use words to remember better than the animals, to be more sagacious and prudent than they, but we do so only as animals; but we may use words to 'conclude universally', and this we do as philosophers, who by definitions make of words instruments of reasoning. In one use language is employed as an extension of sense; in the other it is the instrument (or the creator) of reasoning. And between sense and reason, the particular and the universal, there is no bridge. On the one side lies perception, memory, fancy, prudence; on the other philosophy or reasoning. The first is indeed 'knowledge', and may provide profit and delight, and Hobbes certainly does not despise it; but it is by reasoning that power comes. 'To conclude, the light of humane minds is Perspicuous Words, but by exact definitions first snuffed, and purged from ambiguity; *Reason* is the *pace;* Encrease of *Science*, the *way*; and the benefit of man-kind, the *end*' (*Lev.*, p. 37). The 'Light of Human minds' is not in sense, memory and the rest; and Hobbes says in the first chapter of *De Corpore*, 'we must consider that although Sense and Memory of Things, which are common to man and all living creatures, be knowledge, yet because they are given us immediately by nature, and not gotten by ratiocination, they are not philosophy' (E.1. p. 3).

VI

Experience and philosophy, particular and universal, are thus sundered. But where, we ask, are we to place history and poetry? But if we trouble to ask the question, we can hardly have much doubt about Hobbes's answer. They fall in the world of 'experience', not of philosophy. Let us take history first. 'And therefore', says Hobbes in

Leviathan (p. 50), 'when the Discourse is put into Speech, and begins with the Definition of Words, and proceeds by Connexion of the same into generall Affirmations, and of these again into Syllogisms; the End or last summe is called the Conclusion: and the thought of the mind by it signified, is that Conditionall Knowledge, or Knowledge of the consequence of words, which is commonly called SCIENCE. But if the first ground of such Discourse, be not Definitions; or if the Definitions be not rightly joyned together into Syllogismes, then the End or Conclusion, is again OPINION . . .' Now history is therefore opinion and relies on faith; for then 'wee believe any saying whatsoever it be, to be true, from arguments taken, not from the thing it selfe, or from the principles of naturall Reason, but from the Authority, and good opinion wee have, of him that sayd it' (p. 51). It is therefore of a piece with sense-knowledge. That is not to say that Hobbes despises it; indeed history may be instructive and give rise to the characteristic virtue of 'Experience', namely, prudence. But, founded in 'faith', it must rely on 'Præsumtion of things past' and be conjectural; and if history instructs us as to our own future, it is again conjectural only.

I go on now to speak of what Hobbes has to say about poetry, which, like history, must fall on the side of 'sense'. Before doing so, I wish to make a few observations about his doctrine of 'sense' or 'experience'. It will be clear to the reader that he packs a great deal of human experience into this sub-rational activity. It is, he is at pains to point, in its essential nature, something shared with the animals; what is distinctively non-animal in us, the 'Light of the humane mind', is reasoning and reasoning alone, the power of deducing effect from cause. Now Hobbes is perfectly aware that few men employ their powers of reasoning; 'men that know not what it is that we call *causing*, (that is, almost all men) have no other rule to guesse by, but by observing, and remembering what they have seen to precede the like effect at some other time, or times before, without seeing between the antecedent and subsequent Event, any dependance or connexion at all: And therefore from the like things past, they expect the like things to come . . .', he says in *Leviathan* (p. 84). Thus it is that the great bulk of human experience falls below the level of reasoning; and it contains sense, memory, imagination, sagacity, prudence, merely inductive science, history, poetry.

Now it is clear from this that Hobbes is placing a huge burden upon 'sense', whatever extensions of it speech may supply. For in sense we are passive; sense is 'caused by the pressure, that is, by the motion, of externall things upon our Eyes, Eares, and other organs thereunto ordained'; imagination and memory are but 'decaying sense'; and sagacity, prudence, history, poetry are but the children of memory. But let us consider but one of these children, the one he calls 'sagacity'. 'The Discourse of the Mind, when it is governed by designe, is nothing but seeking, or the faculty of Invention, which the Latines call *Sagacitas*, and *Solertia*; a hunting out of causes, or some effect, present or past; or of the effects, of some present or past cause' (*Lev.*, p. 20); and of 'the seeking of causes' Hobbes declares explicitly that 'it is common to Man and Beast'. Now it is, in fact, very hard to see how this can be the child of memory; or how design can occur in the mere motion of sense. Hobbes quite fails to make intelligible how all this can occur out of mere motions set up in us by sense-objects; he is, surreptitiously, giving to 'Traynes of Imaginations' (p. 18) creative powers which his premisses strictly deny him.

Also, I make this observation, which follows on that I have just made. In speaking of 'Traynes of Imaginations' Hobbes frequently, if implicitly, acknowledges that they require conceptual thought, or the employment of 'universalls'. He says on p. 22 of the *Leviathan*, where he speaks of prudence, that 'A *Signe*, is the Event Antecedent, of the Consequent; and certainly, the Consequent of the Antecedent, when *the like Consequences* (my italics) have been observed before . . .'' Now it is true that Hobbes set up for an extreme nominalist; but he also was not consistent in it. But I only remark now that he clearly gives us to understand that at the level of sense and imagination conceptual thought, though not of course reasoning, is active.

Now in view of these two observations, first, that memory and imagination take on a creative rôle in Hobbes's doctrine, however inconsistently; and second, that conceptual thought is active in 'Experience', I ask: Can Hobbes maintain his sharp separation of sense and reasoning? Ought not so absolute a dichotomy of particular and universal to be abandoned? Is there no continuity between the animal and the God in man? Is the seeking out of causes by sagacity to be regarded as a wholly different thing from the discovery of causes by reasoning? Hobbes himself at times suggests these questions to us: in Chapter 5 of *Leviathan* (p. 38) he says that the great virtue of 'Experience' is *prudence*, that of science, *sapience*; and he goes on, 'But to make their difference appeare more cleerly, let us suppose one man endued with an excellent naturall use, and dexterity in handling his armes; and another to have added to that dexterity, an acquired

Science, of where he can offend, or be offended by his adversarie, in every possible posture, or guard: The ability of the former, would be to the ability of the later, as Prudence to Sapience; both usefull; but the later infallible . . .' But the illustration is not a happy one. The sapient fencer may all too readily fall through an excess of rules; and in any case, are not the rules of the sapient the fruits of the experience of the prudent? And if here Hobbes suggests to us the opposite of what he urges, we shall see that there is another place in his writings where he seems to acknowledge that imagination and reason are not so far apart after all.

VII

Let us now go on to speak of those 'Traynes of Imagination' which make up poetry. Hobbes says on p. 14 of *Leviathan* that 'Imagination being only of those things which have been formerly perceived by Sense, either all at once, or by parts at severall times; the former, (which is the imagining the whole object, as it was presented to the sense) is *simple Imagination*; as when one imagineth a man, or horse, which he hath seen before. The other is *Compounded*; as when from the sight of a man at one time, and of a horse at another, we conceive in our mind a Centaure. So when a man compoundeth the image of his own person, with the image of the actions of another man; as when a man imagins himself a *Hercules*, or an *Alexander*, (which happeneth often to them that are much taken with reading of Romants) it is a compound imagination, and properly but a Fiction of the mind.'

'Romants' are compound imaginations and *properly* but fictions of the mind. Now the serious matter here (serious, that is, for Hobbes), is that he must admit that there *are* fictions of the mind; and having formerly told us that the mind is tied in memory to the succession of things in sense, he now tells us precisely that we are capable of *not* being so tied, but may freely compound, disregarding the order of succession in sense. Fancy is memory; but it also creates fictions of its own. And it is clear that even if Hippolytus, Dido and Iago were only, as he says, 'compounded imaginations', Hobbes cannot possibly, on his showing, explain the 'compounding'; and here he is inconsistent in a way which lets him manifest his dislike of 'romants' (to which he himself, in earlier days and before a mathematical light had broken upon him, had been addicted). They are properly fictions; and if he is here willing to envisage the mind as apparently denying the laws of motion, it is only to make clear to us that it does so only to create fictions, aberrations and what is *not* in the mathematical world to which alone serious attention is due. The mind may, he allows, fly off freakishly from the world and indulge itself; and he embraces his inconsistency in mathematical physics to show his contempt for poetry, or at least for 'romants'. But where are we to draw the line between the fictions created by romances and the figures created by a Homer? Let us, if we will, put Ariosto and Spenser out of court; but can we then keep Shakespeare? Is not Lear as much a fiction as Caliban? We can fairly allow that recollection plays its part in poetry; but we do not travel far in poetry without the attendance of fictions. And if fiction is to go, can Hobbes seriously imagine that imagination, which is memory, which in turn is but decaying sense, *is* poetry?

So Hobbes seems to lay hold on poetry and wring its neck. Or so we might think. But in fact this bold spirit will not be so bold. Neither Hobbes in England nor Descartes in France will have done with poetry. There had been a time in Descartes' life when he was, as he tells us, in the *Discours 'amoureux de la Poesie'*; and sometime between 1616 and 1620, when his mind was in a ferment, he was capable of writing: 'mirum videri possit quare graves sententiae in scriptis poetarum, magis quam philosophorum. Ratio est quod poetae per enthusiasmum et vim imaginationis scripsere: Sunt in nobis semina scientiae, ut in silice, quae per rationem a philosophis educuntur, per imaginationem a poetis excutiuntur magisque elucent.' Truly, he here sharply opposes reason to enthusiasm, inspiration to imagination; and that he does so means that a choice of one or the other will be inevitable. Nor will there be any doubt which he will choose. 'Je me plaisais surtout aux Mathematiques, à cause de la certitude et de l'évidence de leurs raisons';[1] and he says this in the *Discours* after speaking of poetry in a way very different from that we see in the Latin I have just quoted. Poetry, he says, is a natural gift, unteachable; but if it is only a gift at its best for 'les inventions les plus agréables', and poets are those who can express these 'avec le plus d'ornement et de douceur'. Poetry has lost the day as a serious thing; it becomes something pleasing, elegant and sweet; and as such it survives. Yet it survives; and Descartes himself continued to have lively literary ambitions, and composed poetry. So it was with Hobbes. He will not grossly carve poetry out of human experience. He too will compose poetry and translate Homer.

---

[1] Descartes, *Discours de la Méthode*, ed. Gilson, Paris, 1925, p. 7.

There will then be a theory of fancy which will somehow justify poetry. But what kind of a theory can it be? 'Romants' and presumably therefore all 'fictions' are condemned; we are left with 'decaying sense'. What is left for Hobbes to say?

Now in Chapter 8 of *Leviathan*, Hobbes distinguishes between 'Naturall' and 'Acquired' wit. Natural wit belongs to 'Experience', the level of mind below that at which reason operates; acquired wit belongs to reason. Natural wit is an intellectual virtue which corresponds to prudence; acquired wit one which coresponds to sapience. This is what he says on (pp. 52–53): 'By Naturall, I mean not, that which a man has from his Birth: for that is nothing else but Sense; wherein men differ so little from one another, and from brute Beasts, as it is not to be reckoned amongst Vertues. But I mean, that *Wit*, which is gotten by Use onely, and Experience; without Method, Culture or Instruction'; and on p. 56 he says, 'As for *Acquired Wit*, (I mean acquired by method and instruction,) there is none but Reason; which is grounded on the right use of Speech; and produceth the Sciences'. Natural wit then is what shows itself, in varying degrees, in all discourse which is made at the level of 'Experience'; it is exhibited in the sagacious man, the prudent man, the historian and the poet. Hobbes had said earlier (p. 53): 'This NATURALL WIT, consisteth principally in two things; *Celerity of Imagining*, (that is, swift succession of one thought to another;) and *steddy direction* to some approved end'.

Celerity of imagining, he says, is one of the two factors which make up the difference between a man of wit and a dull man. Now is this a difference in congenital endowment of an intellectual or imaginative kind? The answer is definitely, no. The difference in quickness of wit is 'caused by the difference of mens passions; that love and dislike, some one thing, some another: and therefore some mens thoughts run one way, some another; and are held to, and observe differently the things that passe through their imaginations' (p. 53). Therefore the stream of thoughts passing through a man's imagination (which however in strictness we may recall, is but memory) is determined by his passions. We must take Hobbes to mean that the passions decide both the direction of a man's imagination and the quickness of his imagining. This is highly disputable, no doubt; but let is be as Hobbes says. He then says (p. 53): 'and whereas in this succession of mens thoughts, there is nothing to observe in the things they think on, but either in what they be *like one another*, or in what they be *unlike*, or *what they serve for*, or *how they serve to such a purpose;* Those that observe their similitudes, in case they be such as are but rarely observed by others, are sayd to have a *Good Wit;* by which, in this occasion, is meant a *Good Fancy.* Now I pause in the exposition to emphasize that Hobbes here uses 'fancy' in a sense different from that in which he has earlier employed the word in *Leviathan.* Earlier, as in Chapter 2, 'fancy' was synonymous with 'imagination' and with 'memory'; it was 'decaying sense'. But here it has a quite distinct significance, it is a perception of similitudes; and to be quick in perceiving similitudes unperceived by others is to have a good fancy, and, to that extent, a good wit. Then he goes on to oppose, to the fancy, *judgement,* which is quickness in seeing the 'differences, and dissimilitudes . . . between thing and thing' (p. 53). Therefore, fancy and judgement alike, so far from being mere 'sense' or mere 'imagination', are activities of the mind, bearing down on the images of sense, seeing similitudes and dissimilitudes between them.

Now Hobbes has a good deal more to say about fancy and judgement. He has said that a good fancy is one which is quick to observe novel similitudes. But he hastens to explain that 'a great Fancy is one kind of Madnesse'; to have quick and powerful fancy without corresponding strength of judgement is to be, in strict truth, not a great wit, but a sort of madman. Fancy is mad; judgement is sane. 'Great wits' means men of powerful fancy; in general, fancy is naturally chaotic and wild, and constantly requires the control of judgement; and in his *Answer to the Preface to Gondibert* (E. 4. p. 449) Hobbes declares that 'judgement begets the strength and structure, and fancy begets the ornaments of a poem', from which we may further gather that judgement makes for order, design, structure; fancy only, at best, agreeable ornament. Again, he says in *Leviathan* (p. 54) that 'In a good History, the Judgement must be eminent: because the goodnesse consisteth, in the Method, in the Truth, and in the Choyse of the actions that are most profitable to be known. Fancy has no place, but onely in adorning the stile'; method and truth are yielded by judgement, adornment by the fancy. If fancy is pre-eminent over judgement in poetry (and Hobbes says that it should be), it is only because, in poetry, we look for and are pleased by 'Extravagancy' (p. 54). We are here at the centre of Augustan orthodoxy. It is judgement which ensures design and order to a poem, and which gives to poetic discourse (as to every other kind of discourse) *'steddy direction* to some approved end'.

VIII

Now this doctrine, which here, in the eighth chapter of *Leviathan*, is given a classic exposition, was so powerful throughout the Augustan period, that I venture now to make a number of observations upon it. Judgement, he has said, observes differences, fancy similitudes; also, judgement constructs a poem, fancy supplies the ornaments in the form of simile. But strictly, where the mind creates 'fictions' it does so, Hobbes tells us in Chapter 2, through the power of fancy where 'fancy' is identical with 'imagination'; 'Fictions of the mind' (p. 15) are 'compounded imaginations'. Here the fancy is constructive, however inconsistent Hobbes may be in saying so. He also sees the fancy as the power which discerns similitudes and gives rise to metaphor and simile. These two powers of the fancy are intrinsically wild and unrestrained and require the check of the judgement; and when he says, as in the *Answer to the Preface of Gondibert*, that 'judgement begets the strength and structure . . . of a poem', we must take him to mean not that judgement is responsible for the 'fictions' which make up the story, but that judgement by its restraining and ordering power gives shape and unity to what otherwise would be confused and wild. But Hobbes wavers and is unclear about all this. For in *Leviathan* fancy creates fictions, in the *Answer* the judgement *begets* the structure and fancy begets the *ornaments;* and it is plausible to believe that Hobbes is trying to maintain a sharp dichotomy between fancy and judgement analogous to that he upholds between sense and reason, and will not be drawn into recognizing that, in fact, fancy and judgement *co-operate* in designing the structure of a poem. Fancy creates the fictions, as Hobbes explicitly declares in Chapter 2 of *Leviathan;* but judgement 'begets the strength and structure of a poem', as he explicitly declares in the *Answer*. But the truth is that each alike is involved in the making of the 'fictions'. I suggested that Hobbes himself sometimes implies that sense and reason, prudence and sapience, 'dexterity' (or untaught ability), and rules are not to be regarded as wholly different in kind; and in the same way, it is only by a violent and false act of abstraction that we can thus seek altogether to oppose fancy and judgement; they do not meet from the ends of opposed winds, but are from the start somehow intimate with each other. They are friendly enough; and if tensions grow up between them, they are family tensions only. But Hobbes was unwilling (for much the bigger part) to think so.

I can set out the same point in another aspect. For let us consider

Hobbes's doctrine that fancy discerns similitudes, the judgement differences. But how does the fancy, which is 'one kind of Madnesse' hit at all on similitudes, some of which presumably the judgement, though looking always for differences, will allow? Is not the discernment of a similarity, if it *is* a similarity, an act of judgement? Is not to compare and see similitude as much an act of judgement as to compare and distinguish? Is it possible to see similitude without *also* seeing differences? And if it must come to that, does not the lunatic exercise as fine a sense of difference, within his own world, as he does of similitude?

We can, I think, see Hobbes's motive in speaking in this way, and what blinded him from seeing the error in what he said in these matters. He consistently exalts reason above experience; he consistently exalts, within the world of 'experience', judgement over fancy, setting up sharp oppositions between the two pairs; judgement is the representative, so to speak, of reason in the world of 'Experience'. His inclination is always to the more intellectual side of knowledge. And we have therefore a philosopher who roots everything in sense, and declares that everything 'we conceive has been perceived first by sense'; but who also consistently depresses sense in the interest of higher intellectual faculties which however, he must also say, *are* sense. This is the paradox of all his thinking. And the result of it is that the 'originall fancy' from which all comes and on which all depends is also made the source of 'one kind of Madnesse'; all derives from fancy, and fancy is mad. The impetus of Hobbes's philosophy is to deliver us from sense and fancy; he also declares that we are entirely tied to it. Hobbes's thought is everywhere a masterpiece of exquisite paradox. Hence, in his philosophy of knowledge, sense is but 'originall fancy'; and in his æsthetic, fancy is a wild and lawless thing, needing the sternest control.

I can further illustrate the difficulties of Hobbes's opposition of judgement and fancy in this way. The reader will recall that he says in *Leviathan* (p. 53) that 'naturall wit' consists chiefly in two things: celerity of imagining, 'that is, swift succession of one thought to another', and 'steddy direction to some approved end'. Then, after speaking of how the passions affect the speed of imagining, he says that those who observe the similitudes of their thoughts '*in case they be such as are rarely but observed by others* [my italics] are sayd to have a *Good Wit*; by which, in this occasion, is meant a *Good Fancy*'. Here, a sign of 'good' fancy is, not merely celerity, but seeing novel similitudes; a similitude is a sign of a 'good' fancy when it is rarely observed and is unusual. But we say, the question about any similitude is not, Is it rare? but, Is it indeed *good*, or *true*, or *apt*? Let us grant that a man may be quick in seeing similitudes, and that the similitudes he observes are entirely novel. But the fact remains that he may be a lunatic. And of course Hobbes declares, before the paragraph is finished, that the fancy, 'without Steddinesse, and Direction to some End . . . is one of kind of Madnesse'. But it is clear that Hobbes felt the impulse to define *goodness* of fancy; he saw that mere 'celerity' and 'steddinesse' do not explain this; but he shied off from acknowledging that the fancy may be said to discern truly, or aptly, or well; he was not willing to talk of truth of imagination. As it is, in order to avoid doing this, he goes in for the curiously un-Augustan test of novelty; at the centre of this classic exposition of Augustanism there is a lively Romantic heresy.

But we have still to put the strongest objection to what Hobbes says here of poetry. It is not only that he cannot consistently allow 'designe' in discourse, whether the discourse deal in the 'fictions' of poetry or seeks out causes; also, it is not only that he cannot rightly explain the 'fictions'. What is still more serious is *that he cannot and does not so much as begin to give a serious account or doctrine of æsthetic experience.* 'But without Steddinesse, and Direction to some End, a great Fancy is one kind of Madnesse', he says; and if so, poetic discourse must be steady and have direction to an end. Now with the question, What is the 'end' of poetry in Hobbes's doctrine? I shall deal later. I remark now only that Hobbes conceives that poetic discourse has an end out-side itself; but I am here more concerned to point out the consequences of the following statement, which he makes in Chapter 8 of *Leviathan* (p. 54): 'In a good Poem, whether it be *Epique* or *Dramatique;* as also in *Sonnets, Epigrams*, and other Pieces, both Judgement and Fancy are required. But the Fancy must be more eminent; because they please for the Extravagancy; but ought not to displease by Indiscretion'. Then he goes on to say that there is 'no place' for fancy in history, but 'onely in adorning the stile'; and when it comes to 'Demonstration', 'Councell, and all rigourous search of Truth, Judgement does all; except sometimes the understanding have need to be opened by some apt similitude; and then there is so much use of Fancy. But for Meta-phors, they are in this case utterly excluded. For seeing they openly professe deceit; to admit them into Councell, or Reasoning, were manifest folly' (p. 54). From all this it is clear that the fancy is never to be taken seriously. In Councell or Reasoning, it may be put to limited employment; in history it may adorn style; in poetry it pleases for its 'Extravagancy'. In poetry we do not expect truth; we are only entertained by a not unreasonable amount of untruth.

Now if we are at all disposed to attribute to poetry any considerable importance, and to give weight to the *Oresteia* and to *King Lear*, we will not be likely to accept Hobbes's doctrine of Æsthetic. It gives the arts no chance; they are damned from the start. If the poets listen to Hobbes, what will they do? How can they raise their spirits to start writing, and if they make a start, how will they proceed? Hobbes was a rationalist. Locke, who comes after him, was a rationalist only in a very limited degree; but he will have less to say for poetry than even Hobbes. Locke was, as we shall see, a more temperate, modest and catholic mind than Hobbes; but because he was less literary and had less feeling for words, he will not even suffer poetry to exist. Hobbes will have poetry for 'Extravagancy'; Locke will hardly admit it as a source of amusement. The outlook for the arts in general, and for poetry in particular, is grim indeed.

But for our part, we wish to give to the arts a notable place in human experience; and therefore we add a final objection to Hobbes's scheme. Hobbes allows sense, and judgement and reason; he allows fancy only as either 'decaying sense' or as 'one kind of Madnesse'. But it is clear that somewhere in our philosophy of human life, we must allow for a power which is neither sense, nor intellect, which is, however, the crucial factor in our æsthetic experience. This power is what is best called imagination, a power closely related to both sense and intellect, acting as intermediary between them, but to be identified with neither. Of this power I shall speak in the last section of this chapter.

IX

And yet Hobbes himself cannot rest in this form of the distinction between fancy and judgement. There is at least one notable occasion when he sees clearly that it is not so simple. It is his *Answer to the Preface to Gondibert*. In *Leviathan*, Fancy sees similitudes, Judgement discerns and distinguishes. In the *Answer*, the Judgement registers both differences *and* resemblances. This is what he says: 'For memory is the world, though not really, yet so as in a looking-glass, in which the judgement, the severer sister, busieth herself in a grave and rigid examination of all the parts of nature, and in registering by letters their order, causes, uses, differences and resemblances . . .' This is already, without looking ahead, a statement of considerable interest. Memory is a mirror in which the world is reflected. And yet, Hobbes says, it cannot be so simple. Sense cannot, in strictness be said to *reflect* the world; for the world needs to be sorted out by the judgement, discerning order, causes, uses, differences and resemblances. There is here more than a possibility of a different way of thinking from what we have found in *Leviathan*, which was published in 1651, the year after that in which the *Answer* appeared. But leaving this aside, Hobbes then goes on to say: 'Whereby the fancy, when any work of art is to be performed, finds her materials at hand and prepared for use, and needs no more than a swift motion over them, that what she wants, and is there to be had, may not lie too long unespied'. That is to say, her material has been sorted out; differences and similitudes have been observed by the judgement; she has only to move quickly and pick and choose. But he goes on: 'So that when she seemeth to fly from one Indies to the other, and from heaven to earth, and to penetrate into the hardest matter and obscurest places into the future, and into herself, and all this in a point of time, the voyage is not very great, herself being all she seeks. And her wonderful celerity, consisteth not so much in motion, or in copious imagery discreetly ordered, and perfectly registered in the memory; which most men under the name of philosophy have a glimpse of, and is pretended to by many, that grossly mistaking embrace contention in her place. But *so far forth as the fancy of man has traced the ways of true philosophy* [my italics], so far hath it produced very marvellous effects to the benefit of mankind. All that is beautiful or defensible in building; or marvellous in engines and instruments of motion; whatsoever commodity men receive from the observations of the heavens and from the description of the earth, from the account of time, from walking in the seas, and whatsoever distinguisheth the civility of Europe, from the barbarity of the American savages; is the workmanship of fancy, but guided by the precepts of true philosophy . . .' (E. 4. p. 449).

Now there are things in this remarkable passage which I find obscure. But I so far understand it (or think I do) as to agree with an American scholar, Mr. Clarence DeWitt Thorpe, of Michigan, who sees in it a doctrine in some respects not at all in accordance with what was to be the Augustan orthodoxy; but instead, an approach to a quite different doctrine of the imagination. For it seems clear that Hobbes now gives to fancy a leading rôle in 'true philosophy' and in the application of science to human needs and in the making of civilization; and if this is so, it seems hardly possible to sustain, what he does in *Leviathan*, the

sharp dichotomy of reason and sense, judgement and fancy. Truly, he
still says that judgement deals with 'order, causes, uses, differences and
resemblances'; but the fancy is capable of tracing the ways of 'true
philosophy' and is a necessary agent in devising 'engines and instruments of motion' and, indeed, civilization generally. The reader will
recall Hobbes's definition of philosophy—'Knowledge we acquire, by
true ratiocination, of appearances or apparent effects, from the knowledge we have of some possible *production* or *generation* of the same; and
of such production, as has been or may be, from the knowledge we have
of the effects'. But here, in the *Answer*, Hobbes appears to be saying
that fancy can anticipate 'true philosophy' and 'true ratiocination'; and
if so, once again, we might have expected Hobbes no longer to uphold
the violent antitheses on which his philosophy is founded; he might
have seen that the fancy may have a certain rational quality and the
reason owe something to the imagination.

But Hobbes did not do so; and as I have said, it is in the *Answer* that
he remarks that 'time and education beget experience; experience
begets memory; memory begets judgement and fancy, judgement
begets the strength and structure, and fnacy begets the ornaments of a
poem. The ancients therefore fabled not absurdly, in making Memory
the mother of the Muses.' And yet, it is in the paragraph in which
this observation occurs that he speaks of fancy as having 'traced the
ways of true philosophy' (E. 4. p. 449). He then goes on to say that
the 'workmanship of fancy' is shown in the application of science to
use and in the building up of civilization generally; and in this, fancy
has been guided by 'the precepts of true philosophy'. He then says
(p. 450): 'But where these precepts fail, as they have hitherto failed
in the doctrine of moral virtue, there the architect Fancy must take the
philosopher's part upon herself. He, therefore, who undertakes an
heroic poem, which is to exhibit a venerable and amiable image of heroic
virtue, must not only be the poet, to place and connect, but also the
philosopher, to furnish and square his matter; that is, to make both
body and soul, colour and shadow, of his poem out of his own
store . . .' Thus, in poetry which treats of mankind (and 'the description of great men and great actions is the constant design of the poet';
and again, 'The subject of a poem is the manners of men, not natural
causes'), the Fancy is at once an architect and a philosopher. Here, in
moral philosophy, the fancy has been indispensable and has rightly
taken 'the philosopher's part on herself' in constructing heroic poems.
But if so, will it do to speak of judgement as begetting the

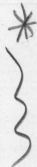

strength and structure and fancy as (only) begetting the *ornaments* of a poem?

From this, I think it certain that there was an uncertainty and vacillation in Hobbes's doctrine of the fancy, and that from time to time he forgot his way of opposing it sharply to reason and judgement.

X

I have suggested, in the course of expounding Hobbes's views on the fancy, that he was very uncertain of his way and falls into contradictions. But I have still to ask, and answer, the question: How did Hobbes envisage the end and purpose of poetry? What did he think it was for? How, seeing that he was at some pains not to obliterate it from experience, did he retain it for useful? It is clear that as a form of knowledge he could think nothing of it. Yet seeing that he retains it as a form of discourse, in which judgement is required, what is the end to which its 'steddinesse' as a form of discourse is directed? And it will be convenient, in asking this question about poetry, to ask it also about historical discourse. What is *its* purpose?

Now to answer these questions, it will be serviceable to look back to the sickly, ill-complexioned humanist scholar who survived up to 1629 and translated Thucydides. In his writings before that year he says, indeed, nothing about poetry. But at least he says something about history; and what he says about it then, and what he says about it later, will help us to understand his attitude to poetry.

Hobbes's only writings before 1629 are the translation of Thucydides with its introduction, and the poem *De Mirabilibus Pecci*. For the rest, our authorities are Hobbes's *Autobiographies*, Blackbourne's *Vitæ Hobbianæ Auctarium* and (what Blackbourne's account is based on) Aubrey's notes. This is not, indeed, very much. But it provides us with enough from which to obtain a reasonably firm impression of Hobbes the Humanist. To this list we may fairly add the two digests he wrote of Aristotle's *Rhetoric*. These indeed he made about 1635 in the course of instructing his young pupil; but we may be sure that he had acquired detailed acquaintance with the *Rhetoric* in the days before he had opened *Euclid*. Let us now briefly review what information he and others give us about this time in his life, which stretches from 1610 to 1629, before he could know how much his mind was to change at the end of the thirties and when he had much Latin and Greek but little science and less mathematics.

Oxford, Aristotle and scholastic logic had meant little to him; he had been more interested in maps and travel, and after leaving Oxford he nearly lost his classics. But a lucky voyage to the Continent made him wish to be a scholar, in days of great classical scholars; and in the years that followed the 1610 tour, he read widely in the Chatsworth Library. How much the library of the Earl of Devonshire meant to him is clear from what he says in the dedication of the translation of Thucydides: 'there was not any, who more really, and less for glory's sake favoured those that studied the liberal arts liberally, than my lord your father did; nor in whose house a man should less need the university than in his. For his own study, it was bestowed, for the most part, in that kind of learning which best deserveth the pains and power of great persons, history and civil knowledge . . .' (E. 8. p. iv). Here, more than at Oxford, was his university. It was Latimer, in Wiltshire, who had taught him classics; and the home of the Cavendishes was to succour his humanist learning as Oxford had not. He found the philosophy he had learnt at Oxford despised on the Continent; and he came home to be, above all, a scholar in ancient history and poetry. In the prose-life he says: 'philosophiam autem logicamque (in quibus praeclare profecisse se arbitrabatur) viris prudentibus derisui esse videns, abjecta logica et philosophia illa vana, quantum temporis habebat vacui, impendere decrevit linquis Graecae at Latinae. Itaque cum in Angliam reversus esset, historicos et poetas (adhibitis grammaticorum celebrium commentariis) versavit diligenter (L. 1. pp. xiii–xiv); and in the verse-life,

> Vertor ago ad nostras, ad Graecas, atque Latinas
> Historias; etiam, carmina saepe lego.
> Flaccus, Virgilius, fuit et mihi notus Homerus,
> Euripides, Sophocles, Plautus, Aristophanes,
> Pluresque; et multi Scriptores Historiarum:
> Sed mihi prae reliquis Thucydides placuit. (L. 1. p. lxxxviii.)

To these it is perhaps worth while adding the statement in the *Vitæ Hobbianæ Auctarium*: 'Reversus itaque, cum jam Candisianæ gentis munificentia tempus atque otium ipsi suppeteret priora studia respiciendi, magno literaturæ Academicæ fastidio affici coepit . . . Aliam itaque philosophandi rationem sibi ineundam ratus, lectioni veterum philosophorum, poëtarum, historicorum, tum e Graecis tum Latinis, diligentes incubuit . . .' (L. 1. p. xxiv). I quote this because it is interesting to observe that Hobbes speaks only of his reading classical historians and poets; Blackbourne says, philosophers too. Here, it is not unlikely that Blackbourne is right. Hobbes, writing out of the days when he scorned Aristotle, might not feel disposed to speak of his reading in classical philosophy. That, as a now confirmed humanist scholar, he would read Aristotle, is extremely likely; and in the preface to his Thucydides he says that 'Homer in poesy, Aristotle in philosophy, Demosthenes in eloquence, and others of the ancients in other knowledge, do still maintain their primacy . . . And in the number of these is justly ranked also our Thucydides; a workman no less perfect in his work, than any of the former' (E. 8. p. vii). Writing in his still humanist days, he is willing enough to speak of classical philosophy and of Aristotle.

Until 1629, when he discovered geometry, he was, then, the humanist scholar; and his work as a humanist was crowned by his translation of Thucydides, which was published in 1628. Besides, when Aubrey says that 'before Thucydides, he spent two yeares in reading romances and playes',[1] it is natural to suppose that the romances and plays were recent or contemporary works; about the same time he composed *De Mirabilibus*; and he counted amongst his friends Bacon, Ben Jonson, Lord Herbert of Cherbury and Sir Robert Aytoun, an admired poet of the time.

We can now turn to the introductions to his *Thucydides*, in which he gives us his views in the writing of history. They are very clear. He says: 'For the principal and proper work of history [is] to instruct and enable men, by the knowledge of actions past, to bear themselves prudently in the present and providently towards the future'; and this task he says, is better performed by Thucydides than by any other historian. It is not, Hobbes is careful to explain, that Thucydides is anywhere explicitly a teacher; 'he never digresses to read a lecture, moral or political'; but the reader by attentive reading may 'from the narratives draw out lessons to himself' (E. 8. p. vii–viii).

History then is justified by its didactic effect; and Hobbes will have nothing to do with history for the sake of the delight it may give. He deals hardly with Dionysius of Halicarnassus who makes the 'scope of history, not profit by writing truth, but delight of the hearer, as if it were a song' (p. xxvi); and he pours contempt on the preference of Dionysius for Herodotus on the ground that he was 'wiser in the choice of his argument' than Thucydides (p. xxiv). Dionysius indeed saw the historian as an artist, and prescribed to the artist rules for the writing of history, the choice and ordering of the material and theme;

[1] Aubrey, *loc. cit.*, p. 361.

but, says Hobbes, Herodotus 'undertook to write of those things of which it was impossible for him to know the truth; and which delight more the ear with fabulous narratives, than satisfy the mind with truth' (p. xxiv). He ends by quoting with strong approval the judgement on Thucydides of Justus Lipsius, who had died some twenty years earlier: 'Everywhere for elocution grave; short, and thick with sense; sound in his judgements; everywhere secretly instructing and directing a man's life and actions' (pp. xxxi–xxxii).

I quote the great scholar from Hobbes's pages to show that Hobbes's views in history carried the authority of the highest Renaissance learning. And if Hobbes was in line with Lipsius, he was also following here in the wake of Bacon. Dr. Strauss, in his valuable essay, *The Political Philosophy of Hobbes*,[1] has rightly reminded us of this. Bacon may not indeed have started Hobbes on his philosophical road; but he may well have been the inspirer of his translation of Thucydides. Dr. Strauss observes that Bacon, like other writers of the Renaissance, did not believe that the precepts of philosophy can win men to virtue; but that what precept and reason fail to do, history, by illustrating, but without stating, precepts, may succeed in doing. This is indeed a part of the thesis of Sidney; who makes the historian say that the philosopher's 'vertue is excellent in the dangerlesse Academie of *Plato*, but mine sheweth foorth her honorable face in the battailes of *Marathon*, *Pharsalia*, *Poitiers* and *Agincourt*'.

I am not now concerned to discuss this view of history; but only to ask, what effects Hobbes's later and mathematical philosophy had on his tenure of it? Dr. Strauss has, happily, asked this question, and has answered it fully. I agree with his answer, and consider that it is fully borne out by Hobbes's writings.

In the introduction to *Thucydides* Hobbes says: 'For in *truth* consisteth the *soul*, and in *elocution* the *body* of history . . . For the faith of this [Thucydides'] history, I shall have the less to say: in respect that no man hath ever yet called it into question. Nor indeed could any man justly doubt of the truth of that writer, in whom they had nothing at all to suspect of those things that could have caused him either voluntarily to lie, or ignorantly to deliver an untruth. . . . In sum, if the truth of a history did ever appear by the manner of relating, it doth so in this history: so coherent, perspicuous and persuasive is the whole narration, and every part thereof' (p. xxi). Thucydides really does, he says, give us the truth; and the tests of truth in history are coherence, perspicuity and

---

[1] Oxford, 1936.

persuasiveness. Now this may strike as rash and unsceptical enough; and all the more so, because, as we have seen, Hobbes is very much on his guard against any control of historical writing by artistic requirements or satisfactions. He knows well enough what the difficulties and dangers are in this matter of historical 'truth'; in some historians, he says, 'there be subtle conjectures at the secret aims and inward cogitations of such as fall under their pen; which is also none of the least virtues in a history, where conjecture is thoroughly grounded, not forced to serve the purpose of the writer in adorning his style, or manifesting his subtlety in conjecturing' (p. viii); and it is because he can say this, that we are all the more surprised that he can swallow Thucydides, quite whole, because he is 'coherent, perspicuous and persuasive'. It seems incredible that he will maintain this ingenousness when he has been sophisticated by mathematics. Nor does he. He will come to see, as he says in the first chapter of *De Corpore*, that 'although Sense and Memory of things . . . be knowledge, yet . . . they are not philosophy'; and in *Leviathan* (p. 22) we have: 'As Prudence is a *Præsumtion* of the *Future*, contracted from the *Experience* of time *Past*: So there is a Præsumtion of things Past taken from other things (not future but) past also. For he that hath seen by what courses and degrees, a flourishing State hath first come into civil warre'—always there is the thought of civil war—'and then to ruine; upon the sight of the ruines of any other State, will guesse, the like warre, and the like courses have been there also. But this conjecture, has the same incertainty almost with the conjecture of the Future; both being grounded only upon Experience.' And on p. 52 we are told that 'it is evident, that whatsoever we believe, upon no other reason, then what is drawn from authority of men onely, and their writings; whether they be sent from God or not, is Faith in men onely'. All this is a very different story from what we find in the preface to *Thucydides*. History has yielded to philosophy.

And yet, in spite of this, we also find this in Chapter 8 of *Leviathan*: 'In a good History, the Judgement must be eminent; because the goodnesse consisteth, in the Method, in the Truth, and in the choyse of the actions that are most profitable to be known. Fancy has no place, but only in adorning the stile'. Here, he speaks like a good humanist enough. He has indeed lost any belief he had that historical truth is possible, and he believes that philosophy alone gives real knowledge; still, what he says in the words I have just quoted, is identical with the doctrine of the preface to *Thucydides*. The humanist is dying hard.

Indeed, he does not die at all. He inconsistently survives even into the philosopher's extreme old age, and translates Homer.

XI

For I have been speaking of Hobbes the historian, not of Hobbes the poet. And I turn now to his views on poetry, and by doing so we shall be able to complete our review of his doctrine about history.

Hobbes the humanist reconciled himself to history only on condition that it was true, and Dionysius of Halicarnassus evoked his lively anger. For Herodotus, whom Dionysius preferred to Thucydides, 'undertook to write of those things . . . which delight more the ear with fabulous narrations, than satisfy the mind with truth' (E. 8. p. xxiv); and Dionysius 'makes the scope of history, not profit by writing truth, but delight of the hearer, as if it were a song' (p. xxvi). But what then of Homer, Virgil and Ovid—not historians indeed but trafficking certainly in fabulous narrations? Hobbes says nothing of them in the prefaces to *Thucydides*. 'For in *truth* consisteth the *soul*, and in *elocution* the *body* of history. The latter without the former is but *a picture of history* . . .' (these last are my italics) he says. Now alongside this let us put this sentence from the *Answer to the Preface to Gondibert*, which was done in 1650, the year before the appearance of *Leviathan*: 'For as truth is the bound of the historical, so the *resemblance of truth* [again my italics] is the utmost limit of poetical liberty' (E. 4. p. 451). So, histories which are not true may picture the truth; and poetry may be historical in this sense, that it may resemble truth. And we find him saying in the preface to his translation of Homer, that Virgil and Lucan 'except in the introduction of their Gods, are but so many histories in verse' (E. 10. p. viii), where, by 'histories' he can only mean histories that are 'pictures of history'. In this way we reach a point where history of the kind which 'pictures' history is indistinguishable from poetry. Poetry on its side, must present what might have happened and must 'resemble' truth; and in a sense may thus be called history.

Now bearing this in mind, we must recall that Hobbes the philosopher must decline to call history knowledge; it is a product of sense and memory, not of ratiocination. But his philosophy, by the employment of reason, affords a plenitude of truth. Why therefore should Hobbes reconcile himself to pictures of and resemblances to truth? As a humanist, before 1629, he had persuaded himself (with difficulty as I have suggested: the rationalist was present, after all, in the humanist) that some history could be true; but as a philosopher he is quite clear that all history is only conjecture. Why then does history survive in his scheme of life and thought? And why, still more, poetry, which is less true, even as a 'picture' of history and truth? Why does he not cut their throats and have done? The answer can only be what he said in the preface to Thucydides, that history instructs men to bear themselves prudently; and this justifies history, though history is now throughout conjecture, and nowhere knowledge. Philosophy has superseded history; and history cannot provide truth. But its conjectures may be useful in teaching virtue; and if the conjectures of history may have this use, so also may the fictions of poetry. For there is little to choose between conjecture and fiction.

If this is so, the answer to our question, How did his later philosophy affect his views on history? seems to be that it reduced history from knowledge to conjecture, but left its value as a teacher of virtue unaffected. But in fact, this is not the whole of the story, as we can easily see if we look to the *Answer to the Preface to Gondibert*.

'The subject of a poem', he says there, 'is the manners of men, not natural causes' (E. 4. p. 445). This is, of course, a drastic truncation of poetry. There must not be another *De Rerum Natura*; nor plays in which a Lear exclaims, 'Is there any cause in Nature that makes these hard hearts?' Causes are for philosophy and science, the manners of men for poetry; and in presenting the manners of men the poet may not go beyond the conceived possibility of nature. Poetic discourse however must, like all other forms of discourse, have steadiness and direction to an end; and the end is 'by imitating human life, in delightful and measured lines, to avert men from vice, and incline them to vertuous and honourable actions' (p. 443).

Now let us bow to mathematical philosophy, and let us acknowledge that it is not for poetry to bother itself with causes, natural or supernatural. But we may perhaps mildly enquire whether, in dealing with the manners of men, poetry may claim to present what is true about human nature? Can it tell us what vice, virtue and honourable actions are? Does it know what they are? or if it does not, can it find out? Is not this, we ask, like everything else, the job of a philosophy suitably ordered by mathematical knowledge? Happily Hobbes supplies us with a reply, which I have already quoted in another connection, in the *Answer*. Where the precepts of true philosophy fail, '*as they have hitherto failed in the doctrine of moral virtue* [the italics are mine], there the architect Fancy must take the philosopher's part upon herself. He,

therefore, who undertakes an heroic poem, which is to exhibit a venerable and amiable image of heroic virtue, must not only be the poet, to
place and connect, but also the philosopher, to furnish and square his
matter . . .' (p. 450).

'As they have hitherto failed in the doctrine of moral virtue.' But it
is now 1650, and next year *Leviathan* will be published, and philosophy
will have given the world the precepts of true philosophy in the doctrine of moral virtue. Until then, poetry must supply its own moral
ideas. Indeed Davenant seems to have done so very well. Davenant's
description of love 'in the person of Bertha, in the seventh canto of the
second book', excels anything, Hobbes tells us, that has been said on
that subject, whether by ancient or modern poets (p. 451). But this
could only have been a hit or miss affair. In the future Dryden will
study and use Hobbes's Ethic in his plays. But in fact, will there be in
the future any real need for plays and poetry? There will not. Listen
to Hobbes in the first chapter of the *De Corpore*, which he completed in
1655: 'Now that which is chiefly wanting . . . is a true and certain rule
of our actions, by which we might know whether that we undertake
be just or unjust. For it is to no purpose to be bidden in every thing
to do right, before there be a certain rule and measure of right established, which no man hitherto hath established. Seeing, therefore, from
the not knowing of civil duties, that is, from the want of moral science,
proceed civil wars, and the greatest calamities of mankind, we may very
well attribute to such science the production of the contrary commod-
ities. And this much is sufficient, to say nothing of the praises and
other contentment proceeding from philosophy, to let you see the
utility of the same in every kind thereof' (E. 1. pp. 9–10).

This is definite enough. What is chiefly wanting is a true and certain
rule of our actions, and this Hobbes's Ethic will now supply. It is
certain, therefore, that he cannot be greatly in earnest with poetry as a
moral teacher; it is the moral philosopher who is the teacher, and what
he teaches is the ethic of *Leviathan*. And if poetry must give way to
moral science, so must history. There is little to choose between conjecture and fiction; it is reason and not imagination which is the source
of truth.

*hence,
Law
see 52*

It is therefore a poor outlook for poetry. Indeed, there is not an
outlook at all. Moral science provides virtue, and a true and certain
rule of action. For the rest, philosophy deals with natural causes. And
supernatural causes? Well, they are ruled out from the scope even of
philosophy; and we may be sure that Hobbes would not suffer their

being treated of in poetry. In ancient days, indeed, poets were divines; 'had the names of prophets; exercised amongst the people a kind of spiritual authority; would be thought to speak by a divine spirit' (E. 4. p. 448). But now there is no reason why a man 'who speaks wisely from the principles of Nature, and his own meditation' should wish 'to be thought to speak by inspiration, like a bagpipe'. He will then, one supposes, write in prose and be content to be a philosopher. But the imaginative exploration by poetry of the universe of experience—that is something Hobbes did not envisage, nor could believe to be either possible or desirable.

And yet, as I have said, Hobbes keeps places for history and poetry in his scheme. Late in the day he thought it worth while, for want indeed, as he tells us, of something to do, to translate Homer. The power of the classics, of Homer above all, did not fade out of his mind. The humanist lived on. But did he ever, in his old age, ask himself if the *Iliad*, which, in the preface to his translation, he commends as giving profit as well as delight to the reader—if the *Iliad* satisfies the ethic of *Leviathan*? Are the heroes images of Hobbist virtue? On the contrary, they are images of 'honour'. The Glaukus who said,

$$\text{Ἱππόλοχος δέ μ' ἔτικτε, καὶ ἐκ τοῦ φημι γενέσθαι·}$$
$$\text{πέμπε δέ μ' ἐς Τροίην, καί μοι μάλα πόλλ' ἐπέτελλεν,}$$
$$\text{αἰὲν ἀριστεύειν καὶ ὑπείροχον ἔμμεναι ἄλλων. . . .[1]}\quad(\textit{Iliad } 6.\ 206\text{–}8).$$

is the very model of 'honour' as Hobbes expounds it in the tenth chapter of *Leviathan*; and, as Dr. Strauss reminds us, what, as a humanist he had called heroic virtue became to the later philosopher not a virtue at all, but a source of evil, the rebellious, illimitable pride and vanity of man.[2] Certainly Homer is no Hobbist tract; and when Hobbes speaks of heroic virtue, as he still does in the preface to the translation of Homer, it is to explain that the hero's 'glory . . . lies in courage, nobility' and other virtues of nature, or in the command he has over other men (E. 10. p. 4). The virtues of the Homeric hero are *virtues of nature*, and are not the virtues required in the Hobbist state. In the *Leviathan* 'honour' is not a virtue, but a passion. There, 'nobility is Power'. In this pride of honour and power Hobbes sees the menace to his state; and Leviathan is 'King of the Proud'. So that it will not do to try to make of Homer a teacher of virtue. He will no more satisfy Hobbes

---

[1] Hippolochus was my father; from him I declare myself sprung. He sent me to Troy and charged me ever to be best and to excel all others.

[2] Strauss, *loc. cit.*, pp. 49–50.

than he satisfied Plato as an instructor of morals. Hobbes will not say so in so many words. In the preface to Homer he speaks indeed of profit to be got in the reading of him; but the emphasis is on delight. This is what he says: 'And the design is not only to profit, but also to delight the reader. By profit, I intend not here any accession of wealth, either to the poet, or to the reader; but accession of prudence, justice and fortitude, by the example of such great and noble persons as he introduceth speaking, or describeth acting. For all men love to behold, though not to practise virtue. So that at last the work of an heroic poet is no more but to furnish an ingenuous reader, when his leisure abounds, with the diversion of an honest and delightful story, whether true or feigned' (E. 10. p. iii). The last sentence gives away the game; we shall read Homer for the reason that Hobbes translated him— because he 'had nothing else to do'. And as for the 'prudence, justice and fortitude' of the preceding sentence, on the next page they have become the 'glory of courage, nobility and other virtues of nature'. It was hard to keep up the pretence.

So the wheel turns its circle. And the ardent humanist who would not suffer history to give delight 'as if it were a song' gives place to the impassioned and reforming philosopher who commends Homer to an 'ingenuous reader, when his leisure abounds'.

XII

I wish next to make some observations on the philosophy which I have now briefly but not, I trust, inaccurately or unfairly, expounded. I have tried to explain the rôle of reason in Hobbes's philosophy, and then the rôle of sense, imagination and fancy. I do not propose to speak further of Hobbes's rationalism. My motive in speaking of it at such length was to give the reader as lively an impression as I could of the pride of reason which animated the first of the great Augustan philosophers, and also how easily it went along in his mind with an aggressive naturalism. We speak frequently of the years from 1650 to 1780 in England as the Age of Reason; and it is well therefore to be informed on what reason was and how its tasks and possibilities were envisaged at the outset. Here, in regard to Hobbes, 'reason' may fairly be taken to mean rationalism. But at a later stage, indeed before the seventeenth century was out, rationalism in England, as Hobbes set it forth, was a lost cause. And if we speak of an age of reason, it is necessary to bear in mind that, after Hobbes, Augustan philosophy is *not* rationalist. With Locke, English Empiricism comes in, and was to continue in different forms in the two greatest succeeding philosophers, Berkeley and Hume.

But if I shall say little more about Hobbes's rationalism, I wish to speak further of Hobbes's theory of sense-knowledge, and of imagination. Locke broke drastically away from the rationalism of Descartes and Hobbes; but Hobbes's doctrines of sense-knowledge were based on certain assumptions, or errors, which were to continue through Augustan philosophy; and it is convenient therefore to speak of them here both before speaking of Locke, Berkeley and Hume and before speaking of Augustan poetry. Trying to expound Hobbes's views of sense, memory and fancy, I was drawn naturally into observing certain contradictions in what he says. I wish now briefly to remark on certain fundamental misconceptions which animate and misdirect his reflections, and which continued into later Augustan philosophies; and the reader will bear in mind that in a highly intellectual age, in which there existed, in all cultivated society, the greatest respect for the labours and findings of the intelligence in philosophy and science, these errors were bound to react on the attitudes of poets to their composition and be shown in the compositions themselves.

The prime error in Hobbes's theory of sense-knowledge is what may be called the confusion between sensation and imagination. In his doctrine, they are one thing; in fact they are two things. Hobbes (and his successors in differing degrees agree with him) believes that for a grown-up to open his eyes and see a patch of colour is sensation. In fact, it is imagination. No doubt a newly born child, on opening its eyes, may be said to have sensation, or as near to it as can be come by; but a grown child on seeing a patch of colour, discriminated by him in and against a sensory background, carries out an act of imagination. In the remainder of this chapter, I shall speak only briefly of this matter. In a later chapter, I shall have occasion to speak of it at greater length.

Now philosophical terms, we know, are grossly misleading, and not least to philosophers. The philosophy of Hobbes (and no philosopher was ever more suspicious of words or more critical of their abuse by others) illustrates it.

It is very important therefore to employ the terms 'sense', 'sensation' and (I add) 'sense-data' with great circumspection. Hobbes says (what I have already quoted) in the *De Corpore*: 'we must consider that although sense and memory of things, which are common to man and all living creatures, be knowledge, yet because they are given us immediately by nature, and not gotten by ratiocination, they are not philosophy'. Here is in all truth a *locus classicus* for the Augustan exaltation of ratiocination and misunderstanding of sense-knowledge. 'Sense of things' is given us immediately by nature; it is something we share with the animals and is therefore slightly ignoble. But in fact, things are not so simple; and if 'sense of things' is something we share with the animals, to give some play and importance to sense-knowledge is to remind ourselves that we are at least as much animals as we are angels, and that still less are we God himself. It may be less agreeable to our pride; but we shall be less likely to bring trouble, both of a philosophical and of a more drastic kind, on ourselves.

For the 'sense of things' is not in fact 'given us immediately by nature'. What is provided 'by nature' are certain stimuli which act upon our organisms in such a way as bring about what, if our sense-organs and nervous systems are healthy, we call sensation. But sensations are not discriminated objects; they are mere feelings saturated in emotion; and they are in and of the ever-changing flux of consciousness. So far we have no 'sense of things'; nor, if we wait till Domesday, will sensation provide 'things' for our contemplation. If the sensations 'given us immediately by nature' are to be moved, however slowly, and however partially, out of feeling and into knowledge, it can only be through the growing power of the mind, which elevates mere sense into idea. Now the power thus exerted by the mind, however mysterious its origin may be, is best called imagination, which, in a dawning self-consciousness, labours to lift out of the flux in which there is neither self nor world but only a drift of sensation and feeling, something firm and fixed. Imagination indeed fails to do this; the fixing and making firm of which I have spoken requires, indeed, the aid of the intelligence, through which alone the flux can be arrested or at least made to look as if it were not a flux; still, it is the at first half-blind imagination which instigates the first movements to knowledge. Much of this blindness, in all truth, the imagination never loses; and the bright refining light of the intelligence is always painful to its eyes. And yet what the intelligence judges to be the poor half-lights of imagination are those in which the self is born, and in which at the first, it must see as best it can; in this half-light the mind stirs out of its trance of feeling. The imagination cannot indeed be said to provide to it objects for its scrutiny; there is yet no occasion for mere curiosity. At most there is something which is barely beyond the frontier of the self. It is truly idea; but it is hardly conceptualized.

It is then, the imagination which stimulates the mind to attend to or contemplate what it learns increasingly to select from a mass of feeling; and along with this, another side of this process, the mind begins to attend to itself, to be aware of itself as beholding. And yet, so far, we have not yet reached what may fairly be called a world. What is beheld and that which beholds are, so to say, at a slight enough remove from each other; the object is hardly known, and little more than felt; it is no longer of the very stuff of the mind and is idea; but still it is shot through with subjectivity.

But this is not a state in which there is rest. For the imagination produces a chronic unease which the imagination cannot cure; and thought comes to the aid of imagination, bringing its innumerable categories and concepts wherewith to hold and encompass what otherwise might have fallen back into the flux of subjectivity. Thought distances further what have barely been disjoined; it changes a state of blank beholdment into an asking of questions; and tries to replace mystery with understanding. And it is only at this stage that objects are clearly present to our minds, in a world apprehended with the aid of the intelligence. They are in increasingly greater number pushed further off into objectivity; and what is in them of subjectivity the mind, under the pressure of its many tasks, may learn to disregard. There is thus a great simplifying of the life of the mind; thought selects carefully and omits much; and it achieves a refined and economical order in which the mind can move skilfully and adroitly, and be relieved of the full burden of imaginative experience.

Now whether thought, by the application of its processes to experience, can finally bring to the mind the ease and freedom which it wants, is another matter, into which we need not now go. My only, and very limited, concern is to emphasize what Hobbes wholly omits, namely, an order of experience which is not sensation and not thought, but which yet grasps sensory unities; and this prehension, which is imaginative, is the condition of intellectual activity. Moreover, this imaginative prehension is not something which may be said to yield place to thought; it continues as the condition of thought; it prehends that on which thought may conduct its labours. What now is merely imaginative idea may fall under the analytic scrutiny of thought; but it does so without falling beyond the scope and grasp of the imagination; being conceptually known, it is also imaginative idea.

There is therefore a constant tension between imagination and thought. Because what is imagined is not complete or perfect, imagination invokes the aid of thought; and in this way the mind achieves what are properly objects. And yet a price is paid; for a greater objectivity is gained at the expense of a certain shrinking of the mind and of the content of knowledge. The abstractions of the intelligence seek to remove much of the inexhaustible individual reality; and a rift is set up between its cold conceptual order and the warm personal unity of what is imagined. The imagination requires the intelligence, but is also jealous of it; while the intelligence, conscious of its power and easier articulation, seeks in vain to outstrip the imagination. And out of this tension symbol is born; for symbol is the difficult compromise in which the two come to some kind of terms, the agreed mode of expression which at once avoids conceptual ordering and definition and yet precipitates the mind into the search for them.

The imagination then is not sense, whether decaying or not, but a power which prehends elements 'given by sense' and grasps them in unities and as ideas upon which the abstracting intelligence may then work its refinements and economies. As the child's mind grows, imagination must precede intelligence; yet a facilitating environment quickly evokes through language the play of abstraction. Even so, it is not difficult to see, in what we can piece together of the history of the language of our race, the long labour with which language passed from being predominately an imaginative expression to being predominately an instrument of conceptual explication. But our purpose now is only to say that both imagination and thought are necessary to what we ordinarily call perception of objects; and their great play is blandly ignored by Hobbes when he says that the 'sense of things' is given us immediately by nature.

Certainly in what I have said there is nothing new. But what is strange is how disinclined the English philosophical mind has been to acknowledge its truth. Hobbes speaks of perception as if the world marches into the mind self-declared and self-explained, or is contained in the motion of sense-stimuli, which acts as a vehicle to carry it into the brain; and if the mind is indeed Locke's blank paper (though Locke never said it was merely that), the world can at most inscribe on it the scrawlings of mere sense. This failure is continued in Berkeley and Hume; in Mill; and in our own day the unceasing talk about sense-data has shown an unbelievable imperviousness to philosophical learning. For sense-data are an abstraction of philosophers who will not fairly inspect the act of perception, and what is involved in it; and they are left, and rightly, as Hume was, in a nightmare of meaningless and chaotic sense-data from which they are helpless to wake up.

For it is not wrong, but right, to begin philosophy by studying perception; and to study it with fairmindedness is to discern in it a fundamental imaginative power which, rightly understood, leads on to the study and understanding of artistic power. To fail to acknowledge what is not intellectual in sense-knowledge is naturally to attribute the 'strength and structure' of poetic works to intelligence and mere ornamentation to fancy or imagination; it is also, in Pope's words, to deplore that description should hold the place of sense in poetry, where Pope uses 'sense' in a manner that came in only late in the seventeenth century and had extensive use in the eighteenth, to mean 'natural understanding, intelligence, especially as bearing on action or behaviour'. In this way the nature of poetry and its relation to morals is profoundly misconceived, and the true place of art in the economy of the human spirit ignored. But of this I shall speak later, and of its consequence for poetic art. Immediately, there are two other matters, arising out of Hobbes's philosophy, on which I wish to remark.

Now, it may be said that little good purpose can be served by using the word imagination as I have used it in the preceding paragraphs. 'To imagine', it may be said, 'is to be aware of what is not present to us, as in memory, or again, of what we ordinarily call the 'imaginary'; to say that we *imagine* what is before us must be at best misleading and is in fact foolish. The objects of the imagination are strictly either what have been present to us in the past and are not so now, or what have never been present to anyone at any time and are fictitious. But to object in this way is to miss the intention of our use of the word. As I use it, it is not relevant that what is imagined is fictitious; to speak of our imagination of objects is to speak of the activity of the mind in holding a unity before it for beholdment and then for intellectual analysis; whether what is known be the desk on which I write or Hamlet whom I 'imagine', does not affect the nature of the mental act; in either case there is entertainment of a whole of perception, and it is this sense which informs our use of the word 'imagination'.

But even if this be agreed, it may still be objected that we are compelled to find, within the universe thus imaginatively prehended, a criterion by which we may distinguish what is imagined and seen, from what is imagined and fictitious; so that, acknowledging that all objects are imaginative objects, we may know what we mean when we speak of 'imaginary' objects. Now certainly we must look for such a criterion.

But it is not, in fact, easy to find, as the history of philosophy from Hobbes to Hume clearly shows. For if we make it a criterion that 'imaginary' objects are created at will, and that in waking perception of things certain sense-features (which, so considered, can only be abstractions) are offered us, as it were, 'by nature' and not created by us at will, it may fairly be replied that we do not make our dream-objects at will, nor the bears which are 'really' bushes. And little inspection is necessary to show that it is very difficult to put down the colours of Tamburlaine's banners for unreal, and to put up the colours of the local cricket club for 'real'. Hobbes himself confirms this. 'Sense', he says, 'is but originall fancy'; and again, 'This decaying sense, when wee would express the thing itself, (I mean *fancy* it selfe), wee call *Imagination*, as I said before: But when we would express the decay, and signifie that the sense is *fading*, old, and past, it is called memory. So that *Imagination* and *Memory*, are but one thing which for divers considerations hath divers names.' He has no means of discriminating between the 'real' and the 'unreal' of sense, what is 'seen' and what is 'imaginary'; and what he failed to find, Locke, Berkeley and Hume failed to demonstrate, for all the attempts they made.

But, it may still be argued, what is 'seen' comes to us more clearly, vividly, bearing as it were a certificate of its objectivity; what we remember, what we 'make-up', are in comparison faded and fluctuating. But alas, though this has been tried out by at least one very bright intelligence, it is fairly obvious that it will not work. For it simply is not true that what is remembered, what is dreamed, what is 'imaginary' is always dim, obscure, fragmentary. The recollections of youth, summoned to the sweet silent sessions of old age, have, we are told, an unbelievable vivacity and brightness and seem to blot out the years between; dreams certainly can be lively and leave us helpless, in spite of our struggles, to wake up; and Hamlet saying to Horatio, 'Thou wouldst not think how ill all's here about my heart' is carried more alive into the heart than a hundred people we meet of a morning.

In denying in this way that we can distinguish between 'sense' and 'imagination' Hobbes will come along with us. And yet he says that certain 'imaginary' things are 'unreal'. These are 'compound imaginations' and properly but fictions of the mind—as when from the sight of a man at one time, and of a horse at another, we conceive in our mind a centaur. Now we saw that Hobbes's philosophy can give him no means of explaining how we can do this. But leaving this aside, it is certain that no one in earnest with artistic creation can be disposed to think that the 'fictions' of poetry are made in this way, by a putting together of bits and pieces.

Now in order to consider fairly what Hobbes has to say in this matter, we must have in mind artistic creation typical of our own civilization. For what may have been the genuine imaginative creations of earlier civilizations acquire for us a certain fanciful note, if I may now use the distinction between imagination and fancy which Coleridge, following Kant, rightly insisted is necessary. For what is properly to be called fancy is precisely illustrated by the instance of the centaur, if we have in mind the centaur as he is for us and not as he was for the Greeks, to whom the centaur may well have been serious imaginative idea. It is for us a mechanical and unrealized union of man and horse in one ; but typical imaginative ideas of our civilization are Iago and Imogen, whose creation and existence are very different from that of the centaur. Hobbes illustrates the power of the mind to create so-called 'fictions' from the fancy; but if we think of Hamlet, Cordelia, Satan, Mr. Micawber, there is another and very different story to tell. Now Shakespeare had better reason than Hobbes to know how 'fictions' are created; and the Friar in *Much Ado* says of Hero, then being put out for dead, that

> The idea of her life shall sweetly creep
> Into his study of imagination;
> And every lovely organ of her life
> Shall come apparell'd in more precious habit,
> More moving-delicate and full of life,
> Into the eye and prospect of his soul,
> Than when she lived indeed . . .

Shakespeare is here speaking of an act of memory, but also of imagination; and we have here not only, in this matter, inestimably higher authority than Hobbes, but also what, to everybody's experience, rings truer. It is of the *life* of Hero that the friar speaks, and of the vitality of the idea of her life as it will come to Claudio; and he uses the word 'life' three times in the seven lines. He does not speak of an image of her face or body, but of the life which animates the body; and in Claudio's idea she will be more moving-delicate and full of life than when he knew her living. This idea shall creep into his study of imagination; that is, into his imagination intent and dwelling on her; it will inhabit his mind and be there a living thing. The imagination of Claudio will be *studious*, concentrated, active, (with the suggestion, that frequently hangs about Shakespeare's use of 'study'—'to study help', 'to study fashions to adorn my body of devising'); and yet the idea comes with its own life and power of entry into the mind; it will come filled with life into the eye of the soul. Shakespeare only three times uses the word 'idea'; here it is near to Newman's favourite use of the word; as in the *Essay on Development*, where he speaks of ideas as like 'bodily substances, which are not apprehended except under the clothing of their properties and results, and which admit of being walked round, and surveyed on opposite sides, and in different perspectives, and in contrary lights, in evidence of their reality'; definition of them is not possible; we are 'forced to enumerate properties and accidents by way of description'; and ideas are not 'brought home to the intellect as objective except through this variety'.[1]

As I have said, Shakespeare here speaks of the recollection of a loved woman. But the memory of her, as Shakespeare represents it, is not a piece of 'decaying sense'. It is neither sense nor decaying, but an idea more 'moving-delicate and full of life' than when it was 'sense' indeed. But if this is so of the ideas which enter the study of imagination from the memory, what shall we say of those ideas which cannot be derived from the memory? The centaur, as I have said, will not serve; Beatrice and Cordelia too are moving-delicate and full of life; and it is as 'certain as anything most true' that the idea of Beatrice moved into Shakespeare's study of imagination with every appearance of her own power; and that Cordelia entered into the eye and prospect of his soul under the impulse of her own heavenly grace. They are not figures of paper and gum, but of life; and it is philosophical enough, or scientific enough for that matter, to appeal away from a philosopher obsessed with geometrical concepts to the greatest of all creators of living ideas—

> And as imagination bodies forth
> The forms of things unknown, the poet's pen
> Turns then to shapes, and gives to airy nothing
> A local habitation and a name.

No doubt, to appeal to Shakespeare's poetry from his own prose, would have irritated Hobbes acutely. 'Metaphors openly professe deceipt'; and 'to admit them into Councell, or Reasoning were manifest folly'. But it is an ill philosophy which will, in seeking an Æsthetic, go to Hobbes's narrow and closed mind before seeking out the openness and candour of Shakespeare's.

Now in this brief and dogmatic section, I am very conscious that I

---

[1] Newman, *Essay on the Development of Christian Doctrine*, London, 1897, p. 34.

have barely approached certain great and difficult problems. But in what follows I shall hope to be more precise and to attempt answers to questions barely raised here. In speaking of Locke, I shall find convenient occasion to speak at greater length on what I have called the imagination and to illustrate its workings; I shall also find occasion to speak of its relation to the intelligence (for the reader may well judge that in what I have said so far I have merely pushed in a *tertium quid* between sense and thought and thereby solved no problem); and sooner or later, we shall need to explain how, if all things are, as I have suggested, 'imagined,' we can at all claim that in perception we know what is 'real.'

CHAPTER TWO ... *The Humble Heart*

I

IN 1703 Rev. Mr. Richard King, writing to Locke, enclosed a letter from a friend requesting Locke to set down his recollections of Edward Pococke. Pococke, who had died in 1691, had been the greatest Oriental scholar in the Kingdom, Laudian Reader in Arabic and Regius Professor of Hebrew at Oxford, and a friend of Laud, Selden and Locke. He was a firm Anglican and Royalist; yet, during the Commonwealth, he was not required to declare allegiance to the Long Parliament and Cromwell; and when in 1650 a move was made to dispossess him of his living of Childrey in Berkshire, John Owen, the puritan Vice-Chancellor of Oxford, came warmly and effectively to his help. This is what Locke wrote about him. I do not apologize for quoting it at length, for it is an incomparable portrait of a scholar, and is not well known.[1]

'. . . So extraordinary an example, in so degenerate an age, deserves, for the rarity, and, as I was going to say, for the incredibility of it, the attestation of all that knew him, and considered his worth.

The christian world is a witness of his great learning, that the works he published would not suffer to be concealed. Nor could his devotion and piety lie hid, and be unobserved in a college; where his constant and regular assisting at the cathedral service, never interrupted by sharpness of weather, and scarce restrained by downright want of health, showed the temper and disposition of his mind.

But his other virtues and excellent qualities, had so strong and close a covering of modesty and unaffected humility; that, though they shone the brighter to those who had the opportunities to be more intimately acquainted with him, and eyes to discern and distinguish solidity from show, and esteem virtue that sought not reputation; yet they were the less taken notice, and talked of, by the generality of those to whom he was not wholly unknown. Not that he was at all close and reserved; but, on the contrary, the readiest to communicate to any one that consulted him.

Indeed he was not forward to talk, nor ever would be the leading man in the discourse, though it were on a subject that he understood better than any of the company; and would often content himself to sit still and hear others debate matters which he himself was more a master of. He had often the

[1] *Works of John Locke*, 10 vols. London, 1801, vol. x, p. 300 ff. All quotations from Locke are made from this edition.

silence of a learner, where he had the knowledge of a master; and that not with a design, as is often, that the ignorance any one betrayed might give him the opportunity to display his own knowledge, with the more lustre and advantage, to their shame; or censure them when they were gone. For these arts of triumph and ostentation, frequently practised by men of skill and ability, were utterly unknown to him. It was very seldom that he contradicted any one; or if it were necessary at any time to inform any one better, who was in a mistake, it was in so soft and gentle a manner, that it had nothing of the air of dispute or correction, and seemed to have little of opposition in it. I never heard him say any thing that put any one that was present the least out of countenance; nor ever censure, or so much as speak diminishingly, of any one that was absent.

He was a man of no irregular appetites. If he indulged any one too much, it was that of study, which his wife would often complain of, (and, I think, not without reason,) that a due consideration of his age and health could not make him abate.

Though he was a man of the greatest temperance in himself, and the farthest from ostentation and vanity in his way of living; yet he was of a liberal mind, and given to hospitality; which considering the smallness of his preferments, and the numerous family of children he had to provide for, might be thought to have out-done those who made more noise and show.

His name, which was in great esteem beyond sea, and that deservedly, drew on him visits from all foreigners of learning, who came to Oxford, to see that university. They never failed to be highly satisfied with his great knowledge and civility, which was not always with expence.

Though at the restoration of king Charles, when preferment rained down on some men's heads, his merits were so overlooked or forgotten, that he was barely restored to what was his before, without receiving any new preferment then, or at any time after; yet I never heard him take any the least notice of it, or make the least complaint in a case that would have grated sorely on some men's patience, and have filled their mouths with murmuring, and their lives with discontent. But he was always unaffectedly cheerful; no marks of any thing that lay heavy at his heart, for his being neglected, ever broke from him. He was so far from having any displeasure lie concealed there, that whenever any expressions of dissatisfaction, for what they thought hard usage, broke from others in his presence, he always diverted the discourse; and if it were any body with whom he thought he might take that liberty, he silenced it with visible marks of dislike.

Though he was not, as I said, a forward, much less an assuming talker; yet he was the farthest in the world from being sullen or morose. He would talk very freely, and very well, of all parts of learning, besides that wherein he was known to excel. But this was not all; he could discourse very well of other things. He was not unacquainted with the world, though he made no show of it.

His backwardness to meddle in other people's matters, or to enter into debates, where names and persons were brought upon the stage, and judgments and censure were hardly avoided; concealed his abilities, in matters of business and conduct, from most people. But yet I can truly say, that I knew not any one in that university, whom I would more willingly consult, in any affair that required consideration, nor whose opinion I thought it better worth the hearing than his, if he could be drawn to enter into it, and give his advice.

Though in company he never used himself, nor willingly heard from others any personal reflections on other men, though set off with a sharpness that usually tickles, and by most men is mistaken for the best, if not the only seasoning of pleasant conversation; yet he would often bear his part in innocent mirth, and, by some apposite and diverting story, continue and heighten the good-humour. . . .

I do not remember that, in all my conversation with him, I ever saw him once angry, or to be so far provoked as to change colour or countenance, or tone of voice. Displeasing actions and accidents would sometimes occur; there is no help for that; but nothing of that kind moved him, that I saw, to any passionate words; much less to chiding or clamour. His life appeared to me one constant calm.

How great his patience was in his long and dangerous lameness (wherein there were very terrible and painful operations) you have, no doubt, learnt from others. I happened to be absent from Oxford most of that time; but I have heard, and believed it, that it was suitable to the other parts of his life.

To conclude, I can say of him, what few men can say of any friend of theirs, nor I of any other of my acquaintance; that I do not remember I ever saw in him any one action that I did, or could in my own mind blame, or thought amiss in him.

We cannot doubt that the impression made on Locke by Pococke was profound. Locke says in a letter which he wrote to King on the very day on which he set down the recollections I have quoted, that he had never known 'a fitter person than he, to be preserved as an example, and proposed to the imitation of men of letters';[1] and if the impression was profound, it was also lasting, for Locke was writing within a year of his own death and bitterly deplored his failing memory. Here, in all truth, was Newman's gentleman; and the idea of him passed into Locke's mind and was potent in fashioning him.

It is very important to see Locke in this light. We must see him as the confidant of Shaftesbury and William, as one who shared in the planting of Carolina, was secretary to the Council of Trade and Plantations in the time of Charles and Commissioner of Trade in the

---

[1] *Works*, vol. x. p. 299.

time of William; more than this, we must see him as the great theorist of constitutional monarchy, and as the philosopher of the human mind. But above all, we must see him moved by the image of virtue and piety which he beheld in Pococke. In Locke there is little of the pride of mind which animated Hobbes, or, if we wish, made of Hobbes, as we must sometimes feel, a repulsive mask; instead, there is a humble and quiet heart which hides no obscure and unacknowledged motives and fears.

To read the life and the letters of Locke is not at all, in the first place, to confirm in us the thought of Locke as one of the great founders of English rationalism. This, in one sense of the word 'rationalism' he was, no doubt. But if we contemplate him rightly, we shall see him in the light, not of what came after him, but of what went before him. Behind Locke there stretches a line of famous and good men, of temperate spirit and free mind, of a rare sweetness and gentleness: Hooker, John Hales, Chillingworth, Falkland, Whichcote, Cudworth. Locke inherits the temper of these men, and it is a temper of unusual grace and beauty. Hooker was one of Locke's acknowledged masters; he recommended Chillingworth as a master of right reasoning; of Falkland he must have heard a great deal from Shaftesbury, who was his friend at the time of the Civil War, as Locke tells us in his notes on the life of Shaftesbury;[1] Cudworth he knew, and of Whichcote, if he never was acquainted with him, he must have talked with their mutual friend Mapletoft. We understand Locke much better by reading Walton's *Lives* (which it is hard to believe Locke himself had not read) than by reading deistic discourses. Locke was very far from deism; he was near to, indeed he was of a piece with, the spirit of the men who frequented Great Tew in the thirties of the century, and of whom Clarendon has given us his masterly portraits; and the temper of all these men enabled them to avoid the bitter dogmatism alike of High Church and of Puritan to the increase of their piety and charity. It was pre-eminently their temperate mien of reasonableness and faith which made possible, after the coming of Descartes and Hobbes, the greatest of English philosophers. Descartes and Hobbes were able, by prodigious intellectual gifts, to give the world highly organized systems of rationalism. Locke ever hated systems and distrusted the intellect; and this he was able to do because he inherited from the Chillingworths and the Pocockes a piety which made him humble in the face of what was more than human and more than human reason. Yet, if he was no apostle of rationalism, he was that incalculably better

---

[1] *Works*, vol. ix. p.266.

thing, an apostle of reasonableness; and his reasonableness sprang, not
from a doctrine, but from an indefinable temper which, because it was
inspired by faith in God, declined to despise and tried temperately to
employ, the powers of the reason. 'If you ask', he wrote in his epitaph,
'what manner of man he was, he replies that he was happy in his mediocrity';[1] and it was his mediocrity and his belief in mediocrity, in the
older and better sense of the word, as we shall have many occasions to
see, which best explains his excellence.

II

He went to Westminster School in 1646 and was drilled in Latin and
Greek. At Oxford, where he went in 1652, John Owen was beginning
to reform the University and was Dean of Christ Church, Locke's own
college, as well as Vice-Chancellor. Even Clarendon was to acknowledge that Owen's rule at Oxford 'yielded a harvest of extraordinary
good and sound knowledge in all parts of learning'. Still, it was not
the harvest Locke wanted; the Puritans did not change the matter of
the teaching, and Locke was to complain bitterly of the Peripatetic
philosophy, obscure terms and useless questions peddled in the
schools. Oxford gave him very much what it had given Hobbes, which
was very little. Lady Masham, writing to LeClerc after Locke's death,
says he was no hard working student and sought out the company 'of
pleasant and witty men' as a refuge from useless learning; and we are
told too that he did what Hobbes had done: he spent much time 'in
reading romances from his aversion to the disputations then in fashion'
and read widely in books of travel. It is of great interest to observe the
refuge from the schools the two men found in 'romances'.[2] Hobbes,
Aubrey tells us, regretted the two years which he had given to such
reading; and though Esther Masham was to entertain some of Locke's
leisure in his old age by reading romances to him, imaginative literature
was never, as we shall see, to be more than a source of recreation and
amusement to him. 'Should children', Coleridge was to write, 'be permitted to read romances, and relations of giants and magicians and
genii? I know all that has been said against it; but I have formed my
faith in the affirmative—I have known some who have been *rationally*
educated, as it is styled. They were marked by a microscopic acuteness,
but when they looked at great things, all became black and they saw

[1] *Life of John Locke*, by H. R. Fox Bourne, 2 vols., London, 1876, vol. ii. p. 561.
[2] *Ibid.*, pp. 53–4.

nothing . . . and called the want of imagination judgment and the never being moved to rapture philosophy'.[1] Wordsworth when a boy would lie a whole day together reading *Arabian Nights* by 'Derwent's murmuring stream'. Newman was to read Mrs. Radcliffe, Miss Porter, and find life-long delight in *Thalaba*. The maturity of all three was to endorse and even nourish their boyish delights. The trials of their undergraduate life drove Hobbes and Locke to these or similar pleasures; but Hobbes, we may be sure, indeed we know, reacted sternly from excursions of the fancy; Locke perhaps did so more reluctantly, and humanly enough to leave him a kindly and condescending listener to young Esther's reading of 'the romance of *Astraea*'.[2]

In 1658 he became Senior Student at Christ Church. He welcomed the Restoration and was to stay in Oxford until 1667. During these years he decided not to take orders, in spite of the persuasion of his friends, and not to get married, in spite of a serious attack of love. Had he taken orders, we cannot doubt he would have been one of the great thinkers and (no less) administrators of the English Church; as it was, he was for the greater part of his life in close touch with the greatest figures in Church thought and politics. Through Pococke he knew many of the High Church party; he was a friend of Wilkins and the intimate friend of Simon Patrick, Isaac Barrow and above all of Archbishop Tillotson ('a man so much superior to every theologian whom I know, both in character and in abilities'), all Latitudinarians; and of those outside the Anglican Commission he was the friend of Baxter. Had he married, we can only say that it would have been no fault of his had his marriage not been one of rare happiness; he had, Fox Bourne says, and rightly, 'a lover's heart'. As it was, he was something of a match-maker, and when his friend LeClerc married, and for a time wrote to Locke only irregularly, Locke bowed before a demand superior to friendship; 'love does and should engross all the attention of a lover', he said. Besides, he was in love all his life, with children, with his friends, with Betty Clarke, Esther Masham, Damaris Masham. His correspondence is a feast of passionate friendship, seasoned with his unique banter and archness. As he grew older his love and his need for love became still greater; and his letters to Molyneux and Anthony Collins are the letters of one for whom friendship is one of the two supreme values of life. To this we shall return.

---

[1] S. T. Coleridge, *Letters*, ed. E. H. Coleridge, vol. i. p. 16.
[2] Fox Bourne, vol. ii. p. 297.

In 1666 he met Shaftesbury; and his life took a new and surprising turn. In 1667 he went to live at Exeter House, Shaftesbury's London home. Shaftesbury had liked Locke at their first meeting, and until Shaftesbury's death in 1683, but for the years 1675 to 1679 when he travelled in France for his health, Locke was to be near Shaftesbury, an adviser in medicine, in education, in politics, in religion and philosophy. I shall not attempt to recount the fortunes of Shaftesbury during these years. I remark only that prudence requires that we form our opinion of him more in accordance with what Locke has to say about him than with what Dryden had to say in *Absalom and Achitophel*. Locke was a better man and a better judge of men than Dryden; and his friendship with Shaftesbury was long and close, too long and too close to make it possible for us to see in the epitaph Locke wrote for him the mere hollow praise it is easy to give to the great and famous.

In 1668 Locke became a Fellow of the Royal Society and was already intimate with two illustrious scientists, Boyle and Sydenham. But in spite of his quick curiosity in many fields of scientific learning, science always held a modest enough place in the economy of his mind. He never played, or sought to play, any great part in the Royal Society. Fox Bourne quotes[1] from Birch's *History of the Royal Society* a story which shows Locke, ordinarily scrupulous in fulfilling his undertakings, in an unusual light. At a meeting of the Society in Gresham College in November 1672 it was said that a sulphur ball showed powers of attraction, and 'Mr. Locke intimated that himself had made some experiments with such a ball, and promised that he would bring it to the society at the next meeting'. But when, a week later, 'Mr. Locke, being called upon for his sulphur ball, which he had promised at the last meeting to produce at this, excused himself that he had forgot it, promising to bring it at the next'. But at the next meeting, it was Boyle and not Locke who exhibited the attractive powers of a sulphur ball. Locke's 'mediocrity' shows itself in his temperate addiction to science; and though he was learned and skilled in medicine he never practised except in private and desultory ways. That he was not drawn wholly into scientific work was no doubt a happy thing for philosophy; but it is probably more important to remark that the scepticism which he directed at scientific knowledge in the *Essay* was always at work in him and inhibited him from exclusive devotion to scientific pursuits. He was content to be a lively amateur of science; or even a journeyman, to

[1] Fox Bourne, vol. i. p. 318.

judge by his readiness to pass on to Boyle information on matters he had occasion to investigate.

Besides, perhaps because he was 'critical', as Kant (in a different way) was to be, of the scientific understanding, he showed signs of interest in history, in an age remarkable for its interest in antiquities. It was the age of Dugdale, Hickes and Hearne; and Locke enjoyed a long and intimate friendship with Tyrrell, who occupies an honourable place among the historians of the time. Tyrrell was the author of *A History of England*, and we are told that 'his introduction on Anglo-Saxon Government may still be read with interest'.[1] Locke must have talked with Tyrrell on these and such matters; a letter to Richard King on 25 August 1703 shows the extent of his reading in early English history; and we are not therefore surprised that when Locke's friend William Allestree became Secretary to the English Ambassador in Sweden, he was asked to send back all the information he could get about Scandinavian antiquities. So far as he was a scientist, Locke was an experimental one, not, like Hobbes, a rationalist and deductive one; and his theory of mathematical knowledge as knowledge strictly 'of our own ideas' quite denied him the intoxication Hobbes felt at the sight of a page of Euclid. Now deductive and mathematical science, scorning experiment, drove history out of Hobbes's scheme of things. But Locke can give high place to historical knowledge; if mathematics provide certainty, it is certainty only about things of our own making; and history can provide probability so great as to be, for all time or purposes, certainty.

It was in 1671 that there occurred, at Exeter House, what is, one supposes, the most celebrated meeting in English philosophical history. Locke was thirty-nine at the tine, and one of his friends at the meeting was Tyrrell, the historian. Locke himself tells us of the meeting. The plain, historical method was not, in its concern with the human mind in general, above telling us about the history of Locke's own mind and masterpiece. 'Were it fit to trouble thee', he says to the Reader, 'with the history of this Essay, I should tell thee, that five or six friends meeting at my chamber, and discoursing on a subject very remote from this [Tyrrell tells us they were discussing morality and revealed religion], found themselves quickly at a stand, by the difficulties that rose on every side. After we had a while puzzled ourselves, without coming any nearer a resolution of those doubts which perplexed us, it came into my thoughts, that we took a wrong course; and

---

[1] David Douglas, *English Scholars*, London, 1943, p. 169.

that before we set ourselves upon inquiries of that nature, it was necessary to examine our abilities, and see what objects our understandings were, or were not, fitted to deal with. This I proposed to the company, who all readily assented; and thereupon it was agreed, that this should be our first inquiry. Some hasty and undigested thoughts on a subject I had never before considered, which I set down against our next meeting, gave the first entrance into this discourse . . .'[1] The meeting took place early in 1671, and in the course of the year he wrote two drafts of the essay, the second and longer unfinished. These two drafts have now been published, the first in England, by Professor Aaron and Mr. Gibb, the second in America, by Professor Rand; and we can now see clearly how Locke's mind moved in this momentous year in English philosophy. In the first draft he moved rashly, as we might expect, to deal with what were, for him, final matters, that is, the limits of knowledge, what he treats of in Book 4 of the finished *Essay*; but he saw that he was moving too quickly, and in a second draft he studied 'sensation' and 'reflection', which he saw he must deal thoroughly with before setting out his last conclusions; and he treats therefore in it of the matters which we find in the first two books of the *Essay*. But the *Essay*, which was not to be finished until 1689 and to be published until 1690, naturally differs in many ways from the drafts.

But until 1675 he was very busy with other and practical matters. In 1673 he had been appointed Secretary to the Council of Trade and Plantations. Hard work told on his health. He came of a consumptive family, and he had to be careful. He went therefore late in 1675 to France and spent there three happy years, making many acquaintances among scholars and scientists, to return to England in April, 1679. The year 1678 had been of great importance in English history. As late as November there had been a bitter and historic debate in which Sacheverell asked if Parliament might not change the succession? Whigs and Tories were being defined under the stress of events, and in the same month Oates proclaimed the plot to poison the King. Shaftesbury was playing to the City, and, a nobleman, he stumped the country to create a radical party. Danby fell in December, and in the January of 1679 the long Cavalier Parliament was dissolved. February saw the Whigs triumph at the polls and March the Parliament meet. But the speed of events was slowed up; the Exclusion Bill was not brought in till May, a month after Locke landed back in England; and

[1] *Works,* vol. i. *Epistle to the Reader.*

by that time Charles was able to prorogue and then dissolve the Parliament, to the furious exasperation of Shaftesbury.

So Locke returned, to an England not far from civil war. The threat of civil war had helped to make of Hobbes a believer, not indeed in what may fairly be called the Divine Right of Kings, but, on secular and practical grounds, in the absolute authority of the monarch; but Locke's line in politics had been laid down before he met Shaftesbury and when civil war was certainly not threatening, in the days of Clarendon's power in the sixties, and he never swerved from it. After his return to England in 1679 Locke spent the greater part of the time before 1683, when he fled to Holland, in Oxford. How much he knew of Shaftesbury's intrigues with Monmouth at this time, we do not know. Locke was prudent and cautious by nature; and that his ill-health should keep him out of London at this desperate and, as it was to prove, decisive time for Shaftesbury, was perhaps something he did not regret. We do not know Locke's opinions of Shaftesbury's designs for Monmouth; but he was certainly spied on in his Oxford retreat; and in 1683, seven months after Shaftesbury had died in Holland, Locke left for Amsterdam.

Here he was to be until 1689, when he returned to England in the company of the new Queen. Holland was to prove a blessing to his health; he made lasting friends there and was to leave Holland for England with deep reluctance. Here he wrote on education and toleration; but above all he was able to finish, or nearly finish, the *Essay*. He had always worked at it, when the pressure of administration relaxed, since 1675; but it was his stay in Holland, in a good air and with the love of friends, that gave him his chance to complete it. Tyrrell and other friends sent him the news from England. In 1687 he had gone to live in Rotterdam; and, as news from England came to a head, he was able there to be in touch with what was going on in the Hague. During the last crisis of Shaftesbury's life he had been in Oxford, not in London; and now, at a time of still greater crisis, he was at some remove from the centre of plotting, while yet in touch with it. This strain of caution and timidity is the least agreeable thing in Locke's character; or, better, it is the only disagreeable thing in it. He had this at least in common with Hobbes; and yet, unlike Hobbes, he did not stand outside what was going on; his sympathies were by no means shown only in his writings. But even here, in his writings, he was frequently glad to shelter behind anonymity; and he was cross, what he rarely was, with Limborch for letting out the secret of his authorship of the *Letter concerning Toleration*. Locke was by nature irascible; but ordinarily he disciplined his anger, and only his timidity could let it escape his control. We are not then surprised that Locke crossed over to England only when James had fled. But however that may be, he was in no hurry to leave Holland; it had become very dear to him; and at a time when Holland has again become especially dear to Englishmen, it is right to quote some words Locke wrote to a Dutch friend a few days before he left for England. 'I almost feel as though I were leaving my own country and my own kinsfolk; for everything that belongs to kinship, goodwill, love, kindness—everything that binds men together with ties stronger than the ties of blood—I have found amongst you in abundance.'[1]

Locke was to live until 1704. He was urged to become an ambassador soon after his return; but his health and his inclination sent him into the country, and from 1691 he was to live at Oates in the home of Lady Masham, a daughter of Cudworth. In 1696, indeed, he became a Commissioner to the newly formed Board of Trade and Plantations; his ill-health made his work a heavy burden, and he would have escaped from it, if he could, in the following year; but he was not to be released until 1700. The *Letter concerning Toleration* was published soon after he returned to England, and in 1690, the year of the *Essay*, appeared, also anonymously, *Two Treatises of Civil Government*. In 1692 came the first of his writings on money; in 1693 *Some Thoughts concerning Education*; and two years later *The Reasonableness of Christianity* appeared. Towards the end of the decade came the long controversy with Stillingfleet, Bishop of Worcester. Stillingfleet too had been a protégé of Shaftesbury's, and occupies an honourable place in the history of Anglican theology; and what he had to say about the *Essay* came out of no thoughtless conservatism. He was one of the most brilliant men of his day; and if he could rouse Locke to lengthy defences of his philosophical views, he could also, in a very different kind of controversy, which raged in the seventies and eighties on the origin of episcopacy in England, make an impressive contribution to early English Church History. Therefore, to dispute with him was no light undertaking for Locke, who had, in any case, little of the polemical and contentious spirit which animated Stillingfleet. We cannot fail to be amazed at Locke's industry during these last years; for to all this he added long commentaries on and paraphrases of the letters of St. Paul. That he was able to do so many and so varied things, in his old

[1] Fox Bourne, vol. ii. p. 85.

age and in poor health, is the most potent of testimonies to the quietness and assurance of his spirit as he grew older.

Locke had known Damaris Masham since early in the eighties. In
1685 she became the second wife of Sir Francis Masham, one of whose
children by his earlier marriage was Esther, who was a favourite of
Locke's. Soon after he settled in her home Locke, writing to Limborch, said of her that she 'is so well versed in theological and philosophical studies, and of such an original mind, that you will not find
many men to whom she is not superior in wealth of knowledge and
ability to profit by it. Her judgment is excellent, and I know few who
can bring such clearness of thought to bear upon the most abstruse
subjects . . .'[1] The affection they felt for each other was as strong as
their intellectual companionship; and Locke's discretion, orderliness
and cheerfulness must have made him an ideal guest. Lady Masham
tells us that Locke thought that civility was 'not only the great ornament of life' which 'gave lustre and gloss to all our actions'; it was also
'a christian duty'. And, she goes on, 'I believe it not easy to say whether
his penetration and the solidity of his judgment in subtle and abstruse
speculations, or the agreeableness of his wit in common conversation,
were the most extraordinary; but the reputation of the one made the
other more admirable, these two so seldom meeting. So that many who
sought his acquaintance from a real desire to learn of him what might be
expected from a great philosopher . . . were much surprised, when they
saw him first, to find not only a well-bred gentleman, but a man that
was master of all the talents belonging to the polite conversation of
the world.' 'Mr. Locke', said one of his visitors, 'is not at all the grave
philosopher, able to be nothing but a philosopher, that I pictured to
myself; he is a perfect courtier, and his obliging and civil behaviour is
as admirable as the profoundness and delicacy of his genius'.[2]

The love and interest he gave to children were as great as his judgement in dealing with them. His *Thoughts on Education* is a mighty monument of good sense; and he could speak as both doctor and philosopher.
In his letters to Esther and to Betty Clarke there is plenty of facetious
grace and fancy. Esther called herself Laudabrilis and him Joannes,
and Laudabrilis was shortened to Dab, or sometimes Dib. To a letter
she wrote him when, in the nineties, he was Commissioner of Trade,
he replied:

DEAR DAB,—Your letter the last week, after so long silence, looks as if you
had been bottling up kindness for your Joannes, which at last you have let

[1] Fox Bourne, vol. ii, p. 213.   [2] *Ibid.*, p. 532-3.

run to the rejoicing of his heart more than if you had overflowed to him sack and sugar or cherry brandy. I was not a little dejected in being so long out of your thoughts, as appeared to me by your no words, which is a very ill sign in a prattle-box of your age. But in good sooth you have now made me amends, and, if what you say be but true, Joannes will perk up again and will not give place to the finest powdered spark in town. I think you know my heart pretty well, but you are a little mistaken about my head. Though it belongs now to a man of trade, and is thwacked with sea-coal and fuller's earth, lamp black and hobnails and a thousand such considerable things, yet there is a room empty and clear kept on purpose for the lady, and if you did but see how you sit mistress there and command all the ambergris and pearls, all the fine silks and muslins which are in my Storehouse, you would not complain of the filling of a place where you would sit mistress.[1]

His love for children was a sign of how readily he gave himself in friendship. In 1696 King William wished to know something of Quakers at first hand, and went, in Locke's company, incognito, to a meeting at which Rebecca Collier preached. They had liked the service and after it Locke had talked with Rebecca Collier and Rachel Bracken. A little later Locke sent them this letter.[2]

MY SWEET FRIENDS, — A paper of sweetmeats by the bearer, to attend your journey, comes to testify the sweetness I found in your society. I admire no converse like that of Christian freedom, and fear no bondage like that of pride and prejudice. I now see acquaintance by sight cannot reach the height of enjoyment which acquaintance by knowledge arrives unto. Outward hearing may misguide, but internal knowledge cannot err. We have something here of what we shall have hereafter, to 'know as we are known.' This we, with other friends, were at the first view partakers of; and the more there is of this in this life, the less we need inquire of what nation, country, party or persuasion our friends are, for our own knowledge is more sure to us than another's. These we know when we have believed. Now the God of all grace grant that you may hold fast that rare grace of charity and choose that unbiassed and unbounded love which, if it decay not, will spring up mightily, as the waters of the sanctuary, higher and higher, until you with the universal church swim together in the ocean of divine love. Women, indeed, had the honour first to publish the resurrection of the Lord of Love; why not again the resurrection of the Spirit of Love? And let all disciples of Christ rejoice therein, as doth your partner,

JOHN LOCKE.

This letter manifests Locke's own 'sweetness' and 'rare grace'; that he should have gone to the meeting as the chosen companion of the King

[1] Fox Bourne, vol. ii, p. 455.   [2] *Ibid.*, p. 453.

of England was little enough to a man whose mind was fast in such humility. This is a spirit far removed from Hobbes, and as far again removed from what 'rationalism' was to end in, the spirit of Hume.

I referred earlier to Locke's friendships with Molyneux and Collins. The correspondence with Molyneux was conducted before the two friends met; for very soon after his visit to Locke at Oates, in 1698, Molyneux died suddenly. Molyneux was a much younger man than Locke, and when they first made acquaintance by correspondence, in 1692, he was thirty-six years of age. In *A Treatise of Dioptrics*, published in that year, he complimented Locke with evident sincerity on the *Essay*, and Locke at once wrote to him, saying that he saw in what Molyneux had said 'great advances of friendship' towards him. Molyneux replied with delight, and Locke promptly wrote again, and in a manner completely typical of him in all his personal relationships. 'You must, therefore', he said, 'expect to have me live with you hereafter, with all the liberty and assurance of a settled friendship. For, meeting with but few men in the world whose acquaintance I find much reason to covet, I make more than ordinary haste into the familiarity of a rational inquirer after and lover of truth, whenever I can light on any such. There are beauties of the mind, as well as of the body, that take and prevail at first sight: and wherever I have met with this, I have readily surrendered myself and have never yet been deceived in my expectation.'[1] 'I am convinced', he said at a later time, 'that you love your friends extremely, where you have made choice of them',[2] uttering his own way in friendship; 'a rational free-minded man, tied to nothing but truth, is so rare a thing, that I almost worship such a friend';[3] and he can begin a letter in a blaze of love with: 'You look with the eyes, and speak the language of friendship, when you make my life of much more concern to the world than your own'.[4] To love truth 'with a clear-thinking head' and with a free mind, and to share that love with another was Locke's incomparably greatest pleasure; for it, what he calls the pursuit of wealth and power, fortune and interest may go by unheeded; in the double love of truth and friends, Locke's spirit glows with passion. It would be a sad error to think of Locke as dull or cold in mind or heart. 'Friendship, I see, takes no measure of any thing, but by itself: and where it is great and high, will make its object so, and raise it above its level.'[5]

Molyneux died in 1698. There was much at Oates to comfort Locke

---

[1] *Works*, vol. ix. p. 293. [2] *Ibid.*, p. 312. [3] *Ibid.*, p. 348.
[4] *Ibid.*, p. 354. [5] *Ibid.*, p. 386.

in his grief; but in his last two years Anthony Collins filled Molyneux's place in Locke's heart. 'It is no small advantage to me, to have found such a friend', Locke wrote in May 1704, 'at the last scene of my life; when I am good for nothing, and am grown so useless, that I cannot be sure that, in every good office you do me, you can propose to yourself no other advantage but the pleasure of doing it'.[1] He was to die in October. In August he wrote a letter to Collins, to be delivered to him after his death; he asked him to transact certain matters of business, and ended the letter in this way:

May you live long and happy in the enjoyment of health, freedom, content, and all those blessings which providence has bestowed on you, and your virtue entitles you to. I know you loved me living, and will preserve my memory now I am dead. All the use to be made of it is, that this life is a scene of vanity, that soon passes away; and affords no solid satisfaction, but in the consciousness of doing well, and in the hopes of another life. This is what I can say upon experience; and what you will find to be true, when you come to make up the account. Adieu: I leave my best wishes with you.[2]

Lady Masham wrote that 'all the faculties of his mind were perfect to the last; but his weakness, of which only he died, made such gradual and visible advances that few people, I think, do so sensibly see death approach them as he did. During all which time no one could observe the least alteration in his humour, always cheerful, civil, conversible, to the last day; thoughtful of all the concerns of his friends, and omitting no fit occasion of giving Christian advice to all about him.'[3] On the day before he died he told Lady Masham that he had lived long enough, thanking God for a happy life; and that after all, this life was only vanity.

III

In the preceding chapter I reviewed the life of Hobbes for the reason that his life and work show a violent departure from the earlier renaissance humanism to a new and rationalist outlook, a sudden falling away from former values to novel disciplines and hopes. Hobbes's early interests in literature and history and the humanism that went with them, declined; and a new philosophy, which reduces all to matter and motion, takes its place. Rationalism came in, with Hobbes, suddenly and completely; and the world is reduced to what reason (or so Hobbes believed) can wholly understand. So far from all things going forth into mystery, mystery goes out from all things, and reason is

---

[1] *Works*, vol. ix, p. 288.   [2] *Ibid.*, p. 298.   [3] Fox Bourne, vol. ii. p. 556.

King. Hobbes's personality, as this change in his outlook and values
came about, is transformed. From being a miserable dependent, he
acquires a certain jauntiness, a certain inexpressible assurance. He
becomes not at all the despondent, cynical and crusty creature he is
sometimes described as being; on the contrary, he is very much on
top of things; he has something impregnable about him, a metallic
quality which puts him beyond the ills and failures of men. This makes
him vaguely repellent; his philosophy gives him an eccentric air, an
oddity which ordinary flesh and blood beholds with a curious mixture
of amusement, fascination and revulsion. Also, it makes him an isolated
figure; he is friendless, through a certain inhumanity, something
diabolical which can even, and calmly, use Christianity for its own purposes. And this *use* of Christianity, by a spirit of rationalist materialism,
we cannot see as a cynicism; for Hobbes seems to have passed beyond
us into a world of values where he cannot be expected to understand
that such pride of the mind is the least forgiveable of sins. There is no
scepticism in him; he is sure; and to be without scepticism is as
dangerous for a mortal soul as to be without faith.

But I have also told something of the life and personality of Locke,
in order to show that when we speak of the age of reason, we must be
on our guard against flaccid generalizations and impressions. Hobbes
and Locke are alike great figures of an age of reason. But Hobbes
breaks sharply from what had gone before, has no continuity with the
past; Locke grows out from it and continues its spirit creatively. In
the thirties Hobbes had known Falkland and the Convivium at Great
Tew. But he learnt nothing from them. He was by that time becoming
impervious to influences, and the minds of Hammond, Falkland,
Chillingworth, Sidney Godolphin, were lost on him. Locke was born
in those thirties. But the clear and fair temper of mind which these men
helped to create was renewed in him and advanced by him. For I have
said enough to show that the humility and sweetness of the Christian
temper was Locke's outstanding quality. There are beauties of the
mind, as well as of the body, that take and prevail at first sight; and the
beauty of Locke's mind was of this kind. Humility above all distinguished him as a man and a friend; and it was inevitable that this
humility should show itself in his intellectual work. It is in this that
he is most different from Hobbes. His life is therefore rich in simple
but profound human relationships; and in deed and thought he is content with a human mediocrity. He is a humanist. System-making he
will have nothing of. 'It will be no excuse', he says in the Introduction

to the *Essay*, 'to an idle and untoward servant, who would not attend his business by candlelight, to plead that he had not broad sunshine. The candle, that is set up in us, shines bright enough for all our purposes.' It is clear to him that there must be much, the very greatest things, we cannot understand; but, having a sense of those things, we may yet live out our human life, if we have humility enough, with dignity, without shame of its peculiar pleasures and joys, and in expectation that in another world than this it will be given us to know what is here denied us. This is the true and abiding humanism, which is simply the modesty of our appointed station; and Christianity, so far from diminishing it, amplifies and confirms it. This is the golden centre of Locke's mind. He has a human normalcy. His quietness, patience, kindliness, love, toleration and forbearance, all flow from it; and these qualities he comes by not easily, but in spite of a hot-tempered and passionate nature.

Locke was saved from the exasperation which comes of seeking absolutes, and from the hideous complacency which comes of thinking one has found them. This is his 'contentment with mediocrity.' How this temper showed itself in his life can be shown from a letter he wrote to Denis Grenville from Paris in 1678. He writes:

I conceive, then, that the great difficulty, uncertainty, and perplexity of thought you complain of in these particulars, arises in great measure from this ground, that you think a man is obliged strictly and precisely at all times to do that which is absolutely best; and that there is always some action so incumbent upon a man, so necessary to be done, preferable to all others, that, if it be omitted, one certainly fails in one's duty, and all other actions whatsoever, otherwise good in themselves, yet coming in the place of some more important and better that at the time might be done, are tainted with guilt, and can be no more an acceptable offering to God than a blemished victim under the law.

I confess our duty is sometimes so evident, and the rule and circumstances so determine it to the present performance, that there is no latitude left; nothing ought at that time to come in the room of it. But this I think happens seldom, at least I may confidently say it does not in the greatest part of the actions of our lives, wherein I think God, out of his infinite goodness, considering our ignorance and frailty, hath left us a great liberty.[1]

And later in the letter, he adds,

I have often thought that our state here in this world is a state of mediocrity, which is not capable of extremes, though on one side there may be

[1] Fox Bourne, vol. i. p. 390.

excellency and perfection. Thus we are not capable of continual rest or continual exercise, though the latter has certainly much more of excellency in it. We are not able to labour always with the body, nor always with the mind; and, to come to our present purpose, we are not capable of living altogether exactly by strict rule, nor altogether without one . . . But this being but an odd notion of mine, it may suffice only to have mentioned it . . . Only give me leave to say, that if it holds true, it will be applicable in several cases, and be of use to us in the conduct of our lives and actions.

But Grenville did not catch Locke's temper and wisdom; he ended up as Catholic Archbishop of York in the exiled James II's England. Locke himself, indeed, did not, in his ethical doctrine, live up to the good sense of this letter. We shall have occasion later to consider the rationalist in Locke. I remark now only that he entertained the idea of a deductive system of ethics, and that this is surprising and contrary to what we might have expected, contrary to the spirit of what I have just been quoting. It is true that Locke certainly gives the impression of holding his rationalist ethic half-heartedly. He once resolved, at Molyneux's request, to work out his ethical system in detail, what he certainly does not do in the *Essay*; but he never did so. No doubt he felt that his head was here leading him (under what impulse we shall need to investigate) away from his good sense and practical judgement.

I said that Locke's humility was bound to show itself in his intellectual work. It does so. And in this we can show further the difference of his spirit from that of Hobbes. Hobbes, it will be recalled, was not good at quick replies to 'a serious quaere'. And we may surmise the reason. He needed to meet all problems and questions from, as it were, the very headquarters of his system. Hobbes's mind was fundamentally intuitive and imaginative; his argumentation is a façade which cannot hide his passionate perception, his peremptory ordering of experience into a fixed pattern. Therefore, to meet a question, he must first retire into his headquarters to get it into perspective; he must retreat before he can advance to it, like a spider moving from the centre of its web to consume a fly caught somewhere in his outworks. A problem to Hobbes was not so much a problem, as something to be caught and apprehended into an overriding perception; or perhaps we might say that 'a serious quaere' for Hobbes needed only his own restatement in order no longer to be, for him, 'a serious quaere'. This is, perhaps, also to say that Hobbes was an artist, before he was a philosopher. But Locke was not like this. It is an interesting experience to pass from reading Hobbes with his swift, dogmatic, economical manner to

Locke's slower, rambling and repetitive procedure. Hobbes is sure of himself; he sees clearly what he wishes to see, and goes ahead with a firm, brief statement. Locke is not so sure, does not see so clearly, goes over the matter again, as it were to persuade himself he can have left nothing out and is being fair and clear. A problem is genuinely a problem; it needs to be considered on its own merits; it makes its own demand, and Locke is patient before it. It must then, no doubt, after consideration, be related to other problems and the answers to them; but nothing is foreordained and inevitable; there is no pattern clamouring to be imposed on the new material; all is fair and open. This only means that Locke begins with no system, no perception of ineluctable power, and that he ends with no system. Philosophy is not for Locke a kind of conquering, subduing march; it is little more than a skirmish; and if the result is not wholly unsatisfactory, there is nothing for it but to draw off one's forces for a while and be content. Hobbes was a Tamburlaine of philosophy; Locke was more like his own William, winning few victories, but sticking to it faithfully. 'I pretend not to publish this Essay for the information of men of large thoughts, and quick apprehensions' he says in *The Epistle to the Reader*. Unlike Hobbes, he loves truth more than power, and must be content to wrestle with what he knows he cannot conquer utterly. 'The true philosopher', he says again in *The Epistle to the Reader* with which the *Essay* opens, 'will have reason to think his time not ill spent, even when he cannot much boast of any great acquisition'.

IV

I have spoken of Locke's humanism, having in mind his sense of the modesty, but none the less, of the dignity also, of man's place in the world. But Locke was also a humanist, though a temperate one, in his addiction to classical studies. Here too I may be permitted to point the contrast with Hobbes. Until he was forty Hobbes was a typical Renaissance scholar, and translated Thucydides for the benefit of seventeenth-century public men. But he changed his note. We have studied his attitude to Homer; and we see in *Behemoth* how far, under the stress of his hatred of Rome and of Nonconformity, he went in rejecting classical studies. Aristotle became hateful to him for the service he had been made to render to Catholic philosophy. 'For none of the ancient philosophers' writings are comparable to those of Aristotle, for their aptness to puzzle and entangle men with words, and to breed

6

disputation, which must at last be ended in the determination of the Church of Rome.'[1] Ancient history became hateful to him for the services it had rendered to the Rebels. 'For it is a hard matter for men, who do all think highly of their own wits . . . to be persuaded that they want any ability requisite for the government of a commonwealth, especially having read the glorious histories and the sententious politics of the ancient popular governments of the Greeks and Romans . . .' (p. 193). It is no longer the translator of Thucydides who is speaking; and Aristotle, Plato, Cicero and Seneca all come under the ban, for they all 'furnish arguments for liberty'. 'As for the Latin, Greek and Hebrew tongues, it was once, to the detection of Roman fraud, and to the ejection of the Romish power, very profitable, or rather necessary; but now that is done, and we have the Scripture in English, and preaching in English, I see no great need of Greek, Latin and Hebrew. I should think myself better qualified by understanding well the language of our neighbours, French, Dutch, and Spanish' (p. 276).

Now Locke is sometimes represented as an enemy of classical studies. This is a great mistake. All he did was to bring common-sense to bear on the teaching of the classical tongues. In the *Thoughts on Education* he is sensible enough to consider the classics in relation to the use to which they will be put by the boys and young men who spend a great deal of time in acquiring them; and he comes to the conclusion, a conclusion which can scarcely be doubted, that many of them will put their classics to no use whatever, and that the deadly grammatical and pedantic grind to which they are submitted is wasteful and foolish, productive of neither enjoyment nor utility. 'Can there be anything more ridiculous, than that a father should waste his own money, and his son's time, in setting him to learn the roman language, when, at the same time, he designs him for a trade, wherein he having no use of latin, fails not to forget that little which he brought from school, and which it is ten to one he abhors for the ill-usage it procured him?'[2] There is only one answer to this question. 'Would not a Chinese', he asks, 'who took notice of this way of breeding, be apt to imagine, that all our young gentlemen were designed to be teachers and professors of the dead languages of foreign countries, and not to be men of business in their own?' (p. 162). Locke's only concern is to stop classical studies being made an occasion for producing pedants; and in our own time classical scholars are at last willing to talk in this strain. Yet he thought Latin 'absolutely necessary to a gentleman' (p. 152). and 'a man

[1] Hobbes, E. 6. p. 215.   [2] *Works*, vol. ix. p. 152.

can have no place amongst the learned, in this part of the world, who is a stranger' to either Greek or Latin.

In writing the *Thoughts on Education* Locke had chiefly in mind the education of a 'gentleman'. A gentleman must have Latin; and Locke would have him regularly practised in Latin composition; the ancient classic authors, he says, provide plenty of examples of 'skill and grace' in composition which should be used as 'patterns for . . . daily imitation'. Here Cicero, who was easily Locke's favourite classical author, is chiefly in his mind. He would have the *De Oratore* and the *Institutio* of Quintilian studied, and what he calls 'Boileau's *Traité du Sublime*'.[1] But it is true that he heartily grudges the time given to becoming proficient in the classical tongues; he is conscious of the neglect of our own tongue and wants what is, in effect, a new rhetoric for a discipline in English. 'There can scarce be a greater defect in a gentleman,' he says in the *Thoughts on Education*, 'than not to express himself well, either in writing or speaking' (p. 179). There are many gentlemen having this defect which he thinks is 'not so much their fault, as the fault of their education . . . They have been taught rhetoric, but yet never taught how to express themselves handsomely with their tongues, or pens, in the language they are always to use; as if the names of the figures, that embellished the discourses of those who understood the art of speaking, were the very art and skill of speaking well. This, as all other things of practice, is to be learned not by a few or a great many rules given, but by exercise and application, according to good rules, or rather patterns, till habits are got, and a facility of doing it well' (p. 179). I emphasize this notion of Locke's. Locke talked good sense about the teaching of classics, and was not listened to; he is here talking good sense about the teaching of English, and again has not been listened to. 'To write and speak correctly, gives a grace, and gains a favourable attention to what one has to say: and, since it is english that an english gentleman will have constant use of, that is the language he should chiefly cultivate, and wherein most care should be taken to polish and perfect his style. To speak or write better latin than english, may make a man be talked of; but he would find it more to his purpose to express himself well in his own tongue, that he uses every moment, than to have the vain commendation of others for a very insignificant quality. This I find universally neglected, and no care taken any where to improve young men in their own language, that they may thoroughly understand and be masters of it. If any one among us have a facility

[1] *Works*, vol. iii. *Some Thoughts concerning Reading and Study*, p. 271.

or purity more than ordinary in his mother tongue, it is owing to
chance, or to his genius, or any thing, rather than to his education, or
any care of his teacher' (p. 181). University teachers of English have
yet to take account of what Locke says here; and we at least know that
what he calls a 'plain easy sense, without any incoherence, confusion,
or roughness' does not come to us by nature.

But my purpose in speaking of Locke's view in these matters is to
show that he was deeply concerned with the literary aspect of education,
and how much of a humanist he remained. A gentleman without
Latin, or a scholar without Greek, is unthinkable; and he has no doubt
that it is better for a gentleman, to be 'well versed in greek and roman
writers' than to be a 'good peripatetic or cartesian: because those
ancient authors observed and painted mankind well, and give the best
light into that kind of knowledge' (p. 84). Here he takes his stand
firmly with classical humanism against scholasticism and, no less,
cartesianism; he equates cartesianism and scholasticism, and puts above
them both the kind of knowledge provided by the ancient authors,
namely, an understanding of mankind. I have said something earlier
of his interest in history. In the *Thoughts on Education* and in the
Thoughts concerning Reading and Study for a Gentleman, on both of which I
have drawn in what is above, he gives a high place to historical study.
History he says is 'the great mistress of prudence and civil knowledge';
and 'as nothing teaches, so nothing delights more than history'.

His own reading and learning, not only in philosophy, science and
theology, but also in politics, history and travel, were very wide. But
I have seen nothing to make me believe Locke read habitually or much
in imaginative literature. In *Thoughts on Education* he speaks of the
'most difficult and sublime of the Latin authors, such as are Tully,
Virgil and Horace'. I have said that Cicero seems to be easily his
favourite Latin author, both for his style and his matter; and though
he here mentions Virgil, he gives, in *Thoughts concerning Reading and
Study*, the impression that he puts the satirists above Virgil.[1] He says
there that the prime thing in a gentleman is knowledge of men. This
must be got chiefly from experience. But of books which help to give
this knowledge he mentions the *Rhetoric*, where Aristotle 'hath admir-
ably discoursed' of the passions, and La Bruyère's *Caractères;* and he says,
'Satyrical writings also, such as Juvenal and Persius, and above all
Horace; though they point the deformities of men, yet they thereby
teach us to know them' (p. 275). Such works, he thinks, have a clear

[1] *Works*, vol. iii. p. 275.

use. Then he goes on, 'There is another use of reading, which is for diversion and delight. Such are poetical writings, especially dramatic, if they be free from prophaneness, obscenity, and what corrupts good manners; for such pitch should not be handled.' This puts the poetry of the imagination in its place. And I quote now a paragraph from the *Thoughts on Education* in which he speaks of 'verses'. I quote at length, for it is an astonishing statement.

If these may be any reasons against children's making latin themes at school, I have much more to say, and of more weight, against their making verses of any sort: for, if he has no genius to poetry, it is the most unreasonable thing in the world to torment a child, and waste his time about that which can never succeed; and if he have a poetic vein, it is to me the strangest thing in the world, that the father should desire or suffer it to be cherished or improved. Methinks the parents should labour to have it stifled and suppressed as much as may be; and I know not what reason a father can have to wish his son a poet, who does not desire to have him bid defiance to all other callings and business; which is not yet the worst of the case; for if he proves a successful rhymer, and gets once the reputation of a wit, I desire it may be considered, what company and places he is like to spend his time in, nay, and estate too: for it is very seldom seen, that any one discovers mines of gold or silver in Parnassus. It is a pleasant air, but a barren soil; and there are very few instances of those who have added to their patrimony by any thing they have reaped from thence. Poetry and gaming, which usually go together, are alike in this too, that they seldom bring any advantage, but to those who have nothing else to live on. Men of estates almost constantly go away losers; and it is well if they escape at a cheaper rate than their whole estates, or the greatest part of them. If therefore you would not have your son the fiddle to every jovial company, without whom the sparks could not relish their wine, nor know how to pass an afternoon idly; if you would not have him waste his time and estate to divert others, and contemn the dirty acres left him by his ancestors, I do not think you will much care he should be a poet, or that his school-master should enter him in versifying. But yet, if anyone will think poetry a desirable quality in his son, and that the study of it would raise his fancy and parts, he must need yet confess, that, to that end, reading the excellent greek and roman poets, is of more use than making bad verses of his own, in a language that is not his own.[1]

He keeps a warm place in his heart for the classical poets; but there is not a word about Spenser, Shakespeare and Milton; and if he would have his way, English poetry would cease to be. In 1688, he wrote to his friend LeClerc, who had proved to his own satisfaction, and to

---

[1] *Works*, vol. ix. pp. 167–68.

Locke's, that Hebrew poetry was rhymed. This monstrous notion
seemed to Locke the most natural in the world; he was clearly puzzled
that any one should write unrhymed poetry. He explains to LeClerc
that the Greeks had a great variety of dialects and had therefore to
avoid rhyme. The Romans imitated the Greeks in this, as in other
ways. And, he goes on: 'However you have quoted the English for
writing verses without rhyme, yet I know but one man that has done
so, and he, too, one much versed in and addicted to the Greek and
Roman polite learning, whose admiration of their poetry put him, as I
imagine, in that way of writing'.[1] It is possible, of course, that Locke
was excluding dramatic poetry from his consideration. He here shows
no enthusiasm for Milton, though indeed this was not the occasion for
his doing so, had he felt it; but his interest in the history of English
poetry must have been light enough for him to take no account of
blank verse before Milton.

We have therefore this situation. It may be said that Locke is one
of the two greatest figures in our English 'classical' or 'Augustan'
period. He is but a temperate apostle of reason, sceptical of enthusiasm,
but of a passionate heart, of a fine grace and temper in thought, conduct
and religion. He is the greatest of English philosophers, and there is
not in the history of English culture a more attractive person. He is a
humanist in two important meanings of the word, having a strong
sense of all properly human values and appraising highly the literatures
of Greece and Rome. Yet he shows little interest in the past of English
poetry, and will do what he can to see that it has no future. His philosophy, which we must now turn to study, will give the imagination
little enough place. Poetry will have small territory in his map of the
mind. That Locke should thus see the imagination and all its ways,
may well be more alarming than that Hobbes should. Hobbes was
curiously inhuman, Locke agreeably and warmly human; Hobbes an
extreme rationalist, Locke a sober and temperate one. Hobbes had a
great influence, Locke a still greater. In Locke the best spirit of the
age was embodied; and it was a fine, tender and noble spirit, strong
in intellect and warm in feeling. But he thinks that poetry has at best
a pleasant air, and is a barren soil.

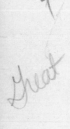

V

The reader will recall what I said of Hobbes's rationalism, that it
everywhere exalts the creative rôle of reason. We make geometrical

[1] Fox Bourne, vol. ii. pp. 76–77.

figure in a space which is a phantasm only; and motion and body, subject to phantasmal space, are thus made transparent to our intelligence. Geometry is the clue to all; given space and motion, with body represented as strictly quantitative and a vehicle of motion merely, nature is deducible throughout; nothing need escape us, nor fail to take its place in a 'science of the διότι'. We should, therefore, be able wholly to understand the coming-to-be of anything whatsoever. We, as it were, re-enact its creation; we re-make it in our own minds; its causation becomes wholly intelligible to us; and whether the intelligible cause we discover was in fact the cause employed by God in creation is indifferent to us. It may be that the universe as by philosophy we come to understand it is intelligible in a way quite different from the way in which it is intelligible to God; and in this sense man becomes a re-creator of the universe.

And if there really be body, motion and an unphantasmal space, that can only be a fortunate accident; and they enjoy their reality only on condition that they submit themselves to a space and time (for time too is phantasmal) of our imposing. In this way Hobbes ensures validity to the eternal laws of reason in their application to the real world. But it is hard to deny, and Hobbes must have found it hard not to see, that in such a philosophical state of affairs, there is a lively possibility that body, motion and space are *not* real. And if they are not, we are left with a world, wholly translucent to reason, which exists within the confines of the mind. Hobbes had, as any one would have, good reason for avoiding this conclusion. But at least, in taking the other way, he made the human reason lord of all it surveys by imprisoning body and motion and 'real' space within a phantasmal space and time. Truly, it will not do to think of Hobbes as an idealist. Reading Hobbes's exposition of a subjective space and time, we look ahead to Kant's celebrated doctrine of space and time as ideal forms of perception. But Kant used this notion for purposes not at all rationalist; and in any case Hobbes was a materialist. Still, it is plausible to think that moving in Hobbes's mind, though unclearly, was the motive that, by subjecting real space, motion and body to subjective time and space, he was ensuring the complete and irrefragable control of the world by the geometrical reason. For in the purposes of true philosophy body is considered as extended merely and as a vehicle of motion; and all other qualities of body issue wholly from motion.

But Locke takes us far from any such doctrine. He declared, in the course of his controversy with Stillingfleet, that he was not 'well read' in Hobbes. But if he had not read him 'well', he had read him; and it is impossible not to feel that he frequently writes with Hobbes in mind, as one against whom he is throwing the whole weight of his argument and beliefs. It may well be that when, in the *Epistle to the Reader*, he says he is not publishing the *Essay* for men of 'large thoughts and quick apprehensions' he is giving a sidelong glance at Hobbes and all his ways. The first thing to do, he says in the Introduction, is 'to take a survey of our own understandings, examine our own powers, and see to what things they were adapted'. Therefore in vain we seek satisfaction if 'we let loose our thoughts into the vast ocean of being; as if that boundless extent were the natural and undoubted possession of our understandings, wherein there was nothing exempt from its decisions, or that escaped its comprehension'. Here is the chief difference between Locke and Hobbes. It is the difference between humility and pride, and between two minds the one naturally religious, the other naturally irreligious. It is also the difference between a dogmatic and a critical intention, and between a mind which sees knowledge as the end of philosophy and one which looks hopefully to establish a reasonable assent or faith. Hobbes sees philosophy as an imitation of creation; reason will move on the surface of the deep and will establish its light; the world will be re-made and man made new in a new society. But in Locke's imagery, the world is not a deep above which we move but an ocean on which we voyage, and which is illimitable. Locke does not wish to fasten the world into a geometrical pattern in which man too will have an ordained design; 'our business here is not to know all things, but those which concern our conduct.' Locke, like Hobbes, will have philosophy be useful; but it can be *useful* only to a rational creature who *conducts* himself; it cannot be *useful* to a creature whose responsibility it reduces to motion. Hobbes makes reason a light lighting up a chaos which then undergoes an ordering; Locke makes it a candle bright enough for 'all our purposes' which illumines only a small part of a God-created world.

Throughout his philosophy, Locke gives the mind a humble rôle enough. It is right to see him as profoundly anti-rationalist. And his anti-rationalism is shown as clearly in those parts of his philosophy which may, in a superficial way be judged 'rationalist' as in those parts which are 'empiricist'. To see this, we need only consider his theory of mathematical knowledge. 'I doubt not', he said in 4. 4. vi,[1] 'but it will

---

[1] The *Essay* is contained in the first three volumes of the *Collected Works* of the edition of 1801. In quoting from the *Essay* in this edition, I give the numbers of the book, chapter and section, respectively.

be easily granted, that the knowledge we have of mathematical truths, is not only certain, but real knowledge; and not the bare empty vision of vain, insignificant chimeras of the brain: and yet, if we will consider, we shall find that it is only of our own ideas'. The mathematician deals with ideas of his own making; he is quite sure of what he knows about them, 'seeing that they have barely an ideal existence' in his mind; if a triangle studied by the mathematician in an ideal existence, happens also to exist in nature, that is lucky and by good chance enables mathematical knowledge to overflow its ideal world and so far to illumine the real world. We *make* the figures and quantities with which we deal in mathematics, and therefore we have certain knowledge of them. Mathematical ideas are, like other complex ideas (excepting of course those of substances) a combination of ideas 'which the mind, by its free choice, puts together, without considering any connexion they have in nature' (4. 4. v.). Such ideas are their own archetypes; they are not required to conform to anything; and in treating of these ideas, 'we intend *things* [the italics are mine] no further than as they are *conformable to our ideas*'.

Now it is not difficult to observe what difficulties appear in this doctrine. For we can press a clear dilemma upon Locke, and address him in this way: if mathematics can be said, as you argue, to provide 'real knowledge', then its ideas are surely 'real': but if mathematical ideas are 'combinations of ideas, which the mind, *by its free choice* puts together', are they not fictions which are properly objects of fancy? Can fancy and knowledge thus meet and embrace? Why does the fancy provide in poetry only 'a barren soil' and in mathematics a loam yielding a prodigious harvest?

But as in speaking of Hobbes we are less concerned with doctrine and the objections that may be urged against it than with the motive that animates; and when we see Locke both elevating mathematics into one of the very few sources of absolute knowledge in a world in which certainty, on his own showing, is a rare gift to the human mind, and at the same time humiliating it into something on a level with a poetaster's scribbling, our imaginations are stirred, and we look to the causes, which can only be motives, of this surprising paradox. That he should acknowledge the certainty of mathematics is not surprising; what is surprising is that he accords it certainty on the condition of its being acknowledged for a creation of fancy. Yet the reason is not far to seek: he will not risk a universe to which mathematics is the key. Give Descartes and Hobbes extension and motion and they will make a universe; give them to Locke, and he insists he can only construct in them an apodictical fairyland. Locke, in other words, is too reasonable to be a rationalist. He knows, to use his own word, that there is that whose existence he knows 'sensitively', substantial things; but they escape mathematics. Mathematics, he said in effect, may make a world, but it is not the world of all of us; it is a world of fancy, and it is none the less a world of fancy for being constructed by irrefragable reasoning. Hobbes had said: We make geometrical figure, and in a subjective space to which the physical world cannot fail to be subject; and therefore our minds are masters of the world. Locke said: the ideas of mathematics are of our own making; and therefore if they supply knowledge at all, it is knowledge about themselves and only by good fortune about the world. Hobbes the rationalist assumes that fancy rules the world; Locke, too reasonable to be either a rationalist or a poet, assumes that fancy can govern nothing but the fanciful.

No doubt Locke's view of mathematics will not do; and in his anxiety to humble it, he did not trouble to puzzle himself by asking how and why things in fact conform at all to mathematical ideas, any more than Hobbes puzzled himself by asking how and why the real world of space and motion becomes subjected to phantasmal time and space— they were both content with these agreeable accidents. Kant, writing with a longer and clearer view of what mathematics had done in physical science, was to take a different view of it and to explain how and why the world is patient of mathematical truth. But we can hardly blame Locke if his view is too simple. He was writing against Descartes and Hobbes. And in any catholic view of things he was far nearer the truth than they.

The intention, then, which enlivens his rationalism in mathematics is not rationalist at all. And it is for similar reasons that he insists on the reality of body and will not suffer it to be given a merely mathematical expression. Hobbes had said that body is a 'mere name'; and 'in it no form or any other accident but quantity are at all considered'. Locke will not have this. 'I appeal to every man's own thoughts, whether the idea of space be not as distinct from that of solidity, as it is from the idea of scarlet colour?'(2. 13. ii); and in substance, which is a mystery to us, is vested 'powers'. Extension is *not* the essence of body, and what that essence is we do not and shall not know. But there are qualities and 'powers' (which are not, as Hobbes would have us believe, reducible to motion, but genuine accidents) inhering in what is impenetrable both by other matter and by our minds. At the centre, so to speak, of the physical world and of our own being Locke firmly and without apology plants substance; and substance is a mystery. 'If it be demanded (as usually it is) whether this space, void of body, be substance or accident, I shall readily answer, I know not; nor shall be ashamed to own my ignorance, till they that ask me show me a clear distinct idea of substance'(2. 13. xvii). Philosophy plays with symbols, and is literary. A Descartes and a Hobbes, infused with the spirit of mathematics, dissolve substance into extension by the hot light of their reason and all must be transparent to it; but Locke insists on the mystery of things, and the most potent symbol of it is what he affirms to be the impenetrability of matter. We know only the outsides of things, the simple ideas given in experience; within, things are dark and inscrutable.

But the obscurity which Locke places within all things is at the cost of clarity and consistency in his philosophy. One cannot traffic thus in darkness without oneself entering into it. And Locke, with his abstract idea of substance in general and his ideas of substances in particular, brings his empiricism into trouble. For where does the idea of substance or of substances come from? And where for that matter the idea of 'power' and 'cause'? Not certainly from sensation, which provides only simple ideas; and it is easy therefore to say 'Here at least we catch Locke out! Here empiricism is at bay!' But if we do so, we mistake the spirit of his philosophy. For what animated it was not a mere empiricism. Instead, it was precisely a wish to assert what transcends experience, to insist on what lies about and within the mind, unknown and mysterious to it. We have barely begun to understand Locke if this is not clear to us. And if I do not exaggerate here (as I think I do not), we shall find no special satisfaction in flogging Locke with his inconsistencies; instead, we shall keep in mind his high and serious intention. The gift of the great philosophers to us is no mere bag of intellectual tricks and opportunities of showing how clever we are when one or other of them fails to work; and when we read Locke, it is an error to fail continuously to realize that what made him, as we say, 'an empiricist', is the piety and humility of his mind before the world and its creator. 'We stand', his empiricism says, 'outside the things of this world, and our ideas of them leave us in ignorance of their essence; and if we do not understand the finite things of the world, how much more shall we not understand ourselves, and the still higher spiritual beings which God has created, and above all, God Himself?'

Locke's empiricism then must be seen not as a doctrine which he can hope to make consistent but as a literary expression of his sensibility, of his sense of life and the world. He cannot, in any case, make it consistent; and Locke knew this perfectly well. I have been at some pains to show that his mind was eminently fair, and could not easily delude itself; and he must have known that his empiricism could not be elevated into a neat and watertight doctrine. To have carried it to the lengths required in all consistency would have been to go ahead into a phenomenalism. Locke saw this; he knew well enough that sensation does not provide us with our ideas of substance, of cause, of 'power'; and when he talks of any one of these ideas his embarrassment is obvious. But he prefers intellectual embarrassment to the defeat of his fundamental purpose. He will not assume that what we do not see with our senses or understand with our minds does not exist. He will not evacuate the world, after the manner of Hobbes, of what eludes mathematical physics; but no more will he, after the manner of Hume, reduce the world to a succession of inexplicable sense-data. He is content to say that there are matters about which philosophers must talk like children. The child is father of the philosopher; and 'thus here', he says, talking of substance, 'as in all other cases where we use words without having clear and distinct ideas, we talk like children: who, being questioned what such a thing is, which they know not, readily give this satisfactory answer, that it is something: which in truth signifies no more, when so used, either by children or men, but that they know not what; and that the thing they pretend to know, and talk of, is what they have no distinct idea of at all, and so are perfectly ignorant of it, and in the dark' (2. 23. ii). There are things about which he is in the dark; and it is the purpose of his philosophy to show this and to exhort us to be content to remain in the dark. There are matters about which his mind can rest, with good sense, in agnosticism. His essay is an *Essay concerning Human Understanding*; it is also an *Essay concerning Human Ignorance*.

Our knowledge being so narrow . . . it will perhaps give us some light into the present state of our minds, if we look a little into the dark side, and take a view of our ignorance; which, being infinitely larger than our knowledge, may serve much to the quieting of disputes, and improvement of useful knowledge; if, discovering how far we have clear and distinct ideas, we confine our thoughts within the contemplation of those things that are within the reach of our understandings, and launch not out into that abyss of darkness (where we have not eyes to see, nor faculties to perceive anything) out of a presumption that nothing is beyond our comprehension. But to be satisfied of the folly of such a conceit, we need not go far. He that knows anything, knows this in the first place, that he need not seek long for instances of his ignorance. The meanest and most obvious things that come in our way, have dark sides, that the quickest sight cannot penetrate into. The clearest and most enlarged understandings of thinking men find themselves puzzled and at a loss, in every particle of matter.

So he writes in 4. 3. xxii. There is a surrounding and illimitable darkness; the candle of knowledge burns small and gives a little, gloomy light. This, as I have said, is the thought that actuates his philosophy from beginning to end. And he can therefore go on, in Book 4, to his cool critique of scientific knowledge. Scientific knowledge cannot be *scientific*, it cannot supply 'adequate ideas'. 'We are not capable of scientifical knowledge' of bodies (4. 3. xxvi); 'nor shall ever be able to discover general, instructive, unquestionable truths concerning them.' And if understanding of body is denied us, the same, or rather a still greater, ignorance conceals from us, 'in an impenetrable obscurity, almost the whole intellectual world; a greater certainly, and more beautiful world than the material' (4. 3. xxvii).

Now no reader of the *Essay* can fail to notice how often Locke speaks of superior spiritual beings, and of angels. He has himself little doubt of their existence. We have indeed, he says, 'no certain information' even of their existence 'but by revelation'. 'That there are degrees of spiritual beings between us and the great God, who is there by his own search and ability, can come to know?' (4. 3. xxvii). We know of their existence, or in strictness give assent to it, only through revelation. But Locke does not hesitate, again and again, in the *Essay* to illumine his perception of the powers and range of the human mind by speaking of angels who both enjoy superior power of sense and entertain 'as clear ideas of the radical constitution of substances, as we have of a triangle' (3. 11. xxiii). Revelation is the source, he says, of our knowledge of the existence of such beings. But it is clear that had Locke not been able to appeal to the authority of revelation, his imagination would yet have played abundantly about his idea of them; though he quotes revelation for authority, his real authority is in his own imagination of the world. In that imagination man is *not* an angel, and substances are opaque to him; and although to think, in company with Descartes and Hobbes, that they are not opaque is the height of hubristic folly, he can vaguely envisage an order of mind for which the opacity of our world may be changed to a transparency. Man is neither God nor angel; but the candle-light of his mind may, in another world than this, and at the hand of the Father of Lights, increase to a power of which now we can have the barest 'idea'. Around about *us* certainly is darkness; but it is *our* darkness and not God's nor the angels'. Keats used to speak of his 'favourite speculations'. One of them was that one of the 'grandeurs of immortality' will be that 'there will be no space and consequently the only commerce between spirits will be by their intelligence of each other—when they will completely understand each other—while we in this world merely comprehend each other in different degrees—the higher the degree of good so higher is our love and friendship'. So Locke 'must necessarily conclude that separate spirits, which are beings that have perfecter knowledge and greater happiness than we, must needs have also a perfecter way of communicating their thoughts than we have . . . But of immediate communication, having no experiment in ourselves, . . . we have no idea how spirits, which use not words, can with quickness . . .' (2. 23. xxxvi).

VI

Locke's doctrine of 'sensitive' knowledge is a peculiar and striking part of his doctrine of sense-knowledge. We have 'sensitive' knowledge, he says in 4 .2. xiv. about the 'particular existence of finite beings without us'. We may be said to know, he thinks, that physical objects exist with a knowledge that goes beyond probability and possesses certainty, though not indeed the certainty of either intuition or demonstration. We have ideas of things 'in our minds', but cannot certainly infer the existence of anything without us 'which corresponds to that idea'; no certain inference is possible; and we also have no intuition of its existence. But objects affect us, he holds, with such force, and there is so great a difference between seeing the sun by day and thinking of it by night, that we may say that we have knowledge of existence of things 'by that perception and consciousness we have of the actual entrance of ideas from them' (4. 2. xiv). We have 'assurance' of their being, not indeed the assurance of inference or intuition, but a feeling, an inner satisfaction that things exist.

Now this kind of knowledge, if it exists as Locke holds, is an irrational enough sentiment. Locke calls it knowledge and accords it a degree of certainty. But if it is supplied neither by sense (for Locke can hardly say it is a sensation), nor by intuition nor by demonstration, what is it? No one in his senses would deny we have a feeling of certainty on these matters, what I suppose Mr. Santayana would call animal faith; and indeed it is best called a faith, so strong as not to be ordinarily questioned; for as Locke says, objects act on us briskly. Still, as a form of knowledge, its nature is not clear to us; it is not an intellectual process like intuition or demonstration, nor again a sensation.

Now Locke explicitly limits this knowledge (or faith, if we will, which he thinks merits the name of knowledge) to the existence of things in nature. Indeed he limits it to objects actually present to our senses, and to objects which have been present to our senses of whose existence at the time we saw them we feel 'assured' in memory. Beyond this, we can have 'sensitive' certainty of nothing else outside us. He does not make room, in his doctrine, for what we may call 'sensitive' certainty or assurance of the existence of God. Instead, he rests belief in God on demonstration. But if the 'sensitive soul' in us may have faith, so strong as to be certainty, in the existence of things, might not the 'intellectual soul' in us have faith too, in the existence of God? Why does Locke make belief in God something completely rational, and belief in things an affair of a feeling of assurance? He protests the complete certainty of his proof of God's existence. 'It is plain to me, we have a more certain knowledge of the existence of a God, than of anything our senses have not immediately discovered to us. Nay, I presume I may say, that we more certainly know that there is a God, than that there is anything else without us. When I say we know, I mean that there is such a knowledge within our reach which we cannot miss, if we will but apply our minds to that, as we do to several other inquiries' (4. 10. vi). That is to say, the certainty of our knowledge of God's existence, gained by demonstration, is stronger than the certainty of our 'sensitive' knowledge.

Now in reading through the tenth chapter of the Fourth Book in which Locke is so emphatic that proof of God's being is so entirely sure, it is, I think, certain that Locke is not being true to his own experience. Here, certainly, he is being very rational, and at great pains to show us the complete rationality of belief in God. In fact, his proof is not a proof, if only because his own doctrine of causation was much too vague and fluctuating to be used in this way. But apart from that, we think that Locke is forcing a false pace and for once falling from his normal fairness and detachment of mind. It is not by such a doubtful proof that he, so critical of the powers and range of human knowledge, came to be religious; and he must have known that at least the great majority of religious men do not come to religion by demonstration and proof. Locke is here using reason in the interests of what is really a faith, but making himself blind to its fairly obvious inefficacy. His own beauty and piety of spirit did not spring from doubtful argument of this kind; it sprang far more from his rearing, and from his knowledge of Pococke and of men like him.

But it may be replied that Locke does not deny that religious faith may come about by other means than demonstration. And this is true. He does not. Still, he is curiously shy of speaking of belief in God as faith merely. What he is prepared to say of our faith in the existence of things, he will not say of our faith in the existence of God. Yet, if he is shy of speaking of it, he is not altogether silent about it. There are one or two passages in the *Essay* where his own religious experience is manifested. There is a passage in 4. 7., to which Locke's latest and most authoritative expositor, Professor Aaron, has called attention, which I quote. Locke is speaking of what he calls Maxims, and he says: 'When we find out an idea, by whose intervention we discover the connexion of two others, this is a revelation from God to us, by the voice of reason: for we then come to know a truth that we did not know before. When God declares any truth to us, this is a revelation to us by the voice of his spirit, and we are advanced in our knowledge. But in neither of these do we receive our light or knowledge from maxims. But in the one the things themselves afford it, and we see the truth in them by perceiving their agreement or disagreement. In the other, God himself affords it immediately, to us, and we see the truth of what he says in his unerring veracity' (4. 7. xi). He here clearly affirms his belief in revelation immediately to the soul, in the sense the soul may have of God's presence to it and of His imparting to it new truth. In speaking of our 'sensitive' knowledge of things, he had said that it gives us knowledge of 'the existence of particular external objects, by that perception and consciousness we have of the actual entrance of ideas from them'; and we are not, I think, stretching the sense of the passage I have just quoted from 4. 7. if we say that Locke is here near to saying that the soul, in religious experience, may have knowledge of the existence of God, 'by that perception and consciousness we have of the actual entrance of ideas from' Him. We catch here the reality of Locke's *faith* in God and his sense of God's existence and presence, which is much more than, and is not derived from, demonstration that God exists.

But it is necessary, in order to come by a full and fair impression of Locke's religion, to turn, for the present, from Locke's belief that

God's existence can be proved, to his doctrine of assent and of assent to divine revelation. I shall then return to make some further observations on the 'mathematical certainty' of God's existence. For Locke was not a deist, but a Christian.

VII

Locke treats of reason and revelation in their relation to each other in 4. 18. of the *Essay* and in the *Reasonableness of Christianity*. Now in the *Essay* he says that reason must exercise itself in considering whether revelation is authentic; and it is clear to him that anything purporting to be revealed may not be accepted if it is 'contrary to, and inconsistent with the clear and self-evident dictates of reason.' Revelation may not set aside either the intuition or the demonstrations of the intelligence; and he is right in saying, in the tenth section of the chapter, that 'there can be no evidence, that any traditional revelation is of divine original, in the words we receive it, and in the sense we understand it, so clear and so certain, as that of the principles of reason . . .' This is perfectly good sense, and no Christian, I imagine, would wish to dispute it; if we look for *proof* of the Christian revelation, it is certain we shall not find it. But, of course, to say this is by no means to rule out assent to revelation. Faith may not run counter to certain reason; but it may rightly secure assent where our knowledge can at best only come by what is probably true, and where we deal, as in so much of our knowledge, in ideas that are neither clear nor distinct. Now Locke's philosophy has, for its purpose, I think it is not too much to say, to supply philosophical ground for religious assent. We have heard so much of Locke the empiricist, and of Locke the rationalist, that we have overlooked the most important Locke of all, the philosopher of assent. Truly, he believed that rational demonstration of God's existence can be made out. He would not let *that* be made a matter of assent, what we think it was, in reality, to him and to all other religious souls. But for the rest, he was at pains to put a limit to our certainties and to insist on what are, to us, the mystery of things; he will not, by any philosophical sleight of hand, conjure out of the world what is intransigent to our understandings. 'In this fleeting state of action and blindness we are in', we are driven to assent, in the most momentous matters of faith, as in the humblest presuppositions of our daily lives. Science may not come by 'certainty and demonstration' and rests on assent; and we do not comprehend the substance of bodies and of minds, the nature of superior spiritual beings, and of God. Therefore Locke's philosophy is, for much the bigger part, a preparation for assent; the temper and tenor of his mind incline him to belief in matters of religion which the mind is helpless to discover, and having discovered, encompass. Locke is, first and last, a *Christian* philosopher. We everywhere mistake him, if we do not discern that this is so.

Assent, then, must move in the world of probability. In mathematics we have certainty; but here we are not dealing with the world. In matters where the use of the senses is involved, we may have universal assent, to the uniform succession of one event by another, to the testimonies on which the bulk of historical knowledge is based, though even here, no doubt, we must allow for varying degrees of assent in different men. But as we pass from matters on which widespread assent is possible and natural, to matters where probability is harder to assess, there occurs, in the making of assent, the play of what Locke calls *judgement*. And in judgement there is a certain indefinable exercise of personality; what is individual in a man shows itself in his assents. In the opening paragraph of iv. xvi., *Of the Degrees of Assent*, speaking of the right formation of assents in men's minds, he says: 'It suffices that they have once with care and fairness sifted the matter as far as they could; and that they have searched into all the particulars, that they could imagine to give any light to the question; and with the best of their skill cast up the account upon the whole evidence: and thus, having once found on which side the probability appeared to *them* [the italics are mine], after as full and exact an inquiry as they can make, they lay up the conclusion in their memories, as a truth they have discovered . . .' It is, I think, clear from this, that Locke sees (and of course rightly sees) that in assessing what is probably true, a man's personal and peculiar qualities of mind and personality are exercised. Judgement he says, in effect, has its idiom, its style, and issues at once and both from fair assessment of evidence and from the history and quality of the man who judges.

But the range of 'judgement' in mortal life is very great. Let us agree that mathematics gives certainty, that immediate intuition certainly shows us that we exist, that an irrefragable argument demonstrates that God exists. This is a great deal. And yet it is little enough. For in all forms of intellectual enquiry which are not merely mathematical, in experimental science and in history alike; in innumerable matters which occur every day in a man's life; in his general conduct and dealing with his fellows; in all this and more, judgement is ever exercised; and

above all, judgement is exercised in accepting or rejecting Divine
Revelation. And in all these things a man's assent comes from *him*; 'on
which side does the probability appear' to *him*? and his assent will be
his assent, and will be determined by what he *is*.

Besides, in all these things, he does not advance by the steps of
syllogism. Locke's attack on the 'schools' and syllogistic reasoning is
famous; at least, one sentence of it is famous: 'But God has not been so
sparing to men to make them barely two-legged creatures, and left it
to Aristotle to make them rational' (4. 17. iv). Syllogism, he says, is not
only not necessary where strict knowledge is possible, for 'by its own
penetration, where it is strong and exercised, reason usually sees
quicker and clearer without syllogism'; but it is *'of far less or no use at
all in probabilities'* (the italics are mine). Judgement does not and cannot
act through formal inference; it is a *seeking* for truth, where 'syllogism,
at best, is but the act of fencing with the little knowledge we have,
without making any addition to it' (4. 17. iv–vi). Where the mind is
creatively employed in discovery, the cumbrous machinery of explicit
argument is not used; and it is not used because the mind, moving in
the probable, is not trafficking in generalities; instead it is moving
amongst particulars, relating particular to particular, and whole to
whole. 'As if', says Locke (4. 17. viii), 'we could not reason, and have
knowledge about particulars: whereas, in truth, the matter rightly considered, the immediate object of all our reasoning and knowledge, is
nothing but particulars'; so that reason, where it is the act of a living
mind, is a prehension of a state of affairs, a new ordering of a situation.
And thus it is that, if judgement has a personal quality, a style, it is
because it acts upon and orders what is concrete and novel; it is creative
and living. But explicit argumentation is a machinery of restatement
which turns only when the action of discovery is done; and if it is not
content to be that, it will 'manacle' thought in its 'chain' of syllogisms.
For thought, as Hobbes might say, is quick. Locke acknowledges
indeed that syllogistic inference may act as a check upon thought and
that 'right reasoning may be reduced' to Aristotle's 'forms of syllogism'.
'But yet I think, without any diminution to him, I may truly say, that
they are not the only, nor the best way of reasoning, for the leading of
those into truth who are willing to find it, and desire to make the best
use they may of their reason, for the attainment of knowledge' (4. 17. iv).

Now I have said that Locke limits assent and judgement to the at
best probable. It cannot give certainty. In inductive, analogical and
experimental thinking, and in assessing the value of testimony in

history, we cannot advance beyond the very probable. But, Locke says, in 4. 16. xiv., 'there is one sort of propositions that challenge the highest degree of our assent upon bare testimony, whether the thing proposed agree or disagree with common experience and the ordinary course of things, or no. The reason whereof is, because the testimony is of such a one, as cannot deceive, nor be deceived, and that is God himself. This carries with it an assurance beyond doubt, evidence beyond exception. This is called by a peculiar name, revelation, and our assent to it, faith . . .' Has *this* assent, then, *certainty?* Locke does not say so. At least, he said so in the first four editions of the *Essay*; for the concluding sentence of what I have just quoted continued, in those editions, as follows: 'This is called by a peculiar name, revelation, and our assent to it, faith, which has as much certainty as our know-ledge itself . . .' But in the fifth edition the sentence was changed to ' . . . faith, which as absolutely determines our minds and *as perfectly excludes all wavering, as our knowledge itself* [the italics are mine]; and we may as well doubt of our own being, as we can whether any revelation from God be true. So that faith is a settled and sure principle of assent and assurance, and leaves no manner of room for doubt or hesitation.'[1] Now I think it is clear, from the change Locke made in the text, that he felt he could not raise faith to the certainty of knowledge. It may 'absolutely determine our minds' and 'perfectly exclude wavering'; but (what I have previously quoted from 4. 18. x.) 'there can be no evidence that any traditional revelation is of divine original, in the words we receive it, and in the sense we understand it, so clear and so certain as that of the principles of reason'; and in 4. 16. xiv., where he is not speaking specifically of traditional revelation but of all revelation what-soever, he says, that our assent 'can be *rationally* [my italics] no higher than the evidence of its being a revelation . . .' Considering therefore what we believe by revelation, it cannot have the certainty of the 'prin-ciples of reason', of knowledge. And yet, Locke says, faith may 'abso-lutely determine our minds' and be a 'settled and sure principle of assent and assurance'. Faith therefore may give perfect 'assurance', but not *knowledge*.

Now so far, I think we cannot quarrel with Locke. He is saying, however paradoxical it may appear, that in faith we may have certitude, where we have in knowledge uncertainty, or at best strong probability; faith may give us complete assurance, reason only strong but inconclu-sive evidence. That this is so is shown I think by experience. And yet,

[1] See A. C. Fraser's edition of the *Essay*, Oxford, 1894, vol. ii. p. 383.

at this point, *Locke loses his nerve*. He will not hold firmly to this paradox out of a right loyalty to experience; he lets it go out of a false loyalty to reason.

He says, rightly, that in assent to revelation our assent can be 'rationally no higher than the evidence of its being a revelation'. And yet, he is committed to justifying a full 'assurance', in faith, in the truth of revelation. But Locke will not commit himself unmistakably to this two-fold and paradoxical doctrine. Instead, he runs away from it. For in the chapter *Of Enthusiasm*, which was added in the fourth edition, he was explicitly to condemn faith which goes in the least beyond the evidence, and to condemn that 'assurance beyond doubt' of which he spoke in 4. 16. as 'enthusiasm' which any lover of truth must eschew. Before I quote what he says in 4. 19, I make two observations. First, that the change in the text to which I referred a few paragraphs ago was made in the fifth edition, published in 1706, two years after his death and showing changes made by him between 1700 (when the fourth edition was published) and 1704, the year of his death. But that change was intelligible, and so far from being inconsistent, increased the consistency of his doctrine. He was only insisting that faith, rationally considered, cannot take us outside the bounds of probability. Second, that Locke wrote the chapter *Of Enthusiasm* between 1695 (when he wrote to Molyneux announcing his intention of writing it) and 1700, the year in which the fourth edition was published. And during these years, Swift was at Moor Park and busy writing *A Tale of a Tub*.

This is what Locke says in the first section of 4. 19. It is Locke's great (and inconsistent) retractation. I shall quote at some length because of its importance.

He that would seriously set upon the search of truth, ought in the first place to prepare his mind with a love of it. For he that loves it not, will not take much pains to get it, nor be much concerned when he misses it. There is nobody in the commonwealth of learning, who does not profess himself a lover of truth; and there is not a rational creature that would not take it amiss to be thought otherwise of. And yet for all this, one may truly say, that there are very few lovers of truth for truth-sake, even amongst those who persuade themselves that they are so. How a man may know whether he be so in earnest, is worth inquiry: and I think there is one unerring mark of it, viz. the not entertaining any proposition with greater assurance, than the proofs it is built upon will warrant. Whoever goes beyond this measure of assent, it is plain, receives not truth in the love of it, loves not truth for truth-sake, but for some other bye-end. For the evidence that any proposition is true (except such as are self-evident) lying only in the proofs a man has of it, whatsoever degrees of assent he affords it beyond the degrees of that evidence, it is plain that all the surplusage of assurance is owing to some other affection, and not to the love of truth: it being as impossible, that the love of truth should carry my assent above the evidence there is to me that it is true, as that the love of truth should make me assent to any proposition for the sake of that evidence, which it has not, that it is true; which is in effect to love it as a truth, because it is possible or probable that it may not be true. In any truth that gets not possession of our minds by the irresistible light of self-evidence, or by the force of demonstration, the arguments that gain it assent are the vouchers and gage of its probability to us; and we can receive it for no other, than such as they deliver it to our understandings. Whatsoever credit or authority we give to any proposition more than it receives from the principles and proofs it supports itself upon, is owing to our inclinations that way, and is so far a derogation from the love of truth as such: which, as it can receive no evidence from our passions or interests, so it should receive no tincture from them.

Now if Locke is to stand by this, how can faith 'as absolutely determine our minds and as perfectly exclude all wavering' without being condemned for enthusiastic? We cannot have 'assurance beyond doubt' in revelation without a 'surplusage' not warranted by the degree of evidence; and if we have such a surplusage, we can have it only out of a disloyalty to truth, for a 'bye-end' and on account of a base servitude to 'passions or interests'. In the interests of 'reason' Locke will now run plain contrary to experience; a right empiricism is yielding to claims of reason which ignore fact and experience. As it is, he has moved far, in this chapter, which saw the light in 1700, from the temper of Book 4 as it originally appeared in 1690. For in 4. 18. viii., he had even gone so far as to write that '*revelation*, where God has been pleased to give it, *must carry it against the probable conjectures of reason*. Because the mind not being certain of the truth of that it does not evidently know, but only yielding to the probability that appears in it, is bound to give up its assent to such a testimony; which, it is satisfied, comes from one who cannot err, and will not deceive'; and in the same chapter in a passage I have already quoted, he emphatically explains that evidence of a traditional revelation cannot take us beyond probability. Besides, if he must now speak in this way of revelation, what must he now, in consistency, say of 'sensitive' knowledge of the external of physical things? There is certainly not proof of their existence; and must we therefore lose the full 'assurance' which in fact we have of it? Therefore Locke's chapter on enthusiasm is crucial; it is a triumph of 'reason', but a defeat of plain openness and fairness of mind; and its consequences for the eighteenth century will be deep and heavy. For Locke had some sense of another road he might have taken. At the end of his chapter on assent (4. 16. xiv), he said that faith is in truth 'nothing else but an assent founded on the highest reason'. What did he mean by this, and by 'highest reason'? Many years were to pass before an Englishman, like Locke a man of catholic interests and unlike Locke a poet as well, would say that 'Christian faith is the perfection of human intelligence', and would set out the nature of the 'highest reason' which Locke mentions but does not explore.

I have said that Locke's chapter on enthusiasm was crucial in the spiritual history of the eighteenth century. It was written in the very closing years of the seventeenth century, and was published in 1700. The die was now cast; and cast by a man who was himself no deist or rationalist, but one in whom the best and deepest piety of the seventeenth century lived on. When Locke said, in 4. 19, in the chapter on enthusiasm, that 'reason must be our last judge and guide in everything', the new age had indeed come; and it was announced by one who in saying this was untrue to his own experience. It was a solemn moment enough in history. Ahead lie the wastes of deism, and the detestable cocksureness of Bolingbroke's 'free-thinking' and Pope's *Essay on Man*. For neither of these can we exempt Locke from responsibility. 'God when he makes the prophet does not unmake the man', said Locke. But it was a dangerous half-truth. Wesley was to be necessary, renewing not only true faith and piety but also unhealthy excitement, hysteria and superstition; and this, had Locke been able to sustain the fine balance of faith and reason which animates the greater part—much the greater part—of the *Essay*, might not have been necessary; for Locke's influence and prestige were very great. The rarest spirits in religion and philosophy alike walk a knife-edge; and maintain, in tension, a wonderful repose. Locke was one of these; he had an exquisite finesse and delicacy in the spiritual life, which showed itself in all his many friendships and responsibilities, as well as in his writings. Therefore, that his was the voice which more than any other finally inaugurated the age of 'reason' is a surprising and tragic irony.

Yet Locke's influence was not singlefold. If he helped (in spite of being no deist) to strengthen deism, he had other influences. I have spoken of what I take to be the animating motive of his empiricism; it was to set limits to the range of our knowledge, to show the necessity of assent, throwing up, as it were, before men's eyes, the encompassing darkness of the world, in which, without revelation, we are lost. And this, his strongest intention, was certainly not wholly lost in the eighteenth century. Of the men who followed, early in the next century, it was Addison and Butler who had most of Locke's temper and fairness of mind. Addison's papers on the Pleasures of the Imagination and others of the *Spectator* papers are near to Locke's sensibility; and *The Analogy of Religion* bears certain and extensive marks of Locke's influence.

VIII

Now bearing all this in mind, I wish, before I leave Locke's doctrine on knowledge and faith, to do two things. First, to make some observations on his Christian beliefs; and, secondly, to revert to his belief that we can prove, and with 'mathematical certainty', that God exists.

I have said that Locke was no deist. What he says in 4. 19 certainly came as an encouragement to deism, and deist theologians were encouraged by it to let go their hold on anything that lay beyond natural religion. But I have also said that the chapter on enthusiasm does not agree with the main tenor of the teaching of Book 4; and that we must see it as a late and regrettable disturbance of Locke's fine balance, in the rest of the *Essay*, of faith and reason. Besides, if he was no deist, he was also no Socinian.

Now it is generally thought that his essay, *The Reasonableness of Christianity as delivered in the Scriptures*, which was published in 1695, shows a slight enough hold on the mysteries of Christianity; and that if his critic, Edwards, exaggerated in calling it 'all over Socinianized', his charge is still intelligible or at least is not, as Professor Aaron says, 'altogether surprising'. I only wish, in speaking of this essay, to say and to give grounds for saying, that we must be careful clearly to understand Locke's intention in composing it; and that if we do not do this, we shall rush into a quite excessive sympathy with the attack which Edwards made on it. In order to do what is in my mind, I do not need to expound the content of Locke's essay; I need only expound the purpose which he wrote it to serve; and this purpose is made abundantly clear in his replies to Edwards.

'I must confess', says Locke, in his first reply to Edwards, 'discourses of this kind, which I met with, spread up and down, at first amazed me; knowing the sincerity of those thoughts, which persuaded me to publish it, not without some hope of doing some service to decaying piety, and mistaken and slandered Christianity.'[1] Certainly, of the sincerity and piety of Locke's intention, there can be no question; and this, it can be said, can be heartily agreed to without, by doing so, acquitting Locke of grave unorthodoxy. But even here, at the outset, it is well to remember that we speak of *Locke's* sincerity and piety, which were exceptional; and we shall be wise if we assume that Locke will not speak rashly and without the most careful thought of what he is doing, and that if he says that Edwards's attack surprised him, he is only saying what is true and that without exaggeration.

What then causes Locke to be surprised? The answer is, that Edwards taxes him with saying nothing of the first words of the Fourth Gospel. Edwards is smelling out Socinianism. But then, Locke had not quoted Matthew i. 18. 23, an omission Edwards had not noticed. But the omission of these verses did not mean that Locke denied the Virgin Birth; and Locke had no more intended to deny the Divinity of Christ than his miraculous birth. In other words, the mistake Edwards made was to take Locke's essay as a statement of Locke's Christian beliefs; but this, says Locke, it was never intended to be. Were it intended for that, it would have been a very different document. As it is, 'there is not one word of socinianism in it', Locke says.

What then was its intention? It was designed 'as the title shows, chiefly for those who were not yet thoroughly, or firmly, Christians, proposing to work on those, who either wholly disbelieved, or doubted of the truth of the christian religion'.[2] He addresses it to unbelievers and half-believers who are also men of some education (for it is clear that the essay is addressed only to people accustomed to systematic argument); and, he says '*as the title shows*', because, when he speaks of the 'reasonableness of Christianity' he is not speaking of Christianity as wholly rational and an affair of natural religion; he is implying only that Christianity demands, at the least, the most earnest consideration of men accustomed to think about human life and its destiny. For in all truth, if Christianity were not reasonable, but affronted the reason of men, it would not be worth a moment's consideration; but to say this, as any Christian must be prepared to say, is not at all to remove mystery out of Christian belief; and Locke declares on the second page of *The Reasonableness of Christianity* that to make 'Jesus Christ nothing but the restorer and preacher of pure natural religion' is to make nonsense of the Gospels and to do 'violence to the whole tenour of the New Testament'.

[1] *Works*, vol. vii. p. 165.   [2] *Ibid.*, p. 164.

We must be clear then of this: that Locke is only maintaining the spirit and poise of Book 4 at its best, in speaking of the reasonableness of Christianity; he for his part wholly accepts the authority of the Gospels; and only says that what a fair examination of the Gospels shows is demanded of every one capable of fairly employing his mind, and that if this is given, no one will find in the Gospels what is contrary to reason. Now in expounding what he judges to be the central truths taught by the Gospels, he sees the Messiahship of Jesus for most important; his teaching and miracles; his resurrection and rule and his gift of eternal life; and in the Christian, belief, 'beyond doubt', in these things; repentance, baptism, love of righteousness in Christ's Kingdom and belief in his saving grace. These are the most important things, he says; he will not be drawn into systematic, theological discussion; he writes in the first place not as a scholar or philosopher but as a 'sober, good man' capable of reading the Gospels with a fair and open mind. No doubt questions arise on all sides; but he will not be drawn into systematic discussion of the Trinity, of the sonship of Christ, of the Resurrection, of Grace.

Now these things he sets out, so far as his purpose requires, not as a complete exposition of Christian belief. There can be no question whatever of Locke's strict belief in the articles of the English Church; his essay gives no ground for doubting it. But the intention of the essay is that it should be a propaedeutic merely; Locke offers it for no more than that; he is setting forth the least that is required of any one who may with any propriety be called a Christian. But with these accepted by the learning soul, that is not the end. Locke is only helping him to make first and essential steps. He says that he is setting out only the least that can make a man a believer; but 'this excludes not the belief of any of those other truths contained in the scriptures of the Old and New Testaments, which it is the duty of every Christian to study, and thereby *build himself up in our most holy faith*'.[1] He was aware that Christianity is not built in a day in the soul, which must advance, and slowly, into its mysteries. But at the outset, and in an age not disposed to faith, it is right to emphasize its 'reasonableness'. But nowhere does he suggest that the revelation made in Christ can be proved; and nowhere is Christianity made 'natural'. He is opening to his readers articles of *faith*; and only says that they outrage no man's reason.

Amongst the most impressive pages of *The Reasonableness of Christianity* are those in which Locke explains the 'reasonableness' of divine

[1] *Works*, vol. vii. p. 176. The italics are mine.

revelation being made to man and of the necessity of *authority* in religion. His prose, when he speaks of these things, is more impassioned than is usual with him; and this is all the more interesting, because he is here on ground which his own beliefs (namely, that God's existence can be proved and that the body of ethics can be rationally deduced) made difficult to cross.

Now Locke holds that God had by the light of natural reason 'revealed to all mankind, who would make use of that light, that he was good and merciful . . . He that made use of this candle of the Lord, so far as to find what was his duty, could not miss to find also the way to reconciliation and forgiveness, when he had failed of his duty . . .' But if so, he asks, 'What need was there of a Saviour? What advantage have we by Jesus Christ?'[3] Was it true, after all, what he said in the Introduction to the *Essay*, that the candle 'burns bright enough for all our purposes'? I quote the paragraph which follows, Locke's 'general answer', with which he begins his discussion of the need which required that natural religion be superseded by revealed religion.

It is enough to justify the fitness of anything to be done, by resolving it into the 'wisdom of God,' who has done it; though our short views and narrow understandings, may utterly incapacitate us to see that wisdom, and to judge rightly of it. We know little of this visible, and nothing at all of the state of that intellectual world, wherein are infinite numbers and degrees of spirits out of the reach of our ken, or guess; and therefore know not what transactions there were between God and our Saviour, in reference to his kingdom. We know not what need there was to set up an head and a chieftain, in opposition to 'the prince of this world, the prince of the power of the air,' etc. whereof there are more than obscure intimations in scripture. And we shall take too much upon us, if we shall call God's wisdom or providence to account, and pertly condemn for needless all that our weak, and perhaps biassed, understanding cannot account for.

Now here, at the outset, is the note of authority, or of willingness to accept it, the need for faith arising from our necessary ignorance. This 'general answer', he says, is reply enough to the question, and 'such as a rational man, or fair searcher after truth', will acquiesce in. But he adds that there are other considerations which show 'that it was not without need' that Christ 'was sent into the world'. I do not propose to expound in detail what Locke thinks these considerations to be. He says that the great mass of men was lost in ignorance, sense and lust; and 'reason, speaking ever so clearly to the wise and virtuous, had never

[3] *Works*, vol. vii. p. 134.

ıthority enough to prevail on the multitude'.[1] The rational and think-
ıng part of mankind, it is true, when they sought after Him, found
the one supreme, invisible God; but if they acknowledged and wor-
shipped Him, it was only in their minds. Therefore Christ found the
world in a state of 'darkness and error'; the knowledge of one God of
goodness and mercy was slight and uncertain; and what there was
brought with it no passion of worship. The candle of the Lord had
been weak and impotent enough.

And if it had given too little knowledge of God, it had not given a
clear and certain morality. 'Natural religion, in its full extent, was nowhere, that I know, taken care of, by the force of natural reason. It
should seem, by the little that has hitherto been done in it, that it is
too hard a task for unassisted reason to establish morality in all its parts,
upon its true foundation, with a clear and convincing light.' The
candle gives light, but dimly; revelation gives a light 'clear and convincing'. Locke does not despise 'natural reason' and what reason may
do in religion and morality. He says simply that history and experience
show that it is not enough. 'The philosophers, who spoke from reason,
made not much mention of the Deity in their ethics. They depended
on reason and her oracles, which contain nothing but truth: but yet
some parts of that truth lie too deep for our natural powers easily to
reach, and make plain and visible to mankind; without some light from
above to direct them'. And then he adds,[2] 'when truths are once known
to us, though by tradition, we are apt to . . . ascribe to our own understandings the discovery of what, in reality, we borrowed from others
. . . A great many things which we have been bred up in the belief of,
from our cradles, . . . we take for unquestionable obvious truths and
easily demonstrable . . . And many are beholden to revelation, who do
not acknowledge it.' This last observation is in all truth one of great
moment, and is all too readily forgotten.

I have quoted enough to show the tenor and temper of Locke's
thoughts in this essay. But I add this quotation: 'Did the saying of
Aristippus, or Confucius, give it an authority? Was Zeno a law-giver
to mankind? If not, what he or any other philosopher delivered, was
but a saying of his. Mankind might hearken to it, or reject it, as they
pleased; or as it suited their interest, passions, principles or humours.
They were under no obligations; the opinion of this or that philosopher
was of no authority. And if it were, you must take all he said under the
same character. All his dictates must go for law, certain and true; or

[1] *Works*, vol. vii. p. 135.   [2] *Ibid.*, p. 144.

none of them . . . A body of ethics, proved to be the law of nature, from principles of reason, and teaching all the duties of life; I think nobody will say the world had before our Saviour's time.'[1] I need quote no more to show the note and depth of Locke's Christianity. There is no deism here; but instead a fair balance which avoids the error both of fideism and deism. I have said that Locke's philosophy, almost everywhere, keeps a fair balance between the value to us of our reason and the limitations of our knowledge; this balance is fairly kept in *The Reasonableness of Christianity*; and it can have this title, and rightly have it, and be no less rightly called Christian in its temper and sensibility. Besides, I have also said that Locke's philosophy gave room for history and contingency. And this, united with his sense of human ignorance, gave further inclination to his mind to embrace a historical revelation.

IX

Let us now then go back again, and in view of what I have said in the two preceding sections, consider again Locke's doctrine that God's existence can be demonstrated with 'mathematical certainty', and (what it is also convenient to do now) to his doctrine that ethics can be shown to be a deductive system of knowledge. We assent to revelation in faith, however fully faith may determine our minds; but we *know* that God exists. We may have assurance, complete even, and wholly 'settled', in revelation, yet not certainty; but God's existence is completely demonstrable. Revelation is still within the realm of probability; that God exists is certain.

Now I have said that what is shown in Locke's use of the cosmological proof is more his faith than his reason; it issues more from assent than from syllogism. Why should Locke, of all men, the end and motive of whose philosophy is to give reasonable ground for assent, drive syllogism hard in religion? If syllogism manacles thought, is no instrument of discovery, and at best restates and checks what has been found by the living reason, can it be important in religion? It is Locke himself who has said: 'A man knows first, and then he is able to prove it syllogistically. So that syllogism comes after knowledge, and then a man has little or no need of it' (4. 17. vi). He also said that syllogism is 'more adapted to catch and entangle the mind, than to instruct and inform the understanding' (4. 17. iv), and is 'abundantly liable to fallacies'. Locke's *Christianity*, what is the heart of him, sprang from

[1] *Works,* vol. vii. p. 141.

assent; had he not been wiser to leave proofs and demonstrations to deists?

For my part, I do not doubt that he had. We can certainly advance important reasons why we should conclude that God exists, or which must make us think it probable; but it is not given us to prove it. But Locke will not risk making God's existence something only assented to; something 'reasonable' enough to believe, but unproved. Besides, he said at length, as we have seen, how wavering and of how little avail natural religion was in the ancient world. Why then does he not simplify his philosophy, accept the implicit requirements of common experience and have also more consistency? He says that we have 'sensitive' *knowledge* of the existence of things, 'demonstrative' *knowledge* of the existence of God and *assent* only to the Christian revelation. But why not assent to all three, 'reasonably enough', and along with assent to all three, certitude, though not certainty? It would have been better for Locke's philosophy, truer to his own experience, and better for the eighteenth century, had he taken his courage in both hands and said so.

In the *Essay* he declares his rationalist doctrine of ethics: ethics is deducible like mathematics. But he will not, because he cannot, work it out; the theorems are not forthcoming; or what theorems he offers are absurdly false. And in *The Reasonableness of Christianity* he is at pains to tell us that the unaided intellect had *not* deduced an infallible system of ethics. Locke knew well enough that the ancient world was certainly lacking in neither powerful intelligence nor passionate interest in ethical matters; but 'philosophy seemed to have spend its strength, and done its utmost: or if it should have gone farther, as we see it did not, and from undeniable principles given us ethics in a science like mathematics in every part demonstrable [he is still clinging to his philosophical fiction]; this yet would not have been so effectual to man in this imperfect state, nor proper for the cure'.[1] And he goes on to say that if such a deductive ethic came about, it would be of use (if indeed it were of use at all) only to the learned and clever; the mass of mankind would still be groping in the dark.

It is clear therefore that the argument for the 'reasonableness' of Christianity cuts across the proof of God's existence and a deductive ethic; and Locke can hardly have it both ways. If revelation is to be 'reasonable', natural religion is not enough; but if you attach great weight in religion to what the unaided intellect can prove, you are

---

[1] *Works*, vol. vii. pp. 145–46.

likely, and quickly, to attach little weight to revelation. If authority there is to be, it cannot, by its nature, be demonstrated. Or, if you want only the authority of what you judge to be demonstrable, and imagine you have proved to your complete satisfaction that God exists and that you possess a deductive ethic, you quickly find yourself at home with the vulgar and commonplace sensibility of the deists.

No doubt Locke is not happy here, and his balance of mind not easy. But I think we can fairly say two things. First, that the quality and temper of his mind is not true to itself in his proof of God and his proposed deductive ethic; he was a man of assent and not of apodictic doctrine. Second, that he asserted his proof and the possibility of a rationalist ethic out of a certain timidity, in which he was encouraged by the growing spirit of the age. He wanted to do what he could, speaking out of a deep Christian piety, to help the cause of religion; and some things he wanted to put beyond doubt. He temporized therefore, from the highest and most pious motives, with his time. Certainly, he misjudged here; this was not the way. And no doubt it was his yielding, so far in the *Essay*, to the spirit of the age that later made it possible for him to write the chapter on enthusiasm and break what had been previously, for much the bigger part, the excellent balance in his mind of faith and reason. For him to have so far yielded to proofs in the *Essay* as it first appeared was an opening of the flood-gates; and in the later chapter *Of Enthusiasm*, the deist flood is pouring into and undermining his philosophical building.

X

I have only one thing to add before I turn to his theory of knowledge: it is to suggest that it is profitable to compare Locke with Pascal. Locke refers to Pascal in the *Essay*, in 2. 10. ix, a paragraph which was added in the second edition. The Port Royal edition of the *Pensées* had been published in 1670 and had aroused great interest. In the autumn of 1672 Locke went on holiday to France. While there he read Nicole's *Essais de Morale* and soon after his return translated them. Now Nicole was a friend of Arnauld and Pascal. He had retired to Port Royal five years before Pascal and Arnauld; and on the expulsion of the Jansenists from the Sorbonne engaged in the resulting controversy. In 1656 he helped Pascal with the *Lettres Provinciales* and two years later translated it into Latin. In 1670 and 1671 he published his own *Essais*, which, says Fox Bourne, 'excited an interest only, though greatly, surpassed by that aroused by the *Pensées*'.[1] Locke translated three of them. The first was a proof of God's existence and of the soul's immortality, written in a very Cartesian point of view; and Locke was later to disclaim any sympathy with it. But the second, on the weakness of man, in body and in mind, contains an attack on Descartes' Presumption, and is near in temper and argument to much that we find in both Pascal and Locke. Now it is very likely that in Paris in 1672 Locke not only read Nicole, but Pascal's *Pensées* also; indeed, it is hard to believe that he could have missed them. Not only this. Mme Perier's *Life* of her brother was published in Amsterdam in 1684. Locke had left England for his exile in 1683 and was in Amsterdam for the bigger part of the first half of 1684 and was back there by November of that year. Again, it is certainly not rash to think it very likely that Locke read the *Life*.

Locke's reference to Pascal in the *Essay* has to do with his prodigious memory, which he had no doubt read of either in Etienne Perier's introduction to the Port Royal edition or in Mme Perier's *Life*; nothing is said of Pascal's beliefs. Now I think that Locke and Pascal had a great deal in common; and that Locke does not speak of the *Pensées* in the *Essay* is in itself not evidence that Locke had not read them. It was not his practice to refer frequently to writers who were clearly and frequently in his mind; the name of Descartes is mentioned only twice throughout the *Essay;* Hobbes is not mentioned at all, though we once find the word 'Hobbist'; and if he disliked explicit controversy, it was also not his manner to mention (and we may be sure that it was not out of ingratitude) the names of writers who had helped him and with whom he was in sympathy; he does not, for example, mention Chillingworth or Tillotson in the *Essay*.

In any case, it is no essential part of my purpose to prove that Locke had read the *Pensées;* and if he had not, that does not make any less interesting any comparison between the two men and their writings. Now I should say that the sensibility of both writers is organized about their sense of the 'mediocrity' of man's nature. I have spoken earlier of Locke's 'mediocrity' and of his contentment with it; and Pascal comes back frequently to the same thought. 'Nothing is good but mediocrity. The majority has settled that, and finds fault with him who escapes it at whichever end. I will not oppose it. I quite consent to put myself there, and refuse to be at the lower end, not because it is low, but because it is an end; for I would likewise refuse to be placed at the top. To leave the mean is to abandon humanity. The greatness of the soul consists in knowing how to preserve the mean. So far from

[1] Fox Bourne, vol. i. p. 295.

greatness consisting in leaving it, it consists in not leaving it.'[1] This is the wisdom, simple but profound, which animates Pascal and Locke. And then Pascal goes on in the next section but one (that is, in Brunschvicg's arrangement) to say: 'All good maxims are in the world. We only need to apply them. . . . It is true there must be inequality among men; but if this is conceded, the door is opened not only to the highest power, but to the highest tyranny. We must relax our minds a little; but this opens the door to the greatest debauchery. Let us mark the limits. There are no limits in things. Laws would put them there, and the mind cannot suffer it.' The reader will recall what Locke said in his letter to Grenville: 'I have often thought that our state here in this world is a state of mediocrity, which is not capable of extremes, though on one side there may be great excellency and perfection. Thus we are not capable of continual rest or exercise, though the latter has certainly more of excellency in it. We are not able to labour always with the body, nor always with the mind; and . . . we are not capable of living altogether exactly by strict rule, nor altogether without one—not always retired, nor always in company.'

It is the same thought; and it sets the temper, and the temperateness, of both men. Always there is a middle way, a balance, a knife-edge; and to be human is fairly to judge that balance and creatively to live it. This is true of behaviour; it is true also of philosophy; one spirit is required in both, and to leave the mean in action or in thought is to 'abandon humanity'. Let is mark the limits. But there are 'no limits in things', 'strict rules' are not to be had. There is an art, a judgement, which consists 'in knowing how to preserve the mean'; and *that* is the 'greatness' of the human soul.

Now both Locke and Pascal try to work out such a balance in their doctrine. There is, says Pascal (in 392), a 'doubtful ambiguity' and a 'certain doubtful dimness, from which our doubts cannot take away all the clearness nor our own natural lights chase away all the darkness'. There is a little light, which we must trust, and there is much darkness, which we cannot dispel. Philosophy must begin from this sense of things; without it philosophy may show much intelligence and little humanity. Therefore, 'the last proceeding of reason is to recognise that there is an infinity of things, which are beyond it. It is but feeble if it does not see so far as to know this. But if natural things are beyond it, what will be said of supernatural?' So Pascal in 267; and it is, as the reader will see from all I have said of Locke and quoted from him, the very note of Locke's philosophy. Therefore also, there are 'two

---

[1] W. F. Trotter's translation of Brunschvicg's edition, Temple Classics, London, p. 378.

8

extremes: to exclude reason, to admit reason only'; and, 'if we submit everything to reason, our religion will have no mysterious and super-natural element. If we offend the principles of reason, our religion will be absurd and ridiculous' (273). It is true that neither Pascal nor Locke succeeded in keeping the balance here; sometimes Pascal seems to go over to a fideism, or again, to the *Il faut parier*, and Locke misjudges the balance with his cosmological proof and in the chapter on enthu-siasm, tipping the scales on the opposite side; still, at their typical and best, they both represent the highest spiritual achievements of the seventeenth century in Western Europe, and give to reason its rightful place in the economy of the spiritual life.

There are other ways in which it would be instructive to compare Pascal and Locke. I have said (with Professor Aaron's authority to support me) that we can see, in the *Essay*, clear enough evidence that the 'reasons of the heart' were active in Locke's life. Faith, Pascal said, is 'God felt by the heart, not by the reason' (278); and Locke, guarded as he everywhere is in the *Essay*, would not have dissented; at the end even of the chapter on enthusiasm, where he seems to overlay the life of faith with safeguards and inhibitions, he yet speaks of the 'immediate influence and assistance of the Holy Spirit' as something he is 'far from denying'. Or again, we might compare Pascal's spirit of *finesse* and intuition with Locke's doctrine of individual judgement, of assent, and his attack on 'syllogism'. But to do this is not now to my purpose. I only wish, in concluding my account of his general philosophical thinking, to suggest that Locke is best understood if we see him near to, if not in the company of, Pascal, and least understood if we see him as near to, or in the company of, the 'rationalists' and deists. It may seem a far march from the inchoate and impassioned thoughts and ejacula-tions of the *Pensées* to the cool, diffuse and cautious explorations of the *Essay on the Human Understanding*. But we must not be deceived by appearances. Locke too, as I was at pains earlier to explain, had a warm and passionate heart. The *Pensées* moreover is not a book written, as it stands, for the public; much, no doubt, would have been cut out or changed. And Locke was not the man to parade his deepest feelings.

The reader will understand that I do not offer what I have said above as a full-length comparison of the two men. They were, in some important respects, very different from each other. But I think the comparison just so far as it goes; and my concern has been only to show that we are nearer the mark if we think of Locke as near to Pascal than as near to the deists.

I

WE must now turn from Locke's general philosophical doctrine to speak of his theory of sense-knowledge; and in doing so, I shall be able to develop further what I said, in the course of criticizing Hobbes, in the last sections of Chapter One.

To think of Locke's theory of knowledge is perhaps to think first of the *tabula rasa*, of the ideas which are the object of the understanding when a man thinks, and of other pieces of apparatus which together may be composed into a dull and lifeless epistemological machine. But I have spoken of the spirit and intention of Locke's philosophy; and it is not at all a dull or lifeless spirit and intention. It looks, from the beginning, to a spiritual and Christian end; and not to see this aim, animating the organism of Locke's doctrine, is to make it insignificant, unless to pedants. Locke certainly speaks, in *The Epistle to the Reader*, of the scientific master-builders, of Boyle, Sydenham and 'the incomparable Mr. Newton', and goes on to say that he is content to be 'an under-labourer in clearing the ground a little, and removing some of the rubbish that lies in the way to knowledge'; but I have said enough to make clear, if indeed it needed to be made clear, that Locke is at best a very temperate gospeller of science; from the beginning he was more disposed to see the limits of knowledge than to extend them; and his empiricism was not, like the empiricism of our time, actuated first and chiefly by a desire to find a basis for scientific knowledge, though this was part of his legitimate intention. His motive, in all his thought, is pious; and the *tabula rasa* and the 'ideas' spring far more from a religious than from a scientific intention, from a mind more passionately religious than it was intemperately 'scientific'. He is to deal, he says, in the *Introduction*, first with ideas, then to consider what *knowledge* they may afford, and lastly with *faith, opinion*, or *assent*. The end of it all is the reasonable assent which he expounds in Book 4; and no doubt Book 4 is the spirit and inspiration of Books 1 and 2. 'If we can find out', he says again in the Introduction (iv), 'how far the understanding can extend its view; how far it has faculties to attain certainty, and in what cases it can only judge and guess; we may learn to content ourselves with what is attainable by us in this state'. He begins from a prejudice, a sense of 'this state'; and this 'sense' is a religious sense.

Now the mind, he says, is 'void of all characters, without any ideas'.
It has everything to learn, is wholly docile, has no powers of dictating
to experience, has no laws to impose. It has frequently been thought
that Locke, beginning from this dogma, was striking a blow at the
spirit of man; here, it has been thought, from the beginning, is an un-
spiritual philosophy, condemned from the outset to being incapable
of any of those higher flights beloved of some philosophers. T. H.
Green merits great respect. But no reader of his introduction to Hume
can fail to observe how much Locke irritates him, and that what
irritates him is Locke's persistently modest way of speaking about the
human mind. 'He speaks of his own mind, it is to be noticed, just as
he might of his body' says Green, obviously shocked. 'It meant something born with, and dependent on, the particular animal organism that
first saw the light at Wrington on a particular day in 1632.'[1] So indeed
Locke did speak; and he also said that the coach that carried his body
from London to Oxford also carried his soul. And so, beyond all
question, it did. But Locke thought nobly of the soul, all the same;
it had, in his eyes, if I am not mistaken, a higher destiny than it had in
the eyes of Green; Green may have believed in Mind, but Locke believed in the Mind of God, which, in another world than this, the soul
may know and enjoy. Certainly such a faith animated Locke from the
beginning, and is to be discerned in the modesty of his thinking about
the mind and in his declaration that the soul at its beginning knows
nothing whatever.

II

Now it is true that Locke's theory of knowledge is by no means,
from the outset, satisfactory. But it is not as unsatisfactory as it is
is frequently made out to be; and it is very important not to hurry into
neat interpretations of what Locke says, which do not fairly take into
account the many sides of his inevitably complicated doctrine. It is
certain, in the first place, as I have sufficiently shown, that Locke is
no sensationalist or phenomenalist. So far from saying that things are
fully shown to us in sense, that their nature is fully disclosed to us in
seeing and hearing, Locke is anxious above all *not* to say any such thing.
On the contrary, there is much, much the greater part indeed, in the
physical world which we know neither in sense nor in any other way.
But still, it will be said, Locke was a sensationalist in another sense;
namely, that he says, or speaks as if he believed, that not only is the

[1] *Works of T. H. Green*, London, 1885, vol. i. p. 6.

mind a *tabula rasa*, but that it is also wholly passive in its knowledge of the world; so that the mind has only to suffer, as it were, the impact of stimuli in order to become aware of a world of objects. This certainly is Hobbes's way. But it is not so simple a matter in Locke, and we have need to be careful. That he was an empiricist, or rather, set himself to be one, is true; there is nothing in the *Essay* to show that Locke would disagree with Hobbes when he says in *Leviathan*, chapter 1, that 'there is no conception in a mans mind, which hath not at first, totally, or by parts, been begotten upon the organs of *sense*. The rest are derived from that originall'; but whether he was a consistent empiricist is another matter, to which I have referred earlier, and shall, no doubt, refer again, but which for the present we may leave. I confine myself now to saying that Locke nowhere asserts that the mind is wholly passive in knowledge of objects. It is true that he sometimes speaks as if he believed this; and the *Essay* is frequently unsatisfactory and vague where it speaks of sensation and perception. For example, in the first chapter of Book 2 he speaks of the 'Senses, conversant about particular sensible objects' as *conveying* 'into the mind several distinct perceptions of things . . . And thus we come by those ideas we have, of Yellow, White, Heat, Cold . . . and all those which we call sensible qualities . . .' (iii). So far, there is nothing, or very little, to choose between him and Hobbes on sense-knowledge. But Locke goes on to say, '. . . which when I say the senses convey into the mind, I mean, they from external objects convey into the mind what produces there those perceptions. This great source of most of the ideas we have, depending wholly upon our senses, and derived by them to the understanding, I call SENSATION.' Now here, Locke is clearly distinguishing between sensation and perception; and in the second part of what I have just quoted, he is at pains to restate what he has said in the first part in order to avoid misunderstanding. In the first part the senses convey perceptions into the mind; in the second he speaks of the senses conveying into the mind what *produces* perceptions. Now that Locke was hazy and uncertain in this matter is further shown in 2. 1. xxiii, where he says that he conceives 'that ideas . . . are coeval with sensation; which is such an impression or motion, made in some part of the body as *produces some perception* in the understanding'. But the words I have italicized were not in the first three editions; in them we find: '. . impression or notion. made in some part of the body as *makes it to be taken notice of* in the understanding'.[1] Still, whichever of these two expressions we choose,

[1] A. C. Fraser's edition of the *Essay*, vol. i. p. 141.

it is clear that Locke is suggesting that the understanding actively apprehends, and does not merely have something 'conveyed' into it; knowledge is not an affair of motion and mechanical, and the mind not merely passive. And in the French edition, which was published in Amsterdam in 1700, he added, after what I last quoted, 'It is about these impressions made on our senses by outward objects that the mind seems *first* to employ itself, in such operations as we call perception, remembering, consideration, reasoning, etc'.[1] From this it is clear that sensation may give 'impressions', in receiving which the mind is passive; but perception is an operation of the understanding and upon 'impressions'. And if this is so, the mind may be a *tabula rasa*; but to say that Locke holds that the mind is passive in sense-knowledge is to misrepresent him. It is undeniable that he sometimes uses 'perception' to mean 'sensation' and that he does not sort these things out as clearly as we may wish. But that what I have said represents what he intended in the *Essay*, is, I think, certain.[2] An 'idea' is an object of *perception*, not of sensation, and perception is an action of the mind.

In 2. 9, which is called *Of Perception*, he is capable of speaking of the 'ideas we receive by sensation' (in section viii). This is one of those places where he does not maintain a steady distinction. But in much of the chapter he speaks of the ways in which the mind, active in knowledge, affects sensations. 'A sufficient impulse there may be on the organ; but if not reaching the observation of the mind, there follows no perception . . . Want of sensation, in this case, is not through any defect in the organ . . . but that which uses to produce the idea, though conveyed in by the usual organ, not being taken notice of in the understanding, and so imprinting no idea in the mind, there follows no sensation' (2. 9. iv). Now this passage illustrates how Locke will write uncertainly and inconsistently in these matters; he speaks of an idea being 'imprinted in' the mind; still, the main intention of the passage is to show the activity of the mind's understanding in knowledge, and its selectiveness; and so far from the mind being passive, even in mere *sensation*, it can obliterate the impressions of sense. Again, he speaks of the effect of 'judgement' in sense-perception. 'When we set before our eyes a round globe, of any uniform colour, e.g., gold, alabaster, or jet; it is certain that the idea thereby imprinted in our mind is of a flat circle variously shadowed, with several degrees of light and brightness coming to our eyes. But we having by use been accustomed to per-

---

[1] A. C. Fraser's edition of the *Essay*, vol. i. p. 141.
[2] See R. I. Aaron, *John Locke*, London, 1937, pp. 100–101 footnote and pp. 124–25.

ceive what kind of appearance convex bodies are wont to make in us, what alterations are made in the reflections of light by the difference of the sensible figures of bodies; the judgement presently, by an habitual custom, alters the appearances into their causes; so that from that which is truly variety of shadow or colour, collecting the figure, it makes it pass for a mark of figure, and frames to itself the perception of a convex figure and an uniform colour; when the idea we receive from thence is only a plane variously coloured, as is evident in painting' (2. 9. viii). Now here again Locke writes uncertainly. For he speaks of the 'flat circle variously shadowed' being indeed an 'idea', but as 'imprinted in our mind'; but the 'convex figure and an uniform colour' is a 'perception' which the judgement 'frames to itself'. This is a tangle and needs to be sorted out. For on Locke's own showing, the idea of the 'flat circle, variously shadowed' is not mere sensation; in the passage in 2. 1. xxiii, from which I quoted, he says that 'ideas are *coeval with* sensation; which is such an impression or motion made in some part of the body as produces some perception in the understanding'. Now a thing coeval with another is not identical with it; and he speaks of sensation as giving an impression which stimulates the mind to perceive and to apprehend 'idea'. But if this is so (and there can be little doubt that it is so), the 'flat circle, variously shadowed' is not sensation or impression, but genuinely idea, something perceived, and the 'convex figure and an uniform colour' a more complex idea arrived at by more complex perception; both are ideas and apprehended by perception. Locke's vacillation and uncertainty are unmistakable; still, again, the main burden of the passage about the convex figure is to show that perception is certainly not a mechanical patiency of the mind. He is only in error because he seems to decline to carry his analysis below the level at which we perceive objects in three-dimensional space.

I have said enough to show that Locke's view of perception is fuller and more accurate than Hobbes's. But he did not firmly grasp and set out the doctrine that what the mind apprehends in perception, which is necessarily active, is always idea; where the mind perceives an object, however much that object may be changed by later and more advanced perceiving, we are beyond, far indeed beyond, the mere impressions received from sensation; or again, we may, if we are well enough trained to acquire the simplicity of the eye, unburden ourselves of the very complex idea of the convex figure and revert to the simpler idea, which is yet genuine idea, of the 'flat circle, variously shadowed'. Now I suggested, in writing about Hobbes, that we may call this activity of the mind imaginative; the act of perception is in the first place an act of imagination, a bringing together and ordering into wholes of what, following high authority, we may fairly call the 'manifold of sensation'. Locke speaks of the *understanding* 'taking notice of' impressions; it would have been better to speak of the *imagination* taking notice of impressions and forming them into ideas. In what sense such acts of imagination may be called acts of *knowing* is another matter; and on the face of it at least, it seems senseless to call imagining and knowing the same thing; it is one thing to have ideas, another to *know*. Locke, unlike Hobbes, was fully aware of this problem; and in a moment I shall recount what he has to say about it. Before doing so, I wish to remark further on what he says about perceiving as an action of the mind.

In the illustration of the convex figure Locke speaks of the 'ideas we receive by sensation' being altered by 'the judgement'. Now I have said that what he here calls an 'idea we receive by sensation' is in fact an idea of perception. But it is with his use of 'judgement' that I am now especially concerned. What does he mean by 'judgement'? Not, certainly, what he means by judgement where, in Book 4, it is equivalent to assent or belief as opposed to certain knowledge. There, judgement is a form of knowing; it is not indeed, in strictness, knowing, for it can provide only probability; still, in it the mind is active in perceiving the agreement or disagreement of its ideas; and in this, knowledge in the broadest sense, according to Locke, consists. No, by 'judgement' here he means the faculty of discerning, of which he he speaks in 2. 11. He there distinguishes between wit and judgement; and he does so precisely on the lines laid down by Hobbes. Wit sees the 'resemblance or congruity' between ideas, and brings such similar ideas together, thereby making up 'pleasant pictures, and agreeable visions in the fancy'. But judgement 'lies quite on the other side, in separating carefully, one from another, ideas, wherein can be found the least difference; thereby to avoid being misled by similitude, and by affinity to take one thing for another' (2. 11. iii). This is certainly 'Hobbist' enough; and we shall need to come back to this in another connection. I observe now only that judgement, as Locke uses the word here, is the intellectual act of discrimination.

Now I ask, does this mean that, in Locke's doctrine, the mind, in what he calls perception, discriminates as much as it does in its apprehension of the convex figure so that perception may not exist without very developed and explicit discrimination? At first sight, we might answer, Yes. The flat circle is an 'idea received by sensation'; the convex figure a properly perceived object, an idea of perception; and I do not doubt that there was that in Locke which strongly inclined him to think in this way, to require in what he thought might rightly be called perception a high degree of explicit analysis; so that although he speaks of the flat circle as an 'idea', he yet goes on to call it an 'idea of sensation'; and if this is so, he seems to think that there is perceiving proper only where there is judgement, which 'alters the appearances into their causes' (2. 9. viii), and thereby treats the appearances as *signs* of a *thing*.

But that we must be careful is shown precisely by his use of the phrase 'ideas of sensation'. As I have said, he is careful to speak of ideas as distinct from, though coeval with, sensation; and the fact that he speaks of 'ideas of sensation' does not mean that he goes back on this distinction. By 'idea of sensation' he means not an idea provided by sensation, what he clearly affirms to be impossible; he means an idea not accompanied by 'judgement' but distinguishable from sensation. It is, if we will, a lowly form of perception, at a level below which appearances are read as signs; but it is still a level at which we apprehend ideas. Now if this is so, Locke uses 'sensation' dangerously. He uses it to mean barely what external objects may be said to convey to the mind, impressions which the mind does, in all truth, receive passively; he also uses it to mean perception unaccompanied by judgement or explicit analysis, the action of the mind on mere impressions whereby impressions are raised into 'ideas' without however the aid of what may properly be called 'judgement'.

Therefore we must say that Locke does not require that 'judgement' must accompany perception; and I think I can show further that I am interpreting Locke justly. In 2. 9. xi, the chapter *Of Perception*, he speaks of perception in animals. The 'faculty of perception seems to me to be that, which puts the distinction betwixt the animal kingdom and the inferior parts of nature'. In the Sensitive Plant, there is 'bare mechanism'; but 'perception, I believe is, in some degree, in all sorts of animals; tho' in some possibly, the avenues provided by nature for the reception of sensations are so few, and *the perception they are received with* [my italics] so obscure and dull, that it comes extremely short of the quickness and variety of sensation which is in other animals . . .' (xii). That is, there are degrees of perception, or of the liveliness of the perceiving with which sensations are received. An old and decrepit man may lose his memory and his senses may be decayed; so that, 'if there be some of the inlets yet half open, the impressions made are scarcely perceived, or not at all retained' (xiv); and in some such way we must envisage the mental life of the lower animals. In general, the impressions of sense must 'be taken notice of', he says in 2. 9. iii; and 'if they are not taken notice of within; there is no perception'. But this perceiving may range from 'some small dim perception' to the liveliest perception of which men are capable. I think it therefore certain that by 'ideas of sensation' he means ideas of a lowly order of perception; they are impressions erected, by however dull powers of perceiving, into ideas, but without being accompanied by enough analysis to justify our use of the word 'judgement'.

The reader must judge if I have misinterpreted Locke. I do not think I have. At the most I think I have only brought out a speculation which is certainly in the *Essay* and which most represents Locke's belief. Besides, it is a speculation which, to the best of my judgement, is true, and is necessary if we are to deal adequately with our experience in knowing. The impressions of sense do not give ideas; they are the mere matter of experience. It is perceiving which may or may not be accompanied by 'judgement', which can, in proportion to the amount of intellectual analysis in the mind's act, hold and retain for *contemplation* (the word is Locke's in 2. 10. i) what else would be in an unformed flux of impression merely.

III

Still, it will be said, 'There is another serious charge which may be brought against him. You are trying to make us believe in a Locke after your own heart; and even if you are right so far, you have now to take account of what no less a person than Mr. Alexander said about him. He said that Locke "falls short of his own ideal of describing the contents of experience. He overlooks the fact of continuity. The objects of experience are to him fragmentary and disconnected. . . . Qualities are grouped together by the mechanical bond of an underlying support or substance. . . . To all intents and purposes, in spite of his urging the inter-relatedness of things, the world is to him a number of isolated atoms grouped together in the last resort by the good pleasure of God".[1] Is not this at least true?'

It is only partially true. Certainly Locke gives reason to speak as Alexander does. Here, as in the doctrines we have just been discussing, he frequently hesitates or is unclear. But if study of the *Essay* gives reasonable ground for what Alexander says, it certainly also gives ground for saying that there is in it much more than the beginning of a

[1] S. Alexander, *Locke*, London, 1908, pp. 65–67.

quite different doctrine. We must now consider the theory of simple and complex ideas.

The 'atomistic' doctrine sometimes attributed to Locke consists in this: that in perception we obtain impressions through the various senses which by 'being taken notice of' became ideas; and that these 'simple' ideas, of white and sweet and hard, are put together (with other simple ideas of space, of a substance, etc., with which we need not now trouble ourselves) to make up a 'complex' idea of, say, a lump of sugar. Now here is the kind of passage in which Locke gives reason for thinking he believed something like this, which I quote from 2. 2. i:

> Though the qualities that affect our senses are, in the things themselves, so united and blended, that there is no separation, no distance between them; yet it is plain, the idea they produce in the mind enter by the senses simple and unmixed. For, though the sight and touch often take in from the same subject, at the same time, different ideas; . . . yet the simple ideas, thus united in the same subject, are as perfectly distinct as those that come in by different senses: the coldness and hardness which a man feels in a piece of ice being as distinct ideas in the mind, as the smell and whiteness of a lily; . . . And there is nothing plainer to a man than the clear and distinct perception he has of those simple ideas; which, being each in itself uncompounded, contains in it nothing but one uniform appearance, or conception in the mind, and is not distinguishable into different ideas.

And he then goes on in the next paragraph to say:

> These simple ideas, the materials of all our knowledge, are suggested and furnished to the mind only by . . . sensation and reflection. When the understanding is once stored with these simple ideas, it has the power to repeat, compare and unite them, even to an almost infinite variety; and so can make at pleasure new complex ideas.

(At this point, let us not trouble ourselves by what is intended by 'suggested' and 'reflection' in the last sentence but one.)

Now the question is, When Locke writes in this way, is he giving us a genetical definition of complex ideas to which he is once and for all and clearly committed? Is the 'plain historical method' here a historical method in our usual sense of the word 'historical' and not in the old Greek sense of ἰστορία? At first sight we may hardly know what to answer. Certainly, the words suggest that he is speaking of the coming-to-be of complex ideas in the mind; on the other hand, it seems incredible that a mind so fair and sensible should commit itself to a doctrine so obviously wrong. And it is therefore necessary to cast about in the *Essay* for evidence which will decide us how to answer.

But we have not to cast far and long. If what I have said in the preceding section of this chapter rightly expounds Locke's intention, it is certain that he is not here explaining how we come to know objects. He has said that the mind, whether of men or animals, may have ideas by 'taking notice' of impressions of sense, and this without 'judgement'. But if so, it is inconceivable that at this modest level of perceiving we carry out so complicated a process as he describes in the passages I have quoted above; 'perception in the lowest degree of it' (2. 9. xv), cannot possibly traffic in analysis and synthesis on such a scale. Locke knows this. In 2. 9. vii, he writes of comparison and composition, and says of animals: 'though they take in, and retain together several combinations of simple ideas, as possibly the shape, smell, and voice of his master make up the complex idea a dog has of him, or rather are so many distinct marks whereby he knows him; yet *I do not think they do of themselves ever compound them, and make complex ideas*' (my italics). This is clear enough. When Locke speaks of lowly perceiving, the jig-saw of simple and complex ideas is thrown to the winds ; and if so, we have weighty evidence that in the passages I quoted from 2. 2, he was thinking analytically and not genetically. He says that the ideas a dog has in perceiving are grasped in their complexity; he can hardly also hold that children begin with simple ideas and proceed to complex ideas by analysis and compounding. And neither a fair inspection of experience nor consistency can allow him to say so.

Besides, there is much other evidence. In 2. 12. i, where he begins his discussion of complex ideas, he says: 'As simple ideas are *observed to exist in several combinations united together* [my italics], so the mind has a power to consider several of them united together as one idea; and that not only as they are united in external objects, but as itself has joined them together'. This can only mean that some ideas are first apprehended as not 'simple'; they are first grasped as 'one idea', as a unity of what may afterwards be analysed into 'simple' parts. Professor Aaron says that 'such distinctions as [Locke] was able to make between simple and complex ideas broke down in the course of his argument' (p. 100); he refers to the passage I have just quoted, along with some others, and then remarks on what Locke says of space and time. In Locke's view space and time are simple ideas; and yet he says: 'Though they are justly reckoned amongst our simple ideas, yet none of the distinct ideas we have of either is without all manner of composition; it is the very nature of both of them to consist of parts' (2. 15. ix); but if this is so, we must conclude that each is first known, in its complexity, as *one* idea; only later may analysis discriminate the parts within the whole. Professor Aaron further rightly says that the notion of complex idea cannot be applied, as Locke wishes, to our idea of relation and to our general ideas; and he concludes his discussion by saying that 'Locke begins with the compositional theory in Book 2, but as his argument proceeds it becomes less and less useful. He is not greatly perturbed at this however, precisely because he does not think compositionalism fundamental to his argument' (p. 102). And indeed, it is not; the jig-saw doctrine is not at all indispensable to empiricism.

Finally, I remark that in 2. 7. vii, Locke says: 'Existence and Unity are two other ideas that are suggested to the understanding by every object without, and every idea within. When ideas are in our minds, we consider them as being actually there, as well as we consider things to be actually without us; which is, that they exist, or have existence. And whatever we can consider as one thing, whether a real being or idea, suggests to the understanding the idea of unity.' Now again, I am not concerned with the word 'suggest' which he here uses ; nor am I concerned to criticize his doctrine here. I observe only that if existence and unity, which Locke says are simple ideas, accompany all other ideas whatsoever, it follows that no idea comes to the mind in naked simplicity; it must come at least garbed in the vestures of existence and unity. But if so, Locke cannot possibly have thought he was ever committed to believing that the mind first apprehends simple ideas, one by one, and then composes them *into* unity. On the contrary, every idea is for the mind already a *unity;* unity is essential to every idea; and perception is a perceiving of unities.

I think this evidence is conclusive. He certainly and frequently speaks of simple and complex ideas as units and joined units respectively; but this is only part of his machinery of exposition. We may sometimes feel, and reasonably, that he becomes the slave of his machine. But there is plenty to show that he does not do so for long. Campbell Fraser, Locke's most exhaustive commentator, says rightly, in his footnote to the first section of 2. 2. i: 'In distinguishing *simple* from *complex* ideas, Locke does not assert that the former are, or can be, received, or represented, *in their simplicity;* nor does he deny that a "simple" idea of sense, *as such*, is an abstraction from our actual experience'.[1]

---

[1] A. C. Fraser's edition, vol. i. p. 144.

IV

I am submitting to the reader the view that, in those parts of his doctrine about knowledge which we have so far considered in this chapter, Locke is in all essentials right. His empiricism is right; all knowledge comes from experience, and the mind at the beginning is a *tabula rasa*. It is also an active thing, changing impression into idea and a formless manifold into unity.

But I remarked, in section II of this chapter, that Locke attributes the first step in knowledge to the 'understanding'; but I suggest he might well have attributed it to 'imagination'. Now this is not an affair of names merely; it makes all the difference as to what place we shall give to the æsthetic in our map of human experience. Indeed, on it depends whether we shall give it any place at all; and if we give it no rightful room we shall misrepresent the nature and scope of *all* human activities. Words, even when used by philosophers, are the instruments of prejudice as well as of thought. Locke's use of 'understanding' shows he is blind to the æsthetic; and this is perhaps the cardinal error of the *Essay*.

At the end of the Introduction occurs the celebrated statement that 'idea' is the term which 'serves best to stand for whatsoever is the object of the understanding when a man thinks'. Now Locke used the word 'idea' very widely; and no doubt, when he said that an 'idea' is the 'object of the understanding when a man thinks', he was concerting a sentence which might cover our apprehending of general ideas as well as of the ideas we entertain of sensible objects. Still, he holds that the perceiving of ideas of sense is the action of the *understanding;* and it is clear that he was aware that in using the word 'understanding' in this way, he was putting it to an unusual use. For we find this in 2. 21, v: 'The power of perception is that which we call the understanding. Perception, which we make the act of the understanding, is of three sorts: 1. The perception of ideas in our mind. 2. The perception of the signification of signs. 3. The perception of the connexion or repugnancy, agreement or disagreement, that there is between any of our ideas. All these are attributed to the understanding, or perceptive power, though it be the two latter only that use allows us to say we understand', or, as he had it in the first edition, 'though it be only to the two latter that, in strictness of speech, the act of understanding is usually applied'.[1] Now at present we are concerned only with per-

[1] A. C. Fraser's edition, vol. i. p. 314.

ception of the first of the three kinds; and Locke acknowledges that ordinarily we would not speak of it as the action of the understanding. But it is precisely his extension of the word to cover this kind of perception which is significant, which shows the prejudice of his mind, and may fairly be criticized.

Now, in Locke's view, as we shall have occasion to observe in greater detail a little later on, the imagination, the first sort of understanding, considered in and by itself, cannot be said to give knowledge. It is the third sort of understanding, he said, which gives knowledge. The first kind of understanding is only, on his doctrine, an envisagement of ideas, without question of their agreement or disagreement, truth or falsity; and he is therefore aware that to speak of it as an action of the *understanding* is not only not to accord with everyday usage, but also to misrepresent the action which the mind employs in it.

Now, that this kind of perception of which we now speak might be called 'imagination' was a thought not far from Locke's mind. And to show this I shall quote the opening sections of 4. 4. I do not think there are any paragraphs in the whole *Essay* so interesting or so important. They show how well Locke knew that we have slight enough assurance that our 'knowledge' is 'real'. The chapter is called *Of the Reality of Knowledge*, and this is how he speaks:

I doubt not but my reader by this time may be apt to think, that I have been all this while only building a castle in the air; and be ready to say to me, 'To what purpose all this stir? Knowledge, say you, is only the perception of the agreement or disagreement of our own ideas; but who knows what those ideas may be? . . . If it be true, that all knowledge lies only in the perception of the agreement or disagreement of our own ideas, the visions of an enthusiast, and the reasonings of a sober man, will be equally certain. It is no matter how things are: so a man observe but the agreement of his own imaginations, and talk comformably, it is all truth, all certainty. Such castles in the air will be as strong holds of truth, as the demonstrations of Euclid. That an harpy is not a centaur is by this way as certain knowledge, and as much a truth, as that a square is not a circle.

But of what use is all this fine knowledge of men's own imaginations to a man that enquires after the reality of things? It matters not what men's fancies are, it is the knowledge of things that is only to be prized: it is this alone gives a value to our reasonings, and preference to one man's knowledge over another's, that it is of things as they really are, and not of dreams and fancies.

To which I answer, that if our knowledge of our ideas terminate in them, and reach no farther, where there is something farther intended, our most serious thoughts will be of little more use than the reveries of a crazy brain; and the truths built thereon of no more weight than the discourses of a man, who sees things clearly in a dream, and with great assurance utters them. But, I hope, before I have done, to make it evident, that this way of certainty, by the knowledge of our own ideas, goes a little farther than bare imagination: and I believe it will appear, that all the certainty of general truths a man has, lies in nothing else.

Locke, then, knows well enough how alarming the position is. 'Extravagant fancy', 'castles in the air', 'men's own imaginations', 'chimeras', 'dreams and fancies'; and the ending is prodigiously lame and halting: the 'way of certainty, by the knowledge of our own ideas, goes a little farther than bare imagination'; as for 'general truths', they are admittedly fanciful. Fancy and enthusiasm are above all the enemies, in this Augustan world of reason; but the way of certainty goes only 'a little farther than bare imagination'. How weak a hold Reason and Common Sense had upon the world!

I am not now chiefly concerned to go on to show that Locke's 'way of certainty, by the knowledge of our own ideas' is anything but a way of certainty. I remark only in passing that in the next section he shows that he is completely aware of the problem of 'representative perception'; and that he so clearly states the problem as to show that he knows it cannot be solved. If we know only our ideas, how can we know that 'they agree with things themselves'? Then, in the next section (iv) he speaks of our simple ideas, and says that they are the 'product of things operating in the mind . . . producing therein those perceptions which by the wisdom and will of our maker they are ordained and adapted to. From whence it follows, that simple ideas are not fictions of our fancies . . .' It may indeed 'follow', if we have certain knowledge of God's existence; but we have seen that of God's existence we have only a very imperfect proof indeed.

Now the difficulty which here confronts Locke confronted Hobbes also. But Hobbes had been more masterful, bolder; he had also been less fair. 'And though at some certain distance, the reall, and very object seem invested with the fancy it begets in us; Yet still the object is one thing, the image or fancy is another. So that Sense in all cases, is nothing els but originall fancy, caused (as I have said) by the pressure, that is, by the motion, of externall things upon our Eyes, Eares, and other organs thereunto ordained.' Sense is original fancy, and fancy decaying sense. This is certainly bolder and more dashing than anything we have in Locke; bolder, I mean, in its language and in the pleasure it takes in paradox and irony. But Hobbes had not stopped fairly to face the problems this doctrine created; he had swept on. Locke, haunted by the thought that sense may be, in all truth, only 'originall fancy', stops to treat of it and to find means to dispel it. He does not find the means, and casts himself on the goodness of God.

But there is this difference between the doctrines of Hobbes and Locke. Locke's doctrine is more accurate than Hobbes's. Locke distinguished between impression and idea, what the mind patiently receives and what it actively prehends; he makes room for perceiving. But Hobbes had represented perception as a mechanical thing and an affair of motion merely. And it was his materialism which made him bold enough to speak of sense as 'originall fancy'; he could rest in what he felt to be the pure and unimpeachable intentions of matter and motion; *they* could hardly deceive. But the mind, if it is active in perception, *may* deceive; it may play tricks. Can we rightly believe it does not? And if we say, the mind's apprehending of ideas is imaginative, are we not lost, from the very beginning, and without hope of finding a way?

Here, no doubt, is the mystery of knowledge. Idea is not impression, and is all we have. To apprehend impression is to change it into idea; and idea, while it is set over against the mind for an object, is also of and from the mind; it is and it is not mental; and the more it is distanced in knowledge from the mind, or the more knowledge is added to imagination, the more it becomes a creature of the mind. We give form to what comes to us without it; imagination and understanding are but the form-giving powers of the mind without which we cannot know a world, or without which a world cannot be in idea; to know is to change. And yet what we know must also come with authenticity and in its own objective power; it must come as a revelation, and be disposed for our inspection. It is all, in all truth, paradoxical enough. But we shall get farthest by candidly acknowledging the paradoxical facts and by declining to begin with the party-cries of a fashionable reaction.

But with this problem we are not to deal immediately. For the present, my intention is to remark that Locke said that we perceive ideas by the understanding; but that, in the light of the paragraphs I quoted from the opening of the fourth chapter of Book 4, Locke could hardly have complained had someone insisted that it would be more satisfactory if we said that we perceive ideas by the imagination. But Locke was frightened of 'the fancy'; and he fought off his fears by speaking

9

of the understanding where he might naturally have spoken of the imagination. It made him feel more comfortable; but it did not change the facts. And for our part, we are committed to saying that in this kind of perception it is indeed our imaginations which are active. We are animated, as Locke was not, by a wish to find living-space for the æsthetic in the human spirit, and are less disposed to feel frightened by the words 'fancy' and 'imagination'.

V

We shall return to the problem, How can the imagination be fairly said to play its part in giving us knowledge? But before treating it, we must further consider the relation of Locke's first 'sort of perception' to the third, of what we prefer to call the imagination to that kind of perception which issues into statement of the relations of ideas. We must, I think, reflect further on this matter than Locke, if only to understand why he both calls his first sort of perception an act of the understanding and apologizes for doing so. There was presumably a vagueness and uncertainty in his mind here; and we need to look to understand its causes and, if possible, its cure.

I quote again the statement in 2. 21. v:

The power of perception is that which we call the understanding. Perception, which we make the act of the understanding, is of three sorts: 1. The perception of ideas in our mind. 2. The perception of the signification of signs. 3. The perception of the connexion or repugnancy, agreement or disagreement, that there is between any of our ideas. All these are attributed to the understanding, or perceptive power, though it be the two latter only that use allows us to say we understand.

Now of the second kind, our understanding and use of language, I shall now say nothing. Later, I shall have something to say of Locke's view of language; but for the present, we concern ourselves with the first and third kinds.

Now on this statement I remark two things. First, I think we may safely say that in speaking of the three sorts of understanding, Locke is not setting himself to describe the stages in the growth of the human understanding. We have no authority, here or in any other part of the *Essay*, by which we may interpret him in this way. Instead, he is here speaking of the three aspects of a single process which acts at the adult human level; and he does not envisage the first sort of understanding (what we prefer to call imagination) acting without an accompanying, even if rudimentary, action (as in 'small dim perceptions'), of the third sort of understanding. *'Existence* and *Unity'*, he says (2. 7. vii), 'are two . . . ideas that are suggested to the understanding by every object without and every idea within'. The imagination does not and cannot act in an existential vacuum. Truly, it is, and is only, the indispensable agent for the envisagement of sensuous unities; but it also always carries along with it, or perhaps contains in it, from the outset of experience, the beginnings of judgement and is therefore a labour to prehend what is then and there; there is always that which claims the ideas of the imagination for real. At lowly levels of perception, where we have what Locke calls 'ideas of sensation' in the sense which I explained a little earlier, there may be little enough analysis; 'contemplation' may exceed discrimination and comparison. Still, where the imagination bodies forth ideas, at whatever level, there is also the claim that those ideas are real, and not imaginary. It is the fancy, and not the imagination, which traffics in the imaginary; and we are left to regret that Locke, who had to his hand the means for making this vital distinction, declined to make it, and left it to Kant and then Coleridge to preach and labour it. Now if this is so, the imagination is never without its claim to *know;* it is not the *fancy*.[1] The bush which I see as a bear is not *supposed* to be a bear; it *is* to me, through my imagination, a bear. Children may well *suppose* a hollow bush to be a pirate's lair; but we all know how easily their fanciful supposal may embarrass them if a grown-up comes suddenly upon them.

But so far as we think along these lines, and so far as we find authority (and we certainly find some) in Locke for doing so, we may feel some justification for calling the 'first sort of perception' an act of the understanding; for to claim to know must be, if only in slight measure, a claim to 'understand'. (We are therefore committed to denying that the distinction, which has been made so much of in our time, between knowledge by acquaintance and knowledge by description can be sustained; and we shall argue later that in fact our experience does not disclose to us either the mere particular or the mere universal: we know

[1] In saying this, I do not wish to imply, what would clearly be false, that fancy, which is a very advanced and cultivated form of mental activity, can be said to exist in separation from judgement; it consists only in trying to behave as if the distinction of true and false, real and imaginary, did not exist. But this is sophisticated, and a form of play (for all play is highly sophisticated); it is an enticement of the mind into a willing suspension of disbelief; and elaborately to carry on as if the fatal distinction did not exist is only to acknowledge it as a prison from which one can only *play* at escaping. About the fancy and its rôle in Augustan literature, I shall have much to say at a later stage.

only varying degrees of each.) And yet Locke quite clearly affirms in
another place (4. 1. i), that knowledge seems to him 'to be nothing but
the perception of the connexion of and agreement, or disagreement and
repugnancy of any of our ideas'; and if this is so, he must decline to call
the 'first sort of perception' a form of knowledge.

Still, we need not be censorious at Locke's expense. For we can
fairly take him as speaking in 4. 1. i, of our ordinary usage of the word
'knowledge', in accordance with which we may be said to know only
when an act of mind contains conceptual analysis and synthesis and
then issues into express judgement. He here writes of human knowledge as it ordinarily is; and it is natural that he should say that we have
knowledge only when thought (however dependent on the mind's
imagination and acquaintance with systems of word-signs) proceeds to
explicit analysis and judgement. We shall not therefore be disposed
to quarrel with Locke or to think him unreasonable in speaking of
knowledge as he does in 4. 1. i. Still, he does not trouble to enquire
at any length into the kind of knowledge the imagination may be said
to have and into its relation to the third kind of perception; and that
he did not do this is typical of Locke and his age, and shows the blindness of the time to the æsthetic as a region of human experience.

I have said that the imagination always claims to be knowledge, and
is a beholdment of what is taken as being. But I said also that we can
well understand Locke's saying that only those acts which issue into
express judgement can be said to have and to give knowledge. For
Kant, who was not afraid of the word imagination (at least, he was less
afraid of it than Locke), repeated this doctrine. 'Synthesis', he said, 'in
general . . . is the mere result of the power of imagination, a blind but
indispensable function of the soul, without which we should have no
knowledge whatsoever, but of which we are scarcely ever conscious.
To bring this synthesis *to concepts* is a function which belongs to the
understanding, and it is through this function of the understanding that
we first obtain knowledge properly so called.'[1] And later on the same
page we read that the 'synthesis of the manifold by means of the
imagination . . . does not yet yield knowledge'. So far Locke and Kant
seem to be agreed. But we saw, in section II of this chapter, that Locke
is not consistent here; I set out evidence for saying that he did not deny
that we may have perception, which so far as it goes, is knowledge,
though it is certainly unaccompanied by explicit conceptual analysis;
such knowledge may be said to be 'obscure and dull', but it is yet

---

[1] Kemp Smith's translation of *The Critique of Pure Reason*, London, 1929, p. 112.

knowledge. Locke shows here that he is uncertain; but Kant shows that he is uncertain too. And it is not hard to illustrate Kant's uncertainty. In the Introduction to the *Critique of Pure Reason*, he says that there are 'two stems of human knowledge, namely, *sensibility* and *understanding*, which perhaps spring from a common, but to us unknown, root. Through the former, objects are given to us; through the latter, they are thought.'[1] On the one hand sense impressions; on the other, conceptual analysis and synthesis. But there is perhaps a common and unknown root. So he says in the Introduction. But in the Transcendental Deduction the 'common root' is clearly identified as imagination. 'And while concepts', he says (I quote from the first edition), 'which belong to the understanding, are brought into play through relation of the manifold to the unity of apperception, it is only by means of the imagination that they can be brought into relation to sensible intuition. A pure imagination, which conditions all *a priori* knowledge, is thus one of the fundamental faculties of the human soul. . . . The two extremes, namely, sensibility and understanding, must stand in necessary connection with each other through the mediation of this transcendental function of imagination, because otherwise the former, though indeed yielding appearances, would supply no objects of empirical knowledge, and consequently no experience.'[2] Here indeed imagination is not so much a root as a mediator; and this difference of image shows an uncertainty and vacillation in Kant's mind when it tries to envisage the relationship of imagination to the discursive understanding. Philosophers do not contrive to do without metaphors; and the difference between his *Wurzel* and his *Vermittler* is also a difference between doctrines. For if the understanding is a development from the imagination, a stem from a root, it can only be because the imagination is from the beginning what Kant ordinarily calls the understanding, namely, a faculty of knowledge; the understanding and its categories must be, in a sense, *in* the imagination. Thus, when the understanding develops, it is but certain features of the imagination become explicit and fully conscious; the categories have been, in the earlier activities of the imagination, embedded or implicit; so that, as Professor Kemp Smith observes, 'the productive imagination is . . . viewed as rendering possible the understanding, that is, the conscious apprehension of the *a priori* as an element embedded in objective experience'.[3] If we accept the image

---

[1] Kemp Smith's translation of *The Critique of Pure Reason*, London, 1929, pp. 61–62.
[2] *Ibid.*, p. 146.
[3] Kemp Smith, *Commentary to Kant's Critique of Pure Reason*, London, 1923, p. 264.

of the root, the imagination is the primordial, fundamental power of knowledge in the soul out of which the understanding grows.

But if, instead, we envisage the imagination as a *Vermittler* between sense and understanding, what are we to say? Clearly, we must say that imagination may so act as mediator only because it has something in common with the two parties concerned. But if so, what has the imagination in common with understanding? And to this question there can only be one answer, namely, that imagination, like understanding, is a faculty of knowledge. What else could they have in common which would make the mediation possible? Kant must therefore no longer accumulate in the understanding all the sources of knowledge, and must not say that it is through the 'function of the understanding that we first obtain knowledge properly so called'. But even here, we notice the 'properly so called'; even here, where he places the whole burden of knowledge on the understanding, it is yet clear that he has a mind for a knowledge other than that given by the conscious understanding; and this can only be that knowledge given by the imagination. The imagination may not be said to give knowledge 'properly so called' or 'as we ordinarily understand the word'; but there is in Locke and Kant the sense that it gives a kind of knowledge, and even that the kind of knowledge it gives is primordial and the womb of the knowledge to which the growing understanding may come. In *The Critique of Judgement* Kant speaks frankly and habitually of the 'cognitive powers' (*Erkenntnisvermögen*) by which he means imagination and understanding; and we have seen that Locke places his 'perception of ideas', which we have called imagination, in a list of the sorts of understanding, even if he does so with a puzzled apology.

VI

There is then here a striking and two-fold similarity between Locke and Kant. Locke in the *Essay* and Kant in the *Critique of Pure Reason* both seem to speak of the imagination as a form of knowledge and also seem to deny that it can properly be said to give knowledge. But there is also a difference. Kant went on, as I said, to accept the imagination as a cognitive power in its own right, and to write the *Critique of Judgement* in which he composed an Æsthetic based on it. Locke had no interest in Æsthetic; nor did what he had come to in his 'first kind of understanding' arouse such interest in him.

I do not propose to expound Kant's *Critique of Æsthetic Judgement*.

It is not necessary to my purpose. But in the course of what I go on now to say in this section, my debt to Kant's Æsthetic is very great, as any student of Kant will see. What I shall now try to do is to make clearer what is intended when we speak of imagination as a kind of knowing, or, if one will, of understanding. Locke called what we call the imagination an act of understanding, and left it at that. But I can best exhibit the shortcoming of Augustan philosophy, indeed of the greatest Augustan philosopher, by outlining a doctrine about art which follows naturally enough on what we find in the *Essay*, but which Locke had not interest or motive for constructing. His analysis has been fair, and incomparably more accurate than Hobbes's; he has laid down the essentials of the right doctrine of the rôle of imagination in knowledge, even if he has sedulously avoided using the word; and he has therefore to his hands the clue to an adequate Æsthetic, which, had he gone on to develop it, might have changed the face of the eighteenth century. But he did not go on with it; and he did not go on with it because he felt no impulse to justify the æsthetic in human experience. With all his breadth and fairness of mind, here he was blind and without catholicity. For an Æsthetic (which is where philosophy must begin) must look above all to the varying proportions of the imagination and understanding, or cognitive powers, in response to the world, and to the strains and tensions which must exist, in varying strengths, between them.

Now we say, It is necessary to be in earnest with imagination as a form of knowledge. But it will be replied: Surely Locke and Kant were right in saying that knowledge is possible only by means of the concept, through thought proper; and in asking us to believe in imagination as a power of knowing you are inviting us to try to envisage a knowing which is nearly or wholly below the conceptual level. But we cannot do this; we cannot divest ourselves of intellectuality in the interests of so-called symbolism; you are asking us to contract our minds into a primitive sensualism which, if we could achieve it, would in any case be very distasteful. You are appealing to a supposed form of mental activity which lies beyond our experience; and really, are you not therefore bombinating in a sort of speculative vacuum?

To this reply, That if indeed I were making appeal to something beyond our experience, the case would be hopeless; but that in fact I am doing nothing of the kind. I appeal only to that part of our experience which I am concerned to try to explain, namely, the artistic; and we are certainly advised to look to our own mature experience, drawing from that, so far as we can, an impression of early stages in the life of mankind and the child before intellectuality had come to its full height.

I shall speak of artistic experience in literature, for it is with literary history that we are chiefly concerned; and if we look to the acknowledged masterpieces of literature we shall not find it difficult to mark down their most striking qualities as works of imagination. Now in the first place we shall agree that in *King Lear* we neither expect nor get any *doctrine* about human life. But that *King Lear* has to do with human life, its fortunes and destiny, and that it deals with them in a high and serious way, we also all agree; no work of art can be more serious, or more important. Now on reflection it is strange that we should all readily agree about both these things; to treat human life with the highest seriousness and yet to communicate no doctrine about it, is to do something whose nature is as elusive to define as it is surprising to observe.

It may be said that it is misleading to say that *King Lear* communicates no doctrine. But in fact, if we asked to set out what doctrine, what belief or body of beliefs about human life may be found in the play as clearly Shakespeare's own, we shall find ourselves hard put to it. Certainly, some of the personages of the play state their beliefs; but it is also not certain that any one of them is Shakespeare's own. We cannot say with any confidence that the play is the work of a Christian or even of a religious man; nor again that it is the work of an unbeliever; and Dr. Johnson, a pious Christian and a fervent moralist, wrote in his *Preface to Shakespeare* these words about Shakespeare as a moralist: 'His first defect is that to which may be imputed most of the evil in books or in men.' This is a serious charge enough; and he goes on to explain what he means:

He sacrifices virtue to convenience, and is so much more careful to please than to instruct, that he seems to write without any moral purpose. From his writings indeed a system of social duty may be selected, for he that thinks reasonably must think morally; but his precepts and axioms drop casually from him; he makes no just distribution of good or evil, nor is always careful to shew in the virtuous a disapprobation of the wicked; he carries his persons indifferently through right and wrong, and at the close dismisses them without further care, and leaves their examples to operate by chance. This fault the barbarity of his age cannot extenuate; for it is always a writer's duty to make the world better, and justice is a virtue independant on time or place.

And yet no one has been more impressive and eloquent in praise of Shakespeare than Johnson:

The effects of favour and competition are at an end; the tradition of his friendships and his enmities has perished; his works support no opinion with arguments, nor supply any faction with invectives; they can neither indulge vanity nor gratify malignity, but are read without any other reason than the desire of pleasure, and are therefore praised only as pleasure is obtained; yet, thus unassisted by interest or passion, they have passed through variations of taste and changes of manners, and, as they developed from one generation to another, have received new honours at every transmission . . . The stream of time, which is continually washing the dissoluble fabricks of other poets, passes without injury by the adamant of *Shakespeare*.

This is praise indeed, which I quote to show that we must not think Johnson unaware of Shakespeare's transcendent merits. But there is something of a mystery here. Shakespeare does not satisfy Johnson's Christianity; he does not even satisfy certain rudimentary requirements of Johnson the moralist; he writes to support no argument or opinion: he is unassisted by interest and by passion; yet he is adamant and immortal. But why? The plays are read, says Johnson, 'without any reason but the desire for pleasure'. Only, unluckily, this will not do, so far, at least, as *King Lear* is concerned. For the death of Cordelia so distressed Johnson when he first read the play, that as he said, 'I know not whether I ever endured to read again the last scenes of the play till I undertook to revise them as an editor'. So, unless we are prepared to follow Johnson in condemning out of hand the ending of *King Lear*, we are hardly likely to rest the greatness of Shakespeare on his power of communicating pleasure; or if we do, it will be pleasure of a curious kind whose nature and source we should wish to know.

It seems then that the 'greatness' of Shakespeare's play has not to do with religious and moral doctrine, with opinion, interest and purpose; it serves no end and propagates no truth. I think we all agree in this. We cannot catch the play in a metaphysical or moralistic scheme; there is no formula to which it may be reduced, nor purpose in the light of which we may understand it. At the end as at the beginning, we have only the play, and there is nothing in terms of which we can express it; it is inexpressible, monadic, absolute. There is no generalizing it; or if we try to generalize it, we arrive at what is so thin, bloodless, trite even, that we readily give up the task.

Still, this is only one side of a many-sided situation. We may say that the play has no meaning we can set out in prose; that if by significance we mean something susceptible of statement, the play is insignificant, signifying nothing; that it has no purpose. But this leaves us uneasy. The play *has* meaning, significance, purpose; it *is* a treating of life with all possible high seriousness. And we can only resolve our unease by saying that it means, without meaning anything in particular, signifies but signifies nothing we can be said to know, has a high purpose but seems neither to prescribe nor realize any specific intention. I say 'resolve our unease'; but in reality we do not thus find a resolution of our discomfort. We may, indeed, have found something in the nature of a formula; and formulæ are gratifying. But it is a formula which has merit, if it has merit, only because it is as baffling and paradoxical as the play itself. It is a good formula not because it explains anything, but only because it reflects the teased mind which can find satisfaction only by hitting on a proposition which outrages logic and is no proposition at all. For it barely carries us any further. We are only saying that the play certainly means something, and that that something is the play itself. Here meaning is not an affair of the concept but, by an insoluble contradiction, of the individual. We pass from the play to no statement of meanings but assert that its meaning is real enough by dumbly pointing to the play. Individuality is meaningful; but because it is individuality, it will not be resolved into all the concepts in the world. Its meaning is an effluent light which vestures it, and not an articulated theorem which expresses it.

Let us now return to what I said earlier, that Æsthetic must take a special interest in the tensions between imagination and intelligence. What I have now said will, I trust, make this clearer. In a work of what I may call pure imagination, we see what defies conceptual explication; and yet the work is also a temptation to explicate it. It cries out for and defeats explanation; it is animated by purpose, of a most serious kind, which also eludes us; it is filled with interest and passion which are yet for nothing we can state. This state of affairs comes about because the play exhibits imagination and intelligence in certain proportions, and in a certain sustained tension; and these proportions and this tension are here such as not to give release to the understanding which is yet employed and in a high degree. That intelligence went into the making of *King Lear* no one will doubt; it is wonderfully organized and internally adapted; and its language considered merely as meanings is that of a man of powerful intellectual gifts. But all this, and much else, is, as it were, *within* the play, employed in the building of its structure and fabric; and when we contemplate the play as a whole, the intelligence fails to move successfully *without* and around it. There are no rules of which it is an instance and no concepts which it illustrates. As a totality it encloses and is not enclosed by the understanding. For this reason we may, in speaking of the play, expound its structure and inner adaptation, the shape of the plot, the parallels of incident and the contrasts of character. But when we are asked, what is it, the whole play, for, and what does it signify? we have little or nothing to say. For it is animated by no opinion and has no philosophical origin.

For this reason we may say that in the making of the play the intelligence was there, and active, but was *freely* active, having no end or purpose and being guided in accordance with no rule or precept; and its freedom, its release from religion, morals, interest or passion (as Johnson said) is given it by the imagination, which is also free, a spontaneous activity of the soul. The imagination imparts its freedom to the understanding by keeping it in a certain servility. Only in bondage to the imagination is the intelligence ever free.

But this is not a state natural or agreeable to the understanding. And in the work of art, in our case in *King Lear*, its subordinacy to imagination, its containment *within* the work of art, is enforced only by effort. Even so, it so far contaminates the imagination as to impel the mind to ask questions; and with the trying to answer them we have gone over from the world of imagination into that of understanding. 'Is there any cause in nature that makes these hard hearts?' is Lear's question; but we cannot fail to hear it as the play's question also, as Shakespeare's and as ours. Still, the play refrains from answer; so does Shakespeare; and so, in the contemplation of the play, do we. But if we seek to answer the question we secede from the artistic into the philosophical; and we may, no doubt, upbraid the work of art for inducing us to try to become philosophers. Thus it is that some of the greatest works of art walk a knife-edge; there is a suspense between imagination and understanding; and thus it is that when I speak of *King Lear* as a work of *pure* imagination, I do not mean that it is uninfected by metaphysical curiosity, but only that in it the imagination just manages to keep its supremacy. It is in those works where this tension is almost intolerable, and where the artistic consciousness comes near to breaking and to losing its autonomy, that we are aware of the very highest artistic power; it is precisely there that imagination needs to be strongest.

But it will be said, 'Admitting that there is something in all this, how is it connected with Locke's first and third sorts of understanding; and if, as you say, the imagination is a kind of knowing, which has to safe-guard itself against the kind of knowing which the understanding enjoys, what sort of knowing is it, and what does it know?

The imagination 'takes notice' of impressions and makes them ideas. We may, if we are very tired or very nervous, fail to focus our eyes readily; and what is then before our eyes, little more than a blur, corre-sponds to impression (I say 'corresponds', for so long as we take notice of it all, the blur is strictly idea); but, with the eyes focused, what was blurred becomes clear and, as it were, *held* by the mind for the coloured patch it is. Ordinarily, these patches of colour (to speak of sight only, for convenience) are held by the mind as parts or aspects of more complicated ideas, as things related in innumerable ways to other ideas of things in space and time, all of which together make up our world. Now our world is imagined, in the sense I have explained; all in it is idea, by the elevation of impression into object, what is held by the mind. But in our experience as human beings our ideas are not merely imagined; they are related, in an indefinitely large number of ways, to each other; and this is possible through the power of comparison and discrimination exerted by thought which acts through concepts. Therefore our ordinary experience is a compound of imagination and thought, and each is never without the other. But in our everyday life it is naturally the conceptual aspect of our knowledge which is more obvious and predominant, for we are conducting, so long as we are awake, a life in varying degrees intelligent and moral; and our funda-mental imaginative activity, of which we are rarely aware, habitually serves the purposes of our intelligences. Locke's first sort of under-standing is certainly there, but overlooked; what is present to our minds is the agreement and disagreement of our ideas, not at all our coming by them. And we said that we can well understand Locke saying that the 'third sort' unmistakably merits the name of under-standing and gives knowledge, but that the first sort, for ordinary human experience, is hardly a knowing, still less an understanding.

Yet, in our experience of *King Lear* we are aware of an object which we do *not* know through the concept. It is beheld and not understood; it is single and unrelated; it serves no purpose; and neither supplies information of fact nor illustration of meaning. It is, in short, the per-ception of an idea merely; and of an idea that seems to float detached from our everyday world and is a world to itself. But all the time, like all other ideas of the imagination it makes an insistent claim to be, in a sense we can hardly catch, *real*. Now this is imaginative experience; and by it we can perhaps envisage the imagination as a primitive thing which grasps an idea without as yet the intellectual power to *relate* it to what is round and about it, to what is before or after, and thereby *place* it and, as it were, *master* it. For it is the habit of the intelligence to be above and to look down on its object, in a context which explains it; it is the habit of the imagination to look up to its object and to behold it, inexplicated and ununderstood. Now what the imagination affords may not be knowledge as Locke and Kant and we ordinarily understand by the word; *that* is knowledge through the explicit concept. Still, it is a knowing, an apprehending an idea.

The reader will recall that in section VII of chapter 1, I said that it is the imagination which first stimulates the mind to awaken out of its trance of feeling and to distance objects from itself, at however little remove. I said too that, at this stage, the object occupies a sort of no-man's-land between what is subjective and what is objective; it is idea and therefore object, but is also shot through with feeling and still saturated in the mind. Now something of this our artistic experience has also; we are at a remove from the idea, because it is idea; but it is also of the very stuff of our feeling; we, as it were, overflow into it and it overflows into us; it is removed from us, but still very near to us; the gap, and therewith the mystery of knowledge has occurred, and yet only barely. That is why we hesitate to call the imagination a knowledge or an understanding. The imagination is certainly not blind, as Kant sometimes said, but we can perhaps adopt Macbeth's words and say of it what he said of Banquo's ghost, 'There is no speculation in those eyes'. 'Speculation' in Shakespeare's sense there is; 'speculation' in our modern sense, there is not.

Now we should not think of the understanding as a faculty distinct from the imagination; but more wisely follow Aristotle's way of thinking which is also one of Kant's ways of thinking and see it as an outgrowth and development from the imagination. It comes to the assistance of the imagination, still further mitigates feeling and puts the object, through its concepts, at a greater remove. It comes to its assistance in the conduct of life and its morality, in science and philosophy. It comes to the assistance, too, of art; but in the worlds of art, it is held in a certain subservience. It is there employed and even extensively employed; but its mitigation of feeling and removal of idea is controlled and restricted. Here there occurs a conscious and sustained antagonism between the more primitive form of knowledge which we call the imagination and that development from it which we call the understanding or intelligence. Here the more primitive resists that sophistication to which it itself gives rise; and art arises out of this situation.

VII

I have spoken of tensions between imagination and understanding, and of the resistance of imagination to understanding. I shall now try to illustrate this; and in doing so, I shall hope to throw more light on the nature of symbolism in knowledge.

If the concept is to be refused and the idea not conceptually analysed, there remains only to show the idea; it must be exhibited. And an idea can be exhibited only by means of an idea; there can be no other choice. Now this employment of idea to convey idea is the practise of symbolism, and in this artistic creation consists. Yet there is here an obvious difficulty. For how can one idea exhibit another unless that other idea is already known? And if it is known, why exhibit it by means of another? Or, if it is not known, how can the idea, employed to show it, begin to be effective? Or again, does not what I may call the equivalencing of ideas require proposition? It is hard to see how the proposed symbolism can work or begin to work.

Now in reflecting on this, and in explaining further what is in my mind, I shall again use *King Lear*. But first I shall illustrate some of the more obvious and limited forms of symbolism in literature. I take this passage of Shakespeare for analysis. I take it because it is neither better nor worse than many other passages from Shakespeare's work and is, I think, thoroughly typical. At the beginning of *The Merchant of Venice*, Salarino speaks to Antonio in this way:

> Your mind is tossing on the ocean;
> There, where your argosies with portly sail,
> Like signiors and rich burghers of the flood,
> Or, as it were, the pageants of the sea,
> Do overpeer the petty traffickers,
> That curt'sy to them, do them reverence
> As they fly by them with their woven wings.

Now I exclude from consideration in this passage the first, fourth and last lines; the first is not required for my purpose; and the fourth and the last I think to be flaws in it, illustrations, if I may say so, of a certain excess in Shakespeare of which some of his critics have complained. If then we look to the remaining lines, we observe Shakespeare conveying an idea of the splendid vessels of Antonio. 'Your argosies with portly sail' he says; and the word 'portly', applied to the bellied sails, also helps to lead in the idea of the burgher. The burgher no doubt is the London merchant-prince; and we come to him, by Shakespeare's adroitness, *via* the Venetian Signior. The sails are portly; but so are the London burghers, the idea of whom is no doubt the symbolizing idea through which we are to prehend the idea of the great vessels. Here then are the two ideas, the ships and the merchants. Let us see how Shakespeare proceeds. 'The rich burghers of the flood', he says. If our minds have moved to portly London merchants, they are not allowed to dwell, as it were, in London only; our minds must inhabit the seas as well as the streets of London; for we read of 'burghers *of the flood*'. Now the rich burghers of the flood 'do overpeer the petty traffickers'; and the three words 'overpeer', 'petty' and 'traffickers' all play crucial rôles in Shakespeare's symbolizing. For 'overpeer' may mean to look down over onto; and so far belongs to the idea of the great ships from whose decks one may peer down to the decks of the lesser trading vessels. So 'petty', which still carried, in Shakespeare's time, the meaning of physically small; and so 'traffickers' which meant coasting vessels of burden. But the three words also belong to the idea of the merchants; as belonging to this idea, 'overpeer' means 'to be greater than', 'be more than the peer of'; 'petty' means 'humble, unimportant'; and 'trafficker' means 'tradesman in a small way'. Now in this line, by this two-fold valency or the ambiguity of the words, the two ideas, that of the ships and of the wealthy merchants, are, as it were, run into each other; they are inextricably mixed up with each other or fused; and the effect is not of an equivalence, of the conveyance of one idea by means of another, but of a single and richer idea of a trader which is ship and merchant in one. But Shakespeare has not finished yet. He goes on with 'that curt'sy to them, do them reverence'. The curtsy no doubt is the curtsy of the little trader to the merchant prince; but it is also the dipping and rising of the small vessels as they ride in the wake of the great argosies as these fly by them. The last line however, with its bird-imagery is inconsistent with what has gone before; and in the last line but one we have the final touch in the building of the symbol.

In this passage, which is quite typical of Shakespeare's usual manner, there is indeed statement, which is in the formal simile. But the movement of the passage is to overcome the separateness of the two ideas; the two ideas must not stand alongside each other for comparison by the intelligence; they must merge; so that one idea does not so much *show* the other as *become* it. Now this fusion of idea with idea, of fact with image, *is* symbolism in its perfection; it shows the working of the pure imagination. The passage may be said to state a comparison; but it also labours to overcome statement and simile and to defeat the logic of proposition by the making of a single, if richer and more complex idea. In this way, the second idea does not stand for comparison with the first; it acts as an enrichment or expansion of the first. In a word, we have not, for the end to which the imagination labours, a symbol *for* something. Instead, the symbol *is* the clarification of idea by a process of fusion. The symbol is not *of* an idea; it *is* the idea changed, defined and made precise. Symbolism is not a process of comparison but of definition; not of vicarious function, but of development. For this reason the making of symbol *is* perception as it moves from being relatively passive to being more active in prehension and to grasping and holding its idea.

I speak in this way of 'symbol' for this reason. I use the word in accordance with its original meaning in the Greek verb and noun respectively. συμβάλλειν signified in the first place to throw or put together; and τό σύμβολον was 'each of two halves or corresponding pieces of an ἀστράγαλος (bone or dice) or other object, which two ξένοι or any two contract parties, broke between them, each party keeping one piece, in order to have proof of the identity of the presenter of the other'.[1] Thus the thought was of something which was due to be joined to another to make a single thing, two halves of a whole; the thought was not, in the first place, of a thing which stood for another, or even of a thing which was like another. Now where the pure imagination works, symbol has this quality; and this is illustrated in the passage I quoted, in which Shakespeare will not tolerate the quick passage of our minds back and fore between two ideas, but unites, instead, the two ideas into one. The second idea acts as an amplification or development of the first; or again, it becomes a way of apprehending the first.

Understanding the word in this way, we can see how the questions I put a little way back can be answered; or rather, may be removed. Those problems arose because our statement of the nature of symbol was inaccurate; because, that is to say, we were representing the artist as trafficking in two ideas which he held apart. But in fact we have not two ideas, where one is the symbol of the other; instead, the one enters into and qualifies the other; it *shows* the other by *changing* it. But also, this qualification is mutual and acts both ways; each gives vigour and

---

[1] *Liddell and Scott.*

life to the other as it becomes unified with it; in fusing with the other, each brings its peculiar value to the idea which results.

Still, it will be said, there are, at the beginning, two ideas which the simile ('like signiors or rich burghers of the flood') holds apart in the very act of its comparison. We have certainly spoken as if this were so. But we must observe the following fact. I spoke some time ago of the blur we perceive if our eyes are unfocused as corresponding to impression, in contrast to the idea we may clearly apprehend when our eyes are rightly focused. But I added that the blur, so far as perceived at all, is idea, however confused it may be. Now we have to take account of degrees of clarity in our ideas; and when we find 'symbol' for an unclear idea, that unclear idea is to the idea clarified and sharpened by the action of the 'symbol' much as the blur is to the object clearly perceived. The coming of the 'symbol' is the act whereby, as it were, the eyes of imagination are focused.

Besides, as I have said, the labour of the passage is to try to overcome whatever of separation there is; and it is just here that we observe an example of that tension between imagination and intelligence of which I spoke. For if we say, x is like y, we contrast the two in the act of discerning something in common between them; this is the two-fold action of the intelligence, habitually at work. But it is this state of affairs, the situation provided by the intelligence in which we think differences as well as identity, which the imagination must overcome. *Its* impulse is to apprehend a single idea and to run one idea into another with no residue of differences; and the intellectual act which discerns both sameness and difference through the concept must be mitigated. The intelligence may agree that an argosy is like a rich merchant, and in doing so must also see differences between them; but the labour of the imagination is, so far as it can, to apprehend an idea which somehow consists of the idea of both ship and trader; it seeks a unified perception which requires that discrimination and, no less, unification through the concept merely, be made as powerless as may be. The intelligence is employed so far as it is necessary to state the comparison, 'like signiors'; but from then on, the effect of the intelligence, which is to think sameness and differences alike, must be combated. And, for much the bigger part, poetry proceeds by the direct road of metaphor; it scouts an introductory simile; it proceeds straight to see one thing in terms of another; it does not invite a weighing of similarities and differences, and employs metaphor as a way of seeing things. A metaphor acts so as, not to adorn, but to clarify, a perception.

Now in the light of this, we recall how the Augustans habitually distinguished between judgement and fancy. We have seen how Hobbes and Locke made this distinction, and how they were agreed that it was valid. They spoke, both of them, as if discernment of difference were the act of the understanding, discernment of sameness that of the fancy. In fact the intelligence discerns both sameness and difference, through the concept. But the imagination (which they ordinarily called the fancy) avoids conceptual analysis and synthesis so far as it can; it is the perception of an idea, as Locke says of his 'first sort of understanding'; and, to have this, it merges one idea into another, overcoming disparity and making unity, so that the intelligence is side-tracked and its methods dropped. The agreement as well as the disagreement, the connexion as well as the repugnancy between our ideas, is perceived by the third sort of understanding, the understanding properly so called; but this is not the job of the first sort, which grasps an idea in its singleness and without reference to others. Had Locke reflected a little more, he would have seen that what he called the fancy, when he contrasted it with the judgement, was but an aspect of his third sort of understanding, and an intellectual act; and he would then have seen that what requires to be distinguished is the imagination, which tries to perceive its complex but single ideas merely, and the intelligence which proceeds by the method of the concept to both analysis and synthesis at once. We see therefore how confused and misleading was this crucial Augustan distinction, which could only provide a poor foundation for reflection on and for the practise of poetry.

I conclude this section with this observation. We all know the difficulties into which philosophers get when they reflect on what the concept really is. If I think the concept 'man', I am asked, what am I thinking of? I must not think this or that race of mankind, or this or that individual man. But if I exclude the less general and the particular, can I be said to be thinking of man at all? The concept of 'man' becomes in this way emptied of content and a mere nothing. Now this state of affairs is the ineluctable end of the understanding's procedure. It must both analyze and synthesize at once, bring together and hold apart; as it advances in abstraction it must both leave out and retain. But this it cannot do; and its processes stand in self-contradiction. As the concept takes more in, it leaves more out; it seems to progress towards inanity.

But at the level of the imagination's percepts, a different thing happens. The imagination will not abstract, and be involved therefore in the increasing tenuity of the understanding's concepts. Instead, it sets about dissolving its percepts into each other, and resists the play of the understanding's habits. The understanding unites, but only to dis-unite; the imagination unites. This is a curious and even mysterious thing. But it happens, as any page of Shakespeare will demonstrate. The concepts of the understanding have what Bradley called a 'blood-lessness'; but the ideas of the imagination have a life in them; they grow in concreteness, not abstraction; they acquire the raciness and force of living things, and the 'warm and breathing beauty of the flesh'.

VIII

Let us now return to *King Lear*. First, I confirm that the manner of writing which we found in the passage from *The Merchant of Venice* is typical of Shakespeare, by quoting these lines from *Lear*. They occur in Act III, where Lear insists that the Fool go before him into the hovel out of the storm., He then apostrophizes the poor in this way:

> Poor naked wretches, wheresoe'er you are,
> That bide the pelting of this pitiless storm,
> How shall your houseless heads and unfed sides,
> Your loop'd and window's raggedness, defend you
> From seasons such as these? (III. iv. 28–32)

If the reader will read the last three lines carefully, and will bear in mind that 'house' is two words and not one, having in its second and little known meaning the sense of 'textile covering'; if also he will consider the phrases 'unfed sides' and 'loop'd and window'd raggedness', he will see what a fusion of ideas is here; the body as the house of the soul and the house as protection for the body are ideas fused in the way I have spoken of.

But I am concerned now with the play as a whole. I spoke earlier of the tension of imagination and understanding in it; and I have said that in general it is in the play of this tension that symbol occurs. Now *King Lear* is a single idea. It is not indeed simple, but a unity of many personages, events and situations. Now if we look to this complex unity, we ask, Where here is symbol? What meaning is there in speak-ing of the play, as a whole, as symbol?

The answer to this question will be, that in the composition of the play Shakespeare made clear to himself the unclear idea of life which was active in his experience at the time. In the face of the multi-tudinous elements in his life and knowledge his mind was plastic and sought order and pattern; to these he could come only by the process of symbolizing what he knew, but knew too vaguely and in too fluc-tuating a way; and the bringing to clarity and (so far as he could) to order was also the finding of symbol. The symbol is the play. Only, we must not say that it is a symbol of what exists outside it for us or existed outside it for Shakespeare. For, to take first our experience of the play, it will not do to say that for us *King Lear* is a symbol of the life and fortunes of man. For what is the life of man? We do not know; and we can find no symbol for that of which we have already no idea. Or if we claim to know, we shall hardly let our scheme of belief inter-fere with our apprehending of Shakespeare's play. When we read or see the play, it is the play's idea of human life which fills our minds; but it is not an idea which is communicated by the play; it *is* the play. There is no scheme of belief, or other idea, standing without the play by which or in terms of which we grasp the play; it is complete and entire within itself, or not at all.

Besides, if we consider the play, not in our own point of view as wit-nesses, but as the creation of Shakespeare, we have the same result. For of what, in Shakespeare's mind, was the play an idea? We may per-haps reply, Of human life. But then, does this mean that Shakespeare had his idea of human life formed in his mind before he wrote *Lear*; and that *Lear* is, as it were, a translation of that idea into another? But a little reflection shows that this will not do. The mind of art does not work like this. Instead, what Shakespeare did, in composing his play, was to work his multitudinous impressions into an idea, or to evolve an unclear idea into a clear one; and that idea is the play we know. If so, *King Lear* was Shakespeare's idea of life as he then perceived it; and we cannot rightly say that he had another and previous one which he chose to put into the form of *Lear*. Shakespeare beheld life and beheld it only (at that time), in the form of the play; in it life became for him clear idea. The making of the play was not a supernumerary act which added nothing to his knowledge; instead, it was the making of his knowledge and the forming of his idea. Now if this is so, the play may in truth be said to *be* human life as Shakespeare knew it when the play was made. It was, we may say, his idea of life; and in seeing the play we see nothing less than human life as Shakespeare, at the time of the composition of the play, saw it.

But if this is so, we must say of it that it is what it symbolizes; it *is* life as we see and find it nowhere else; and to say this is only to say what every reader of Shakespeare discovers in his reading. We look, in the pages of Shakespeare, into the face of nature; we behold no allegory, or parable, or other system of signs or tokens; instead, life moves before us in all its complexity as good and evil, joy and catastrophe; so that, as Dr. Johnson said, 'he who has mazed his imagination, in following the phantoms which other writers raise up before him, may here be cured of his delirious extasies, by reading human sentiments in human language; by scenes from which a hermit may estimate the transactions of the world, and a confessor predict the progress of its passions'; and so that again, as Coleridge said, Shakespeare is like 'Nature, the prime genial artist', himself a 'nature humanized, a genial understanding directing self-consciously a power and an implicit wisdom deeper even than our consciousness'.[1]

Few readers of Shakespeare can fail to feel that what Johnson and Coleridge say is true; and the reason is not far to seek. Lear, Goneril and the rest occupy indeed no part of the space of history; they are in a world whose frontiers do not touch ours and which we cannot invade; it is self-enclosed and monadic. And it is so precisely because it is a creation of a man's mind. This is a paradox; but it is true. Shakespeare *makes* his Lear, Cordelia, Regan and sets them in a world which is a world of its own; he is a 'nature humanized' and must therefore make a world, other than and not contiguous with his and ours. Still, it is of his making; in watching Lear and the rest we watch the mind of Shakespeare; and we see the creator in the creation. For the characters of the play *are* Shakespeare; and they *are* us so far as we apprehend the play. Lear was contained in the Shakespeare who gave him birth; his passions, and the passions of the other characters, were felt and realized in Shakespeare who suffered in them. Therefore, the idea of *King Lear* we have is also the life of Shakespeare as he was then; and in contemplating the play we become what we behold; as he was what he created.

(The reader will recall that Hobbes took pleasure in the thought of the mind as a creator, through the power of reason. The complete intelligibility of mathematics, he thought, comes from this, that the mind makes its mathematical ideas; and he played with the idea that nature too, because, as he believed, a deductive system, was also of our making. In this last notion, at least, he was certainly wrong. But it is curious that he took no interest in what William James called the

[1] *Lectures and Notes on Shakespeare*, Bohn edn., London, 1904, pp. 229-30.

sub-universes of art. They may only be sub-universes. But they are at only least, somehow, contained in *the* universe; and in any case they are the worlds mortal mind can make claim to create. Had Hobbes looked, for the key to the mystery of human knowledge, to the making-power of the imagination and less to what he believed to be the making-power of the intellect, he would have seen more clearly than he did. Mathematics may be indeed our creation, as Hobbes and Locke believed; but it deals only in abstractions and is at a remove from the mystery of life itself.)

It is therefore no mere figure of speech to say that in *King Lear* the symbol is also the symbolized, the idea and the symbol one and the same. And this state of affairs has its origin in a feature of the imagination to which I have already called attention. The imagination is at a small remove from its objects; they are not distanced by the concept; and are saturated in the mind. Lear was not merely thought by Shakespeare, but imagined; and he could thus be imagined because he was not other than Shakespeare but a part of him, his passions felt, in all their range and force, in Shakespeare's mind. The knowledge which the imagination has enjoys a certain *identity* with its object.

But it will be said, if this is so, we should expect to see the evidence, in the products of the poetic mind, of this co-called saturation of the idea in the mind. And we reply, That is what we do find; the world and the mind are inextricably involved in each other in the universe of poetry. Shakespeare suffers in his characters; but also, in poetic ideas of the physical, we see the physical personalized at every turn. The galleons of Antonio are burghers; and everywhere in Shakespeare the physical and the less than human is penetrated by human feeling. There is barely need to give illustrations of this; there are few lines of Shakespeare which do not show it. I give this example, which is entirely typical, Titania's

> Therefore the winds, piping to us in vain,
> As in revenge, have suck'd up from the sea
> Contagious fogs; which, falling in the land,
> Have every pelting river made so proud,
> That they have overborne their continents:
> . . . and the green corn
> Hath rotted ere his youth attain'd a beard;

or this, Antony's

> and tonight I'll force
> The wine peep through their scars;

or this, Iachimo's

> The flame o' the taper
> Bows towards her, and would under-peep her lids
> To see the enclosed lights.

I specially call the reader's attention to the presence everywhere in Shakespeare of what the grammar books call the 'personal metaphor'. For the Augustans had strong views about it; and I shall have good occasion to speak of it at some later stage.

The reader will now see the natural conclusion of what has gone before. Symbolism is the mark of the 'first sort of understanding' in its resistance to the 'third sort'; it is the effort of the mind to *assimilate* its objects and its reluctance to 'understand' them; or, it is the prehension of them, so far as is possible, in terms of its own feeling and experience. In the imagination's action the mind, so far as it can be, *is* its ideas; in their turn the ideas are expressive of the mind. The ideas, indeed, because they are ideas, are raised above and out of mere experience; but they rise up drenched, as it were, in feeling. The intelligence works upon them, but never wholly removes their imaginative being. The infection by the mind of what is known is never altogether taken away; the sharp separation of the self from its object in conceptual analysis never destroys the intimacy between them from which knowledge begins and without some persistence of which it could not continue. This identity and assimilation are essential to knowledge, and a condition of the action of the intelligence. Knowledge is indeed a *prehension* by the mind, a taking of the object into itself; and for this reason knowledge is also a living process in which the mind expresses itself in what it nevertheless may rightly be said to know.

We may summarize what we have now said by returning to a paragraph which occurs earlier in this chapter, on p. 129. I said there that if our knowledge is of what is only imagined, it is difficult to see how we can be said to come to have knowledge at all. And in saying this, I was only repeating Locke, who had asked 'But what use is all this fine knowledge of men's own imaginations to a man that enquires after the reality of things?' I said that 'to apprehend impression is to change it into idea'; and that an idea is of the mind however much it may seem to come with authenticity and from without. How now, in the light of what I have just been saying, shall we answer this question? How can an idea be a revelation of things; be of the mind and yet a knowledge of objects? How, if an idea be imagined, can it be true?

Now we have been saying that in perception the idea turns out to be symbolical in its nature and shot through with the mind; what we know is assimilated to the mind and the mind to it; and this occurs in the change of impression into idea. In our perception, definition is a symbolizing; the making of symbol *is* perception, I said, as it moves from being relatively passive to being more active in prehension and to grasping and holding its idea; the coming of the 'symbol' is the act whereby, as it were, the eyes of imagination are focused; the idea and the symbol are one. Now if this is so, can we better answer the questions I reiterated in the preceding paragraph? The answer is that we can. For when we see that the idea is symbolical, our way is, if not clear, at least clearer. So long as we speak of ideas, we are left with a dichotomy between idea and object, the idea and that of which we have the idea; and the problem of representative perception is upon us. But if the idea be a symbol, the position is different. An idea is of something; but a symbol, as we have employed the word, is not *of* anything but only the means by which an object is grasped. A symbol does not stand alongside the object; it is a means of apprehending it; or better, it *is* the object as we come to know it in perception. Therefore, there is no question of *representative* perception; the object comes to us as and only as symbolized; it appears, and only appears, in this form. For this reason what we have been calling the idea is indeed of the mind; but it is no less an appearing of the object.

But it will be said, this is only dodging the difficulty, or at best postponing it. For if the object becomes symbolized by us, is it not, at the best, hopelessly distorted like things seen in the toy mirrors of children at the seaside? You still have no ground, it may be said, for saying that the imagination gives us things truly. Now to this we can only reply that it may be that things are distorted in our perception of them. Our perception of things is inadequate and partial; Locke bears witness how little we know of the things we see. Still, though partially or distortedly appearing, it is still the object appearing; it is a manifestation of itself in the medium of our minds. Besides, we have no authority beyond question for thinking that in any essentials we misrepresent the being of things. Thus it is true, for example, as we have seen and shall have occasion to see again a little later, that the imagination grasps the things of the world as animated, however vaguely, by activity and will like our own: we cannot, in imagination, devitalize the world. But it requires a special metaphysical demonstration to show that in doing so, the imagination grasps the being of things in a wholly false way; and such a demonstration has not yet, so far as I know, made its appearance.

Few, certainly, are going to take the materialism of so-called 'scientific' philosophy seriously.

IX

I have spoken of symbol and idea as one, and of the unity of the symbol and the symbolized. But the 'one' and the 'union' is, after all, an exaggeration. The imagination is, when all is said and done, at a remove from its object; if it were not so, there would be no idea, nor any need of symbol. The idea is shot through by the mind which beholds it; but it is still also object; and as ideal object it is held back from unity with the mind. But then symbolism comes with its power of resisting the action of the understanding, and will not suffer the object to be pushed away in thought, to become a dead thing suspended somewhere before the mind. Instead, it holds it as near as may be; and tries to penetrate it with its own life. Symbolism is, negatively, the resistance of the imagination to the understanding, the labour of assimilating the object to the mind.

But then, it is only a *resistance*. It is not indeed by any means an unsuccessful one. But it cannot overcome and destroy that which it resists. The coming-to-be of idea, the metamorphosis of impression into what is held by the mind, is the act of imagination; but it is also, by the fundamental paradox of our knowing, the starting-point of the understanding's life. It initiates the existence of the object; it holds before the mind what is not itself; and it is a condition of the imagination's action that in its labour to assimilate what it knows, it should, in the end, be defeated. There is always that, by the very existence of the idea, which is not the self, and which eludes and transcends it. Therefore the symbol cannot swallow and digest it, or the mind in all truth become what it beholds. Assimilation there is; still, the mind cannot, in strictness, assimilate what is for ever its *object*.

I have said, and it is fundamental to all I am trying to say, that the idea is imaginative object; but it is also fundamental that the imagination is also the matrix of the intelligence and offers to the intelligence that on which it may, and indeed must, work. Therefore, if tension there is, it is essential to the imagination's life; and it is folly to carry on polemics against the understanding. Anti-intellectualism is the attempted suicide of the mind; and it is neither in the imagination nor in the intelligence alone (for they cannot act, indeed, in total isolation from each other) that the mind will, in the end, be known as it is known.

The reader will see therefore that the development of the symbol, the union of the symbolized and the symbol, is never, in fact, made complete; and there is a limit to assimilation. Now because this is so, it will not do to say that the idea is identical with its expression. The mind may be in imagination 'near' its object, and feel its community with it. Still, the fact of knowledge commits the mind to a restlessness from which it cannot escape, so long as knowledge, as we have it, remains. To say that idea and expression are one is to say that known and knower are one; and it is certain that they are not. Certainly there is here a paradox. On the one side, the idea is mental, of the mind; but there is always that which is there, and, as known, beyond us. So far as it is idea, it is wholly expressible; so far as it is known, it eludes complete expressing, and leaves the mind baffled and distressed.

I do not see how, unless we are prepared to accept this state of affairs, we can explain our experience. Before articulation comes, we must assume that idea is somehow operative and goads the mind to express it. We may naturally exaggerate and say of the idea that before it has expression, it is without form and void, and therefore not idea. But our experience has a way of kicking down the walls which thought constructs. Thought is absolute, and wants things one side of the fence or the other; and here, it tells us that what we are speaking of is either idea or not idea, it is either expressed or unexpressed. But experience tells us that it is not all as clear-cut as this; and there is a sort of hinterland before, and no less, after, articulation. Always there is that which *transcends* the mind, which is not yet fully idea, but is yet an ineluctable accompaniment of the idea; and that this is so, the mind feels.

Out of this state of affairs neither the life of thought nor the life of imagination can escape. The mind may indeed, confronted with the idea, seek the help of thought and its conceptual explication. But it cannot leave the idea, which is the condition of the mind's intellectual action; sooner or later it will wish to return to perception merely; and then it is confronted with what is, in principle, the old situation. But if the mind resists the powers of the intelligence and clings to the æsthetic, there is still no solution. We may say that the work of art is nomadic and complete. There is a sense in which this is true. But there is also a sense in which it is not. For we have to consider the life of the artist as a whole. And then we see his life as a progress from one creation to another. There is that in any one work of his art which draws him on to the making of the next. He cannot indeed develop his work of art; it is done and there is nothing more that can be done with it; he can only start afresh and make another. But to this progress there is no end. And if we contemplate the work of Shakespeare, we see him in the end trying to overcome the very conditions of his art, in a region where his art has become curiously unexpressive, where, less than ever, the idea may be said to be expressed.

This matter is so important that I venture to say a little more about it. And lest I be misunderstood, I wish to say that I am not denying that the idea finds expression, or that expression is not a necessary aspect of the coming of the mind to its idea. I only say that when we have come to the idea, no doubt by way of expressing it, there goes along with it and present to our minds, the possibility, if you will, of a better, or still clearer, or more ample idea; and the sense of this possible development is an unavoidable part of our experience. We hardly cease, in our sense-experience, to be aware that our ideas of the sensuous fail us, that they could be stronger and more satisfying than they are; in intellectual work we have a sense of an ordering and clarity from which we fall short; a historian, learned in his chosen period, knows how much he loses in his imagining of the time's history; and we feel that our idea of a person we know and love misses a certain brilliance through our own failure of vitality and feeling. In all these instances, and in innumerable others we might take, the something beyond the idea is *there*; nor would we have what idea we have, if it were not. But, it may be said, What you say may be true; but this vague something which eludes us is simply not idea, and that is all there is to it. And yet, we reply, is it not our experience that we know that it *is* idea, and that it is real, though our minds have not yet matched up to it? For it is certainly not mere experience, a blind suffering of feeling; instead, we know that it is there, a possibility open to us to realize. We know it for idea, and yet fail to bring it within the scope of our minds; it exists, as it were, on the edge of our imagination. Besides, we feel about it not that it is another idea, between which and that which we have there is no community whatever; instead we are aware of it as a further stage in the development of the idea we have.

For we have, in these matters, to be careful not to erect the idea into a kind of 'thing'; it is not something fixed, atomic and self-complete. We must not commit the error commonly ascribed to Locke which we discussed earlier. It might be truer to see the idea as a stage in the mind's development, or as a stage in the development of more adequate idea. And all I am saying is that in our experience we are aware that this is so, and that the idea is always inadequate, and always will be. Reality stretches out beyond and behind it; and this transcendence by reality of the idea is a part of our knowledge of the idea. It is easy to hypostatize the idea, to sever it from our living experience of it, and then to say, it *is* its expression; but if we decline to commit this philosophical error, we shall acknowledge that there is that in our knowledge which remains inexpressible but which is also dynamical in the mind's growth. To say that idea is always susceptible to full expression or *is* its expression is dogmatically to traffic in abstractions.

To illustrate this further, let us recall how Locke said that there are some things in which philosophers must be content to talk like children. There are ideas, he said, that are neither clear nor distinct; substance was an 'I know not what'. In saying this, he was saying something true enough. But philosophers are jealous for language and expression; they will not be beaten. Hence the urge to phenomenalism, which has been felt by philosophers who differ in other respects from one another; the Berkeleys and the Russells are here prepared to join hands. But Locke's 'mediocrity' saved him from this impulse; and though Descartes, animated by the spirit of mathematics and its abstractions, contented himself only with what he judged to be clear and distinct, the philosophical spirit of Locke was wiser. Locke certainly sought clarity; and no doubt it was precisely because of this that he would not bluff himself into believing that his thought was clear when it was not. Less animated by intellectual ambition, he was less liable to illusions, and stuck closer to the experience of mankind. For it is easy enough no doubt to resolve things into congeries of sense-data, and to tell us that if we try to make out that things are anything but these, we are babbling nonsense. But if it be a choice between this nonsense, which is, after all, only the nonsense of men everywhere, and the nonsense of philosophers, we shall be wise to go for the former. It is true enough that we and the world are mysteries to ourselves; but we shall not exterminate what we do not understand by neat philosophical campaigns. And when, from a different quarter, we are told the idea and the expression of it are one and the same, we discern the same spirit at work, though under a very different guise. But to this campaign also, the world and our experience will not yield. There is that which may have only meagre expression or none; but it is none the less there, and known for being there.

This limitation of our knowledge is our mortal lot, and there is an ideal of knowledge which it is not given to us to realize. Father D'Arcy has written eloquently of this ideal. In ideal knowledge, he says on pp. 49–50 of *The Nature of Belief*,[1]

the rôle played by the various parts which we distinguish in an act of cognition—the subject thinking, the thinking, and the object thought of—would be altered. The object would not lose its colour and characteristic, but it *would* cease to be just an object cut off from the act of thinking, a *pensiero pensato*, to use Gentile's phrase, a corpse hanging on the gallows of the mind. Instead of being a limit to our thought the object would be fused with the experience and have the right to be called the self-expression of the subject. The lover in the Persian tale, when asked who he was, replied 'It is thou!'

In complete knowledge [he goes on], the mind is absorbed in what is near and dear to it, and this absorption is its own life expressed and enjoyed. Introspection is no longer needed, because in the realisation of all things we ourselves have also become fully alive. When an actor or an artist is engaged upon his work, self-consciousness acts as a hindrance; yet perfect acting and perfect art are as truly self-expression as the expression of the part played; which shows that ultimately the two fuse. The flame shows its force and its brightness in consuming its object; were that object to stamp the flame with its own colour and the flame to live consuming but not destroying, we should have something like an adequate picture of the life of the mind at its highest. Activity, that is, without anything left over, everything turned into live experience or expression, nothing in my thought which is not wholly mine, as much mine as the 'I' in my thinking—this is the epiphany of the soul's life, when all within becomes light, and there is no longer the shadow of division between the subject and the object, the 'I' and the 'me,' the thinker and his thought. The soul sees itself in the very seeing, and all else which its nature comprehends in the one saturating exhaustive experience. Gone now are those half lights, the chequered glimpses of our nature seen through the foliage of sense, those projections of the self, the mists which lie around the objects of our thought, making them remote and vague. The nature of the self, like the bow of Ulysses, sings at the touch of the master, and in that singing are to be heard the forms of all known things re-echoing. [And he adds a little later:] In human knowledge at the present moment there is incompleteness, whether we look without or within; in perfect human knowledge there will be no more mysteries within, and what is without will shine in the light of the soul's lamp, so far as that light can comprehend it. But all human thought, even the highest, has its horizons; there are realms which it cannot encompass and mirror in its nature, be it the most candid and clear. God alone measures reality by what He is, and in His essence sees all things vividly or faintly resembling His truth.

[1] London, 1945.

Such an ideal could not occur to us if idea and expression were one. But that it occurs Locke, once again, no less than Father D'Arcy, bears witness. He insists that we can know only nominal essences of things; but always in his mind is the thought of superior intelligences to whom the real essenses of things lie open. (I do not however imply that Locke's doctrine of nominal essences is a necessary formulation of the sensibility of which I am speaking here.) I only add to what Father D'Arcy says, that the mode of knowledge of which he speaks could not be envisaged, still less be an *ideal* of knowledge, were it not, in a measure however slight, realized in all our knowledge whatsoever.

X

Now in speaking hitherto, I have spoken too much as if in knowledge we were bodiless minds, and I have referred too little to the rôle of the body. For in fact we are embodied minds; and this is a truth, however easily forgotten by philosophers, which we must bear in mind.[1] What I shall now go on to say will throw further light on what has gone before; it will also give us further opportunity to illustrate the action of symbolism in poetry.

Now it is certain that self-consciousness and the world disclosed to the mind occur together. The mind comes to be aware of itself; at the same time, and as part of the same process, the mind comes to be aware of objects. But there are two things here to remember. First, that it is misleading to say that 'the mind becomes aware of itself'; what becomes aware of itself is an embodied self. Second, that as the embodied self becomes aware of itself it becomes aware of itself only as a part of a wider context, a world in which it is.

But now, how is this world, of which the embodied self becomes aware and in which the embodied self is aware of itself as existing, represented in knowledge? The answer is, that it is represented as consisting of things which are imagined to be like the embodied self, at least in certain important respects. It would, indeed, be strange if this were not so. The strong wind against which we force ourselves is represented as analogous, however vaguely, to one of our hands if we press it hard against the other; the swift movement of a shell from a gun is 'like' the swift movement of our fist when we 'shoot out' an arm in attack or self-defence. This is not at all to say that we endow the

---

[1] See, on the matters I shall speak of here, G. F. Stout's *Mind and Matter*, Cambridge, 1931.

wind or the shell with mind. We do not represent the wind or the shell to ourselves as embodied selves, as Mr. Stout explained in chapter 2 of his book. We only represent their movements as like the movement of those parts of our bodies which are under our control. Still, if we do this, we imagine the world, as vaguely as you wish, as 'animated' by activity and will like our own. Whether this has any valid implication for metaphysics is another matter. But the fact is that the imagination grasps the things of the world as of a piece with our own experience of ourselves; and if it did not, if there were not, as it were, this continuing penetration of the world by the experience of the embodied mind, the world could be no more than a show of discrete 'sense-data,' a disorder of phantasmal sensualities.

Now to say this is, I think, only to state an undeniable fact of our experience; and I think it certain that nothing that science (which after all is not philosophy) can say will disabuse us of this way of imagining the world. I only add, further, that to say this is not all to set out any doctrine of 'self-projection' such as some thinkers have propagated. 'Self-projection' will not do, and for the good reason that we do not begin with a self-conscious self which then sets us off discovering and making worlds. The world, envisaged as I have suggested, is already there when the embodied self comes to any idea of itself; it has been part and parcel of the discovery to itself of the embodied mind.

If this is so, our bodies play a momentous rôle in our imagination and knowledge of the world. For we not only see colour and hear sound; we resist and press and force objects and in turn are 'resisted' and 'pressed' and 'forced' by them; and our tactual and motor experience of our own bodies enter, as it were, into the objects we resist or suffer. Our sense of ourselves as active overflows into the world; and this activity is never merely of mind or of body, but of both. Indeed we may be sure that anything approaching a clear distinction between body and mind came only very late in the growth of human self-consciousness; and even now, to realize the distinction requires a labour of introspection. The trouble has been that when the distinction became at all clear, it encouraged philosophers to forget how 'bodily' our minds are. We forget that we know things as much by our motor and tactual sensation as by our visual.

The reader will therefore see that when I spoke, at an earlier stage, of the 'contamination' of the imagination's object by the mind, it would have been better to say, 'by the embodied self'. He will also see the source of the fundamental symbolism of poetry which is active in those passages from Shakespeare I have quoted. I have already described symbolism in a number of ways; I now add that it is nothing more nor less than the felt community of the embodied self with what it imagines and which is maintained against the action of the intelligence.

Now language is an activity neither of the mind nor of the body, but of the embodied mind; and we have to remember that language is not words written or in print; it is a speaking of sounds.

And to give one example of the importance of this, I take some lines from *Paradise Lost*. They are lines in Book IV (l. 724 ff), where Adam, in his prayer, speaks of the Garden of Eden as

> this delicious place
> For us too large, where thy abundance wants
> Partakers, and uncropt falls to the ground.

Dr. Johnson once criticized these lines, and said that they were 'remarkably inharmonious'. He had in mind, in particular, the last of the lines I have quoted. Now we may be sure (though Jonnson indeed was not) that if the line is inharmonious, it is so only because Milton intended it. Milton was, if anything, a most deliberate artist and certainly knew what he was doing. Why then is the line inharmonious? The answer is that the poet was less concerned with 'harmony' than with communicating an idea of an event or of events, the falling of the fruit from the trees of Paradise. To do this, he wrote 'and uncropt falls to the ground'. 'And uncropt' with its consonant groups and open vowels, with the awkward hiatus (if we give 'and' its full value) between the 'and' and 'uncropt' may be said (to speak for the present crudely and as we shall see, unsatisfactorily) a 'picture' of the round and weighted fruit; in 'falls' there is release; there is movement, which is short and brief and fast, in 'to the'; and this movement reaches its certain and final end in the all-receiving four-consonanted and round-vowelled 'ground'. I think we may be sure this was what Milton intended. Now *Paradise Lost* calls, more perhaps than most poems, to be read aloud. It has been said that Milton's poetry fails in the visual, and this 'discovery' has been widely hailed. But we cannot, perhaps, expect everything; and there is God's plenty in Milton. However this may be, supposing I have rightly divined his intention, let us further consider this inharmonious line.

It is, I think, clear that in it Milton employs two 'symbolisms'. They are first, a symbolism of sound; the second is what I shall call a motor symbolism. In the first, there is the complicated set of sounds in 'and uncropt', then fast, easy sounds in 'falls to the', then the large, round, conclusive, continuing 'ground'. Besides, the pitch of the voice falls with the apple; it declines steeply as we move from the first to the last word. But the motor symbolism is perhaps even more important. This consists in the disposition of our mouths, in the changes in these dispositions and in the rates of these changes, what we apprehend through kinæsthesis; we have to frame our mouths and breath and speak as the poet dictates; and this is a great part of the means whereby he conveys his idea. Now we may say that in these ways he creates two 'pictures' or 'models' (these words have been used, in recent years, in a context not far away from that in which we are now moving)—two 'pictures' or 'models' of the apple and then of its movement and coming to rest.

I said that in speaking, in this way, of 'pictures' or 'models', I was speaking crudely. And this is so because, as we read the lines, we are not aware of the models *as* models; we do not *compare* them with that of which we have said they are 'models'. To do this is to carry on an intellectual action, and is the sort of thing which literary critics do, after the event of reading the line. A model may stand alongside that of which it is a model; these 'models' do nothing of the kind. And they do not do so precisely because they are symbols, and neither models nor signs. Both model and sign stand apart from what the one copies and the other signifies. But these symbols enter into their object; they help to make what they symbolize; they define and give detail to the idea, not by being, in our reading of the line, *like* the object spoken of (though to reflection at least they are that) but by, if I may so speak, their likeness to the object becoming a factor in the very occurrence of the idea. It is this that makes the difference. The model does not at all make that of which it is a model; nor a sign make that of which it is sign. But the symbol is constituent of what it symbolizes. It may be that, as we are told by some modern logicians, the proposition is a model of the state of affairs spoken of; but 'poetical proposition', as we see it in these lines of Milton, is not a model or copy but constituent of the idea; it is a symbol.

Here then, the reader will see, the body is assimilated to the object; it becomes like it; and in becoming like it becomes also an agent in the knowing of it. Like the sensible species of Aristotle it acts unknown, or almost so, to disclose the known. I only add that I do not wish to suggest that the body, with that symbolizing power I have described, is not also employed in lines appealing more directly to the eye than the lines of Milton I have quoted. In the passage from *The Merchant of Venice* the line

As they fly by them with their woven wings,

with its open vowels for breadth and the smoothness of the muscular action in our speaking of it, employ the visual, the auditory and the kinæsthetic. And in general, onomatopœia is far less effective in poetry than kinæsthetic symbol.

XI

Before I go on to speak of Locke's second kind of understanding, and to his views on language, I wish to illustrate further, what will also serve to lead on to some discussion of Locke's opinions about language, what I have called the tensions between imagination and intelligence. I have said that there are degrees of tension between imagination and understanding; the proportions of each in an act of the mind may vary. And what I mean will be clear if the reader will consider, after *King Lear*, these three works: *De Rerum Natura*, the *Divina Commedia*, *The Faerie Queene*. No one will deny the poetical quality of these three works; they are genuinely works of the imagination. Still, *De Rerum Natura* is an exposition of a philosophy; the *Divina Commedia* is based upon another and uses it explicitly; *The Faerie Queene* is an allegory.

Now to speak at length of these three works, in the point of view in which I have mentioned them, is far beyond the scope of this essay. But the reader will see what is in my mind; we can only define the difference between them as works of art in terms of the differing proportions of imagination and intelligence in the creative acts that went to their making. Now in allegory, which I comment on because of the long tradition it enjoyed in European literature, the intelligence and its concepts are present explicitly; there runs as it were alongside the narrative a more or less clear conceptual scheme or system of meanings, which we are required to grasp, and do grasp, as we go along. *The Faerie Queene* serves here well enough. It is said sometimes that it is possible to read *The Faerie Queene* as pure story and to find it delightful; but in fact this is not true; we would find the story baffling without knowing what it is all about; and what it is *about*, what it *means*, we need to know. In allegory therefore, we have indeed poetry; but it is an inferior poetry, splendid as it may be and as *The Faerie Queene* is.

In it the imagination and the intelligence come to terms; here indeed is a concordat entered into by the two; and the concordat comes about because allegory is didactic and has an end outside the poetry.

I am here skirting a large field of enquiry and definition. But, before leaving it altogether, I take, to illustrate further my meaning, a work of art small enough to be spoken of in fairly small compass. Here is a sonnet of Shakespeare.

> Poor soul, the centre of my sinful earth,
> Starv'd by these rebel powers that thee array,[1]
> Why dost thou pine within and suffer dearth,
> Painting thy outward walls so costly gay?
> Why so large cost, having so short a lease,
> Dost thou upon thy fading mansion spend?
> Shall worms, inheritors of this excess,
> Eat up thy charge? is this thy body's end?
> Then, soul, live thou upon thy servant's loss,
> And let that pine to aggravate thy store;
> Buy terms divine in selling hours of dross;
> Within be fed, without be rich no more:
> > So shall thou feed on Death, that feeds on men,
> > And Death once dead, there's no more dying then.

Now it is possible for the reader of this sonnet to state, with reasonable accuracy, the *meaning* of this poem. He may state it, no doubt, in a number of ways. He may choose a Christian or a Platonic idiom in expounding it, or he may avoid both. Still, he will not find it very difficult to set out what it says. Now the fact that we can *say* what it says, signifies that it has an intellectual quality, which makes it different from *King Lear*, and which may even be said to make it less poetical than *King Lear*. But before we say more, let us analyze it.

The 'poor' of the apostrophe we take in the first place as expressing pity, a sense in which we still use the word. But it becomes clear that the usual meaning of the word is also intended; the 'suffer dearth' of the third line shows this. The soul, which may be pitied and which is poor, is the centre of the 'sinful earth' of the body, where 'centre' no doubt suggests the heart as the seat of the soul, for Harvey's discovery of the circulation of the blood was not to come until 1616. But 'centre' serves also to lead on to the military image of the next line, with the thought of the soul as invested, surrounded by rebels. The 'rebel powers' are

---

[1] I take Steevens's reading for the first word of this line. I think it suits, better than any other suggested reading, the surrounding imagery.

the powers of the sinful body, which 'array' the soul. Now 'array' carries two meanings; first, that of 'attiring' and 'clothing'; second, that of 'afflicting', 'discomfiting' (a use of which the Oxford Dictionary gives examples up to 1600). There is the suggestion, too, of 'array against', what is arrayed in battle against the soul. In the first two lines, therefore, we have the idea of the spiritual, the soul, expressed as the heart, the centre of the body; and around it is the body, which clothes, discomfits and attacks its rightful and life-giving lord. The reader will see how intricate here is the fusion of ideas, which taxes analysis.

But in the next two lines, the imagery changes, apparently inconsequentially. But, in careful reading, the connexions with what has gone before are there. We pick up, now, the second sense of 'poor' of which I spoke; we also continue the first sense of 'array', that of 'clothing'; and if 'starv'd' is right, there is a third connexion. Indeed, the third line is near enough, in imagery, to the first two, with only this difference: that it is suggested that the state of the soul, thus held in the power of the rebel-body, is unnecessary; the soul is now upbraided for weakness. But in the fourth line, there is indeed a change of image: the body now becomes the house of the soul which 'pines within'; still the transition to it is brought about by the connexion in our minds of 'poor' with 'pine' and 'dearth', and of 'array' with 'costly gay'. I call attention to the second of these two. So long as 'array' is in our minds, we have the idea of the body as the clothing of the soul. But in the fourth line the body has become the *walls* of the soul, its house. How can Shakespeare ease this jump in the imagery? He does it, partly I think, by the two adjectives, 'costly' and 'gay', which are of a kind to keep alive the image of clothing in our minds; but also, I suspect that the 'painting' suggests the use of cosmetics; and this calls up the image of the actual flesh of the body; so that the thought of the body itself is used to act as the transition between the image of fine clothes and that of the brilliant exterior of the house. In this way, the fact, the literal, is employed by the art of the metaphorical.

Now in the next four lines (5–8) the imagery of the body as house and of the soul as dwelling in it, is developed. And now, the soul is a *tenant*, and with a short lease. We have come a long way from the opening imagery of the poem; but only by very subtle fusion of imagery. And as we go further into line 6, we read that the house, on which the soul, its tenant, has only a short lease, is, in any case, only a 'fading mansion'. Now this phrase requires our attention. We observe two things about it. In the first place, Shakespeare catches the two meanings of 'fade'. First, there is that which is connected with the word 'painting' earlier; the house loses the former brilliance of its fresh paint, however costly. But there is also the sense of decay, decline, falling into ruin, passing away; and it is this second sense which he will develop in the lines that follow. In the second place there is 'mansion'. Now 'mansion' is indeed a rich word. There are at least four meanings. They are: (a) a place of abode, where one dwells; (b) the chief residence of a lord or great man; (c) its figurative use for the body, frequent in the sixteenth century (Tindale writes of 'oure erthy mancion wherein we now dwell'; and Shakespeare in *Cymbeline* of 'The innocent Mansion of my Love'); (d) a halting-place in a journey. All these meanings can find their place in the imagery of the poem.

But now there comes another change. 'Shall worms, inheritors of this excess, eat up thy charge?' Of the dwelling-place of the soul, worms are the heirs. Here, indeed, the idea of tenancy seems to have been quietly dropped; the body, after all, *was* the property of the soul. But it was, inevitably a 'fading' property; and on property which must necessarily fall into ruin no one can have more than a lease; so that, after all, there is no disparity in the imagery. Still, with 'worms' we come back to the literal, to the flesh; and this return has been eased by 'fading', for 'fade' in one of its first meanings was and is used of *living* things. But this return to the literal is at once countered by fresh imagery. Shall the worms 'inheritors of this excess', 'eat up the charge' of the body? Here is a further example of what I have remarked on earlier, Shakespeare fusion of fact and 'symbol'. In fact, worms eat the body as they may consume the timbers of a house; but into this is run, as it were, the image or 'symbol' of the greedy heirs devouring the legacy; and the worms *are* the heirs. Besides, the body is now spoken of as the 'charge' of the soul; and 'charge', too, is a many-sided word. It is a load or burden; therefore a source of trouble and distress; a thing of moral weight or moment; an expense, cost (archaic now, but alive enough in Shakespeare's time); a task or duty laid upon one; custody, superintendence; and accusation. All these senses are alive in the poem and have been active in the making of its imagery; and yet the word is here used of something that is eaten up by the inheriting worms.

I have not so far, I trust, exaggerated in showing how complicated and subtle great poetry is; in eight lines there has been a swiftly changing but wonderfully continuous development in imagery. Through these lines have played what may be called the themes of the soul's helplessness, poverty and brief tenure of the body; the soul has been wrongfully rebelled against by its inferiors, been a poor tenant, a prodigal spender, having prodigal heirs. And the body has been, in turn, a rebellious power, the brilliant front of a house, a mansion doomed to decay and worm-eaten. But the octet ends with a brutal and unmitigated return to the literal: 'Is this thy body's end?' We have passed from, at the poem's beginning, pity and commiseration, to gentle rebuke, to upbraiding, and now to the harsh question which can have only one answer.

And now the sonnet turns; and we pass to the putting of stern charge upon the soul. The 'argument' of the first eight lines is complete, its 'demonstration' unanswerable. What follows is injunction, which picks up, as it goes, the imagery of what has gone before, setting it in a new context of the possible. In line 9 the body becomes a servant, not a rebel, and *he* must pine, to make wealthy the soul. Line 10 picks up the imagery of property with its 'buy terms divine', where 'term' both belongs to the property-imagery and also means 'period of time'. Still, the term which the soul must come by must be in fact no term, but life endless—*interminabilis*, in the famous sentence of Boëthius describing eternity; and Shakespeare must therefore counter the idea of limited time by the adjective 'divine'. But 'divine' not only overcomes the idea of a limit in time; it may carry also the idea of perfection and purity; and as such it is set over against the 'dross' of the end of the line. Then in line 12, we return to the idea of food and of wealth. And finally in the couplet which concludes the poem, it is the idea of eating which is developed. The soul must feed on death. It is the soul, not worms, which must consume the body; and *then* the body is a food to the soul and a nourishment. The soul lives precisely through the body's dying; nothing less than a dying life will do. We began with the starving of the soul by the body; but we end with the soul coming to health by making the body its very food. Besides, in this way, death, now identified with the body, itself dies; and it can die only by starvation. The body is, as it were, spiritualized by its death; it must die that the soul may live. For the soul has obtained terms divine; it is only the body which knows the 'hours' of time; and the death of the body is at once the end of death and of time.

I have written at some length of this poem for two reasons. Chiefly, I have done so to illustrate what may be called imaginative thought. It may indeed be said that the poem contains much and profound thought; there is indeed doctrine in it. It is an intellectual poem, and is philosophical. Still, nowhere is the thought allowed to escape the domination of the image; it is a poem in which thought is, so to speak, carried on by the senses. Now the reader will recall Kant's saying that the imagination is 'one of the fundamental faculties of the human soul', and that senses and understanding are brought into relation with each other through and by it; and he thought that perhaps imagination is the 'common root' of both. Something of what was in his mind we may understand from study of Shakespeare's poem as well as from what he says of the schematism of the categories, a schematism which he called an art (*Kunst*) hidden in the depth of the soul. Thus it is that by the mediating (or perhaps originating) power of the imagination knowledge may be had and enjoyed by the total personality; for in it sense and intelligence are brought together. Now my purpose in this chapter has been to show where the æsthetic occurs and lives. It does so in the many tensions which may exist between imagination and understanding. There are indeed many differing tensions. One of them is well illustrated in Shakespeare's sonnet. But there are innumerable others. The imagination must live in and through the senses; and in art the understanding is compelled to live, in varying degrees, in the imagination.

My second purpose in speaking at length of Shakespeare's sonnet was to show how the 'argument' of poetry may be said to move. It is a movement from image to image; and in doing so it must endeavour to overcome discontinuity and jumps. It does so, above all, by fusing and joining its images; but it also proceeds by deliberate and elaborate equivocation. This fusion of imagery teases and baffles the intelligence; and equivocation, which is a fallacy in logic, is one of the nerves of poetry.

XII

Shakespeare's sonnet will serve for preface to what must be only a few observations about what Locke says, in Book 3 of the *Essay*, concerning words and language. Now I said, before making this long diversion from expounding him, that Locke's analysis of the kinds of understanding, in particular his distinction of the first kind from the third, put in his hands the means whereby he might have gone on to lay the true foundations of Æsthetic; and that if he did not do so, it was because he was unaware of the æsthetic. But it would, no doubt, be better to say that he was not wholly unaware of it; and that he saw it in such a way and in such a point of view, that he naturally takes what opportunity comes his way of disparaging and maligning it. For so far as he was aware of it, he was aware of it as ornament only; and because it is only ornament, it is at the best a mere distraction from the pursuit of knowledge; and at the worst, it misleads and falsifies. Book 3. 10 is a chapter on the abuse of words; and in his list of the abuses to which he thought words are put, the seventh and last is their figurative employment. 'Since wit and fancy find easier entertainment in the world, than dry truth and real knowledge, figurative speeches and allusion in language will hardly be admitted as an imperfection or abuse of it. I confess, in discourses where we seek rather pleasure and delight than information and improvement, such ornaments as are borrowed from them can scarce pass for faults. But yet if we would speak of things as they are, we must allow that all the art of rhetorick, besides order and clearness, all the artificial and figurative application of words, eloquence hath invented are for nothing else but to insinuate wrong ideas, move the passions, and thereby mislead the judgment, and so indeed are perfect cheats: and . . . are certainly, in all discourses that pretend to inform or instruct, wholly to be avoided; and where truth and knowledge are concerned, cannot but be thought a great fault...' (3. 10. xxxiv). This is altogether in the manner of Hobbes's: 'In Demonstration, in Councell, and all rigourous search of Truth, Judgement does all . . . But for metaphors, they are utterly excluded. For seeing they openly professe deceipt; to admit them into Councell, or Reasoning, were manifest folly'. 'Men of letters' (a contemptuous phrase in Locke's use of it) are welcome to metaphors; but what we want is dry truth and real knowledge; and for this, metaphors will not serve.

Now the reader will understand that if our concern is indeed with demonstration, counsel, reasoning, dry truth, there can be no question of disagreeing with either Hobbes or Locke; they are right in what they say; here, no doubt, metaphor is to be avoided, though it may be less easily avoided than they were disposed to think. Besides, they do not condemn figurative language in itself; figurative writing and speeches have their place, and metaphor its rightful rôle, as ornament. For the reason that the æsthetic is ornamental, they condemn it only when it feigns a function it may not fairly have. But they cannot be said to condemn the æsthetic, as we have tried to set it out; and they do not do so because they show no signs of being aware of its existence. They are not aware of symbol as a feature of knowledge; and there can therefore be no question of *arguing* with Hobbes and Locke about the æsthetic, as there can be no question of arguing with a colour-blind man that there is a range of colours he does not discern. Certainly, no purpose would be served by trying to convince a Hobbes and a Locke that Shakespeare gives us 'dry truth and real knowledge', for it is clear that Shakespeare does nothing of the sort; and because Shakespeare does nothing of the sort, they are not interested in him. We have only to accept, with the piety of the historian, the fact that in these writers the sense of the æsthetic was atrophied. And we can only ask, if they are typical of their age, and if they influence the 'men of letters', what will happen to poetry? The question is interesting. It is also a large one. And later we must try to supply the answer.

Locke's second kind of understanding is 'the perception of the signification of signs'; and it is only the second and the third kinds 'that use allows us to say that we understand'. Accordingly, he sees language as only an affair of understanding, and its efficient use is to be judged wholly in that light. 'The use of language is, by short sounds, to signify with ease and dispatch general conceptions', he says in 3. 5. vii; again, in 3. 6. xxxiii, he speaks of 'the true end of speech, which is to be the easiest and shortest way of communicating our notions'; and again in 3. 10. xiii, 'language . . . was given us for the improvement of knowledge and bond of society'. Therefore Locke considers language only as the articulation of thought proper; it expresses notions and the relations between them. He is here in agreement with Hobbes, who says early in the fourth chapter of *Leviathan:* 'The most noble and profitable invention of all other, was that of SPEECH, consisting of *Names* or *Appellations*, and their Connexion; whereby men register their Thoughts; recall them when they are past; and also declare them one to another for mutuall utility and conversation; without which, there had been amongst men, neither Common-wealth, nor Society, nor Contract, nor Peace, no more than amongst Lyons, Bears and Wolves. The first author of Speech was *God* himself, that instructed *Adam* how to name such creatures as he presented to his sight . . .' Language is to both of them the instrument of intelligence and social utility, 'the great instrument and common tie of society', as Locke says. Both are further agreed that language has two uses; first, 'for the recording our thoughts for the help of our memories', second, 'for the communicating of our thoughts to others'. This is Locke's way of putting it, and it is hardly different from Hobbes's. The only notable difference between them is that Hobbes will allow us to call words 'signs' only when being used in the second way.

Now there is between us and these writers this difference, that their

minds felt no invitation to stumble their way back through unimaginable tracts of time during which, as man's mind moved beyond the
animal, organs of speech slowly developed. And because their thoughts
were not habituated to these indefinitely long vistas, they took less
interest in childhood and the growth of language in childhood than we
do now. No doubt, childhood is an unsafe guide enough to us, when
we try to piece out the early mind of man; but it is a help; and we are
right to use it, so long as we are reasonably critical. But neither Hobbes
nor Locke troubled, in their thinking about language, to consider the
child's advance in speech. When Locke speaks of children, it is to say
that they frequently know a word before they know its meaning; and
where we may perhaps see this state of affairs (which certainly exists)
as throwing light on the 'dark backward' of our mental lives, Locke
sees it only as illustrating a defect which he observes in adult life, the
use of words without knowing what they mean; he uses it as a point
from which to look inwards into the habits of the grown mind. This
is what we should expect in a theorist of language who is concerned to
make language as intellectual as may be, a precise expression of concepts clearly grasped, and for each of which there is one word and no
other.

It will be clear to the reader, if he is at all disposed to agree with
what has gone before, that Locke's view of language does not meet the
facts. If there is indeed a wide and important range of experience in
which the imagination holds the intelligence in subordinacy, we must
allow for an employment of language predominantly imaginative as
well as for its employment in a predominantly intellectual way.

Now language is strictly an expression of idea and cannot occur at
the level of experience merely. There must be, if only dimly, an idea
of both self and object before those sounds which we call language can
come into being. An idea, I have said, is something so far 'held', with
however great difficulty, by the mind; and it is language which sig-
nalizes the occurrence of the idea, a something 'held'. Only as lifted,
however briefly, above the flux of experience, can what is known evoke
language; and as known, it is already idea. It may be indeed, only one
of Locke's 'ideas of sensation', or a 'some small dim perception'; yet,
it is not sensation merely. Sensation may evoke cries, sounds merely;
only what is imagined can evoke sounds spoken.

Still, we must not make the mistake of thinking that, at a level of
mental life which, considered as intellectual, is poor and primitive,
imaginative ideas of great clarity and brilliance may not occur. The

drawings recently discovered in French caves show that to think this would be quite wrong; nor need we think that the tribal songs in which language may well have had its origin were artistically crude. They may have been 'meaningless' enough; but they were not therefore necessarily bad art. Now that language began when man's intellectual powers and his conceptual analysis of his ideas were very slight is not only shown by what we know of the history of language as a movement to analytic from synthetic forms; it is only what we cannot forbear to think quite inevitable. That he was capable of imaginative idea of great power and clarity we know; that he was even a blundering scientist or philosopher is incredible. And it was in this world where idea might be brilliant, and thought certainly meagre, that language began. Man did not begin his history as a little philosopher or a little scientist; he was much nearer to being an artist. Hobbes and Locke were unaware of the length of man's history; but had they been aware of it, it is quite credible that they would have thought of him, as writers on primitive man are still capable of thinking of him, as themselves writ small. If Sir James Frazer could so profoundly misrepresent the nature of magic, we need not be censorious towards Locke's views on language. Language, we may be sure, was not, in the first place, something merely used or intellectual; nor did society begin when language was first used to communicate thought. The last chapter of Jespersen's *Language, its Nature, Development and Origin* is necessarily only tentative; but that the line which his speculations follow is the right line, we may reasonably believe. Thought has evolved, over unimaginable periods of time, out of a matrix which was imaginative and lyrical.

Everything, to say nothing of their inevitable ignorance of the history of language, disposed Hobbes and Locke not to contemplate this possibility. Still, they were writing, Hobbes in the middle, Locke towards the end, of the century in which Shakespeare had written his greatest plays; and had they been capable of lively response to poetry, they would have reflected that language may be adapted to express refined conceptual analysis, and also have a different but legitimate employment. Hobbes's mind indeed had a hard, metallic quality which was all against such response and such speculation; but we might have expected Locke to be different. Certainly, Shakespeare's poetic practice ignores all those requirements which Locke looked to have in a satisfactory language; his poetry abounds in equivocation and is all the greater because of it. And that Locke, whose mind was, I have said, pre-eminently fair and open, could not see this, is, perhaps, surprising.

But it is not less surprising that he, of all people, the philosopher of assent and judgement who set small store by syllogisms, should imagine that thought can divest itself of what is individual and idiomatic. How could he fail to see philosophy as a form of literature, if assent and judgement are indeed to have room in it? And if this is so, it is not only that he was simply unaware of language used in a predominantly imaginative way; he opposed his theory of language, which gives space to man considered only as intelligent, to his sense of the individuality of thought itself. I said at an earlier stage that thought is, as it were, surrounded by imagination; it works upon and within imaginative idea, however unconscious it may be of this. There was much in Locke's philosophy which was calculated to make him see this. But he just falls short. He just fell short, in another matter, in the chapter *Of Enthusiasm*; he is also not true to himself in setting out a theory of language which makes it a mere tool of thought. In man's early days language began as an imaginative thing; and it continues in our own day as, in varying degrees, an imaginative as well as an intellectual thing. It is vain to think that the scientist or the philosopher escapes from what is imaginative; so far as he does so, he disqualifies himself from discovery and becomes the equivalent of the Grub Street hack. Besides, there is an unbroken line along which the mind may move from the bleakest generalization to ideas deeply realized, from 'All men are mortal' to

> Thou'lt come no more,
> Never, never, never, never, never;

and we may in youth acknowledge a general statement for true which in later years has for us the force of overwhelming idea. And thus it is, also, that between the scientist and the poet there is no gap or discontinuity of mind; their union is always an ideal which beckons, or should beckon, the poet of a scientific age. The heart of scientific generalization is idea; and without it science could not exist. This is as true of philosophy as of science. Somehow or other (and I am not now concerned to explore it in detail) there is a certain community between the percept and the concept. It is hard indeed for thought to see how this may be; but that it is so, we cannot reasonably doubt.

The reader will recall that I left off expounding Locke in order to consider the implications of his 'first kind of understanding'. Some of these implications I have now sketched; and I have done so partly in order to suggest a significant shortcoming in Locke's reflection, and partly in order that I might, what I owed to the reader, outline something of the doctrine in whose light this narrative is recounted. In doing so, I have raised questions which I have not yet answered. Some of these I shall try to answer at later stages, as the progress of the narrative requires or gives occasion.

I have tried to suggest a point of view in which knowledge and being may be brought closer together than they could hope to be in Augustan philosophy, and in this *rapprochement* imagination plays the crucial rôle. For it takes a place, as I have said, midway between sense and understanding, or better, partakes of both, while being neither; and it is that by which the community and intimacy of the knower and the known is maintained. This intimacy is also the 'assimilation' of the knower to the known, and of the known to the knower, and is the condition of all knowledge. This intimacy shows itself in poetry, in symbolism; and symbolism is not a device of poetry but a fundamental feature of knowledge which poetry unquestioningly acknowledges. At least, much poetry does. But not all. For Augustan philosophy took little account of it; and Augustan poetry behaved, to no small extent, as if it did not exist. And this is perhaps the most important fact about the poetry written in England in the period of which in this work we are speaking. To say this is not, in anticipation, to condemn Augustan poetry; it is only necessary in order to understand it.

I

MY purpose in speaking about Bolingbroke's philosophical writings is to show in what form Locke's *Essay* and *Reasonableness of Christianity* passed into the mind of the succeeding age. Bolingbroke's essays in philosophy hold no high place in the history of English philosophy. They are indeed finely composed by a master of English prose. But the ideas in them are not philosophically conceived, and issue not from fair reflection but from prejudices and passions. This indeed is what chiefly strikes a reader. Bolingbroke writes out of an age of reason. But animating his 'rationalism' is a strength of feeling which surprises and shocks us; and rationalism is here a gospel which is held with a force of feeling of which the gospeller himself seems curiously unaware. What this feeling and play of prejudice was we shall have need to enquire. But I only remark now that Bolingbroke serves our purposes because he acknowledged Locke for his master and because he may be said to represent, and with considerable brilliance and accomplishment, the more or less deistic ideas which were taken up by the men of the time who made little enough pretensions to systematic thinking but liked to be 'up' in ideas and abreast of the time. In Bolingbroke we see the mind of the time as it dwelt in a man of great talent, a brilliant writer, a friend of the best literary men of the time and a statesman who played, for a short time, a spectacular, if in the end a not very influential rôle, in the politics of a most important period in English history. Besides, he was the admired guide, philosopher and friend of Pope and provided most of the ideas amongst which Pope lived and which he expressed in *The Essay on Man* and elsewhere; and what I have now to say about Bolingbroke is very relevant to the study of Pope's philosophical and ethical writings. I shall first briefly recount the main events in Bolingbroke's career and endeavour to give some impression of his personality. I shall then turn to his philosophical writings.

II

Readers of Lecky's *History* will recall the impressive pages in the first chapter in which Lecky speaks of the continuing belief, through the later years of the seventeenth century and on through the reign of

Anne, in the monarch's miraculous powers of healing. William III, indeed, a stranger, had not the power; the Revolution could not claim these extraordinary endowments for the foreign King; but Anne's coming to the throne was a restoration both of the Stuarts and of miraculous royal powers. Everybody knows that Johnson was touched by the Queen; but we may be more impressed when we read in the *Journal to Stella* that Swift urged the Duchess of Osmond 'to get a lad touched for the evil'; but 'the Queen has not been able to touch, and it now grows so warm, I fear she will not at all'. If Swift could thus think and feel, to what excesses of Royalist superstition could not the masses come? Addison's paper in *The Spectator* of 1711 on the superstitions of the times is an exquisite expression of the transition, in the mind of a Whig and a reader of Locke, to our modern ways of feeling. His humour and banter were no doubt more telling than violent denunciation; but they were so because they were an accommodation to the still strong sense of outrageous possibilities; Addison himself has not a mind made up about a number of these things; and Sir Roger needed the restraint of his chaplain to prevent his going witch-hunting. Belief in the kinds of superstition about which Addison wrote was of a piece with those feelings which gathered round the person of the sovereign of lineal descent. The effect of Sacheverell's sermon in 1709 expressed modes of feeling which were destined, indeed, to swift decline; but Lecky could say that 'had the Queen died during the excitement of the Sacheverell agitation, it is more than probable that the Pretender would have at once been summoned to the throne'. In fact, what put the return of the Pretender out of the question was the one thing for which we may honour him: his complete loyalty to his faith; this was the supreme irony of the situation. But if James Edward made it clear that he would not change his religion for a throne, there were plenty of men in England who were still willing to consider him for Anne's successor. Loyalty to him would die hard. Still, it is true that the Church Party were put in an impossible position; they were bound to be divided, falter and fail; and it is interesting to observe the religious background of its two chief leaders as the crisis drew on. Harley came of nonconformist stock, and the most powerful religious influence on St. John's youth was that of his Puritanical grandmother who set him to read theological treatises under the guidance of a nonconformist divine. Harley indeed was no extremist, and trimmed in religion as in politics. But St. John was extreme enough; it was he who voiced the views of Church and Tory as things were drawing to a head.

St. John had reason to dislike Puritanism, perhaps; but he was certainly not a convert to High Church Anglicanism. What sort of religion and what sort of God he believed in we shall see at a later stage; and his morals were as loose as the philosophical thinking with which he advanced, in later days, his egregious deism.

Henry St. John was born in 1678, of two ancient families. He seems to have been brought up by his grandparents, both of them persons of great worth and piety. But St. John's father, a man of his time, passed his lifetime in idleness and pleasure. Writing to Stella on the very day in November 1710 on which he first dined with St. John, Swift said that the Secretary's father 'is a man of pleasure, that walks the Mall, and frequents St. James's Coffee-house, and the chocolate-houses; and the young son is principal Secretary of State. Is there not something very odd in that?' Perhaps there was; but what is certain is that young St. John as he grew up, lacked the guidance of a responsible father, what his excellent grandparents could not hope to make up for.

He was at school at Eton; and from there (as is likely) went to Christ Church. It is unlucky that there is uncertainty about his having resided at Christ Church, and indeed in general about his time at Oxford; Hobbes and Locke had got little enough from their Oxford days; and whether Christ Church was more to St. John's taste than to Locke's we do not know. But in 1702 he was made an Honorary Doctor of Oxford and his name was entered on the books of the college. He thus became, if he had not been before, a Christ Church man. In 1711 Atterbury, the most accomplished High Churchman of his time, was made Dean of Christ Church by the Tory Government in which St. John was Secretary of State; and writing to Stella in March 1712 Swift says: 'I missed the Secretary, and then walked to Chelsea to dine with the Dean of Christ Church, who was engaged to Lord Orrery with some other Christ Church men. He made me go with him whether I would or not, for they have this long time admitted me a Christ Church man'. The Government—Christ Church axis was to become strong, whatever Christ Church thought of Atterbury. But this is to look ahead. Whatever the truth about St. John's residence at Oxford may be, there can be no doubt that when we find him in London in 1697 and then going off, in the same year, on the grand tour, he had a wide knowledge of classical literature; he had great literary gifts and a prodigious memory; he was indeed to have two years of leisure from affairs from 1708 to 1710, when he read extensively; but his reading and knowledge, by the time he was only nineteen, in 1697, must have been truly surprising. The bigger part of the time he was abroad he spent in Paris; and there, he made himself intimate with the French language and acquainted with Matthew Prior. Both his knowledge of French and his friendship with Prior were to bear fruit in later days.

At this time, in his early twenties, he was already a pretty typical rake of the time. But if being a cousin of Rochester was a help to being a rake, it may also have encouraged his literary interest; and we know that he was friendly with Dryden in these last years of Dryden's life. He married in 1700, and in the following year entered Parliament for Wootton Bassett. He at once started to play the High Tory and made a brilliant mark as an orator and debater; his learning, oratorical gifts and personal beauty made him shine out in his party; and his association with Harley, his 'master', began now. But if he was a Tory, he was at this time willing enough, with the other Tories, to put the Act of Settlement on the Statute Book; there was no question in the Tories' minds, now, about the Hanoverian succession; and they were to look back, from 1714, with dismay at what they did in 1701. In 1701 Bolingbroke might conduct his brilliant oratorical campaigns against Whigs; but he was then wholeheartedly a Hanoverian.

William dissolved Parliament late in 1701, and early in the following year the Whigs came back strengthened in their representation in the Commons. William won the hatred of the Tories for thus dissolving a Parliament in which they were so strong; but he passed beyond hatred in March, 1702; and the accession of the new sovereign did not at all affect the will of the new Parliament to make war with Louis; the war about the Spanish successor was declared in May. William's last act, however, had been to sign the Abjuration Bill, by which all holders of office in Church and State were required to swear loyalty to William, then to Anne, and to abjure the Pretender and his heirs as having no right or title to the throne. Some Tories voted in the Bill's favour; most did not, and amongst these was St. John.

Anne's first Parliament, which met in the autumn, was very Tory. The country had been willing to accept the Royal lead. Ministerial changes had been made, since William's death, in favour of the Tories; Godolphin had been made Lord Treasurer and Marlborough Commander of the English and Dutch armies; and this administration, in spite of becoming predominantly Whig as the years passed, was to continue until 1710. In it St. John was to play a brilliant rôle. Now, in 1702, he continued to display his consummate gifts as a Parliamentary performer; and in so predominantly Tory a House, he played the High

Church part to the top of his bent. In the winter of 1702–3 the Occasional Conformity Bill was brought in, and St. John took the lead in getting it through the Commons. Harley, sensible as ever, did not like the Bill; St. John, all too willing to be extremist and doctrinaire for doctrines he did not believe in, got it through the House. Here was an anticipation of what was to happen, in 1714, with the Schism Act, with this difference: that in 1714 Bolingbroke, as he was then to be, was not only being violently and hypocritically doctrinaire, but was also fighting the fairmindedness and fundamental decency of Oxford (as he was then to be) by grossly embarrassing him in order to secure his resignation. It is the part that St. John played, now in 1702 and then in 1714, that marks him down as lacking the commonest honesty. Swift's admiration for St. John was great; but he does not disguise his contempt for just that in St. John to which I have referred; writing to Stella in November 1711, he said: 'I was early with the Secretary today, but he was gone to his devotions. and to receive the Sacrament: several rakes did the same; it was not for piety, but employments; according to Act of Parliament'. The Occasional Conformity Bill was thrown out in the Lords; the execrable Schism Bill was to become law.

The Tories were well in the ascendant till 1704. But there was too little unity amongst them. The Occasional Conformity Bill was again passed in the Commons, and again, with a greater majority than before, thrown out by the Lords. The pendulum was swinging again; and the prosecution of the war, about which the Whigs were wholehearted and the Tories in part unhappy, was bound to weaken the High Tories in the administration. The crisis came in 1704. The High Tories, or most of them, went out; the Administration became a moderate Tory one, the chief architect of which was Harley, always the expert behind the scenes. But it was in this government of mild Toryism that St. John first obtained office. He was made Secretary at War.

We may well be amazed that he should hold such office, when he was only twenty-five. With Marlborough he was to control the military destinies of England for four years in one of its greatest wars. But we may also be surprised that he could take a place in a Ministry from which most of his High Tory friends had been extruded and which the squires certainly had no love for. But he contrived, apparently to his complete satisfaction, to accept office. And here we ought not, perhaps to be censorious: he was still devoted to Harley, and he adored Marlborough; and if he was dazzled by the glitter of high office, he might well also feel called to a labour of high patriotism in taking over the administration of the war. In any case, he kept his office till 1708, to the satisfaction of his colleagues, Marlborough and the nation at large; he bent his great powers, mental and physical, to the detail of his work; his industry and capacity for detail were prodigious; and during his four years of office Blenheim and Ramillies changed the face of the war. His High Toryism was bound, under these circumstances, to suffer some abatement: late in 1704, the High Tories were for tacking the Occasional Conformity Bill to a money bill; but their move was defeated, and St. John voted against it.

In these years Harley was St. John's good genius. Harley was essentially a trimmer, a disbeliever in party-government, a hater of extremes, a maker of balances and tensions; and during these first years of office, St. John was looking, in the manner of Harley, beyond the apparent differences of party, to party-less and therefore faction-less government. This doctrine he was to preach again, in his retirement, in *The Idea of a Patriot King*, at a time when the course of events had made it altogether unpracticable; but now, between 1704 and 1708, it was very much what he believed, taking it over from Harley. 'The real foundation of difference between the two parties', he wrote to Marlborough in 1705, 'is removed, and she (the Queen) seems to throw herself on the gentlemen of England, who had much better have her at the head of 'em than any ringleaders of fashion. Unless gentlemen can show that her administration puts the Church or State in danger, they must own the contest to be about persons: and if it be so, can any honest man hesitate which side to take?'[1] This was his political temper in these years, and it is one we can respect. But he was not to keep it; he had not the steadiness and quietness of mind to sustain it in himself; it was he who above all was to make of Toryism a faction in the last years of Anne's reign, and to ruin Toryism for years to come. Had he stood loyally by the great man whom he now ackowledged for master, and continued to learn from him, it might all have been a different story. But at the heart of him was a vicious and doctrinaire ebullience which he never, except for these four years, tamed. He had every opportunity of learning political wisdom, and chose faction.

So long as the war went on, with all the demands it inevitably made in money, patience and perseverance, the Whigs were bound to loom larger in the administration. With the details of the shiftings of power and the play of intrigue which went on, we need not concern ourselves. Harley intrigued, with the help of Mrs. Masham, to reduce

---

[1] Quoted by Mr. Feiling in *A History of the Tory Party*, 1640-1714, Oxford, 1924, p. 387.

the growing Whig influence; he wanted an administration neither Tory nor Whig, and played his cards accordingly. The Whigs took alarm as they saw a new direction being given to affairs from the Court; Marlborough and Godolphin, above all jealous for the war, felt themselves between the Deep Sea of the Tories and the Whig Devil. St. John must have viewed the situation that was coming about with alarm and dismay: it was likely he would have to choose between his two heroes, Harley and Marlborough. When the crisis came, early in 1708, events turned against Harley; he resigned, and St. John went with him. The Government was now, for all practical purposes, a Whig Government; only Godolphin and Marlborough remained to show that it was in any sense what it had been in 1702.

Harley had come very near to success in his Bedchamber intrigues: but his failure and loss of office, along with the imminent danger to his life in which he stood on account of the discovery of the treason of Greg, one of his secretaries, who might well have bought his life by incriminating Harley however falsely, left him calm. St. John, one supposes, could hardly not resign. Yet Swift, in his letter to Archbishop King on February 12, written after Harley's resignation and before St. John's, does not appear to take it for granted that St. John will go. 'Mr. St. John designs to lay down in a few days, as a friend of his told me, though he advised him to the contrary; and they talk that Mr. Brydges, and Mr. Coke the Vice-chamberlain, with some others, will do the like.'[1] However that may be, he stood by Harley, who was still his better self. But he could not, for some reason, again contest Wootton Bassett; and the Tories went to little trouble to help him to find another seat. He was out and was to remain out until October 1710. His politics then were soon to take another tone. But in the meanwhile, he retired to his country house at Bucklersbury in Berkshire.

At the beginning of his second exile, in 1735, he wrote a letter, addressed to Lord Bathurst, *On the True Use of Retirement and Study*. He wrote it having in mind the last phase of his life on which he was now entering.

This love (of study) and this desire (of knowledge) [he says], I have felt all my life, and I am not quite a stranger to this study and application. There has been something always ready to whisper in my ear, whilst I ran the course of pleasure and of business,

'Solve senescentem mature sanus equum.'

[1] Elrington Ball, *Correspondence of Swift*, London, 1910, vol. i. p. 74.

But my Genius, unlike the demon of Socrates, whispered so softly, that very often I heard him not, in the hurry of those passions by which I was transported. Some calmer hours there were: in them I hearkened to him. Reflection had often it's turn, and the love of study and the desire of knowledge have never quite abandoned me. I am not therefore entirely unprepared for the life I will lead, and it is not without reason that I promise myself more satisfaction in the latter part of it, than I ever knew in the former.'[1]

And he goes on a little later to say:

In short, my lord, he who retires from the world, with a resolution of employing his leisure, in the first place to re-examine and settle his opinions, is inexcusable if he does not begin with those that are most important to him, and if he does not deal honestly by himself. To deal honestly by himself, he must observe the rule I have insisted upon, and not suffer the delusions of the world to follow him into his retreat. Every man's reason is every man's oracle: this oracle is best conducted in the silence of retirement; and when we have so consulted, whatever the decision be, whether in favor of our prejudices or against them, we must rest satisfied: since nothing can be more certain than this, that he who follows that guide in the search of truth, as that was given him to lead him to it, will have a much better plea to make, whenever or wherever he may be called to account, than he, who has resigned himself, either deliberately or inadvertently, to any authority upon earth.

He must, in composing these sentences, have thought of his time of leisure from 1708 to 1710 and have asked himself whether he ought not, then, to have found principles which would have guided him more wisely through the years from 1710 to 1714. We could hardly expect his genius to speak in the manner of the genius of Socrates; but it might have prepared him to stand loyally by his political 'master'. We may fairly complain about St. John that these quiet years did not save him from the passions which animated him during the last years of the reign. He was to say a good deal in his philosophical writings of reason and passion. In fact he was himself, in Chesterfield's words, 'a most mortifying instance of the violence of human passions, and of the weakness of the most improved and exalted human reason'.[2]

The apparent endlessness of the war, the financial strain it involved, and then the Whigs' impeachment of Sacheverell made it possible for Harley, with the help of Shrewsbury, another of the great Trimmers, to play, in the course of 1710, for a redressing of the balance of the parties in the Administration. They worked their subtle way behind the

[1] *Letters on the Study and Use of History*, London, 1770, pp. 414–15.
[2] *Letters of Chesterfield*, ed. Lord Mahon, London, 1845, vol. ii. p. 449.

scenes. The Duchess of Marlborough had been dismissed in April; and moves were now made to strengthen the Tories in the Government. Harley wanted a coalition and no more; and he plotted Godolphin's dismissal in August to that end; but the General Election of October, which showed the folly of the impeachment of Sacheverell, made a Tory Government inevitable. The year 1710 saw, whether for good or evil, a most important stage in the growth of Party government in England; it was the turn of the Tories now; it would be the turn of the Whigs before long.

In such a purely Party administration Harley, who became Lord Treasurer, virtually Prime Minister, in 1711, was bound to be unhappy. He did not want thus to be committed and would have preferred coalition. St. John, on the other hand, fired by this Tory victory as he had been fired by the Tory victory of 1702, swung with zest into the Party game. He became one of the two Secretaries of State; and it was soon clear that Harley was no longer his 'master' in politics. He was to say frankly, at a later date, in his *Letter to Sir William Wyndham*, what it was that animated him at this time:

I am afraid that we came to court in the same dispositions as all parties have done; that the principal spring of our actions was to have the government of the state in our hands; that our principal views were the conservation of this power, great employments to ourselves, and great opportunities of rewarding those who had helped to raise us, and of hurting those who stood in opposition to us. It is however true, that with these considerations of private and party interest there were others intermingled, which had for their object the public good of the nation, at least what we took to be such.

A little later he says:

. . . From hence we judged it to follow, that they [the Whigs] had been forced, and must continue so, to render the national interest subservient to the interest of those who lent them an additional strength, without which they could never be the prevalent party. The view, therefore, of those amongst us, who thought in this manner, was to improve the queen's favor to break the body of the whigs, to render their supports useless to them, and to fill the employments of the kingdom, down to the meanest, with tories. We imagined that such measures, joined to the advantages of our members and our property, would secure us against all attempts during her reign; and that we should soon become too considerable, not to make our terms in all events which might happen afterwards: concerning which, to speak truly, I believe few or none of us had any very settled resolution.

All this is at least frank enough; and describing the respective reputations in the House of Commons of himself and Harley as time went on, he says a little later:

In the house of commons his credit was low, and my reputation very high. You know the nature of that assembly: they grow, like hounds, fond of the man who shews them game, and by whose halloo they are used to be encouraged.

The image was all too apposite. St. John went back to be what he had been from 1702 to 1704. It was here, during the first session of the new Government, that St. John made the blunder of his life, in beginning to drift from Harley; his flight from England in 1715 was only secondary to this. It was early in 1711 that Harley and St. John began to move apart; and Harley was convinced that St. John's wish to send an expedition to Quebec, which they discussed in March, arose, in part at least, from St. John's need to obtain money quickly by illicit commissions. Things were not made better by the events which then occurred. Harley was stabbed by Guiscard, a treacherous spy, in March, and bore himself calmly and nobly in the event and during his illness. His popularity revived in the national anxiety; on his recovery he was made Earl of Oxford; and St. John's jealousy was all the greater for his failure to manage the House of Commons in the place of Harley during his illness. It would not be long before he too would be in the Lords, but, to his bitterness, a Viscount only, not an Earl. Had he been steadier, and been urged by reason and not by insensate passion, he might now, acting in loyalty to Oxford, have led the Commons while Oxford led the Lords. But this would have required a diminution of his High Toryism in the interests of sanity; it would also have needed a greatness and an insight he did not possess. He preferred the Lords and disloyalty to his chief. 'He had', said Chesterfield, 'noble and general sentiments, rather than fixed, reflected principles of good-nature and friendship; but they were more violent than lasting, and suddenly and often varied to their opposite extremes, with regard even to the same persons'.

To follow the events of these four years up to the death of Anne is not necessary for our purpose. Three things may be said. First, the Master of Trinity has told us[1] that we must not exaggerate, after the fashion of St. John's contemporaries and of later historians, the part St. John played in the negotiations which led finally to the Peace of

[1] G. M. Trevelyan, *The Peace and the Protestant Succession*, London, 1934, p. 177

Utrecht in 1713. 'Already, . . . before St. John had been admitted into
the secret, the broadest outline of the Peace had been agreed on between
England and France', says Mr. Trevelyan. But during Harley's absence
from business after the stabbing, St. John came to know of what was
going on, and from this time it was he who took over the negotiations. That Harley should so long have kept the secret from St. John
surprises us the less, because it seems that during all the play of intrigue
in 1710, after the impeachment of Sacheverell and before the election,
to reduce the number of the Whigs in the Cabinet, St. John does not
seem to have been in Harley's confidence. However that may be, there
can be no doubt of the vigour, single-mindedness and courage with
which St. John conducted the negotiations from this time on. No one
can like the duplicity whereby the Peace was finally brought about; but
it seems certain that if it was to be brought about so soon, duplicity
was inevitable; and in any case, in the last resort, Harley had initiated
the discussions and must, with the rest of the Government, share the
responsibility. On the terms of the Treaty history has given a favourable verdict; we are not likely to have a better informed or more im-
partial verdict than that which Mr. Trevelyan gives in the preface to
The Peace and the Protestant Succession; and on p. 230 he says that Bolingbroke 'stands in history as the man who, by courses however devious
and questionable, negotiated a Peace which proved in the working
more satisfactory than any other that has ended a general European
conflict in modern times'.

Secondly, we said that the conduct of foreign affairs passed, early in
1711, into St. John's confident hands. Here was something satisfactory enough: it made for jealousy, but on the issue of the Peace,
Oxford and Harley had no differences. But it was domestic affairs and
the matter of the Succession which were most troublesome. The latter
indeed was not a thing wholly separate from the peace-making: in
August 1712 Bolingbroke (he had been made Viscount Bolingbroke
in July) went to Paris, was lionized by Parisian society and received by
the Grand Monarch; and this was bound to fan in him the smouldering
Jacobite fires. (We have come far from the day, in September 1651,
when Evelyn stood with Hobbes at the window of Hobbes's apartments
in Paris to watch 'the whole equipage and glorious cavalcade of the
young French Monarch, Louis XIV, passing to Parliament, when first
he took the kingly government on him, now being in his 14th year,' as
Evelyn tells us in the *Diary*. Hobbes was there an exile, with Charles II;
now Bolingbroke came, in the days of another Stuart exile, and when

he entered the Paris theatre (where *Le Cid* was being performed) the whole house rose to him; but he was to be back, in 1715, himself an exile.) Certainly the visit to Paris must have encouraged doubtful ideas; and to negotiate a Peace with and be thus acclaimed by France might be wise for the nation and bad for the negotiator. Besides, such a peace could hardly be desirable in the eyes of the Hanoverian heir.

But in fact Harley had been engaged in doubtful intrigue with the Pretender since the autumn of 1710, and it was to continue as long as he held office. Harley had been indeed vague enough in all that went on, and the French agents despaired of getting anything definite from him; he was always saying that everything must wait upon the Peace; and after the Peace he continued to be vague and inscrutable. Bolingbroke, on his side, was deeply engaged in the Peace negotiations from 1711 to 1713 and had little to do with the Pretender before the Treaty was signed. He had, indeed, in October 1712, been in correspondence with Gaultier, one of the agents; but in general there is little before March 1713 to justify thinking of him as deeply involved; and up to a few months of Oxford's dismissal in July 1714 the Pretender and those with him inevitably attached more importance to Oxford than to Bolingbroke.[1] Then indeed, as Oxford's position in the Administration grew weaker, Bolingbroke looms larger in the eyes of the Pretender and those around him; but always Bolingbroke insisted, as Oxford also insisted, that James Edward must abjure Catholicism. It is clear that Bolingbroke never questioned that a Catholic king was unthinkable.

Still, the difference between Oxford and Bolingbroke, as we see it in the record of their political lives, certainly encourages us to believe that Bolingbroke, altogether more impetuous, daring and doctrinaire than Oxford, must have entertained the thought of a Restoration with more warmth than Oxford; and we know that he wished systematically to place High Tories and Jacobites in the public service and the Army. This plan Oxford, supported by the Queen, steadily resisted; and when Oxford went, in July 1714, the Queen would not give the leading place in the Administration to Bolingbroke. She had only a few days to live; but she was too like Oxford in her political judgement and too different from Bolingbroke to entrust Bolingbroke with the highest power. She had at last let Oxford go; she would not let Bolingbroke succeed him. Bolingbroke had only a few days in which to act. He set about making a High Tory Administration; he also suggested to

[1] *English Historical Review*, vol. lii. H. N. Fieldhouse, "Bolingbroke's Share in the Jacobite Intrigue of 1710–14," pp. 449–51.

the Whigs that they form a coalition with him: what Oxford would always have liked and what Bolingbroke had done his best to make impossible. Had the Queen lived, and had Bolingbroke succeeded in contriving a High Tory Government, it is incredible that he would have tried to ensure that England have a Catholic king; and Queen or no Queen, the Whigs could have nothing to do with Jacobites or would-be Jacobites. As it was, the Queen lasted only a few days; and she nominated Shrewsbury, a Whig and one of the great and indispensible Trimmers of the age, to be Lord Treasurer; and the Hanoverian succession was assured. It seems certain that despite all the intrigue they had carried on with the Pretender, neither Oxford nor Bolingbroke had really wanted a Stuart Restoration. Oxford was only keeping issues open, and was certainly only concerned for the welfare of the nation as a whole; Bolingbroke was thinking of himself, his career and a section of the nation, and therefore could be less trusted not to do rash and disastrous things. Had Bolingbroke kept Oxford for his 'master', they might well together have held the Tory party firmly to the Act of Settlement and saved it from collapse.

But (thirdly), Bolingbroke's conduct had made this impossible; he had done everything to make Oxford's habitual moderation ineffective. It is natural to contrast Bolingbroke's brilliance during these last years of the reign with the increasing ineffectiveness of Oxford. Oxford was indeed in an impossible position. He was the leader of what he had always wished to avoid, a Party administration, with an altogether too great majority behind it. Given, over against him, a man of brilliant powers all too ready to show the hounds the game and to encourage them with halloos, his life was bound to become wretched and his position desperate: as the years passed, he could only hang on, allay what mischief he could for as long as he could, and hope that his own temperate attitude would finally win. There is a profound sense in which he was indeed successful: he clung to office to within a few days of Anne's death; and then it was to Shrewsbury, like himself an eminently temperate and disinterested spirit, that the Lord Treasurership passed.

But it is true that from early in 1712 Oxford became a sad figure. In December 1711 the Government had been defeated in the Lords on their Peace policy: a temporary alliance of High Tories and Whigs passed, at last, an Occasional Conformity Bill, and a motion forbidding the Government to leave Spain to a Bourbon. But in reply, Oxford advised the Queen to create twelve Tory peers, and this she did; he

dished the Whigs and created a mighty precedent. We may assume
that however effective the decision was, it was not one after Oxford's
heart. It was too much a manœurve in the Party game; and Bolingbroke, in his exile, when he returned to the mind of his 'master', deplored it. Oxford must have roused himself in some bitterness to make
this decision; and though he saved the Peace by it, he afterwards
deteriorated. His health became bad; he drank too much; and he fell
into irresolution and inertia. He felt himself beaten; but he would still
carry on as long as he could. But in the meantime St. John was at his
best in the Peace negotiations, and at his most powerful and factious
in the House of Commons. The hounds were in full cry, and he led
attacks on Walpole and Marlborough for corruption: Walpole was
imprisoned and Marlborough dismissed. These were the days, late in
1711 and early in 1712, when *The Conduct of the Allies* was selling by its
thousands and when Addison brought Sir Roger to town; they were
also St. John's greatest days: we can perhaps sympathize with him for
his bitterness when in July he became only a viscount. But he was
bound to be consoled by his reception in Paris in the following month.
Now, in all truth, he was at his apogee. But it was all at the expense of
his friendship with Oxford; feeling between them became worse.
Swift tried hard in the autumn to make them friends, but he was not
successful.[1]

In April 1713 the Queen announced in Parliament the signing of the
Treaties of Peace; but the Commercial Treaty with France, in which
Bolingbroke passionately believed and which was later to be judged
far-sighted, was defeated. Oxford showed little enthusiasm for them,
and Bolingbroke's bitterness towards him was further exacerbated.
Besides, Oxford was dealing with the Whigs; with the Peace through,
he was willing enough to entertain the thought of an alliance with them
to save the Act of Settlement. But Bolingbroke led a counter-move-
ment of the High Tories: there were too many Whigs, they said, in the
Army and Public Services. Now, more than ever, Oxford's position
was intolerable: he could neither effect a coalition nor suffer High Tory
mischief to go unchecked; and in the autumn he nearly resigned. In
that autumn, also, the Tories came back from the General Election
with their power little reduced; and it had generally been thought that a
victory for them would mean an attack on nonconformity. Certainly
Oxford was now, as ever, for moderation. But Bolingbroke was for
faction. Could Bolingbroke now, after this fateful election, have

[1] *Journal to Stella*, September 15, 1712.

recovered something of the political sensibility he possessed from 1704 to 1708, he and Oxford could easily have decided the Tory party to be clearly for the Hanoverian succession; that they did not do so is far more the fault of Bolingbroke than of Oxford. Instead, Bolingbroke took violent measures against both Oxford and the nonconformists. The Schism Act, designed to destroy nonconformist education, was brought in and passed in June 1714. It stood for everything in life and politics which Oxford loathed; it stood for nothing that Boling-broke loved, except selfishness, intolerance and hypocrisy. There can hardly be a spectacle in English history more nauseating than this of a profligate deist pleading for the destruction of nonconformity in the name of the Established Church. But in fact, it was the spirit of Harley which was, for much the bigger part, to survive; and Bolingbroke was to pay for his mingled stupidity and hypocrisy with long years of bitter exile which, to crown the justice of the course of events, he brought upon himself by his unnecessary flight in 1715. The irony of history is nowhere more clearly shown than in the summer of 1714. The Schism Act was to come into force on August 1. On that day the Queen died, and the White Staff was in Shrewsbury's hands.

III

The story of Bolingbroke's life after 1715 is, for obvious reasons, less complicated, and may be told more briefly. Bolingbroke was only thirty-six when Anne died, and he was not again to be a minister of the Crown, nor even, indeed, except for a few days in 1715, again to sit in Parliament.

If Bolingbroke hoped, in 1714, that he might yet find a place for himself in the government of England, he was soon to be disillusioned. He got no mercy. At the end of August he was dismissed from his secretaryship and was succeeded by Townshend. George I showed no signs of playing the Patriot King: there was no question of an all-party Cabinet. In the elections of January 1715, a royal proclamation asked for a Whig majority and got it. Walpole made it clear that the members of the former Government would be punished; and when, in March, the two ambassadors, Strafford and Prior, who had negotiated the Peace, were recalled for examination, Bolingbroke took fright. Marl-borough added to his fears by warning him that serious trouble was bound to come; and on March 28th Bolingbroke crossed to Calais. Oxford, for his part, set about collecting documents to prove his innocence and showed no signs of panic; when Bolingbroke suggested to him that they should take joint action in their defence, he declined the offer.

Bolingbroke's flight has always been thought to be a prime blunder; he himself could not fail, in due course, to judge it to be so. Oxford stayed quietly where he was, and after being impeached and imprisoned in the Tower for two years, was acquitted. But had all the correspondence with France in 1713 and 1714 been available, it would have been seen that Bolingbroke was in no worse case than Oxford.[1] But Oxford's staying where he was and Bolingbroke's flight showed again a fundamental difference between the two men. As it was, he was attainted of high treason in September and his property confiscated. It was not until 1723 that he was pardoned and allowed to return to England.

Before the Act of Attainder was passed, he joined the cause of the Pretender, and became his Secretary of State. But his relations with the Pretender were unhappy and were not to last long. The '15 was entered on against Bolingbroke's wishes; and when James Edward returned to France from the Rising, he dismissed him from his service. No doubt this was chiefly an act of anger, done in disappointment; but it looked, for a time, as if it might do Bolingbroke some good; there was a chance that he might now be pardoned; but he would not inform against others; and the Government hardened its heart. There were to be seven more years of exile. It was now, in 1716, that he wrote his *Reflections on Exile* and the famous *Letter to Sir William Wyndham*, a brillaint composition, in which he reviewed the politics of the years from 1710 to 1715. From 1720 to 1723 he lived on his small estate of La Source, near Orleans; here he gave himself up to study and here Voltaire came to meet and admire him. But his heart was in England and politics, and he made advances for his pardon. He obtained it at last early in 1723. In June he made a short visit to England, passing Atterbury, who was on his way to banishment in France. In 1714, when Anne died, Atterbury had wanted to proclaim James III at the Royal Exchange; Bolingbroke told him then that they would only get their throats cut. But Atterbury had remained a fervid supporter of the Pretender and had helped to plot trouble the year before. Now the two Christ Church men were changing places, 'being exchanged', as Atterbury said. But Walpole saw to it that Bolingbroke did not take his seat in the Lords; in 1725 a Bill enabled him to enjoy his estates, but he might not sit in Parliament or hold public office.

[1] G. M. Trevelyan, *The Peace and the Protestant Succession*, p. 248.

From now, in 1725, until 1742 (when he still had nine years to live) he was to be active in opposition to Walpole. He bought an estate near Oxbridge, called Dawley, which was to be a shining centre for literature and politcal opposition. Pope was not far away, in Twickenham, and they were to see a great deal of each other in these next years: they were to be very important in Pope's literary career.

> That not in Fancy's Maze he wander'd long,
> But stoop'd to Truth, and moraliz'd his song,

was something he had to thank Bolingbroke for. He says, himself, addressing his guide, philosopher and friend in the last lines of the *Essay on Man*,

> That urg'd by Thee, I turn'd the tuneful art
> From sounds to things, from Fancy to the heart.

He was to enter now, under Bolingbroke's tuition, on what he was to consider, when writing the *Epistle to Arbuthnot* in 1735, his greatest period. He had in fact wandered for quite a long time in 'Fancy's Maze'; but soon, after *The Dunciad*, would come *The Essay on Man*, *The Moral Essays*, and the *Imitations of Horace*, all composed under Bolingbroke's influence. The great bulk of these were written between 1730 and 1735; and in these years Bolingbroke was writing those philosophical letters and essays addressed to Pope which we shall study in the succeeding sections of this chapter, but which are undated in Mallet's edition. There are four completed essays: *Concerning the Nature, Extent and Reality of Human Knowledge; On the Folly and Presumption of Philosophers, especially in matters of the First Philosophy; Containing some further Reflections on the Rise and Progress of Monotheism; Concerning Authority in matters of Religion*. These four *Essays* are followed, in the *Philosophical Works*, by a considerable number of what Bolingbroke calls *Fragments or Minutes of Essays*; they occupy the last third or so of the third volume, the whole of the fourth and about a half of the fifth and last, in Mallet's edition of the *Philosophical Works* (1754). These are preceded by an *Advertisement*, written by Bolingbroke, which I shall quote from (vol. 3, p. 334):

The foregoing Essays, if they may deserve that name, and the Fragments or Minutes that follow, were thrown upon paper in Mr. Pope's lifetime, and at his desire. They were all communicated to him in scraps, as they were occasionally writ. But the latter not having been connected and put together under different heads, and in the same order as the former had been, before his death, if that may be called order; I have contented myself to correct and extend them a little, and to leave them as Fragments, or Minutes, in the form in which they appear, tho they might be styled Essays with no more impropriety than those which precede them. They are all nothing more than repetitions of conversations often interrupted, often renewed, and often carried on a little confusedly. The opinions I held are exposed as clearly, as they ought to be by a man who thinks his opinions founded in truth. I thought, and I think still, that mine were so . . .

This is an interesting statement. It declares the manner of their composition; the Essays, he says, are 'scraps' put together and the Fragments are scraps which he could not conveniently arrange into 'Essays'. But in the spring of 1731, writing to Swift, he says:

In the mean time Pope has given me more trouble than he or I thought of; and you will be surprised to find that I have been partly drawn by him, and partly by myself, to write a pretty large volume upon a very grave and very important subject: that I have ventured to pay no regard whatever to any authority except a sacred authority, and that I have ventured to start a thought which must . . . render all your metaphysical theology both ridiculous and abominable.[1]

This suggests that he is setting out to write a systematic treatise; and this indeed is the impression we get from the Introductory Letter which precedes the first Essay. But in fact the bulk of the philosophical works as we have them certainly look like something composed after the fashion spoken of in the Advertisement. If so, it is interesting to remark that it was in much the same way that Pope composed the Essay on Man: 'I have many fragments which I am beginning to put together, but nothing perfect or finished, nor in any condition to be shown, except to a friend at the fireside', he told Caryll in December 1730.[2]

Besides we observe that the Essays and Fragments were written down after conversations with Pope, at Pope's wish and sent along to him piecemeal. We may assume that the crucial conversations occurred from 1729 to 1731; for writing in November 1729, Bolingbroke told Swift that Pope was at work on the 'Ethic Epistles',[3] the name of the proposed entire work which would include the Essay on Man and the Moral Essays; Pope told Swift[3] the same thing; and in October 1730 Bolingbroke told Lord Bathurst that he and Pope were 'deep in metaphysics'.[4] In August 1731, he writes to Swift: 'Does Pope talk to you

---

[1] Works of Swift, ed. Scott, Edinburgh, 1824, vol. xvii. pp. 377–78
[2] Elwin and Courthope's The Works of Pope, vol. ii. p. 273.
[3] Ibid., vol. vii. pp. 175–6.   [4] Ibid., vol. viii. p. 340.

of the noble work, which, at my instigation, he has begun in such a manner, that he must be convinced by this time, I judged better of his talents than he did?'[1] And he goes on to say that the first three epistles are finished. These were the first three parts of the *Essay on Man*, which were not however to be published until 1733. In the Introductory Letter to Pope which precedes the first Essay, Bolingbroke refers to Pope's having begun the 'Ethic Epistles';[2] in the first Essay itself the 'Third Ethic Epistle' is spoken of (vol. 1, p. 35); and in the second Essay (vol. 1. p. 309) Bolingbroke quotes from the closing lines of the fourth epistle of the *Essay on Man* on which, he declares, in the letter of August 1731 from which I have just quoted, Pope was at that time working hard. These facts confirm what Bolingbroke says in his Advertisement, that the Essays and Fragments were written after their long and frequent conversations: it was on the conversations, not on the Essays, that Pope chiefly drew for the *Essay on Man*; the Essays and Fragments were only, says Bolingbroke, 'repetitions of conversations'. But it seems likely that it was after 1735, when he withdrew to France, that he revised and extended the Fragments; he may also have worked on the Essays; and in the fifth of the Letters in *The Study and Use of History*, which he wrote at that time, we find him quoting the *Essay on Man* on self-love and saying: 'So sings our friend Pope, my lord, and so I believe. So I shall prove too, if I mistake not, in an epistle I am about to write to him, in order to complete a set that were writ some years ago.' Whether he did as he says, we do not know; nor, if he did, what part of the *Philosophical Works* it constitutes. Nor can we know how much he revised the Fragments and Essays.

There is however reason to believe that Bolingbroke did more for the *Essay on Man* than talk to its author. Boswell quotes, in the *Life of Johnson*, a letter from Blair in which Blair declares that he was told by Lord Bathurst that the *Essay on Man* 'was originally composed by Lord Bolingbroke in prose, and that Mr. Pope did no more than put it into verse'.[3] Johnson would not have this; it was, he says, 'too strongly stated'. No doubt it was. But Spence records that Pope told him that 'beside their frequent talking over that subject together, he had received, I think, seven or eight sheets from Lord Bolingbroke in

---

[1] Elwin and Courthorpe's *The Works of the Pope*, vol. vii. p. 247.
[2] *Works of Bolingbroke*, London, 1777, vol. iii. p. 312.
In the 1754 edition of the *Philosophical Works* this introductory letter to Pope is not printed. All other references to the philosophical works of Bolingbroke are to Mallet's 1754 edition.
[3] Birkbeck Hill's edition of Boswell's *Life*, vol. iii. p. 402.

relation to it (as I apprehended by way of letters), both to direct the plan in general, and to supply the matter for the particular epistles'.[1] It may be that it was these sheets Bathurst saw. But we may well follow Johnson and agree that he exaggerated.

The *Essays* and *Fragments* were published in 1754, three years after Bolingbroke's death. Johnson's observation on them and their author is well known: 'Sir, he was a scoundrel, and a coward: a scoundrel, for charging a blunderluss against religion and morality; a coward, because he had not the resolution to fire it off himself, but left half a crown to a beggarly Scotchman, to draw the trigger after his death'. Their publication followed soon upon Bolingbroke's death. But if they were published as late as the fifties, after being written in the early thirties, there can be little doubt that they set out what had been Bolingbroke's beliefs from a much earlier time. In the letter of August 2, 1731, to Swift, when he was writing hard, he said: 'As far as I am able to recollect, my way of thinking has been uniform enough for more than twenty years'.[2] This takes us back to the years he spent at Bucklersbury from 1708 to 1710, when, as in 1731, he was at leisure to read and study. It was then, in that brief interlude between his two periods of office, that he laid the foundations, for what they were worth, of his philosophy.

But it is not only in the *Essay on Man* that we see chiefly the influence of Bolingbroke on Pope. It is to be seen also in the *Moral Essays*; it was Bolingbroke who suggested the idea of the *Imitations of Horace*; and it was he who inspired the patriotism of the *Epilogue to the Satires*. If these were indeed the days of Pope's greatest work, Bolingbroke certainly had a lot to do with it. At the end of the letter, *On the True Use of Retirement and Study*, to which I have already referred, and which was written after he returned again to France in 1735, he said: 'In the mean time, let me refer you to our friend, Pope. He says I made a philosopher of him: I am sure he has contributed very much, and I thank him for it, to the making a hermit of me'.

In 1735 he left England. He was disappointed and exasperated by the course of English politics and went to France where he was to stay until June 1738. From 1725 to 1735 his aim in politics had been to unite all elements of opposition to Walpole. Dawley and his London house were meeting-places of diverse factions which were united only in their dislike of Walpole. There were Whigs 'malcontent' with Walpole, whose leader was the accomplished William Pulteney; there

[1] Elwin and Courthope, vol. ii. p. 275.
[2] *Ibid.*, vol. vii. p. 243.

were Hanoverian Tories led by Sir William Wyndham; and there were Jacobites led by William Shippen. All these Bolingbroke sought to bring together; and as the years passed Whigs kept coming over to them. Cartaret came in 1730, Chesterfield in 1733; and in that year also the 'Boy Patriots', amongst whom was young Cornet Pitt, joined the ranks. They were a brilliant assortment, and on their side were the literary men, Swift, Pope, Gay, Arbuthnot, Fielding. To crown it, Frederick, Prince of Wales, became after 1728 their nominal leader. Bolingbroke and Pulteney joined forces in 1725; and in December 1726 the first number of *The Craftsman* appeared. It was to run for ten years, with Bolingbroke and Pulteney its most powerful contributors: the former's *Remarks on the History of England* and *Dissertation on Parties* appeared in its pages. But Walpole had other means than literature of maintaining his power. *The Craftsman* was by no means ineffective; it played a notable part in compelling Walpole to withdraw the Excise Bill of 1733, and ultimately in bringing about war with Spain in 1739; but when, in 1734, in spite of the defeat of the Excise Bill, Walpole's power was proved unshaken by the election, Bolingbroke lost heart. In 1735 he dropped his connexion with Pulteney; the alliance had inevitably been a superficial one; Bolingbroke's ideas about government at this time, which he was soon to set out in *The Patriot King* and which were really those of his old political 'master', were not shared by Whigs, whether in power like Walpole or out of it like Pulteney; and he and his ideas were bound to be, in the last resort, more of an embarrassment to the Opposition than a help. Walpole had won; but from now on he became increasingly aware of the power of Pitt in whom much of the spirit and thought of Bolingbroke was to live on. In the forties, when Bolingbroke was old and fretful, Pitt would go down to Battersea to talk with him.

Bolingbroke was to take little more part in politics. It was now, in retiring to France that he wrote *On the True Use of Retirement and Study*, *On the Spirit of Patriotism*, in which he attacked Whigs and Tories for their feebleness in opposition, and *On the Study and the Use of History*. He returned to England in 1738 for two months. His writings in France were those of a man who had done with politics. But in 1737 Queen Caroline, who had supported Walpole so faithfully, died, and Bolingbroke's political hopes rose again, building themselves up around Frederick, Prince of Wales. It was now he wrote *The Idea of a Patriot King*, in its first draft, which he passed to Pope. But so long as the malcontent Whigs were only set on changing one Whig ministry for another, there was little Bolingbroke could do; and when, in 1740, Sir William Wyndham died, any lingering hopes of a coalition which Bolingbroke still cherished were destroyed. In 1742 Walpole fell at last. Bolingbroke came over from France; but Pulteney and Carteret went into alliance with members of Walpole's ministry to form another Whig Administration. It was only what he had expected. But hope had died hard.

In 1744 he settled finally in England and went soon to live in the old Manor House in Battersea in which he had been born and brought up. He was in touch with the 'Boy Patriots', and his interest in politics did not flag. But it was in 1744 that Pope died; and in the following year the Rebellion must have given Bolingbroke long thoughts. In 1745, too, Swift died, dying, as he had feared he would, like a rat in a hole; he had gone back to Ireland, in 1723, for the last time. It must have seemed a long time to Bolingbroke since Swift had come over in 1726, with the manuscript of *Gulliver* in his pocket, and Pope had had him, Bolingbroke, Congreve and Gay to dinner at Twickenham. Since then, of the Triumvirate, as Swift had called them, only Pope had had lasting success. And when, in 1749, Bolingbroke published *The Idea of a Patriot King*, he prefaced it with a virulent attack on Pope who had, he found, published in 1741 the draft of the essay which he had given him in 1738. Pope had then been dead five years; Bolingbroke had been at his death-bed and was inexpressibly grieved. It was a pity that so memorable a literary friendship should end in this way. In March 1751 Bolingbroke's wife, to whom he had been devoted, died; and he himself died in the following December, when he was seventy-three years old. He bore his final and terrible illness 'with firmness', Chesterfield tells us. 'A week before he died', Chesterfield goes on, 'I took my last leave of him with grief; and he returned me his last farewell with tenderness, and said, "God who placed me here, will do what he pleases with me hereafter; and he knows best what to do. May he bless you."'

There is no doubt about the immense fascination which Bolingbroke had for his contemporaries. The praise of him by the two greatest writers of his age is almost unqualified. This is what Swift said, writing to Stella in November 1711,

I think Mr. St. John the greatest young man I ever knew; wit, capacity, beauty, quickness of apprehension, good learning, and an excellent taste; the best orator in the House of Commons, admirable conversation, good nature, and good manners; generous and a despiser of money. His only fault is talking to his friends in way of complaint of too great a load of business, which looks a little like affectation; and he endeavours too much to mix the fine gentleman and man of pleasure with the man of business. What truth and sincerity he may have I know not: he is now but thirty-two, and has been Secretary above a year. Is not all this extraordinary?

And Pope, writing to Swift in 1736 after reading the *Letters on History*, said: 'Nothing can depress his genius. Whatever befalls him, he will still be the greatest man in the world, either in his own time, or with posterity.'[1] Of all his gifts, it was his gift of speech, whether in conversation or in oratory, that most dazzled his contemporaries. Chesterfield said that 'he adorned whatever subject he either spoke or wrote upon by the most splendid eloquence; not a studied or laboured eloquence, but such a glowing happiness of diction, which (from care perhaps at first) is become so habitual to him, that even his most familiar conversations, if taken down in writing, would have borne the press, without the least correction, either as to method or to style'; and Pitt used to say that of all lost works, ancient or modern, he would choose first to have a speech of Bolingbroke.

Bolingbroke himself wrote about oratory; and he did so, in *The Spirit of Patriotism*, in a way which recalls Cicero in the *De Oratore*. It may well be that in doing so, he had Cicero in mind. Cicero had been exiled in 58 B.C., and had returned in 57 B.C. to the acclamation of Rome. But then came the meeting of Pompey and Caesar at Luca, and Cicero decided that opposition would be useless; he withdrew from the Courts and the Senate, and composed the *De Oratore*. Bolingbroke had been exiled, for a longer time indeed than Cicero; but he had come back, also with acclamation. Then came his long struggle in opposition, but now, in 1736, he had despaired of it and came into retreat, and to write. Like Cicero he might now say, *refero ad mansuetiores Musas, quae me maxime sicut iam a prima adulescentia delectarunt*. And here, where he speaks of eloquence we cannot forbear to think he had the argument of Cicero in the first book of *De Oratore* in mind. I have the less hesitation in quoting this passage at length, because the philosophical writings, written 'scrappily', do not give a fair impression of Bolingbroke's eloquence and commanding powers of composition.

Eloquence has charms to lead mankind, and gives a nobler superiority than power, that every dunce may use, or fraud, that every knave may employ. But eloquence must flow like a stream that is fed by an abundant spring, and not spout forth a little frothy water on some gaudy day, and remain dry the rest of the year. The famous orators of *Greece* and *Rome* were

---

[1] Elwin and Courthope, vol. vii. p. 342.

the statesmen and ministers of those commonwealths. The nature of their governments, and the humour of those ages made elaborate orations necessary. They harangued oftener than they debated; and the *ars dicendi* required more study and more exercise of mind, and of body too, amongst them, than are necessary among us. But as much pains as they took in learning how to conduct the stream of eloquence, they took more to enlarge the fountain from which it flowed. Hear DEMOSTHENES, hear CICERO, thunder against PHILIP, CATILINE, and ANTHONY. I chuse the example of the first, rather than that of PERICLES, whom he imitated, or of PHOCION, whom he opposed, or of any other considerable personage in *Greece*; and the example of CICERO rather than that of CRASSUS or of HORTENSIUS, or of any other of the great men of *Rome*; because the eloquence of these two has been so celebrated, that we are accustomed to look upon them almost as *mere orators*. They were orators indeed, and no man who has a soul can read their orations, after the revolution of so many ages, after the extinction of the governments, and of the people for whom they were composed, without feeling, at this hour, the passions they were designed to move, and the spirit they were designed to raise. But if we look into the history of these two men, and consider the parts they acted, we shall see them in another light, and admire them in an higher sphere of action. DEMOSTHENES had been neglected, in his education, by the same tutors who cheated him of his inheritance. CICERO was bred with greater advantage: and PLUTARCH, I think, says, that when he first appeared the people used to call him, by way of derision, the *Greek*, and the scholar. But whatever advantage of this kind the latter might have over the former, and to which of them soever you ascribe the superior genius, the progress which both of them made in every part of *political knowledge*, by their industry and application, was marvellous. CICERO might be a better philosopher, but DEMOSTHENES was no less a statesman: and both of them performed actions, and acquired fame, above the reach of eloquence alone. DEMOSTHENES used to compare eloquence to a weapon, aptly enough; for eloquence, like every other weapon, is of little use to the owner, unless he have the force and the skill to use it. This force and this skill DEMOSTHENES had in an eminent degree. Observe them in one instance among many. It was of mighty importance to PHILIP, to prevent the accession of *Thebes* to the grand alliance that DEMOSTHENES, at the head of the Athenian commonwealth, formed against the growing power of the Macedonians, PHILIP had emissaries and his ambassadors on the spot, to oppose to those of *Athens*, and we may be assured that he neglected none of those arts upon this occasion, that he employed so successfully on others. The struggle was great, but DEMOSTHENES prevailed, and the Thebans engaged in the war against PHILIP. Was it by his eloquence alone that he prevailed, in a divided state, over all the subtilty of intrigue, all the dexterity of negotiation, all the seduction, all the corruption, and all the terror that the ablest and most powerful prince could employ? Was DEMOSTHENES wholly taken up with composing orations, and haranguing the people in this remarkable crisis? He harangued them, no doubt, at *Thebes*, as well as at *Athens*, and in the rest of *Greece*, where all the great resolutions of making alliances, waging war, or concluding peace, were determined in democratical assemblies. But yet haranguing was, no doubt, the least part of his business, and eloquence was neither the sole, nor the principal talent, as the style of writers would induce us to believe, on which his success depended. He must have been master of other arts, subserviently to which his eloquence was employed, and must have had a thorough knowledge of his own state, and of the other states of *Greece*, of their dispositions, and of their interests relatively to one another, and relatively to their neighbours, to the *Persians* particularly, with whom he held a correspondence, not much to his honor in appearance, whatever he might intend by it: I say, he must have been master of many other arts, and have possessed an immense fund of knowledge, to make his eloquence in every case successful, and even pertinent or seasonable in some, as well as to direct it, and to furnish it with matter whenever he thought proper to employ this weapon.[1]

IV

This is not the place in which to speak of Bolingbroke's historical writings. '*Who now reads Bolingbroke?* asked Burke scornfully. And the right answer is, so far as regards, at any rate, the historical writings of Bolingbroke: "Far too few of us; the more's the pity!" ' So Matthew Arnold in his essay on Falkland. And of all his writings it was the historical ones which Chesterfield wanted his son to read. But I wish only to speak of Bolingbroke's attitude to history and of the value he placed on it.

He says that what alone justifies the study of history is that it instructs us in virtue. 'The true and proper object of this application is a constant improvement in private and public virtue';[2] and he goes on: 'An application to any study, that tends neither directly nor indirectly to make us better men and better citizens, is at best but a specious and ingenious sort of idleness, to use an expression of TILLOTSON: and the knowledge we acquire by it is a creditable kind of ignorance, nothing more'. It is a story we have heard before: 'Such is the imperfection of human understanding, such the frail temper of our minds, that abstract or general propositions, tho ever so true, appear obscure or doubtful to us very often, till they are explained by examples' (p. 15). So, also, Hobbes had written, as the reader will recall. But we saw, in speaking of Hobbes's views about history, that he was more completely addicted

---

[1] *On the Spirit of Patriotism*, London, 1752, pp. 48–53.
[2] *Letters on the Study and Use of History*, London, 1770, p. 14.

to this doctrine after he had come by his philosophy than in his earlier humanist days. In those earlier days he had indeed accepted this doctrine; but he had also upheld history as something which provides truth. But Hobbes the philosopher, as in *Leviathan* and elsewhere, emphasizes to us that history is very conjectural and he speaks less of its truth; he now stakes everything on its didactic value. But, as we saw, if this is all the value history has, on what grounds should it be preferred to poetry? Indeed, is it not, considered as a teacher of morals, inferior to poetry, as Sidney argued it is? Poetry can play the didactic game better than history; it can create a golden world of its own.

Now this is precisely the difficulty into which Bolingbroke gets himself. He will turn history into moral philosophy. 'We ought always to keep in mind, that history is philosophy teaching by examples how to conduct ourselves in all the situations of private and public life; that therefore we must apply ourselves to it in a philosophical spirit and manner; that we must rise from particular to general knowledge . . .' (p. 48). But if this is so, we are all too likely to lose the sense that history may give us truth; and we are not at all surprised when Bolingbroke pours unlimited contempt on historical research. Nothing can show better how impossible his position is than this passage, in which, in the first *Letter*, he speaks (pp. 7–9) of those men whom he places in his fourth class of historical scholars:

There is a fourth class . . . Men of the first rank in learning, and to whom the whole tribe of scholars bow with reverence. A man must be as indifferent as I am to common censure and approbation, to avow a thorough contempt for the whole business of these learned lives; for all the researches into antiquity, for all the systems of chronology and history, that we owe to the immense labours of a Scaliger, a Bochart, a Petavius, an Usher, and even a Marsham. The same materials are common to them all; but these materials are few, and there is a moral impossibility that they should ever have more. They have combined these into every form that can be given to them: they have supposed, they have guessed, they have joined disjointed passages of different authors, and broken traditions of uncertain originals, of various people, and of centuries remote from one another as well as from ours. In short, that they might leave no liberty untaken, even a wild fantastical similitude of sounds has served to prop up a system. As the materials they have are few, so are the very best, and such as pass for authentic, extremely precarious; as some of these learned persons themselves confess . . . In short, my lord, all these systems are so many enchanted castles; they appear to be something, they are nothing but appearances: like them too, dissolve the charm, and they vanish from the sight . . .

But it is clear that Bolingbroke cannot have it both ways. He complains that the scholars guess, join, construct. But if so, the only way to reduce conjecture is more research into and accumulation of materials. And yet Bolingbroke now denies that there are more materials to be obtained (a piece of dogmatism springing from his prejudice against scholarship), and now expresses his contempt for 'the whole tribe of scholars', 'pedants', 'monkish annalists', 'nuisances to society', to give only a few of his names of abuse. Historical study, as a means of coming by the *truth* of the past does not interest him; it is merely a 'specious and ingenious sort of idleness'. Will he then accept a thorough 'Pyrrhonism' towards historical knowledge? Or will he count 'history' as a sort of poetic story which has dropped from the skies which we may use as we will for moral instruction? We might expect that so lordly a contemner of scholarship might do so. But no; in the fourth *Letter* he argues against this. But if we are to believe that we may come by historical truth at all, must we not have scholars? No, he says, we do not want 'mere antiquaries and scholars', 'forward cox-combs and prating pedants' (p. 48). The plain fact is that Bolingbroke's attitude to history will not bear a moment's serious inspection; because he is not in earnest with historical truth but only with 'making us better men', he makes havoc of both history and any philosophical foundation for it. It is right, no doubt, to want to be 'philosophical'; but you are no more a philosopher for denying that historians have a right to exist.

And yet Bolingbroke's life had been lived in a great age of English historical scholarship. The years from 1660 to 1730 are classical in the history of English history. Hobbes, who lived well on into this time, was untouched by it; Bolingbroke who survived it, wrote, at its ending, the egregious *Letters* of which I have been speaking. Only Locke, through Tyrrell, came into touch with it; and we have seen evidence of his antiquarian interests.[1]

Bolingbroke could write in a spirit of contempt for all that Hickes, Dugdale, Wanley, Brady and Hearne stood for; and he could also preach the value of history for private and public virtue, without being himself conspicuous in either. But there was one contemporary of his who was at the centre of the great movement of the time in historical study, and whose life was not, like Bolingbroke's, overruled by passion. This was Robert Harley, Earl of Oxford. Speaking of the scholars of the early eighteenth century, Mr. David Douglas says in *English*

[1] For further evidence of Locke's interest in historical scholarship see *Thoughts concerning Reading and Study, Works*, vol. iii. p. 275.

Scholars (p. 341) that the whole company of them 'looked up to the first Earl of Oxford as the great Maecenas of English mediaeval learning, and they were right to do so, for he was the correspondent and bene-factor of very many of them, and he deserved their gratitude as surely as he earned the thanks of posterity'. Throughout the years of Anne's reign Oxford was building up the great Library. Before Anne had come to the throne, he was in touch with Humphrey Wanley; it was through Wanley that the D'Ewes collection was bought, in 1706; and in a few years Oxford made him Library-Keeper of the Harleian library. Wanley and all he did for Old English Scholarship could win little more than contempt from Bolingbroke; but Oxford saw to it that he had every possible facility. This is not the least of the differences be-tween these two men. History was to Bolingbroke something to preach about, from which lessons might be drawn, which however he himself did not study to learn and practice; to Oxford, the past was something which dwelt and lived in the present, and gave a certain deliverance from passion, narrowness and meanness of mind. We can-not separate their respective attitudes to history and scholarship from what they were, as men and statemen. Chesterfield says of Bolingbroke that he was 'a most mortifying instance of the violence of human passions. . . . Impetuosity, excess and almost extravagancy, character-ized not only his passions but even his senses. . . . Even a difference of opinion upon a philosophical subject would provoke, and prove him no practical philosopher';[1] but when Swift speaks of Harley in the *Journal*, it is always to give an impression of a man pleasant, dis-interested, incorruptible, calm.[2] It is one thing to preach that reason must overcome passion; it is another to live it.

V

I turn now to speak of Bolingbroke's philosophical writings. I said early in chapter 2 that Locke's religious sensibility is best understood as one that belongs to the seventeenth century; he was not a deist but a figure of seventeenth-century piety; and I hope that I have been able to show clearly to the reader that this was so. But I also tried to exhibit certain ways in which he expressed a new and growing sensibility and in which he nourished and strengthened it. Above all, the chapter *Of Enthusiasm*, more than any other single document, set the tone of the

[1] *Letters*, ed. Mahon, vol. ii. pp. 448–49.
[2] *Journal*, ed. Aitken, see e.g., pp. 220–21, 248, 298, 354, 365.

new age. I do not mean, of course, that Locke alone, or Locke's chapter on enthusiasm alone, were decisive in these things. At least, it is doubtful if we can accord to any one man or to any one book such conclusive influence. But, when we bear in mind how widely Locke was read and was to be read, and by how many different kinds of readers, we may fairly put down his writings for more decisive than most. For his empiricism and intellectual caution were bound to win the respect of his fellow countrymen; he carried therefore all the more responsibility; and had he been able to restrain himself from an excessive intellectualism in certain parts of the Fourth Book of the *Essay*, and remained more consistently loyal to the fundamental notion of assent which animates the bigger part of that Book, he would have greatly reduced the power of the deistic movement, and have made it impossible for accomplished but shallow-minded men of the world to invoke him for their master. It was fatally easy for Bolingbroke to find in Locke what he wanted; and at crucial points Locke played into his hands or declined to speak out strongly enough. Matthew Arnold was to complain about Gray that he never 'spoke out'. But it was very hard, at the place in the century where Gray was, to do so. It would have been easier for Locke. Instead, he temporized with the age. The gentleness of his nature, his caution, and even timidity helped to make possible his deep and tender piety; they did not arm him to combat the growing danger of the time. For much the bigger part he represented a reasonable and pious Anglicanism, and sustained the tensions necessary for a healthy and sane religion; and it is all the more pity that he failed to ensure that the succeeding generations would sustain a right balance of reason and faith, and that the Wesleys and Blakes, with their several excesses, should become necessary.

I now go on to show Locke's influence on Bolingbroke, and how Bolingbroke used some of the chief notions which Locke put out in the *Essay*. In the third volume of the *Philosophical Works*[1] Bolingbroke calls Locke 'my master, for such I am proud to own him' (p. 355); and in the second section of the first Essay he declares that his intention and method are those of Locke.

I . . . shall content myself to observe, in Mr. Locke's method and with his assistance, something about the phaenomena of the human mind, by which we may judge surely of the nature, extent, and reality of human knowledge. I say, we may judge surely of them; because our ideas are the foundations, or

[1] *The Philosophical Works of Henry St. John, Lord Viscount Bolingbroke*, 5 vols., London 1754, from which all quotations are made.

the materials, call them which you please, of all our knowledge; because, without entering into an enquiry concerning the origin of them, we may know so certainly, as to exclude all doubt, what ideas we have; and because, when we know this, we know with the same certainty what kinds, and degrees of knowledge we have, and are capable of having (1. p. 18).

This is certainly in the manner of Locke. In the preceding section, which opens the first long essay addressed to Pope, Bolingbroke has unfolded his standard and declared his polemic; Plato, Malebranche and Berkeley are set up for the enemies of all reasonable philosophical counsel; and upon them, and others like them, he will conduct, again and again through the five volumes, his dashing attacks. But this we can leave for a moment. Having said what I have quoted from the beginning of the second section, he goes on to speak of how we come by our knowledge and what prescribes the limits of its range.

I do not propose to try to conduct the reader through the details of the pages that follow. But I shall outline it, and try to say what it comes to. There are, he says, ideas of sensation and ideas of reflection. He says (1. p. 18) of ideas of sensation that they are 'received from without' and are 'caused by such sensations, as the presence of external objects excites in us according to laws of passion and action, which the Creator has established'. We do not know what these laws are, nor by what method the Creator contrives to make external objects produce so singular an effect; we may not know *how*, but we certainly know *that*. 'But this I know, that a leaf of wormwood conveys to my mind, by the sense of sight, and that of touch, for instance, the ideas of color, extension, figure, solidity . . . as certainly as I know that the act of my mind, called volition, produced the motion of my hand which gathered the leaf. Our ignorance of causes does not hinder our knowledge of effects. This knowledge has been thought sufficient for us, in these cases, by infinite wisdom: and nothing can be more ridiculous than to hear men affirm dogmatically, when they guess at most, and that very wildly, and very precariously' (p. 19). Now the reader will recall that Locke spoke in one place of the senses as '*conveying* into the mind several distinct perceptions of things'; but I was at pains to point out that Locke was clearly unhappy about this use of the metaphor of conveyance, and used a number of alternative expressions which make clear that he wished not to be misunderstood. In particular, he spoke of the 'impressions made on our senses by outward objects'; he did not indeed sufficiently develop the difference between 'impression' and 'idea'; but it is certainly there in the pages of Book 2. Bolingbroke shows no such uneasiness about the metaphor of conveyance. 'This I know', he says, 'that the leaf of wormwood conveys to my mind . . . the idea of color . . . as certainly as the act of my mind, called volition, produced the motion of my hand . . .' The reader of Boling-broke must quickly get the impression that he is a dogmatist; and that in the sense that disqualifies him from being a philosopher. That is to say, he is quite determined not to acknowledge that there are, in these matters, problems to be solved; he will not *think*. All is plain and clear; and if all does not appear to be plain and clear, it is altogether the fault of philosophers. Nowhere, in discussing our knowledge of the external world, does he raise and consider the inevitable problems; he will not begin to consider what these ideas are of which he speaks; he nowhere speaks of the problems created by memory, error, dream and hallucina-tion; there are never any signs that he acknowledges the difficulties of representative perception. He does indeed, in one place, far on in the fourth volume (p. 356) recognize that 'our most simple ideas are some-times fallacious'; but this is a place in his writings where he is not speaking of perception but wishes to minimize our knowledge of God and is ready to adduce any evidence, however inconsistent, with what else he has said, to combat metaphysical knowledge. 'Nothing can be more ridiculous than to hear men affirm dogmatically, when they guess at most, and that very widely, and very precariously.' It is against this ridiculous behaviour that Bolingbroke's writing is directed; it is also what his writings exhibit to a more than ridiculous degree. There was no need for him to tell us, at the end of the second Essay, that he con-sidered that there would be 'more real knowledge, and more true wisdom among mankind, if there was less learning, and less philo-sophy' (2. p. 142); it has become very manifest to the reader, before he has read so far, that Bolingbroke's Essays are essentially anti-philo-sophical; he wishes to put an end to philosophical thought; and in his own writings it can scarcely be said to exist.

Now to this, the significant motive of these writings, we shall return. But I go on to say something more of what Bolingbroke declares about human knowledge, lest the reader may consider that I am rushing hotly to condemn him. He considers that in perception of sense, the mind is passive; in perception of its own processes, Locke's ideas of reflection, it is active. 'We conceive passively the ideas of sensible qualities from without' (1. p. 22); but then 'the activity of the soul, or mind, commences, and another source of original ideas is opened: for we then acquire ideas from, and by the operations of our minds'. But having spoken of external sense as passive and internal sense as active, he is content to leave it so, and to pass on. He follows Locke in calling the ideas so obtained the 'materials' of all knowledge. He adds (1. p. 24) that as material for building, they are poor stuff; they 'will appear like mud, and straw and lath, materials fit to erect some frail, and homely cottage; but not of substance, nor value sufficient for the construction of those enormous piles, from whose lofty towers philosophers would persuade us that they discover all nature subject to their inspection, that they pry into the source of all being, and into the inmost recesses of wisdom'. This, again, is very much in the manner of Locke. But we shall see that it is not Locke's motive which animates Bolingbroke's sustained depreciation of human knowledge.

He then goes on (p. 28) to speak of complex ideas. Here he is chiefly concerned with 'complex ideas of substances' to use Locke's description; later he will speak of modes. Now there is at once a difficulty for him: does the mind *compose* its complex ideas of things? Locke certainly said it did; the mind frames the idea by uniting the simple ideas of sense in a supposed substratum. But will Bolingbroke say so? He knows very well that there are risks, in his point of view, in speaking in this way; the thought that the mind has such powers alarms him; and he says boldly that 'as soon as we are born, various appearances present themselves to the sight, the din of the world strikes our ears, in short a multitude of impressions made on the tender organs of sense convey to the mind a multitude of ideas simple and complex, confusedly and continually, into the mind'. So that complex ideas, too, are *conveyed* into the mind. He is not, indeed, wholly happy about this. On the preceding page (p. 28) he has said that 'the composition, and comparison of ideas is plainly a lesson of nature: this lesson is taught us by the first sensations we have'. It is a difficult lesson for so young a pupil. But the pupil is apt and 'acts conformably to the suggestions it receives from these impressions, and takes with its first ideas the hints how to multiply, and improve them. If nature makes us lame, she gives crutches to lean upon . . . she takes us by the hand, and leads us by experience to art.' The mind has indeed its 'arts'; but in our earliest infancy at least, we are wise beyond our days and do what Nature tells us. If, in later days, we abuse these 'arts', it is the fault of learning, philosophy and 'over-heated imaginations'; when we are infants and without minds of our own, we accept Nature for our guide and may not go wrong. What Bolingbroke, with his Nurse Nature, requires of us is that we become as infants again; our adult perversity and the follies of philosophers and scholars consist in our declining to act conformably with the suggestions we receive from impressions. But how impressions (which after all is what 'Nature' comes to here) can assume this pedagogic and suggestive rôle, Bolingbroke does not begin to consider. Besides, the lesson of Nature (whereby we come to apprehend complex ideas of things and people) does not end here; 'she carries it on to all the different compositions of our simple ideas, and to all the different combinations we frame of our simple, and complex ideas; from substances to modes, the dependencies and affections of substances; and from them to the relations of things one to another; that is, she carries it on to all the operations of the mind, and to all the objects of our thoughts in the acquisition of knowledge' (p. 30).

The 'lesson of nature' then is learnt by us not only in forming complex ideas of substances, but in our apprehension of modes. Bolingbroke takes over from Locke the doctrine of modes, simple and mixed. But before speaking further of this, I wish to emphasize that Bolingbroke shows plenty of signs of feeling embarrassed by our complex ideas of substances. Locke had found them difficult enough; but with his characteristic fairness he had been content to talk about the I-know-not-what of substance; we have a vague idea which goes along with sensible ideas to compose our ideas of things and people. Bolingbroke, with *his* characteristic disingenuousness and *un*fairness says (on p. 30) that Nature 'obtrudes' the complex ideas of substances on us. This is his alternative way of saying that in perception we act on the hints provided us by our instructive impressions. But does Nature obtrude any idea of an I-know-not-what? Can Nature, so kindly and wise a nurse, be guilty of introducing us to an idea which is so troublesome and has led to so much nonsense being talked? But Bolingbroke will not discuss the matter, and Nature speaks with no clear voice. He acknowledges that he must refer qualities to that of which they *are* qualities; nor can he 'consider a substance otherwise than relatively to its modes'. Then he says (also on p. 30), 'the complex idea we have of every substance is nothing more, than a combination of several sensible ideas which determine the apparent nature of it to us'. Is he then making of our complex ideas only aggregations of ideas conveyed by sense? This certainly would be a theory to consider, and certain eighteenth-century philosophers were willing enough to consider it. But can Nature tolerate such notions? Hardly. And that Bolingbroke will not consider the notion in earnest is shown by the last part of his sentence, where he says of sensible ideas that they determine the 'apparent nature' of a substance to us; sensible ideas *do* show us something of the nature of the substance of which they are qualities. But it is only the 'apparent' nature; and we are setting up a fine distinction between real and apparent substances. Now in the face of these metaphysical difficulties and refinements, what does Bolingbroke do? Will he now begin to think and honestly try to resolve what seems to be a genuine enough problem? The answer is, No. What he goes on to write is this (p. 31):

'on the whole, it will appear, whenever we consider this matter further, that the far greatest part of what has been said by philosophers about being, and substance, indeed all they have advanced beyond those clear and obvious notions, which every thinking man frames, or may frame without their help, is pure jargon, or else something very trite, disguised under a metaphysical mask, and called by an hard name, ontology, or ontosophy.'

What those 'clear and obvious notions, which every thinking man frames or may frame without their help' is precisely what Bolingbroke has not told us, and it is only because he has thought so far as to see that clear and obvious notions are not forthcoming that he escapes into abuse of philosophy.

Now it is undeniable that these passages, in which Bolingbroke speaks of complex ideas of substances, are written under the direct influence of Locke; at no point can we say that he is far from the teaching of the *Essay* in 2. 23. In saying that the sensible ideas we have in our complex idea of a substance do not reveal the real nature of things, he is still following his master. Besides, it may be said that in endowing sensations with a certain pedagogic function, so that they suggest to the mind how it should proceed, he is at least very near to Locke. Locke himself uses the word 'suggest' in just such contexts; in 2. 7. vii, for example, he says that unity is an idea 'suggested to the understanding by every object without'; and in his discussion on substance in 2. 23, it is clear enough that he regards the idea of substance as suggested to us when we see 'certain simple ideas co-existent together'. All this is true. Still, the reader need not read far in the twenty-third chapter of the second Book and then look through Bolingbroke's few hurried pages, to feel the difference of tone between the two writings; it is the difference between dogmatism which takes refuge in abuse and fair-minded enquiry which, if it does not solve its problems, at least exposes them and opens the way for succeeding generations, if only they believe in the power of thought, to advance further. Everywhere in Bolingbroke there is a greater violence than in Locke; he is determined to set out quickly conclusions which indeed are not at all conclusions in the sense that they issue from his own thinking and to which Locke, for whom they were genuine conclusions, came only slowly and laboriously. This haste and dogmatism goes along with two intentions which are not to be discerned in Locke: the extreme playing down of the rôle of the mind's action in knowledge and the corresponding elevation of 'Nature' into a semi-mythological figure. I may perhaps remark further on these two features of Bolingbroke's writing. I have already pointed out his uncritical talk of the conveyance of ideas into the mind and of their obtrusion upon us; and I need only quote, against Bolingbroke's statement that Nature obtrudes on us complex ideas of substances, this section from Locke: 'Hence, when we talk or think of any particular sort of corporeal substances, as horse, stone, etc., though the idea we have of either of them be but the complication or collection of those several simple ideas of sensible qualities, which we used to find united in the thing called horse or stone; yet because we cannot conceive how they should subsist alone, nor one in another, we suppose them existing in, and supported by some common subject; which support we denote by the name substance, though it be certain we have no clear or distinct idea of that thing we suppose a support' (2. 23. v).   No doubt this statement may readily be criticized; it is a too simple and intellectualized version of how we come to knowledge of things; still, it is open and clear, and represents the mind as struggling to do the best it can with a situation which mere 'experience' does not order of itself. Locke makes no effort to hide the difficulties of his empiricism. Besides, he makes no attempt to escape from these difficulties by invoking a personalized 'Nature' who everywhere instructs us and helps us along. To help out the difficulties of doctrine with vague analogies of this kind was not at all to Locke's taste. We shall have occasion again to speak of the readiness of Bolingbroke to employ metaphor readily enough when it served his purpose.

He is quite sure that in the growth of our knowledge we are everywhere 'assisted, directly or indirectly, by the lessons of nature'. But a still greater crisis is bound to loom up before him when he speaks of modes and relations. He has obliged the mind to receive complex ideas of substances willy-nilly; Nature may be a kindly nurse, but she pushes these ideas down our throats. But what of the modes of which Locke speaks and which he declares, beyond any doubt, are of the mind's making? What will Bolingbroke, in his obvious wish to extend empiricism beyond what Locke will allow, make of this situation?

He accepts the doctrine of modes. 'I understand . . . what Mr. Locke understands by simple and mixed modes, the various combinations that our minds make of the same simple idea, and the various compositions that they make of simple ideas of different kinds' (p. 31). Now in the doctrine of Locke, the modes, whether simple as in mathematics or mixed as in ethical concepts are the free creation of the mind. Mathematical ideas, Locke says, are 'combinations of ideas, which the mind, by its free choice, puts together'; and he says that names of mixed modes 'stand for ideas perfectly arbitrary' (3. 4. xviii). Now if Bolingbroke is at all uneasy at Locke's treatment of complex ideas of substances, what will he say of these arbitrary powers with which Locke endows the mind in its knowledge of modes? This is how he writes (1. pp. 31–32):

Ideas of things computable, and measurable, are the objects of mathematics. Ideas of moral, and immoral actions are the objects of ethics. From whence has the mathematician his first ideas of number, or his first ideas of solid extension, of lines, surfaces, and figures? From whence has the moralist his first ideas of happiness, and unhappiness, of good and evil? The mind can exercise a power, in some sort arbitrary, over all it's simple ideas, that is, it can repeat them at it's pleasure, and it can frame them into complex ideas without any regard to actual, tho with a regard to possible existence; which regard will be always preserved, unless the mind be disordered. The mind then has a power of framing all the different compositions, and combinations of ideas, about which these sciences are conversant: but yet these operations are not performed by the native energy of the mind alone, without any help, without any patern. Nature lends the help, nature sets the patern, when complex ideas of these modes and relations force themselves on the mind, as the complex ideas of substances do.

This passage is interesting and shows a further important departure from Locke's teaching. The disciple is here in great alarm; and here at least he must certainly say things for which there is no authority in the *Essay*. 'These operations', he says, 'are not performed by the native energy of the mind alone'; Nature is at hand still, helps the mind and provides a pattern on which the ideas of the modes are modelled; 'Nature lends the help, nature sets the patern, when complex ideas of these modes and relations force themselves on the mind, as the complex ideas of substances do'. So the ideas of modes are not less forced on us than those of substances. We might think that, if so, it is hard to see the rôle of the 'patern', and that Bolingbroke might tell us further how and why he can speak now of Nature's help and now of Nature's

14

compulsion. This sort of metaphor smacks too much of caprice, or is too much a way of avoiding thinking carefully about the event. But my point now is to emphasize to the reader that Bolingbroke will not allow the mind the apparently genuine creativeness which Locke attributes to it in its 'arbitrary' creation of modes. Bolingbroke says that the mind can 'exercise a power, in some sort arbitrary'; but yet it always acts with a regard to 'possible existence'; unless, indeed, it be 'disordered'; and he ends up by saying that the complex ideas of modes are forced on the mind, or rather, 'force themselves on the mind'. It is therefore becoming increasingly clear to us what Bolingbroke is doing. He is taking over the scheme of Locke's theory of knowledge; but at every step he is reducing, indeed he endeavours to destroy, the mind's initiative, power and resources. The mind only entertains ideas which are thrust into it; naturally, therefore it cannot go wrong; if it departs from what is put into it by 'nature', it is 'disordered'. And yet it has powers 'in some sort arbitrary'. At every stage Bolingbroke is employing Locke's philosophy as an instrument of an extreme empiricism for which there is no authority in the *Essay*. Now had Bolingbroke used Locke's doc-trines as a point from which to develop and, so far as he could, demon-strate a more violent empiricism, no reasonably objection could have been made out against him; and this was, of course, to be done later in the century. But our amateur philosopher will not do this; he does little more than set out his gospel of 'nature' without either declaring or examining his differences from Locke. On p. 37 he says:

Modes are the affections and dependencies of substances; relations are the affections and dependencies of substances and modes; and no one of them can exist any longer than both the ideas that produced it, or by the comparison of which it was framed, subsist. It might seem therefore the less likely that outward objects should communicate such ideas to the mind, or even in-struct the mind to frame them; and yet so it is.

Now if we here leave on one side what is said about relations, I em-phasize that Bolingbroke is grossly misrepresenting Locke so far as simple and mixed modes are concerned. Locke says (2. 13. i) of simple modes that they come about through 'modifications of the same idea, which the mind either finds in things existing, or is able to make within itself, without the help of any extrinsecal object, or any foreign sug-gestion'; and of mixed modes he says that the mind 'exercises an active power in making these several combinations: for it being once furnished with simple ideas, it can put them together in several compositions, and so make variety of complex ideas, without examining whether they exist so together in nature' (2. 22. ii). This freedom of the mind in the making of ideas Bolingbroke is unwilling to allow; or rather he allows it, only adding that it is a freedom only to be compelled by 'nature'. Bolingbroke's discipleship to Locke is much more superficial than real. (It should be added that later [1. p. 185] he delivers a wholesale attack on Locke's view of modes as ideas which are their own archetypes.) He is employing Locke's scheme of thought for purposes which are not Locke's at all. The *Essay in the Human Understanding* is in all truth a curious mixture of rationalism and empiricism, and is a highly individual synthesis; it cannot be captured within any formula or simple statement. Bolingbroke, insensitive to its individuality as he must have been to the qualities of Locke's personality, destroys its balance and compromise at many places and makes it a servant of his own unreflective and crass empiricism.

It is in the spirit of this empiricism that Bolingbroke speaks of invention. 'Nature', he says on p. 34, 'that urged men, by necessity, to invention, helped them to invent . . . Nature set the example, example begot imitation, imitation practice, practice introduced speculation, and speculation in it's turn improved practice. I might easily run through . . . examples . . . to shew how the first principles of arts and sciences are derived from ideas furnished by the productions, and operations of nature, such as our senses represent them to us; nay, how instinct instructs reason, the instinct of other animals the reason of man'; and he concludes by saying then there is no need for him to tell Pope of all this, who has written of it in the third Ethic Epistle. Now running through this is the vague metaphorical way of writing we have already noticed in his writings, with its talk of 'Nature' instructing us. Ideal construction goes beyond perceptual experience. But it adds nothing and it explains nothing, to say that 'Nature' instructs us to make new combinations of ideas. Something genuinely novel is brought forth, and is certainly brought forth by our minds. Now what is true of ideal construction is no less true of the actions of comparing and abstracting; they too are productive of something new and no amount of mere revival can explain them. No more can any talk of 'Nature' explain them. To perceive two things to be similiar is to do something which neither objects nor anything else can do for us. Bolingbroke says of relations that it seems 'the less likely that outward objects should communicate such ideas to the mind, or even instruct the mind to frame them; and yet so it is'. But in fact, so it is not, nor can ever intelligibly

be so. And if comparing is a genuinely productive process of the mind
(and Locke acknowledged that this was so by saying (2. 25. viii) that it
is an operation of the mind about its ideas and even that relations are
'extraneous and superinduced' upon things), imaginative and fanciful
constructions carry their novelty more certainly upon their face; to
speak of 'Nature' in Bolingbroke's fashion is only to flee into unintelligible mythology. Hobbes would have scorned to employ such
devices. He preferred what to us is clearly the grossest inconsistency.
But he earns a greater respect from us in all his inconsistency than
Bolingbroke with his maudlin poetry of 'Nature'. Now it is true that
Locke says very little about invention and fancy. In one place in the
Essay (2. 10. viii) he says that 'invention, fancy and quickness of parts'
depend on strength and serviceability of memory. Here he recalls the
manner of Hobbes in speaking of these things. But if he is unsatisfactory and brief here, he grants to the mind powers and operations far
beyond anything to be found in Hobbes and Bolingbroke.

Now Bolingbroke is speaking here of the inventions that come of
applied science. Of invention in art, what Locke, in common with the
other Augustans, called the fancy, he says, neither here nor anywhere
else, nothing at all. 'Nature' helps us to invent what is useful for us in a
civilized life; but whether 'Nature' helps in the production of works of
art, we are not told. Now the views of other Augustans, in particular
of Pope, as to what 'Nature' requires of the artist, we shall have occasion
to discuss in a later part of our history. I remark here only that Bolingbroke does not speak of the matter. He does not tell us whether 'Nature'
obtrudes ideas into the mind of the artist, or otherwise instructs him.
But we gather something of what he would have said about it from the
paragraph which I quoted earlier in speaking of his view of the way in
which the mind comes by the modes. 'The mind', he said, 'can exercise
a power, in some sort arbitrary, over all it's simple ideas, that is, it can
repeat them at it's pleasure, and it can frame them into complex ideas
without any regard to actual, tho with a regard to possible existence;
which regard will always be preserved, unless the mind be disordered.'
No doubt he would require that the artist have regard to 'possible
existence'. But presumably 'Nature' will be called in to instruct us in
what may fairly be judged to be 'possible existence'; and here there may
be plenty of disagreement and doubt; it will be easy to judge minds to
be disordered; and 'Nature' will prove a stick with which to beat many a
back. But in fact, as Bolingbroke employs 'Nature', it is itself as unnatural a notion as can be; it is a pretty piece of fancy employed only

to defeat the natural processes of thinking as carefully and precisely on human knowledge as we clearly ought. This world of Bolingbroke's, in which there is to be no nonsense, and all is to be sensible and well-suited to the 'coffee-houses and taverns', hangs from a halting enough bit of mythology.

There are only two other doctrines, of those to be found in Bolingbroke's exposition of the nature of human knowledge in the first *Essay*, on which I shall comment before going on to reflect further on the spirit and intention of these writings. They are, Bolingbroke's view of the validity of our complex ideas of substances, in which he follows Locke; and secondly, his view of general ideas, in which he deserts the master.

The reader will recall that in speaking of Locke, I emphasized that he does not allow that our ideas of substances carry us far in knowledge of substances. What we know are nominal essences only; simple ideas of sense, joined together in the something of substance, give us no knowledge of the essential constitution of things. Our knowledge is knowledge very much from the outside, an observing that certain qualities go together in a thing, and it is little more. 'Let our complex idea of any species of substances be what it will, we can hardly, from the simple ideas contained in it, certainly determine the necessary co-existence of any other quality whatsoever' (4. 3. xiv). In this sense the world is opaque to our gaze; we can only generalize with probability. Science can give us no certainty. This doctrine Bolingbroke entirely accepts. Here is one of his statements. 'Our real knowledge goes no further than particular experiment: and as we attempt to make it general, we make it precarious. The reason is plain. It is a knowledge of particular effects that have no connection, nor dependency one on another, even when they, or more properly the powers that produce them, are united in the same substance: and of these powers considered as causes, and not in their effects, we have no means of attaining any knowledge at all' (1. p. 48). We observe here, then, Bolingbroke's complete agreement with Locke; here he need not depart from the letter of what Locke says. But I must quote further from Bolingbroke in order to show the reader how different a rôle this doctrine plays in the economy of his mind from that which it plays in Locke's.

Sense and intellect, [he says on p. 48] must conspire in the acquisition of physical knowledge; but the latter must never proceed independently of the former. Experiment is that pillar of fire, which can alone conduct us to the promised land; and they, who lose sight of it, lose themselves in the

dark wilds of imagination. This many have done from the infancy of philosophy, which has lasted longer than we are apt to imagine; and which, one
might be tempted to think on some occasions, continues still, by a fondness
to retain some of the rattles and baubles of early ages. These rattles and
baubles have been laid aside, however, by no philosophers so much, as by
those who have applied themselves to cultivate experimental physics; and
therefore as imperfect as our knowledge of nature is, and must be always, yet
has it been more advanced within less than two centuries, than it had been in
twenty that preceded them.

There is in all this an enthusiasm, a 'heat of imagination' even, to
which Locke was not moved in his review of scientific knowledge.

VI

I turn now to speak of Bolingbroke's doctrine of the general idea.
In his discussion of these ideas (which occupies the fifth section of the
first Essay) he opposes the master. In those doctrines of his of which I
have already spoken he does not mention his differences from Locke,
though, even in the ardour of his empiricism, he can hardly fail to be
aware of them. But with general ideas, it is different; he is compelled
openly to disagree. He does so with mingled reproach and praise; he
upbraids his teacher, and also apologizes by declaring him (1. p. 127)
the author of 'surely the most complete work of this kind that any
language can boast'. He is speaking of one of the views of the general
idea that Locke puts out in the *Essay*, and says: 'If Mr. Locke could
dream he had such a power as he describes this of abstracting to be (a
power to form, with "some pains and skill,[1] the general idea of a triangle", for instance, "neither oblique, nor rectangle, neither equilateral,
equicrural, nor scalenon, but all, and none of these at once") let writers
learn to be less dogmatical, and readers to be less implicit. It is undeniable that there is such a thing as philosophical delirium. Men of
the coolest tempers, we see, are liable to be seized by it; and when they
are so, even their minds are apt to flatter, to deceive, and to debauch
themselves. I quote this as an instance of the mind's being debauched,
as well as flattered, and deceived . . .' (1. pp. 120–21). This is strong
language. As we shall see, there is far more violent abuse of other
philosophers strewn up and down these writings; but that he could
speak in this way about Locke shows the strength of his feelings when
he comes to speak of general ideas.

[1] The passage is in 4. 7. ix of the *Essay*.

Now the passage of which Bolingbroke here speaks is especially famous because Berkeley (whom Bolingbroke had read) seized on it to attack it sharply. Mr. Aaron (p. 193) has observed about it that it occurs in a chapter where Locke is not treating specifically of the theory of universals but is showing that the mind can come to its general ideas only with labour and difficulty. And in any case, Locke does not say here, what Berkeley takes him to say, that in apprehending a general idea we somehow entertain an image of a triangle which is oblique and rightangled and scalene and equilateral all at once. Mr. Aaron rightly declares that Locke could not have believed anything so silly. From what he says here, we are not required to conclude that Locke believed that the general idea is an image. An idea is 'the object of the understanding when a man thinks'; and he is nowhere committed to saying that an idea must be a sensuous image. We cannot fairly attribute to him anything more than this belief: that a general idea, which is not an image, whatever else it may be, somehow 'covers' all the different kinds of triangles. And he acknowledges, in effect, that it is hard to see how it can do this, can both be general and have genuine relevance to the many kinds of particulars. For we must notice what Locke goes on to say after writing the lines which Bolingbroke quotes.

In effect, it [the general idea] is something imperfect, that cannot exist; an idea wherein some parts of several different and inconsistent ideas are put together. It is true, the mind, in this imperfect state, has need of such ideas, and makes all the haste to them it can, for the conveniency of communication and enlargement of knowledge. . . . But yet one has reason to suspect such ideas are marks of our imperfection . . .

I shall return to this quotation, which is taken from Book 4 of the *Essay* (7. ix). But at early stages in the *Essay* Locke has had some things to say about general ideas of which I wish now to take notice. In 2. 11. ix, he had certainly spoken of the general idea as an image. 'The mind makes the particular ideas, received from particular objects, to become general . . . Ideas taken from particular beings, become general representatives of all of the same kind . . . Such precise, naked appearances in the mind . . . the understanding lays up (with names commonly annexed to them) as the standard to rank real existences into sorts . . .' Now this was Locke's first statement about general ideas. But a mind as sensible as his was bound not to retain it through the course of the *Essay*; for clearly such a doctrine cannot explain its own employment of the words 'representative' and 'sorts'. Had Locke retained this doctrine, and had the statement in Book 4 which Berkeley criticized been made by one who held this doctrine, Berkeley's criticisms would have been justified. But Locke did not retain it; and the passage in Book 4 was composed in the light, not of the doctrine propounded in Book 2, but of one propounded in Book 3. It is true that some things which we find in Book 3 (3. vi) are very near to, if not identical with, what is to be found in 2. 11. ix. There, in Book 2, he had spoken of abstraction, and said that we come to what is 'general' by means of it; the images which became 'representative' are got by a process of stripping from an image 'all other existences, and the circumstances of real existence, as time, place, or any other concomitant ideas'; and what is left is what he calls 'precise, naked appearances in the mind'. It is these naked ideas which are 'representative'. And in Book 3 he continues, for a time, in this vein. He repeats in 3. 3. vi–vii very much what he has said in Book 2. 11. ix; and the representative ideas, he explains further, are 'such abstract and partial ideas of more complex ones, taken at first from particular existences'; that is, we lop off from our idea of John all those features which he does not share with Peter and James; and the coming to what is general is wholly an affair of leaving out, of abstraction. Now this doctrine will not do, and for a number of reasons. For if what is left, when we have carried out our abstraction of the peculiarities of John, is, in any sense, still John, however naked, it is still impossible to see how he can be representative of a 'sort'; the idea of a sort, a general, and not at all particular, idea is taken for granted all the time. But if he is not, in any way, still John (and he certainly is not, for 'naked' is an understatement of what he has been reduced to), he has been metamorphosed into something quite general; and we must acknowledge a genuinely general idea.

Now Locke seems to have been aware, if not clearly, of this dilemma. For as the chapter advances, it becomes clear that he increasingly envisages the general idea as, in all truth, general. He comes to speak of 'abstract ideas' in a way that suggests that they are genuinely abstract, and not mutilated particulars. And in 3. 3. xiii, he says that the sorting of things 'under names is the workmanship of the understanding, taking occasion from the similitude it observes amongst them to make abstract general ideas, and set them up in the mind, with names annexed to them as patterns or forms . . .' He adds that 'the word form in that sense has a very proper signification'. This, no doubt, is by way of apology for using the word at all. But he can hardly fail to be aware that he is now coming near to adopting an ancient tradition which the thought and feeling of his time is not at all disposed to adopt; still, he goes on in xiv to say that 'in truth, every distinct abstract idea is a distinct essence'; and (in xv) that 'the essence of each genus, or sort, comes to be nothing but that abstract idea which the general, or sortal . . . name stands for'. Now it seems certain that this is a very different doctrine from that from which he started. It is equally certain that he does not regard these essences as full Platonic forms existing in their own right and manifesting themselves in particular things; for he goes on to explain that they are only nominal essences, not real ones. They do not disclose the inner constitution of things; they are man-made, and are that in which science, which can give only probability, deals. This, at least, is the position so far as empirical science goes. It is different in mathematics, where our ideas, wholly and arbitrarily contrived by us, are their own archetypes; here, presumably, we know real essences, for mathematical ideas have no necessary relevance to reality; they are our free creation. It is then, I think, clear that Locke, disposed as he was to believe that we can apprehend only what is particular, gave up, with all his characteristic openness of mind, his doctrine of the mutilated particular, and came to rest in the belief that we apprehend genuinely general ideas which arise out of our observation of the similitudes of things. In general ideas we apprehend an identity, shared by many things, and which makes particulars what, so far as known to mortal mind, they are.[1]

Now it is in the light of all this, that we must read the passage in Book 4 (7. ix) which Bolingbroke and Berkeley criticized. The 'general idea of triangle' of which Locke speaks there is not an image or particular; it is of an essence present in all kinds of triangle; and Locke is only observing that such ideas, which must have relevance to all possible kinds of triangles, 'carry difficulty with them, and do not so easily offer themselves, as we are apt to imagine'. Impressed by the difficulty they carry with them, the intrinsic difficulty of seeing how this can be, he adds that such ideas are 'marks of our imperfection'.

Now Berkeley criticized the passage in 4. 7. ix in which Locke speaks of the general idea of a triangle as 'neither oblique nor rectangle, neither equilateral nor scalenon' on the grounds, as he believed, that Locke envisaged the general idea as a particular triangle which somehow had all those shapes at once. In fact Locke did not suggest this. Bolingbroke however did not take the passage in this way; he took it as

---

[1] In *John Locke*, p. 192 ff, Mr. Aaron writes at length on the subject of Locke's treatment of universals, and what I have written owes much to what he says.

suggesting that Locke held that there is a general idea of triangle distinct from any particular triangle. That this is how he took it is, I think, made clear by the fact that he in one place (1. p. 114) misquotes the passage, declaring that he had no idea of triangularity 'abstracted with pains and skill "from the special species of triangles, and present to the mind independently of them".' This is Bolingbroke's version of Locke's sentence, given without turning over Locke's pages; but it is a version which shows, I think, that Bolingbroke had at least the merit of having divined Locke's position more accurately than Berkeley. Berkeley saw in the passage a folly which was not there at all; Bolingbroke saw in it a folly, if folly it be, which *was* there.

Bolingbroke distinguishes between our knowledge of the particular and our knowledge of the 'general' by speaking again of 'Nature.' 'Nature' teaches us, so long as we are aware of the particular; she obtrudes ideas, even complex ideas of substances, into our minds; and even modes are constructed in accordance with her 'lessons'. But from that point on, we are left to our own devices. That is what, on 1. pp. 106–107, he says: 'The lesson of nature, as I have called it, that is, the information and instruction we gain by observing the constitution of our physical and moral systems, and the state and course of things that exist constantly, or transiently in them, ends with our complex ideas and notions. When nature leaves us, we are forced to put ourselves, in our ulterior progress towards general knowledge, under the conduct of her mimic, art; so that if our feet are apt to slip, if we totter in the way, and are subject to ramble out of it, whilst nature is our guide, all this must needs happen much more when we have no other guide but art, and when we are reduced to supply natural imperfection by expedients.' Nature leaves us to our own devices, or art; and 'knowledge, particular by nature, becomes in some degree general by art'. But how does our 'art' work? Art is said to be the 'mimic' of nature. But how in this crucial matter nature can be mimicked it is hard to see; for 'nature,' says Bolingbroke, 'shows us men, but not man in general'; and if so, and so far as we come by general ideas at all, our art must be unnatural.

Bolingbroke's doctrine is in fact Locke's first doctrine, the one propounded in Book 2 of the *Essay*. The general idea is a particular one which becomes so far general by being representative. Ideas are 'all particular and have no generality but that of application. They represent to the mind that which does or may exist ... The ideal man, or the ideal horse, which the mind perceives, is a particular idea that represents all the men, and all the horses that exist, or ever did exist; and the ideal triangle is as truly a particular idea that represents all the triangles that exist, or can exist in the mind, or out of it.' So he writes in the long footnote which begins in 1. p. 116. This footnote he adds, we think, because what he has written above in the text may appear to be hopelessly inconsistent; and he writes to support his page with a strong footnote which will leave no doubt in the reader's mind of what he believes. Only a little earlier in the text (p. 115) he has gone so far as to say that 'I know the general nature, the real essence, of justice, and am able to define it in very clear propositions, tho I am not able to frame any general idea or notion of it abstracted from all particulars, and containing them all'. This certainly looks like a descent into deep waters; and it is little wonder if he thinks a firm statement in a footnote is called for. There he says, again: 'Particular ideas of actual, or possible existence, are made general in some sort, that is, in their effect. . . . But the power of generalising ideas is so insufficient, that it goes no further. We make one phantasm of a man stand for all men, and one of an horse for all horses; but here our progress by ideas, that is, by single perceptions of the mind, stops' (p. 118). And here Bolingbroke stopped also. He would think about it no more. But this was where Locke began, and whence, by keeping his eyes open, he moved to a very different place.

VII

I have now said enough to show the reader the way in which Bolingbroke treats the work of Locke. He declares himself to accept it only to change it, and for the most part to change it without acknowledging that he is doing so. Only in the matter of general ideas, does he openly break with his 'master'; and there, he reproaches even him with philosophical delirium and a debauchment of his mind. But no one, looking back across two centuries, are likely to judge Locke's mind delirious and debauched; instead, we are aware of the fanaticism which animated Bolingbroke's. Fanaticism is none the less fanaticism for seeing its own quality in others; and beneath the 'cool temper' of mind of which Bolingbroke imagines himself to be fairly possessed there is an unreflecting urgency which suggests an unacknowledged passion and prejudice greater by far than any that touched the mind of Locke. Locke was always cool enough, and confident enough, to continue in thinking; there was that in Bolingbroke which consistently inhibited philosophical thought. But before I continue to compare the two men and to reflect further on the positivism (to use a modern term) which Bolingbroke abstracted from the body of Locke's writings, I wish to make some observations on the topic of the preceding section. In discussing Locke in the preceding chapter I did not at all discuss his view of general ideas; I confined myself largely to his doctrine of perception and to developing a feature of it which he left unregarded. I shall try now to suggest a view of the universal and the general idea which may accord with the view of perception which I sketched in the last chapter. Besides, it is necessary that we should do so in order to review at all adequately the metaphysic of deism (if metaphysic it can be called) which Bolingbroke sets out later in his writings. What we have to say therefore in the next two sections looks onwards to matters we shall treat of later, in addition to looking backwards to matters we treated of formerly.

The reader will recall that I argued in the last chapter that we must acknowledge the power best called imagination, which lies between sense and intelligence and also partakes of both. Imagination is not sensation but is a changing of the impressions of sense into ideas; it is an envisagement of ideas which, in spite of the name we are obliged to give it, is always an envisagement of what is taken to exist; and it is therefore to be distinguished from the fancy. Because this is so, we cannot represent it as operating without the rudiments of intellect; or rather, we see it as the matrix out of which all knowledge, however advanced to highly intellectual levels, develops and from which it never separates itself; and therefore, also, the imagination is not a blind faculty; but is, in the activity of prehending the individual, the starting point of the life of the intellect. Now if this is so, it is clear that we are committed to saying that the universal is present in what is imagined; however much we may speak of the imagination's grasp of the particular, it is an exaggeration to say that the imagination lays hold of the particular as a mere and unmitigated particular. This would be impossible; such an action could not be an act of knowing; it would not be an action at all, and could be only a passivity in sensation.

Now in order to meet the objection which naturally occurs to meet doctrine of this kind, I suggested that we have to make resort to artistic experience where, if anywhere in our adult life, we become very aware of what is individual and rest, as it were, in that awareness without irritable reaching after conceptual explanation and ordering. Certainly, in the enjoyment of the work of art, there is an extensive, yet also a subdued, play of the intelligence; and in what way this occurs, I tried to explain. Perhaps in order to recall more sharply into the reader's mind what I said in the preceding chapter, I may perhaps give a brief illustration of what was intended; it is also an illustration which will lead us on to speak of the universal for thought. I think that if we reflect on *King Lear* we may very well contemplate the King as standing, as in an allegorical manner, for humanity. In the figure of Lear we see humanity, in its folly, pride, humility, greatness; and also as learning the lesson of love and humility through suffering. In addition we may see the children, Goneril and Regan on the one side, and Cordelia on the other, all *his* children and sprung from *his* loins, as standing for the evil and the good in him. The drama is the struggle between the evil and the good in him. The good triumphs; it is Cordelia who wins his soul into a new life; and this is no less so because the price of the struggle is the death of all. Now I say that in reflecting in this way on the play, we may see it thus allegorically and exhibit it in terms of concepts. We do not indeed ordinarily do so; but I think that to 'interpret' the play in this way is not, at the lowest, absurd. And I suggest that this conceptual scheme, or something like it, is a part, though not a distinct part, of our experience; it is not articulated in our minds, but is caught up in or immersed, in our total experience. A work of the 'pure imagination' secures that this is the state of affairs in our minds, and, in spite of a burden of thought, declines to be allegory.

Now it is perhaps better to try to set out the phase of experience we have in mind by appeal to adult experience than to the experience of the child in his perception of objects. But I think that we are driven to believe that there must be a phase in the growing life of the child when he is aware of sounds, colours and things as sounds, colours and things without also being in possession of general ideas or apprehending the strictly universal as universal. It is incredible that he should not pass through such a phase, and that he should not enjoy the acutest perceptions in which the sensuous features of the world are brilliantly exhibited to him without his also apprehending the universal. No doubt we can all remember being caught out of ourselves, when small children, by the sight of a piece of coloured paper or some such object, and becoming, as we say, 'lost' in contemplation of it; or again, we can see some such thing happening half-a-dozen times a day to any small child we may know. We must acknowledge that the child knows 'what it is'; but the sense of it as a 'member of a class' is simply not there. Still, on the other hand, thought is yet present. It seems nonsense to say that the universal is 'imagined'; and yet it is there, an element in an activity which is quite predominantly imaginative, not intellectual.

Now I have thus recalled matters of which I spoke at some length in the preceding chapter not only for what may be the convenience of the reader but in order, also, to suggest to him the implications of what we have said for the doctrine of universality. Lear is himself; but he is also mankind. The flower which absorbs the child is none the less to him a flower, and no mere particular; besides, it is known as existing and as a unity, at a time when these, as general ideas, can hardly be before the child's mind.

Now I suggest that it is in situations like these we have what may help us to understand our knowledge of universals; and in what way this is so, I shall try to explain. When the child is absorbed in its flower, or we in *Lear*, we are, in some sense, aware of the universal, for knowledge of the sheer particular is impossible. We are aware, in watching the character and fortunes of Lear enacted on the stage, of humanity, of man; but it is *this* humanity, Lear's humanity. The child is aware of florality; but it is *this* florality, the florality of *this* flower. The universal is there, but it is, however much a paradox it may be, a particularized universal; and it is only, as thus particularized, that in these cases it occurs. To say this seems to me to be only to record fact, to observe what in fact happens in these cases; and the philosopher's first duty is to acquire what Professor Alexander called the 'natural piety of the historian'; we must observe as fairly as we can what is in the situation before assaulting it with battering rams of doctrine.

But it will be said that, however desirable natural piety may be, in the philosopher or anyone else, doctrine lays it down that to talk about a universal being particularized is to talk nonsense. To which it can only be replied that if it is nonsense, it is yet what occurs, and that no other statement of the state of affairs will bear inspection. And I can only ask that at this stage we be allowed to talk our 'nonsense' in the hope that a fuller statement of our intention will be able to explain, if only in some measure, the necessity of this 'nonsense', if nonsense it is. In any case I am now speaking not of what would be judged to be typical cases of perception, our normal perception of things in every day life. I am speaking of artistic experience and of the experience of a child; though, indeed, I am suggesting that these will help us, later on, to understand normal adult experience.

There is no need for me to urge the very familiar objection to the abstract universal represented as wholly cut away from the particular. We do not know the universal abstracted from sense; we simply cannot think it; cut thought away from the particular and it seems to perish. But if so, we are yet not at all committed to denying the universal element in knowledge; we have seen that to do this is to destroy knowledge. But if we declare our knowledge of the abstract universal a logician's myth and precisely the myth he might be expected to produce, are we not back in the position of Locke in the first doctrine he propounded (in Book 2) and which Bolingbroke (and Berkeley too, for that matter) held when he declares that the universal is a particular idea 'representative' of ideas like it? And are we not identifying ourselves with Bolingbroke in his attack on what Locke says about general ideas in Book 4. of the *Essay*? We have certainly said that Bolingbroke's doctrine will not serve; for it represents knowledge as trafficking in particulars only, while tacitly admitting that it cannot exist without the universal. This way of retreat we cannot take. We are committed both to denying that we know an abstract universal and an abstract particular. The one surreptitiously employs images of sense and tries to look as if it does not employ them; the other surreptitiously employs universals and tries to look as if it does not employ *them*. There must be a middle way if we are, in doctrine, to square up to the facts of our experience in knowledge.

We must say therefore that there are indeed universals; but that we know them only as they inhabit and are exhibited in particulars. But if we say so, we must beware of thinking that all is now clear and intelligible; for it obviously is not; and we are in danger of so particularizing the universal and universalizing the particular as to cast natural piety to the winds after a fashion of our own and of flying in the face of the facts.

Now I suggested that in the child's absorption in the flower and in our absorption in Lear we may be said to grasp the universal in the form of the particular; it is *Lear's* humanity and *this* florality which is known; the universal seems to be exhibited in the guise of a particular so far as it is exhibited at all. It is difficult to see how this can be so. But let us consider now what we have called more normal perception, perceptions of things in the course of the business of life or of scientific study by adults who would be said to possess general ideas, where general ideas would be said to be explicitly apprehended. What shall we say of this? We shall indeed acknowledge that here there seems to have occurred a gap between what is general and what is particular; and the particular is seen as exemplifying or sharing something which seems to claim some separate kind of existence. But in fact, we are committed to denying that that gap exists; and are also suggesting that the universal is in fact never known for abstract, but only as in the particular. But how can we show that this is so? Was not Locke right when he said that we form 'with pains and skill' the general idea of a triangle which is 'neither oblique nor rectangle, neither equilateral, equicrural nor scalenon; but all and none of these at once'?

Now I spoke, in the preceding chapter, of what I called the tensions between imagination and intelligence; and I tried to illustrate to the reader what I intend by speaking in this way. The imagination is indeed the seed-plot or nursing-ground of the intelligence; and the intelligence grows in and out of the imagination. But as it grows, indispensable as it is to the imagination, and acquires greater strength, it 'distances' the object from the mind. In doing this it is resisted by the imagination which shares something of the nature of sense; and the symbolism which is essential to the imagination tries to maintain itself against the systematizing and impersonalizing intelligence. I said that in works of art the imagination holds the intelligence in a certain subordinacy, with whatever difficulty. Yet, the conceptual analytical intelligence is not to be held down; and the requirements of practice and civilization ensure that it is not. Now in art we can, indeed, sometimes feel that the universal is in danger of breaking out from the union in which it is held with the senses and the imagination. In the greatest art, this does not happen. In some art, even very great art, it does; the imagination and the understanding fall apart. It is the difference between Shakespeare and Milton. But where the imagination does not sustain its autonomy and the union of the mind is lost, the intelligence goes forward to its systematizing and explanatory labours and its pursuit of principles; in this, it tries to shed sense and imagination and to apprehend forms and principles, the suggestions of which come indeed from the particulars, but the full apprehension of which the contemplation of particulars finally impedes and hinders. Now this was, and is, the significance of Plato in the history of the human mind: his philosophy represents the intelligence which has now fully defined its aims and ambitions and is ready enough to forget its earlier breeding. Plato is still the most illustrious enemy of art; and as everybody knows he exerts all the more power as an enemy of the æsthetic because his own senses and imagination were brilliant and quick. Besides, when the intelligence has come to this pitch, its objects are declared to be no mere manufacture of the mind; but rather compose an intelligible world, eternal and unaware of a temporal existence below.

But the plain fact remains that we cannot apprehend a pure 'idea' or 'form'; to think of triangularity which is not the triangularity of this triangle or of that is to have a mind quite blank. We must therefore be content to say that the general idea, through which we labour to grasp a 'universal', occurs with the effort of the intelligence to break out from its association with sense and imagination, and that the universal is an ideal of the intelligence, necessarily vague and unformed, which it represents as the goal of its labours. It is true that the life of the mind is impossible without the universal. Still, when the intelligence tries to break out from the unity of the mind and to state the universal for an independent entity, it at once begins to deal in what eludes it, an I-know-not-what, which it judges to be there, in the particulars, but which it is unable to disengage from them. To 'disengage' it is to destroy it, or to destroy the mind's power to apprehend it. And for this reason the life of the intelligence is maintained in a singular unease; it is aware of the universal in the particular; it is not and is more than the particular; without it the particular cannot be the particular. And yet, considered in itself it is an *ignis fatuus* which ever eludes and transcends the mind. The movement of the intelligence is towards the pure universal, the essence; but it is a movement that may not come to its end. Hence the knife-edge on which the intelligence walks; to fall back into the imaginative and æsthetic will not do and is a kind of suicide; wholly to shed the imaginative is impossible, and the effort to do so is to reduce the mind, so far as possible, to nullity. The imagination, altogether without the intelligence, is blind; but so is the intelligence without the imagination.

This is obscure; or it may be trite. But I shall try to explain further what I mean. And it is at this point that I invoke the aid of Locke, and quote again what he says in 4. 7. ix, where after saying what Boling-broke quoted, he goes on with: 'In effect, it [the general idea] is something imperfect, that cannot exist; an idea wherein some parts of several different and inconsistent ideas are put together. It is true, the mind, in this imperfect state, has need of such ideas, and makes all the haste to them it can, for the conveniency of communication and enlargement of knowledge; to both of which it is naturally very much inclined. But yet one has reason to suspect such ideas are marks of our imperfection...' The general idea, says Locke, is 'something imperfect that cannot exist'; the mind has need of them and cannot do without them; but they are condemned to a certain imperfection and unintelligibility and are framed in a paradox. They are certainly somehow there; and yet, as wholly general ideas, we cannot grasp them. And to explain this state of affairs, which Locke characteristically accepts as a part of his plain historical method, he falls back on his pervasive thought of the mediocrity of our nature. He is predisposed enough to think what Bolingbroke thinks; but unlike Bolingbroke he is also disposed to think about what he is predisposed to think, and comes to the solution of his problem, not indeed by solving it, but at least by perceiving its necessity, the necessity of its being insoluble.

I have spoken at some length, in a previous chapter, of Locke's notion that we are 'mediocre' creatures; and everywhere in the *Essay* is the thought of 'superior beings' with powers of knowledge greater than our own, and to whom particular substances are known, not through any superficial nominal essence, but in their real essences. To us the object is a limit of our knowledge as well as an object of it; to them it may be known intelligibly, become wholly transparent and, as it were, received into the mind or the mind into it. In the same vein, Locke writes of memory. He remarks, it will be remembered, on Pascal's unusual powers of memory (2. 10. ix); and says that some of the angels may 'be endowed with capacities able to retain together, and constantly set before them, as in one picture, all their past knowledge at once'. Now when he speaks, in the passage of Book 4 which I have quoted and which Bolingbroke and Berkeley criticized, that the general idea is 'something imperfect that cannot exist' he has in mind the limits of our powers; we are dealing, in general ideas, with what is indeed indispensable for our life, which yet, however, is an enigma to us. At the one end of our experience is the particular, with its I-know-not-what of substance; at the other is the universal which an inspection also shows to be an I-know-not-what. With these mysteries we must remain content; we cannot explain them; much less must we try to explain them away. And as we cannot dispense with the mystery of the universal if we are to apprehend the particular, we also cannot dispense with the mystery of the particular if we are to apprehend the general. Our minds inhabit a terrain between the merely particular and the wholly general; and we may not pass the frontiers of either. We are only aware that they are frontiers.

What shall we say, then? We must say that the historic theories of the universal are intelligible to us, but that we have no 'theory' ourselves, nor in the nature of things is a satisfactory 'theory' possible.

We can understand realism, for it is certain, as we have said many times, that we cannot know mere particulars, and we seem to apprehend the identity of many particulars. Yet the fact remains that this pure and abstract identity is unthinkable by us; we labour to grasp it but it eludes us. It is the inevitable end of our thought, but we fail to reach it. It is the ideal of thought, which, being what we are, we shall never realize. But, on the other hand, we can well understand nominalist positions. Here at least we can even indulge a soft spot for Bolingbroke and complain of him here only that he did not read his passage from Locke carefully enough, in particular where Locke says that the general idea is 'something imperfect that cannot exist'; for we do not know the general idea abstracted from particulars, and to think of triangle is to think of the triangularity of some one triangle. Still as against Bolingbroke, we certainly think of the *triangularity* of some one triangle; and to make any one triangle representative of others is to assume what is denied or to deny that knowledge is possible at all. For these reasons, we are ourselves left in a philosophically unmanageable state of affairs; and we may perhaps find satisfaction in reflecting that the purpose of philosophy is not merely that of solving what problems we can; it is also that of acknowledging that there are problems we cannot solve, and that our minds are in many ways teased by what we cannot, in any strict sense, be said to know. Here, by the problem of the universal, we are 'teased out of thought'; but it may be that in this way our darkness is more lightened for us than it can be by some masterful handling of elements in our experience which in fact remain when all our theories have had their say and have gone.

VIII

But lest the reader think that all this is a poor enough result of a great deal of pother; and lest he think this conclusion, if conclusion it can be called, is of no value for and of little relevance to our argument in this book, I wish to make the following further observations.

First, the imagination, confronted with the individuality of its objects, attempts to master them, as it were, by the procedure of symbolism. There is always indeed something which eludes and must elude it, the we-know-not-what which may not be penetrated and consumed; reality is certainly not exhausted by it; the very fact of knowledge, our knowledge being what it is, ensures that this is so. But at the level of the intellectual life, we have a situation in certain respects similar. Here, the intelligence tries to pluck itself out of the economy

of the mind, that is, to seize upon the universal as an object of its thinking. But here too there is failure, and the universal eludes the general
idea, as the particular is never mastered by the symbol. Thus it is that,
say what we will, the universal is known, so far as it is known at all,
only with the aid of imagination: it is *this* triangularity, *this* florality, *this*
humanity we know. The objects of both imagination and intelligence
stand at a remove; imagination and intelligence go so far towards their
objects, but only to reach a gap which they cannot cross.

Now we tried to show how the imagination in poetry proceeds by
the way of symbolism, whereby one idea, somehow run into another,
defines it. *Here*, unless our doctrine is quite mistaken, *is* a fusion of
imagery and one image dissolved into another. But in the life of the
intelligence, this is not the way. Berkeley took Locke to mean that a
general idea is a composite image which is made up, somehow, of
images of all kinds of triangles. Locke did not intend this. But yet,
it may be that we can take some steps in this direction, of joining, at
least, parts of different images. But even if we do so, the requirements
of the intellectual life are not met. The image before the mind, whether
composite or not, must point (to use an unsatisfactory metaphor for
the moment) not to other particulars but to something general; it is
nothing less than the universal which thought is out for. If the image
is indeed necessary, it must 'represent', not other particulars, but
nothing less than the universal. But the question is, can the particular
'represent' the universal? And the answer is clear and certain; by the
very nature of things it cannot. For such 'representation' to be possible
we should necessarily be able to hold the two ideas, the one particular,
the other general, alongside each other, and then allow the particular
to stand for the general. But this is impossible. We do not know the
particular divorced from the general, or the general divorced from the
particular.

It is certain therefore that the rôle of the image in thought is different
from its rôle in poetry. But, in our distress, we may find consolation
and even help in observing this fact. We said that in poetry one image
does not 'stand for' another; instead, it is a symbol in the sense that it is
somehow fused with and thereby sharpens or defines the other. The
symbol and the symbolized are united, so far as may be. Now we have
observed that whatever else it may or may not do, the image in the play
of thought cannot 'stand for', or 'represent' the universal; and we might
perhaps reflect that if indeed the image is vital to the general idea, it may
be that it is so as a symbol in the sense we have defined. But against

this, there seems to be an insuperable objection. In the lines in *Venus and Adonis*,

> Look! how a bright star shooteth from the sky,
> So glides he in the night from Venus' eye.

the image of the star may be fused with that of the falling goddess; but there is, between any image and a universal an inherent disparity. The universal must *resist* the image.

And yet, on further reflection, we may be disposed to try further this way of enquiry. For it seems to be most true that we cannot apprehend the universal without the aid of imagination. And if this is so, we must ask further whether the images of sense may somehow be 'fused into' the universal? The facts seem to suggest it; for the universal and the image seem to require each other. We cannot grasp either, so far as we grasp them at all, without the other. And if so the image *does* symbolize the universal, not as an *example* of it, for to say that is to revert to 'representation', but as an intrinsic part of it so far as it is known to us. But it will be said, to speak in this way is to remove from under our feet any ground we may have for distinguishing between art and science. And so, indeed, it may appear at first sight. But in fact, in saying that the particular is not example, I am only saying that it is never *merely* an example. Truly, the intelligence seeks to make it that; but the burden of our argument is that it can never wholly succeed. Symbol is the life of art, and in symbol art rests; but the intelligence must be ever striving to transform symbol into illustration or example, and to do this it tries always to make it abstract. Science, that is to say, is the attempt to allegorize, so to speak, the symbol, or to sunder it from the universal, so that it may stand for it. But that it can altogether succeed in this, the facts of experience conclusively deny. We legitimately speak of symbol in art and of example in science; but in doing so, we have in mind, in all strictness, only that art embraces the symbol, and that science labours to slough it off, but without success. I only add before going on, and to avoid possible misunderstanding, that in thinking in this way I am not at all falling back from what I have previously said, namely, that the universal is not to be resolved into particulars; I am now only concerned with the way in which we know it and with the rôle of the image in our knowledge of the universal. I am only trying to elucidate a very trying state of affairs; I am not trying to explain it away.

In the experience of the child, as we have spoken of it, and in our

experience of a work of art, we have said that the distinction of particular from universal is not attempted; the universal is known and is
there, but indissolubly with the particular. But when we come to adult
perception and to the play of free ideas, we seem to be confronted with
a new situation. Here the universal seems to be loosened from the
thing perceived, or from the image employed, and to be labouring to be
wholly free from imagination. That this is so is shown in a number
of ways. It is shown, in actual perception, by the slightness of our
imaginative responses to innumerable things; objects are, as it were,
ticked off by the mind as this, that or the other; their pecularities fall
away from our imaginations in the course of an interest which is predominantly practical and conceptual. But when we advance further to
free trains of ideas, we see that the imagery which 'goes along' with our
thinking is frequently slight, changeable and fragmentary; it varies
from mind to mind and seems to be quite unpredictable and not infrequently freakish. And here, it is clear that as copies, where copies are
at all possible, images are poor indeed; but that frequently nothing in
the nature of copies is possible at all. Most frequently images of words
alone seem to represent the world of imagination in the world of
thought; and in general, it simply will not do to say that thought relies
on the presence to the mind of mental reproduction of objects as 'instances' of the universal. For these reasons it will not do to say that in
order to think we must necessarily envisage a particular which 'exemplifies' the universal.

Now the chief difference between 'free' thought of this kind, what
occurs when we think independently of what is presented to us in
sense, and on the other hand perception, whether the child's or the
grown up's, seems to be this: that in sense perception we have, or may be
thought to have, before us, an 'example' of the universal; we seem to see
the particular as 'sharing in' or illustrating the universal; but that in free
ideas, we very frequently cannot be said to have a picture of a particular
and therefore of an 'example' of the universal in and before our minds.

And yet, we have seen reason to believe that we must be on our guard
against this way of thinking. For we have denied that we are capable
of thinking the universal in its abstractness; and for this reason we are
committed to denying that when we see an object we see it as an
example of the universal, and that for the reason that we cannot hold
the particular and the universal apart in our minds; let us try to, and
they both disappear. We have said of the child's perception and of our
experience of Shakespeare's *Lear* that in them we appear to grasp the

universal in the very form of imagination; and if we consider normal adult perception, we must conclude that fundamentally we have in it the same state of affairs. Here too we grasp the universal as it is in the particular. And if this is so, what is particular, the thing seen, is part and parcel of the universal as we know it; it is an aspect of a total idea in which, we are compelled to conclude, universal and the particular are united and are run into each other, so that we cannot sunder the apprehension of one from that of the other. This means that in perceiving objects we are not perceiving a particular which exemplifies a universal (for we cannot thus hold the two apart); we are instead, apprehending a particularized universal and a universalized particular. And if this seems a flight into nonsense, I can only reply that it is not such nonsense as to talk about the particular as exemplifying the universal, as if we were capable to knowing particulars as mere particulars, and universals as pure universals. Now if this is so, the position in normal perception is not fundamentally different from what we have in the perception of a child or in our perception of Lear and his fortunes. There is indeed a difference: it is that in ordinary adult perception, the tension between imagination and intelligence is greater; the intelligence is trying to assert its freedom, as the structure of language shows. But the fact remains that it cannot have it.

Now this is significant for our doctrine of what happens in free ideation. In ordinary perception, what the imagination grasps through sensation is not a particular exemplifying the universal; it is the symbol through which the universal is grasped, so far as it is grasped at all. It is the universal brought down into images of sense; and the universal is grasped in the symbolical guise of the sensuous. Now because this is so, we need be less disturbed that in free ideation we can hardly be said, at least frequently, to apprehend any close copy of objects. Our perception of objects may be dim and fragmentary enough; but that our imagery is fragmentary in free ideation need not trouble us. 'Horse is to me', said Titchener, 'a double curve and a rampant posture, with a touch of mane about it'.[1] If Titchener is here saying that 'horse' is only this imagery, he is certainly wrong; but what he describes is about as much imagery as the average person entertains when he thinks of 'horse'. But that the imagery is sketchy does not matter; it is still the symbol which is of a piece with what is symbolized.

[1] Quoted in Brand Blanshard, *The Nature of Thought*, London, 1939, vol. i. p. 272: a book which contains an admirable discussion of the idea in relation to the image, as well as many other excellent discussions.

Now it may be that there are 'universals' enough, which may seem wholly cut off from imagery of any kind, if by 'imagery' we mean anythink which is at all a copy, however fragmentary. For one thing there is the play of word-imagery. We cannot indeed be sure that words perform their work in entire independence of the images of sense whose place they have so largely come to take; and it is not, I think, rash to think that they do not. No doubt clear imagery falls away to be replaced by words; but it is exceedingly difficult to be sure that imagery of this kind falls entirely away. Even when, for example, we are reading quickly, it is presumptuous to concluded that no imagery, dim as we will, of things is not present. Introspection cannot catch the mind as we should like, and we need to be careful not to be too sure. But let us grant that thinking can proceed wholly without imagery of things and situations, (I say situations, for we have to bear relations, as well as things, in mind; and may well think of 'togetherness' through envisaging a group of things), and can act only by the use of words, and images of them written or spoken. But even here, we need to remember that we can hardly cut off the word from our individual being. It is not only that, when I think of 'tree' the very form of the letters as I see them composing the word in my image of it may be expressive; but also, we can hardly deny that there go along with words innumerable kinæsthetic reactions, again obscure enough, and so obscure as not ordinarily to be caught by introspection. For language, as we have seen, cannot wholly shed its nature as an act of the embodied self; and the word is not something entirely divorced and distanced from what we are. I think that we cannot think the words 'but' or 'however' without some amount, however much a remnant, of a bodily posture or gesture.

We must then acknowledge that 'copies', however poor, are not indispensable to thought; but it seems certain that in apprehending the universal, the world of sense is never lost to the mind. Something in the world of sense, whether a copy or not, is retained and is expressive as an intrinsic part of what the mind knows in its thinking. For this reason, we may say that all thought is imaginative thought and does not dispense with symbol; and for this reason also we were right in suggesting that in the perception of young children and in our own æsthetic experience we have the clue to the general problem of the relation of imagination to thought. There is, indeed, a good deal of difference between the child's perception and the thought required in reading a historical or political or scientific work; indeed we have illustrated, within the confines of artistic experience itself, the many tensions that occur between the imagination and the intelligence and the varying powers which they respectively acquire. Still, the union of the two is never wholly destroyed. Imagination is intellectual; and thought is always, in some degree, imaginative. As I suggested in the preceding chapter, there is an unbroken line by which we pass to the proposition 'all men are mortal' from the words of the heart-broken Lear.

We have moved far away, as it may appear, from Bolingbroke. But we shall return to the problem of universals when, in the sections following the next, we consider Bolingbroke's metaphysics and what he has to say about the Platonic tradition in European philosophy.

IX

I return briefly now to compare Bolingbroke further with Locke. I have compared them in certain points of doctrine. I wish to speak in this section of the motives of Bolingbroke's way of thinking. To do this will also be to show the distance of his mind from Locke's in spite of a professed discipleship and of certain similarities of doctrine.

That Bolingbroke wished to play down, far more than Locke, the initiative and creativeness of the mind in treating the ideas of sense, is I think clear. Besides, Locke's system, if system it may be called (and Locke certainly would not care to hear what he had to say called a system), contains a surprising amount of rationalism. This rationalism Bolingbroke disliked; but he did not think hard enough to evolve a considerable body of doctrine which would have no rationalism in it; instead, he kept it after a fashion, and disingenuously made what he called 'Nature' remove its thrust and potency. How he did this, we have seen. But there can be little doubt that Bolingbroke would have liked a more thoroughly empiricist doctrine, in which 'experience' might explain all our knowledge; and indeed what he gives us is, in effect, a much more empirical doctrine than we find in Locke; only, it is given unphilosophically and, in large part, resorts to crude mythology.

But again, there were things in Locke's *Essay* altogether to Bolingbroke's taste. Certainly there was a strong empiricist strain in Locke; and his disciple was clearly very pleased to see the *Essay* imposing rigorous limits on our knowledge of the physical world, and of the soul. Or again, Locke's pervasive way of giving the mind a very modest rôle indeed in creation was agreeable to Bolingbroke; and, like Locke, he delighted to think of an infinite wisdom whose ways we cannot make out and whose methods in the creating and ordering of the world are beyond our scrutiny. That we come into the world beggars in knowledge and ought not to carry on as if we were princes was an idea for which he found plenty of authority in Locke; and in general, even if he found it necessary to rebuke and upbraid Locke for his doctrine of universals, there were plenty of other stores in the *Essay* to be rifled, suggestions to be taken up, and so developed as to merit being given the vague authority of the great philosopher.

All this we have seen, and it may be summed up by saying that Bolingbroke's philosophy represents a development of Locke's philosophy in the direction of Hume's. The century was to produce a writer who took Locke's empiricism and developed it stringently, what Bolingbroke had the impulse but not the ability (or perhaps only the patience) to do. And between Bolingbroke and Locke there was, for all practical purposes, a much greater distance than between Bolingbroke and Hume. For Locke's empiricism directly expressed a deep piety; Bolingbroke's empiricism expressed no piety whatever and was animated by no religious motives. And we observe happening, when we read Bolingbroke, what we can see happening in our own time: logical positivism may be the instrument of a deeply religious consciousness, and may also be the instrument of hasty and ill-considered judgement. The empiricism of Bolingbroke springs from a very different motive and sensibility from that which animates Locke's. Locke's empiricism sprang from a profound sense of human ignorance and of the need of light which the human mind cannot itself come by; Bolingbroke's came from assurance and certainty. It makes no difference that what Bolingbroke was sure of was that he knew little enough, if only because he obviously found great pleasure and satisfaction in belittling the mind. Cocksureness is none the less a deplorable and unphilosophical thing for being cocksureness that one knows, once for all, that one can know little. Hobbes was sure that reason can penetrate the world and thoroughly understand it; and the pride of his mind is obnoxious to us. But it was at least a pride which came of a certain greatness of spirit and not from satisfaction in whipping an already miserable enough thing. Certainly, the wheel is coming to its full circle as we move on from Hobbes to Locke and thence to Bolingbroke; it will not complete its circle till we come to Hume; but there is irony enough to be enjoyed in observing the satisfaction of Hobbes, with his rationalist materialism, and Bolingbroke, with his empiricism, in their respective assessments of the powers of the mind.

Besides, they are both men of reason. But Locke, who stands between them, with his individual mixture of empiricism and rationalism (though his rationalism, as we saw, is not without its empirical motives) is alone, of the three, in his piety.

Bolingbroke, then, employs the *Essay* primarily as a source-book of positivism and then extends and amplifies this positivism. And in urging it he is at once very anxious and very assured. In doing so, Bolingbroke is in effect conducting, as I have already suggested, a campaign against philosophy itself. He was impatient, indeed he was angry, with the whole business of philosophy. Philosophers were anathema to him: we shall later on have plenty of opportunity to notice the violence of his hatred of them. I have already quoted his observation that there would be 'more real knowledge and more true wisdom among mankind, if there was less learning and less philosophy'; and in another place (1. p. 97), after speaking of the passion and amour-propre which, in place of the calm love of truth, goes along with human disputation, he writes this:

Will it be pretended that the schools of religion and learning have, in this respect, any advantage over other public assemblies, over coffee-houses and taverns? If it is, we may safely deny it; because we can easily prove the contrary. In vain will it be urged, that men who have much learning, and who are accustomed to investigate, and to fix the most abstruse and momentous truths, must of course, and even without superior parts, be better able nicely to discern, to determine, and to compare and to connect ideas and notions, than those who neither possess the same learning and the same habits, nor have the same art of reasoning. This may be in some respects true, but upon the whole it is not so: and a plain man would overwhelm the scholar who should hold this language, by shewing, in numerous instances, the weakness of the human mind, that of this very scholar perhaps in some; the narrow confines, and in them the instability, of our ideas and notions, the impertinence of logic, the futility of metaphysics, the blasphemy of divinity, and the fraud of disputation.

This is not, in all truth, a model of dispassionate dispute; and in the next page he says that we have 'a right to abominate those who do their utmost to render the discovery of truth impracticable, to perpetuate controversy, and to pervert the use and design of language. I prefer ignorance to such learning, Swift's bagatelle[1] to such philosophy, and the disputes of a club where it does not prevail, to those of an academy or university where it does.' He goes on: 'It is, in truth, in those places,

---

[1] 'Vive la bagatelle!' was a favourite cry of Swift.

and wherever metaphysics and theology have been made sciences, that
the arts of controversial legerdemain are practised with most license,
dexterity and success.' I have made these lengthy quotations to show the
reader that when I speak of the violence of Bolingbroke's feelings in
these matters, I am not at all exaggerating. We can certainly make allow-
ance for a natural and strong reaction from mediaeval scholasticism and
from the 'peripatetic' teaching in the universities which had afflicted
Hobbes and Locke; we can also allow for a healthy reaction from the
pedantry and unnecessary displays of learning which went on in the
seventeenth century. But even then, we are faced with a residue of
passion which requires other explanation.

No doubt it is not possible for one who hates philosophy as much as
this to be consistent. He must practise it to some extent; and this is
bound to land him in trouble. If he genuinely philosophizes, he gets
into genuine difficulties; he can only deny that these exist by a sacrifice
of candour; and he must choose between dishonesty and a cool acknow-
ledgment that all is not plain sailing. If he chooses neither, he will go
off into abuse; and this is precisely what Bolingbroke frequently and
vehemently does. Besides, *all* philosophers are not bounders, cheats
and mountebanks. There is Locke, apparently indeed, apart from
Bolingbroke himself, the single exception; but even he from time to
time, cool as he was, went off into attacks of philosophical delirium and
let his 'imagination' get 'heated'. In fairness to Bolingbroke, he himself did not write philosophical books; he wrote only letters and essays
for the edification of Pope; and it was Mallet and not he who finally
fired the blunderbuss. Still, what he wrote represents a good deal of
philosophical industry of a kind; and so far we may mildly upbraid him
with inconsistency. In addition, he was so far metaphysically-minded
as to believe that it is possible to prove that God exists; and this is a
piece of philosophical ambition which has not animated at least some
of the thinkers whom Bolingbroke would put down for logic-choppers,
dreamers and fanatics. But all this we can let pass. We wish only to
find out what it was in him which made it so easy for him to become a
victim of inconsistency, and to browbeat philosophers, with a violence
and abuse they could not hope to rival, for faults which he himself
exhibits in the extreme; and what it was which impelled him to do at
least some philosophizing without any notable attempt to show the
commonest openness of mind.

I have said that it was not piety. I shall speak later of the kind of God
in whom Bolingbroke believed; but it is no secret that He was chiefly a

stick with which to beat the heads of philosophers in particular and of mankind in general. Certainly, no one is going to find religious faith in Bolingbroke's pages; and there are few enough signs of it in his life. Nor, on the other hand, are there signs that his many beliefs caused him dismay at any time. We all know that Hume, at the end of the *Essay on Human Nature*, confessed that his philosophy dismayed and chilled him; there is nothing of the kind in Bolingbroke, only an apparent complacency and a lively cocksureness. It is true that Bolingbroke had by no means gone so far on the road to scepticism as Hume, and he contrived to give himself a good deal of philosophical comfort; but we might have expected that *some* alarm and despondency, in his dreary deistic universe, might *sometimes* have shaken him.

Besides, it cannot be said that Bolingbroke was a notable devotee of scientific knowledge and methods. I did, indeed, earlier on in this chapter quote a passage from p. 48 of the first volume in which, in a burst of eloquence, he calls experiment 'the pillar of fire which can alone conduct us to the promised land'; but here he is using scientific knowledge as a stick with which to beat the philosophers; for this purpose he would employ any stick that came his way, God or science or whatever else; and in this place it is not so much that the thought of scientific knowledge fires him as that he is pleased to be able to observe that science had made certain and observable progress where philosophy had made (as he believed) none at all. That he was not in general a notable devotee of science is, I think, clearly shown by this passage which occurs in vol. 1. pp. 74–75:

There is no study, after that of morality, which deserves the application of the human mind so much, as that of natural philosophy, and of the arts and sciences which serve to promote it. The will of God, in the constitution of our moral system, is the object of one. His infinite wisdom and power, that are manifested in the natural system of the universe, are the object of the other. One is the immediate concern of every man, and lies therefore within the reach of every man. The other does so too, as far as our immediate wants require, and far enough to excite awe and veneration of a Supreme Being in every attentive mind. But farther than this, a knowledge of physical nature is not the immediate and necessary concern of every man; and therefore a further enquiry into it becomes the labor of a few, tho the fruits of this enquiry be to the advantage of many. Discoveries of use in human life have been sometimes made; but these fruits in general consist chiefly in the gratification of curiosity. Their acquisition, therefore, is painful: and when all that can be gathered are gathered, the crop will be small. Should the human species exist a thousand generations more, and the study of nature be carried on through all of them with the same application, a little more particular knowledge of the apparent properties of matter, and of the sensible principles and laws of motion might be acquired: more phaenomena might be discovered, and a few more of those links, perhaps, which compose the great immeasurable chain of causes and effects that descends from the throne of God. But human sense, which can alone furnish the materials of this knowledge, continuing the same, the want of ideas, the want of adequate ideas would make it to the last impracticable to penetrate into the great secrets of nature, the real essences of substances, and the primary causes of their action, their passion, and all their operations; so that mankind would cease to be, without having acquired a complete and real knowledge of the world they inhabited, and of the bodies they wore in it.

This is certainly chilly enough. Bolingbroke, after all, is no great gospeller of science. He approves that some few people should satisfy their curiosity in these matters, and acknowledges that 'discoveries of use in human life have been sometimes made'; but here at least he does not see science precipitating us into any promised land. Where, earlier, he had spoken of the promised land, we can only assume he suffered an attack of what he would call delirium.

The truth appears to be that Bolingbroke was repelled by the spectacle of intellectual enquiry which went beyond what might be heard in the 'coffee-houses and taverns'. We should not however say so in too strong a tone of contempt, if only because his great friend and fellow writer and Tory, Swift, seems to have felt very much the same in these matters. It is a curious feature of the life of these times, which we are accustomed to call the age of reason, that in them strenuous intellectual enquiry was frequently despised or at least regarded as a departure from what may rightly be expected of man's conduct of himself in the world; and there is certainly no more powerful statement of this feeling than in Swift. We think of Laputa and the ninth section of *A Tale of a Tub*; for my part, I do not get the impression from Swift's writings that he was attacking only abuses of the intellectual life in science and philosophy; his writings seem, to me at least, to convey a certain exasperation with speculation and enquiry in all their forms. And if so, what fires this anti-intellectualism and contempt for the intellectual life, whether in science or philosophy?[1] 'For the brain', says Swift (also in section ix, *A Tale of a Tub*) 'in its natural position and state of serenity, disposeth its owner *to pass his life in the common forms*

---

[1] Of course, I am not suggesting that we find these things in all the literary men of the time. The mind of Addison, for example, was eminently fair and interested in intellectual inquiry.

[my italics], without any thought of subduing multitudes to his own power, his reasons or his visions'. To depart from the 'common forms' is to depart from sanity; and if Bolingbroke must tolerate science, it must be only as a pursuit by the few.

Now it may well be that we have to take into account the continuing influence of stoicism in the eighteenth century. It had been a powerful force since the Renaissance. It had deeply influenced Shakespeare as well, we may say, as Chapman, who is most quoted to show how readily the men of the late sixteenth and early seventeenth centuries had listened to stoical doctrines; I do not doubt that Horatio and Edgar owe a good deal of their characters to the ancient teaching, and embody a great deal of the ideal of the man who in suffering all suffers nothing. And the influence continued. Marcus Aurelius was well read in the seventeenth century; he was even more read in the eighteenth. The eighteenth century brought forth no less than fifty-eight editions of the *Meditations*; and we do not read far in Swift, Pope and Bolingbroke before discerning, in spite of many differences, what shows that stoicism was still a potency in England. Something of the belief in 'nature' comes from it; the dogmatic belief in the pervasion of the order of the world by a perfect reason; and not least the strong aversion to philosophical and scientific enquiry in the interests of the human, rational living of life. But to say all this is not to say very much. The tracing of influences and debts is, in itself, a wearisome business, frequently enough of that pedantic kind which would win (and here with some justification) the contempt and mockery of Swift. What is important is to ask, why should the men of this age feel this distrust of the intellectual life, whether or not they were reinforced in it by the Stoics? There must be, presumably, a reason why they chose to read stoic authors; the editions of Marcus did not fall from the skies. Why did they share, with Marcus and other Stoics, a singular antagonism to the intellectual life?

Now it is certain that no two things could be more different than the exquisite sensibility of Marcus Aurelius and the crude feeling of Bolingbroke. But this at least may be said: that stoicism was a religion (if religion it may be called) of withdrawal and defeat; and was a phenomenon of failure and 'loss of nerve'. It had indeed nobility; but all the same, there can hardly be a book in human history sadder than the *Meditations*. It is, in all truth, surprising to find ourselves speaking in the same breath of Marcus and Bolingbroke or of Marcus and Swift; but we do so only because we know that there was a widespread interest in stoicism, and especially in Marcus Aurelius, at the time; and because we observe in the Roman Emperor a disregard for the intellectual life and in Bolingbroke (and in Swift) a savage hate of it, or at least of certain of its manifestations. Now if this is so, it is, we opine, because there was in Bolingbroke and Swift, as there was in stoicism, different as Bolingbroke and Swift were from Marcus Aurelius, a certain failure of confidence. From the later fourth century onwards, philosophy is largely a story of scepticism and dogmatism; and stoicism both made very strong affirmations, and, as if in a certain fear, expressed a lively disapproval of the speculative intelligence. I do not wish to exaggerate the importance of considering the Bolingbrokes and the Swifts in the light of the continuing interest in stoicism; my chief concern is only to suggest that here, with Bolingbroke and Swift as elsewhere, to attack the speculative intelligence is to show a certain panic in the face of life, and a loss of nerve, which are none the less great because there goes with them plenty of affirmation that Reason orders the world and that everything that happens is in accordance with it. Such affirmations may be said to be, in a sense, religious; but they represent religious belief being itself employed only to beat the human into a cringing acceptance of a brutal cosmic authoritarianism; it is religion become a tool in the hands of faithlessness. For it is not only that Bolingbroke's thought is not animated by piety; his thought is animated by as much hatred of religion as of the speculative intelligence; the two things issue from the same source. Bolingbroke's depreciated the powers of the mind and abused religion and philosophy in what was, in essence, a despairing and frenzied rending and tearing of life itself; and we see, in Swift, how the spectacle of human life filled him with loathing and horror. We observed that Hobbes knew how brittle civilization is, and how easily man's life might become again nasty, brutish and short; Swift saw that human life was only that, even in its civilized state, and a life of yahoos merely. 'Although reason', he said, 'were intended by providence to govern our passions, yet it seems that, in two points of the greatest moment to the being and continuance of the world, God hath intended our passions to prevail over reason. The first is, the propagation of our species, since no wise man ever married from the dictates of reason. The other is, the love of life, which, from the dictates of reason, every man would despise, and wish it at an end, or that it never had a beginning.' This is what underlies the cult of reason in Hobbes, Bolingbroke and Swift. I shall return to this a little later. I only remark now that it is no accident that they were in varying degrees for intolerant regimes in government, nor that Hume, later on, was to study Bolingbroke's *Patriot King* and admire it. Only Locke, of these men of whom we speak, had real assurance in the face of life and a belief that tolerance was possible as well as desirable.

X

I go on now to speak of Bolingbroke's deistic metaphysics and of what he was accustomed to say of those philosophers who in the past and at that time had ventured to take a view different from his own. I have, in the sections preceding this one, looked ahead to Bolingbroke's metaphysics; we must now speak of it in more detail.

I said, at the beginning of this chapter, that we do not read more than a few of the first pages of Bolingbroke's philosophical writings before it is clear that he entertains a very violent hatred and contempt for Plato, Malebranche, and Berkeley. It is true that in his references to Berkeley his dislike of his doctrine (or of the bigger part of it) goes along with a clear affection for him; one of the pleasantest things in Bolingbroke's pages is a certain liking he shows for the Bishop, even when he disapproves virulently of what he has to say. In particular, St. Augustine, in whom we see, more than in any other figure, the historic synthesis of Platonism and Christianity, is hateful to him. Plato, St. Augustine, Plotinus and, in his own day, the Cambridge Platonists and Samuel Clarke, stand for what Bolingbroke will not have, at any cost; he comes back again and again to vilify and befoul their names and works. Plato above all is the source of philosophical evil; and that his doctrine should have at all influenced and succoured Christianity is the principal catastrophe the human mind has suffered.

This virulent and impassioned hatred of Platonism in all its forms is of great interest and significance. To express it was Bolingbroke's chief aim in his writings. I shall now make some quotations to ensure to the reader that I am not misrepresenting him, or exaggerating.

What man, he asks (in vol. 2, p. 111), who was not in the delirium of a metaphysical fever, and who turned his eyes coolly and soberly inward, has not seen that we know nothing of sensible objects but what our senses discover to us, and our memory retains of them after they are discovered; and that all those ideal entities, the abstract forms of them, are the bold fictions of imagination? Who ever reflected on the operations of his mind, and did not perceive that all his ideas, or complex notions of mixed modes and relations, ere the creatures of the mind, who puts them together for her use as experience

16

and observation direct, nay arbitrarily if she pleases; that he never discerned them any where but in his own mind; that they are of mere human production; and that as they are often variously combined or compounded by different minds, so they are seldom preserved in any mind steadily and invariably? Shall we be afraid then to say that the doctrine of ideas in Plato is absurd and false, and that he has by reaching it corrupted the first elements of knowledge? It is manifest that he has done so, too manifest to be denied: and for this reason his admirers have endeavoured rather to accustom mankind to the absurdity, by their constant imitations of it, than to defend it.

Notwithstanding all that has been observed, and much more that might have been observed, to shew the fallacy and impertinence of a philosophy that has been so long admired, this philosophy has rolled down a torrent of chimerical knowledge from pagan and christian antiquity, with little opposition, and scarce any interruption, to the present age; for which reason it is as necessary to expose the futility of this philosophy now, as it would have been many centuries ago. Not only pagan, but christian theology has been derived from Plato in great measure; and, as strangely as that may sound, even from Homer too, if he imitated Homer as much, and borrowed as much from him, as Longinus and others of the antients affirm. There is a certain marvellous which dazzles and seizes the mind, the philosophical as well as the unphilosophical; and the man who thinking he understands, admires his own understanding, as well as the man who admires, because he does not understand. This gave a great lustre to the platonic philosophy: and is employed in season and out of season, so as to run through almost every part of it.

He goes on, on p. 114, to say:

The profane assumption we speak of here, which had it's foundation in the platonic and pythagoric systems, tends to lessen our admiration and adoration of the Supreme Being, or at least the humiliation of ourselves, by taking our thoughts off from the sensible connection between us and other animals, and by applying them to an imaginary connection between the divine and human nature. There are no anthropomorphites I think left: but there have been men among the most devout theists of paganism, and there are those among christian philosophers and divines, who join God and man as absurdly by a supposed similitude of intellect, knowledge, and manner of knowing, as those heretics did by a supposed similitude of figure. Vanity has not only maintained this absurdity among the followers of Plato, but spread it among those of different sects. I will not turn to the extravagant passages of this sort, that are to be found in the writings we have of the latter pythagorician Platonists. I will mention one only from those of St. Austin, which happens to occur to my memory, and may serve instar omnium. Nothing is superior to the human soul, says that father, but God. 'Nihil est potentius—nihil est sublimius. Quicquid supra illam est jam creator est.' This doctrine the saint learned, as he learned that of the divine Logos, from Plato, or from those madmen the disciples of Pythagoras and Plato. In short, the vanity of the human heart indulged itself in this kind of flattery so much, that even the Stoics borrowed the same notions.

Later in the same volume (p. 358) he says that

Since the works of Plato are in our hands, we may speak of him and his theology with more assurance, than of those who went before him, or of their doctrines. Those of Orpheus, or those that passed under such a name in ancient Greece, were chiefly mythological; those of Pythagoras, symbolical; and those of Plato, metaphysical, with a mixture of the other two. Nothing could be more proper, not effectual, to promote fantastical knowledge, than a method of philosophising by fables, symbols, and almost a perpetual allegory. But the founder of the academy did more. He poisoned the very source of all real knowledge, by inducing men to believe, that their minds are capable of abstracting, as no human mind can abstract, and of acquiring ideas, that it is impossible any human mind should perceive. He pretended to raise a mystic ladder, on which we might not only clamber up by dint of meditation to a region of pure intellect, wherein alone is knowledge, and leave sensible objects behind us, concerning which nothing better than opinion is to be had; but find at the head of it incorporeal essences, immaterial forms, spiritual beings, and perhaps the Logos or second god: as the supreme God is supposed to have been at the head of the ladder Jacob saw in his dream. Angels went up and down one: philosophers were to go up and down the other.

This philosopher dealt little in physics: and he was in the right to neglect them. Metaphysics served his purpose better. Hypotheses of the former kind must be founded in some real knowledge: how high soever the top of the ladder reaches, the foot must stand firm on the earth. But hypotheses of the other kind are more easy to be framed, and less easy to be controlled. Thus, for instance, an intellectual world being once assumed, wherein the ideas, the forms, the patterns of all that exist in the sensible world reside, it was easy to people it with numberless intellectual, that is, spiritual, that is, immaterial, that is, simple beings without extension or solidity, that is, beings of which these refiners had negative, but no positive ideas. They were at liberty afterwards to suppose whatever relations they pleased between these beings, and between them and men. Metaphysical hypotheses, in short, are not content to account for what may be by what is, nor to improve science according to the conditions of our nature, by raising probability on the foundations of certainty: but the makers of them affect to range in the immense void of possibility, with little or no regard to actuality; and begin very often, as well as end, in supposition. Not only their systems are hypothetical, but the first principles of them, and the very ideas and notions which compose them, are hypothetical too.

Such a philosopher, such a teacher of imaginary and fantastic knowledge, Plato was.

Finally, I quote this passage (vol. 2. pp. 332–33):

Christianity, as it stands in the gospel, contains not only a complete, but a very plain system of religion; it is in truth the system of natural religion: and such it might have continued, to the unspeakable advantage of mankind, if it had been propagated with the same simplicity with which it was originally taught by Christ himself. But this could not have happened, unless it had pleased the divine providence to preserve the purity of it by constant interpositions, and by extraordinary means sufficient to alter the ordinary course of things. Such a constant interposition, and such extraordinary means, not being employed, christianity was left very soon to shift for itself, in the midst of a frantic world, and in an age when the most licentious reasonings, and the most extravagant superstitions, in opinion and practice, prevailed universally under the respectable names of theology and metaphysics; and when the Jews themselves, on whose religion, and on the authority of whose scriptures, christianity was founded, had already gone far in corrupting both by oral traditions and cabalistical whimsies, by a mixture of notions taken from the chaldaic philosophy during their captivity, and from the Grecian philosophy since the expedition of Alexander. The traces of these mixtures are discernible: those of Greek origin most manifestly; and among them, those of platonism are so strongly marked, that it is impossible to mistake them. This philosophy was the very quintessence of the theology and metaphysics which Plato, and Pythagoras before him, had imported into Greece. It had been extracted by the intense heat of the warmest imagination that ever Greece produced, and had contributed more, than any other system of paganism, to turn theists into enthusiasts, and to confirm that fondness for mystery, without an air of which no doctrine could pass for divine.

I have quoted at such length in order to convey to the reader unmistakably what it is that Bolingbroke is above all anxious to clear out of the way: it is nothing less, as I have said, than the major European philosophical tradition. Locke had said, in his *Epistle to the Reader*, that it was 'ambition enough to be employed as an under-labourer in clearing the ground a little, and removing some of the rubbish that lies in the way to knowledge'. Locke was certainly no Platonist; but we can see (and he could hardly have foreseen) how quickly his words would instigate his professed disciples to put Plato and St. Augustine on the rubbish-heaps of history.

XI

Before speaking further of this polemic of Bolingbroke's, its significance and detail, I wish to remark on a feature of the abuse it employs. I mean Bolingbroke's habit of calling the philosophers whom he dislikes, of whom Plato is the chief and head, *poets* and creatures of *imagination*. No terms of contempt seem to him stronger, or more telling, than these. He departs, we observe, from the widespread Augustan practice of speaking of the 'fancy'; 'imagination' is his word. In raising 'an immaterial, intellectual world' Plato and his followers 'knew little, imagined much, built beyond nature' (2. p. 386); again, 'I do not believe that Plato was an enthusiast in any other sense, than you poets affect to appear such when you call for inspiration, and boast of the divine fury' (2. p. 102); and, 'it is a strong instance of the perversity of the human will, but it is true in fact, that men attempt often to go beyond nature, for no better reason than this, because they cannot go up to it; or than this, because they do not find that to be, which imagination had told them might be. These men are metaphysicians . . .'

Now in speaking of poetry and imagination (and as he uses these terms in these essays they mean philosophical speculation), he opposes to them nature, reason, judgement, plain common sense, all of which seem to mean very much the same thing. 'I will follow no man out of the high road of plain common sense. In that, the philosopher may lead me to all real knowledge for common sense does not exclude uncommon discoveries in the search of truth' (1. p. 160); 'to know things as they are is to know truth. To know them as they may be is to guess at truth. Judgement and observation guide to one, imagination and speculation to the other. To know them as they are, the mind must be constantly intent to frame it's ideas and notions after that great original, nature . . .' (1. p. 84); 'imagination submitted to judgement will never go beyond knowledge founded on experience, or high probability immediately deducible from it' (1. p. 85). In these and many other sentences like them, he explains to us what he means by imagination. I have observed earlier that Bolingbroke is, in all this talk about 'Nature,' walking, to say the least, on very thin ice. For our complex ideas are, in fact, of our own making, and our minds have arbitrary powers. Only, nature 'obtrudes' them on us, and if we are 'natural' and sensible and use our common sense, we shall not entertain an idea which nature has not induced us to frame.

But it is obvious that this does not give us the shadow of a criterion whereby to judge what is 'natural'; 'Nature' itself here becomes an instrument of the wildest prejudice and, to use the term ourselves, of 'imagination'. Nature, we are told again and again, will declare to us what is only possible and what is probable and real; there is no need for us to guess at truth. But who is judge between the voice of 'Nature' in a Plato and in a Bolingbroke? I wish not to weary the reader by reiterating this; but the Augustans played with the idea of Nature so extensively; and it is necessary to emphasize that the employment of the idea by a Pope and a Bolingbroke was only arbitrary; it arose out of their own forms of enthusiasm and guesswork.

We remark Bolingbroke's use, for abuse, of the word 'imagination', and observe that he is using it in a sense somewhat different from that in which Hobbes and Locke used the word 'fancy'. I explained earlier that they intended by fancy what observes identities and similarities, and this in contrast to judgement which, they said, maintained the sense of differences in the mind. I said that this doctrine will not serve; for the two processes are part and parcel of each other, and are not at all different in kind. Locke however wrote, in the *Essay* (2. 30), about what he called 'fantastical' or 'imaginary' ideas. Simple ideas, he says there, are all 'real'; we receive them, and that is all there is to it. But it is different with our complex ideas, which the mind frames. But which of them, he asks, 'are real, and which barely imaginary combinations?' The answer is that ideas of mixed modes and relations are their own archetypes; that (iv) 'there is nothing more required to this kind of ideas to make them real, but that they be so framed, *that there be a possibility of existing conformable to them*' (my italics); then Locke adds, aware, no doubt, that this is a difficult position to hold, 'they cannot be chimerical, unless *any one will jumble together in them inconsistent ideas*' (again my italics). No good purpose is served in criticizing these statements; Locke advances the two different criteria out of clear embarrassment. And, so far as complex ideas of substances are concerned, the position is little better; 'those are fantastical,' he says in v, 'which are made up of such collections of simple ideas as were really never united, never were found together in any substance: e.g. a rational creature, consisting of a horse's head, joined to a body of human shape, or such as the *centaurs* are described: or, a body yellow, very malleable, fusible and fixed; but lighter than common water ... Whether such substances as these can possibly exist or not, it is probable we do not know: but be that as it will, these ideas of substances, being made conformable to no pattern existing that we know ... ought to pass with us for barely imaginary . . .' Locke acknowledges with all his characteristic frankness, that in these things we cannot judge what possible existences are; and it is clear that if we were indeed bound to combinations of simple ideas actually found, there could be no play for the scientific imagination. Besides, we observed at an earlier stage (p. 127) how honestly Locke recognizes the possibility that all our ideas, in apprehending the agreement or disagreement of which our knowledge consists, may compose only a 'castle in the air'; and on his showing this applies not only to our knowledge of substances, but no less to our ethical and mathematical knowledge and to our knowledge of God.

But the fairness of mind Locke shows here, as everywhere else, does not at all manifest itself in Bolingbroke's writings. Locke knows well enough how difficult it all is; Bolingbroke succeeds only in giving the impression that it is all perfectly simple and that any one not a purblind idiot knows quite well what is 'real' and what is not. Therefore he can use the word 'imagination' for abuse merely. But he can do so only because, here as elsewhere, he will not take the trouble to *think*. Instead, he resorts to his mythological 'Nature', our nurse and instructress, a piece of crude machinery to which Locke would never resort; and then puts down metaphysics to 'imagination'.

XII

We now must consider what it is in Platonic metaphysics which is put down for 'imagination' by Bolingbroke. The quotations I gave provide the answer; it is of course the Ideas. Plato 'poisoned the very source of all real knowledge, by inducing men to believe, that their minds are capable of abstracting, as no human mind can abstract, and of acquiring ideas, that it is impossible any human mind should perceive. He pretended to raise a mystic ladder, on which we might not only clamber up by dint of meditation to a region of pure intellect, wherein alone is knowledge, and leave sensible objects behind us . . .' (2. p. 359). In this way, he says (2. p. 114), our thoughts are applied to 'an imaginary connection between the divine and human nature', and we 'join God and man . . . absurdly by a supposed similitude of intellect, knowledge and manner of knowing'. As I have said, Bolingbroke is above all anxious to rule out any notion that many may share in or enjoy the Divine Nature. He saw that Platonism, more than any other doctrine, has provided a philosophical basis for Christianity. And hence his violent attack on Plato and all his influence and disciples.

We have seen that Bolingbroke believed that our general ideas are ideas of a particular only which is somehow 'representative' of other particulars. This doctrine will not do. We cannot deny, without flying in the face of the facts, that we know what is universal; we only added that in knowing it, we know it imperfectly, and cannot shed the imagination, which always provides us with the symbol in and through which it is apprehended. To know the universal is indeed to transcend the imagination; but it is not to dispense with it. Knowledge of the universal is imaginative thought; and the image and the universal are not two things but, in our experience, are inextricably joined. Bolingbroke believed that to say that we know, in any sense, what is universal is to be 'imaginative'; we say that we do indeed know what is universal, and that our imaginations (but not only our imaginations) are indeed employed.

Now Locke, as I have said, was no Platonist. It is true, as we have seen, that in the end he came to think of universals as 'essences': 'for whatever becomes of Alexander and Bucephalus, the idea to which man and horse [he means the names] are annexed are supposed nevertheless to remain the same, and so the essence of those species are preserved whole and undestroyed, whatever changes happen to any, or all, of the individuals of those species' (3. 3. xix). But, also, these are only nominal essences and are framed by us; the essences may be 'whole and undestroyed' and rest 'safe and entire' (and in speaking thus Locke seems to be nearing Platonic ideas); but in fact they do not exist outside our mind. They may be fixed; but they are fixed by us. And what is true of our general ideas of 'sorts' of things is true also of our general ideas in mathematics and morals, except that these are not like the former, created out of our experience of things but out of our minds merely. Locke seems to have been on the way to a more Platonic doctrine; but he was checked, and for obvious reasons. Had he said that the 'essences' of the 'sorts' were objective and genuine apprehensions he would have found it difficult to sustain his distinction between real and nominal essences. Had he said that mathematical essences were objective, his empiricism would have been in all truth a lost cause; and he can be as rationalist as he is only because he also denies that those ideas we have which are not derived from experience do not have to do with reality. Bolingbroke denies, in effect, the universal element in knowledge. Locke asserts it, only to say that it is something mind-made with little footing in reality. Bolingbroke's denial is denied by the facts; Locke's assertion demolishes both mathematics and morality as claimants to disclose what is real. Bolingbroke assumes the universal in denying it; Locke implies that in mathematics and morality we are at best playing with counters of our own making.[1]

Bolingbroke's doctrine is negligible. Locke's is not; and I shall make a few observations about it, from which I shall be able to pass to speaking further about universals in the light of what I have formerly said in Section VIII of the present chapter. In a preceding chapter I said that while we can easily understand Locke's motives in speaking of mathematics as a mere play of (as he might have said) 'fancy', the doctrine is hardly credible. It is so, if only because it reduces mathematical physics to being an altogether unintelligible accident. The great fruitfulness of mathematics in their application to the physical world may not be left for a mystery; we can only, out of regard for the facts, assume that in mathematics we have a genuine key to the understanding of the physical world. Now if this is so, we must further move on to reject Locke's neat and clearcut distinction between nominal and real essences, or between ideas of nominal and of real essences. It is no doubt true that we have not and never shall wholly comprehend the physical world; but to say that is not to reduce scientific knowledge to mere observation and the putting together into complex ideas of what are seen to exist alongside in nature; instead, scientific knowledge is, so far as it goes, an exposure of intelligible elements in the natural world; it is an *understanding* of the natural world, so far as it goes. Now if this is so, it is no less unsatisfactory to make of our moral ideas and judgements what contains no necessary relevance to what is real. It was agreeable to Locke to give to morality a 'deduction' as clear as we can have in mathematics, and accordingly he classified the mixed modes of ethics with the simple modes of mathematics as man-made; but to do this is both to ignore the obvious difference between mathematics and morals, that of fact and value, 'is' and 'ought', and to give no metaphysical footing to morality. Locke's doctrines of our general ideas match up to our experience better than do Bolingbroke's; but still, they are certainly not adequate to it.

Now we for our part can only class ourselves with those who bring down Bolingbroke's anger on their heads. We have said that in knowledge we know the genuinely universal, 'symbolized' indeed in the medium of the imagination, but, still, the universal. I wish only to say this in addition: we have not said that we know the pure universal; we

---

[1] There is, of course, another doctrine of morals in Locke's work, a hedonist and empiricist one. It was this, of course, which Bolingbroke accepted.

do not, just as we do not know the 'pure' individual; for we cannot move in a merely imaginative or in a merely intelligible world. What we know is the universal mediated by imagination; and therefore, the universal is at once transcendent of our minds and brought down to them and thereby made impure. The universal is transcendent because, in our coming to know it, it is made imperfect; or better, we cannot encompass it; it defeats us, and escapes us. But it is also immanent; for we do know it, as the facts clearly require us to believe, in and through the images of our imaginations. Or again, we might say that what is universal in the objects we know is not the absolute universal, but something in between what is imagined and what is intelligible, an 'inferior universality' which is known by imagination and thought in concert, and which however seeks to draw the mind off to the universal which wholly transcends sense. Here, at the very limits of our knowledge, the tensions between thought and imagination are strong and deep, and give no rest to the mind. For we are cast, and left, in the paradox of which we spoke earlier: namely, that the universals which we know are *these* or *those* universals, *this* humanity and *that* florality, *this* circularity and *that* triangularity, *this* goodness and *that* injustice. This is, as we said, an unpleasing and teaseful situation for us. But it seems to be our case. Beyond the universals as they are shown in the images of imagination, there are the universals themselves, in their purity, unsymbolized in sense; but as such they are indeed transcendent. Yet, it is they which are shown to us in the symbols amongst which we move; the eternity of the ideas is imaged to the imagination in the symbols of time; and the universe we know is a symbolical universe.

Alles Vergängliche
Ist nur ein Gleichnis;

and it was Goethe who also declared that we see 'the real symbolism' in the particular representing the universal not as 'a dream or shadow but as a living, instantaneous revelation of what cannot be searched out'. Thus, these symbols are not symbols *of* the universal; they are part and parcel of our knowledge of the universal. Once again, the symbol and the symbolized are fused in our idea. I have said that the ultimate individuality of the particular retains within itself something inviolable by our minds; and the ultimate generality of the universal lies no less beyond us.

We must therefore turn to meet and counter the fury and contempt of Bolingbroke. We are guilty, it seems, of his charges, philosophical delirium and all the rest. But we seem only to be meeting the facts; and our best plan will be not to suffer abuse, but to consider how Bolingbroke himself gets along in his universe of plain common sense.

XIII

For far as Bolingbroke has gone, and would like to go, in empiricism, in reducing the world to the merest particulars and in destroying speculative philosophy, he is also committed to far-reaching metaphysical doctrines. Above all, he has no doubt that the universe is a system devised by a deity of perfect wisdom. Indeed the wisdom of his deity is so perfect that to make question of it is the purest human insolence. We may not be able to see or understand much of its workings; but this is additional proof of its perfection. That God's wisdom transcends ours in an infinite degree puts him beyond the doubt of all reasonable men. 'Infinite wisdom', he tells us in the fourth volume at p. 326, 'appears everywhere. Every new discovery . . . is a new proof of this wisdom, as well as of the power of God. The power of executing is seen in every instance; and tho we cannot discern the wisdom of contrivance and direction, which are more remote from our observation, in every instance, yet we see them in so many, that it becomes the highest absurdity not to acknowledge them in all. They, who do not acknowledge them so, judge of the proceedings of an all-perfect Being . . . as they would not judge of those of a prince or minister of state, who had acquired and deserved, by a long course of political conduct, the reputation of wisdom'. This, no doubt, was not Bolingbroke's way of thinking about Walpole. But then, Bolingbroke knew what political wisdom was, and was in a position to judge the English, as well as the cosmic, direction of affairs. 'Two things are then evident', he had said a few pages earlier (p. 323), 'one, that since infinite wisdom determined to call into existence every being that does exist, and to constitute that universal system, which we call the system of nature, it was right and fit that infinite power should be exercised for this purpose. The other, that, since infinite wisdom not only established the end, but directed the means, the system of the universe must be necessarily the best of all possible systems . . .' All this is bold speculation in one who is at pains precisely to demolish the idea of any 'supposed similitude of intellect, knowledge and manner of knowing' (2. p. 114) between man and God; and who tells us (4. p. 316) that the 'distance between them (i.e. divine and human intelligence) . . . is so immense, as to admit in reality no degree of comparison'. On the one side, God is altogether transcendent; on the other, we are in a position to approve of his proceedings as completely wise. And clearly, Bolingbroke may give this approval, not out of faith, philosophical delirium, or other 'building beyond nature'; he is thinking and arguing, he tells us (4. p. 322), 'from knowledge, not from imagination'.

There is little good purpose served in belabouring this argument. Bolingbroke may not consistently talk in this way. To say this is not at all to diminish the value of the argument from design. The cosmological argument has a value which philosophical theology in our time has perhaps underrated; and if so, it is perhaps because religious philosophy has not forgotten the rôle it played in the doctrine of irreligious theorists like Bolingbroke. But whatever its past history, it is certainly not to be despised; on the contrary, it remains a potent argument for the existence of God. But what strikes us in Bolingbroke's pages is the rashness and affrontery with which he holds that it proves that there is an *omnipotent* and *all-wise* Divine mind. An omnipotent Divine mind there may well be; but that such a mind is proved by the considerations Bolingbroke advances, is certainly not clear. But again, it is not that his argument will not do, but his motive in insisting that it does, which is interesting. It is obvious to both theist and atheist that Bolingbroke is not fairly facing the evidence. But why not? The answer is, in all truth, that he is enthusiastic and delirious, and animated by unphilosophical passions; and his enthusiasm and passion can only be, we think, for diminishing our human heads; God is infinitely great and wise in order that we may be shown up for the wretched foolish things we are. In all true religion God is indeed great, and man indeed small and humble; yet our manhood may be taken up into God. But Bolingbroke's God is made infinitely great and our humanity infinitely small in order that they may be completely and for ever sundered. This is the irreligion of Bolingbroke.

There is no 'similitude of intellect' between man and God. But man can somehow know the truth about the world's origin and that it is the 'best of all possible worlds'. This is speculative and inconsistent doctrine enough; and one might have thought Bolingbroke had given away the game. So, indeed, he has. Only he has not seen it. 'A close affinity between the divine and the human mind, and a certain sameness of ideas and notions, is the common boast of metaphysical theology', he says in the third volume, at p. 371; and one might have thought that in judging, 'from knowledge and not from imagination', that God is all-great, all-wise, all-powerful and acts always for the best, Bolingbroke had joined in the boastful clamour. Indeed, he had. But he did not know it; and goes on, in a spirit of assumed and (by him) undoubted consistency, to wage a campaign against attributing to God our moral values. To call God perfectly wise will do; to call him good is philosophical delirium at the top of its bent.

But it is necessary, and only fair to Bolingbroke, to observe how he tries to maintain that God is wholly transcendent while also saying that we can be sure that He is all-wise. God is, he affirms, the omnipotent and wholly wise creator of the world. But he is at great pains to point out that we have no knowledge of the manner of God's knowing. God is omniscient; but his knowing is an altogether different knowing from ours; and 'how he knows, or what knowledge is in him, we are unable to say' (3. p. 378). This, certainly, the whole direction of Bolingbroke's thinking would incline him to sustain; he wants a God who is wholly transcendent. But here, even Bolingbroke acknowledges, in effect, that he cannot be consistent; and he is driven to declaring an affinity between the human and divine in knowledge. Or rather, he does not declare it, but goes only so far, under what was for him always the mollifying influence of Berkeley, to say, 'I see no inconveniency in speaking of the divine ideas, when we speak of the divine knowledge. On the contrary, I see much conveniency in it; because I apprehend that we can neither conceive anything, nor explain our conceptions on many occasions, concerning God's knowledge, without ascribing to him hypothetically the sole manner of knowing that is known to us (3. pp. 375–6). He only adds, 'But I think it, however, both absurd and profane to pronounce dogmatically that this is God's manner of knowing, that he has no other . . .' But to say all this is to come a long way to meet his opponents; and he is in danger of being judged enthusiastic when he says (p. 379) that 'we may frame dark and confused notions of knowledge vastly superior to our own in kind, as well as in degree . . .' Here, against what he considers the excesses of Cudworth's Platonism, he says he is a 'modest and humble theist, who is far from all metaphysical presumption and theological arrogance', and who thinks that 'we are shut up in one of those dark caverns of the universe mentioned in the Phaedo; that there we grope about after knowledge, not by the light of the sun, but by that of a small and dim taper. This light, whatever it is, was bestowed on us by God. He gave us our light. He did not give us his own' (3. p. 374). But to say so much is to be on the highroad to Platonism. Our light may be only a taper's; still, it is light, and given us by God; and in saying that 'God did not give us his own' he can only fairly mean that God's light is more powerful than ours, what no one would wish to deny.

It is only fair to Bolingbroke to point out all this. He attacks Cudworth and Clarke with great violence; but if he is to have his God, he has to acknowledge 'affinity' between Him and us in knowledge. This he acknowledges, with occasional touches of modesty rare in him. It is none the less agreeable to point them out. But they on their side are none the less inconsistencies. The prevailing intention of his philosophy is to remove God to the extreme end of a chain of influences establishing his existence, and to keep Him there. But the chain is also a connexion; and if Bolingbroke is to have his God, he cannot merely be a demonstrated one. A wholly transcendent God is a contradiction in terms, and the motive for believing in Him can only be irreligious. The effect of Bolingbroke's nominalism, again, was to keep apart the human and the Divine; the universal is a myth, and there are only particulars. But if so, the Divine is ruled out from the beginning and community destroyed; it will not do to clamour for system and to deny the universal.

But if Bolingbroke wavers by admitting some little affinity between God's knowledge and ours, he seems far more determined not to admit affinity in moral values between God and man. But here it seems certain from the outset that Bolingbroke is in as great difficulty as before. For his God has perfect wisdom and acts always for the best; the world of his making is the best of all possible worlds. But to say this is to prescribe identity of value; to acknowledge the wisdom of anyone and that he has acted for the best assumes that he and we have certain ideals in common. So, at least, we should have thought. But Bolingbroke is nowhere fiercer than in this matter. 'The presumption of those, who pretend to reduce our moral obligations from the moral attributes of God, has so much theological authority on it's side, that the absurdity of it cannot be too often exposed and censured ... Tho we rise from the knowledge of ourselves, and of the other works of God, to a knowledge of his existence and his wisdom and power, which we call infinite ... yet we cannot thus rise to a knowledge of his manner of being, nor of his manner of producing those effects which give us ideas of wisdom and power; and as little, or less if possible, can we rise from our moral obligations to his supposed moral attributes.' Then he goes on at once to say, 'I call them supposed, because, after all that has been said to prove a necessary connection between his physical and his moral attributes, the latter may be all absorbed in his wisdom. It is even more agreeable to the phaenomena, to believe that they are so, and that, his wisdom determining him to do always that which is fittest to be done upon the whole, of which fitness we are in no degree competent judges, the effects of it give us sometimes ideas of those moral qualities, which we acquire by reflection on ourselves or by our dealings with one another, and sometimes not' (4. pp. 18–19). This remarkable passage sets out well enough both Bolingbroke's doctrine and the difficulties he is up against. He will not allow that God and man are 'of the same mind' (4. p. 21). His fundamental motive in thinking so, we have discussed. But he finds it easy to advance arguments against attributing moral qualities to God: 'How shall we deduce fortitude from the attributes of God, or ascribe this virtue to him who can endure no pain, nor be exposed to any danger?' (4. p. 21); and he can accordingly set up for a virtuous opponent of crude anthropomorphic notions of the Deity. At the same time, the passages I have quoted show his embarrassment. He speaks of God's moral attributes being absorbed in His wisdom; of His wisdom determining him to do always that which is fittest to be done; and of the effects of what He does giving us sometimes ideas of His moral qualities.

Like his knowledge and manner of knowing, God's moral qualities, if he can be said to possess any, lie beyond us. Here too, if Bolingbroke can have his way, the divine and the human cannot meet. We have indeed moral obligations, which may be said to be ordained by God in His wisdom. But our morality flows only from our nature as social beings which God has given us; it is therefore contrived by God and extrinsic to His own nature; to do certain things is to achieve happiness, and thus the wishes of God, and the law He commands us to obey, are manifested; but in these obligations, which we may or may not observe, nothing of God's nature shows through; morality is wholly mundane and secular, however much commanded by God. Here, too, God and man have not 'one mind'. There is nothing peculiarly moral, so to say, about morality. It is the result of God's command merely, and a creature of time; it does not express what is eternal; Cudworth and Clarke were altogether wrong in thinking things to be good or bad by nature; things are so only by what must be for us the arbitrary (though no doubt the perfectly wise) will of God. In addition, it is nonsense to speak of God's love for us; to believe that God loves us is only to make fantastic knowledge minister to self-love (4. p. 307). Reason will not indeed deny that the soul is immortal; but reason cannot demonstrate that it is, and to believe that it is may well be a vulgar error (4. p. 348). Certainly

Bolingbroke's disposition is to think it an error designed to raise man, 'in imagination, above corporeal nature' (4. p. 206). There is a form of prayer which may be approved by what Bolingbroke calls a 'theist'; but as a mode of 'access to the Supreme Being', prayer is only flattery of humanity. Bolingbroke gives us, on pp. 333–34 of the fourth volume, a model 'theistic' prayer; and it is well worth study.

The reader will see from all this that Bolingbroke's metaphysics is both very extensive and hardly consistent. I shall say no more of its inconsistency; of its extensiveness I remark only that, great as it is, its animating motive is negative. Bolingbroke's thought takes a wide sweep. But not because he thinks metaphysical construction desirable, but because, by playing boldly, he hopes to put a stop to metaphysics of the usual kind. He makes to the metaphysicians the gift of God's existence. But he gives little more. God may exist, and Bolingbroke thereby, indeed, ensures to us a systematic universe; but for the rest, it is cold comfort. God is evacuated of any taint of humanity and the human of any taint of the divine; we are left very near to the animals and at an infinite remove from Him; and we must accept the wisdom of an omnipotent Mind with whom we have nothing in common. This is Bolingbroke's 'theism'; but it is a theism which for all practical purpose asserts God's existence in order to destroy religion. It is, so far as one can have such a thing, a positivistic metaphysic. Positivism, as we now know it, denies that metaphysics is possible; Bolingbroke's positivism goes in for a metaphysic which makes of God a fact cut free from our values. It is indeed a poor enough piece of philosophizing; but it is less its inconsistencies than its motive which interests us and which is significant.

XIV

I ask now: What will such a thinker make of Christianity? When I have briefly answered this question, I shall speak of the significance of deism in the history and philosophy of religion; and then I shall sketch a doctrine which, in the light of what I have said earlier, may do justice to the rôle of the imagination in religion.

Little good purpose is served nor any great need fulfilled by speaking at any length of Bolingbroke's attitude to Christianity. It is certain that, however he may choose to express himself, he can have little use for it; he is really content with what he thinks is the simplicity and clearness of natural religion. It is however only fair to Bolingbroke to say, at the outset, that there are places in his pages where he writes like a Christian. The places are few; but it is right to refer to them as it was right to speak earlier of his occasional modesties in the matter of God's knowledge. One of the places I have in mind is at pp. 4–5 of the third volume where he speaks sympathetically even of St. Augustine. He has spoken of St. Augustine's repentance for his earlier Manichæism and of his discovery of Platonism, 'wherein he found the divinity of the Word established by many arguments. Of the incarnation of the Word, indeed, he found nothing. But he found it afterwards in the Scriptures, and he remained persuaded that God had prepared him, by this accidental information, for what he was to learn, when he should study the scriptures, concerning the humiliation of the Word made flesh . . . Thus you see how Plato, in the wanderings of a wild imagination, had discovered, in part at least, one of the greatest mysteries of Christianity; and how God made use of this truth, which he who published it did not know to be such, for the conversion of one of the greatest doctors and saints of the church.' This is not Bolingbroke's usual tone and manner. He had said, immediately before what I have quoted, that here we see the 'frantic mother of a frantic offspring', by which he means Plato, being made a vehicle of grace to the world; but he at once adds that he (Bolingbroke) has 'no conception' of grace. Still, he admits its operation here; and we are surprised that he, of all people, is capable of speaking in this way.

He is certainly committed to believing that Christianity 'as it stands in the gospel . . . is in truth the system of natural religion' (2. p. 332). This Locke had denied; his disciple affirms it. He may not of course in truth believe this. What is in the gospel manifestly asserts what Bolingbroke elsewhere denies, that God is good, loves man, and may be approached in a form of prayer of which Bolingbroke could not approve, to mention nothing more. But Bolingbroke will have it that what is set forth in the teaching of the gospels is 'natural' only; and his Christianity consists in believing, in addition to this 'natural' gospel, that Christ was the Messiah promised to the Jews, that he wrought miracles to show his divine mission and thereby enforce his 'natural' religion, and that he promised rewards and punishments when he should come again to judge the world (2. pp. 328–29). This is the substance of Bolingbroke's Christianity. The coming of Christ and his miracles were a device for emphasizing what had no intrinsic novelty, and was discoverable by reason; and this coming and these miracles would surely have been wholly effective had not St. Paul and innumerable other Saints and theologians overlaid the simplicity of the original

17

gospel with false accretions of mystery. No doubt Bolingbroke is willing to add belief in Christ's promises of rewards and punishments as an essential part of Christianity in order to bolster himself up in his own belief that but for St. Paul and the rest the mission of Christ would have been wholly successful; his belief in the rationality of man was not so strong as all that after all. However that may be, 'the gospel of Christ is one thing, the gospel of St. Paul, and all those who have grafted after him in the same stock, another' (2. p. 328). Of the rôle of the death of Christ in Christianity Bolingbroke can speak only harshly. Locke had, in all truth, been silent enough about it; Bolingbroke declares it quite unnecessary to God's scheme of salvation; to believe it is both to humanize and brutalize the divine (4. p. 268 ff). To enforce his view, he is willing enough to be inconsistent with what he has said elsewhere: 'Surely our ideas of moral attributes will lead us to think that God would have been satisfied, more agreeably to his goodness and mercy, without any expiation, upon the repentance of the offenders, and more agreeably to his justice with any other expiation, rather than with this'. Here, he is willing enough to let it be known that he has closer knowledge of God's moral being than the Cudworths and the Clarkes.

In truth, Bolingbroke has no need to believe in a revelation. He accepts, he tells us, the Messiahship of Christ and his miracles as divine reinforcements of natural religion; but his natural religion and ethic provide him with an abounding optimism which must have made any supernatural revelation gratuitous.

We are designed to be social, not solitary creatures. Mutual wants unite us: and natural benevolence and political order, on which our happiness depends, are founded in them. This is the law of our nature; and tho every man is not able for different reasons to discern it, or discerning to apply it, yet so many are able to do this, that they serve as guides to the rest. . . . Pleasures are the objects of self love: happiness that of reason. Reason is so far from depriving us of the first, that happiness consists in a series of them: and as this can be neither attained nor enjoyed securely out of society, a due use of our reason makes social and self love coincide, or even become in effect the same. The condition wherein we are born and bred, the very condition so much complained of, prepares us for this coincidence, the foundation of all human happiness; and our whole nature, appetite, passion, and reason concur to promote it (4. pp. 388–89).

So runs Bolingbroke's cheerful view of human nature and of God's providence in so designing it. Hobbes's state of nature in which man is vile, is a myth; man is naturally good, and only the coming of 'political' society destroyed that perfection, so far as it can be destroyed, by removing man from his original and happy family life. It is little wonder that Burke, in his preface to his splendid parody of Boling-broke, *A Vindication of Natural Society*, said bluntly that Bolingbroke's design was to show that 'the same engines which were employed for the destruction of religion, might be employed with equal success for the subversion of government'.[1] But in fact, it is not just to charge Boling-broke with any such 'design'. The fact is that he did not think so far or so clearly.

What is certain is that Bolingbroke tries his best to make the ethical life of humanity as 'natural' as possible. What he does with knowledge he will do, so far as he can, with conduct. Here, indeed, he does not invoke a mythological nature at every stage; he talks instead about 'the author of our nature' and 'the will of God'. And the author of our nature has made us all sociable. To this 'general sociability' we are all led by instinct, 'by a sense of pleasure'; 'and reason, that, recalling the past, foresees the future, confirms us in it by a sense of happiness.' He continues:

Instinct is an inferior principle, and sufficient for the inferior ends to which other animals are directed. Reason is a superior principle, and suffi-cient for the superior ends to which mankind is directed. The necessities, the conveniencies of life, and every agreeable sensation, are the objects of both. But happiness is a continued enjoyment of these, and that is an object proportioned to reason alone. Neither is obtained out of society; and socia-bility therefore is the foundation of human happiness. Society cannot be maintained without benevolence, justice, and the other moral virtues. These virtues, therefore, are the foundations of society; and thus men are led, by a chain of necessary consequences, from the instinctive to the rational law of nature, if I may speak so. Self love operates in all these stages. We love ourselves, we love our families, we love the particular societies to which we belong, and our benevolence extends at last to the whole race of mankind. Like so many different vortices, the center of them all is self love, and that which is the most distant from it is the weakest.

This will appear to be in fact the true constitution of human nature. It is the intelligible plan of divine wisdom. Man is able to understand it, and may be induced to follow it by the double motive of interest and duty. As to the first, real utility and right reason coincide. As to the last, since the author of our nature has determined us irresistibly to desire our own happiness, and since he has constituted us so, that private good depends on the public, and

[1] Burke, *Works*, London, 1815, vol. i. p. 5.

the happiness of every individual on the happiness of society, the practice of all the social virtues is the law of our nature, and made such by the will of God, who, having determined the end and proportioned the means, has willed that we should pursue one by the other. To think thus, is to think reasonably of man and of the law of his nature, as well as humbly and reverently of the Supreme Being. (4. pp. 10–11).

It is little wonder that if instinct and reason thus operate in us,

the divine institution of the law of nature, the conscious certainty we have, and the plainness and simplicity of it, are in their full force, and superior to those of the same kind which any other revelation contains. (4. p. 28).

I do not propose to follow Bolingbroke through the twists and turns he makes to reconcile this doctrine with the facts which stared him in the face. My purpose is only to show further, if it is at all necessary, the inexpressible superficiality of his thinking and to emphasize further the motive which prompts it. I spoke earlier of Swift's loathing and contempt of humanity. But his Houyhnhnms were but humanity living that law of nature which Bolingbroke describes. 'The word *Houy-hnhnm*, in their tongue, signifies a horse, and in its etymology, *the perfection of nature*'.[1] Again: 'As these noble Houyhnhnms are endowed by nature with a general disposition to all virtues, and have no conceptions or ideas of what is evil in a rational creature, so their grand maxim is to cultivate reason, and to be wholly governed by it. Neither is reason among them a point problematical as with us, where men can argue with plausibility on both sides of the question; but strikes you with immediate conviction';[2] and again: 'Friendship and benevolence are the two principal virtues among the Houyhnhnms, and these are not confined to particular objects, but universal to the whole race. For a stranger from the remotest part is equally treated with the nearest neighbour . . .' The Houyhnhnms, living their family lives and meeting in a representative council of the whole nation once every four years, is a portrait of that human nature described in these passages I have just quoted from Bolingbroke; and it is amusing to see stoicism coming together with the fierce naturalism which animated Swift and Bolingbroke. But in fact, as we all know, what Swift saw was not Houyhnhnms but Yahoos; neither he nor Bolingbroke saw 'the perfection of nature', but reason abused by passion, and untold misery and evil. And thus it is that their dream of 'a perfection of nature', indulged only at the expense of dissolving reason into instinct, was of a

[1] *Gulliver's Travels*, part 4. chap. 3.

piece with their hatred, contempt and despair of human life. Hobbes
had said bluntly that man is a Yahoo without freedom, and could be
saved from destruction and violent death only by absolute monarchy;
Swift and Bolingbroke dream a silly dream of natural perfection, and
are at a loss to explain the Yahoodom of the world. The visions of 'the
perfection of nature' and of the Yahoo are neither of them *sane*. Only
Locke, of them all, had the sanity to see man as a decent and good
creature enough, with his passions all too often too strong for his reason,
but who could yet fairly hope to be saved from himself.

XV

I turn now, before bringing my essay to its end, with a brief retrospect and with some conclusions that may be drawn from it, to make
some further observations on Bolingbroke's 'religion' and 'christianity'.
I shall do this by means of speaking of the rôle of the imagination in
religion. For poetry and religion are never far away from each other;
and an age which gave no room to the æsthetic properly conceived was
inevitably disastrous for religion. Locke indeed, I have said, was a man
of true Christian piety. But he allowed a so-called rationalism so to
influence him as to make him open to the charge of being a maker of
deism; and for poetry he had no use whatever. Of the arts Bolingbroke
speaks little in his pages; and there is little anywhere in what he
writes to make us think that poetry and other forms of the imagination
meant anything to him. In Bolingbroke we see religion and Christianity
disembowelled by 'reason'; and although Bolingbroke wrote comparatively late in the deistic period and although his papers were published when interest in deism had steeply declined, he was representative
enough of his age. We must, indeed, be careful of making any man
'representative of his age'; and writing in view of the towers of the
Cathedral in which Joseph Butler lies buried, I am not, I trust, likely to
forget that there were other and incomparably more catholic voices in
the land in Bolingbroke's time. But at least, they were few enough;
and there is no need to emphasize how much religion and morality
deteriorated in the first half of the eighteenth century.

Bolingbroke raged against the 'frantic' imagination which 'builds
beyond nature'. But religion is, when all is said and done, a building
beyond nature by the imagination. It is not, indeed, only that, nor can
it be. But it is idle to deny that to empty religion of what is imaginative
is to destroy it; it is indeed precisely to reduce it to what it becomes in

the hands of a Bolingbroke. Now the outcome of the Bolingbroke's theology is, as I said, to make of God a fact severed wholly from values; Bolingbroke contrives to remain, as he says, a 'theist', but in such a way as to ensure that we share no values with God and that He is not, and cannot be, an end for the spiritual life. Our knowledge of Him is and can be only knowledge of an inferred fact; and His meaning for us is to be construed as something extrinsic to His own nature. Bolingbroke cannot indeed be consistent in all this; but the intention of all his writing is to establish some such doctrine. To say this is only that he tries to make of God what we may call a scientific object in a chain of causation; and God is therefore made, or would be made if Bolingbroke could or would be consistent, of no human importance, and one thing amongst others.

But that God is not thus to be captured by the positivistic or scientific intelligence and allowed an existence on terms dictated by it, is shown in a number of ways from Bolingbroke's writings. What is specially relevant for our present purposes is that Bolingbroke is not able, as the other deists were not, to dispense with what is ordinarily called analogy. It is, I believe, in his essays, that the image of the clockmaker first makes its appearance.

We are forced [he says on p. 59 of the second volume] to help our conceptions of the divine nature by images taken from human nature, and the imperfections of this nature are our excuse. But then we must take care not to make humanity the measure of divinity, and much more not to make the last the least of the two. When we have raised our idea of any human excellency as high as we are able, it remains a very limited idea. When we apply it to God, we must add to it therefore our negative idea, our notion of infinity; that is, we must not confine it by the same, not suppose it confined by any limitations whatever. Thus when we speak of the world the work of God, we must not conceive it to have been made by a laborious progression, and to have remained at last imperfect like the works of men. We must conceive on the contrary, as well as we can, that God willed it to exist, and it existed; that he wills it to continue, and it continues, distinct from the workman, like any human work, and infinitely better fitted by the contrivance and disposition of it to answer all the purposes of the divine architect, without his immediate and continual interposition. To think otherwise is to measure divinity by a more scanty measure than humanity; and, because we cannot conceive how the operations of this vast machine are performed, to account for them by supposing it, in this instance, less perfect than a machine of human execution.   Carry a clock to the wild inhabitants of the Cape of Good Hope. They will soon be convinced that intelligence made it: and none but the most stupid will imagine that this intelligence is in the hand that they see move, and in the wheels that they see turn. Those among them, who pretend to greater sagacity than the rest, may perhaps suspect that the workman is concealed in the clock, and there conducts invisibly all the motions of it. The first of these hottentot philosophers are, you see, more rational than atheists; the second are more so than the heathen naturalists; and the third are just at a pitch with some modern metaphysicians.

The imperfections of our nature drive us to employ 'images taken from human nature'; and Bolingbroke proffers what he judges a permissible one, taken not from human nature, but from a piece of 'machinery of human execution'. He does indeed speak here of raising 'our idea of human excellency as high as we are able' and of applying it to God; but it turns out that the 'excellency' is only the excellency of a maker of a machine, and that human excellency in such a matter cannot hope, as indeed it cannot, to equal a divine excellency which can call a machine, and a very big one, out of nothing and leave it to work, and perfectly, for ever. Still, here is the imaginative theology of deism, and it is an imagination mastered by the mechanical concepts of Newtonian science.

Now what is wrong here is not that Bolingbroke falls back on an image to help him to convey what is in his mind. He says, rightly, that we are forced to help our conceptions of the divine nature by images taken from human nature; and religion cannot shed the imagination any more than any other form of our experience. What is wrong is only and precisely that Bolingbroke chose an image derived from the applications of physical science and *not* from human nature and from those modes of human experience which are not expressible mechanically. We may excuse Bolingbroke for not realizing that Newtonian physics were not the last and final physics and that all was not as scientifically simple as it then seemed; but it is still true that the image he employed showed a cosmological imagination which went along with little philosophical criticism and was animated by prejudice of a quite peculiarly interested kind. But my present point is only that Bolingbroke acknowledges that our knowledge of ultimate things requires imagery, and that the imagination must, in some degree at least, 'build beyond nature'. If religion does anything at all, it builds beyond nature; ordinarily, it discerns, or thinks it discerns, a spiritual world stretching out beyond the world we see and touch and yet manifesting itself in this world. Bolingbroke recognizes that this is so, however grudgingly; and in order to communicate his sense of it, he employs an imagination which he ventures to think is not 'frantic'. 'Frantic' it certainly was not; instead, it was chilly and designing enough. But it was none the less mistaken; for necessary and ineluctable as the imagination is in religion, it may not dispense with fair and open-minded philosophical criticism. And Bolingbroke, attacking what he judged to be the crude and vain anthropomorphism of a Clarke, did not stop to ask whether he was not himself employing a still cruder and vainer one. Symbolical apprehension of the Divine there must be. But it may not act in disregard of philosophical reflection.

That Bolingbroke's thought in this matter was rash, prejudiced and weak is certain; but what is equally certain, is that, in disputing with Clarke, Bolingbroke was dealing with problems as difficult as they are important; and that this is so, great tracts in the history of philosophy show clearly. How can we attribute to the Divine and Eternal that goodness, justice, mercy, love which we know in human life? And must not the Divine, if it is to mean anything in any human sense to humanity, undergo a crude anthropomorphizing? Or, how can we escape the agnosticism into which a Bolingbroke is thrown about God's nature if we are not to express Him in terms of mortal imagination?

I cannot, within the scope and purpose of the present essay, treat this great topic fully and systematically. I can only suggest in what way, in the light of the argument that has gone before, it may fairly be approached. This way will already have suggested itself to the reader, if he has felt any sympathy with what we have said, at earlier stages, about human knowledge. For our argument has been that our knowledge does not and cannot escape symbolism. The imagination in knowledge acts as an assimilation of the object to ourselves and of ourselves to the object, and without this action it is impossible to see how knowledge could occur at all; and, as we also saw, thought in its highest reaches acts from a base in imagination.

What then shall we say of our knowledge of divine things? We must say what was said by two theologians of later days, Coleridge and Newman. Newman said in one of his university sermons that the 'metaphors' by which we speak of divine things as when we speak of the person of God or of the Incarnation, are not 'mere symbols of ideas which exist independently of them, but their meaning is coincident and identical with the ideas. When, indeed, we have knowledge of a thing from other sources, then the metaphors we may apply to it are but accidental appendages to that knowledge; whereas our ideas of

Divine things are just co-extensive with the figures by which we express them, neither more nor less, and without them are not . . .'[1] Here indeed, we observe, Newman says 'merely symbols', using the word in a way not in accordance with our usage in this essay. But as he goes on, he employs precisely the notion which we have expressed by the word 'symbol.' The divine things we know only in and through symbol, as we have used the word. So Coleridge in the first *Lay Sermon*:[2]

It is among the miseries of the present age that it recognises no medium between literal and metaphorical. Faith is either to be buried in the dead letter, or its name and honours usurped by a counterfeit product of the mechanical understanding, which in the blindness of self-complacency confounds symbols with allegories. Now an allegory is but a translation of abstract notions into a picture-language, which is itself nothing but an abstraction from objects of the senses. . . . On the other hand a symbol . . . is characterised by a translucence of the special in the individual, or of the general in the special or of the universal in the general. Above all by the translucence of the eternal in and through the temporal. It always partakes of the reality which it renders intelligible: and while it enunciates the whole, abides itself as a living part in that unity, of which it is the representative.

So Coleridge and Newman. And what they say here, applied to divine things, has been our prevailing thought throughout this essay; and this thought reaches its consummation in affirming of our knowledge of the Divine what we have said of all our knowledge whatsoever. If we are right in this, we may say that the most important fact about the English Augustans is that symbolism had no active meaning for them; and that the fortunes of Christianity in their hands were only a manifestation, though the most important manifestation, of their antagonism to symbolism in all its forms, artistic and religious. The symbolism which is everywhere in the writing of Shakespeare is deplored by the Augustans (though Dryden at times put up a defence of it); it was judged to be against 'Nature'. Bolingbroke, indeed, employed an image to express his idea of God; but it was an image dictated by what Coleridge called the 'mechanical understanding'.

Now to say all this is certainly not to show that the Divine exists. It may be that in our apprehension, shot through with our human experience, of the Divine, we are the victims of illusion. I am not now concerned to try to show that this is not so. I only observe that the

---

[1] Newman, *University Sermons*, London, 1890, pp. 338–39.
[2] Bohn edition, London, 1894, p. 322.

phase of Augustan philosophy of which we have been speaking comes to a way of imagining God which issues from a predominance of mechanical categories in the representation of ultimate things which critical reflection cannot accept. It is indeed possible to throw up theism altogether; a 'theism' such as Bolingbroke's which cuts apart, as far as any sort of belief in God can tolerate, fact and value, is an intolerable compromise in which it is impossible to stay. So far to humanize God as to make of Him an amoral machine-maker is to indulge anthropomorphism with a view to mortifying our humanity merely: it issues from a philosophical sadism which is as disagreeable to contemplate as it is difficult to sustain by reflection. If we are at all to believe in God, anthropomorphize in a measure we must; and if so, we must *anthropomorphize*; we must see God in the image of *Man*. There is no reason why our imagination of the Divine should not be rational; there is a rational imagination which need not resist the play of intellectual criticism; and if so, we shall see that fair reason will not suffer us, if we are to believe in God at all, to select for divine honours only the scientific consciousness and its capacity for scientific contrivances.

But if the symbolism in terms of which we apprehend the Divine anthropomorphizes the transcendent, it does not and cannot be something in which we rest with acquiescence. I have said, in speaking of our knowledge of finite objects and of what is universal, that we are aware of what we cannot reduce to idea and which resists expression in symbol. There is always that which defeats us in our knowledge of the sensible and of the intelligible; for our station in the universe is one of mediocrity. But always there is an ideal of which we are aware: an ideal in our knowledge of particulars and of the intelligible to which we are continuously summoned and towards which we endeavour to move. And in religion there is a sense of a transcendent perfection, of that which is perfect, of which we cannot be said to have an idea, which yet seems to be of a piece with all our ideas, a background from which we may not sever what ideas we possess. Whatever we may say of the ontological argument as an argument merely, it will never fail to have its value as expressing our feeling that, if we have or can have no faith in an ultimate metaphysical perfection, we are lost in a wilderness of scepticism and despair. It is true enough that we anthropomorphize the Divine and that we can do no other. But it is also true that religion has never *merely* done so. Always there is that which lies beyond the human, what is different from the human; for without this there could not be the worship without which there is no religion. No doubt the being of God comes to us, in our symbolism, distorted and partial; and this we know, somehow, well enough. But we may still say that, under the conditions provided by our mediocre nature, it is yet generally shown to us in our symbols. To say this is certainly not to warn off metaphysics from religion. It may be that the highest function metaphysics can perform is to purify us from the passions for metaphysical system; a 'finished' system of metaphysic is a fascinating but dangerous thing. But to say this is not at all to despise the activity of metaphysics; and we ought not to be content to rest uncritically in the religious imagination; for that, too, has innumerable dangers. But in the last resort we are driven to contemplate the Divine, however inadequately, in the image of the best that human nature has it in it to be, of the taking of the manhood into God; and metaphysical reflection will, I think, confirm that the rôle of symbolism in religion is as justified as it is inevitable.

Conclusion

WE have now completed our survey of three Augustan philosophers, all of them deeply influential in their time. The reader will have seen how different they are from one another. Hobbes is indeed a rationalist; but along with his rationalism there goes a materialism; and his mind is set fast in this hopeless contradiction. Locke will have little to do with rationalism (except in Mathematics and Ethics) and was certainly no materialist; he saw the human mind as set in a world which it can little understand; and along with this sense of our ignorance there went, in him, a profoundly religious sense of a transcendent spiritual world. Hobbes would have the human mind above the world, understanding it, and controlling it in the interest of power; Locke sees it as placed within the world which is lit, faintly indeed, but adequately for our purposes, by the Candle of the Lord. Hobbes makes of religion not, as he says, philosophy, but law; religion, too, becomes an instrument of power; and the Kingdom of God becomes a civil government in which God becomes a civil sovereign. But this is far away from Locke's view of religion, as it is far from his politics.

But if Hobbes removed God from philosophical discourse, Locke held firmly that we can prove that He exists. Using the word in another sense, Locke was here the rationalist, and Hobbes was not. Here, Locke held that reasoning could do things which Hobbes denied; and he would not leave belief in God to be an affair of assent. He should, we think, have done so; thereby he would have made religion reasonable, though not demonstrable. And in the chapter *On Enthusiasm*, as we saw, he helped the cause of deism. Hobbes, with his unlimited intellectual ambition, made of God a political ruler; Locke, incomparably more modest, demonstrated His existence only to help the deists to make Him into a cosmic and inhuman despot. This is what He becomes in Bolingbroke's pages. His existence is held to be beyond question, and his inhumanity beyond doubt; He is acceptable only if his transcendence of us is absolute and his unimportance complete. Hobbes had been chiefly interested in God as a political power; Bolingbroke was interested in him as authorizing the Schism Act.

We see an analogous state of affairs in the Theory of Knowledge. Hobbes had declared that there was no conception in our minds not originally furnished by sense; in sense the mind is passive, and memory and the children of memory are ultimately 'decaying sense'. Locke would not have this, and gave to the mind powers and freedom not spoken of in Hobbes. But in Bolingbroke's writings, mere sense recovers much of the importance it had in Hobbes's; without Hobbes's rationalism, Bolingbroke plays down the powers of the mind, and 'Nature' becomes a miraculous power to save us from philosophical embarrassment.

Finally, in all three writers, the imagination, or the fancy as they most frequently called it, is either not to be taken seriously or is an enemy of the mind's health. Hobbes exalts reason above all, and then, within the world of 'experience', the judgement. Sometimes, indeed there occurs in his mind the thought that perhaps the fancy is not so irresponsible nor so trivial as he ordinarily believed. But his considered opinion, if we are to judge by *Leviathan*, was that the fancy was troublesome to the serious mind, and might only in poetry be given some rein, pleasing us then for its very extravagancy. But Locke would have done with poetry; its soil is barren. This is all the more surprising because Locke's philosophy, more accurate and catholic than Hobbes's, offered him the occasion of contriving an important place in experience for the æsthetic, as I tried to show; but he was not disposed to see and to take it. Bolingbroke pours all his scorn on the imagination as it shows itself, according to his doctrine, in philosophy; it went along with unhealthy heats and disorders of the mind; and in poetry, it was he who turned Pope from sound to sense, from fancy's maze to moralized song. Bolingbroke and Hobbes indeed compromised. They were literary men as well as philosophers: Hobbes's philosophy is itself literature and he wrote verse and translated Homer; while Bolingbroke was literary to his finger tips and liked to think of the profound influence he exerted on the greatest poet of the time. But the influence of all these men was antagonistic to much that is ordinarily considered to be legitimate and desirable in poetry. Only Hobbes, of the three, was a rationalist; but all three were men of reason, which they sharply opposed to the imagination.

Under these circumstances, there was created a difficult situation for poetry. Writers such as these created a problem for the Augustan poets. But it was not to prove an insoluble problem. The poets and literary men found a number of brilliant ways of dealing with it; and there was at least one consummate solution of it.

I have suggested certain respects in which the Augustan philosophers fell short. I have urged that they failed to state the rightful place of the imagination in human experience; that when they spoke of it, they wrongly opposed it, in its essential nature, to the intelligence; and that, though it is abundantly true that the imagination and the intelligence create tensions in our experience, that does not mean that both alike may not take their places in the life of reason. For in truth, each requires the other and is helpless without it; and they come to an accommodation with each other in symbol, without which our experience would be incomparably poorer. But if I have urged these and suchlike reflections and criticisms against the Augustan philosophers of whom I have spoken, I have not done so with any foolish view to preparing the ground for any sort of 'attack' on the Augustan poets. On the contrary, I have done so more with a view to exhibiting the quality of the performance of these poets under difficult circumstances. In any case, we are not *chiefly* concerned to carry on what is called 'literary criticism', but to come by some sort of historical understanding of literature.

Index

PATHOLOGY IN GYNECOLOGY AND OBSTETRICS

FOURTH EDITION

PATHOLOGY IN GYNECOLOGY AND OBSTETRICS

CLAUDE GOMPEL, MD, FIAC

Emeritus Professor and Chairman
Department of Pathology
Institut Jules Bordet and Hôpital St. Pierre
Free University of Brussels
Brussels, Belgium

STEVEN G. SILVERBERG, MD

Professor of Pathology
Director of Anatomic Pathology
The George Washington University Medical Center
Washington, D.C.

with eight contributors

J. B. Lippincott Company • PHILADELPHIA

Acquisitions Editor: Richard Winters
Sponsoring Editor: Jody Schott
Associate Managing Editor: Elizabeth A. Durand
Indexer: Alexandra Nickerson
Art Director: Susan Hermansen
Interior Designer: Arlene Putterman
Cover Designer: Robert Freese
Production Manager: Caren Erlichman
Production Coordinator: Kevin P. Johnson
Compositor: Graphic Sciences Corporation
Printer/Binder: Arcata Graphics/Kingsport
Color Insert Printer: Princeton Polychrome Press

4th Edition

6 5 4 3 2 1

Library of Congress Cataloging-in-Publication Data

Gompel, Claude.
    Pathology in gynecology and obstetrics / Claude Gompel,
Steven G. Silverberg, with eight contributors. — 4th ed.
        p.   cm.
    Includes bibliographical references and index.
    ISBN 0-397-51226-0
    1. Pathology, Gynecological.   2. Pregnancy—
Complications. I. Silverberg, Steven G., 1938-   . II. Title.
    [DNLM: 1. Genital Diseases, Female—pathology.
    2. Pregnancy Complications—pathology. 3. Genitalia,
Female—pathology.   WP 140
    G634p 1994]
    RG77.G65   1994
    618—dc20
    DNLM/DLC
    for Library of Congress   93-25778
                                            CIP

The authors and publisher have exerted every effort to
ensure that drug selections and dosages set forth in this text
are in accord with current recommendations and practice at
the time of publication. However, in view of ongoing research,
changes in government regulations, and the constant flow of
information relating to drug therapy and drug reactions, the
reader is urged to check the package insert for each drug for
any change in indications and dosage and for added warnings
and precautions. This is particularly important when the
recommended agent is a new or infrequently employed drug.

To Marie and Kiyoe

Contributors

Janice M. Lage, MD
Associate Professor
Department of Pathology
Georgetown University School of Medicine
Director of Surgical Pathology
Georgetown University Medical Center
Washington, DC

Hernando Salazar, MD, MPH
Senior Member
Chief of Surgical Pathology
Fox Chase Cancer Center
Philadelphia, Pennsylvania

Hironobu Sasano, MD
Assistant Professor
Department of Pathology
Tohoku University School of Medicine
Sendai, Japan

Shinji Sato, MD, PhD
Assistant Professor
Department of Obstetrics and Gynecology
Tohoku University School of Medicine
Sendai, Japan

Richard J. Stock, MD, MPH
Clinical Associate Professor
Department of Obstetrics and Gynecology and
    Pathology
Eastern Virginia Medical School
Norfolk, Virginia
Obstetrics and Gynecology Program Director
Naval Hospital
Portsmouth, Virginia

Alain P. Verhest, MD, PhD
Associate Professor
Department of Pathology
Free University of Brussels (U.L.B.)
Faculty of Medicine
Chef de Clinique
Department of Pathology
Hôpital Universitaire Erasme
Brussels, Belgium

Akira Yajima, MD
Professor and Chairman
Department of Obstetrics and Gynecology
Tohoku University School of Medicine
Sendai, Japan

Charles Zaloudek, MD
Professor of Clinical Pathology
University of California, San Francisco
School of Medicine
San Francisco, California

Preface

As in our three previous editions, the purpose of this edition of *Pathology in Gynecology and Obstetrics* continues to be to provide a concise and practical reference, with thorough bibliographic documentation, of the complex field of gynecologic and obstetric pathology for practitioners and trainees in both pathology and obstetrics and gynecology. We have also found that our previous editions have been useful in the education of those undergraduate medical students who desire more than the very brief introduction to this field provided by most textbooks of general pathology, and we hope that this edition will continue to serve that purpose.

The present edition, like its predecessors, devotes one chapter to each of the organs of the female genital tract, beginning with the embryology, gross anatomy, and normal histology and then progressing to the malformations, inflammatory lesions, hormonal disturbances, and benign and malignant neoplasms that may be responsible for clinical and subclinical variations from the normal state. Because of the close pathophysiologic relations between the genital tract and the breast, and the frequency with which diseases of the breast are encountered in gynecologic practice, we have continued to devote a chapter to the pathology of the breast. This chapter has been greatly expanded in the current edition in order to encompass the dramatic changes that have taken place in breast pathology in recent years, including new biopsy techniques resulting in specimens very different from those seen only a few years ago, an ever-expanding array of therapeutic options for malignant and premalignant lesions, and a vast menu of diagnostic and prognostic tests available to complement standard histopathologic evaluation.

In an attempt to summarize these currently available and emerging techniques as they apply to gyne-

cologic and breast pathology, we have added a new chapter by Drs. Alain Verhest, Hironobu Sasano, Shinji Sato, and Akira Yajima on new technologies in gynecologic pathology. This chapter also further widens the international scope of the book by adding experts from Japan to those from North America and Europe who have already participated in previous editions. Drs. Charles Zaloudek, Hernando Salazar, and Richard J. Stock have revised their chapters, and Dr. Janice Lage has capably taken over the chapter on the placenta and its adnexa. We have continued to expand the integrated coverage of cytologic findings together with clinical, macroscopic and histopathologic ones, and have increased the number of color plates to that end.

Any understanding of obstetric and gynecologic pathology, whether at the level of an individual case or in the writing of a textbook, is always the result of a close collaboration between the clinician and the pathologist. We who practice gynecologic pathology are particularly fortunate in being able to work daily with dedicated clinicians who are especially interested in the pathologic findings in their cases and who are eager to share their clinical knowledge with us. Our clinical colleagues in Brussels and Washington have offered many helpful suggestions in the preparation of this volume.

The late Drs. Fred W. Stewart and Frank W. Foote, Jr., both Chairmen Emeritus of the Pathology Department of Memorial Hospital for Cancer and Allied Diseases of New York, have given both of us the opportunity to study the most varied aspects of gynecologic pathology and to use the vast resources of their histologic collections. We mourn the passing of both of them since the publication of our third edition. We have also been privileged to be able to use the material and expertise of Drs. Saul Kay and

William J. Frable of the Medical College of Virginia in Richmond, Robert H. Fennell of the University of Colorado School of Medicine in Denver, and the late Professor Albert Claude of the Institut Jules Bordet in Brussels. One of us also wants to thank all his colleagues in Chalon-sur-Saône, France, where he acted as consultant pathologist for a few years. The many other excellent clinicians and pathologists with whom we have interacted over the years have provided a constant source of intellectual stimulation and of friendly and helpful advice, as have our residents in pathology at the Institut Jules Bordet and the George Washington University Medical Center.

Some histologic and photographic documents have been communicated obligingly to us by our colleagues whose names appear in the captions beneath the reproductions. The photomicrographs and electron micrographs were produced by Miss Barbara Neuburger, Mrs. M. L. Simonet, Mr. A. Demeire, Mr. Howard Mitchell, Mr. Phil Rutledge, and Mr. Seth Honig. Many of the diagrams and drawings are the work of Mr. Robert Fauconier. Mrs. I. Chorowitz and Mrs. Dorothy Molero contributed their expert services in transcribing the manuscript and aiding us in reviewing it. Our collaboration with J. B. Lippincott Company is now well into its second decade, and Mr. Richard Winters, Ms. Jody Schott and Ms. Elizabeth Durand are the latest of a series of Lippincott professionals who have provided invaluable assistance in the production of these volumes.

Last but certainly not least, none of this would have been possible without the constant encouragement, assistance, and love provided by our wives, Marie and Kiyoe.

Claude Gompel, MD
Steven G. Silverberg, MD

Contents

Color Plates

Chapter 7 (following page 432)

Chapter 10 (following page 432)

Chapter 12 (following page 432)

Pathology in Gynecology and Obstetrics, Fourth Edition, edited by Claude Gompel and Steven G. Silverberg. J. B. Lippincott Company, Philadelphia © 1994.

1

The Vulva

EMBRYOLOGY

The external genital organs originate from three protuberances: the genital tubercle and the genital pads, also known as the labioscrotal swellings, all of ectodermal origin.[1,2] After passing through an undifferentiated stage during the first 2 months of embryonic life, the genital tubercle forms the clitoris, to which is appended a mesodermal fold, the prepuce of the clitoris (Fig. 1-1). The genital pads give rise to the mons pubis, the labia majora, and the posterior commissure. The pads surround the urogenital orifice, whose borders or genital folds are transformed into the labia minora. All these structures form the boundaries of the vestibular orifice, which becomes the vestibule, into which the vagina and the urethra open. The junction of ectoderm and entoderm is at the level of the free border of the labia minora. Bartholin's glands, which originate in the vestibule, probably are of entodermal origin. Frequently, there is a vestigial persistence of the wolffian (mesonephric) ducts, the excretory ducts of the primitive kidneys, in the form of culs-de-sac of variable length opening under the urethral meatus (Gartner's duct; Fig. 1-2). These ducts can give rise to wolffian duct cysts or Gartner's ducts cysts, which are covered with a columnar epithelium.[3–5]

ANATOMY AND HISTOLOGY

The female external genital organs are composed of the labia majora, labia minora, vestibule, hymen,

mons pubis, urethral meatus, vulvovaginal glands (notably Skene's glands),[6] and an erectile apparatus comprising the clitoris and vestibular bulbs (Fig. 1-3). The mons pubis is a fatty structure that contains elastic fibers and is covered by a pigmented epidermis overlying hair follicles and sebaceous and sweat glands.

The *labia majora* form a cutaneous fold rich in adipose tissue and sebaceous and sweat glands. They contain some smooth muscle fibers and are covered by a pigmented hair-bearing epidermis (Fig. 1-4). The internal surface is smooth, whereas the external surface contains numerous hair follicles. The two surfaces join anteriorly to form the anterior commissure of the vulva; posteriorly, they continue into the posterior commissure. Their size depends on the amount of fatty tissue. Like the labia minora, they do not develop fully until the onset of genital activity.

The *labia minora* are covered by a pigmented epidermis that lacks hair follicles and rests on a stroma rich in blood vessels, elastic fibers, and sebaceous glands that secrete the vulvar smegma. They are devoid of adipose tissue. Anteriorly, they originate at the prepuce. They fuse posteriorly to form the fourchette.

The *hymen*, which limits the inferior orifice of the vagina, is composed of connective tissue rich in elastic fibers and thin-walled vessels and covered by nonkeratinized squamous mucosa. A depression, the navicular fossa, separates the fourchette from the hymen.

The *clitoris* is an erectile apparatus covered by keratinized squamous mucosa (Fig. 1-5). It is completed by two other erectile structures, the *vestibular*

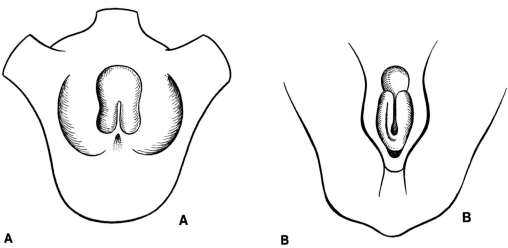

FIGURE 1-1 Embryologic appearance of the vulva. **(A)** Genital tubercle and pads. **(B)** Formation of the clitoris and labia minora.

bulbs, situated on either side of the vulvovaginal orifice. It is half encircled toward the front by the prepuce, formed by the junction of the labia minora. Histologically, it is composed of vascular lacunae separated by connective tissue septa that are rich in collagen and in elastic and smooth muscle fibers. They are lined by an endothelium that is in continuity with that of the blood vessels.

Bartholin's glands, or the *vulvovaginal glands,* are two mucous glands of tubuloalveolar type carpeted with columnar mucus-secreting cells (Fig. 1-6). Their excretory ducts are lined by a noncornified squamous epithelium and are open at the union of the anterior two thirds and posterior third of the groove separating the labia minora from the hymen. The glands produce a clear mucoid secretion.

Skene's glands form a network of glandular canals situated laterally and posteriorly to the urethra. Their number and disposition vary, but the two periurethral ducts described by Skene are always present (Fig. 1-7).[7] These ducts are covered by columnar epithelium containing foci of mucous cells. The glands, on the other hand, possess a pseudostratified columnar epithelium. These structures represent homologues of prostatic glands.

The superficial perineal artery and its branches arise from the internal pudendal artery. The numerous and well-developed veins empty into the internal pudendal and saphenous veins. The lymphatics drain into the superficial and deep inguinal nodes or the external iliac nodes.

The nerves are derived from the perineal branch of the internal pudendal nerve. The sensory innervation is well developed.

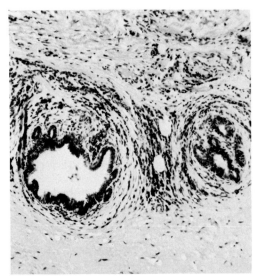

FIGURE 1-2 Gartner's duct: embryonic wolffian residua lined by columnar epithelium and situated in the connective tissue of the clitoral region.

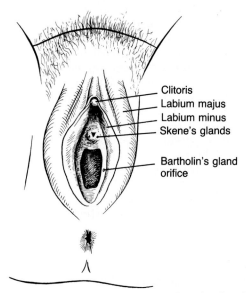

Clitoris
Labium majus
Labium minus
Skene's glands

Bartholin's gland orifice

FIGURE 1-3 Anatomic diagram of the vulva, showing the clitoris, labia majora, labia minora, glands of Skene, and orifices of Bartholin's glands.

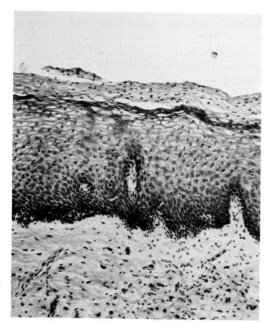

FIGURE 1-4 Squamous epithelium of the labia majora.

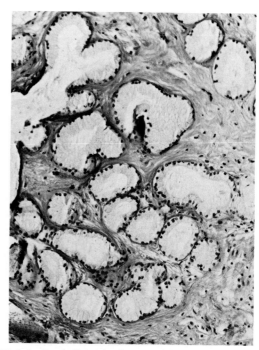

FIGURE 1-6 Bartholin's gland: normal histology.

MALFORMATIONS, HYPOPLASIAS, AND HYPERTROPHIES

Vulvar malformations are not frequent. Total aplasia is extremely rare and is encountered only in certain nonviable fetal monsters and in association with extrophy of the bladder. Hypoplasia is more frequent. When it is pronounced, one finds an infantile vulva with thin and poorly developed labia majora and minora. The clitoris is small, and the mons pubis

is almost nonexistent. Any degree of hypoplasia can be encountered, but it is always symmetrical. Duplication of the vulva is a rarity and is accompanied by duplication of the rectum and müllerian structures. Congenital hypertrophy can be partial or total; acquired hypertrophy of the labia minora is encountered in some women who practice masturbation. Total atresia or absence of the vulvar orifice is extremely rare.[8] A partial atresia characterized by stenosis of the vestibular orifice due to partial fusion of the labia is sometimes encountered.[9]

Aplasia of the clitoris is rare.[10] Hypertrophy of the clitoris most often depends on hormonal stimulation. It usually results from prolonged treatment with androgens or progesterone or from a tumoral

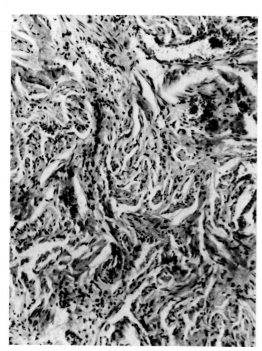

FIGURE 1-5 Clitoris: normal erectile tissue.

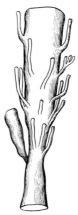

FIGURE 1-7 Anatomic disposition of the paraurethral glands. (Redrawn from Huffman JW: The detailed anatomy of the paraurethral ducts in the adult human female. Am J Obstet Gynecol 55:86–101, 1948)

virilization. Clitoral hypertrophy also is encountered in male pseudohermaphroditism, in which the clitoris may attain a size sufficient to permit penile–like function. Partial removal of the clitoris may correct the anomaly.

Another malformation is anovulvar atresia, which is represented by the opening of the rectum into the vulva due to the absence of the septum of the primitive cloaca. Pseudophimosis occurs when the prepuce, which partially covers the clitoris, hypertrophies and adheres to the clitoris, causing retention of smegma.

Persistence of the peritoneal diverticulum that is found in the elastic sac of the labium majus can give rise to a hydrocele of the canal of Nuck (an inguinal cyst) in the superior part of the labium.[11] The hydrocele is constant or transitory depending on whether it forms a sac that is completely closed or one that is in communication with the peritoneal cavity.

Aplasia of the urethral orifice is extremely rare and is encountered in some nonviable fetal monsters. If it is partial, it results in slight or marked stenosis. Aplasia of Bartholin's glands is very rare.

INFLAMMATORY DISEASES

Bacterial Infections

Many of the inflammatory diseases of the vulva belong to the realm of dermatopathology, but they merit description here as well. They acquire particular characteristics resulting from the symptoms that they cause in the vulvar region, such as abundant perspiration, contamination of adjacent structures, and hormonal influences. Their *histologic appearance* is not always familiar to the pathologist; the tissues are rarely biopsied because their macroscopic appearance usually is sufficient for diagnosis. Bacterial, viral, and parasitic infections may be encountered.[12–14]

Follicular Vulvitis

In follicular vulvitis, the hair follicles and sebaceous glands are invaded by bacterial colonies, most often of staphylococci. Macroscopically, the lesions present as small, red, tumefied, tender papules that transform into pustules. The disease can spread to involve the entire region of the labia majora and mons pubis.

Furuncle

Furuncles are caused by *Staphylococcus,* and the risk for a furuncle is increased by poor hygiene, diabetes, anemia, inoculation from other affected areas of the body, or general debility. It is a pyogenic folliculitis, with edema, vascular congestion, diapedesis of polymorphonuclear leukocytes, and formation of a purulent exudate with necrosis of the hair follicle. Elimination of the hair shaft is usually curative. Several furuncles can fuse to form a carbuncle; they are mostly localized to the labia majora.

Tuberculosis

Vulvar tuberculosis is the rarest localization of genital tuberculosis, representing less than 1% of all genital cases.[15] The lesion is situated at the level of the labia majora or minora. Contamination is effected by the lymphatic system or bloodstream, by direct contact, or rarely by sexual relations secondary to a tuberculous lesion of the male kidney or epididymis.

Macroscopic Appearance. The lesion presents as a nonindurated ulcer with torpid borders that is continuous with a subcutaneous yellow-brown nodule or a lupoid lesion.

Microscopic Appearance. There is an epithelioid cell granuloma containing Langhans' giant cells, surrounded by a peripheral zone of lymphocytes and plasma cells. Caseation necrosis is not common (Fig. 1-8). Other granulomatous lesions with giant cells should not be misinterpreted as tuberculosis. They are more frequent and result from reactions to suture material after surgery or from rupture of an epidermal inclusion cyst.

Gonorrhea

The etiologic agent in gonorrhea is the gonococcus, a Gram-negative encapsulated diplococcus first demonstrated by Neisser in 1879. The transmission is almost entirely by venereal exposure.

The lesion appears as an acute purulent inflammatory reaction at the level of the urethra, Bartholin's or Skene's glands, or the cervical glands. The squamous vulvar and vaginal mucosae are rarely involved. Vulvar localization is more frequent in young children, because the epidermis is thin and nonkeratinized.

The infection may sometimes spread to the endometrium, the fallopian tubes, and the rectum.[16] It can cause articular and cardiac lesions (endocarditis) when spread through the bloodstream.

Macroscopic Appearance. In the acute stage of gonorrhea, the vulvovaginal glands are congested and edematous. The urethra and the excretory ducts of the vulvar glands exude purulent material. If the infection becomes chronic, the sequelae are frequent at the level of Bartholin's glands, with fibrosis, obstruction of the excretory ducts, and cyst formation. The chronic disease can exhibit periods of acute exacerbation, with formation of new abscesses.

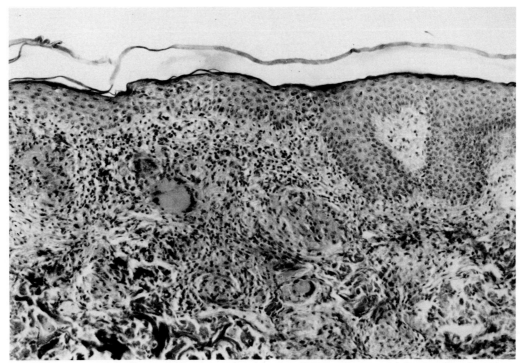

FIGURE 1-8 Vulvar tuberculosis: photomicrograph of a dermal granuloma containing Langhans' giant cells.

Microscopic Appearance. Histologic examination reveals an acute purulent infiltrate with polymorphonuclear leukocytes, the etiology of which can be determined only by culturing the microbe. In chronic gonorrhea, the microscopic structure of Bartholin's glands undergoes pronounced changes: the ductal epithelium is flattened and sometimes reduced to a single layer, and the acini are deformed by the surrounded fibrosis and infiltrated with lymphocytes and plasma cells (Fig. 1-9).

Chancroid

Chancroid is a very rare venereal disease that is more common in men than in women. It is caused by *Haemophilus ducreyi,* the Gram-negative, non-motile, pleomorphic rod discovered by Ducrey in 1889. Chancroid is also known as *soft chancre, soft sore,* and *Ducrey's chancre.*

Clinical Manifestations. After an incubation period of 3 to 10 days, a painful ulcer with a granulomatous purulent surface appears. The pain is often severe and differentiates this disease from syphilitic chancre. It is accompanied by bilateral inguinal lymphadenopathy.

Diagnosis. The diagnosis is made from the appearance of the lesion, from the microscopic demonstration of *Haemophilus ducreyi* in smears of material from scrapings of lesions, from culture, and from serologic identification.

Macroscopic Appearance. The chancre of inoculation is localized on any portion of the external genitalia. It begins as a red macule and is transformed into a pustule. The latter ulcerates and gives rise to multiple purulent granulomatous lesions with sharply defined projecting margins; their nonindurated borders differentiate them from syphilitic lesions. Regional adenopathy develops within 2 weeks after inoculation, becomes voluminous, and ulcerates.

Microscopic Appearance. The lesion is characterized by a granuloma with marked infiltration by lymphocytes and plasma cells. There is edema and superficial ulceration. Acute endarteritis and periarteritis may be present.[17] There may be secondary infection by luetic spirochetes. If disease involves the urethral region, it may provoke a cicatricial stenosis.

Differential Diagnosis. The differential diagnosis must be made with syphilis, lymphogranuloma venereum, and granuloma inguinale.[18]

Granuloma Inguinale

Granuloma inguinale is a rare chronic infection whose etiologic agent is *Calymmatobacterium granulomatosis,* a Gram-negative, non-motile, encapsulated bacillus first mentioned by Donovan in 1904 and demonstrated by Giemsa or Warthin-Starry stains.[19] Synonyms are *granuloma venereum, Donovan's granulomatosis,* and *Donovan's disease.* The diagnosis is made by direct examination of smears, tissue sec-

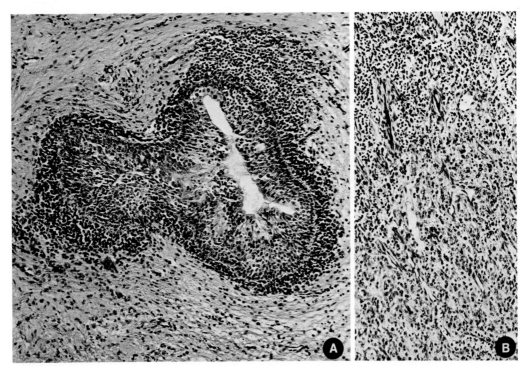

FIGURE 1-9 Gonococcal bartholinitis. **(A)** Periglandular leukocytic infiltrate. **(B)** Inflammatory cells invading the stroma.

tions, culture, or complement fixation test. This granulomatous, ulcerating infection is often associated with venereal diseases.[20,21] It is found more frequently in tropical countries and in the southern states of the United States. Granuloma inguinale is not a venereal disease; the organism is considered to be of fecal origin and may become pathogenic in patients with poor hygiene. There is a risk of developing carcinoma, as in any chronic granulomatous infection.[22]

Macroscopic Appearance. The lesion begins as a nodule or a papule and is localized to the genitalia, the inguinal region, and the anal region. The lower abdominal wall and inner aspects of the thighs may be involved. The original papular lesion ulcerates and forms a dark red, rough-surfaced granulation tissue with well-defined margins, which progressively extends peripherally. Several ulcers may grow separately and become purulent. When the cervix is involved, the process may extend to the endometrium, the ovaries, and the tubes. Uterine lesions are more common in pregnant women, in whom they provoke abortion and are accompanied by a high fetal mortality rate. Lymphatic extension and blockage are frequent and are associated with elephantiasis. Atrophic or sometimes hypertrophic scarring follows.

Microscopic Appearance. The initial papulonodular lesion shows edema of the papillae, epithelial hypertrophy that may progress to the stage of pseudoepi-

theliomatous hyperplasia, and a neutrophilic infiltrate in the subjacent dermis. The ulcer is covered by a granulation tissue rich in lymphocytes, plasma cells, and histiocytes. Among the latter are large vacuolated macrophages measuring 25 to 90 μm, with nuclei compressed by cellular inclusions known as *Donovan bodies*.[23] They may be detected with methylene blue or in paraffin sections with argentaffine stains.[24] There is proliferation of capillaries and acute endarteritis obliterans. When inguinal nodes are involved, parasite-laden macrophages and polymorphonuclear leukocytes are present.

Differential Diagnosis. The differential diagnosis must be made with the chancre of syphilis.

Syphilis

Syphilis is caused by a spirochete, *Treponema pallidum*, which was discovered by Schaudinn and Hoffman in 1905. The different types of cellular lesions result from combinations of the following elementary alterations:

Lymphoplasmacytic infiltration, with perivascular predominance
Inflammatory vascular and capillary lesions
Necrotic inflammatory granulomata (gumma)
Sclerosis.

None of these microscopic pictures is pathognomonic of syphilis. These cellular modifications are combined and integrated in the three clinical forms of the disease: the primary period of inoculation, contamination and dissemination; the secondary period of generalization, appearing about 6 weeks later; and the tertiary period of localization, becoming manifest after months or years.[25] In women, the infection can be clinically occult in the primary and secondary stages, becoming obvious only in the tertiary stage.

Primary Period (Chancre of Inoculation)

Macroscopic Appearance. The localizations of the primary chancre are the mucosal surfaces of the vulva and vagina and the external portion of the cervix. After a median incubation period of 3 weeks, a macule appears and is transformed into a painless indurated papule that ranges from several millimeters to 2 cm in diameter. This papule then progresses to a round or oval indurated ulcer with elevated borders, covered by a gray-red exudate and surrounded by a zone of congestion (Color Figure 1-1). During this period, the spirochete disseminates widely in the tissues and lymphatics. The chancre disappears spontaneously in 3 to 8 weeks. The inguinal lymph nodes are enlarged and indurated but not tender.[26] This diagnosis should be considered in the differential diagnosis of ulcerated lesions of the vulva and the vagina.

Microscopic Appearance. The chancre of inoculation is an inflammatory granuloma composed of histiocytes, macrophages, plasma cells, lymphocytes, and vessels showing endothelial proliferation and endarteritis. It is situated in the subcutaneous tissue and surmounted by a zone of ulceration. The inflammatory infiltrate begins around the vessels and extends to form a diffuse mass. The presence of the spirochetes proves the luetic etiology. The organism can be demonstrated by dark-field microscopy in the fresh state or by fluorescence or silver impregnation.[27] Regional adenopathy reveals a follicular hyperplasia, histiocytic infiltration with giant cell formation, and lymphocytic depletion. This depletion can be associated with an impairment of cell-mediated immunity.[25] The evolution is by secondary fibrosis.[28]

Secondary Syphilitic Lesions.

Secondary lesions appear 6 to 10 weeks after inoculation. They are disseminated over the entire body and occur in several episodes separated by periods of remission. The lesions contain numerous spirochetes. In the external genital organs, two types of lesions are commonly found: mucous patches and papulohypertrophic syphilids. *Mucous patches* consist of predominantly perivascular lymphoplasmacytic infiltrates, intense neovascularization, and reactive hyperplasia of the surface epithelium (Fig. 1-10). They are disseminated over the entire vulvovaginal mucosa. *Papulohypertrophic syphilids* show marked cutaneous hyperplasia with intercellular edema and leukocytic infiltration. They present in the form of rounded, erosive, slightly elevated brown lesions measuring several centimeters in diameter.

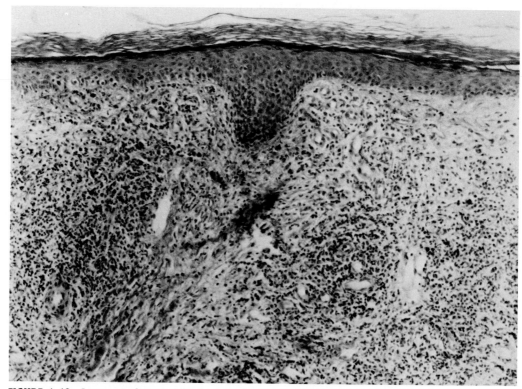

FIGURE 1-10 Late secondary syphilis: lymphoplasmacytic infiltrate principally localized around blood vessels.

Tertiary Syphilitic Lesions. Tertiary lesions become manifest several months or even years after the primary inoculation. Like the other luetic lesions, they are characterized by the presence of lymphocytes, plasma cells, macrophages, and epithelioid cells. The lesions of endarteritis obliterans of arterioles and capillaries are intense and provoke the appearance of zones of necrosis. The *gumma* is a granuloma with a necrotic center surrounded by epithelioid cells, giant cells, lymphocytes, plasma cells, and connective tissue that encloses and limits the lesion. Although the tertiary lesions only rarely involve the genital organs, gumma of the vulva has been described.

Bartholin's Gland Abscess (Bartholinitis)

Bartholin's gland abscess is a frequently occurring lesion. The organisms most frequently responsible are *Neisseria gonorrhoeae*, *Streptococcus*, *Staphylococcus*, *Escherichia coli*, and *Trichomonas vaginalis*.

Macroscopic Appearance. A red, painful tumefaction is found in the inferior portion of the labium majus with or without softening.

Microscopic Appearance. The inflammatory process involves the excretory duct or, less often, the acini. A painful collection of pus is formed and tends to fistulize as a secondary event. The cavity of the abscess may be single or multilocular. The chronic form arises from repeated inflammatory episodes and eventuates in the formation of a cyst. The paraurethral glands (Skene's glands) can be involved by the inflammatory process. Gram-negative diplococci of *Neisseria gonorrhoeae* can be seen in the cytoplasm of neutrophils with a Gram stain. Rare vulvar and vaginal localizations of diphtheria (*Corynebacterium diphtheriae*) have been reported.

Erysipelas

Erysipelas is an acute inflammation caused by β-hemolytic streptococci. It is now a rare infection. Erysipelas is characterized by phlegmonous edema and is seldom localized to the vulva. It begins as a pruritic, erythematous, shiny lesion with an indurated and raised border that may attain a diameter of several centimeters. The microscopic picture shows a diffuse inflammatory lesion extending throughout the epidermis.

Ecthyma

Ecthyma is a pyodermatitis caused by organisms similar to those causing impetigo (*Streptococcus pyogenes*). A debilitated general state or inadequate hygiene often explains the virulence of this infection. Puerperal ulcers are of streptococcal origin. Macroscopically, vesicles or pustules penetrate deeply or spread out on the epidermis. They ulcerate and scar in a few weeks.

The histologic lesion consists of a purulent exudate underlaid by inflammatory granulation tissue rich in neutrophils and newly formed vessels. The vessels often demonstrate endarteritic and phlebitic lesions. Pseudoepitheliomatous hyperplasia sometimes develops in the overlying epidermis.

Chronic Hypertrophic Vulvitis

Chronic hypertrophic vulvitis shows lesions similar to cheilitis granulomatosa (Miescher-Melkersson-Rosenthal syndrome).[29,30] It is characterized by a chronic swelling of the vulva. Microscopic findings include inflammatory infiltrates with epithelioid cell granulomas. The histogenesis is unknown.

Vulvitis Circumscripta Plasmacellularis

Vulvitis circumscripta plasmacellularis is a rare clinicomorphologic entity characterized by a thinned and flattened epithelium accompanied by a dermal inflammatory infiltrate with numerous plasma cells.[31]

Ulcus Vulvae Acutum (Acute Ulcer of Lipschütz)

The labia majora and minora may be sites of chronic and acute ulcers.[32] These ulcers accompany systemic infections such as typhoid fever, amebiasis, brucellosis, and viral pneumonia or are associated with oral ulcers and uveitis (*Behçet's syndrome*).[33,34] In young women, the acute stage of the infection is sometimes confused with a venereal disease. Systemic manifestations such as pneumonitis, gastrointestinal ulcerations, and lesions of the central nervous system have been observed.

Etiology. The etiology of these ulcers is not definitely established. A virus has been suspected, but its existence has not been confirmed. Most likely it is an autoimmune disorder; elevated levels of immune complexes, circulating antibodies against epithelial cells, and deposition of immunoglobulins around vessels are in favor of a humoral mechanism.[35] The *Bacillus crassus* described by Lipschütz is no longer considered the causative agent.

Macroscopic Appearance. These ulcers measure 1 to 3 cm in diameter and have well-defined borders. They are painful, nonindurated, and covered with a gray purulent exudate (Color Figure 1-2). The peripheral skin or mucosa is red and appears edematous. Spontaneous healing is the rule.

Microscopic Appearance. Nonspecific inflammation and small abscesses accompany a vasculitis that is characterized by a lymphocytic infiltrate and marked endothelial swelling. Secondary fibrosis with scarring may occur.[36]

Differential Diagnosis. The differential diagnosis includes syphilitic chancre, chancroid, and herpes.

Viral Infections

Condyloma Acuminatum

Condyloma acuminatum or venereal wart is a contagious viral infection caused by human papillomavirus (HPV), a DNA virus that belongs to the family of *Papovaviridae*.[37,38] The prevalence of condylomata and related intraepithelial lesions has increased significantly in recent decades.[39] The presence of HPV DNA has been demonstrated in the nucleus and cytoplasm of infected cells after passing through the plasma membrane. More than 60 HPV types have been identified by molecular hybridization and restriction enzymes techniques.[40,41] Types 6, 11, 16, 18, 31, and 35 are the types most commonly associated with lesions of the human female genital tract. HPV types 6 and 11 are observed in condyloma and some low-grade dysplasias, whereas types 16, 18, 31, and 35 are found in most intraepithelial neoplasias. HPV infections are frequent in the population and may not always be associated with a neoplastic process. Highly sensitive techniques used to detect HPV, such as the polymerase chain reaction, may be associated with two difficulties: they may detect inadvertent DNA contamination or unrelated latent infection.

Clinical Appearance. Clinically, the lesion presents as multiple hyperkeratotic budding papillomata that have a tendency to agglomerate (Color Figure 1-3). The lesions are situated in the vulva and in the perianal region, urethra, perineum, vagina, and cervix.[40] Transmission occurs mostly with venereal contact. Pregnancy favors the appearance of voluminous lesions, which may be transmitted to the newborn in rare cases. The exophytic condyloma is not the only form of the disease; flat lesions are also described (flat condyloma). They are observed less frequently on the vulva than on the cervix.[37,41] See Chapter 3 for more details on HPV infection and carcinoma.

Microscopic Appearance. Microscopically, the papillomatous formations develop on a fibrovascular stroma, forming a support for the epithelium, which shows papillary acanthosis, hyperkeratosis, parakeratosis, and hyperplasia of the rete pegs. Perinuclear haloes with nuclear atypia and binucleate cells, predominantly in the granular layer, are the morphologic indicators of the presence of HPV. These cells were called *koilocytes* by Koss and Durfee in 1956.[42] The same cellular lesions are found in the flat condyloma and were related to HPV by Meisels and Fortin and by Purola and Savia.[43,44] Table 1-1 summarizes the typical cytologic and histologic features recognized in condyloma.

Ultrastructural or immunohistochemical studies are necessary to demonstrate the intranuclear viral particles. The epithelial changes are accompanied by chronic inflammation and vascular congestion of the underlying dermis. Flat condyloma is characterized by the same cellular anomalies without the formation of exophytic papillary structures.

TABLE 1-1.
Morphologic Features of Condyloma

Koilocytosis
Binucleation
Parakeratosis (incomplete or abnormal keratinization) with nuclear pleomorphism and hyperchromasia
Acanthosis
Papillomatosis

Differential Diagnosis. Differential diagnosis must be made macroscopically with the condyloma latum of secondary syphilis, granuloma inguinale, and verrucous carcinoma. The so-called giant form of condyloma, often associated with HPV-11, is probably a verrucous carcinoma because it can invade adjacent tissues. A similar giant condyloma (condyloma of Buschke-Löwenstein) of the penis has been described.[45]

Microscopically, intraepithelial neoplasms can be differentiated from HPV infection by marked cellular atypia, disorganization of the cellular layers of the epithelium, atypical mitotic figures, and an increased mitotic index. When the histologic anomalies are equivocal for condyloma, analysis for HPV DNA by in situ hybridization may help demonstrate the presence of the virus.[46,47]

Treatment. Treatment of vulvar condylomata ranges from local podophyllin, trichloroacetic acid, and 5-fluorouracil to local excision, cryocautery, electrocautery, and carbon dioxide laser vaporization. When podophyllin is used, one should be careful not to misinterpret podophyllin-induced cellular anomalies as carcinomatous changes. Podophyllin changes regress after 2 weeks. More recently, antiviral agents such as interferon have been used. Cases that do not respond to any type of treatment may eventually progress to (or may already be) vulvar intraepithelial neoplasia (VIN).

Molluscum Contagiosum

Molluscum contagiosum is a contagious viral disease characterized macroscopically by small round elevated papules of several millimeters in diameter. The papules are firm and white-gray, with dark umbilicated centers. They are pruritic and usually are multiple but may be solitary. They appear in the genital region and on the face and arms. The development and multiplication of these lesions take place rapidly. The disease is common in infants, in whom it is often seen in epidemic form. Sexual transmission has been suggested.[48,49] The etiologic agent is a poxvirus containing DNA. The lesions resolve spontaneously.

The histology is that of an acanthotic epithelium extending deeply into the dermis to form the characteristic lobules (Fig. 1-11). In the stratum germinativum, the epithelial cells become strongly eosinophilic and may contain large cytoplasmic viral inclusions

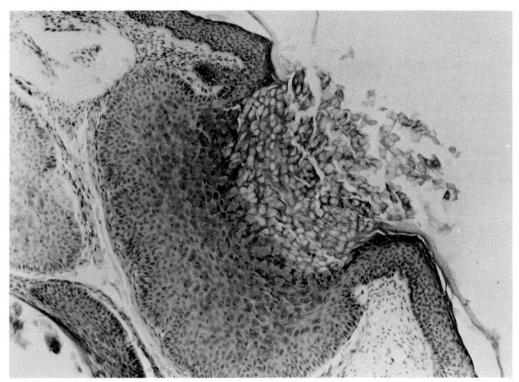

FIGURE 1-11 Molluscum contagiosum: eosinophilic cytoplasmic inclusions agglomerate to constitute a Lipschütz body.

that push aside the nucleus and form eosinophilic masses surrounded by keratohyaline granules (Lipschütz bodies). These masses agglomerate and constitute a molluscum corpuscle, which desquamates on its arrival at the surface of the epithelium. Differential diagnosis must be made with hyperkeratotic verruca, in which the eosinophilic granules found in the stratum granulosum are smaller than those found in molluscum contagiosum.

Contagious pustular dermatitis (ORF) is a rare infection caused by a virus from the same poxvirus group. It occurs in people who are working with sheep. A vulvar localization was diagnosed in a child living in the country.[50]

Herpes Simplex

Herpesvirus hominis infection is caused by two distinct types of DNA virus: herpes simplex virus 1 and 2 (HSV-1 and -2). They can be differentiated by viral culture but cannot be differentiated morphologically. HSV-1 more frequently affects the perioral and ocular regions and upper respiratory tract, and HSV-2 is found predominantly in the genital area (vulva, vagina, and cervix), but both types may be observed at any site.[51–54]

HSV-2 is a common sexually transmitted genital infection and its prevalence is increasing.[55] It is characterized by periods of remission and recurrence. The primary infection is accompanied by constitutional symptoms such as fever, myalgia and headache. The incubation period is 3 to 7 days, and the infection evolves in 2 to 7 days. It causes the appearance of groups of 2- to 5-mm vesicles containing clear fluid that later becomes cloudy. After a few days, one or several painful ulcers appear along the labia majora and minora, which become covered with yellow scabs and finally eventuate in scars.[56] The regional lymph nodes develop inflammatory reactions.

During pregnancy, the transmission of the virus to the newborn may result in a disseminated herpetic infection that can be fatal.[57] HSV infection is, in certain cases, an indication for delivery by cesarean section.[58] Studies show that the prevalence of infection is significantly greater in groups of patients with cervical and vulvar carcinoma, both in situ and invasive.[59] The relation to cervical carcinoma is discussed in more detail in Chapter 3.

The histologic appearance consists of the formation of an intraepithelial vesicle by ballooning degeneration of the epidermal cells, which hypertrophy, degenerate, and desquamate into the vesicular cavity. Intranuclear eosinophilic inclusions are found in variable numbers; they are nonspecific and are seen in herpes zoster and varicella.[60] Lymphocytes and polynuclear leukocytes infiltrate the epidermis and the dermis.

Cytology. Smears should be prepared from the bed of ulceration and not from the serosanguineous content of the vesicle, which usually does not contain epithelial cells.[61,62] The virus infects squamous, metaplastic, and columnar endocervical cells, and cytologic lesions can be observed in all these cellular types. Alterations of size and shape of cells and nuclei can be seen, with the subsequent appearance of atypical cells with bizarre shapes. Hydropic degeneration with a homogenized appearance of nuclei (ground-glass nuclei) is a common feature. Nucleoli are not significantly increased in size. Internuclear molding and dense cyanophilic staining of cytoplasm are common findings. When present, intranuclear inclusions are often surrounded by a clear zone. Multinucleation is the result of viral replication. These multinucleated cells should not be confused with the foreign-body giant cells and reactive multinucleated cells observed in chronic cervicitis (Color Figure 1-4).

The cytologic changes are not always present. Nevertheless, the cytologic method is almost as sensitive as virus culture and isolation. Treatment is symptomatic. New drugs seem to hasten healing, but recurrence is the rule, because the virus has not been eradicated.

Herpes Zoster

Rarely described in the vulva, herpes zoster is a disease of viral origin that affects the dermatomes located in the territories of peripheral nerves. It appears as erythematous plaques containing masses of vesicles. There are intranuclear inclusion bodies identical in appearance to those of herpes simplex and of varicella. Only the clinical picture establishes the diagnosis. The disease is accompanied by systemic phenomena.[63] The severity of the infection is greatly increased in patients with impaired cellular immunity. The virus has been seen by electron microscopy but has never been cultured.

Lymphogranuloma Venereum

Lymphogranuloma venereum is a venereal disease caused by *Chlamydia trachomatis*, a Gram-negative, intracellular parasite probably derived from Gram-negative bacteria.[64] Once considered to be a virus, chlamydiae have distinctive characteristics that eliminate a viral nature: the simultaneous presence of DNA and RNA and of ribosomes.[65] The intracellular localization of the parasite is the only characteristic it shares with viruses. Lymphogranuloma venereum is also known as *lymphogranulomatosis, lymphogranuloma inguinale, Nicolas-Favre disease, venereal disease of Hellerström,* and *poradenitis inguinale.*

Demonstration of particles in smears is difficult. The Warthin-Starry silver impregnation stain helps to demonstrate the presence of the organism. Isolation of the agent is possible on yolk sac material and by intracerebral injection in mice. A useful diagnostic skin test is the Frei test, which uses a yolk sac emulsion containing chlamydiae. The development of a papule indicates a delayed hypersensitivity reaction to group antigen.[66] More recently, immunologic methods have been developed that yield sensitive and reliable results.[67,68]

Clinical Manifestations. After an inoculation period of 3 to 21 days, the primary lesion develops in the genital region and is followed within 2 to 8 weeks by a unilateral or bilateral ilioinguinal lymphadenitis; this is the primary bubo complex first recognized by Durand, Nicolas, and Favre in 1913.[69] Among the different localizations described are the conjunctivae, the urethra, the fallopian tubes, the vagina, and the cervix uteri. Generalized dissemination may produce fever and systemic symptoms. The disease may be acute or may progress to the chronic form. It is more common in tropical and subtropical regions.

Macroscopic Appearance. The primary lesion involves the mucosa of the vulva and urethra. It is usually a small papular lesion followed by a nonindurated painless ulcer with elevated jagged borders. It usually heals in a few weeks. The combination of edema, fistulas, and ulcers is called *esthiomene.* The major manifestation of the disease is the appearance of a fluctuant, conglomerate, swollen mass of ilioinguinal lymph nodes (ilioinguinal bubo), which may ulcerate and form sinuses.[66] In the chronic stage, fibrosis and edema may produce stricture of the vagina, elephantiasis of the vulva, massive enlargement of the clitoris, and anorectal and urethral strictures.

Microscopic Appearance. The primary lesion is characterized by a chronic inflammatory infiltrate and epithelial hyperplasia. The typical acute lesion in the regional lymph nodes is the stellate abscess: an irregular focus of necrosis infiltrated by neutrophils and surrounded by histiocytes, fibroblasts, epithelioid cells, plasma cells, lymphocytes, and occasional multinucleated giant cells. Purulent discharge follows the spontaneous rupture of the lymph node. Fibrosis and chronic inflammation develop in a later stage. The epithelial hyperplasia may eventually proceed to carcinoma.[70]

The cytologic changes, if present, consist of coccoid bodies surrounded by a clear and well-limited vacuole.[71,72] Studies have shown no correlation between the presence of the typical cytologic images and the positive culture of the microorganism.[73] Therefore, the diagnosis of *Chlamydia trachomatis* must be confirmed by culture. Immunofluorescence methods using a labeled antibody have been developed and give accurate results.[74]

Differential Diagnosis. Differential diagnosis must be made with tuberculous and syphilitic granulomas, with cat-scratch disease, and with pasteurellosis in lymph nodes.

Accidental Vaccinia

Cases of localized accidental vaccinia of the vulva have been reported.[75,76] This condition is uncommon, but the possibility should be considered because most cases have been referred to erroneously as venereal diseases. Usually the lesion shows typical umbilicated vesicles. The diagnosis may be made on clinical grounds and confirmed by laboratory tests (detection of virus and antibodies).

Mycotic Infections

Mycotic infections of the vulva are known as *mycotic vulvovaginitis, aphthous vaginitis, diabetic vulvitis,* and *fungal infection.* The isolation of multiple mycotic strains in the vaginal flora has shown the importance of this etiologic factor in vulvar and vaginal lesions.[77-80]

About 10% of women are considered to be carriers of vulvovaginal fungi: 1% to 2% of non-pregnant women and 5% to 10% of pregnant women present with frank vulvovaginitis. *Candida albicans* (also called *Monilia*) is by far the most frequent etiologic agent. Many factors predisposing women to mycotic infection have been demonstrated. The increased glycogen content of the vaginal mucosa during pregnancy and the elevation of urinary glucose in the diabetic woman explain the increased frequency of mycotic infections in these conditions. Transitory elevations of vaginal glycogen during the progestational phase of the menstrual cycle are responsible for premenstrual exacerbations. The frequency of candidal vaginitis is higher in underprivileged socioeconomic groups, relating the infection to poor hygiene.

Patients with the acquired immune deficiency syndrome (AIDS) develop severe infestation with *Monilia.* Tetracycline and immunosuppressant drugs favor mycotic overgrowth of the normal flora. The dominant symptom is pruritus of the internal surfaces of the labia minora, later extending throughout the vulva. Dyspareunia and, more often, dysuria are found. Abundant creamy white vaginal secretions result in erythema and edema of the vulva. Demonstration of the organism can be accomplished quickly by phase contrast examination of the vaginal secretions, or by Gram stains. The stains of Papanicolaou and of Shorr are useful. Serologic techniques and a culture that will grow typical white colonies are necessary to identify the species.

Macroscopic Appearance. On the mucosae are found multiple white spots with a blue tint, which can be incompletely removed by vigorous scraping (Color Figure 1-5). Ulceration is rare.

Microscopic Appearance. The vulvar epithelium shows leukocytic infiltration, cellular vacuolization, and edema. The small white spots correspond to masses of desquamated squamous cells in varying stages of necrosis. Among these masses are found secondary bacterial flora, especially Döderlein bacilli; the conidia (yeast forms) and the filaments (pseudohyphae) are intimately intertwined (Fig. 1-12). They are mainly localized in the superfical layers of the epithelium. In eroded zones, the fungi penetrate more deeply into the epithelium. Smears stained by the method of Shorr or Papanicolaou show inflammatory alteration of the epithelial cells (eg, eosinophilia, perinuclear haloes, and variations in nuclear size), numerous polymorphonuclear leukocytes and histiocytes, and cellular debris. In the vaginal secretions, the spores and hyphae are dispersed among the squamous cells.

Prognosis, Evolution, and Treatment. When not treated, mycotic infections pass through phases of remission and exacerbation, depending on local or systemic conditions. When infection appears during pregnancy, the mycosis usually regresses spontaneously in the postpartum period, not necessarily reappearing during the course of a subsequent pregnancy. The use of fungicides and antibiotics has led to great progress in the therapy of these infections. The potential of *Candida* infections for more serious infections should be borne in mind: septicemia after ruptured tubo-ovarian mycotic abscess has been reported.

Other Infections

This section briefly mentions the less frequent inflammatory diseases that are encountered in biopsy or cytologic material, except for *Trichomonas vaginalis* infection, which is discussed in Chapter 2.[81]

An *ulcerative vulvitis* may appear after coitus for unknown reasons.[82] *Verruciform xanthoma,* described mostly in the oral cavity, has been mentioned in the vulvar mucosa.[83] *Contact dermatitis* is characterized by eczematous reactions of the vulvar mucosa attributed to substances such as cosmetics, detergents, deodorants, and synthetic fabrics. Recognition of the causal agent helps in treatment of these lesions.

Torulopsis glabrata, a fungus related to *Candida,* has been isolated in vulvar and vaginal infections.[84] *Enterobius vermicularis* migrates from the perianal region and may cause a pruritic vulvovaginitis or be asymptomatic. The worm can be identified in vaginal smears or in cellophane-tape preparations. Vulvar localization of *schistosomiasis* has been reported by Arean.[85] The parasite provokes a papillomatous or ulcerated lesion, sometimes mimicking neoplasia. The recognition of the ova in the biopsy is diagnostic. *Filariasis* has been mentioned as a cause of vulvar elephantiasis. *Entamoeba histolytica* has been identified in rare cases as the cause of ulcerative lesions of the vulvovaginal region. A clitoral localization has been reported.[86] *Arthropodal* inflammatory reactions may last longer than usual and be misinterpreted as lymphomas. Clinical recognition of the mite of *Sarcoptes scabiei* helps eliminate the diagnosis

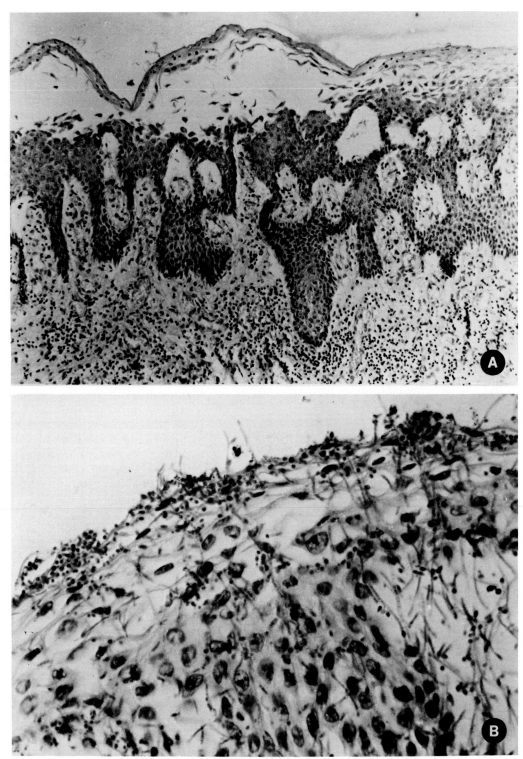

FIGURE 1-12 Mycotic vulvovaginitis showing spores and mycelial filaments.

of a malignant lymphoma. The mite is recovered from the epidermis with a knife blade, mixed with mineral oil, and mounted on a glass slide.[87] *Tinea cruris* and *Tinea versicolor* infections have been noted in the vulva.

Crohn's Disease

Perianal and vulvar lesions such as ulcers, fissures, and enterovaginal fistulas have been described in Crohn's disease.[88,89] In rare instances, they may precede the intestinal manifestations. Microscopically, the lesions consist of inflammatory infiltrates with noncaseating granulomas containing epithelioid and giant cells. Differential diagnosis is made with tuberculosis and foreign body granulomas.

Vulvar Elephantiasis

Vulvar elephantiasis may result from diverse causes. Total or partial obstruction of the lymphatic circulation by inflammatory lesions provokes a subcutaneous proliferation of connective tissue and lymphatics. Chronic infections, particularly lymphogranuloma venereum, tuberculosis, and filariasis, are prominent.[90] Inguinal lymphadenopathy secondary to certain dermatologic conditions of the lower extremity may provoke a homolateral vulvar lymphatic stasis. Vulvar elephantiasis is also referred to as *chronic hypertrophic vulvitis* and *hypertrophic lymphatic stasis.*

Macroscopic Appearance. The appearance is that of hypertrophy and edema of the labia majora and minora. The cutaneous epithelium is thickened, indurated, and hyperkeratotic, explaining the comparison with the skin of an elephant. Ulceration may appear and can be accompanied by pain.

Microscopic Appearance. The most important lesion is lymphatic proliferation and stasis accompanied by chronic inflammatory phenomena. The lymphatic obstruction provokes a secondary proliferation of connective tissue and the development of wide fibrotic zones. The epithelium is hypertrophic with hyperkeratosis and acanthosis; in other foci, the epithelium is thin and ulcerated. One also finds endarteritis, venous thrombi, and perivasculitis. There is a congenital form that is very rarely encountered. Treatment is symptomatic or surgical.

BENIGN TUMORS

Cystic Tumors

Cyst of Bartholin's Gland

Cysts of Bartholin's gland are common and appear at any age before the menopause.[91] The obliteration of the excretory duct of the gland by an acute infection such as gonorrhea later provokes the appearance of cysts measuring up to 5 cm in diameter. The cyst is found in the parenchyma of the inferior third of the labium majus. It presents as a hard, round, slightly tender mass adherent to the surrounding tissues. It is formed by the dilatation of the excretory duct and is therefore lined by squamous epithelium; the compressed glandular tissue is atrophic. The cystic contents are clear or blood-tinged. Clear translucent fluid results from obstruction without inflammatory response. More rarely, dilatations of the glandular acini occur, giving a multicystic appearance.[92] These cysts are lined by a mucus-secreting columnar epithelium. In some cases, the glandular elements are totally replaced by an inflammatory granulation tissue with secondary synechiae of the cystic layers (Fig. 1-13).

Sebaceous Cyst

The sebaceous cyst presents as a small, smooth, subcutaneous nodule associated with the orifice of the pilosebaceous apparatus.[93] The cyst is formed by secondary obliteration and dilatation. It is situated in the labia majora or minora and measures from several millimeters to several centimeters in diameter. The acinar structure of the sebaceous glands disappears because of compression, and the cavity of the cyst is filled with the products of desquamation of the nonkeratinized squamous epithelium of the excretory duct and with fat. The cyst may open onto the surface, ulcerate, and become secondarily infected. These cysts recur easily if they are not completely excised. They are less common than epidermal inclusion cysts.

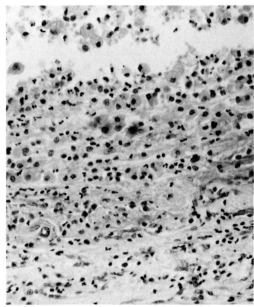

FIGURE 1-13 Cyst of Bartholin's gland: microscopic appearance, showing replacement of epithelial lining by inflammatory cells.

Epidermal Inclusion Cyst

The epidermal inclusion cyst is constituted from fragments of epithelium included in the subcutaneous connective tissue after trauma or surgery (eg, perineorrhaphy, episiotomy). It can also originate from foci of squamous metaplasia in a sebaceous gland.[94] Clinically, it presents the same appearance as the sebaceous cyst and contains a grumous pale yellow substance. It may become inflamed or reach a large volume.

Microscopically, it is lined by a keratinizing squamous epithelium. Fragments of keratin included within the cyst may behave as foreign bodies and provoke a granuloma rich in multinuclear giant cells. These cysts may disrupt or, secondarily, calcify. Rare malignant transformation has been reported. Other postsurgical tumors have been reported, including endometriosis, granulomatous polyps, and fibroepithelial polyps.

Mesonephric Cyst (Cyst of Gartner's Duct)

Cysts of Gartner's duct develop from vestiges of the wolffian duct.[95] They are lined by a columnar or cuboidal, nonmuciparous, and rarely ciliated epithelium. Smooth muscle cells are often identified in the wall.

Cyst of the Canal of Nuck

The persistence of the peritoneal diverticulum of the labium majus gives rise to cysts lined by a flattened mesothelium. They are located near the insertion of the round ligament.[96]

Mucous Cyst

Mucous cysts are predominantly located in the vestibule. Microscopically, they are lined by a mucus-secreting epithelium of cuboidal or columnar cells that stain with Alcian blue and mucicarmine stains. They are probably derived from the urogenital sinus epithelium that forms the vestibule.[97–99]

Cyst of Skene's Glands

Cysts of the paraurethral glands are rare but are occasionally observed in neonates. They are lined by a transitional-type epithelium.[100,101]

Solid Tumors

Squamous Papilloma

The true papilloma is a single verrucous tumor that is slow-growing and appears in elderly women at the level of the labia. It is composed of a connective tissue stroma covered by squamous epithelium showing pronounced hyperkeratosis and papillomatosis. This entity should be differentiated from the fibroepithelial polyp.[102]

Fibroepithelial Polyp

Fibroepithelial polyps of the vulva are common.[103,104] Macroscopically, they are small, papillomatous lesions, large pedunculated tumors, or any intermediate type. The tumors have a soft to rubbery consistency. Microscopically, they consist of loose, edematous connective tissue covered by a hyperkeratotic and acanthotic squamous epithelium (Fig. 1-14). Stromal cells differentiate along two cell lines: fibroblasts and myoblasts. The presence of atypical cells in the stroma should not mislead the pathologist to report the lesion erroneously as sarcoma botryoides.[103] These cells do not invade the overlying epithelium. Immunohistochemical reactivity for vimentin and desmin is present in some cases, supporting the myofibroblastic nature of these polyps.[104] Pigmentation may be abundant, suggesting erroneously the diagnosis of nevus or acanthosis nigricans.

Keratoacanthoma

This rare lesion is a fast-growing proliferation of the squamous epithelium, forming a central mass of keratin that is pushed upward from the surface. Flow-cytometric analysis has shown that this rapidly growing lesion that spontaneously regresses is a true neoplasm and not a reactive hyperplasia.[105,106] Differential diagnosis, as in other more common cutaneous locations, is made with squamous cell carcinoma.

Warty Dyskeratoma

Warty dyskeratoma is a benign tumor occurring as an elevated nodule with a keratotic umbilicated center. It has been reported very rarely in the vulva.[107] Microscopically, it shows an epidermal invagination filled with acantholytic, keratinous material. The bottom of the invagination is covered with elongated dermal papillae lined with a single layer of basal cells. Degenerated cells located in the granular layer (corps ronds), also described in *Darier's disease*, are observed.

Seborrheic Keratosis

The vulvar localization of this flat, pigmented, warty lesion is rare. The microscopic appearance consists of hyperkeratosis, hyperplasia of the parabasal layer, and keratin cysts.

Angiokeratoma

Angiokeratoma looks clinically like a dark red angioma and occurs more frequently on the vulvar mucosa of older patients.[108,109] It is a mixed lesion showing dilated capillaries of the upper dermis associated with hyperkeratosis, papillomatosis, and acanthosis of the overlying squamous epithelium. Some epithelial cords originating from the surface epithelium surround the vascular channels. Erosion of the

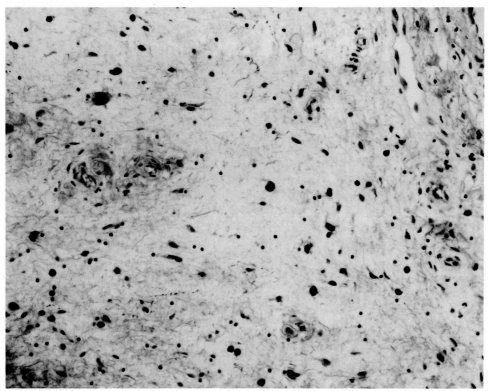

FIGURE 1-14 Stroma of a fibroepithelial polyp of the vulva. The myxoid stroma contains inflammatory cells, variably sized spindle cells, and scattered giant cells with one or more large hyperchromatic nuclei.

superficial mucosa explains the frequent secondary infection. Electron microscopic studies suggest that the lesion is a modified capillary hemangioma.

Urethral Caruncle

The urethral caruncle is a common, nodular, inflammatory rather than neoplastic lesion. It is a single or, rarely, multiple mass, situated at the level of the urethral meatus, in the proximal portion of the urethral wall, or arising from a localized ectropion of the urethral mucosa.[110] It measures several millimeters in diameter and presents as a polypoid or pedunculated mass of bright red color, with a smooth or papillary surface. Microscopically, there is edematous granulation tissue rich in lymphocytes and plasma cells and abundantly vascularized, covered by urethral mucosa (Fig. 1-15). Papillomatous, angiomatous, and granulomatous types are encountered according to the major histologic alterations. The epithelium may ulcerate. This lesion is often asymptomatic or may manifest itself by dysuria or bleeding on contact. Differential diagnosis must be made with carcinoma.

Syringoma

Syringoma is a benign tumor of the eccrine sweat gland duct.[111-113] Clinically, it is constituted by skin-colored or yellow papules situated on both labia majora. Differential diagnosis has to be made with *Fox-Fordyce disease*.[114]

The histology reveals cystic ducts lined by a double layer of epithelial cells of eccrine type with characteristic tail-like strands. The ducts are sometimes filled with keratin. Glycogen accumulation may be observed in tumor cells.

Fibroma and Leiomyoma

Fibroma and leiomyoma are slowly growing, encapsulated benign tumors, situated most frequently at the level of the labia majora or the clitoris. They originate from the connective tissue or from smooth muscle fibers and occur in adults.[115] They are usually small, but in certain exceptional cases may weigh several kilograms.

Microscopic Appearance. The tumor is composed of fusiform connective tissue cells with oval nuclei. In the true fibromyoma, one finds both smooth muscle fibers and collagen fibers. Edema is common. Hyaline or cystic degeneration and calcification may be present. Vascularity varies from one tumor to another. Malignant transformation is extremely rare.

Vascular Tumors

Hemangioma. The hemangioma, or angioma, is seen as a round, wine-red, elevated mass, situated most often in the labia majora. The most common type is cherry hemangioma.

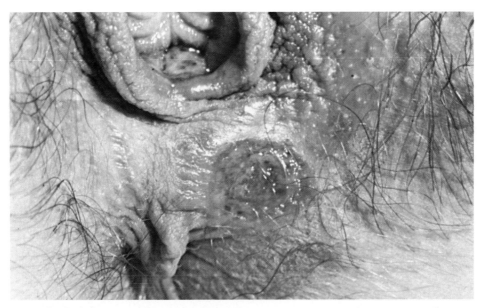

Color Figure 1-1

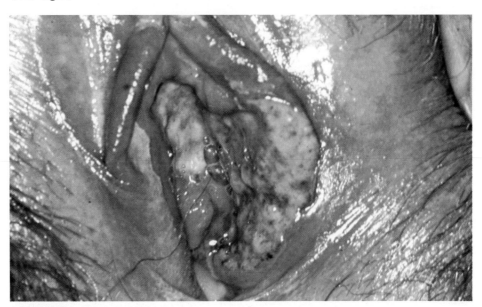

Color Figure 1-2

Color Figure 1-1 Clinical appearance of syphilitic chancre.

Color Figure 1-2 Clinical appearance of ulcus vulvae acutum (Behçet's syndrome).

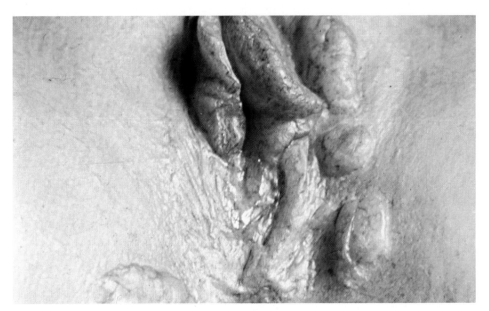

Color Figure 1-3

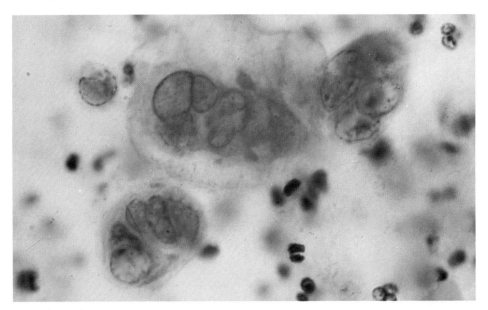

Color Figure 1-4

Color Figure 1-3 Clinical appearance of condyloma acuminatum.

Color Figure 1-4 Vulvovaginal smear showing herpes simplex.

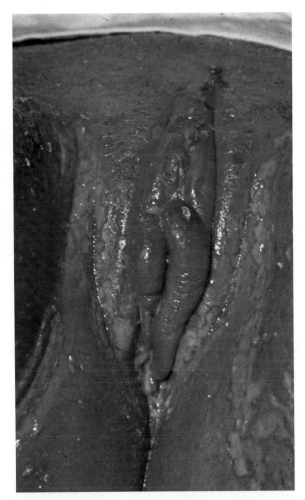

Color Figure 1-5

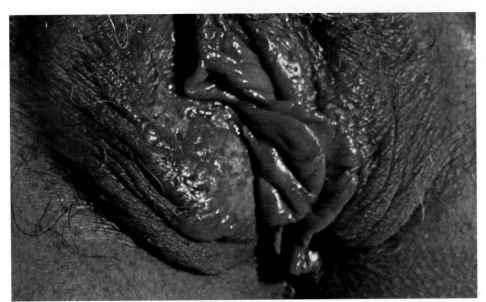

Color Figure 1-6

Color Figure 1-5 Clinical appearance of mycotic vulvovaginitis.

Color Figure 1-6 Clinical appearance of intraepithelial carcinoma.

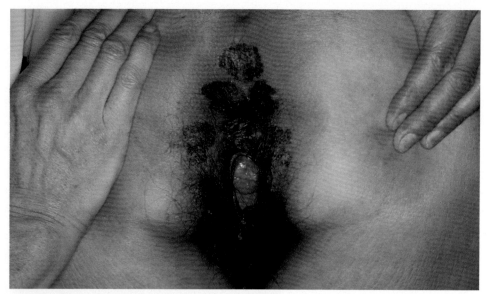

Color Figure 1-7

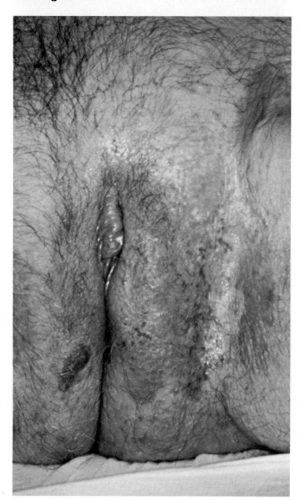

Color Figure 1-8

Color Figure 1-7 Bowenoid papulosis. Multiple pigmented papules of perianal region.

Color Figure 1-8 Clinical appearance of Paget's disease.

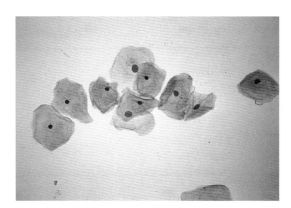

Color Figure 2-1

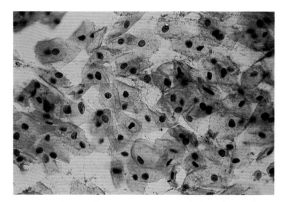

Color Figure 2-2

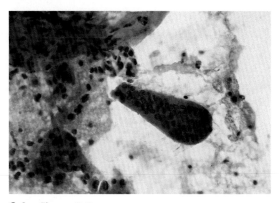

Color Figure 2-3

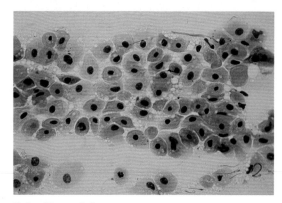

Color Figure 2-4

Color Figure 2-1 Vaginal smear of estrogenic type. Predominantly superficial cells.

Color Figure 2-2 Vaginal smear of luteal type. Mostly intermediate cells.

Color Figure 2-3 Trophoblast in vaginal smear.

Color Figure 2-4 Vaginal smear of atrophic type. Parabasal cells.

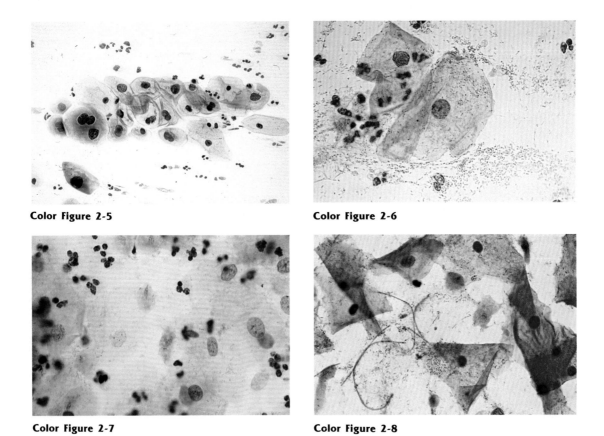

Color Figure 2-5

Color Figure 2-6

Color Figure 2-7

Color Figure 2-8

Color Figure 2-5 Atrophic vaginitis with nuclear atypia. This atypia disappeared after an estrogen injection.

Color Figure 2-6 Clue cells in *Gardnerella* vaginitis: Bacteria partially covering squamous cells.

Color Figure 2-7 *Trichomonas* vaginitis in vaginal smear. Two organisms are seen at center of figure.

Color Figure 2-8 *Leptothrix* organisms in vaginal smear.

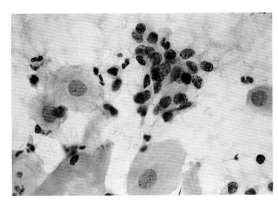

Color Figure 2-9

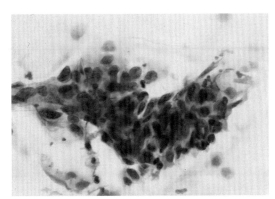

Color Figure 2-10

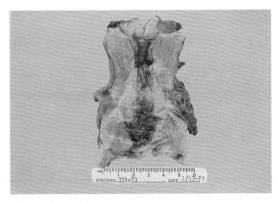

Color Figure 2-11

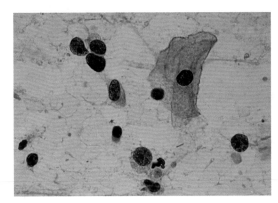

Color Figure 2-12

Color Figure 2-9 Vaginal adenosis. Smear of lateral vaginal wall shows well-preserved endometrial-type cells.

Color Figure 2-10 High grade VAIN in a 54-year-old woman.

Color Figure 2-11 Clear cell adenocarcinoma of vagina and cervix in adolescent girl who was exposed in utero to diethylstilbestrol (DES).

Color Figure 2-12 Clear cell adenocarcinoma of vagina. Malignant glandular cells and one benign squamous cell in vaginal smear from 14-year-old girl who was exposed in utero to DES.

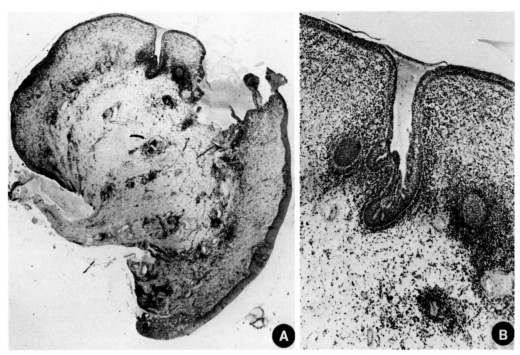

FIGURE 1-15 Urethral caruncle. **(A)** View of the entire lesion. **(B)** Epithelium of urethral type covering an edematous stroma infiltrated by leukocytes.

Histologic examination reveals vascular channels disposed without any order and separated by thin connective tissue septa. The vascular walls are capillary in type. The lesion is not encapsulated. Hemorrhage may take place within the vascular formations and provoke the deposit of hemosiderin within macrophages situated in the stroma. In old lesions, the vessels may become completely sclerosed, leaving only the connective tissue stroma containing these iron-laden macrophages. The evolution of these tumors is benign. *Granuloma pyogenicum,* a lesion composed of lobular arrays of small capillaries in an inflammatory background, may be seen in the vulvar region, most frequently during pregnancy.

Lymphangioma. Lymphangioma, a proliferation of lymphatic vessels, can be encountered but is less common.

Other Vascular Tumors. *Hemangiopericytoma,* a tumor arising from the pericytes, is rarely observed in the vulva. Clinically, it consists of a small mass, easily bleeding and painful. The histology reveals round or spindle-shaped cells proliferating around vascular spaces.[116] Very rare cases of *angiosarcoma* have been cited.[117] A single case of *epithelioid hemangioendothelioma,* a tumor of intermediate malignancy, has been reported.[118]

Lipoma

Lipoma is a benign tumor constituted of adipose tissue. It is soft, encapsulated, and occasionally pedunculated. It is most often found in the labia majora and rarely attains a considerable weight. It is composed of fat cells supported by a more or less abundant connective tissue network.[119,120] When the connective tissue is prominent, it should be called *fibrolipoma.*

Mixed Tumor (Pleomorphic Adenoma)

Mixed tumors are extremely rare. They are histologically similar to their salivary gland counterpart.[121]

Other Benign Soft Tissue Tumors

Among the rare connective tissue tumors are *osteoma, chondroma,* and *myxoma.* The latter is formed by a tissue analogous to the embryonic mesenchyme and is composed of stellate cells anastomosed in a mucoid substance containing collagen fibers. A certain number of fibroepithelial polyps with a loose, edematous stroma have been erroneously labeled *myxomas.*

Glomus tumor has been reported rarely.[122] Single or multiple *neurofibromas* of the vulva are not rare in patients with von Recklinghausen's disease. *Neurilemoma* has been described.[123] Steeper and Rosai described a lesion that they named *aggressive angiomyxoma.*[124] These lesions are usually large, gelatinous, locally infiltrative masses in young women and frequently are related to Bartholin's gland. Histologically, they are characterized by a loose myxoid stroma, prominent thick-walled and often hyalinized blood vessels, and, in some cases, small proliferating benign-appearing glands that probably are entrapped rather than neoplastic (Fig. 1-16). Local recurrence is common, but distant metastases have not been noted.

Angiomyofibroblastoma is a rare mesenchymal tumor.[125] Clinically, it presents in young women as a superficial, small, soft mass of the vulvar region. Microscopically, it may be similar to an aggressive angiomyxoma. It is a circumscribed nodule of irregularly disposed stromal cells with abundant thin-walled vessels. Immunohistochemically, there is reactivity for vimentin and desmin. This benign neoplasm should not be confused with aggressive angiomyxoma, which is locally infiltrating, generally larger, more myxoid, contains larger and thicker-walled vessels, is desmin negative, and frequently recurs.

Other rare benign mesenchymal tumors that have more or less similar structural patterns should be mentioned. The *myxoid epithelioid leiomyoma* is more cellular but lacks the abundant vascularity of aggressive angiomyxoma and angiomyofibroblastoma. The *myxoid peripheral nerve sheath tumor* shows reactivity for S-100 protein and lacks the vascularity of angiomyoblastoma. *Nodular fasciitis* has been reported in the vulva.[126]

Papillary Hidradenoma

Papillary hidradenoma (hidradenoma papilliferum) is a benign, frequently asymptomatic lesion of the sweat glands first described by Pick in 1904; more than 300 cases have been reported.[127-129] This tumor presents as a round or oval, firm, painless, well-encapsulated nodule measuring 0.5 to 2 cm. There is sometimes central ulceration, with a dark red granular area that bleeds easily (umbilication). Papillary hidradenoma is encountered in patients between 30 and 70 years of age and is found in the labia majora

or, more rarely, the labia minora, the interlabial groove, or the posterior commissure. Most cases appear in Caucasian women, and the lesion is rare in black women. It originates in sweat glands that are residua of the embryonic mammary crest. The hypothesis of sudoriferous origin is based on: (1) the histologic similarity of the lesion to sweat glands; (2) localizations corresponding to regions where apocrine glands are found; and (3) histochemical and electron microscopic data. There is a striking resemblance of this lesion to nipple adenoma of the breast, another gland of similar histogenesis.

Histologic Appearance. This tumor is composed of trabecular, tubular, or papillary formations included within a cystic nodule and covered with bistratified epithelium (Fig. 1-17). This epithelium consists of two cell types: (1) large columnar cells with basal nuclei and eosinophilic cytoplasm, showing the picture of apocrine secretion with granules that are periodic acid-Schiff (PAS) positive and diastase-resistant; and (2) external myoepithelial cells, which have the immunohistochemical properties of smooth muscle fibers. These latter cells are themselves bordered by thin connective tissue bundles. Inflammatory reaction of the stroma is minimal.

The hyperplastic, richly papillary appearance and the presence of mitoses have caused this tumor to be confused on occasion with a well-differentiated adenocarcinoma. If the lesion is ulcerated, it must not be confused with a pyogenic granuloma or an epithelioma. Most hidradenomas are cured by local excision. However, one case of hidradenocarcinoma has been reported,[130] and we have seen a metastasizing adenocarcinoma that probably arose in a papillary hidradenoma (Fig. 1-18).

Although not a tumor, *Fox-Fordyce disease,* or "apocrine miliaria" must be mentioned as involving the vulvar apocrine glands.[114] Numerous apocrine

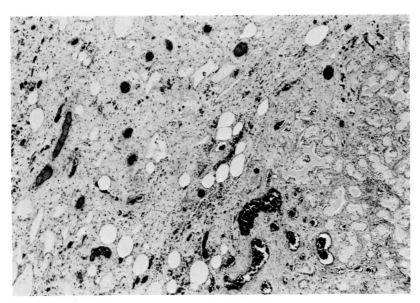

FIGURE 1-16 Aggressive angiomyxoma: myxoid connective tissue containing prominent blood vessels and a cluster of small muciparous glands (*right*) invades pelvic fat in this lesion that recurred clinically at 6 and 9 years after initial local resection.

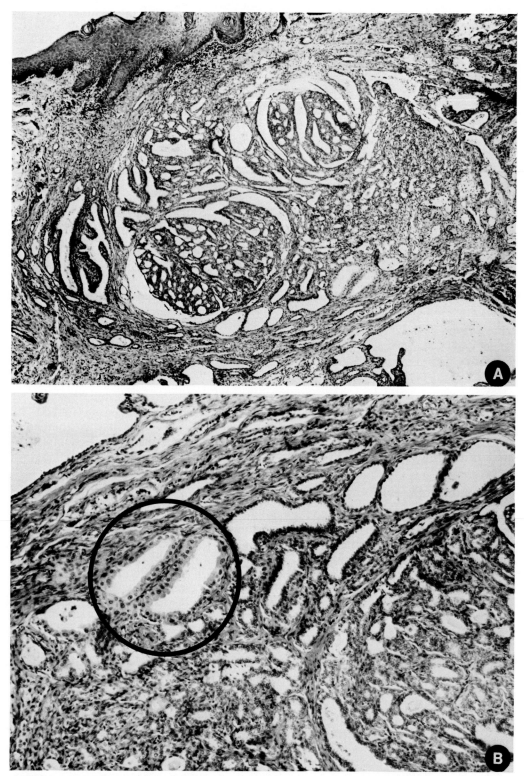

FIGURE 1-17 Papillary hidradenoma: glandular formations covered by bistratified columnar epithelium with foci of apocrine metaplasia.

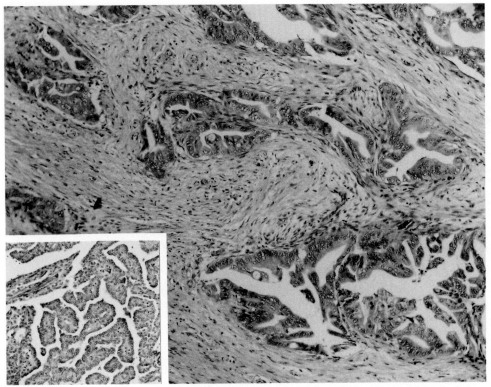

FIGURE 1-18 Invasive adenocarcinoma of vulva in a young woman. This tumor metastasized to the inguinal lymph nodes. Papillary architecture is seen focally in the tumor (*inset*), suggesting possible origin in a papillary hidradenoma or a similar sweat gland tumor.

sweat retention cysts resulting from obstruction of the ducts are seen in this condition; they are accompanied by acanthosis and dermal inflammation, the latter often granulomatous.

Clear Cell Adenoma

Clear cell adenoma is rarely observed in the vulva.[131,132] Presumably derived from eccrine sweat glands, this tumor is composed of solid lobules surrounded by thin collagen bands. Two types of cells are recognized: polygonal cells with small round central nuclei, and round cells with a small dense nucleus surrounded by voluminous clear cytoplasm.

Granular Cell Tumor

Granular cell tumor, a rare tumor described by Abrikosov in 1926, can involve the vulva.[133–135] Rare cases have been reported in prepubertal girls.[134] The tumor is also known as *granular cell myoblastoma* and *Abrikosov's tumor.*

The *histogenesis* of these tumors was subject to debate. According to Abrikosov, they were tumors of muscular origin. A schwannian origin is now widely accepted.[136]

Macroscopic Appearance. The lesion is a firm, well-demarcated, non-tender tumor with smooth surfaces. It measures no more than several centimeters

and is situated on the labia majora. In the vulva, the epithelium may be thinned or may show a reactive hyperplasia.[131] Sectioning reveals a yellow color and a fascicular structure.

Microscopic Appearance. Large collagenous bundles are seen separating solid nests of large cells. There are small, round or oval nuclei and abundant, finely granular, PAS-positive cytoplasm (Fig. 1-19). Often a pseudoepitheliomatous hyperplasia of the overlying squamous epithelium is present and raises the differential diagnosis with squamous carcinoma.[135] The presence of the underlying tumor helps to make the diagnosis. Wide excision is necessary to avoid local recurrence. Rare cases with lymph node metastases have been reported.[137] These do not differ histologically from nonmetastasizing tumors.

ECTOPIC TISSUE

The incomplete regression of the mammary crest, which extends from the axilla to the inner thigh, explains the presence of breast tissue in the vulvar region.[138,139] Another source of ectopic breast tissue may be modified sweat glands.

Different forms of breast lesions can be recognized, such as fibroadenoma (Fig. 1-20), fibrocystic change, lactating tissue, adenocarcinoma, and sar-

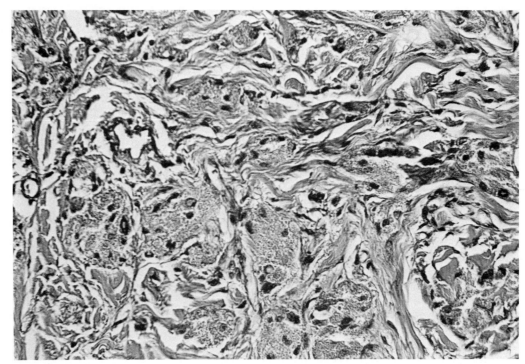

FIGURE 1-19 Granular cell tumor of vulva.

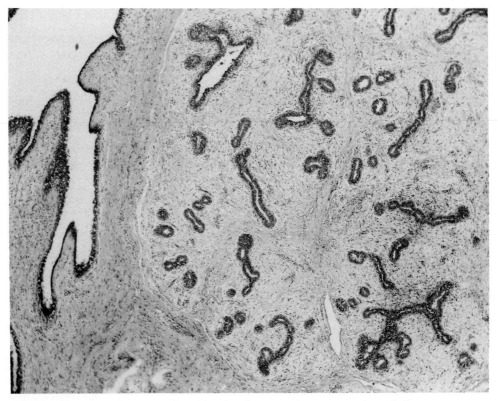

FIGURE 1-20 Fibroadenoma (*right*) arising in vulvar ectopic mammary tissue (*left*).

coma. Some of the benign forms may enlarge with menstruation or pregnancy. Carcinoma arising in vulvar breast tissue has been reported very infrequently.

VULVAR "DYSTROPHIES" OR NONNEOPLASTIC EPITHELIAL DISORDERS AND VULVAR INTRAEPITHELIAL NEOPLASIA (VIN)

Much confusion has arisen in the use of the clinical and histologic definitions that characterize vulvar degenerative and hyperplastic disease. In 1881, Breisky described a progressive atrophy and fibrosis of the vulvar mucosa, which he called *kraurosis vulvae*.[140] This term has since been used to define different atrophic conditions of the vulva, just as the term *leukoplakia* has been popularized by clinicians to characterize white precancerous lesions.

The variety of clinical and morphologic conditions, the different terms used to describe these lesions, the lack of correlations among the findings and opinions of clinicians and pathologists, and the obscure pathogenesis of these conditions partially explain the confusion that has existed in this field. The various terms that have been used for atrophic conditions include *leukoplakia, kraurosis vulvae, white spot disease, sclerotic dermatosis, atrophic* and *hyperplastic vulvitis, neurodermatitis, lichen simplex chronicus,* and *senile atrophy.*

To clarify the situation, the International Society for the Study of Vulvar Disease (ISSVD) proposed the term *dystrophy* in 1976 to qualify atrophic and hyperplastic lesions of the vulvar epidermis and mucosa and the mixed forms resulting from the coexistence of both alterations (Table 1-2).[141] Although this system was preferable to the anarchy that often had prevailed, we found it far from ideal for several reasons:

1. There is little evidence that these lesions are really dystrophic (defective development or degeneration) in the true sense of the word.
2. A term consecrated by long usage and familiar to gynecologists and pathologists alike—*dysplasia*—is available for the most important

lesion: so-called hyperplastic dystrophy with atypia. Following the nomenclature adopted for cervical lesions, the term *vulvar intraepithelial neoplasia* (VIN) has been proposed to replace or coexist with dysplasia.[142,143]
3. Although combinations of more than one of these lesions undoubtedly occur, in our experience they are uncommon and probably are the result of coincidence rather than common causality; the use of the term *mixed dystrophy* promotes the misconception that lichen sclerosus is related to dysplasia and thus to carcinoma.[144]

Responding to criticisms such as these, the ISSVD in 1987[143] revised its classification to separate more clearly those epithelial disorders classified as nonneoplastic (Table 1-3) and those considered VIN (Table 1-4).[145] We prefer this classification and use it routinely in our practices. The "intraepithelial neoplasia" terminology as first applied to cervical lesions by Richart and his colleagues (see Chap. 3) was meant to emphasize the concept that the dysplasias and in situ carcinoma form a continuous spectrum of disease. In the cervix, it was pointed out that the likelihood of cure in an individual patient (not a statistical figure in a population) depended more on the location and extent of the lesion than on its histologic severity. Thus, we believe that the use of "IN" terminology in any organ should philosophically commit the user *not* to divide the lesions included into grades of severity. We can therefore accept "VIN" alone as a diagnosis or a concept, but if clinicians wish the lesions diagnosed to be divided into categories by severity, we then use the "dysplasia" and "carcinoma in situ" terminology that is sanctioned in Table 1-4.

TABLE 1-2.
Classification of Vulvar Dystrophies (ISSVD, 1976)[141]

Hyperplastic dystrophy
  Without atypia
  With atypia
Lichen sclerosus
Mixed dystrophy—lichen sclerosus with foci of epithelial
  hyperplasia
    Without atypia
    With atypia

TABLE 1-3.
Nonneoplastic Epithelial Disorders of the Skin and Mucosa (ISSVD, 1987)[143]

Lichen sclerosus (lichen sclerosus et atrophicus)
Squamous cell hyperplasia (formerly hyperplastic
  dystrophy)
Other dermatoses

TABLE 1-4.
Classification of Vulvar Intraepithelial Neoplasia (ISSVD, 1987)[143]

Grade	Definition
VIN I	Mild dysplasia (formerly mild atypia)
VIN II	Moderate dysplasia (formerly moderate atypia)
VIN III	Severe dysplasia (formerly severe atypia)
VIN III	Carcinoma in situ

Nonneoplastic Epithelial Disorders

Squamous Hyperplasia

Squamous hyperplasia is a benign lesion of adult vulvar skin or mucosa. The clinical appearance varies from red to white and can be thickened and indurated or thin and easily excoriated. Pruritus is a frequent symptom. Scratching provokes fissures, ulceration, and secondary inflammation.

Microscopically, the epithelium shows hyperkeratosis, acanthosis, and eventually parakeratosis. The granular layer is sometimes prominent. There is a chronic inflammatory infiltrate of the dermis, with lymphocytes, plasma cells, and macrophages. No cellular atypia is present.

Lichen Sclerosus

Lichen sclerosus is a chronic, progressive lesion that appears at all ages but is more frequent after the age of 50 years and in parous women.[144,145] The labia minora are most commonly affected. Extravulvar localizations may be present, especially on the trunk. The pathogenesis is obscure. The lesion has been reported in children.[146] Stenosis of the vaginal introitus may be observed.

Macroscopic Appearance. The gross appearance consists of ivory-colored, flat, irregular maculopapules or plaques with a characteristic dry, parchment-like appearance. Ulceration and fissures may complicate the lesion. These are seen on the vulva and on the adjacent perineal and perianal skin.

Microscopic Appearance. Microscopy reveals hyperkeratosis with progressive diminution of the total thickness of the epithelium and flattening of the dermoepidermal junction (Fig. 1-21). There is hydropic degeneration of cells of the basal layer; edema and hyalinization of the upper third of the dermis; swelling and splitting of collagen bundles; disappearance of pilosebaceous apparatus, sweat glands, and melanocytes, with absence of melanosomes in the keratinocytes; and lymphocytic and histiocytic infiltrates below the zone of dermal homogenization. No atypia is observed. The number of elastic fibers is decreased. Their destruction could be due to an elastic-type protease present in dermal fibroblasts.[147]

The major complication of lichen sclerosus is lichenification. Transformation to dysplasia and carcinoma is rare, and the lesion should not be considered a premalignant disease.[144,148] The high metabolic activity of the epithelial cells demonstrated by different methods explains why the qualification *atrophicus*, which was formerly included in the definition of the lesion, has been deleted in recent reports.[149]

Differential Diagnosis. Differential diagnosis is made with scleroderma and lichen planus. The former is extremely rare in the vulva, features dense fibrosis rather than the peculiar dermal homogenization of lichen sclerosus, and is part of a systemic disease. In lichen planus, the inflammatory infiltrate abuts immediately against the epidermis rather than being separated from it by a layer of dermal homogenization (Fig. 1-22).

Other Dermatoses

Other dermatoses such as senile atrophy, lichen planus, other noninfectious dermatitides, and nonspecific hyperplasias and hyperkeratoses are seen from time to time.[145] They should be diagnosed using the histopathologic terminology that is best found in texts of dermatopathology. Terms such as *kraurosis* and *leukoplakia* are perfectly acceptable for the clinical description of atrophic and white lesions, respectively, but should be eschewed by the pathologist because of their lack of histologic specificity.

Dysplasia and In Situ Squamous Carcinoma: Vulvar Intraepithelial Neoplasia (VIN)

Recent advances in understanding the development and progression of premalignant epithelial lesions and preinvasive neoplasia have emphasized many similarities between vulvar and cervical lesions. A nomenclature similar to the one originally used for the comparable cervical lesions has been proposed for the vulva. VIN is characterized according to the histologic definition proposed by the ISSVD as "a disorientation of epithelial architecture that extends throughout the full thickness of the epithelium."[141]

Most authors divide VIN into three grades that correspond to the quality and quantity of cellular anomalies and can be compared with the equivalent grades in the cervix.[150–152] We have already stated our objection to this terminology. VIN appears to be increasing in frequency as a proportion of all cases of preinvasive and invasive vulvar cancer. Although common after the menopause, the lesion is now being found more frequently in younger women, and the association with HPV infection is widely reported, although the HPV detection rate is lower than in cervical intraepithelial neoplasia (CIN).[151,153–155] HPV-16 is the most commonly detected type of virus. HPV-positive cases are more frequent in younger women than in older women and are more likely to be of warty (bowenoid, koilocytotic) or basaloid than of simplex (typical) type, suggesting that there are two different types of VIN in terms of pathogenesis on the basis of the presence or absence of HPV.[154–156]

The lesion may precede invasive carcinoma, as suggested by various epidemiologic, clinical, and pathologic studies.[152,157] The mean elapsed period of time (25 years) is considerably longer than that in the cervix.[158] The continuous spectrum of lesions from mild to severe is not so evident as in the cervix, and the high-grade lesions may be divided into dif-

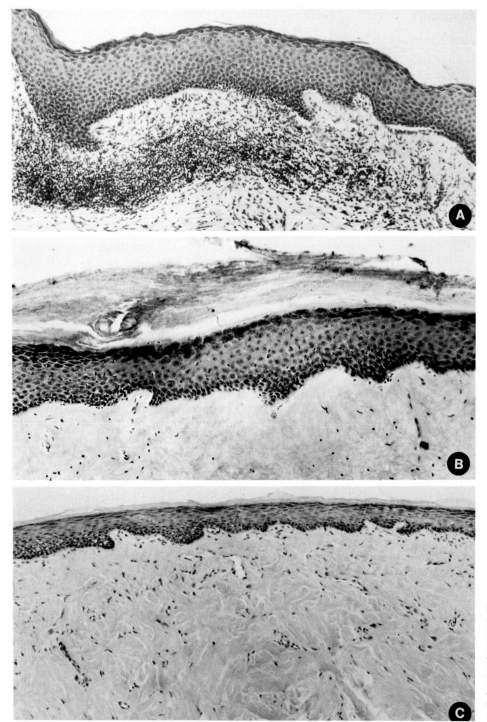

FIGURE 1-21 Lichen sclerosus resulting in kraurosis vulvae. **(A)** Early stage showing moderate hyperkeratosis, edema, and leukocytic infiltration of the stroma. **(B)** Lesion in evolution with distinct hyperkeratosis, alterations in the collagen, and disappearance of the subcutaneous adnexal glands. **(C)** Stage of atrophy.

ferent categories: warty (bowenoid) VIN, basaloid VIN, simplex (typical) VIN, and mixed type. The warty form corresponds to Bowen's disease described in 1912 by that author (Fig. 1-23).[159] The basaloid form resembles the usual carcinoma in situ of the cervix (atypical immature basal cells; Figs. 1-24 and 1-25).[155,158] The simplex type is often confused with squamous hyperplasia without atypia and probably is an uncommon lesion when diagnosed correctly (Fig. 1-26).

Bowenoid papulosis, despite its benign clinical course, should be classified as a carcinoma in situ (see the section on bowenoid papulosis).[160–163]

Vulvar carcinoma in situ is less aggressive than the equivalent cervical lesion. The time between VIN and the development of invasive carcinoma is longer in vulvar lesions than in cervical lesions, and spontaneous regression is more frequent. The presence of VIN in the vicinity of invasive carcinoma is less frequent than the coexistence of CIN and cer-

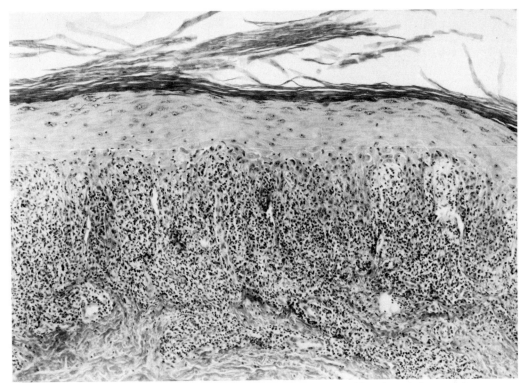

FIGURE 1-22 Lichen planus. An inflammatory infiltrate hugs the epidermis and destroys the basal layer.

vical carcinoma.[158,164,165] The risk of association of VIN with CIN and invasive cervical carcinoma is high (25% in young patients and 15% in older patients)

These differences in behavior between VIN and CIN have not been explained. Normal vulvar epithelium differs from normal cervical epithelium by (among other features) the presence of keratinization, so the threshold for the diagnosis of in situ carcinoma of the vulva is somewhat lower than that in the cervix. In other words, a lesion that might be downgraded to dysplasia in the cervix because of superficial maturation is often acceptable as in situ carcinoma in the vulva. Other factors may intervene,

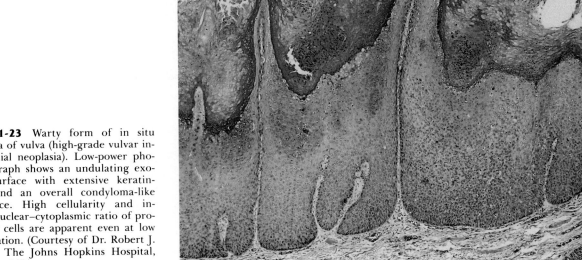

FIGURE 1-23 Warty form of in situ carcinoma of vulva (high-grade vulvar intraepithelial neoplasia). Low-power photomicrograph shows an undulating exophytic surface with extensive keratinization and an overall condyloma-like appearance. High cellularity and increased nuclear–cytoplasmic ratio of proliferating cells are apparent even at low magnification. (Courtesy of Dr. Robert J. Kurman, The Johns Hopkins Hospital, Baltimore, MD).

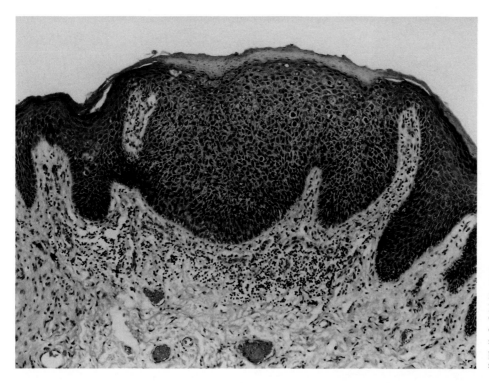

FIGURE 1-24 Basaloid form of in situ carcinoma of vulva (high-grade vulvar intraepithelial neoplasia). The small focus in the center shows a haphazard proliferation of atypical immature basal-type cells extending up to the parakeratotic cells on the flat surface.

such as viral infections, hormonal status, and anatomic localization of the vulvar mucosa.[164]

Macroscopic Appearance. As in the cervix, VIN does not have a diagnostic gross appearance (Color Figure 1-6). Most cases, however, present as *leukoplakia,* or pearly white or ivory, slightly elevated, hyperkeratotic, irregular plaques. Sometimes the lesion exhibits a red-brown surface color. The lesion may be limited to a single focus or may be multicentric. It often involves the perineum, the perianal region, and the vulva. Patients with multifocal disease are found to have a younger age compared with those with unifocal localization. Intra vitam staining

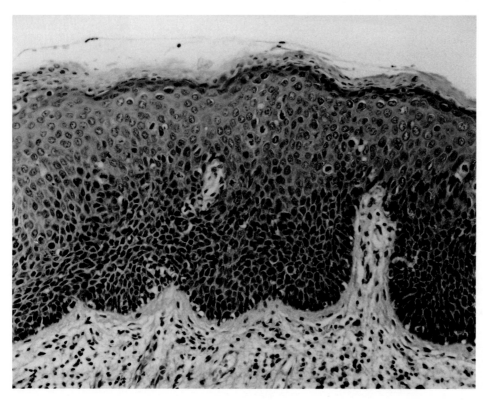

FIGURE 1-25 Basaloid moderate dysplasia of vulva. The atypical immature cells in this lesion proliferate to about the midpoint of the epithelium.

and colposcopic examination may assist in identifying appropriate areas for biopsy or excision.[166]

Microscopic Appearance. The epidermis or mucosa is hyperkeratotic and acanthotic (see Figs. 1-23 through 1-26). A variable degree of atypia (mild, moderate, or severe dysplasia) is present in the deepest epithelial layers, with progression toward the surface but often with some preservation of polarity and maturation in the superficial layers. The atypia consists of the following: disordered polarity of cells; increased nuclear–cytoplasmic ratios; enlarged, irregular, and hyperchromatic nuclei; increased mitotic activity, including abnormal mitoses; and precocious and irregular cellular maturation, with cytoplasmic keratinization and nuclear pyknosis seen focally below the superficial cell layers in which they normally occur. The more diffuse and marked in degree these changes are, and the farther they extend toward the surface, the more severe is the VIN. Sometimes hyperkeratosis is absent. Parakeratosis (with persistence of nuclei in the keratinizing layers) or even focal atrophy may be present, but the sine qua non for the diagnosis is the dyspolarity and cellular atypia. Koilocytes and binucleated cells are generally present in HPV-positive cases. Subjacent stromal inflammation varies from absent to marked, but stromal invasion by neoplastic cells is absent.

Differential Diagnosis. With the increasing experience of pathologists, the diagnostic criteria have become more stringent. If the criteria for dyspolarity and cytologic atypia are adhered to, there should be no confusion with lichen sclerosus, inflammatory dermatoses, or squamous cell hyperplasia with acanthosis and hyperkeratosis. The main problem is the distinction of low-grade VIN lesions from high-grade VIN lesions and of both from bowenoid papulosis (see the section on bowenoid papulosis). Atypias and mitotic figures in the upper third of the epidermis or mucosa usually point toward the diagnosis of in situ carcinoma. Treatment is likely to be similar for dysplasia or carcinoma in situ, so the distinction probably is not of the utmost importance.[166]

Prognosis, Evolution, and Treatment. The evolution is long and may extend over many years with periods of remission. The likelihood of progression to invasive squamous cell carcinoma is small but is far greater in elderly women. The latent period between the appearance of carcinoma in situ and its transformation into invasive cancer is often long, and there is no proof that the former lesion must progress to the latter. Recent studies suggest that the latter, particularly in older women, may not have developed from the former.[158] Patients with multifocal disease are found to have a younger age compared with those with unifocal localization. Occult invasion is more frequently observed in patients of advancing age.[167]

The treatment is predominantly surgical, consist-ing of wide local excision with careful follow-up. Radical vulvectomy with groin dissection is no longer the only treatment. Conservative techniques (cryotherapy, carbon dioxide laser, skinning vulvectomy with skin grafts) have been developed and should be applied when appropriate.

Bowenoid Papulosis

Bowenoid papulosis occurs in male and female genitalia and microscopically resembles Bowen's disease or squamous carcinoma in situ.[160–163,168,169] Its clinical features and its generally benign behavior have suggested to many that it should be considered a distinct clinicopathologic entity, whereas others regard it as a variant of carcinoma in situ. It was first described in 1970 under the name *multicentric pigmented Bowen's disease,*[170] a term that in retrospect probably has not been improved on subsequently.

Clinical Appearance. The lesion is characterized by multiple (usually 5 to 10) small brown-red to violet papules measuring a few millimeters in diameter each. They are located in the vulvar and perineal areas of young adults; almost all patients are younger than 40 years (Color Figure 1-7). Condylomata acuminata and HSV infection are frequently associated with bowenoid papulosis.

Microscopic Appearance. The lesion may be identical to or only slightly different from true Bowen's disease. The cells with uniformly hyperchromatic nuclei are irregularly arranged in a slightly thickened epithelium with no superficial maturation. Atypical mitoses are present. The rete pegs are enlarged and may coalesce with obliteration of the dermal papillae. There is no invasion of the dermis.

The histologic coexistence of this disease with condyloma acuminatum and less frequently with HSV-2 lesions in the same patient has been demonstrated. Immunohistochemical, ultrastructural, and molecular hybridization techniques have clearly established the HPV-16 genesis of the disease.[161,162,168,169]

Differential Diagnosis. The histologic picture is similar to VIN and often is of no help in the diagnosis, although Ulbright and associates have emphasized cellular uniformity and absence of pilosebaceous involvement as useful indicators of bowenoid papulosis.[160] The age of the patient, the multiplicity and small size of the lesions, the verrucoid aspect, and the tendency toward spontaneous resolution are the main reasons to separate bowenoid papulosis from typical Bowen's disease (in situ carcinoma). Furthermore, the frequent coexistence (20% to 50%) of Bowen's disease and CIN or invasive carcinoma of the cervix is not observed in bowenoid papulosis.

The relation of bowenoid papulosis and Bowen's disease remains to be defined. The fact that Bowen's disease (versus nonbowenoid in situ carcinoma) has

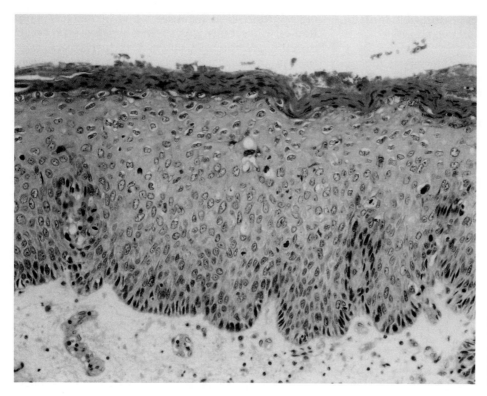

FIGURE 1-26 Simplex (typical) vulvar intraepithelial neoplasia. Large dysplastic cells proliferate toward a parakeratotic but flat surface. Loss of polarity is evident.

been defined in the past as multicentric, occurring in young patients, and less likely to progress to invasive carcinoma suggests that the differences between bowenoid papulosis and "true" Bowen's disease may be more apparent then real. Flow cytometry reveals aneuploid cells with a high DNA content, resulting in a DNA diagnosis of malignancy.[163] Although the typical clinical course is benign, often with spontaneous regression, bowenoid papulosis recurred locally in 20% of cases in one series,[168] and a few reported cases have progressed to or coexisted with invasive carcinoma.[169] Bowenoid papulosis thus should best be considered as a form of carcinoma in situ (VIN) with an unexplained low malignant potential.

VULVAR CYTOLOGY

Techniques of vulvar cytology are direct scraping, imprint of superficial lesions, and fine-needle aspiration of submucosal nodules. The slides should be fixed with 95% ethanol or spray fixative for good preservation. Normal cytology of the vulva is composed of superficial squamous cells and anucleate squames.[171,172]

Vulvar superficial cytology is valuable in the detection of inflammatory diseases and dysplastic or neoplastic lesions of the squamous mucosa and epidermis. The sensitivity of the method to recognize benign, precancerous, and malignant lesions varies according to the severity of the cellular changes. These changes are observed in the cells of the super-

ficial layers obtained by scraping and are characterized by nuclear alterations and modifications of the cell size. Anisonucleosis, hyperchromasia, dyskeratosis, and alterations of the nuclear–cytoplasmic ratio are common features. The anucleate squames present in vulvar imprints are larger in invasive carcinoma than in dysplasia or carcinoma in situ. These diagnoses should always be confirmed histologically.

The classical cytologic manifestation of *condyloma acuminatum* is the presence of koilocytes, sometimes accompanied by parakeratosis in the imprint or scrape smears. *Lichen sclerosus* reveals anucleate squames and parakeratotic cells without cytologic atypia. *Keratinizing carcinoma* is the easiest to recognize: cytoplasmic abnormal keratinization, keratin pearls, apparent intercellular bridges (desmosomes), and nuclear anomalies are evident. *Verrucous carcinoma* imprints or scrapings reveal the presence of hyperkeratotic and parakeratotic cells and slight cellular atypia. Cytology cannot differentiate verrucous carcinoma from pseudoepitheliomatous hyperplasia or condyloma acuminatum in the absence of koilocytes.

Small cell carcinoma shows no sign of keratin maturation, and the cells are small and round with hyperchromatic nuclei. *Paget's disease* exhibits cells with enlarged nuclei and nucleoli and an increased nuclear–cytoplasmic ratio. The nuclei are central or peripheral in location and there is no cytoplasmic keratinization. Mucin vacuoles may be identifiable in the cytoplasm. *Malignant melanoma* and *tumors of Bartholin's gland* can be identified by fine-needle aspiration, as can metastases from vulvar cancers in inguinal lymph nodes. Vulvar cytology is useful in confirming the nature of some *infectious* processes. Fungal and viral infections (especially herpes genitalis and HPV) are particularly amenable to cytologic diagnosis (see Color Figure 1-4). *Endometriosis* of the vulva is extremely rare, but the diagnosis can be made by fine-needle aspiration.[173]

MALIGNANT TUMORS

Primary Tumors

Invasive Squamous Cell Carcinoma

Squamous cell carcinoma of the vulva is seen predominantly in older women and constitutes 4% of female pelvic cancers.[174-180] The age of predilection is between 60 and 90 years (Fig. 1-27).[180] Carcinoma of the vulva is very rare in young women.[181-185] The gravity of its natural history is explained by the early lymphatic dissemination of the tumor cells by the extensive and diffuse network of vulvar lymphatics.[186] This characteristic differentiates vulvar carcinomas from other cutaneous epitheliomas, which remain localized for longer periods of time.

The clinical symptomatology is often simple: the patient presents because of a visible, slow-growing tumor or, more rarely, because of pruritus, pain, bleeding, vaginal discharge, or a burning sensation on micturition. Frequently, the extent of the tumor at the time of diagnosis does not permit the localization of its point of origin. The labia majora and minora are the most common sites of origin of the tumor, followed by the clitoris.

Pathogenesis. The pathogenesis of vulvar carcinoma is not clearly understood. Predisposing conditions are constantly reported: chronic infections such as syphilis and granulomatous venereal diseases are mentioned.[187,188] The occurrence of obesity, diabetes, and hypertension with vulvar carcinoma exceeds the frequency seen in the general population and suggests that some type of endocrinopathy is related to the development of the malignant lesion. Clinical data suggesting a relation between HPV and squamous carcinoma continue to accumulate, although this detection rate is lower than in cervical cancer.[189-191] About 10% of invasive carcinomas show the presence of HPV-16 DNA.[155,192-195] Two groups of tumors can be differentiated according to the presence or absence of HPV (see Microscopic Appearance, below).[155,158,196-198]

Association with other genital cancers, especially cervical lesions, is high (25%).[199] Oncogenic agents such as viruses may operate on different areas of the anogenital epithelium, suggesting a common pathogenetic factor (field response) in the genesis of vulvar, vaginal, and cervical carcinomas and premalignant lesions.

Macroscopic Appearance. The lesion presents as a small, gray, hyperkeratotic, indurated, elevated zone, which has a tendency to become ulcerated and secondarily infected (Fig. 1-28). Alternatively, the tumor may have a papillomatous or multinodular appearance. The labia and clitoris are the most common primary sites. The lesion extends progressively to involve the entire vulva, vagina, and perianal region. In the advanced stages, there is invasion and total destruction of the external genital organs, which are replaced by a large proliferation

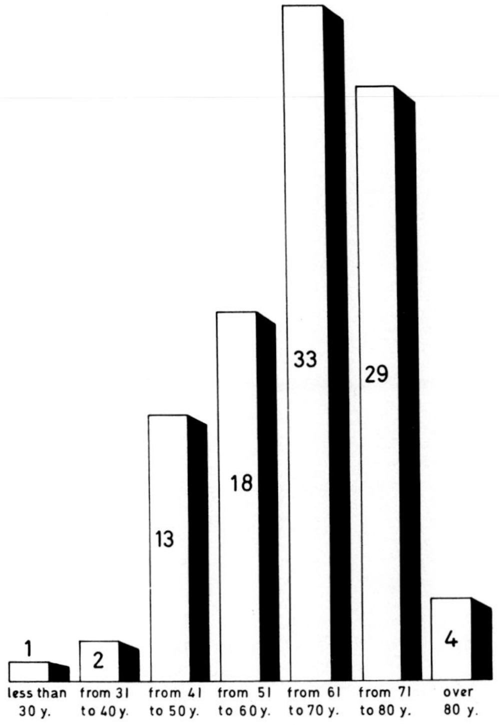

FIGURE 1-27 Frequency (percentage) of carcinoma of the vulva as a function of age (258 cases).

less than 30 y.	from 31 to 40 y.	from 41 to 50 y.	from 51 to 60 y.	from 61 to 70 y.	from 71 to 80 y.	over 80 y.
1	2	13	18	33	29	4

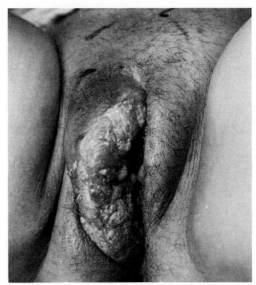

FIGURE 1-28 Squamous cell carcinoma: clinical appearance.

or budding ulceration that is covered with a necrotic fibrinous exudate.

Microscopic Appearance. Vulvar squamous carcinomas are generally better differentiated than those of the cervix and are rich in cornified epithelial pearls (Fig. 1-29). The neoplastic cell cords originate from the basal layers of the epithelium and extend deeply into the dermis and subcutaneous tissue. The squamous cells are large, and their nuclei are irregular, hyperchromatic, and sometimes monstrous. Keratin production is abundant. Mitoses are numerous and atypical (multicentric mitotic figures with aberrant chromosomes). These tumors generally occur in older women, are associated with the "simplex" type of VIN or the lesser grades of dysplasia (or with squamous hyperplasia without atypia), and usually do not contain HPV DNA.[155,158,165,193]

In contrast, squamous carcinomas that contain HPV DNA (usually HPV-16) occur more frequently in younger women and generally are associated with the bowenoid type of VIN (also called *basaloid* by Toki and colleagues), or with warty, condyloma-like lesions, at their periphery.[158] These invasive carcinomas may themselves be of basaloid or warty type. The basaloid type is characterized by large rounded nests or by smaller cords of immature cells with little cytoplasm and little or no keratinization (Fig. 1-30). The warty type has an exophytic condyloma-like appearance at the surface but differs from condyloma or verrucous carcinoma by the presence of a jagged, irregular interface with stroma at the deep invasive border. These two types of invasive carcinoma are associated with the corresponding patterns of VIN (bowenoid or warty) mentioned earlier.[155,158,165,196–198,200]

Other squamous carcinomas may be associated with spindle cell (pseudosarcomatous) metaplasia.[175,201,202] If the entire tumor is of spindle cell type (Fig. 1-31), ultrastructural (desmosomes, tonofilaments) or immunohistochemical (cytokeratin positivity; S-100, HMB-45, desmin and actin negativity) evidence may be required to make the distinction from a spindle cell melanoma or sarcoma.[203]

Grading of vulvar squamous carcinoma is generally performed using a four-grade system, with grade I representing the highly keratinizing tumors with low nuclear–cytoplasmic ratios, little nuclear anaplasia, and few mitotic figures, and grade IV defining the anaplastic spindle cell or small cell tumors.[204] Most of the tumors, regardless of grade, are aneuploid.[205]

Evolution and Prognosis. Early lymphatic dissemination takes place to the inguinal, femoral, and pelvic nodes. Nodal metastases are often bilateral, even if the primary tumor is unilateral. In the absence of inguinal and femoral nodal involvement, deep pelvic nodes are rarely invaded. The necessity of total surgical extirpation of all the nodes is underlined by the fact that an impalpable node is not necessarily a negative node; Way reported that 43% of nonpalpable lymph nodes are microscopically invaded.[202]

The technique of lymphangiography gives some indication of lymph node involvement, as does fine-

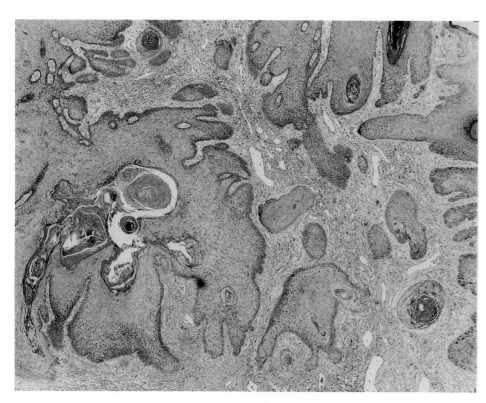

FIGURE 1-29 Squamous cell carcinoma. Microscopic appearance of the typical, highly keratinizing, invasive carcinoma seen predominantly in older women.

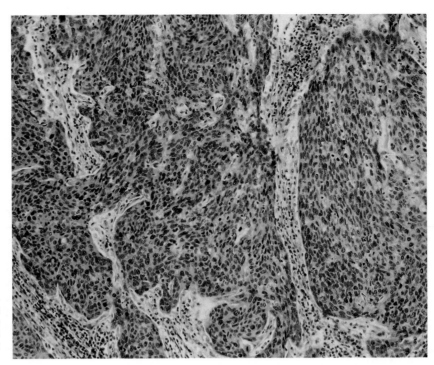

FIGURE 1-30 Squamous cell carcinoma. The basaloid type is characterized by nests of small immature cells showing little clearcut squamous differentiation in this microscopic field. (Courtesy of Dr. Robert J. Kurman)

needle aspiration. Histologic examination of the nodes may reveal not only the presence of a metastasis, but also granulomatous alterations with foreign body multinucleated giant cells, which may be secondary to lymphangiography (in which case fat is seen within the granulomas) or to keratin produced by the tumor cells. Imprint or smear cytology of lymph nodes during surgery may give immediate valuable information to the surgeon, as may fine-needle aspiration cytology before surgery. A relation between the degree of histologic differentiation of the tumor and its clinical malignancy has been proposed by several authors, but this relation is not statistically valid. The prognosis depends much more on the tumor size, the degree of extension of the tumor at the moment of treatment, the integrity of surgical margins,

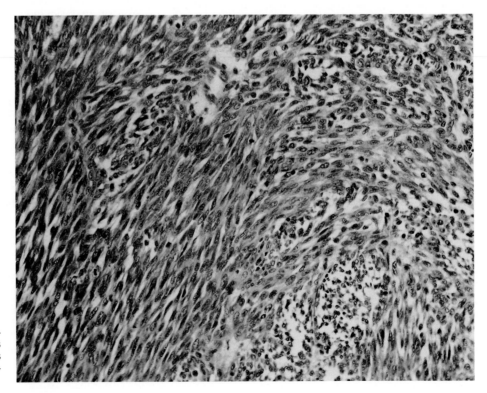

FIGURE 1-31 Spindle cell (pseudosarcomatous) type of squamous cell carcinoma. The tumor cells were immunohistochemically positive for cytokeratins.

and the presence of lymph nodal and distant metastases than on microscopic factors of differentiation.[206-213] The International Federation of Gynecologists and Obstetricians (FIGO) has proposed a classification into four stages that gives a good correlation with 5-year survival (Table 1-5).

The prognosis for cure remains discouraging. The best statistics report from 40% to 60% 5-year survival when there is lymph node invasion, compared with 70% or better in cases with negative nodes.[211] When stromal invasion is limited (less than 1 mm in depth), the prognosis is excellent.[212] Clitoral lesions have a poorer prognosis. Distant metastases occur late to the lungs, liver, and other sites. In summary, long survival depends on early diagnosis, small tumor size, and absence of lymphatic involvement.[213]

Treatment. Vulvectomy with extensive bilateral lymphadenectomy is the usual therapy of choice.[214] The results depend essentially on the precocity of diagnosis and the extent of the surgical resection.[215] The results of radiation therapy do not appear as encouraging, since the classic 5-year survival rates do not surpass 20%, largely because of the difficulty in delivering therapeutic dosages to this highly sensitive region. Newer techniques show more promise, and encouraging results have been reported with chemotherapy using 5-fluorouracil and cisplatin. Chemotherapy acts as a radiosensitizer.[216]

Microinvasive Squamous Cell Carcinoma

Following the observation that squamous carcinomas of the cervix with limited stromal invasion rarely metastasize and are usually cured by conservative therapy, attempts have been made to characterize similar lesions of the vulva.[217,218] As in the cervix, different investigators have used different criteria for the diagnosis of microinvasive carcinoma, with the anticipated different results.[219] Overall, about 12% of patients with tumors characterized as "microinva-

sive" have had lymph node metastases, and a similar proportion have had clinical recurrence.[220] These results are considerably worse than in most series of cervical microinvasive carcinoma, suggesting that this diagnosis should be made with great caution in a vulvar lesion if it will result in more conservative therapy than for other small invasive vulvar cancers. The ISSVD has recently recommended that the designation of microinvasive carcinoma be abandoned, and that "stage IA" be used to designate solitary lesions less than 2 cm in diameter and 1 mm in depth.[141,221]

Other Malignant Epithelial Tumors

Basal Cell Carcinoma. Basal cell carcinoma of the vulva is rare, constituting 2% to 3% of all vulvar cancers.[222-224] Its appearance and clinical behavior are analogous to those observed in other cutaneous regions. It presents as a budding, ulcerated, or papillary lesion and shows multiple localizations. There is no known relation between this tumor and VIN or HPV. There is sometimes local recurrence, but metastases are extremely rare.

Adenoid Squamous Carcinoma. Adenoid squamous carcinoma or adenoacanthoma has been reported in the vulva.[225,226] The tumor is a squamous cell carcinoma with pseudoglandular spaces containing acantholytic and dyskeratotic cells. There is no statistical difference in mortality between this type and the usual squamous cell carcinoma.

Verrucous Carcinoma. Verrucous carcinoma is a large, warty, fungating tumor (Fig. 1-32).[227,228] Ulceration may develop as a late event, with secondary infection and regional adenopathy. Local invasion confirms the malignant nature of the lesion, but it rarely metastasizes. More aggressive behavior has been reported after radiation therapy, so the advised treatment is surgical.

The histologic appearance should be clearly recognized to avoid confusion with well-differentiated squamous carcinoma on the one hand and with giant condyloma acuminatum (if such a lesion exists) on the other. The lesion is characterized by a marked but well-circumscribed acanthosis and papillomatosis, parakeratotic hyperkeratosis, keratin cysts in the centers of the acanthotic rete pegs, and a mild stromal inflammatory infiltrate. The tumor may invade deeply, but always with pushing rather than infiltrative borders. Atypia and mitotic activity are absent or minimal.

The lack of prominent cellular atypia and mitotic figures and the lack of invasion of the stroma by isolated cords of keratinized cells emerging from the rete pegs differentiate verrucous carcinoma from well-differentiated squamous carcinoma. The distinction is important, because the latter tumor metastasizes frequently and does respond to radiation therapy.

TABLE 1-5.
Clinical Staging of Vulvar Carcinoma (FIGO)

Stage	Definition
I	Lesion <2 cm and no suspicious groin nodes
II	Lesion >2 cm and no suspicious groin nodes
III	Lesion extends beyond vulva without grossly positive groin nodes, or
	Lesion confined to vulva with suspicious or positive groin nodes
IV	Lesion extends beyond vulva with grossly positive nodes, or
	Lesion involves mucosa of rectum, bladder or urethra, or bone, or
	All cases with distant or palpable deep pelvic nodal metastases

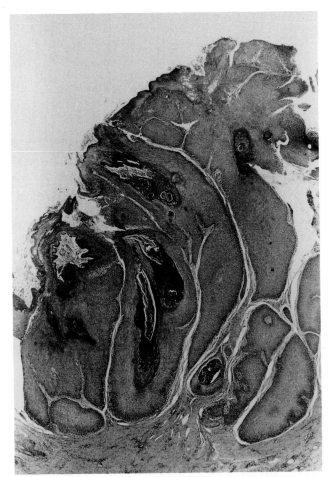

FIGURE 1-32 Verrucous carcinoma. This exophytic papill-omatous tumor contains central keratin plugs in its bulbous tumor nests and invades on a broad "pushing" front. Atypia was minimal at higher magnification.

The giant condyloma acuminatum is differenti-ated by the presence of koilocytotic cells, the exis-tence of fibrovascular cores in the papillae, and the lack of the deep stromal penetration on a broad front that is characteristic of verrucous carcinoma. Many of the lesions initially diagnosed as giant con-dyloma are found on further study to be verrucous carcinomas. This error may occur if the evaluation is made on a small, superficial biopsy that misses the stromal penetration.

Sarcomatoid or Metaplastic Carcinoma. Sarcoma-toid or metaplastic carcinoma was described by Way as a rare type of epithelioma characterized by the presence of giant and spindle cells (see Fig. 1-31).[202] The appearance of this lesion is reminiscent of sar-coma, and it represents an anaplastic form of carci-noma. Each of the five cases that Way studied had an identical evolution: large primary tumor, numerous metastases, and rapidly fatal clinical course. Similar lesions have been described more recently, also with a poor prognosis.[175,229] Ultrastructural findings of desmosomes and tonofilaments in the sarcomatoid cells and immunohistochemical demonstration of keratin are helpful in revealing the true epithelial na-ture of these cells.

Small Cell Carcinoma. Small cell carcinoma is a rare tumor characterized by trabecular structures of small cells with neuroendocrine differentiation. Elec-tron microscopy reveals the presence of neurosecre-tory granules. The origin of the cells is still unset-tled; they are derived from the Merkel's cell (a skin receptor cell) or from some primitive cell with neu-roendocrine differentiation.[214,230]

Sweat Gland Carcinomas. Sweat gland carcinomas are commonly associated with Paget's disease.[231,232] They occur more frequently after the menopause and consist of infiltrating nests of pleomorphic mucicarminophilic cells with inter- or intracellular lumina. Although all these tumors are rare, those showing apocrine differentiation are more common than the eccrine variants.

Paget's Disease. Paget's disease of the vulva is con-siderably rarer than the corresponding lesion of the breast and is found in elderly women.[233–238]

Histogenesis. The histogenesis of the disease re-mains debatable. Different suggestions have been proposed: tumor cells from underlying glandular structures (eccrine,[232] apocrine,[231] or sebaceous glands) colonizing the epidermis; transformed keratinocytes; and endodermal cells of the cloacal region.[233] Casein and carcinoembryonic antigen (CEA) have been identified by immunohistochem-ical techniques.[203]

The diversity of the cellular morphology is un-derstandable if one remembers that the neoplastic cells are derived from the multipotential basal epi-thelial cell of the epidermis.[239] Melanin imbibed from adjacent melanocytes has been observed in some Paget's tumor cells. This should not suggest wrongly the diagnosis of malignant melanoma. Immunostains for S-100 protein and HMB-45 should be negative.[203] Electron microscopic findings have confirmed the concept of an *in situ* carcinoma: neoplastic keratinocytes or squamous cells and secre-tory cells of sweat gland type have been described in Paget's disease of the vulva.[240,241]

Compared with the mammary and perianal localizations, vulvar Paget's disease is less frequently related to an underlying carcinoma; the average fre-quency with which the latter lesion is found is 30%.[238] A careful investigation and histologic exami-nation of all tissue removed by the surgeon is man-datory to exclude the presence of an associated invasive carcinoma.[234,236]

Clinical Appearance. The lesion resembles a chronic dermatitis and is characterized by a well-limited, gray-red zone with white plaques (Color Figure 1-8) that should be differentiated from squamous cell car-cinoma in situ.

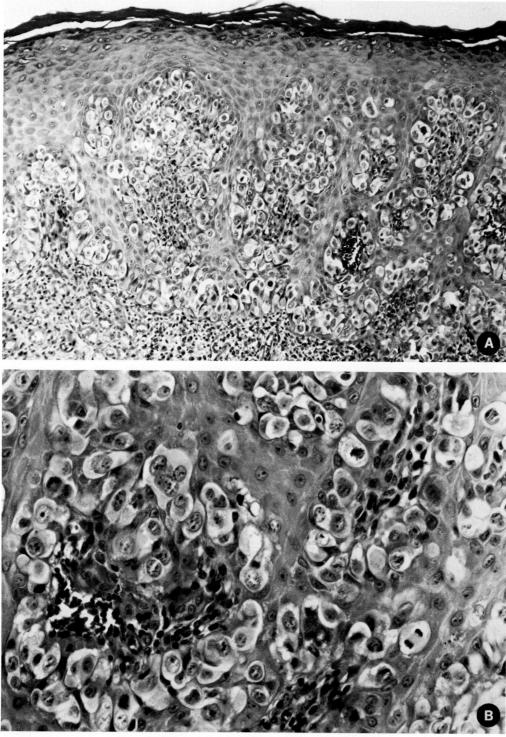

FIGURE 1-33 Paget's disease. **(A)** General microscopic appearance. **(B)** Detail showing large neoplastic cells with clear cytoplasm dispersed throughout the squamous epithelium.

Histologic Appearance. There is a hyperkeratotic and acanthotic epithelium studded with large cells containing clear cytoplasm and voluminous nuclei (Fig. 1-33). They occur singly or in clusters. The tumor cells stain positively with PAS before and after diastase, and most stain with Alcian blue and mucicarmine stains. The subjacent dermis shows a chronic inflammatory infiltrate. Karyotypes from Paget's disease have been reported as normal diploid.[205] Immunohistochemistry is positive for epithelial membrane antigen, CEA, casein, and cytokeratins.[242] Viral investigations have not detected the presence of HPV.[243]

Imprint or abrasive cytology exhibits cells with enlarged nuclei and nucleoli and an increased nuclear–cytoplasmic ratio. The nuclei are central or peripheral, and there is no cytoplasmic keratinization. Binucleation is observed. The cytoplasm has a basophilic stain, and melanin pigment is present in less than 5% of the cells.

Prognosis and Treatment. The type of treatment and the prognosis are determined by the presence of an underlying carcinoma (Fig. 1-34). Lymph node and distant metastases have been reported. Associated extragenital carcinomas (particularly of the breast) are not uncommon.

Adenocarcinoma of Mammary Type. Vulvar mammary tissue (see section on Ectopic Tissue earlier in this chapter) may be the site of malignant lesions.[244,245] These carcinomas are histologically similar to mammary carcinomas arising in the breast.

Carcinoma of Bartholin's Gland. Carcinoma of Bartholin's gland is rare and can be seen at any adult age, with a predilection for elderly women.[246,247] For unknown reasons, the tumor is more frequently localized to the left side. Clinical complaints are nonspecific, and often the first diagnosis is that of an inflammatory lesion or a cyst. Several histologic forms are encountered: adenocarcinoma, squamous cell carcinoma, and, less frequently, adenoid cystic carcinoma, transitional cell carcinoma, mixed and undifferentiated forms. *Adenoid cystic carcinoma* has a distinctive histologic appearance, with epithelial cords scattered through an eosinophilic, often hyalinized, stroma (Fig. 1-35).[248,249] It is identical to the tumor seen in the salivary glands and has a special affinity to invade perineural spaces. *Skene's glands* may be the site of origin of adenocarcinoma in rare cases.[250]

Carcinoma of the Urethra. Although properly belonging to the field of urologic pathology, carcinomas of the urethra are important to this discussion because they usually involve the vulva.[251,252] In the 1952 review by McCrea, 546 authenticated primary urethral malignant tumors were found in the literature: 340 unclassified carcinomas, 116 squamous cell carcinomas, 48 adenocarcinomas, 23 sarcomas, and 19 melanomas.[253] They appear mostly in women older than 50 years of age. The vast majority of these tumors involve the anterior (vulvar) third of the urethra, some involving the entire length of the organ; involvement of the posterior urethra alone is rare. A rare entity is carcinoma arising in a urethral diverticulum.[254,255]

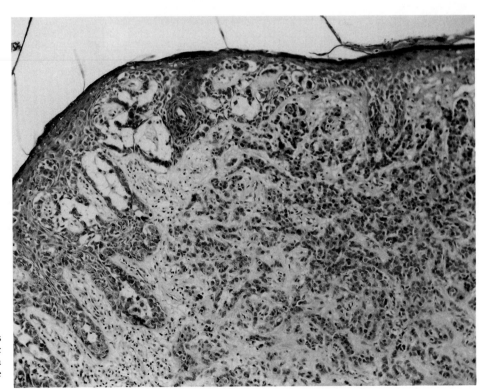

FIGURE 1-34 Invasive Paget's disease. In addition to neoplastic cells in the epidermis, there is a contiguous underlying invasive adenocarcinoma.

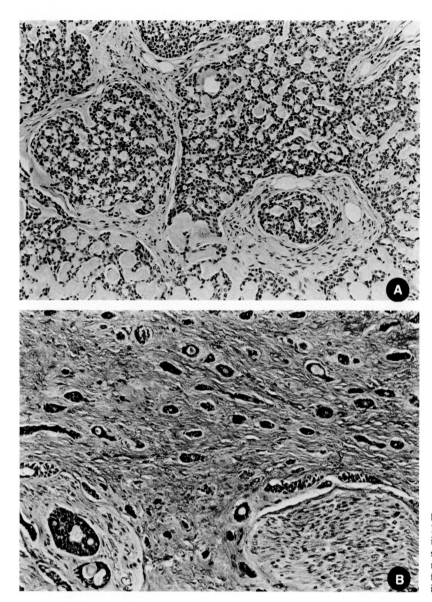

FIGURE 1-35 Adenoid cystic carcinoma of Bartholin's gland. **(A)** Low-power view showing interlacing cribriform glandular formations separated and expanded by hyaline basement membrane-derived material. **(B)** Sclerosing field of tumor with peri- and intraneural invasion.

Macroscopic Appearance. Squamous cell or epidermoid carcinoma begins as a small papillomatous or ulcerated lesion, becoming exophytic when more advanced. Adenocarcinoma, which originates in the paraurethral glands, usually presents as a dark red polypoid mass protruding from the urethral orifice but may be located submucosally.

Microscopic Appearance. The squamous carcinomas are usually well differentiated, resembling other squamous carcinomas of the vulva but with somewhat less keratinization (Fig. 1-36). Spindle cell metaplasia is occasionally present, and inflammatory changes in the stroma are common. The adenocarcinomas are usually composed predominantly of mucin-secreting glands but may contain large cells with clear cytoplasm.[252] Mixed squamous-urothelial (transitional cell) tumors may be observed.

Carcinomas arising in a diverticulum are predom-

inantly adenocarcinomas, followed by transitional and squamous cell tumors. A few cases represent tumors arising from congenital embryonal rests.

Prognosis, Evolution, and Treatment. Small localized tumors have a good prognosis. Pelvic and inguinal lymph node metastases occur predominantly with tumors of the posterior and anterior urethra, respectively. Distant metastases are infrequent, occurring in less than 15% of all cases and possibly more frequently in adenocarcinoma; they have been found in the lungs, brain, liver, and ureters. Squamous cell carcinomas are best treated by surgery or radiation, or both, whereas adenocarcinomas respond poorly to radiation and should therefore be treated primarily by surgery. Five-year survival in most series is in the range of 30%.[256]

The adenocarcinoma type of diverticular origin should be recognized as such, because it appears to

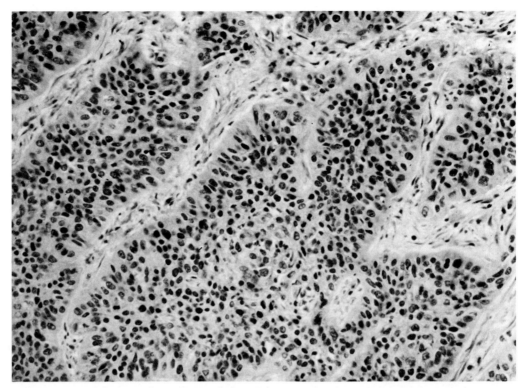

FIGURE 1-36 Squamous cell carcinoma of the urethra.

be less aggressive than the transitional and squamous types.

Malignant Melanoma

Malignant melanoma, a tumor originating from melanin-producing cells, accounts for 2% to 10% of vulvar malignant lesions.[257-261] It affects mainly Caucasians. Lymphatic and bloodstream metastases occur frequently. There is wide hematogenous dissemination to almost all the organs of the body, most notably the lungs, liver, heart, kidneys, and meninges.

Macroscopic Appearance. The macroscopic appearance is that of a black or brown pigmented spot that enlarges and ulcerates (Fig. 1-37A). The tumor is most frequently situated at the level of the labia majora.

Histologic Appearance. The histologic appearance is extremely variable and often is not typical (see Fig. 1-37B). Nodular and superficial spreading types have been reported with equal frequency. The tumor may resemble squamous cell carcinoma, anaplastic adenocarcinoma, or spindle cell sarcoma. Invasion of the surface epithelium by nests of malignant cells, in a manner similar to that of Paget's disease, is one of the characteristic features of malignant melanoma. In the dermis and the fibroadipose subcutaneous tissue, the cells are disposed in bands or large plaques that are separated by thin fascicles of banal stroma.

The nuclei are large, irregular, and hyperchromatic and often contain typical rounded invaginations of cytoplasm (pseudoinclusions). The amount of melanin pigment within the tumor varies from one case to the next, and when it is absent (amelanotic melanoma) the diagnosis is more difficult; in the vulva, this eventuality is rare.

Prognosis. Estimation of the level of invasion of the dermis according to Clark (Table 1-6) and of the thickness of the lesion as suggested by Breslow provides a significant indication of the prognosis. Better 5-year survival rates are correlated with tumors less than 0.75 mm thick and with low levels of Clark classification. Vulvar melanoma is associated with a poor prognosis; the overall survival rate of vulvar melanomas is about 30%.[261] Regional lymph node metastases develop early and rapidly and worsen the prognosis considerably when they are present.

Differential Diagnosis. Differential diagnosis is with Paget's disease for the superficial spreading type and with a metaplastic or sarcomatoid squamous cell carcinoma[229] or sarcoma in the spindle cell nodular type. Immunohistochemistry for S-100 protein (melanoma), carcinoembryonic antigen (Paget's disease), keratin (squamous cell carcinoma), and desmin or vimentin (sarcomas) can be useful, as can special stains for melanin and ultrastructural demonstration of premelanosomes.

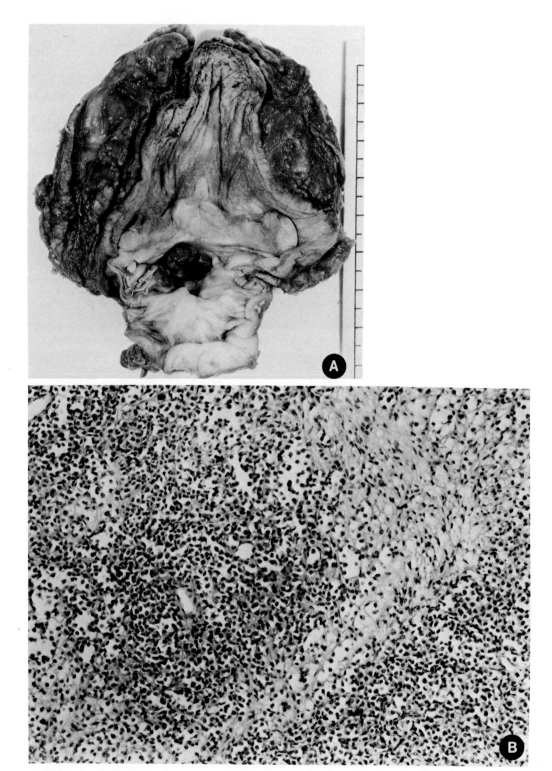

FIGURE 1-37 Malignant melanoma. **(A)** Macroscopic appearance. **(B)** Microscopic appearance.

TABLE 1-6.
Level of Invasion of Malignant Melanoma (Clark Classification)

Level	Definition
I	Intraepidermal involvement only
II	Invasion of the papillary dermis
III	Filling of the papillary dermis with abutment on the reticular dermis
IV	Invasion of the reticular dermis
V	Invasion of the subcutaneous tissue

Malignant Nonepithelial Tumors

Vulvar sarcomas are rare tumors observed at any age but are more frequent among tumors in children and young women.[262–264] *Leiomyosarcoma* is the most common histologic type and appears during the third and the fourth decades.[115] It is characterized by a rapidly growing tumor measuring a few centimeters in diameter and located in the labia majora, the clitoris, or the periurethral region. Important criteria of malignancy are an elevated mitotic count (10 or more mitoses per 10 high-power fields) and the presence of abnormal mitoses. Prognosis is poor if the excision is not complete.[265]

Rhabdomyosarcoma occurs rarely in the vulva, and only a few cases have been reported. It appears at any age, but the embryonal (botryoid) and the alveolar types are more frequently seen in infants and young adults, respectively.[262,266,267] In a study from the Armed Forces Institute of Pathology (1970–1979), 5 of 558 rhabdomyosarcomas were located in the vagina or the vulva.[268] The most difficult cases to recognize are the poorly differentiated round or spindle cell tumors. The presence of rhabdomyoblasts with or without cross striations and the use of immunochemistry will facilitate the diagnosis. Desmin, vimentin, and myoglobulin expression are characteristic. Electron microscopy is helpful.

Rare cases of true *fibrosarcoma* have been reported, if malignant fibrous histiocytoma and malignant schwannoma are correctly distinguished.[269,270] Microscopically, the tumor is a proliferation of fibroblasts arranged in fascicles exhibiting a herringbone appearance and surrounded by abundant reticulin-stained collagen fibers. Immunohistochemistry shows that the cells exhibit reactivity for vimentin and type I collagen.

Malignant fibrous histiocytoma is the second most common vulvar sarcoma in adults.[271] Clinically, one observes a large tumor mass. The microscopic appearance is pleomorphic and reveals a wide spectrum of cellular atypia, ranging from small regular fibroblasts to osteoclast-like giant cells to huge irregular cells with atypical and voluminous nuclei (storiform pleomorphic type). These cells may be accompanied by numerous neutrophils (inflammatory type) or by foci of myxoid transformation of the stroma (myxoid type). Immunohistochemical markers of histiocytes and vimentin are expressed.

Dermatofibrosarcoma protuberans has been rarely reported in the literature.[272,273] This low-grade sarcoma occurs in adults and is characterized microscopically by spindle cells arranged in a prominent storiform pattern. Local recurrence has been mentioned, but distant metastases should not take place.

Epithelioid sarcoma occurs in the labia majora of younger women.[274–276] It is characterized by a combination of spindled and epithelioid cells with bland nuclear features; these cells form multiple nodules with central necrosis. It should be differentiated from *malignant rhabdoid tumor,* another aggressive lesion appearing as a mass in young women.[274] Poorly differentiated squamous carcinoma should not be misinterpreted as epithelioid sarcoma.[201,229]

Liposarcoma is exceedingly rare. We have observed a case involving the labium major in a young woman, and another case has been reported by LiVolsi and Brooks.[277] Rare cases of alveolar soft part sarcoma,[278] malignant schwannoma,[262,279] malignant granular cell tumor,[280] angiosarcoma,[117] and Kaposi's sarcoma[277] have been reported.

Carcinosarcoma of the vulva is very rare. It contains both sarcomatous and carcinomatous elements in variable proportions. The natural history varies from one case to another. The case described by Parham and colleagues showed immunohistochemical positivity for vimentin and desmin as well as for the epithelial markers EMA (epithelial membrane antigen) and keratins.[281]

Malignant lymphomas, when present in the vulvar region, are a manifestation of systemic disease.[282,283] The existence of primary *teratomas* of the vulva has been reported; the rarity permits the omission of further comment. A few cases of *sarcomas of Bartholin's gland* have been described.

Metastatic Tumors

Vulvar metastases represent 10% of vulvar malignant lesions. The most frequent are of cervical or corporeal uterine origin; others include metastases of renal carcinoma or malignant melanoma.[284] *Choriocarcinoma* sometimes invades the vulvar region. The cells often have an undifferentiated appearance that may not recall the histology of the primary lesion. In other instances, the metastases closely reproduce the appearance of the primary lesion, for example, well-differentiated adenocarcinoma of the endometrium or squamous cell carcinoma of the cervix. The latter may be difficult to differentiate from primary vulvar squamous carcinoma; demonstration of an epithelial origin, an in situ component, or a bowenoid appearance favors a vulvar primary, whereas metastases tend to be well circumscribed and limited (at least initially) to the dermis or submucosa. Primary invasive or in situ squamous carcinoma of the vulva frequently coexists with synchronous or metachronous primary squamous neoplasms of the cervix and vagina.

Metastatic melanoma may be differentiated from primary melanoma by the presence of epithelial junctional melanocytic activity in early lesions of the latter; in the later stages, differentiation may be impossible. Melanin is not always present in the metastases of melanoma. The prognosis of these generalized tumors is poor.

References

1. Sternberg SS, ed: Histology for pathologists. New York, Raven Press, 1992
2. Davis J: Human developmental anatomy. New York, Ronald Press, 1963
3. Spaulding MH: The development of the external genitalia in the human embryo. Contrib Embryol Carneg Inst 18:66–88, 1931
4. Wilson KM: Correlation of external genitalia and sexglands in the human embryo. Contrib Embryol Carneg Inst 18:23–30, 1926
5. Hamilton WJ, Mossman HW: Human embryology, 4th ed. Baltimore, Williams & Wilkins, 1972
6. Skene AJC: The anatomy and pathology of two important glands of the female urethra. Am J Obstet Gynecol 13:265–270, 1880
7. Huffman JW: The detailed anatomy of the paraurethral ducts in the adult female. Am J Obstet Gynecol 55:86–101, 1948
8. Dunn JM: Congenital absence of the external genitalia. J Reprod Med 4:66–68, 1970
9. Capraro VJ: Congenital anomalies. Clin Obstet Gynecol 14:988–1012, 1971
10. Falk HC, Hyman AB: Congenital absence of clitoris: A case report. Obstet Gynecol 38:269–271, 1971
11. McElfatrick RA, Condon WB: Hydrocele of the canal of Nuck: A report of two cases. Rocky Mt Med J 72:112–113, 1975
12. Cockerell EG, Knox JM: Dermatologic diseases of the vulva. Am J Obstet Gynecol 84:537–542, 1962
13. Capraro VJ: Vulvovaginitis and other local lesions of the vulva. Clin Obstet Gynecol 1:533–551, 1974
14. Monif GRG: Infectious diseases in obstetrics and gynecology, 2nd ed. Philadelphia, Harper & Row, 1982
15. Brenner BN: Tuberculosis of the vulva: Case reports. S Afr Med J 50:1798–1800, 1976
16. Dans PE: Gonococcal anogenital infection. Clin Obstet Gynecol 18:103–119, 1975
17. Lever WF, Schaumburg-Lever G: Histopathology of the skin, 7th ed. Philadelphia, JB Lippincott, 1990
18. Pund ER, Greenblatt RB, Huie GB: The role of biopsy in the diagnosis of venereal diseases: Histologic differentiation of venereal granuloma and lymphogranuloma and chancroid. Am J Syph 22:495–502, 1938
19. Donovan C: Human piroplasmosis. Lancet 2:714–750, 1904
20. Douglas CP: Lymphogranuloma venereum and granuloma inguinale of the vulva. Br J Obstet Gynaecol 69:871–880, 1962
21. Kuberski T: Granuloma inguinale (Donovanosis). Sex Transm Dis 7:29–36, 1980
22. Sehgal VN, Shyam Prasad AL: Donovanosis: Current concepts. Int J Dermatol 25:8, 1986
23. De Boer A, de Boer F, Van der Merwe JV: Cytologic identification of Donovan bodies in granuloma inguinale. Acta Cytol 28:126–128, 1984
24. Davis CM: Granuloma inguinale: A clinical, histological and ultrastructural study. JAMA 211:632–636, 1970
25. Rudolf AH, Duncan WC: Syphilis: Diagnosis and treatment. Clin Obstet Gynecol 18:163–182, 1975
26. Turner DR, Wright DJM: Lymphadenopathy in early syphilis. J Pathol 110:305–308, 1973
27. Lynch PJ: Sexually transmitted diseases: Granuloma inguinale, lymphogranuloma venereum, chancroid, and infectious syphilis. Clin Obstet Gynecol 21:1041–1052, 1978
28. Hartsock RM, Halling LW, King M: Luetic lymphadenitis. A clinical and histologic study of 20 cases. Am J Clin Pathol 53:304–314, 1970
29. Larsson E, Westermark P: Chronic hypertrophic vulvitis: A condition with similarities to cheilitis granulomatosa (Melkersson-Rosenthal syndrome). Acta Derm Venereol (Stockh) 58:92–93, 1978
30. Westermark P, Henriksson TG: Granulomatous inflammation of the vulva and penis: A genital counterpart to cheilitis granulomatosa. Dermatologica 158:269–274, 1979
31. Mensing H, Janner M: Vulvitis plasmacellularis. Zoon. Z Hautkr 56:728–732, 1981
32. James DG: Behçet's syndrome. N Engl J Med 301:431–432, 1979
33. Behçet H: Uber rezidivierende Aphtose, durch ein Virus verursachte Geschwure am Mund, am Auge und an den Genitalien. Derm Wschr 105:1152–1157, 1937
34. James DG: Behçet's syndrome. N Engl J Med 301:431–432, 1979
35. Gupta RC, O'Duffy JD, McDuffie FC et al: Circulating immune complexes in active Behçet's disease. Clin Exp Immunol 34:213–218, 1978
36. Maciejewski W, Baudmann HJ: Immune complex vasculitis in a patient with Behçet's syndrome. Arch Dermatol Res 264:253–256, 1979
37. Butler EB, Stanbridge CM: Condylomatous lesions of the lower female genital tract. Clin Obstet Gynaecol 11:171–187, 1984
38. Chacho MS, Eppich E, Wersto RP, Koss LG: Influence of human papillomavirus on DNA ploidy determination in genital condylomas Cancer 65:2291–2294, 1990
39. Zur Hausen H: Papillomavirus in anogenital cancer as a model to understand the role of viruses in human cancers. Cancer Res 49:4677–4681, 1989
40. Beeckman AM, Kiviat NB, Daling JR et al: Human papillomavirus type 16 in multifocal neoplasia of the female genital tract. Int J Gynecol Pathol 7:39–47, 1988
41. Tawheed A, Beaudenon S, Favre M, Orth G: Characterization of human papillomavirus type 66 from an invasive carcinoma of cervix uteri. J Clin Microbiol 29:2656–2660, 1991
42. Koss LG, Durfee GR: Unusual patterns of squamous epithelium of the uterine cervix: Cytologic and pathologic study of koilocytotic atypia. Ann N Y Acad Sci 63:1245–1261, 1956
43. Meisels A, Fortin R: Condylomatous lesions of the cervix and vagina. I. Cytologic patterns. Acta Cytol 20:505–509, 1976
44. Purola E, Savia E: Cytology of gynecologic condyloma acuminata. Acta Cytol 21:26–31, 1977
45. Dreyfuss W, Neville WE: Buschke-Löwenstein tumors (giant condyloma acuminata). Am J Surg 90:164-150, 1955
46. Wells M, Griffiths S, Lewis F, Bird CC: Demonstration of human papillomavirus type in paraffin processed tissue from human anogenital lesions by in situ DNA hybridisation. J Pathol 152:77–82, 1987
47. Wang AC, Hsu JJ, Hsueh S et al: Evidence of human papillomavirus deoxyribonucleic acid in vulvar squamous papillomatosis. Int J Gynecol Pathol 10:44–50, 1991
48. Lynch PJ, Minkin W: Molluscum contagiosum of the adult: Probable venereal transmission. Arch Dermatol 98:141–143, 1968
49. Lynch PJ: Molluscum contagiosum venereum. Clin Obstet Gynecol 15:966–975, 1972

50. James JRE: ORF in man. Br Med J 3:804–805, 1968

51. Josey WE: Viral infections of the vulva. Clin Obstet Gynecol 21:1053–1059, 1978

52. Nahmias AM, Roizman B: Infection with herpes simplex virus 1 and 2. N Engl J Med 289:667–674, 719–789, 1973

53. Gardner HL, Kaufman RH: Herpes genitalis: Clinical features. Clin Obstet Gynecol 15:896–911, 1972

54. Amstey MS: Genital herpes virus infection. Clin Obstet Gynecol 18:89–100, 1975

55. Naib ZM, Nahmias AJ, Josey WE: Cytology and histopathology of cervical herpes simplex infection. Cancer 19:1026–1031, 1966

56. Rawls WE, Gardner HL: Herpes genitalis: Venereal aspects. Clin Obstet Gynecol 15:912–918, 1972

57. Ng ABP, Reagan JW, Lindner E: The cellular manifestations of primary and recurrent herpes genitalis. Acta Cytol 14:124–129, 1970

58. Amstey MS, Monif GRG, Nahmias AJ et al: Cesarean section and genital herpes infection. Obstet Gynecol 53:641–642, 1979

59. Cabral GA, Marciano-Cabral F, Fry D et al: Expression of herpes simplex virus type 2 antigens in premalignant and malignant human vulvar cells. Am J Obstet Gynecol 143:611–619, 1982

60. McSorley J, Shapiro L, Brownstein MH: Herpes simplex and varicella zoster: Comparative histopathology of 77 cases. Int J Dermatol 13:69–75, 1974

61. Vesterinen E, Purola E, Saksela E, Leinikki P: Clinical and virological findings in patients with cytologically diagnosed gynecologic herpes simplex infection. Acta Cytol 21:199–205, 1977

62. Morse AR, Coleman DV, Gardner SD: An evaluation of cytology in the diagnosis of herpes simplex virus infection and cytomegalovirus infection of the cervix uteri. Br J Obstet Gynaecol 81:393–398, 1974

63. Brazin SA, Sinkovich JW, Johnson WT: Herpes zoster during pregnancy. Obstet Gynecol 53:175–181, 1979

64. Sweet RL, Schachter J, Lander DV: Chlamydial infections in obstetrics and gynecology. Clin Obstet Gynecol 26:143–164, 1983

65. Sheldon WH, Heyman A: Lymphogranuloma venereum: A study of the primary lesion bubonulus and lymph nodes in cases proved by isolation of the virus. Am J Pathol 23:653–671, 1947

66. Frei W: Venereal lymphogranuloma. JAMA 110:1653–1656, 1938

67. Tam MR, Stamm WE, Handsfield HH et al: Culture-independent diagnosis of *Chlamydia trachomatis* using monoclonal antibodies. N Engl J Med 310:1146–1150, 1984

68. Levy RA, Warford AL: Evaluation of the chlamydiazyme immunoassay for the detection of chlamydia antigen. Am J Clin Pathol 86:330–335, 1986

69. Durand M, Nicolas J, Favre M: Lymphogranulomatose inguinale subaiguë d'origine génitale probable peut-être vénérienne. Bull Soc Méd Hôp Paris 35:274–288, 1913

70. Hanekar AB, Leiman G, Markowitz S: Cytologically detected chlamydial changes and progression of cervical intraepithelial neoplasias. Acta Cytol 29:661–664, 1985

71. Naib ZM: Cytology of TRIC agent infection in the eye of newborn infants and their mothers' genital tracts. Acta Cytol 14:390–395, 1970

72. Gupta PK, Shurbaji MS, Mintor LJ et al: Cytopathologic detection of *Chlamydia trachomatis* in vaginocervical (Fast) smears. Dlagn Cytopathol 4:224–229, 1988

73. Kellogg JA: Clinical and laboratory considerations of culture vs. antigen assays for detection of *Chlamydia trachomatis* from genital specimens. Arch Pathol Lab Med 113:453–460, 1989

74. Shiina Y. Cytomorphologic and immunocytochemical studies of chlamydial infections in cervical smears. Acta Cytol 29:683–691, 1985

75. Hutfield DC: Accidental vaccinia. Br Med J 2:828–829, 1968

76. Humphrey DC: Localized accidental vaccinia of the vulva. Report of three cases and review of the world literature. Amer J Obstet Gynecol 86:460–469, 1963

77. Friedrich EG: Vulvar disease. Philadelphia: WB Saunders, 1976

78. Timonen S, Salo OP, Meyer B et al: Vaginal mycosis. Acta Obstet Gynecol Scand 45:232–247, 1966

79. Heller C, Hoyt V: Squamous cell changes associated with the presence of *Candida* sp. in cervical-vaginal Papanicolaou smears. Acta Cytol 15:379–384, 1971

80. Bibbo M, Wied, GL: Microbiology and inflammation of the female genital tract. In: Compendium on Diagnostic Cytology. Tutorials of Cytology, 6th ed. Chicago, 1988

81. Huffman JW: Vulvovaginitis and other local lesions of the vulva. Clin Obstet Gynecol 20:581–593, 1977

82. Young AW, Tovell HMM, Sadu K: Erosions and ulcers of the vulva: Diagnosis, incidence and management. Obstet Gynecol 50:35–39, 1977

83. Santa Cruz DJ, Martin SA: Verruciform xanthoma of the vulva: Report of two cases. Am J Clin pathol 71:224–228, 1979

84. Kearns PR, Gray JE: Mycotic vulvovaginitis. Obstet Gynecol 20:621–625, 1963

85. Arean VM: Manson's schistosomiasis of the female genital tract. Am J Obstet Gynecol 72:1038–1053, 1956

86. Majmudar B, Chaiken ML, Lee KU: Amebiasis of clitoris mimicking carcinoma. JAMA 236:1145–1146, 1976

87. Muller G, Jacobs PH, Moore NE: Scraping for human scabies: A better method for positive preparations. Arch Dermatol 107:70, 1973

88. Kao M, Paulson JD, Askin FB: Crohn's disease of the vulva. Obtet Gynecol 46:329–333, 1975

89. Lavery AH, Pinkerton JHM, Sloan J: Crohn's disease of the vulva: Two further cases. Br J Dermatol 113:359–363, 1985

90. Bhattacharya P: Hypertrophic tuberculosis of the vulva. Obstet Gynecol 51(Suppl 1):21–22, 1978

91. Rorat E, Ferenczy A, Richart RM: Human Bartholin gland, duct and duct cyst. Arch Pathol 99:367–374, 1975

92. Freedman SR, Goldman RL: Mucocele-like changes in Bartholin's glands. Hum Pathol 9:111–114, 1978

93. Kligman AM: The myth of the sebaceous cyst. Arch Dermatol 89:253–256, 1964

94. Oningbo W: Vulval epidermoid cysts in the Lobos in Nigeria. Arch Dermatol 112:1405–1406, 1976

95. Janovski NA, Weir JH: Comparative histologic and histochemical studies of mesonephric derivatives and tumors. Obstet Gynecol 19:57–63, 1962

96. McElfatrik RA, Condon WB: Hydrocele of the canal of Nuck: A report of two cases. Rocky Mt Med J 72:112–113, 1975

97. Friedrich EG, Wilkinson EJ: Mucous cysts of the vulvar vestibule. Obstet Gynecol 42:407–414, 1973

98. Hart WR: Paramesonephric mucinous cysts of the vulva. Am J Obstet Gynecol 107:1079–1084, 1970

99. Robboy SJ, Ross JS, Prat J et al: Urogenital sinus origin of mucinous and ciliated cysts of the vulva. Obstet Gynecol 51:347–351, 1978

100. Blaivas JG, Pais VM, Retick AB: Paraurethral cysts in female neonate. Urology 7:504–507, 1976

101. Kimbrough HM, Vaughan ED: Skene's duct cyst in a newborn: Case report and review of the literature. J Urol 117:387–388, 1977

102. Knox JM, Freeman RG: Tumors of the vulva and the vagina: Epidermal tumors. Clin Obstet Gynecol 8:925–937, 1965

103. Östör AG, Fortune DW, Riley CB: Fibroepithelial polyps with atypical stromal cells (pseudosarcoma botryoides) of vulva and vagina: A report of 13 cases. Int J Gynecol Pathol 7:351–360, 1988

104. Mucitelli DR, Charles EZ, Kraus FT: Vulvovaginal polyps: Histologic appearance, ultrastructure, immunocytochemical characteristics, and clinicopathologic correlations. Int J Gynecol Pathol 9:20–40, 1990

105. Giltman Ll: Tripolar mitosis in keratoacanthoma. Acta Derm Venereol Suppl (Stockh) 61:362–363, 1981
106. Seidman JD, Berman JJ, Moore GW, Yetter RA: Multiparameter DNA flow cytometry of keratoacanthoma. Anal Quant Cytol Histol 14:113–119, 1992
107. Duray PH, Merino MJ, Axiotis C: Warty dyskeratoma of the vulva. Int J Gynecol Pathol 2:286–293, 1983
108. Imperial R, Helwig EB: Angiokeratoma of the vulva. Obstet Gynecol 29:307–312, 1967
109. Blair C: Angiokeratoma of the vulva. Br J Dermatol 83:409–411, 1970
110. Marshall FC, Uson AC, Melicow MM: Neoplasms and caruncles of the female urethra. Surg Gynecol Obstet 110:723–733, 1960
111. Carneiro SJC, Gardner HL, Knox JM: Syringoma: Three cases with vulvar involvement. Obstet Gynecol 39:95–99, 1972
112. Thomas J, Majmudar B, Gorelkin J: Syringoma localized to the vulva. Arch Dermatol 115:95–96, 1979
113. Young AW Jr, Herman EW, Tovell HMM: Syringoma of the vulva: Incidence, diagnosis and cause of pruritus. Obstet Gynecol 55:515–518, 1980
114. MacMillan DC, Vickers HR: Fox-Fordyce disease. Br J Dermatol 84:181, 1971
115. Tavassoli FA, Norris HJ: Smooth muscle tumors of the vulva. Obstet Gynecol 53:213–217, 1979
116. Reymond RD, Hazra TA, Edlow DW et al: Hemangiopericytoma of the vulva with metastasis to bone 14 years later. Br J Radiol 45:765–768, 1972
117. Maddox JC, Evans HL: Angiosarcoma of skin and soft tissues. Cancer 48:1907–1921, 1981
118. Strayer SA, Yum MN, Sutton GP: Epithelioid hemangioendothelioma of the clitoris: A case report with immunohistochemical and ultrastructural findings. Int J Gynecol Pathol 11:234–239, 1992
119. Lovelady SB, McDonald JR, Waugh JM: Benign tumors of the vulva. Am J Obstet Gynecol 42:309–313, 1941
120. Kaufman RH, Gardner HL: Tumors of the vulva and the vagina: Benign mesodermal tumors. Clin Obstet Gynecol 8:953–981, 1965
121. Rorat E, Wallach RC: Mixed tumors of the vulva: Clinical outcome and pathology. Int J Gynecol Pathol 3:323–328, 1984
122. Katz VL, Askin FB, Bosch BD: Glomus tumor of the vulva: A case report. Obstet Gynecol 67:43S–45S, 1986
123. Huang HJ, Yamabe T, Tagawa H: A solitary neurilemmoma of the clitoris. Gynecol Oncol 15:103–110, 1983
124. Steeper TA, Rosai J: Aggressive angiomyxoma of the female pelvis and perineum: Report of nine cases of a distinctive type of gynecologic soft-tissue neoplasm. Am J Surg Pathol 7:463–476, 1983
125. Fletcher CDM, Tsang WYW, Fisher C et al: Angiomyofibroblastoma of the vulva: A benign neoplasm distinct from aggressive angiomyxoma. Am J Surg Pathol 16:373–382, 1992
126. Gaffney EF, Majmudar B, Bryan JA: Nodular fasciitis (pseudosarcomatous fasciitis) of the vulva. Int J Gynecol Pathol 1:307–312, 1982
127. Schramm G: Diagnosis of a papillary hidradenoma of the vulva by simultaneous cytology and colposcopy. Acta Cytol 23:57–60, 1979
128. Hashimoto K: Hidradenoma papilliferum: An electronmicroscopic study. Acta Derm Venereol (Stockh) 53:22–30, 1973
129. Woodworth J Jr, Dockerty MB, Wilson RB, Pratt JH: Papillary hidradenoma of the vulva: A clinicopathologic study of 69 cases. Am J Obstet Gynecol 110:501–508, 1971
130. Hernandez-Perez E, Cestoni-Parducci R: Nodular hidradenoma and hidradenocarcinoma. J Am Acad Dermatol 12:15–20, 1985
131. Kersting DW: Clear cell hidradenoma and hidradenocarcinoma. Arch Dermatol 87:323–333, 1963
132. Hobbs JE: Tumors of the vulva and the vagina: Sweat gland tumors. Clin Obstet Gynecol 8:946–952, 1965
133. Gifford RRM, Birch HW: Granular cell myoblastoma of multicentric origin involving the vulva: A case report. Am J Obstet Gynecol 117:184–187, 1973
134. Brooks GG: Granular cell myoblastoma of the vulva in a 6-year-old girl. Am J Obstet Gynecol 153:897–898, 1985
135. Wolber RA, Talerman A, Wilkinson EJ, Clement PB: Vulvar granular cell tumors with pseudocarcinomatous hyperplasia: A comparative analysis with well-differentiated squamous cell carcinoma. Int J Gynecol Pathol 10:56–66, 1991
136. Sobel HJ, Marquet E, Schwarz R: Is schwannoma related to granular cell myoblastoma? Arch Pathol 95:396–401, 1973
137. Robertson AJ, McIntosh W, Lamont P, Guthrie W: Malignant granular cell tumor (myoblastoma) of the vulva: Report of a case and review of the literature. Histopathology 5:69–79, 1981
138. Smith Foushee JH, Pruitt AB: Vulvar fibroadenoma from aberrant breast tissue: Report of two cases. Obstet Gynecol 29:819–823, 1967
139. Garcia JJ, Verkauf BS, Hochberg CJ, Ingram JM: Aberrant breast tissue of the vulva: A case report and review of the literature. Obstet Gynecol 52:225–228, 1978
140. Breisky A: Uber Kraurosis Valvae. Z Heilk 6:69–80, 1885
141. International Society for The Study of Vulvar Disease: New nomenclature for vulvar disease: Report of the committee on terminology. Obstet Gynecol 47:122–124, 1976
142. Kaufman RH, Gardner HL: Vulvar dystrophies. Clin Obstet Gynecol 21:1081–1106, 1978
143. Ridley CM, Frankman O, Jones ISC et al: New nomenclature for vulvar disease: International Society for the Study of Vulvar Disease. Hum Pathol 20:495–496, 1989
144. Hart WR, Norris HJ, Helwig EB: Relation of lichen sclerosus et atrophicus of the vulva to development of carcinoma. Obstet Gynecol 45:369–377, 1975
145. McKay M: Vulvar dermatoses. Clin Obstet Gynecol 34(3): 614–629, 1991
146. Flynt T, Gallup DG: Childhood lichen sclerosus. Obstet Gynecol 53:795–815, 1979
147. Godeau G, Frances C, Hornebeck W et al: Isolation and partial characterization of an elastase-type protease in human vulva fibroblasts: Its possible involvement in vulvar elastic tissue destruction of patients with lichen sclerosus et atrophicus. J Invest Dermatol 78:270–275, 1982
148. Friedrich EG: Lichen sclerosus. J Reprod Med 17:147–154, 1976
149. Sideri M, Parazzini F, Rognoni MT et al: Risk factors for vulvar lichen sclerosus. Am J Obstet Gynecol 161:38–42, 1989
150. Crum CP: Vulvar intraepithelial neoplasia: The concept and its application. Hum Pathol 13:187–189, 1982
151. Crum CP, Liskow A, Petras P et al: Vulvar intraepithelial neoplasia (severe atypia and carcinoma in situ): A clinicopathologic analysis of 41 cases. Cancer 54:1429–1434, 1984
152. Andreasson B, Bock JE: Intraepithelial neoplasia in the vulvar region. Gynecol Oncol 21:300–305, 1985
153. Crum CP, Braun LA, Shah KV et al: Vulvar intraepithelial neoplasia: Correlation of nuclear DNA content and the presence of a human papillomavirus (HPV) structural antigen. Cancer 49:468–471, 1982
154. Crum CP, Fu YS, Levine RU et al: Intraepithelial squamous lesions of the vulva: Biologic and histologic criteria for the distinction of condylomas from vulvar intraepithelial neoplasia. Am J Obstet Gynecol 144:77–83, 1982
155. Park JS, Jones RW, McLean MR et al: Possible etiologic heterogeneity of vulvar intraepithelial neoplasia: A correlation of pathologic characteristics with human papillomavirus detection by in situ hybridization and polymerase chain reaction. Cancer 67:1599–1607, 1991
156. Pilotti S, Shah KV, Rilke F et al: HPV-type 16 DNA in carcinoma of the vulva. Mod Pathol 3:442–448, 1990

157. Husseinzadeh N, Newman NJ, Wesseler TA: Vulvar intraepithelial neoplasia: A clinicopathological study of carcinoma in situ of the vulva. Gynecol Oncol 33:157–163, 1989

158. Toki T, Kurman RJ, Park JS et al: Probable nonpapillomavirus etiology of squamous cell carcinoma of the vulva in older women: A clinicopathologic study using in situ hybridization and polymerase chain reaction. Int J Gynecol Pathol 10:107–125, 1991

159. Bowen JT: Precancerous dermatoses: Study of two cases of chronic atypical epithelial proliferation. J Cutan Dis 30:241–255, 1912

160. Ulbright TM, Stehman FB, Roth LM et al: Bowenoid dysplasia of the vulva. Cancer 50:2910–2919, 1979

161. Gross G, Hagedorn M, Ikenberg H: Bowenoid papulosis: Presence of human papilloma virus (HPV) structural antigens and of HPV 16 related DNA sequences. Arch Dermatol 121:858–863, 1985

162. Ikenberg H, Gissman L, Gross G et al: Human papillomavirus type 16-related DNA in genital Bowen's disease and in Bowenoid papulosis. Int J Cancer 32:563–565, 1983

163. Böcking A, Chatelain R, Salterberg A et al: Bowenoid papulosis: Classification as a low-grade in situ carcinoma of the epidermis on the basis of histomorphologic and DNA ploidy studies. Anal Quant Cytol Histol 11:419–425, 1989

164. Zaino RJ, Husseinzadeh N, Nahas W, Mortel R: Epithelial alterations in proximity to invasive squamous carcinoma of the vulva. Int J Gynecol Pathol 1:173–184, 1982

165. Bloss JD, Liao SY, Wilczynski SP et al: Clinical and histologic features of vulvar carcinoma analyzed for human papillomavirus status: Evidence that squamous cell carcinoma of the vulva has more than one etiology. Human Pathol 22:711–718, 1991

166. Jones RW, McLean MR: Carcinoma in situ of the vulva: A review of 31 treated and 5 untreated cases. Obstet Gynecol 68:499–503, 1986

167. Chafe W, Richards A, Morgan L, Wilkinson E: Unrecognized invasive carcinoma in vulvar intraepithelial neoplasia (VIN). Gynecol Oncol 31:154–162, 1988

168. Patterson JW, Kao GF, Graham JH et al: Bowenoid papulosis: A clinicopathologic study with ultrastructural observations. Cancer 57:823–836, 1986

169. Bergeron C, Naghashfar Z, Canaan C et al: Human papillomavirus type 16 in intraepithelial neoplasia (bowenoid papulosis) and coexistent invasive carcinoma of the vulva. Int J Gynecol Pathol 6:1–11, 1987

170. Lloyd KM: Multicentric pigmented Bowen's disease of the groin. Arch Dermatol 101:48–51, 1970

171. Nauth HF, Schilke E: Cytology of the exfoliative layer in normal and diseased vulvar skin: Correlation with histology. Acta Cytol 26:269–283, 1982

172. Dennerstein GJ: The cytology of the vulva. Br J Obstet Gynaecol 75:603–609, 1968

173. Mahmud N, Kusuda M, Khinose S et al: Needle aspiration biopsy of vulvar endometriosis: A case report. Acta Cytol 36:514–516, 1992

174. Podratz KC, Symmonds RE, Taylor WF, Williams TJ: Carcinoma of the vulva. Obstet Gynecol 61:63–74, 1983

175. Copas P, Comas FV, Dyer M, Hall DJ: Spindle cell carcinoma of the vulva. Diagn Gynecol Obstet 4:235–241, 1982

176. Cavanagh D, Praphat H, Ruffalo EH: Cancer of the vulva. Obstet Gynecol Annu 11:303–339, 1982

177. Green TH: Carcinoma of the vulva: A reassessment. Obstet Gynecol 52:462–469, 1978

178. Mabuchi K, Bross DS, Kessler II: Epidemiology of cancer of the vulva: A case-control study. Cancer 55:1843–1848, 1985

179. Menczner J, Voliovitch Y, Modan B et al: Some epidemiologic aspects of carcinoma of the vulva in Israel. Am J Obstet Gynecol 143:893–896, 1982

180. Brinton LA, Nasca PC, Mallin K et al: Case control study of cancer of the vulva. Obstet Gynecol 75:859–866, 1990

181. Rutledge FN, Mitchell MF, Munsell MF et al: Prognostic indicators for invasive carcinoma of the vulva. Gynecol Oncol 42:239–244, 1991

182. Kunschner A, Kanbour Al, David B: Early vulvar carcinoma. Am J Obstet Gynecol 132:599–606, 1978

183. Choo YC: Invasive squamous carcinoma of the vulva in young patients. Gynecol Oncol 13:158–164, 1982

184. Roman LD, Mitchell MF, Burke TW, Silva EG: Unsuspected invasive squamous carcinoma of the vulva in young women. Gynecol Oncol 41:182–185, 1991

185. Hilliard GD, Massey FM, O'Toole RV: Vulvar neoplasia in the young. Am J Obstet Gynecol 135:185–188, 1979

186. Moore DH, Fowler WC Jr, Currie JL, Walton LA: Squamous cell carcinoma of the vulva in pregnancy. Gynecol Oncol 41:74–77, 1991

187. Samaratunga H, Strutton G, Wright RG, Hill B: Squamous cell carcinoma arising in a case of vulvitis granulomatosa or vulval variant of Melkersson-Rosenthal syndrome. Gynecol Oncol 41:263–269, 1991

188. Hay DM, Cole FM: Postgranulomatous epidermoid carcinoma of the vulva. Am J Obstet Gynecol 108:479–484, 1970

189. Hording U, Dangaard S, Iversen AKN et al: Human papillomavirus type 16 in vulvar carcinoma, vulvar intraepithelial neoplasia, and associated cervical neoplasia. Gynecol Oncol 42:22–26, 1991

190. Husseinzadeh N, DeEulios T, Newman N, Wesseler T: HPV changes and their significance in patients with invasive squamous cell carcinoma of the vulva: A clinicopathologic study. Gynecol Oncol 43:237–241, 1991

191. Kaufman RH, Dressman GR, Burck J et al: Herpesvirus-induced antigens in squamous-cell carcinoma in situ of the vulva. N Engl J Med 305:483–488, 1981

192. Korhonen MO, Kaufman RH, Roberts D et al: Carcinoma in situ of the vulva: The search for viral particles. J Reprod Med 27:746–748, 1982

193. Nuovo GJ, Delvenne P, MacConnell P et al: Correlation of histology and detection of human papillomavirus DNA in vulvar cancers. Gynecol Oncol 43:275–280, 1991

194. Park JS, Rader JS, Wu TC et al: HPV-16 viral transcripts in vulvar neoplasia: Preliminary studies. Gynecol Oncol 42:250–255, 1991

195. Pilotti S, Rotola A, D'Amato L et al: Vulvar carcinomas: Search for sequences homologous to human papillomavirus and herpes simplex virus DNA. Mod Pathol 3:442–448, 1990

196. Bornstein J, Kaufman RH, Adam E, Adler-Storthz K: Multicentric intraepithelial neoplasia involving the vulva: Clinical features and association with human papillomavirus and herpes simplex virus. Cancer 62:1601–1604, 1988

197. Rastkar G, Okagaki T, Twiggs LB, Clark BA: Early invasive and in situ warty carcinoma of the vulva: Clinical, histologic and electron microscopic study with particular reference to viral association. Am J Obstet Gynecol 143:814–820, 1982

198. Della Torre G, Donghi R, Longoni A et al: HPV DNA in the intraepithelial neoplasia and carcinoma of the vulva and penis. Diagn Mol Pathol 1:25–30, 1992

199. Hansen LH, Collins CG: Multicentric squamous cell carcinomas of the lower female genital tract: Eleven cases with epidermoid carcinoma of both the vulva and the cervix. Am J Obstet Gynecol 98:982–986, 1967

200. Spitzer M, Chernys AE, Hirschfield L et al: Assessment of criteria used in the histologic diagnosis of human papillomavirus-related disease of the female lower genital tract. Gynecol Oncol 38:105–109, 1990

201. Santeusanio G, Schiaroli S, Anemona L et al: Carcinoma of the vulva with sarcomatoid features: A case report with immunohistochemical study. Gynecol Oncol 40:160–163, 1991

202. Way S: Carcinoma of the vulva. Am J Obstet Gynecol 79:692–697, 1960

203. Nadji M, Ganjei P, Penneys NS, Morales AR: Immunohistochemistry of vulvar neoplasms: A brief review. Int J Gynecol Pathol 3:41–50, 1984

204. Kabulski Z, Frankman O: Histologic malignancy grading in invasive squamous cell carcinoma of the vulva. Int J Obstet Gynecol 16:233–237, 1978

205. Katayama KP, Woodruff JD, Jones HW Jr et al: Chromosomes of condyloma acuminatum, Paget's disease, in situ carcinoma, invasive squamous cell carcinoma and malignant melanoma of the human vulva. Obstet Gynecol 39:346–356, 1972

206. Andreasson B, Nyboe J: Predictive factors with reference to low-risk of metastases in squamous cell carcinoma in the vulvar region. Gynecol Oncol 21:196–206, 1985

207. Franklin EW, Rutledge FD: Prognostic factors in epidermoid carcinoma of the vulva. Obstet Gynecol 37:892–909, 1971

208. Heaps JM, Fu YS, Montz FJ et al: Surgical-pathologic variables predictive of local recurrence in squamous cell carcinoma of the vulva. Gynecol Oncol 38:309–314, 1990

209. Husseinzadeh N, Wesseler T, Schellhas H, Nahmias W: Significance of lymphoplasmacytic infiltration around tumor cell in the prediction of regional lymph node metastases in patients with invasive squamous cell carcinoma of the vulva: A clinicopathologic study. Gynecol Oncol 34:200–205, 1989

210. Krupp PJ, Lee FY, Bohm JW et al: Prognostic parameters and clinical staging criteria in epidermoid carcinoma of the vulva. Obstet Gynecol 46:84–88, 1975

211. Rowley KC, Gallion HH, Donaldson ES et al: Prognostic factors in early vulvar cancer. Gynecol Oncol 31:43–49, 1988

212. Iversen T, Aalders JG, Christensen A, Kolstad P: Squamous cell carcinoma of the vulva: A report of 424 patients, 1956–1974. Gynecol Oncol 9:271–279, 1980

213. Hopkins MP, Reid GC, Vettrano I, Morley GW: Squamous cell carcinoma of the vulva: Prognostic factors influencing survival. Gynecol Oncol 43:113–117, 1991

214. Cliby W, Soisson AP, Berchuck A, Clarke-Pearson DL: Stage I small cell carcinoma of the vulva treated with vulvectomy, lymphadenectomy, and adjuvant chemotherapy. Cancer 67:2415–2417, 1991

215. Thomas GM, Dembo AJ, Bryson SCP et al: Changing concepts in the management of vulvar cancer. Gynecol Oncol 42:9–21, 1991

216. Berek JS, Heaps JM, Fu YS et al: Concurrent cisplatin and 5-fluorouracil chemotherapy and radiation therapy for advanced-stage squamous cell carcinoma of the vulva. Gynecol Oncol 42:197–201, 1991

217. Chu J, Tamimi HK, Ek M, Figge DC: Stage 1 vulvar cancer: Criteria for microinvasion. Obstet Gynecol 59:716–719, 1982

218. di Paola GR, Rueda-Leverone NG, Belardi MG et al: Vulvar carcinoma in situ: Report of 28 cases. Gynecol Oncol 14:236–242, 1982

219. Dvoretsky P, Bonfiglio T, Helmkamp F et al: The pathology of superficially invasive, thin vulvar squamous cell carcinoma. Int J Gynecol Pathol 3:331–342, 1984

220. Wilkinson EJ, Rico MJ, Pierson KK: Microinvasive carcinoma of the vulva. Int J Gynecol Pathol 1:29–39, 1982

221. Kneale BL, Cavanagh D, DiPaola GR et al: Recommendations of the 7th International Congress, International Society for the Study of Vulvar Disease, Task Force and Subcommittee on Micro-Invasive Cancer of the Vulva. Gynecol Oncol 18:134, 1984

222. Breen JL, Neubecker RD, Greenwald E, Gregori CA: Basal cell carcinoma of the vulva. Obstet Gynecol 46:122–129, 1975

223. Merino MJ, LiVolsi VA, Schwartz PE, Rudnicki J: Adenoid basal cell carcinoma of the vulva. Int J Gynecol Pathol 1:299–306, 1982

224. Perrone T, Twiggs LB, Adcock LL, Dehner LP: Vulvar basal cell carcinoma: An infrequently metastasizing neoplasm. Int J Gynecol Pathol 6:152–165, 1987

225. Bannatyne P, Elliott P, Russell P: Vulvar adenosquamous carcinoma arising in a hidradenoma papilliferum, with rapidly fatal outcome: Case report. Gynecol Oncol 35:395–398, 1989

226. Lasser A, Cornog JL, Morris JM: Adenoid squamous cell carcinoma of the vulva. Cancer 33:224–227, 1974

227. Brisigotti M, Moreno A, Murcia C et al: Verrucous carcinoma of the vulva: A clinicopathologic and immunohistochemical study of five cases. Int J Gynecol Pathol 8:1–7, 1989

228. Japaze H, Dinh TV, Woodruff JD: Verrucous carcinoma of the vulva: Study of 24 cases. Obstet Gynecol 60:462–466, 1982

229. Steeper TA, Piscioli F, Rosai J: Squamous cell carcinoma with sarcoma-like stroma of the female genital tract: Clinico-pathologic study of four cases. Cancer 52:890–898, 1983

230. Husseinzadeh N, Wesseler T, Newman N et al: Neuroendocrine (Merkel cell) carcinoma of the vulva. Gynecol Oncol 29:105–112, 1988

231. Plachta A, Speer FD: Apocrine-gland adenocarcinoma and extramammary Paget's disease of the vulva: Review of the literature and report of a case. Cancer 7:910–919, 1954

232. Webb JB, Beswick IP: Eccrine hidradenocarcinoma of the vulva with Paget's disease: Case report with a review of the literature. Br J Obstet Gynaecol 90:90–95, 1983

233. Degefu S, O'Quinn AG, Dhurandhar HN: Paget's disease of the vulva and urogenital malignancies: A case report and review of the literature. Gynecol Oncol 25:347–354, 1986

234. Feuer GA, Shevchuk M, Calanog A: Vulvar Paget's disease: The need to exclude an invasive lesion. Gynecol Oncol 38:81–89, 1990

235. Breen JL, Smith CI, Gregori CA: Extramammary Paget's disease. Clin Obstet Gynecol 21:1107–1115, 1978

236. Hart WR, Millman JB: Progression of intraepithelial Paget's disease of the vulva to invasive carcinoma. Cancer 40:2333–2337, 1977

237. Tsudaka Y, Lopez RG, Pickren JW et al: Paget's disease of the vulva: A clinicopathologic study of eight cases. Obstet Gynecol 45:73–78, 1975

238. Lee SC, Roth LM, Ehrlich C et al: Extramammary Paget's disease of the vulva: A clinicopathologic study of 13 cases. Cancer 39:2540–2549, 1977

239. Fetherson WC, Friedrich EG: The origin and significance of vulvar Paget's disease. Obstet Gynecol 39:735–744, 1972

240. Koss LG, Brockunier A Jr: Ultrastructural aspects of Paget's disease of the vulva. Arch Pathol 87:592–600, 1969

241. Ferenczy A, Richart RM: Ultrastructure of perianal Paget's disease. Cancer 29:1141–1149, 1972

242. Olson DJ, Fujimura M, Swanson P, Okagaki T: Immunohistochemical features of Paget's disease of the vulva with and without adenocarcinoma. Int J Gynecol Pathol 10:285–295, 1991

243. Snow SN, Desouky S, Lo JS, Kurtycz D: Failure to detect human papillomavirus DNA in extramammary Paget's disease. Cancer 69:249–251, 1992

244. Hendrix RC, Behrman SJ: Adenocarcinoma arising in a supernumerary mammary gland in the vulva. Obstet Gynecol 8:238–241, 1956

245. Simon KE, Dutcher JP, Runowicz CD, Wiernik PH: Adenocarcinoma arising in vulvar breast tissue. Cancer 62:2234–2238, 1988

246. Wheelock JB, Goplerud DR, Dunn LJ, Oates JF III: Primary carcinoma of the Bartholin's gland: A report of ten cases. Obstet Gynecol 63:820–824, 1984

247. Leuchter RS, Hacker NF, Voet RL et al: Primary carcinoma of the Bartholin gland: A report of 14 cases and review of the literature. Obstet Gynecol 60:395–396, 1982

248. Rosenberg P, Simonsen E, Risberg B: Adenoid cystic carcinoma of Bartholin's gland: A report of five new cases treated with surgery and radiotherapy. Gynecol Oncol 34:145–147, 1989

249. Rose PG, Tak WK, Reale FR, Hunter RE: Adenoid cystic carcinoma of the vulva: A radiosensitive tumor. Gynecol Oncol 43:81–83, 1991

250. Taylor RN, Lacey CG, Shuman MA: Adenocarcinoma of Skene's duct associated with a systemic coagulopathy. Gynecol Oncol 22:250–256, 1985

251. Benson RC Jr, Tunca JC, Buchler DA et al: Primary carcinoma of the female urethra. Gynecol Oncol 14:313–318, 1982

252. Meis JM, Ayala AG, Johnson DE: Adenocarcinoma of the urethra in women: A clinicopathologic study. Cancer 60:1038–1052, 1987

253. McCrea LE: Malignancy of the female urethra. Urol Surv 2:85–149, 1952

254. Clayton M, Siami P, Guinan P: Urethral diverticular carcinoma. Cancer 70:665–670, 1992

255. Gonzalez MO, Harrison ML, Boileau M: Carcinoma in diverticulum of female urethra. Urology 26:328–332, 1985

256. Moinuddin Ali M, Klein FA, Hazra TA: Primary female urethral carcinoma: A retrospective comparison of different treatment techniques. Cancer 62:54–57, 1988

257. Bastable JH, Gompel C, Verhest A: Malignant melanoma of the vulva. Diagn Gynecol Obstet 2:55–62, 1980

258. Blessing K, Kernohan NM, Miller ID, Al Nafussi AI: Malignant melanoma of the vulva: Clinicopathological features. Int J Gynecol Cancer 1:81–87, 1991

259. Phillips GL, Twiggs LB, Okagaki T: Vulvar melanoma: A microstaging study. Gynecol Oncol 14:80–88, 1982

260. Warner TFCS, Hafez GR, Buchler DA: Neurotropic melanoma of the vulva. Cancer 49:999–1004, 1982

261. Morrow CP, Rutledge FN: Melanoma of the vulva. Obstet Gynecol 39:745–752, 1972

262. Di Saia PJ, Rutledge F, Smith JP: Sarcoma of the vulva: Report of 12 patients. Obstet Gynecol 38:180–184, 1971

263. James GB, Guthrie W, Buchan A: Embryonic sarcoma of the vulva in an infant. Br J Obstet Gynaecol 76:458–461, 1969

264. Nolan RP: Primary non-pigmented sarcoma of the vulva, with report of a case complicating pregnancy. Am J Obstet Gynecol 73:134–140, 1957

265. Audet-Lapointe P, Paquin F, Guerard MJ et al: Leiomyosarcoma of the vulva. Gynecol Oncol 10:350–355, 1980

266. Imachi M, Tsukamoto N, Kamura T et al: Alveolar rhabdomyosarcoma of the vulva: Report of two cases. Acta Cytol 35:345–349, 1991

267. Copeland LJ, Gershenson DM, Saul PB et al: Sarcoma botryoides of the female genital tract. Obstet Gynecol 66:262–266, 1985

268. Enzinger FM, Weiss SW: Soft tissue tumors. St. Louis, CV Mosby, 1983

269. Hall J St E, Amin UF: Fibrosarcoma of the vulva: Case reports and discussion. Int Surg 66:185–187, 1981

270. Hall J, Tseng SCG, Timpl R et al: Collagen types in fibrosarcoma: Absence of type III collagen in reticulin. Hum Pathol 16:439–446, 1985

271. Taylor RN, Bottles K, Miller TR, Braga CA: Malignant fibrous histiocytoma of the vulva. Obstet Gynecol 66:145–148, 1985

272. Agress R, Figge DC, Tamimi H, Greer B: Dermatofibrosarcoma protuberans of the vulva. Gynecol Oncol 16:288–291, 1983

273. Bock JE, Andreasson B, Thorn A, Holck S: Dermatofibrosarcoma protuberans of the vulva. Gynecol Oncol 20:129–135, 1985

274. Perrone T, Swanson PE, Twiggs L et al: Malignant rhabdoid tumor of the vulva: Is distinction from epithelioid sarcoma possible? A pathologic and immunohistochemical study. Am J Surg Pathol 13:848–858, 1989

275. Piver MS, Tsukada Y, Barlow J: Epithelioid sarcoma of the vulva. Obstet Gynecol 40:839–842, 1972

276. Ulbright TM, Brokaw SA, Stehman FB, Roth LM: Epithelioid sarcoma of the vulva: Evidence suggesting a more aggressive behavior than extragenital epithelioid sarcoma. Cancer 52:1462–1469, 1983

277. LiVolsi VA, Brooks JJ: Soft tissue tumors of the vulva. In Wilkinson EJ, ed. Pathology of the vulva and vagina, p 229. New York, Churchill Livingstone, 1987

278. Shen JT, D'Ablaing G, Morrow CP: Alveolar soft part sarcoma of the vulva: Report of first case and review of the literature. Gynecol Oncol 13:120–128, 1982

279. Davos I, Abell M: Soft tissue sarcomas of vulva. Gynecol Oncol 4:70–86, 1976

280. Robertson AJ, McIntosh W, Lamont P, Guthrie W: Malignant granular cell tumor (myoblastoma) of the vulva: Report of a case and review of the literature. Histopathology 5:69–79, 1981

281. Parham DM, Morton K, Robertson AJ, Philip WDP: The changing phenotype appearance of a malignant vulval neoplasm containing both carcinomatous and sarcomatous elements. Histopathology 19:263–268, 1991

282. Labes J, Ring A: Ulcerating cutaneous Hodgkin's disease of the vulva. Am J Obstet Gynecol 89:273–274, 1964

283. Tuder RM: Vulvar destruction by malignant lymphoma. Gynecol Oncol 45:52–57, 1992

284. Dehner LP: Metastatic and secondary tumors of the vulva. Obstet Gynecol 42:47–57, 1973

Pathology in Gynecology and Obstetrics, Fourth Edition, edited by Claude Gompel and Steven G. Silverberg. J. B. Lippincott Company, Philadelphia © 1994.

2 | *The Vagina*

EMBRYOLOGY

The vagina arises from the fusion of the inferior portion of the müllerian ducts and a portion of the endoderm of the urogenital sinus. A solid plug forms at this junction, and this plug is subsequently recanalized. The part played by the mesonephric epithelium, formerly thought to be involved in this formation, is controversial. After the fusion of the lower portions of the müllerian ducts and the urogenital sinus, the squamous cells from the sinus lining invade the fused müllerian ducts and replace the columnar epithelium up to the external cervical os. This phenomenon is completed after the 20th week of embryonic life.[1-4] Experimental studies in rodents tend to suggest that stromal tissue of the vaginal wall induces the differentiation of the squamous epithelium.[5]

ANATOMY AND HISTOLOGY

The vaginal wall consists of several layers. The *tunica externa* is composed of a loose connective tissue containing venous plexus and nerve branches. The *muscularis* is composed of an external layer of longitudinal smooth muscle fibers and an inner layer of circular ones. The *submucosa* is a connective tissue lamina rich in lymphatics, venous plexus, and elastic fibers. Finally, the *tunica interna* is represented by a pluristratified squamous mucosa comprising three parts: the basal, intermediate, and superficial layers.

The relative proportions of these three layers vary according to the hormonal background. The intermediate strata are rich in glycogen (Fig. 2-1). Langerhans cells have been demonstrated in the mucosa.[6] These cells originate from the bone marrow and are involved in the localized immune response. Specific cytoplasmic granules (Birbeck granules) are demonstrated ultrastructurally.[7]

The vascularization of the vagina is richly developed. The *arteries* arise as branches of the uterine artery, inferior vesical artery, middle hemorrhoidal artery, internal pudendal artery, and especially the vaginal artery, a branch of the hypogastric artery. The *veins* form a rich plexus whose branches drain into the internal iliac vein or its tributaries. This vaginal venous plexus is in communication with the uterine, vesical, and hemorrhoidal venous plexus. The *lymphatics* from the upper half of the vagina drain into the internal iliac nodes, notably the obturator, hypogastric, and sometimes the rectal nodes; those of the lower end drain into the inguinal lymphatics and some to the external iliac nodes. Anastomoses exist between the upper and lower halves of the organ and between the left and right sides.[8] The *nerves* issue from the hypogastric and internal pudendal plexus.[9]

MALFORMATIONS

Diverse malformations may be encountered, most of which may be explained by anomalies in fusion of the müllerian ducts.[10] *Absence of the vagina* is rare and oc-

46

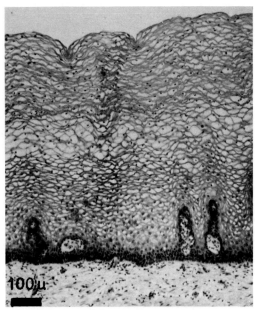

FIGURE 2-1 Functional vaginal epithelium: intermediate cells rich in glycogen.

curs when the müllerian ducts do not come in contact with the urogenital sinus. It is often associated with a rudimentary uterus in otherwise normal females (Rokitansky-Küster-Hauser syndrome).[11] Much rarer is pure vaginal aplasia, commonly associated with hematometra and endometriosis after puberty. Urinary tract anomalies are seen in 15% of cases.[12] Very rare familial cases have been reported.[13]

Solid noncanalized vagina is represented by a massive block of tissue; this malformation is extremely rare. *Transverse* and *diaphragmatic stenoses* are represented by the presence of a transverse septum or regions of stenosis. These may extend over several centimeters. Partial septa or ridges have been noted frequently in young women whose mothers were treated with diethylstilbestrol (DES) during pregnancy.[14]

Double vagina is the presence of a median partition, most often parasagittal, and persistence of internal partitions fused from the müllerian ducts. This septum may occupy the entire vagina or only a portion of its length.[15] One of the normal conduits may be sealed at its inferior end, which will cause hematocolpos at the time of onset of menstruation.

Malformations of the anterior and posterior walls lead to the formation of *diverticula* or urethrovaginal or rectovaginal *fistulas*. Congenital hypertrophy of the mucosal folds (rugae) is rare.

HORMONE-INDUCED VARIATIONS OF THE VAGINAL MUCOSA

Under the influence of estrogen, the vaginal mucosa increases in thickness. The first manifestation is an increase in mitotic activity in the basal layer. Proliferation and growth of cells are stimulated, and the greatest mucosal thickness is noted between days 7 and 14 of a normal cycle. Although it has been thought that mucosal glycogen content increases at this time, quantitative studies disprove this concept.[16]

Thick vaginal epithelia are also seen in the newborn infant (because of the influence of maternal estrogens), in pregnancy (when, under the influence of progesterone, the intermediate layer is most prominent), and in a minority of postmenopausal women (presumably due to residual extragonadal estrogen production). In most postmenopausal women, and between the first few weeks of life and the menarche, when estrogen levels are low, the vaginal mucosa consists of only a few basal and parabasal cell layers, perhaps with a thin cornified layer; this thin epithelium, combined with a neutral to alkaline vaginal fluid at these times, predisposes the vagina to a variety of infections that are discussed later in this chapter.

There are indications that, in addition to epithelial changes, the vaginal vascularization and innervation vary during the menstrual cycle. For several reasons, the most important of which is sampling variation from one part of the vagina to another, biopsy studies often fail to confirm the known cyclic variations of the vaginal mucosa. On the contrary, vaginal smears gather the products of desquamation of large zones of the mucosa and much more effectively reveal the characteristics that vary during the course of a cycle.

Since the historic publication of Pouchet[17] in 1847, and the pioneer work of Papanicolaou[18-20] and Babes,[21] many authors from America and Europe have established the validity of hormonal cytology as an efficient, reliable, rapid and inexpensive method.[22-27] The principle of the method is based on the relation between the degree of cellular maturity and the level of endogenous or exogenous sex steroids present. This relation is mitigated by two factors: (1) the hormonal "climate" is the combination of different specific hormones (estrogens, progestogens and androgens) that have synergic or antagonistic effects, resulting sometimes in nonspecific images; (2) since hormonal cytology depends on accurate clinical data, these must always be correlated with the cytologic image.

Cytosmears for hormonal evaluation should always be prepared from scrapings of the lateral wall of the upper portion of the vagina. If the smears are contaminated with cervical material (indicated by the presence of endocervical cells) or inflammatory infiltrates, a hormonal interpretation should not be attempted.[28]

Hormonal vaginal cytology has lost some of its importance because more accurate methods of measurement of serum or urine hormone concentrations have been introduced (eg, radioimmunochemical assays). Vaginal cytology, however, remains an easy and inexpensive preliminary method of evaluation in daily practice. To obtain better results, four smears should be prepared at different phases of the cycle: two during the proliferative phase governed by estrogen, and two after ovulation during the secretory phase governed by progesterone.

Smears of Estrogenic Type

Estrogens provoke the proliferation and maturation of the squamous cells. A typical appearance, composed of differentiated superficial cells, results; the cells are large, flat, and polyhedral, with eosinophilic cytoplasm and pyknotic nuclei (Fig. 2-2 and Color Figure 2-1). The numerical evaluation of the number of eosinophilic cells with pyknotic nuclei compared with the numbers of other cell types permits an estimation of estrogenic activity. The *karyopyknotic index* is the percentage of superficial eosinophilic and cyanophilic cells with a nucleus whose diameter is less than 6 μm.[25] The *eosinophilic index* is the percentage of eosinophilic superficial cells in the general cell population. Another method of expressing the hormonal activity is calculation of the *maturation index.*[29] This is the count of the different cell types and their expression as percentages based on the evaluation of at least 200 cells (eg, 25% parabasal cells, 35% intermediate cells, and 40% superficial cells). This information must be correlated with the clinical data to have any value in the interpretation of steroid hormonal activity.

Smears of Luteal Type

There is no specific picture reflecting activity of the corpus luteum. The only criteria of luteal stimulation are folding of the superficial and intermediate cells and increased glycogen content of the intermediate cells (navicular cells). Progestational activity in effect favors the proliferation and desquamation of cells before they have arrived at the eosinophilic and pyknotic stage of maturation.[30] This appearance, as we have stated, is not specific: it is seen after suppression of estrogenic activity (by surgical or physiologic menopause) and after stimulation of an atrophic epithelium by estrogens or androgens (Fig. 2-3 and Color Figure 2-2). To be precise and complete, the evaluation of progestational activity should include endometrial biopsy, study of the thermal curve, and a biochemical hormonal study.

Lactobacilli are normally present in abundance in the luteal phase and are observed in more than 50% of healthy women. These Gram-positive, immobile, anaerobic bacilli provoke a cytolysis of the glycogen-rich intermediate cells.

Smears of Gravid Type

The cytologic picture of pregnancy is characterized by the presence of intermediate cells rich in glycogen (navicular cells) and desquamating in plaques.[31–33] Lactobacilli occur in abundance with secondary cytolysis. Endocervical cells are numerous, with an enlarged cytoplasm rich in mucin; rarely, trophoblastic cells are seen and are represented by large, multinucleated cells with an eosinophilic or basophilic cytoplasm (Color Figure 2-3).[34] Decidual cells may be observed when decidual changes occur in the uterine cervix.[35,36] These stromal cells have an abundant, homogeneous, often eosinophilic cytoplasm and a round, centrally located nucleus.

This typical picture does not develop until the end of the third month of pregnancy; before that

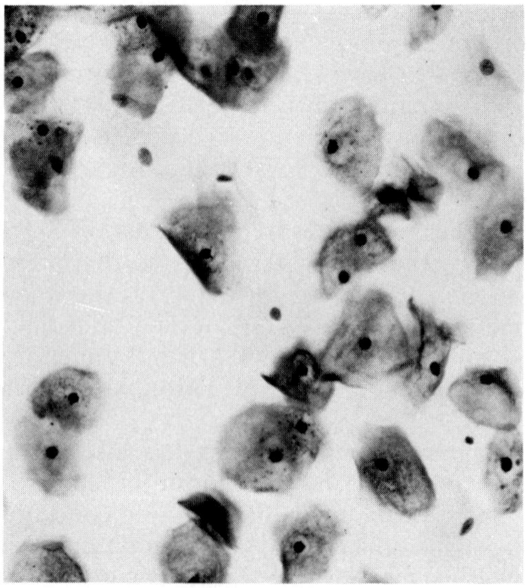

FIGURE 2-2 Vaginal smear of estrogenic type: superficial cells.

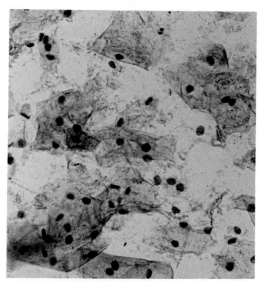

FIGURE 2-3 Vaginal smear of luteal type: folded superficial and intermediate (navicular) cells.

time, the smear is of the menstrual, luteal, or even estrogenic type. The vaginal smear is therefore not a method of diagnosis of pregnancy, but it does permit suspicion of certain anomalies of hormonal equilibrium during pregnancy, notably deficiencies of the corpus luteum. Changes in the smear pattern during the course of a pregnancy are more important than a single abnormal smear.

Smears of Postpartum Type

Immediate postpartum smears show an atrophic pattern, more pronounced in women who are lactating. It is followed by an increase in estrogenic activity after a few weeks postpartum or after cessation of lactation.[37,38]

Smears of Androgenic Type

Androgenic hormones stimulate the proliferation of the basal and intermediate cell layers of the epithelium and provoke the disappearance of the superficial cells. This antiestrogenic effect is clearly visible during the period of hormonal activity. In an atrophic vaginal mucosa, androgens cause the appearance of intermediate and parabasal cells, among which are found cells of a particular type with voluminous nuclei containing scant finely dispersed chromatin (so-called androgenic cells).[39]

Smears of Nonspecific Proliferation

Sex steroid hormones of endogenous or exogenous origin first stimulate the proliferation of the vaginal epithelium. The parabasal cells multiply, and the number of intermediate cells is notably augmented. This cytologic appearance represents a picture of nonspecific epithelial proliferation, composed of plaques of intermediate cells, less numerous parabasal cells, and some superficial cells (Fig. 2-4). If the hormonal activity persists, cytologic changes that are more specific for the hormone administered appear secondarily.[40] This same appearance is found physiologically in women presenting only a modest hormonal activity, such as in the first years of menopause.

Smears of Atrophic Type

Suppression of all hormonal activity produces a progressive atrophy of the epithelium, which then consists of cells of parabasal type (Fig. 2-5 and Color Figure 2-4).[41] In an atrophic epithelium, there are often secondary inflammatory lesions, manifested by nuclear and cytoplasmic alterations and the presence of polymorphonuclear leukocytes and a varied bacterial flora. The picture of atrophy is not always present after menopause; a nonspecific hormonal stimu-

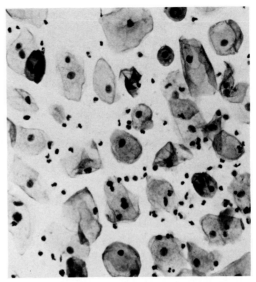

FIGURE 2-4 Vaginal smear of nonspecific proliferation.

lation of ovarian or extraovarian (notably adrenal) origin often persists for a long time.[42] The atrophic picture supervenes more rapidly after surgical castration. Atrophic smears with degenerative cellular anomalies and cellular necrosis may represent problems of differential diagnosis with dysplasia or even carcinoma (Color Figure 2-5). The administration of estrogens for a short period (*estrogen test*) eliminates anomalies of atrophic origin and facilitates the recognition of true neoplasia.[42]

Cell Types Accompanying the Vaginal Cells

A variety of cells may be present in the vaginal smears, which will modify the normal cytologic pat-

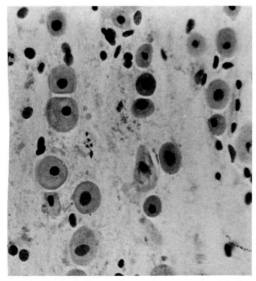

FIGURE 2-5 Vaginal smear of atrophic type: parabasal and inflammatory cells.

tern. Glandular cells of cervical or endometrial origin can be observed. Endometrial cells normally disappear after the 12th day of the cycle. Endocervical and metaplastic cells are more abundant in inflammatory conditions with or without ectropion. Histiocytes, polymorphonuclear leukocytes, and lymphocytes indicate inflammatory reactive changes. Anucleate squamous cells normally are not present; they originate (1) from the lower third of the vaginal mucosa, where they represent, as in the skin, the final step of squamous differentiation; (2) from inflammatory foci of the mucosa (clinical leukoplakia); and (3) from the epidermis of the infant, in pregnant women with ruptured fetal membranes.

INFLAMMATORY DISEASES

A number of inflammatory lesions simultaneously involving the vulva and the vagina are described in detail in Chapter 1. These lesions include those of human papillomavirus (HPV) infection, gonorrhea, diphtheria, chancroid, granuloma inguinale, tuberculosis, syphilis, and mycotic infection. Organisms commonly encountered in association with vaginal lesions include *Trichomonas vaginalis, Herpesvirus hominis, Gardnerelia vaginalis,* and *Enterobius vermicularis.* Among etiologies rarely encountered in temperate climates are amebiasis and schistosomiasis. Some of these organisms may be present without manifestations of clinical symptoms.

In healthy women, the vaginal milieu includes a variety of aerobic as well as obligate and facultative anaerobic organisms that do not necessarily equate with inflammation.[43–45] Predisposing conditions and a trigger mechanism that often is not clearly understood are necessary to modify the saprophytic status of these organisms into that of pathogens. Among the predisposing conditions are variations of the vaginal pH, mucosal injuries during pregnancy and delivery, and absence of the protective squamous maturation in prepubertal girls and postmenopausal women.

Bacterial or Nonspecific Vaginosis

Facultative and anaerobic flora may cause a specific condition called *nonspecific vaginosis*[46] or *bacterial vaginosis.*[47] It is a polymicrobial vaginitis resulting from synergism between these anaerobic bacteria and coccobacilli.[48–51] Cervicovaginal smears reveal the presence of squamous cells covered with bacilli as well as cocci and bacilli diffusely scattered or occurring in clumps. Their identification can be obtained by microbiologic isolation but is not required for the clinical management of this frequent disease. It is common in adolescent girls and may be hormonally dependent.[52]

Gardnerella Vaginitis

This type of vaginitis is characterized by the presence of *Gardnerella vaginalis,* previously classified as *Haemophilus vaginalis.* It was described by Gardner and Dukes[53] and classified by Greenwood and Pickett.[54] The organism is Gram-negative or Gram-variable, catalase-positive, believed to be sexually transmissible, and frequently found in asymptomatic women. It is assumed that it may be responsible for the development of an infection without the interaction of other bacteria. The infection becomes symptomatic when the vaginal pH rises to more than 4.5; other aerobic and anaerobic bacteria may be present. The results should be interpreted with caution because the isolated bacterial agent is not always the etiologic factor responsible for the clinical disease. The vaginal flora identified may vary according to factors such as differences in collecting, transporting, or handling the material and the presence of chemical agents such as contraceptives. The disease is associated with a characteristic vaginal discharge with a fishy odor.

Microscopically, numerous organisms cover over the squamous cells or stick to the cellular edges; these so-called clue cells are observed in stained Papanicolaou smears or under phase contrast (Color Figure 2-6). Some authors believe that in smears the organisms should cover the epithelial cells and spread beyond the cellular margins to avoid overdiagnosis.[55] Culture should confirm the diagnosis. Histologic examination does not reveal any significant alteration, the organism being localized at the surface of the epithelium.

Lactobacillus "Vaginitis"

Lactobacilli are aerobic, Gram-positive organisms that are present in the vaginal flora of most women. They are common in the luteal phase and in pregnancy when glycogen is abundant. Their presence corresponds to a low acid vaginal pH (around 5). The glycogen contained in the cytoplasm of intermediate cells is metabolized and generates lactic acid. The destruction of the cytoplasm explains the presence of naked nuclei. It is still a matter of debate whether lactobacilli can acquire a pathogenic significance.

Atrophic Vaginitis

Atrophic vaginitis is encountered in certain women at the time of cessation of ovarian activity, whether physiologic (menopause) or therapeutic (surgery or radiation). It is accompanied by clinical symptoms: burning sensations, at times painful, purulent leukorrhea, and hemorrhages. The atrophic mucosa becomes ulcerated, often effacing the posterior cul-de-sac and stenosing the bottom of the vaginal canal. Later developments include the formation of adhesions, synechiae, and other cicatricial processes.

Macroscopic Appearance. The mucosa is thin, pale, and smooth; it is the site of small congestive foci, with subsequent ulceration. When the vaginitis is acute, the mucosa is bright red and shiny.

Microscopic Appearance. The epithelium is reduced to a few layers of parabasal and basal cells; it is the site of polymorphonuclear leukocytic infiltration, which is sometimes massive.

The *cytologic pattern* is characterized by the presence of parabasal cells altered by the dryness of the mucosa. The cells are enlarged and the nuclei are discolored, losing their affinity for hematoxylin. A marked eosinophilia of the cytoplasm accompanied by nuclear pyknosis and karyorrhexis characterizes some parabasal cells. When these anomalies are pronounced, they can raise problems of differential diagnosis with dysplasia or carcinoma (see Color Figure 2-5).

The atrophic epithelium shows poor resistance to secondary infection. Local or systemic administration of estrogens brings about a regeneration of the mucosa favorable to cure and "cures" the cytologic abnormalities.

Postpartum Atrophic Vaginitis

Rarely during the period of nursing, one finds a vaginitis that presents the same gross appearance as atrophic vaginitis: bright red congested mucosa covered with ulcers and accompanied by purulent discharge.

Microscopically, there is a thinned vaginal epithelium, reduced to the basal layers and several rows of superficial cells infiltrated with neutrophils. This appearance is comparable to that of an atrophic epithelium, and it is classically considered to be an atrophy of hormonal origin.

The cytologic pattern is similar to the one described in atrophic vaginitis. The administration of estrogens remains efficacious in provoking proliferation of the superficial keratinized layers that protect the epithelium against the bacterial flora.

Fungal Infections

Vaginal Candidiasis

Candida albicans may involve the vaginal mucosa and is the most frequent fungal agent observed in the female genital tract. Vaginal candidiasis is also called *vaginal moniliasis, mycotic* or *yeast vaginitis,* and *vaginal thrush.*

Different candidal types exist; the most common is *C. albicans* followed by *C. glabrata.*[56–60] Some doubts persist about the pathogenic character of the yeast. Clinically, the fungus may not be associated with vaginitis or may produce a white, creamy vaginal discharge with itching. Pregnancy, diabetes, antibiotic agents, corticoids, and immunosuppressive drugs may be related to the presence of the fungus, and it is very common in patients with acquired immunodeficiency syndrome (AIDS). Little is known about the mechanism that provokes the transition from asymptomatic yeast presence to vaginitis. Some strains are refractory to available therapeutic agents, explaining the difficulty of eradicating the causal organism.

Microscopically, the vaginal epithelium is superficially colonized by *Candida,* and it has been suggested that it may penetrate the cells.[61] Acanthosis, intracellular edema, and an inflammatory infiltrate located in the epithelium or in the stroma may be present. Vaginal smears reveal the presence of filamentous structures (hyphae) and/or conidia, which appear as small, oval, encapsulated organisms. Minor epithelial inflammatory changes accompany the fungus, which can be localized in the cytoplasm of squamous cells.[62]

Other Fungi

Vaginal coccidioidomycosis,[63] toxoplasmosis,[64] and blastomycosis[65] have been reported. The organisms can be recognized in vaginal smears but their identification requires cultural characterization.

Parasitic Infections

Trichomonas *Infection and Infestation*

Infection due to *Trichomonas* has been known since Donné, in 1836, published a complete description of these lesions.[66] *Trichomonas vaginalis,* a protozoan, is very common, and 20% to 25% of women undergoing routine gynecologic examinations are revealed to be carriers of the parasite.[67] The practice of exfoliative cytology on a large scale has confirmed the high frequency of this infestation. The parasite is transmitted by sexual contact and can be carried by the male partner.[68] The infection is most frequent during the reproductive years and in pregnancy,[69] is infrequent after menopause, and is rare before puberty.

The trichomonad is a mobile flagellate with four cilia that is refringent on direct examination. The parasites are of various sizes, measuring 10 to 20 μm; giant forms are rarely encountered. Their presence in vaginal secretions is not accompanied by an inflammatory reaction in most cases (infestation).

Clinical Manifestations. The infection is characterized by leukorrhea accompanied by burning sensations and pruritus, dyspareunia, dysuria, and irritation of the adjacent epithelia. The incubation period is between 5 and 28 days. This leukorrhea, pathognomonic of the infection, is yellow-gray and of a foamy or creamy consistency, and it occurs in about 25% of patients. It is very irritating to the tissues. When a bacterial flora coexists, the discharge may be frankly purulent. The vaginal pH is lowered to around 5.0 after the destruction of carbohydrates and liberation of acid radicals. Lower urinary tract infection with dysuria and urethral discharge may be observed.

Laboratory Diagnosis. Laboratory diagnosis relies on the demonstration of the protozoan in the vaginal discharge, which is diluted with isotonic saline solution and examined under the microscope as a wet preparation or is fixed in 50% alcohol and stained with the Papanicolaou technique. The number of trichomonads varies, and a careful examination of the slide is needed before it is recognized. Bare epithelial nuclei should not be misinterpreted as trichomonads.

Macroscopic Appearance. In acute vaginitis due to *Trichomonas*, the mucosa is red, congested, edematous, and granular (so-called strawberry vagina). Small hemorrhagic zones are present, and there may be occasional small superficial ulcers. These alterations involve the vaginal, vulvar, and ectocervical mucosae. Colposcopy reveals a characteristic vascular pattern.[70]

Microscopic Appearance. The vaginal mucosa shows acute or chronic inflammatory lesions, depending on the state of evolution of the infection.

Biopsy of the vaginal mucosa (which is seldom done) reveals a neutrophilic, lymphocytic, and plasmacytic infiltrate, vascular congestion, and stromal edema, as well as disseminated foci of cellular atypia throughout the epithelium. Reserve cell hyperplasia and squamous metaplasia may be present. One finds the organisms on the surface of the squamous epithelial cells or rarely in the epithelium, especially in the superficial cell layers. The parasite shows a pale, cyanophilic cytoplasm and a small, faint, vesicular, eccentric nucleus.

The modifications of the epithelial cells are easily visible in vaginal smears and are manifested by increased eosinophilia and the presence of characteristic perinuclear haloes (Fig. 2-6 and Color Figure 2-7). The nuclei show variation in size, with a general increase in volume, binucleation, karyorrhexis and pyknosis. These cytologic alterations are sometimes so accentuated that they approach cellular abnormalities of neoplastic type. The absence of hyperchromatism and of bizarre nuclei and the presence of the parasite orient the pathologist toward the diagnosis of *Trichomonas* infection. Aggregates of leukocytes called "cannonballs" covering the surface of squamous cells are sometimes recognized and represent *T. vaginalis* located on squamous cells and secondarily phagocytized by leukocytes and macrophages. *Leptothrix* organisms are frequently seen in association with Trichomoniasis, and may be the first clue to the presence of *T. vaginalis* (Color Figure 2-8).

Prognosis, Evolution, and Treatment. *Trichomonas* infection was once considered to be favorable to the

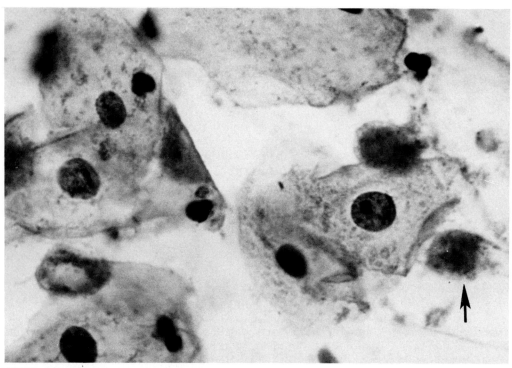

FIGURE 2-6 *Trichomonas* vaginitis: cytologic appearance.

development of cervix cancer. This hypothesis is now discarded, even though a higher incidence of *Trichomonas* infestation is noted in patients with cervical cancer.[71] The essential principles in therapy are the use of local germicides and disinfectants and of local or systemic estrogens over a prolonged period, identification and oral treatment of urinary localizations (urethra, bladder, and Skene's glands), careful search for the parasite in the urogenital tract of the sexual partner, and prophylactic hygiene. Despite apparent cure, even of long duration, the infection often reappears.

Other Parasitic Infections

Enterobius vermicularis, Ascaris lumbricoides, Filaria (nematodes), *Entamoeba histolytica* (protozoan), *Cysticercus, Toxoplasma,* schistosomes, and arthropods have been described as occasional contaminants of the vagina.[72–76]

Desquamative Inflammatory Vaginitis

This entity consists of an atrophic vaginitis, usually limited to the upper half of the vagina, in which desquamation of parabasal cells and neutrophils is prominent despite normal ovarian function. The etiology is unknown, and corticosteroids are the only therapeutic agents that afford relief.[77]

Emphysematous Vaginitis

Emphysematous vaginitis is a rare disease, first described by Huguier, that has been reported most often in association with pregnancy or cardiopulmonary disease.[78] In 1964, Gardner and Fernet found 145 cases in the literature, to which they added 10 of their own.[79] The disease involves the superior portion of the vagina and the ectocervix. Clinically, one observes a red, sometimes superficially ulcerated mucosa. Synonyms are cystic vaginitis, gaseous cysts of the vagina, and emphysematous colpitis.

Macroscopic Appearance. This lesion is characterized by the presence of small liquid- or gas-containing cysts in the mucosa. These cysts may rupture and give rise to ulcers.

Microscopic Appearance. There are cystic cavities with thin walls. They are bordered by giant cells or by an epithelium or endothelium containing multinuclear cells that are surrounded by fibrous cords rich in elastic fibers. This appearance has suggested obliterated and distended lymphatics. The gaseous content of the cysts is probably produced by anaerobic bacteria, but a theory of its production by migrating epithelial cells has been advanced. These hypotheses still demand confirmation, because the inoculation of the cystic contents into the guinea pig

has never been able to reproduce the clinical picture of the disease.[80]

Treatment. There is no specific treatment, but treatment of the accompanying or underlying bacterial infection may be efficacious.

Vaginitis Caused by Physical or Chemical Agents

A variety of physical and chemical phenomena produce acute or chronic inflammatory lesions of the vaginal mucosa. Some examples are pessaries, foreign bodies, contraceptive devices, irradiation, injected products having potassium permanganate as a base, zinc sulfate, and other antiseptics. A local granulation tissue reaction in the vault may be seen after hysterectomy.[81]

Special mention should be made of the mucosal alteration associated with the use of superabsorbent tampons. The lesions include mucosal drying, epithelial layering, and microulcerations. These microscopic lesions may lead to clinically evident mucosal ulcers accompanied by bleeding and discharge.[82,83] The etiology can be explained by cell membrane alterations followed by extracellular fluid transfer and secondarily widened intercellular spaces. Vaginal ulcers represent a portal of entry for *Staphylococcus aureus*, and the relation of this local lesion to the *toxic shock syndrome* has been considered.[84] The syndrome is caused by the release of the staphylococcal toxin into the circulation.[85,86] The syndrome, initially associated with tampon use, is now described with any staphylococcal infection (see Chap. 12).

Macroscopic Appearance. The mucosa is red, congested, and edematous. The surface is often granular.

Microscopic Appearance. There is leukohistiocytic infiltration of the mucosa accompanied by edema or vascular congestion of the subjacent stroma. In places, the mucosa may be ulcerated and replaced by granulation tissue. Nuclear and cytoplasmic anomalies may be found: anisocytosis, anisonucleosis, cytoplasmic vacuolization, and cellular necrosis.

Langerhans Cell Histiocytosis

Langerhans cell histiocytosis is a rare disease that may affect the female genital tract and notably the vagina. Of unknown etiology, it may represent the manifestation of an undefined immunologic disorder. Macroscopically, it is characterized by papular, erythematous, pruritic lesions that sometimes ulcerate. Microscopically, it is a chronic, necrotizing inflammatory lesion with the presence of Langerhans cells with a typical grooved and folded vesicular nucleus. The differential diagnosis is with various inflammatory conditions.[87]

BENIGN TUMORS

Cystic Tumors

Gartner's Duct Cyst

Gartner's duct (mesonephric) cysts are rare; they originate from vestiges of the mesonephric ducts and are found in the lateral vaginal walls. They may attain 2 cm in diameter and may cause dyspareunia.[88]

Histologic Appearance. The cyst wall is lined by a nonciliated, nonmuciparous, columnar or cuboidal epithelium with large pale nuclei (Fig. 2-7). Tension caused by the intracystic liquid may cause flattening or disappearance of the epithelium, making identification difficult. There may be foci of squamous metaplasia. Smooth muscle fibers may be present in the wall. A case of mesonephric carcinoma has been reported.[89]

Cyst of Müllerian Origin

Müllerian or paramesonephric cysts are identical in gross appearance to cysts of Gartner's duct.[88,90,91] Cysts of the inferior third of the vagina are the most frequent, and they may exteriorize at the vulvar orifice. *Histologically,* they are usually lined by muciparous endocervical-type epithelium, but tubal or endometrial features are present in a minority of cases. In the latter instance, the lesion must be differenti-ated from true *endometriosis,* in which endometrial stroma is present as well as epithelium. If the epithelium is tubal in type, with ciliated cells, a *prolapsed fallopian tube* (see below) presents the major diagnostic confusion.

Epithelial Inclusion Cyst

Epithelial inclusion cysts are the most common vaginal cysts.[88,90] They are frequent at the level of the culs-de-sac. They originate from inclusions of fragments of squamous epithelium in the mucosa, often by obstetric or surgical trauma. Of variable size, but never more than a few centimeters, these cysts are lined by squamous epithelium and contain a grumous pale yellow substance that represents products of desquamation (Fig. 2-8). Immunohistochemically, they stain for keratin but not carcinoembryonic antigen.

Urothelial Cyst

Urothelial cysts are rare and usually measure less than 1 cm in diameter. Most of them are localized beneath the mucosa of the vulvar vestibule. They are lined by transitional or stratified columnar epithelium, or by both, confirming the urothelial origin.[92] They may represent remnants of the urogenital sinus or may originate from the mucinous Skene's glands; in this case they are lined by a mucinous epithelium.

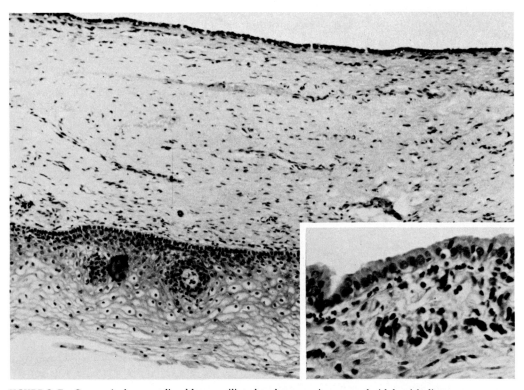

FIGURE 2-7 Gartner's duct cyst lined by nonciliated and nonmuciparous cuboidal epithelium underlain by smooth muscle fibers.

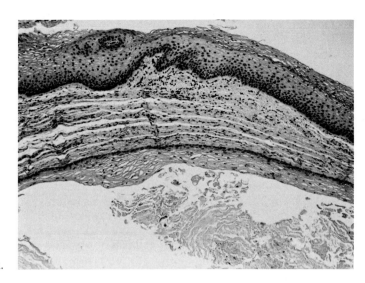

FIGURE 2-8 Epithelial inclusion cyst of vagina.

Solid Tumors

Leiomyoma and Fibroma

Leiomyoma and fibroma are rare tumors.[93,94] They are manifested clinically by the appearance in an adult woman of a mass that produces signs of compression, dyspareunia, and urinary difficulties.

Macroscopic Appearance. There is an ovoid submucosal mass, usually 1 to 5 cm in diameter, which is encapsulated and of firm elastic consistency; the tumor is single or rarely may be multiple. It may on occasion herniate at the vulvar orifice. Rarely, it may attain an enormous volume. Sessile and pedunculated forms exist. When the tumor is large, the overlying vaginal mucosa has a tendency to ulcerate.

Microscopic Appearance. The tumors are composed of connective tissue, smooth muscle fibers, or both. Either of these two elements may dominate. Hyaline degeneration is much rarer than in uterine myomata.

Fibroepithelial Polyp

Vaginal polyps have been described under various names, including *fibroepithelial polyp, sarcoma botryoides-like lesion, pseudosarcoma botryoides,* and *myofibroblastoma.* This benign lesion occurs infrequently in late reproductive life or more rarely during pregnancy.[95–98]

Clinically, it is discovered as a vaginal nodule by the patient, is associated with postcoital bleeding or may be asymptomatic. A history of previous vaginal surgery is mentioned in a significant number of cases.

Macroscopically, it consists of a polypoid nodule usually measuring less than 3 cm in diameter. *Microscopically,* it is covered by a squamous epithelium with foci of hyperkeratosis and parakeratosis. The underlying loose fibrillary stroma is rich in stellate-shaped cells and benign-appearing multinucleated giant cells (Fig. 2-9). The nature of these atypical stromal cells remains obscure. They express vimentin, desmin and receptors for estrogen and proges-

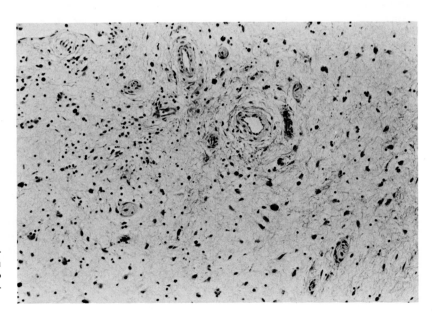

FIGURE 2-9 Vaginal polyp: loose fibrovascular stroma containing scattered cells with large hyperchromatic nuclei. There are no mitotic figures, rhabdomyoblasts, or "cambium layer."

terone, suggesting that they represent stromal cells with a myoid component.[99,100] Numerous capillaries are dispersed in the stroma and numerous mast cells and lymphocytes are present. An alarming degree of atypia may be present in the fibroblastic elements, particularly in association with pregnancy. The absence of a "cambium layer" and the age of the patient should preclude a false diagnosis of sarcoma botryoides, which occurs almost exclusively in infants.

These polyps may represent a localized hyperplasia of the subepithelial zone of the stroma as a result of a granulation tissue reaction after local injury of the mucosa. Physical irritation and hormonal imbalance have been suggested as etiologic factors.[101,102] A few cases with high cellularity, atypical nuclei, and a high mitotic count with abnormal mitotic figures may represent difficulties of interpretation and should be managed carefully.

Vaginal polyps must be differentiated from aggressive angiomyxoma, myxoid neurofibroma, and sarcoma botryoides. Table 2-1 summarizes some characteristics of these different lesions. Local resection is the treatment.

ENDOMETRIOSIS

Endometriosis is the consequence of implantation of endometrial mucosal debris during menstruation or a surgical procedure at the vaginal site. This rare localization appears as a submucosal solid or cystic nodule with a red or blue color. Endometriosis can be localized in the rectovaginal septum; subsequent malignant transformation may occur.[103] Histologic examination reveals characteristic endometrial glands and stroma with secondary hemorrhage or fibrosis.

TABLE 2-1.
Differential Diagnosis of Atypical Stromal Lesions of the Vagina

	Vaginal Polyp	Aggressive Angiomyxoma	Sarcoma Botryoides
Age	Adult	20–30 y	Under 5 y
Size	< 3 cm	Large, ill-defined	Polypoid mass, often large
Localization	Vagina, vulva	Vagina, vulva, pelvis	Anterior wall of vagina
Histology	Loose stroma with stellate and spindle-shaped cells	Hypocellular myxoid stroma with numerous vessels	Myxoid stroma and undifferentiated rhabdomyoblastic cells
Evolution	Benign	Local recurrence	Malignant

POSTOPERATIVE CONDITIONS

Tubal prolapse into the vaginal vault after vaginal hysterectomy has been reported.[104,105] Macroscopically, it is characterized by a granulomatous nodule appearing a few weeks to many years after the operation. Microscopically, the biopsy shows glandular, villous structures covered with a columnar epithelium suggesting a tubal origin (Fig. 2-10); the presence of smooth muscle confirms this impression. An inflammatory infiltrate is common. These glandular structures infiltrated by an inflammatory and granulomatous stroma should not be erroneously interpreted as adenocarcinoma. The presence of smooth muscle and of ciliated epithelium helps to make the distinction. Muscle and the inflammation differentiate tubal prolapse from a benign müllerian cyst.

Postoperative spindle cell nodule, a lesion simulating a sarcoma, has been reported occasionally in the genitourinary tract after surgery. Some cases have been described in the vagina. Macroscopically, it consists of polypoid, hemorrhagic nodules measuring several centimeters in diameter. Microscopically, it is represented by a highly vascularized proliferation rich in spindle cells that have been identified as myofibroblasts. Absence of severe cellular atypia and abnormal mitoses rules out the differential diagnosis of leiomyosarcoma.[106,107]

ADENOSIS

This condition is characterized by the presence of glandular structures in the vaginal mucosa or the lamina propria. The simultaneous involvement of the epithelium and the underlying stroma is present in most cases. Adenosis is caused by a failure of squamous epithelium to replace the original müllerian epithelium that covers the vaginal wall and the ectocervix during fetal life. Adenosis is observed in late fetal life and in infants, children, and adults.

The prevalence of adenosis differs in various published reports.[108,109] Sandberg noted the pres-

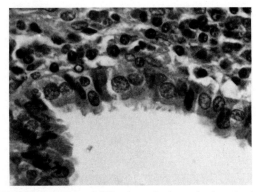

FIGURE-2-10 Prolapsed fallopian tube in vaginal vault: detail of tubal epithelium and inflammatory reaction.

ence of adenosis in 41% of 22 postpubertal vaginas examined by step sections at autopsy, although the lesion was not identified in any of 13 vaginas from prepubertal girls.[110]

More attention has been devoted to this lesion because it was observed with high frequency in young women whose mothers were treated with DES during at-risk pregnancy. The exact prevalence is not known, but Herbst and coworkers[111] have quoted a figure of 38% in routine clinical examination, whereas other authors using colposcopy have suggested that the incidence approaches 100%.[112] About one fifth of the women exposed in utero to DES demonstrate gross structural changes of the vagina and the cervix,[113] and one half exhibit microscopic changes in the vaginal mucosa, consisting of glandular structures and foci of squamous metaplasia.[114–116]

Macroscopic Appearance. The vaginal epithelial changes consist of flat or papillary, iodine-negative, red granular spots detected clinically, on the basis of iodine staining, or by colposcopy. As squamous epithelium replaces the glandular formations, the translucent appearance becomes white and opaque. More rarely, the lesion is confined to the lamina propria and is characterized by a submucosal nodule.

Microscopic Appearance. Glandular formations are lined by mucinous, endocervical-type columnar cells (Fig. 2-11) and more rarely by an endometrial or tubal-type epithelium.[117,118] Squamous metaplasia is frequent and represents the delayed (from fetal life) process of regression and healing of the glandular proliferation.[119–122] The glandular structures originate from the reserve cells of the müllerian epithelium. They progress to immature and mature squamous metaplasia, which finally replaces the columnar cells. Vestiges of the columnar cells are often represented by intracellular droplets of mucin.[118] Increased vascularity and inflammatory infiltrates around the glandular structures in the lamina

propria are commonly present. Immunohistochemically, the columnar cells react positively for carcinoembryonic antigen, notably the cytoplasmic membrane of the luminal cell border. Retained glands may eventually be the origin of neoplastic changes (see the discussion below and in the section on adenocarcinoma).

Cytologic examination contributes to the diagnosis of adenosis under certain conditions: the lesion must be located on the vaginal wall; the mucosa should be involved; and the age of the patient should correspond to the period when adenosis is appearing.[123–127] Direct scraping of the macroscopic lesion avoids cervical contamination. The smears reveal the presence of columnar endocervical-type cells accompanied by squamous metaplastic cells in variable number. The columnar cells have eccentric, basally located nuclei with a finely dispersed chromatin. The cyanophilic cytoplasm may contain numerous small vacuoles or a large single one. Occasionally the glandular cells may be of endometrial or tubal type (Color Figure 2-9). Absence of cellular atypia may help to rule out a malignant lesion, but one has to know that well-differentiated adenocarcinoma may desquamate clumps of regular, small columnar cells with round normochromatic nuclei. One of our cases of clear cell adenocarcinoma revealed the presence of small, very regular columnar cells with dense, round nuclei without atypia.

Squamous metaplasia is represented by parabasal cells with a central, round, bland nucleus and dense cyanophilic cytoplasm with elongated cell extremities.

The cytologic follow-up of adenosis by direct scraping of the lesion shows a decrease or a loss of columnar cells with the presence of an increasing number of metaplastic cells. This reflects the regression of the lesion. False-negative results represent about 25% of the cases and are encountered when the conditions mentioned above are not fulfilled. Cytology is therefore not a screening tool for the diagnosis of adenosis and is not recommended as the sole

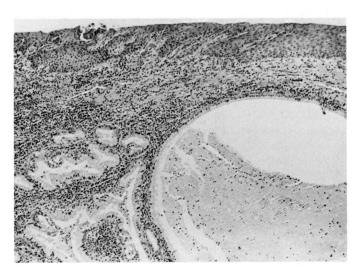

FIGURE 2-11 Vaginal adenosis: submucosal glands lined by endocervical-type epithelium.

tool in monitoring for the possible development of carcinoma.

The *etiology* of adenosis is poorly understood.[128,129] Forsberg has described a probable animal model.[130] Because neonatal estradiol and DES injections in mice induce similar lesions, he postulated an inhibition of mitotic activity in the vaginal columnar epithelium, thereby preventing its transformation to squamous epithelium. Prevention of this change by castration indicates that ovarian hormones are required, which correlates well with the reported absence of adenosis in prepubertal girls.[131] Herbst and associates, however, have reported adenosis in 6 of 73 prepubertal girls at autopsy.[132] More recent studies suggest an important inductive role of the cervicovaginal submucosal stroma. When adenosis is not associated with DES, it has been reported in conjunction with disorders of müllerian development, or after mucosal injury.[133]

The main clinical significance of vaginal adenosis lies in its association with vaginal clear cell carcinomas. A case of vaginal adenosis followed by clear cell adenocarcinoma has been reported after 5-fluorouracil treatment for condyloma.[134] The causal role of viruses or chemotherapy in the development of the lesion remains debatable.

DES and Cervical Intraepithelial Neoplasia

Considering that adenosis shows widened zones of squamous transformation, Stafl and colleagues predicted an increase in cervical intraepithelial neoplasia (CIN) among DES-exposed women.[114] Some further investigations confirmed this contention,[119,135] whereas others did not support it.[120,136] The epidemic of squamous carcinoma predicted by some has not appeared, although DES-exposed progeny are certainly no less likely than other sexually active young women to manifest papillomavirus and other cervicovaginal infections. Different factors can be mentioned to explain the discrepancies: subjectivity in interpretation and grading of dysplastic and metaplastic lesions, absence of evaluation of factors that contribute to the appearance of dysplasia (eg, age of onset of coitus and number of sexual partners and chronic inflammatory lesions), and more biopsy controls in patients who are self- or physician-referred than in patients screened by record review.[137,138] The DESAD project in 1984 provided further data supporting the finding of an increased incidence of CIN in DES-exposed patients.[135]

Squamous carcinomas may eventually prove to be more of a threat than adenocarcinomas, because adenosis heals by squamous metaplasia. Evidence of immune alterations have been demonstrated experimentally, and autoimmune conditions are increased in DES-exposed women, resulting in alterations of development of squamous cell lesions.[139,140]

Microglandular Hyperplasia in Adenosis

Microglandular hyperplasia is more frequently found in the cervix but may appear in the vagina in adenosis lesions. It is most commonly seen after long-term use of oral contraceptives or during pregnancy.[141] *Macroscopically*, there is an elevated, sometimes polypoid, soft, tan-yellow nodule arising on the mucosa. *Microscopically*, there is a proliferation of small mucinous glands with extensive foci of squamous metaplasia. The lesion should not be confused with adenocarcinoma (see Chap. 3 for differential diagnosis).

OTHER BENIGN LESIONS

Other soft tissue tumors such as *hemangioma*,[142] *rhabdomyoma*,[143] *neurofibroma*[144] and *paraganglioma*[145] are occasionally encountered in the vagina. Rhabdomyoma, which is a rare tumor occurring in adults, must be differentiated from embryonal rhabdomyosarcoma (sarcoma botryoides), which occurs in young children (see below). Benign primary vaginal *teratoma* has been reported.[146] Much more common are *squamous papilloma* and *condyloma acuminatum*, the pathologic features of which are described in Chapter 1, because these lesions more frequently occur in the vulva. Benign *nevus* and *blue nevus* are rarely reported.[147] Chen described a polypoid vaginal tumor suggesting the structure of a *Brenner tumor*.[148]

Rare benign *mixed tumors* of müllerian origin have been reported.[149,150] They exhibit epithelial and stromal proliferations reminiscent of ectopic müllerian tissue. A case with local recurrence 8 years after local excision is mentioned in the literature.[151]

MALIGNANT TUMORS

Primary Tumors

Malignant tumors of the vagina are rare. They represent about 1% to 2% of all gynecologic cancers.[152] They are most often squamous carcinomas, more rarely adenocarcinomas or sarcomas. It is important to eliminate the possibility of a squamous cervical carcinoma with vaginal extension before making the diagnosis of a primary vaginal tumor; this applies equally to intraepithelial carcinoma. Similarly, vaginal adenocarcinoma is more frequently metastatic (usually from endometrium) than primary.

Vaginal Intraepithelial Neoplasia

The prevalence of primary vaginal intraepithelial neoplasia (VaIN) is lower than that of similar cervical lesions (CIN).[153–155] A few hundred cases have been reported in the literature.[156] Risk factors include a history of HPV infection (particularly types 16 and 18) and a low socioeconomic status.[157] Coexistence with the human immunodeficiency virus is being increasingly reported.[158] A large number of these lesions are multifocal and are associated with concomitant vulvar or cervical equivalent lesions. Multicentric primaries invoke a "field" concept of carcinogenesis in the lower genital tract. Therefore, it seems coherent to adopt the same classification as the one proposed earlier for cervical lesions and combine under one denomination the different dysplasias (mild, moderate, and severe) and carcinoma in situ (CIS). Now that the new Bethesda nomenclature is becoming widely recognized, it could be extended to the vaginal lesions, which can be divided into low-grade (VaIN I) and high-grade (VaIN II) lesions. Table 2-2 summarizes the different classifications. In practice, one of us (CG) uses the VaIN classification and the other (SGS) the dysplasia/CIS terminology. Whichever system is chosen, its implications should be understood clearly by all pathologists and clinicians in an institution.

Clinically, VaIN is usually asymptomatic and is discovered by routine cytology.[159-162] These lesions appear at a later age than cervical neoplasia, suggesting a different pathogenesis or a longer latency period. HPV DNA is frequently detected and, as in the cervix, high-grade lesions tend to be associated with type 16.[163,164] A case has been reported after immunosuppressive therapy.[165] Colposcopic examination may help to localize the lesion or lesions.

Macroscopic Appearance. When the lesion is single, it consists of a white or pink, slightly elevated, well-limited area. Almost half the lesions are multifocal and localized in the upper third of the organ.

Microscopic Appearance. The lesions are similar to those described in the cervix. According to the severity of the lesion, one observes loss of cell maturation, disorganized stratification of the epithelium with loss of nuclear polarity, hyperchromatic nuclei, increased mitotic activity with or without atypical mitoses, and abnormal keratinization. In mild dysplasia, superficial hyperkeratosis may be present. The notion of the existence of a microinvasive stage has

been introduced,[166] and lesions that penetrate less than 2.5 mm from the vaginal mucosa may have the same chance of survival as noninvasive lesions. This evaluation may be difficult to realize on biopsy material, and the criteria therefore remain controversial.[167] Very few cases with adequate follow-up have been reported.

In *smears,* the cytologic changes can be compared with those observed in cervical scrapings.[168] Koilocytosis is observed in low-grade and, less frequently, in high-grade lesions. Vaginal origin of the atypical cells is suspected if clinical and colposcopic examination of the cervix reveal no lesion. Direct scraping of the vaginal mucosa orients the diagnosis (Color Figure 2-10). If the lesions are located in the lower part of the vagina, the cellular changes have more similarities with vulvar cytologic alterations (marked hyperkeratosis).

Evolution and Treatment. Most cases persist or regress, and some progress to invasive carcinoma. In a series of 23 untreated patients followed for at least 3 years, vaginal carcinoma occurred in 2 cases.[169] Spontaneous regression is more common in low-grade VaIN than in more advanced lesions. The treatment depends on the size, number, and location of the lesions and on the age of the patient. Local excision, cryosurgery, laser therapy, or more extended surgery are the common treatments.

Postirradiation VaIN. Postirradiation VaIN is observed after radiation therapy for invasive carcinoma of the vagina or the cervix. It should be differentiated from postirradiation lesions of benign squamous cells, which can persist in the atrophic mucosa many years after treatment. Postirradiation VaIN is characterized by hyperchromatic, often binucleated nuclei surrounded by a vacuolated cytoplasm. The nucleocytoplasmic ratio is increased, and the presence of very large and atypical cells suggests a postirradiation origin.[170,171] HPV infection facilitated by postirradiation immunodepression may represent an etiologic factor.[172] Postirradiation VaIN may precede a recurrence of invasive carcinoma. The existence of an aneuploid cellular DNA content is associated with a poor clinical prognosis.[173]

Invasive Squamous Cell (Epidermoid) Carcinoma

Primary invasive squamous cell carcinoma of the vagina is rare and represents 2% of all gynecologic invasive cancers.[174-178] It occurs most frequently after the age of 45 (Fig. 2-12). It is a much less common lesion than squamous cell carcinoma of the cervix or vulva.[179] Before this diagnosis is accepted, an extension from one of the latter sites must be ruled out. In addition, multicentric synchronous or metachronous primaries are often present. This pattern is as true of in situ as of advanced invasive tumors.[180,181]

TABLE 2-2.
Classifications of Vaginal Intraepithelial Neoplasia (VaIN)

Mild dysplasia	Moderate dysplasia	Severe dysplasia	Carcinoma in situ
VaIN I	VaIN II		VaIN III
Low-grade intraepithelial lesion		High-grade intraepithelial lesion	

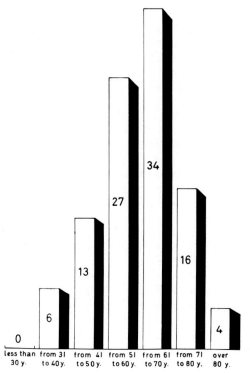

FIGURE 2-12 Incidence of vaginal squamous cell carcinoma (percentage) as a function of age. (Institute J. Bordet, 1925–1960 [118 cases])

Most vaginal cases occur in the upper third of the vagina, usually in the vault, and are more often posterior than anterior or lateral. When cervical cancer is present concurrently, the lesions are usually contiguous and the vaginal focus is then considered to represent secondary extension. In many instances, when only small biopsies are available, the question of second primary versus extension cannot be answered definitively; this is particularly true when the vaginal lesion is detected years after treatment of the cervical cancer. Colposcopy may be helpful in these cases.

HPV DNA, most frequently type 16, is present in a great number of lesions, suggesting, as in the cervix, the role of HPV ·in oncogenesis.[163,164,182] A case has been reported in a DES-exposed woman.[183]

Clinically, the lesion is asymptomatic or may manifest vaginal bleeding or discharge. A palpable mass may be the first manifestation of the tumor.

Macroscopic Appearance. Invasive squamous cell carcinoma presents as an infiltrative, ulcerated, exophytic, or papillomatous lesion measuring a few centimeters in diameter. The International Federation of Gynecologists and Obstetricians (FIGO) adopted in 1961 the following clinical staging system:

Stage I. Carcinoma limited to the vaginal wall

Stage II. Involvement of subvaginal tissues, without extension to the pelvic side walls

Stage III. Extension to one or both pelvic side walls or the pubic symphysis

Stage IV. Involvement of vesical or rectal mucosa or extension beyond the true pelvis

If a tumor involves the vagina and cervix, it is classified as primary in the cervix even if the bulk of the tumor is in the vagina.

Microscopic Appearance. The tumor is composed of neoplastic squamous cell cords originating in the vaginal epithelium. They invade the underlying submucosa and extend under the uninvolved epithelium. These cords are formed of undifferentiated basal-type cells or of differentiated keratinized cells forming cornified pearls (Fig. 2-13). Undifferentiated tumors exhibit atypical spindle cell features that may mimic mesenchymal tumors. The degree of histologic differentiation, based on the amount of keratinization and the number of squamous pearls, does not form a sound basis for estimating the prognosis, the clinical evaluation, or the efficacy of the treatment. Between the differentiated and undifferentiated types, all the intermediate appearances are encountered. The tumor is accompanied by a stromal chronic inflammatory infiltrate, and on occasion one may note the presence of carcinoma in situ at the periphery of the invasive lesion.

Prognosis, Evolution, and Treatment. Extension of the tumor is more often toward the cervix than toward the vulva. It extends even more often outward to the paravaginal and parametrial soft tissues. Direct extension to the rectum, bladder, and urethra takes place. Lymphatic metastases of tumors of the superior portion of the vagina lodge in the iliac, hypogastric, obturator, and sacral nodes; those from the inferior portion go to the pararectal, inguinal, and external iliac nodes.[8] The prognosis is based mainly on the clinical stage of the disease at the time of treatment. Long-term survival depends on early diagnosis, small size of the primary tumor, and absence of lymphatic involvement.[178] The 5-year survival rate is about 20% to 30%, with carcinomas of the upper third of the vagina having a somewhat better prognosis. Treatment may be by surgery, irradiation, or chemotherapy.[184]

Verrucous Carcinoma

Verrucous carcinoma is a distinctive entity that occurs infrequently in the vaginal mucosa (in less than 1% of vaginal carcinomas).[185,186] The same characteristics present in the vulva are encountered in the vagina: a slowly growing fungating mass with a benign histologic appearance and invasion on a broad front. There is frequent secondary ulceration. Microscopically, the lesion is characterized by a warty proliferation of large hyperkeratotic cellular nests extending into the underlying stroma in a pushing fashion (Fig. 2-14). Cellular atypia is very discrete, and the cellular polarity is preserved. It is important that the base of the lesion should be included in the

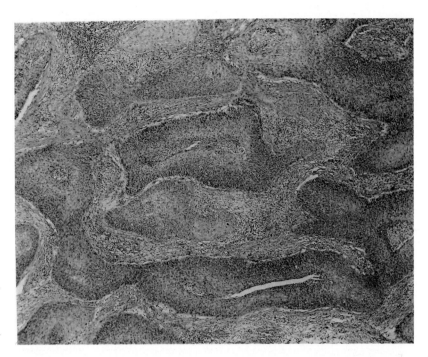

FIGURE 2-13 Squamous cell carcinoma of vagina: microscopic appearance.

biopsy to evaluate the rete pegs extending into the superficial stroma.

Verrucous carcinoma must be differentiated from condyloma acuminatum, pseudoepitheliomatous hyperplasia, and well-differentiated squamous carcinoma. The invasion on a broad front is most important, because invasion is absent in condyloma and infiltrative (with greater atypia as well) in squamous cell carcinoma.

Direct scraping of the lesion shows minimal cellular atypia; hyperkeratotic cells with minimal nuclear changes are abundant. This method is unreliable for diagnosis of this tumor.

Verrucous carcinoma should be properly recognized because it is locally aggressive but rarely metastasizes. Adequate local excision is the treatment of choice. Radiation therapy may result in recurrence of a more aggressive and less differentiated tumor.

Adenocarcinoma

Primary vaginal adenocarcinoma has been recognized since early in this century, predominantly in postmenopausal women and unrelated to exogenous hormonal influence.[132,187–189] It is a rare tumor and is now usually related to adenosis (see above) or orig-

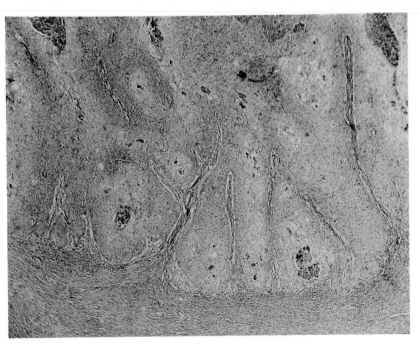

FIGURE 2-14 Verrucous carcinoma. The deep border of this bulky lesion shows the classical pattern of invasion on a broad front. See Figure 1-32 for the exophytic surface of another verrucous carcinoma.

inates from mesonephric duct or Gartner's duct rests.[190,191] A remarkable rise in incidence was first documented by Herbst and associates[192,193] and is attributed to the widespread use from the late 1940s to the 1970s of DES during early pregnancy in cases of habitual or threatened abortion. DES, the nonsteroidal estrogen diethylstilbestrol, was first synthesized in 1938 by the British biochemist Charles Dodds. An estimated 3 to 7 million women had taken the drug by 1971, when the very rare development of clear cell adenocarcinoma of the vagina and the cervix in young female offspring was linked to in utero exposure to the drug.[193–195] More than 500 cases have been recorded, and it is probable that this number is underestimated.[196]

Most recent patients with vaginal adenocarcinoma have been products of DES-treated pregnancies, so that these cases have occurred in young women between the ages of 7 and 33 years, with most cases appearing between the ages of 17 and 21.[196–198]

The risk is higher if the administration of DES was started before 12 weeks of pregnancy. About 60% of the cases originate in the vagina, and the others involve the vagina and cervix or the cervix alone. Most vaginal tumors arise from foci of adenosis on the upper third of the vaginal wall. Adenosis with atypia is often seen adjacent to the tumor and may represent an intermediate lesion (see below). Although we accept that a link between in utero DES exposure and adenocarcinoma is established, it is important to mention that the published series of cases are gathered from retrospective case-control and tumor registry reports that may introduce selection bias affecting the published results. About 25% of the cases have no history of maternal medication,[198,199] and a prospective study revealed no case of invasive genitourinary cancer in the group exposed to DES.[200] These data suggest that DES is not a complete carcinogen and that other factors,

some associated with the onset of puberty, may be involved in the development of the tumor.[201]

Macroscopic Appearance. The tumor is usually superficial, often polypoid, and presents in most cases on the anterior wall of the upper vagina (Color Figure 2-11). Some cases may appear as firm nodules more deeply located in the vaginal wall. Ulceration may occur. Lymph node metastases may be present even when the primary tumor is of limited extent.

Microscopic Appearance. The tumor is an adenocarcinoma that grows in one of three patterns: *tubulocystic, papillary,* or *solid* (Fig. 2-15).

The *tubulocystic* pattern is seen more often in patients older than 15 years and is associated with a better 5-year survival rate. *Papillary, solid,* and *combined* patterns are more often seen in the group of patients younger than 15 years. At high-power magnification, the tumor is seen to be composed of variable proportions of clear and hobnail cells, the former characterized by voluminous clear cytoplasm filled with glycogen and the latter by single-cell apical projections into the central lumina of the epithelial structures.[202,203] Mitoses usually are not abundant. The tumor is histologically, histochemically, and ultrastructurally identical to other clear cell carcinomas of the female genital tract, notably those of the ovary and endometrium.[204–206] Cytoplasmic mucin stains are negative, but mucin is often present at apical cell borders and in lumina. Expression of carcinoembryonic antigen is inconstant. Spectrophotometric DNA analysis of one case has shown an aneuploid chromosomal pattern.[207] Adenocarcinoma in situ is exceedingly rare and may represent an extension of a cervical lesion.[208]

Etiology. The origin of the tumor appears to be müllerian, although tumors of this type were formerly thought to be of mesonephric nature. The

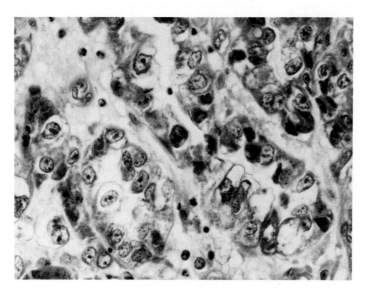

FIGURE 2-15 Clear cell adenocarcinoma of vagina in 17-year-old girl. Tubules are lined by clear and hobnail cells.

müllerian origin is supported by electron microscopic studies.[204-206] The etiology of the cases without any hormonal exposure remains unsettled; the presence of adenosis has been described and may be the origin of the tumor.[110] The precise method by which DES influences the fetal lower genital epithelium is not known, but ultrastructural studies suggest that DES acts on the stroma of the vaginal wall, affecting secondarily the epithelial cells.[209] Most adenocarcinomas arise from foci of adenosis,[203,210] and different morphologic arguments tend to implicate the endometrial-tubal type cell and not the endocervical-type cell as the precursor of the malignant elements. Morphologic similitudes exist between clear cell adenocarcinoma and endometrial carcinoma, and foci of adenosis adjacent to the tumor are composed of endometrial-tubal cells.[211,212] Occasional examples of transitional microscopic images (*atypical adenosis*)[213] have been encountered (Fig. 2-16), some of which have eventuated in carcinoma of clear cell or endometrioid type. The columnar cells of atypical adenosis have hyperchromatic nuclei, large nucleoli, and irregular cytoplasm. An aneuploid chromosomal pattern, a common finding in adenocarcinoma, has been demonstrated by spectrophotometric DNA analysis.[214]

Diagnostic procedures include frequent and thorough clinical examination of DES-exposed patients with cytologic sampling (Color Figure 2-12) and colposcopy with iodine staining. The smears of clear cell adenocarcinoma show isolated elements or aggregates of regular columnar cells with hyperchromatic nuclei and macronucleoli.[215] Very atypical cells may be observed in the solid type of tumor and may be wrongly interpreted as squamous or sarcomatous. The vaginal origin of the cells must be established to suggest the diagnosis. Cytology detects only a fraction of the cases; the Netherlands Registry notes that only 33% of the vaginal tumors were identified in

smears.[216] Absence of routine vaginal sampling, squamous metaplasia covering the tumor, or localization of the lesion under the mucosal surface are tentative explanations of this poor result.[216] Biopsy remains the mandatory procedure in any suspicious area.

The *prognosis* of clear cell carcinoma is relatively favorable, with a 5-year survival rate among cases with adequate follow-up data in the range of 75% to 80%, and about 90% among stage I cases.[197] Poor prognostic factors, in addition to extravaginal extension, include high mitotic activity and lymphatic invasion at the primary site. When recurrence takes place, it tends to be pelvic or intrathoracic, or both. Most cases have been treated surgically, but radiation therapy has also been proved effective.[205]

The *differential diagnosis* comprises other adenocarcinomas of the vagina, the most common of which are metastatic (see below). Carcinomas other than clear cell type, including *endometrioid, intestinal,* and *small cell* types, have been reported as arising on a background of vaginal adenosis.[189,217,218] Adenosis undergoing *microglandular hyperplasia* (see Chap. 3) in women who are pregnant or taking exogenous hormones should not be confused with adenocarcinoma. Rare cases of adenocarcinomas arising in endometriosis of the rectovaginal septum have been reported.[219,220] Another rare lesion is the *endodermal sinus tumor* (yolk sac carcinoma, carcinoma of infant vagina).[221-224] Originally also thought to be a "mesonephroma," this highly malignant tumor of infancy is currently considered to be a germ cell tumor, identical to its more frequent counterparts in ovary and testis. Characteristic histologic features include tubules growing in a loose reticular stroma, papillae with vascular cores projecting into tubules (the so-called glomeruloid bodies of Schiller or endodermal sinuses of Duval), prominent clear cell foci, and intra- and extracellular hyaline globules that are

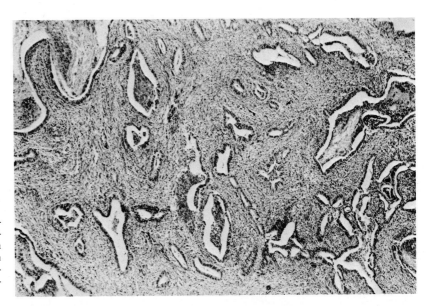

FIGURE 2-16 Atypical adenosis: endometrial-type glands proliferating in anarchic appearance reminiscent of adenomatous hyperplasia of endometrium. This patient (a young woman exposed in utero to diethylstilbestrol) subsequently developed adenocarcinoma at the vaginal site from which this biopsy was obtained.

positive for periodic acid-Schiff (PAS) stain and contain α-fetoprotein (Fig. 2-17). Finally, a prolapsed fallopian tube after hysterectomy (see above) may also enter the differential diagnosis.

Sarcoma

Sarcomas of the vagina are extremely rare and merit only brief commentary. *Leiomyosarcomas*[225-228] are the most common in adults, but variably documented cases of fibrosarcoma,[228] angiosarcoma,[229,230] alveolar soft part sarcoma,[231] synovial sarcoma-like tumor,[232] and various endometrioid sarcomas (Fig. 2-18) also have been reported. They are usually submucosal in origin and ulcerate only as a late event. In children and more rarely in adults, there exists a particular type of sarcoma that merits a more complete description: the *sarcoma botryoides.*

Sarcoma Botryoides (Embryonal Rhabdomyosarcoma).
Sarcoma botryoides presents as a pale red, edematous, polypoid "bunch of grapes" appended to the vaginal wall.[233-236] Two theories have been proposed to explain its nature. It may rise from embryonic rests composed of the mesenchyme surrounding the müllerian ducts, which has retained the ability to differentiate into varied mesodermal tissues, or from tumor cells that secondarily take on an embryonal character. The first hypothesis enjoys the most support. Ninety percent of cases are seen in children under 5 years of age.

Macroscopic Appearance. The tumor exhibits the form of a polypoid mass that owes its red or white color to its richness in myxomatous tissue. It is friable, hemorrhagic, and soft. Cut sections reveal a pale yellow-white, uniform tissue. When it is voluminous, it may be present at the vaginal orifice in the form of nodular clusters of variable size. Some tumors remain localized under the mucosa, eventually herniating into the vaginal cavity and ulcerating.

Microscopic Appearance. The great majority of tumors grow as pure embryonal rhabdomyosarcoma (Fig. 2-19). Beneath the mucosa is a condensed "cambium layer" of small round cells with brightly eosinophilic cytoplasm, in which cross-striations can occasionally be demonstrated; the deeper tissues are edematous and contain fewer tumor cells.

Other histologic patterns may be present: large cells with central nuclei and a clear, abundant cytoplasm containing PAS-positive diastase-soluble material, or small cells with dense nuclei and an elongated eosinophilic cytoplasm. The loosely arranged cells are dispersed in an edematous stroma. Mitoses are numerous. Immunohistochemically, most cases express myoglobin[237] and desmin.[238]

The *clinical prognosis* is poor, with 5-year survival approximating 15%. The evolution is one of local recurrences and extension to adjacent organs, as well as metastases to lymph nodes and lungs. A better prognosis can be expected if the tumor is strictly localized.[235]

Differential diagnosis must be made with the *fibroepithelial polyp,*[95-100] which exhibits the same myxoid stroma but does not have a dense cellular subepithelial layer and reveals no muscular differentiation. This lesion occurs almost exclusively in adults, as does the *fetal rhabdomyoma,*[143,239,240] a rare benign tumor with a myxoid stroma containing strap cells with cross-striations but no cambium layer and no mitotic figures.

Other Malignant Tumors

About 150 cases of primary vaginal *malignant melanoma* have been reported, most often in elderly women.[241-245] They account for less than 3% of all

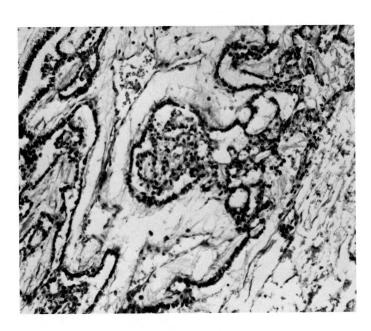

FIGURE 2-17 Endodermal sinus tumor of infant vagina. A Schiller–Duval body is present in the center.

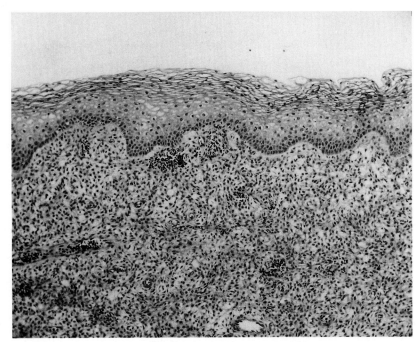

FIGURE 2-18 Low-grade endometrioid stromal sarcoma. The tumor is covered by unremarkable vaginal mucosa.

malignant tumors of the vagina. They appear as blue or black, frequently ulcerated nodules. Histologically, they resemble melanomas in other sites. The depth of invasion (Clark level)[243] and the thickness of the tumor (Breslow method)[246] should be measured, because they represent valuable prognostic factors. The prognosis is poor.

Neuroepithelial small cell carcinoma has been rarely reported in the vagina.[247,248] It is characterized by dense cords of small cells with hyperchromatic nuclei and cytoplasmic argyrophilic granules. The granules are well demonstrated by electron microscopy or immunohistochemistry (chromogranin, neuron-specific enolase). These tumors should be recognized because they have an aggressive nature with rapid recurrences and distant metastases. A case associated with adenosis has been reported.[217]

Among the rarer tumors are *plasmacytoma*,[249,250] *malignant lymphoma*,[251] *basal cell carcinoma*,[252] and *malignant mixed tumor*.[150,253] Seven cases of primary *carcinosarcoma* (malignant mixed mesodermal tumor) have been reported.[228]

Metastatic Tumors

Vaginal metastases are more frequent than primary tumors in this site. They are occasionally the first clinical manifestations of an occult neoplasm elsewhere. They arise most frequently from carcinomas of the vulva, cervix,[180,181] endometrium[254] (Fig. 2-20), or ovary.[255] They are usually found on the posterior vaginal wall. Also encountered are metastases from tumors of the kidney,[256] breast,[257] pancre-

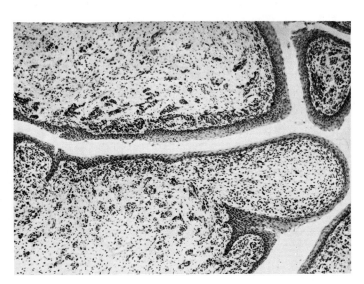

FIGURE 2-19 Sarcoma botryoides: polyps with submucosal "cambium layer" of tumor cells.

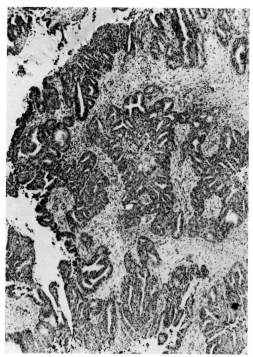

FIGURE 2-20 Metastatic adenocarcinoma of the endometrium in the vagina.

as,[258] and colon and rectum.[259] Metastases of renal clear cell carcinoma may be confused with primary vaginal clear cell carcinoma; the clinical history, tumor location, and ultrastructure are all useful distinguishing features. The metastasis may clinically precede the manifestation of the primary renal lesion.[256,260] Choriocarcinoma not frequently gives rise to blue, very hemorrhagic nodules, the growth of which may be extremely rapid. Uterine sarcomas, like endometrial carcinomas, have a high propensity for vaginal metastases. The prognosis is very poor in these disseminated lesions.

REFERENCES

1. Bulmer D: The development of the human vagina. J Anat 91:490–509, 1957
2. Forsberg JG: Cervicovaginal epithelium: Its origin and development. Am J Obstet Gynecol 115:1025–1043, 1973
3. Ulfelder H, Robboy SJ: The embryological development of the human vagina. Am J Obstet Gynecol 126:769–770, 1976
4. Robboy SJ, Taguchi O, Cunha GR: Normal development of the human female genital tract and alterations resulting from experimental exposure to diethylstilbestrol. Hum Pathol 13:190–197, 1982
5. Cunha GR: Epithelial-stromal interactions in development of the urogenital tract. Int Rev Cytol 47:137–194, 1976
6. Hammar SP, Bockus D, Remington F, Bartha M: The widespread distribution of Langerhans cells in pathologic tissues: An ultrastructural and immunohistochemical study. Hum Pathol 17:894–905, 1986

7. Birbeck MS, Breathnach AS, Everall JD: An electron microscopic study of basal melanocytes and high level clear cells (Langerhans' cell) in vitiligo. J Invest Dermatol 37:51–63, 1961
8. Way S: Primary carcinoma of the vagina. Br J Obstet Gynaecol 55:739–755, 1948
9. Krantz KE: Innervation of the human vulva and vagina. Obstet Gynecol 12:382, 1958
10. Evans TN, Polan ML, Boving RL: Vaginal malformations. Am J Obstet Gynecol 141:910–920, 1981
11. Leduc B, Van Campenhout J, Simard R: Congenital absence of the vagina. Am J Obstet Gynecol 100:512–520, 1968
12. Golditch IM: Vaginal aplasia. Surg Gynecol Obstet 129:361–367, 1969
13. Jones HW Jr, Mermut S: Familial occurrence of congenital absence of the vagina. Am J Obstet Gynecol 114:1100–1101, 1972
14. Jefferies JJ, Robboy SJ, O'Brien PC et al: Structural anomalies of the cervix and vagina in women enrolled in the diethylstilbestrol adenosis (DESAD) project. Am J Obstet Gynecol 148:59–66, 1984
15. Deppisch LM: Transverse vaginal septum: Histologic and embryologic considerations. Obstet Gynecol 39:193–198, 1972
16. Gregoire AT, Kandil O, Ledger WJ: Glycogen content of human vaginal epithelial tissue. Fertil Steril 22:64–68, 1971
17. Pouchet FA: Théorie positive de l'ovulation spontanée et de la fécondation des mammifères et de l'espèce humaine basée sur l'observation de toute la série animale. Paris, Baillière, 1847
18. Papanicolaou GN: New cancer diagnosis. In Proceedings of The Third Race Betterment Conference, p 528. Battle Creek, Michigan, Race Betterment Foundation, 1928
19. Papanicolaou GN: The sexual cycle in the human female as revealed by vaginal smear. Am J Anat 52:519–637, 1933
20. Papanicolaou GN, Traut HF, Marchetti AA: The epithelia of women's reproductive organs: A correlative study of cyclic changes. New York, Commonwealth Fund, 1948
21. Babes AA: Diagnostic du cancer du col uterin par les frottis. Presse Médicale 36:451–454, 1928
22. Gompel C: Atlas of diagnostic cytology. New York, John Wiley, 1978
23. Koss LG: Diagnostic cytology and its histopathologic bases, 4th ed. Philadelphia, JB Lippincott, 1992
24. Meisels A: Computed cytohormonal findings in 3307 healthy women. Acta Cytol 9:328–333, 1965
25. Pundel JP: Précis de colpocytologie hormonale. Paris, Masson et Cie, 1966
26. Wied GL (moderator): Symposium on hormonal cytology. Acta Cytol 12:87–92, 1968
27. Symposium on cytological terminology. Acta Cytol 2:26–27, 1958
28. Wied GL: Importance of the site from which vaginal smears are taken. Am J Clin Pathol 25:742–750, 1955
29. Meisels A: The maturation value. Acta Cytol 11:249, 1967
30. Heber KR: The effect of progestogens on vaginal cytology. Acta Cytol 19:103–109, 1975
31. Lichtfus C, Pundel JP, Gandar R: Le frottis vaginal à la fin de la grossesse. Gynécol Obstét 57:380–398, 1958
32. Von Haam E: The cytology of pregnancy. Acta Cytol 5:320–329, 1961
33. Sammour MB: Vaginal cytology during normal pregnancy: Its role in determination of the approximate date of confinement. Obstet Gynecol 24:682–690, 1964
34. Naib ZM: Single trophoblastic cells as a source of error in the interpretation of routine vaginal smears. Cancer 14:1183–1185, 1961
35. Danos ML, Holmquist ND: Cytologic evaluation of decidual cells: A report of two cases with false abnormal cytology. Acta Cytol 11:325–330, 1967
36. Schneider V, Barnes LA: Ectopic decidual reaction of the uterine cervix. Acta Cytol 25:616–622, 1981

37. Danos ML: Postpartum cytology: Observations over a four year period. Acta Cytol 12:309–312, 1968
38. Butler EB, Taylor DS: The postnatal smear. Acta Cytol 17:237–240, 1973
39. Symposium on androgenic effects. Acta Cytol 1:70–71, 1957
40. Hustin J, Van den Eynde JP: Cytologic evaluation of the effect of various estrogens given in post-menopause. Acta Cytol 21:225–228, 1977
41. Meisels A: The menopause: A cytohormonal study. Acta Cytol 10:49–55, 1966
42. Wied GL, Bibbo M, Keebler CM: Evaluation of the endocrinologic condition by exfoliative cytology. In Wied GL, Keebler CM, Koss LG, Reagan JW, eds. Compendium on diagnostic cytology, 6th ed. Chicago Tutorials on Cytology. Chicago, University of Chicago Press, 1988
43. Spiegel CA, Amsel R, Eschenbach D et al: Anaerobic bacteria in nonspecific vaginitis. N Engl J Med 303:601–607, 1980
44. Bibbo M, Harris MJ, Wied GL: Microbiology and inflammation of the female genital tract. In Wied GL, Keebler CM, Koss LG, Reagan JW, eds. Compendium on diagnostic cytology, 6th ed. Chicago Tutorials on Cytology. Chicago, University of Chicago Press, 1988
45. Eschenbach DA: Vaginal infections. Clin Obstet Gynecol 26:186–202, 1983
46. Blackwell A, Barlow D: Clinical diagnosis of anaerobic vaginosis (nonspecific vaginitis): A practical guide. Br J Vener Dis 58:387–393, 1982
47. Spiegel CA, Eschenbach DA, Amsel R, Holmes KK: Curved anaerobic bacteria in bacterial (nonspecific) vaginosis and their response to antimicrobial therapy. J Infect Dis 148:817–822, 1983
48. Osborne N, Grubin L, Pratson L: Vaginitis in sexually active women: Relationship to nine sexually transmitted organisms. Am J Obstet Gynecol 142:962–967, 1982
49. Van Der Meijden WT, Duivenvoorden HJ, Both-Patoir HC et al: Clinical and laboratory findings in women with bacterial vaginosis and trichomoniasis versus controls. Eur J Obstet Gynecol Reprod Biol 28:39–52, 1988
50. Fredricsson B, Englund K, Weintraub L et al: Bacterial vaginosis is not a simple ecological disorder. Gynecol Obstet Invest 28:156–160, 1989
51. Thomason JL, Gelbart SM, Anderson RJ et al: Statistical evaluation of diagnostic criteria for bacterial vaginosis. Am J Obstet Gynecol 162:155–160, 1990
52. Schneider GT, Geary WL: Vaginitis in adolescent girls. Clin Obstet Gynecol 14:1057–1076, 1971
53. Gardner HL, Dukes CD: Haemophilus vaginalis vaginitis: A newly defined specific infection previously classified as "nonspecific" vaginitis. Am J Obstet Gynecol 69:962–976, 1955
54. Greenwood JR, Pickett MJ: Transfer of *Haemophilus vaginalis* (Gardner and Dukes) to a new genus: *Gardnerella*. Int J Syst Bacteriol 30:170, 1980
55. Schnadig VJ, Davie KD, Shafer SK et al: The cytologist and bacterioses of the vaginal-ectocervical area: Clues, commas and confusion. Acta Cytol 33:287–297, 1988
56. Sobel JD: Epidemiology and pathogenesis of recurrent vulvovaginal candidiasis. Am J Obstet Gynecol 152:924, 1985
57. Monif GRG: Classification and pathogenesis of vulvovaginal candidiasis. Am J Obstet Gynecol 152:935–939, 1985
58. Odds FC: Candida and candidosis. Leicester, Leicester University Press, 1988
59. Horowitz BJ, Edelstein SW, Lippman L: *Candida tropicalis* vulvovaginitis. Obstet Gynecol 66:229–232, 1985
60. Agatensi L, Franchi F, Mondello F et al: Vaginopathic and proteolytic Candida species in outpatients attending a gynaecology clinic. J Clin Path 44:826–830, 1991
61. Merkus JMWM, Bishop MPJM, Stolte LAM: The proper nature of vaginal candidosis and the problem of recurrence. Obstet Gynecol Surv 40:493–503, 1985
62. Schnell M-A, Voigt WH: Are yeasts in vaginal smears intracellular or extracellular? Acta Cytol 20:343–346, 1976
63. Saw EC, Smale LE, Einstein H, Huntington RW: Female genital tract coccidioidomycosis. Obstet Gynecol 45:199–202, 1975
64. San Cristobal A, Roset S: Toxoplasma cysts in vaginal and cervical smears. Acta Cytol 20:285–286, 1976
65. Dryer ML, Young TL, Kaltine AA, Wilson DD: Blastomycosis in a Papanicolaou smear: Report of a case with a possible venereal transmission. Acta Cytol 27:285–287, 1983
66. Donné A: Animalicules observés dans les matières purulentes et le produit des sécrétions des organes génitaux de l'homme et de la femme. C R Acad Sci III (Paris) 3:385–386, 1836
67. Thomason JL, Gelbart SM: *Trichomonas vaginalis*. Obstet Gynecol 74:536–541, 1990
68. Gardner WA, Culberson DE, Bennett BD: *Trichomonas vaginalis* in the prostate gland. Arch Pathol Lab Med 110:430–432, 1986
69. Frost JK: *Trichomonas vaginalis* and cervical epithelial changes. Ann N Y Acad Sci 97:792–799, 1962
70. Kolstad P: The colposcopical picture of *Trichomonas* vaginitis. Acta Obstet Gynecol Scand: 43:388–398, 1964
71. Koss LG, Wolinska WH: *Trichomonas vaginalis* cervicitis and its relationship to cervical cancer: Histocytological study. Cancer 12:1171–1193, 1959
72. Chandra K, Annousamy R: An unusual finding in the vaginal smear. Acta Cytol 19:403, 1975
73. Bhambhani S: Egg of *Ascaris lumbricoides* in cervicovaginal smear. Acta Cytol 28:92, 1984
74. Bhambhani S, Milner A, Pant J, Luthra UK: Ova of *Taenia* and *Enterobius vermicularis* in cervicovaginal smears. Acta Cytol 29:913–914, 1985
75. Braga CA, Teoh TB: Amoebiasis of the cervix and the vagina. J Obstet Gynaecol Br Cwlth 71:299–301, 1964
76. Bellingham FR: Genital bilharzia: A report of 3 cases. Aust N Z J Obstet Gynaecol 12:267–268, 1972
77. Gardner HL: Desquamative inflammatory vaginitis: Newly defined entity. Am J Obstet Gynecol 102:1102–1105, 1968
78. Huguier PC: Mémoire sur les kystes de la matrice et sur les kystes folliculaires du vagin. Mém Soc Chirurgie de Paris 1:241–376, 1847
79. Gardner HL, Fernet P: Etiology of vaginitis emphysematosa: Report of ten cases and review of the literature. Am J Obstet Gynecol 88:680–694, 1964
80. Shenker L, Blaustein A: Emphysematous vaginitis: A theory of its pathogenesis and report of a case. Obstet Gynecol 22:295–300, 1963
81. Montanari GD, Marconato A, Montanari GR et al: Granulation tissue on the vault of the vagina after hysterectomy for cancer: Diagnostic problems. Acta Cytol 12:25–29, 1968
82. Barrett KF, Bledsoe S, Greer BE et al: Tampon-induced vaginal or cervical ulceration. Am J Obstet Gynecol 127:332–333, 1977
83. Friedrich EG, Siegesmund SK: Tampon associated vaginal ulcerations. Obstet Gynecol 55:149–156, 1980
84. Shands KN, Schmid GP, Dan BB et al: Toxic-shock syndrome in menstruating women: Association with tampon use and *Staphylococcus aureus* and clinical features in 52 cases. N Engl J Med 303:1436–1442, 1980
85. Fox H: The pathology of tampon usage and of the toxic shock syndrome. Postgrad Med J 61:31–33, 1985
86. Resnick SD: Toxic shock syndrome: Recent developments in pathogenesis. J Pediatr 116:321–328, 1990
87. Axiotis CA, Merino MJ, Duray PH: Langerhans cell histiocytosis of the female genital tract. Cancer 67:1650–1660, 1991
88. Junaid TA, Thomas SM: Cysts of the vulva and vagina: A comparative study. Int J Gynaecol Obstet 19:239, 1981
89. Hinchey WW, Silva EG, Guarda LA et al: Paravaginal wolffian duct (mesonephros) adenocarcinoma: A light and electron microscopic study. Am J Clin Pathol 80:539–544, 1983
90. Deppisch LM: Cysts of the vagina. Classification and clinical correlations. Obstet Gynecol 45:632–637, 1975

91. Evans DMD, Paine CG: Tumors of the vulva and vagina: Benign cysts and tumors of developmental origin. Clin Obstet Gynecol 8:997–1019, 1965

92. Pradhan S, Tobon H: Vaginal cysts: A clinicopathological study of 41 cases. Int J Gynecol Pathol 5:35–46, 1986

93. Tavassoli FA, Norris HJ: Smooth muscle tumors of the vagina. Obstet Gynecol 53:689–693, 1979

94. Dhaliwal LK, Das I, Gopalan S: Recurrent leiomyoma of the vagina. Int J Gynecol Pathol 37:281–283, 1992

95. Norris HJ, Taylor HB: Polyps of the vagina: A benign lesion resembling sarcoma botryoides. Cancer 19:227–232, 1966

96. Chirayil SJ, Tobon H: Polyps of the vagina: A clinicopathologic study of 18 cases. Cancer 47:2904–2907, 1981

97. Miettinen M, Wahlström T, Vesterinen E, Saksela E: Vaginal polyps with pseudosarcomatous features: A clinicopathologic study of seven cases. Cancer 51:1148–1151, 1983

98. Östör AG, Fortune DW, Riley CB: Fibroepithelial polyps with atypical stromal cells (pseudosarcoma botryoides) of vulva and vagina: A report of 13 cases. Int J Gynecol Pathol 7:351–360, 1988

99. Mucitelli DR, Charles EZ, Kraus FT: Vulvovaginal polyps: Histologic appearance, ultrastructure, immunocytochmical characteristics, and clinicopathologic correlations. Int J Gynecol Pathol 9:20–40, 1990

100. Al-Nafussi AI, Rebello G, Hughes D, Blessing K: Benign vaginal polyp: A histological, histochemical and immunohistochemical study of 20 polyps with comparison to normal vaginal subepithelial layer. Histopathology 20:145–150, 1992

101. Hartmann CA, Sperling M, Stein H: So-called fibroepithelial polyps of the vagina exhibiting an unusual but uniform antigen profile characterized by expression of desmin and steroid hormone receptors but no muscle-specific actin or macrophage markers. Am J Clin Pathol 93:604–608, 1990

102. Halvorsen TB, Johannesen E: Fibroepithelial polyps of the vagina: Are they old granulation tissue polyps? J Clin Pathol 45:235–240, 1992

103. Kapp K, Merino M, LiVolsi V: Adenocarcinoma of the vagina arising in endometriosis: Long-term survival following radiation therapy. Gynecol Oncol 14:271–278, 1982

104. Silverberg SG, Frable WJ: Tubal prolapse into vaginal vault after hysterectomy. Arch Pathol 97:100–103, 1974

105. Wheelock JB, Schneider V, Goplerud DR: Prolapsed fallopian tube masquerading as adenocarcinoma of the vagina in a postmenopausal woman. Gynecol Oncol 21:369–375, 1985

106. Proppe KH, Scully RE, Rosai J: Post-operative spindle cell nodules of the genitourinary tract resembling sarcomas: A report of eight cases. Am J Surg Pathol 8:101–108, 1984

107. Guillou L, Gloor E, DeGrandi P et al: Post-operative pseudosarcoma of the vagina: A case report. Pathol Res Pract 185:245–248, 1989

108. Robboy SJ, Hill EC, Sandberg EC, Czernobilsky B: Vaginal adenosis in women born prior to the diethylstilbestrol (DES) era. Hum Pathol 17:488–493, 1986

109. Scurry J, Planner R, Grant P: Unusual variants of vaginal adenosis: A challenge for diagnosis and treatment. Gynecol Oncol 41:172–177, 1991

110. Sandberg EC: The incidence and distribution of occult vaginal adenosis. Am J Obstet Gynecol 101:322–333, 1968

111. Herbst AL, Kurman RJ, Scully RE: Vaginal and cervical abnormalities after exposure to stilbestrol *in utero*. Obstet Gynecol 40:287–298, 1972

112. Sonek M, Bibbo M, Wied GL: Colposcopic findings in offsprings of DES-treated mothers as related to onset of therapy. J Reprod Med 16:65–71, 1976

113. Hansen K, Egholm M: Diffuse vaginal adenosis: Three cases with imperforate hymen and hematocolpos. Acta Obstet Gynecol Scand 54:287–292, 1975

114. Stafl A, Mattingly RF, Foley DV et al: Clinical diagnosis of vaginal adenosis. Obstet Gynecol 43:118–128, 1974

115. Sandberg EC: Benign cervical and vaginal changes associated with exposure to stilbestrol in utero. Am J Obstet Gynecol 125:777–789, 1976

116. Jefferies JJ, Robboy SJ, O'Brien PC et al: Structural anomalies of the cervix and vagina in women enrolled in the diethylstilbestrol adenosis (DESAD) project. Am J Obstet Gynecol 148:59–66, 1984

117. Antonioli DA, Burke L: Vaginal adenosis: Analysis of 325 biopsy specimens from 100 patients. Am J Clin Pathol 64:625–638, 1975

118. Robboy SJ, Kaufman RH, Prat J et al: Pathologic findings in young women enrolled in National Cooperative Diethylstilbestrol Adenosis (DESAD) Project. Obstet Gynecol 53:309–317, 1979

119. Fetherston WC: Squamous neoplasia of vagina related to DES syndrome. Am J Obstet Gynecol 122:176–181, 1975

120. Burke L, Antonioli D, Rosen S: Vaginal and cervical squamous cell dysplasia in women exposed to diethylstilbestrol in utero. Am J Obstet Gynecol 132:537–543, 1978

121. Noller KL, Townsend DE, Kaufman RH et al: Maturation of vaginal and cervical epithelium in women exposed in utero to diethylstilbestrol (DESAD project). Am J Obstet Gynecol 146:279–285, 1983

122. Bornstein J, Adam E, Adler-Storthz K, Kaufman RH: Development of cervical and vaginal squamous cell neoplasia as a late consequence of in utero exposure to diethylstilbestrol. Obstet Gynecol Surv 43:15–21, 1988

123. Vooijs PG, Ng AB, Wentz WB: The detection of vaginal adenosis and clear cell adenocarcinoma. Acta Cytol 17:59–63, 1973

124. Ng ABP, Reagan JW, Hawliczek S, Wentz WB: Cellular detection of vaginal adenosis. Obstet Gynecol 46:323–328, 1975

125. Bibbo M, Ali I, Al-Nageeb M et al: Cytologic findings in female and male offspring of DES treated mothers. Acta Cytol 19:568–572, 1975

126. Robboy SJ, Friedlander LM, Welch WR et al: Cytology of 575 young women with prenatal exposure to diethylstilbestrol. Obstet Gynecol 48:511–515, 1976

127. Hart WR, Zaharov J, Kaplan BJ et al: Cytologic findings in stilbestrol exposed females with emphasis on detection of vaginal adenosis. Acta Cytol 20:7–14, 1976

128. Robboy SJ: A hypothetic mechanism of diethylstilbestrol (DES)-induced anomalies in exposed progeny. Hum Pathol 14:831–833, 1983

129. Johnson LD, Palmer AE, King NW Jr, Hertig AT: Vaginal adenosis in *Cebus apella* monkeys exposed to DES in utero. Obstet Gynecol 57:629–635, 1981

130. Forsberg JG: Estrogen, vaginal cancer, and vaginal development. Am J Obstet Gynecol 113:83–87, 1972

131. Prins RP, Morrow CP, Townsend DE, DiSaia PJ: Vaginal embryogenesis, estrogens, and adenosis. Obstet Gynecol 48:246–250, 1976

132. Herbst AL, Norusis MJ, Rosenow PJ et al: An analysis of 346 cases of clear cell adenocarcinoma of the vagina and cervix with an emphasis on recurrence and survival. Gynecol Oncol 7:111–112, 1979

133. Sedlacek TV, Riva JM, Magen AB et al: Vaginal and vulvar adenosis: An unsuspected side-effect of carbon dioxide laser vaporization. J Reprod Med 35:995–1001, 1990

134. Goodman A, Zukerberg LR, Nikrui N, Scully RE: Vaginal adenosis and clear cell carcinoma after 5-fluorouracil treatment for condyloma. Cancer 68:1628–1632, 1991

135. Robboy SJ, Noller KL, O'Brien P et al: Increased incidence of cervical and vaginal dysplasia in 3,980 diethylstilbestrol-exposed young women: Experience of the National Collaborative Diethylstilbestrol Adenosis Project. JAMA 252:2979–2983, 1984

136. Robboy SJ, Keh PC, Nickerson RJ et al: Squamous cell dysplasia and carcinoma in situ of the cervix and vagina after prenatal exposure to diethylstilbestrol. Obstet Gynecol 51:528–535, 1978

137. Robboy SJ, Szyfelbein WM, Goellner JR: Dysplasia and cytologic findings in 4,589 young women enrolled in diethyl-

stilbestrol-adenosis (DESAD) project. Am J Obstet Gynecol 140:579–585, 1981

138. Robboy SJ, Prat J, Welch WR et al: Squamous cell neoplasia controversy in the female exposed to diethylstilbestrol. Hum Pathol 8:483–485, 1977

139. Turiel J, Wingard DL: Immune response in DES-exposed women. Fertil Steril 49:928, 1988

140. Noller KL, Blair PB, O'Brien PC et al: Increased occurrence of autoimmune disease among women exposed in utero to diethylstilbestrol. Fertil Steril 49:1080–1082, 1988

141. Robboy SJ, Welch WR: Microglandular hyperplasia in vaginal adenosis associated with oral contraceptives and prenatal diethylstilbestrol exposure. Obstet Gynecol 49:430–434, 1977

142. Bartsch F: Drei Fälle von Haemangioma cavernosum Vaginae in der Schwangerschaft. Zentralbl Gynaekol 81:453–458, 1959

143. Leone PG, Taylor HB: Ultrastructure of a benign polypoid rhabdomyoma of the vagina. Cancer 31:1414–1417, 1973

144. Gold BM: Neurofibromatosis of the bladder and vagina. Am J Obstet Gynecol 113:1055–1056, 1972

145. Pezeshkpour G: Solitary paraganglioma of the vagina. Report of a case. Am J Obstet Gynecol 139:219–221, 1981

146. Kurman RJ, Prabha AC: Thyroid and parathyroid glands in the vaginal wall: Report of a case. Am J Clin Pathol 59:503–507, 1973

147. Tobon H, Murphy AI: Benign nevus of the vagina. Cancer 40:3174–3176, 1977

148. Chen KTK: Brenner tumor of the vagina. Diagn Gynecol Obstet 3:255–258, 1981

149. Buntine DW, Henderson PR, Biggs JGS: Benign müllerian mixed tumor of the vagina. Gynecol Oncol 8:21–26, 1979

150. Sirota RL, Dickersin GR, Scully RE: Mixed tumors of the vagina: A clinicopathological analysis of eight cases. Am J Surg Pathol 5:413–422, 1981

151. Wright RG, Buntine DW, Forbes KL: Recurrent benign mixed tumor of the vagina: Case report. Gynecol Oncol 40:84–86, 1991

152. Bivens MD: Primary carcinoma of the vagina: A report of forty-six cases. Am J Obstet Gynecol 65:390–399, 1953

153. Timonen S, von Numers C, Meyer B: Dysplasia of the vaginal epithelium. Gynecologia 162:125–138, 1966

154. Lenehan PM, Meffe F, Lickrish M: Vaginal intraepithelial neoplasia: Biologic aspects and management. Obstet Gynecol 68:333–337, 1986

155. Aho M, Vesterinen E, Meyer B et al: Natural history of vaginal intraepithelial neoplasia. Cancer 68:195–197, 1991

156. Woodruff JD: Carcinoma in situ of the vagina. Clin Obstet Gynecol 2:485–501, 1981

157. Brinton A, Nasca PC, Mallin K et al: Case-control study of in situ and invasive carcinoma of the vagina. Gynecol Oncol 38:49–54, 1990

158. Schrager LK, Friedland GH, Maude D et al: Cervical and vaginal squamous cell abnormalities in women infected with human immunodeficiency virus. J AIDS 2:570–575, 1989

159. Gallup DG, Morley GW: Carcinoma in situ of the vagina: A study and review. Obstet Gynecol 46:334–340, 1975

160. Hernandez-Linares W, Puthawala A, Nolan JF: Carcinoma in situ of the vagina: Past and present management. Obstet Gynecol 56:356–359, 1980

161. Punnonen R, Grönroos M, Meurman L, Liukko P: Diagnosis and treatment of primary vaginal carcinoma in situ and dysplasia. Acta Obstet Gynecol Scand 60:513, 1981

162. Audet-Lapointe P, Body G, Vauclair R et al: Vaginal intraepithelial neoplasia. Gynecol Oncol 36:232–239, 1990

163. Okagaki T, Twiggs LB, Zachow KR et al: Identification of human papillomavirus DNA in cervical and vaginal intraepithelial neoplasia with molecularly cloned virus-specific DNA probes. Int J Gynecol Pathol 2:153–159, 1983

164. Bornstein J, Kaufman RH, Adam E, Adler-Storthz K: Human papillomavirus associated with vaginal intraepithelial neoplasia in women exposed to diethylstilbestrol in utero. Obstet Gynecol 70:75–80, 1987

165. Bowen-Simpkins P, Hull MGR: Intraepithelial vaginal neoplasia following immunosuppressive therapy treated with topical 5-FU. Obstet Gynecol 46:360–362, 1975

166. Eddy GL, Singh KP, Gansler TS: Superficially invasive carcinoma of the vagina following treatment for cervical cancer: A report of six cases. Gynecol Oncol 36:376–379, 1990

167. Peters WA, Kumar NB, Morley GW: Microinvasive carcinoma of the vagina: A distinct clinical entity? Am J Obstet Gynecol 153:505–507, 1985

168. Spitzer M, Chernys AE, Hischfield L et al: Assessment of criteria used in the histologic diagnosis of human papillomavirus-related disease of the female lower genital tract. Gynecol Oncol 38:105–109, 1990

169. Aho M, Vesterinen E, Meyer B et al: Natural history of vaginal intraepithelial neoplasia. Cancer 68:195–197, 1991

170. Bourg R, Gompel C, Pundel JP: Diagnostic cytologique du cancer génital chez la femme. Paris, Desoer, Liège, Masson et Cie, 1954

171. Wentz WB, Reagan JW: Clinical significance of post-irradiation dysplasia of uterine cervix. Am J Obstet Gynecol 106:812–817, 1970

172. Fujimura M, Ostrow RS, Okagaki T: Implication of human papillomavirus in postirradiation dysplasia. Cancer 68:2181–2185, 1991

173. Okagaki T, Meyer AA, Sciarra JJ: Prognosis of irradiated carcinoma of cervix uteri and nuclear DNA in cytologic postirradiation dysplasia. Cancer 33:647–652, 1974

174. Benedet JL, Murphy KJ, Fairey RN, Boyes DA: Primary invasive carcinoma of the vagina. Obstet Gynecol 62:715, 1983

175. Johnston GA, Klotz J, Boutselis JG: Primary invasive carcinoma of the vagina. Surg Gynecol Obstet 156:34, 1983

176. Andersen ES: Primary carcinoma of the vagina: A study of 29 cases. Gynecol Oncol 33:317–320, 1989

177. Manetta A, Gutrecht EL, Berman ML, Di Saia PJ: Primary invasive carcinoma of the vagina. Obstet Gynecol 76:639–642, 1990

178. Davis KP, Stanhope CR, Garton GR et al: Invasive vaginal carcinoma: Analysis of early-stage disease. Gynecol Oncol 42:131–136, 1991

179. Henson D, Tarone R: An epidemiologic study of cancer of the cervix, vagina, and vulva based on the Third National Cancer Survey in the United States. Am J Obstet Gynecol 129:525–532, 1977

180. Choo YC, Anderson DG: Neoplasms of the vagina following cervical carcinoma. Gynecol Oncol 14:125–132, 1982

181. Yokoyama Y, Wada A: Vaginal involvement of early carcinoma of the cervix uteri. Acta Obstet Gynaecol Jap 18:65–73, 1971

182. Ikenberg H, Runge M, Goppinger A, Pfleiderer A: Human papillomavirus DNA in invasive carcinoma of the vagina. Obstet Gynecol 76:432–438, 1990

183. Faber K, Jones M, Tarraza HM: Invasive squamous cell carcinoma of the vagina in a diethylstilbestrol-exposed woman. Gynecol Oncol 37:125–128, 1990

184. Ball HG, Berman ML: Management of primary vaginal carcinoma. Gynecol Oncol 14:154–163, 1982

185. Ramzy I, Smout MS, Collins JA: Verrucous carcinoma of the vagina. Am J Clin Pathol 65:644–653, 1976

186. Crowther MG, Lowe AG, Shepherd JH: Verrucous carcinoma of the female genital tract: A review. Obstet Gynecol Surv 43:263–280, 1988

187. Mawad RM, Latour JPA: Primary adenocarcinoma of the vagina. Obstet Gynecol 44:889–893, 1974

188. Kaminski PF, Maier RC: Clear cell adenocarcinoma of the cervix unrelated to diethylstilbestrol exposure. Obstet Gynecol 62:720–727, 1983

189. Yaghsezian H, Palazzo JP, Finkel GC et al: Primary vaginal adenocarcinoma of the intestinal type associated with adenosis. Gynecol Oncol 45:62–65, 1992

190. Yousem HL: Adenocarcinoma of Gartner's duct cyst pre-

senting as a vaginal lesion: A case report. Sinai Hosp J 10:112, 1961

191. Hinchey WW, Silva EG, Guarda LA et al: Paravaginal wolffian duct (mesonephros) adenocarcinoma: A light and electron microscopic study. Am J Clin Pathol 80:539–544, 1983

192. Herbst AL, Ulfelder H, Poskanzer DC: Adenocarcinoma of the vagina. N Engl J Med 284:878–881, 1971

193. Herbst AL, Kurman RJ, Scully RE, Poskanzer DC: Clear-cell adenocarcinoma of the genital tract in young females: Registry report. N Engl J Med 287:1259–1264, 1972

194. Kinlen LJ, Badaracco MA, Moffett J, Vessey MP: A survey of the use of estrogens during pregnancy in the United Kingdom and of the genitourinary cancer mortality and incidence rates in young people in England and Wales. Br J Obstet Gynaecol 81:849–855, 1974

195. Turiel JS: Social impact of diethylstilbestrol exposure on women in the United States. Clin Pract Gynecol 2:125–140, 1990

196. Melnick S, Cole P, Anderson D, Herbst A: Rates and risks of diethylstilbestrol-related clear cell adenocarcinoma of the vagina and the cervix. N Engl J Med 316:514–516, 1987

197. Herbst AL, Cole P, Norusis MJ et al: Epidemiologic aspects and factors related to survival in 384 registry cases of clear cell adenocarcinoma of the vagina and cervix. Am J Obstet Gynecol 135:876–886, 1979

198. Sharp GB, Cole P, Anderson D, Herbst AL: Clear cell adenocarcinoma of the lower genital tract: Correlation of mother's recall of diethylstilbestrol history with obstetrical records. Cancer 66:2215–2220, 1990

199. Herbst AL: Clear cell adenocarcinoma and the current status of DES-exposed females. Cancer 48:484–488, 1981

200. Lanier AP, Noller KL, Decker D et al: Cancer and stilbestrol: A follow-up of 1,719 persons exposed to estrogens in utero and born 1943–1959. Mayo Clin Proc 48:793–799, 1973

201. Vessey MP: Epidemiological studies of the effects of diethylstilbestrol. In Napalkov NP, Rice JM, Tomatis L, Yamasaki H. Perinatal and multigeneration carcinogenesis, pp 335–348. Lyon, International Agency for Research on Cancer, 1989

202. Puri S, Fenoglio CM, Richart RM et al: Clear cell carcinoma of cervix and vagina in progeny of women who received DES: Three cases with scanning and transmission electron microscopy. Am J Obstet Gynecol 128:550–555, 1977

203. Robboy SJ, Scully RE, Welch WR et al: Intrauterine DES exposure and its consequences: Pathologic characteristics of vaginal adenosis, clear cell adenocarcinoma, and related lesions. Arch Pathol Lab Med 101:1–5, 1977

204. Gompel C, Horanyi Z, Simonet ML: Ultrastructure of clear cell carcinoma of the vagina and the cervix: Report of a case with unusual ultrastructural findings. Acta Cytol 20:262–265, 1976

205. Silverberg SG, DeGiorgi LS: Clear cell carcinoma of the vagina: A clinical, pathologic and electron microscopic study. Cancer 29:1680–1690, 1971

206. Dickersin GR, Welch WR, Erlandson R, Robboy SJ: Ultrastructure of 16 cases of clear cell adenocarcinoma of the vagina and cervix in young women. Cancer 45:1615–1624, 1980

207. Fu YS, Reagan JW, Richart RM et al: Nuclear DNA and histologic studies of genital lesions in diethylstilbestrol-exposed progeny. II. Intraepithelial glandular abnormalities. Am J Clin Pathol 72:515–520, 1979

208. Cullimore JE, Luesley DM, Rollason TP et al: A case of glandular intraepithelial neoplasia involving the cervix and vagina. Gynecol Oncol 34:249–252, 1989

209. Roberts DK, Walker NJ, Parmley TH, Horbelt DV: Interaction of epithelial and stromal cells in vaginal adenosis. Hum Pathol 19:855–861, 1988

210. Sander R, Nuss RC, Rhatigan RM: Diethylstilbestrol-associ-

ated vaginal adenosis followed by clear cell adenocarcinoma. Int J Gynecol Pathol 5:362–370, 1986

211. Robboy SJ, Welch WR, Young RH et al: Topographic relation of adenosis, clear cell adenocarcinoma and other related lesions of the vagina and cervix in DES progeny. Obstet Gynecol 60:546–551, 1982

212. Robboy SJ, Welch WR: Selected topics in the pathology of the vagina. Hum Pathol 22:868–876, 1991

213. Robboy SJ, Young RH, Welch WR et al: Atypical vaginal adenosis and cervical ectropion: Association with clear cell adenocarcinoma in diethylstilbestrol-exposed offspring. Cancer 54:869–875, 1984

214. Fu YS, Reagan JW, Richart RM, Townsend DE. Nuclear DNA and histologic studies of genital lesions in diethylstilbestrol-exposed progeny. II. Intraepithelial glandular abnormalities. Am J Clin Pathol 72:515–20, 1979

215. Taft PD, Robboy SL, Herbst AL et al: Cytology of clear cell adenocarcinoma of genital tract in young females: Review of 95 cases from the Registry. Acta Cytol 18:279–290, 1974

216. Hanselaar AGJM, Van Leusen NDM, De Wilde PCM, Vooijs GP: Clear cell adenocarcinoma of the vagina and the cervix: A report of the Central Netherlands Registry with emphasis on early detection and prognosis. Cancer 67:1971–1978, 1991

217. Prasad CJ, Ray JA, Kessler S: Primary small cell carcinoma of the vagina arising in a background of atypical adenosis. Cancer 70:2484–2487, 1992

218. Ray J, Ireland K: Non-clear cell adenocarcinoma arising in vaginal adenosis. Arch Pathol Lab Med 109:781–783, 1985

219. Kapp DS, Merino M, LiVolsi V: Adenocarcinoma of the vagina arising in endometriosis: Long-term survival following radiation therapy. Gynecol Oncol 14:271–278, 1982

220. Granai CO, Walters MD, Safaii H et al: Malignant transformation of vaginal endometriosis. Obstet Gynecol 64:592, 1984

221. Norris HJ, Bagley GP, Taylor HB: Carcinoma of the infant vagina—a distinctive tumor. Arch Pathol 90:473–479, 1970

222. Allyn DL, Silverberg SG, Salzberg AM: Endodermal sinus tumor of the vagina: Report of a case with 7-year survival and literature review of so-called "mesonephroma." Cancer 27:1231–1238, 1971

223. Rezaizadeh MM, Woodruff JD: Endodermal sinus tumor of the vagina. Gynecol Oncol 6:459–463, 1978

224. SenGupta SK, Murthy DP, Martin WM, Klufio C: A rare case of endodermal sinus tumour of the vagina in an infant. Aust N Z J Obstet Gynaecol 31:381–382, 1991

225. Malkasian GD, Welcht JS, Soule EH: Primary leiomyosarcoma of the vagina: Report of 8 cases. Am J Obstet Gynecol 86:730–736, 1963

226. Timonenbon H, Murphy AL, Salazar H: Primary leiomyosarcoma of the vagina: Light and electron microscopic observations. Cancer 32:450–457, 1973

227. Tavassoli FA, Norris HJ: Smooth muscle tumors of the vagina. Obstet Gynecol 53:689–693, 1979

228. Peters WA III, Kumar NB, Anderson WA, Morley GW. Primary sarcoma of the adult vagina: A clinicopathologic study. Obstet Gynecol 65:699–704, 1985

229. Prempree T, Tang CK, Hatef A, Forster S: Angiosarcoma of the vagina. Cancer 51:618–622, 1983

230. Tohya T, Katabuchi H, Fukuma K et al: Angiosarcoma of the vagina: A light and electron microscopy study. Acta Obstet Gynecol Scand 70:169–172, 1991

231. Kasai K, Yoshida Y, Okumura M: Alveolar soft part sarcoma in the vagina: Clinical features and morphology. Gynecol Oncol 9:227–236, 1980

232. Okagaki T, Ishida T, Hilgers RD: A malignant tumor of the vagina resembling synovial sarcoma: A light and electron microscopic study. Cancer 37:2306–2320, 1976

233. Salm R: Botryoid sarcoma of the vagina. Br J Cancer 15:220–225, 1961

234. Friedman M, Peretz BA, Nissenbaum M, Paldi E: Modern

treatment of vaginal embryonal rhabdomyosarcoma. Obstet Gynecol Surv 41:614–8, 1986

235. Hays DM, Shimada H, Raney RB et al: Clinical staging and treatment results in rhabdomyosarcoma of the female genital tract among children and adolescents. Cancer 61:1893–903, 1988

236. Hilgers RD, Malkasian GD Jr, Soule EH: Embryonal rhabdomyosarcoma (botryoid type) of the vagina. Am J Obstet Gynecol 107:484–502, 1970

237. Kindblom I, Eidal T, Karlsson K: Immunohistochemical localization of myoglobin in human muscle tissue and embryonal and alveolar rhabdomyosarcoma. Acta Pathol Microbiol Immunol Scand (A) 90:2167, 1982

238. Altmansberger M, Osborne M, Treuner J et al: Diagnosis of human childhood rhabdomyosarcoma by antibodies to desmin: The structural protein of muscle specific intermediate filaments. Virchows Arch B Cell Pathol 39:203–315, 1982

239. Di Sant'Agnese PA, Knowles DM II: Extracardiac rhabdomyoma: A clinicopathologic study and review of the literature. Cancer 46:780–789, 1980

240. Hanski W, Hagel-Lewicka E, Daniszewski K: Rhabdomyomas of female genital tract: Report on two cases. Zentralbl Pathol 137:439–442, 1991

241. Hasumi K, Sakamoto G, Sugano H et al: Primary malignant melanoma of the vagina: Study of four autopsy cases with ultrastructural findings. Cancer 42:2675–2686, 1978

242. Leer B, Buttoni L, Dhru K, Tamini H: Malignant melanoma of the vagina: A case report of progression from preexisting melanosis. Gynecol Oncol 19:238–245, 1984

243. Chung AF, Casey MJ, Flannery JT et al: Malignant melanoma of the vagina: Report of 19 cases. Obstet Gynecol 55:720–727, 1980

244. Levitan Z, Gordon AN, Kaplan AL, Kaufman RH: Primary malignant melanoma of the vagina: Report of four cases and review of the literature. Gynecol Oncol 33:85–90, 1989

245. Borazjani G, Prem KA, Okagaki T et al: Primary malignant melanoma of the vagina: A clinicopathological analysis of 10 cases. Gynecol Oncol 37:264–267, 1990

246. Breslow A: Tumor thickness, level of invasion and node dissection in stage I cutaneous melanoma. Ann Surg 182:572–575, 1975

247. Chafe W: Neuroepithelial small cell carcinoma of the vagina. Cancer 64:1948–1951, 1989

248. Ulich TR, Liao SY, Layfield L et al: Endocrine and tumor differentiation markers in poorly differentiated small-cell carcinoids of the cervix and vagina. Arch Pathol Lab Med 110:1054–1057, 1986

249. Doss LL: Simultaneous extramedullary plasmacytomas of the vagina and vulva: A case report and review of the literature. Cancer 41:2468–2474, 1978

250. Osanto S, Van Der Valk P, Meijer CJLM et al: Solitary plasmacytoma of the vagina. Acta Haematol 66:140–144, 1981

251. Prevot S, Hugol D, Audouin J et al: Primary non Hodgkin's malignant lymphoma of the vagina: Report of 3 cases with review of the literature. Pathol Res Pract 188:78–85, 1992

252. Naves AE, Monti JA, Chichoni E: Basal-cell like carcinoma in the upper third of the vagina. Am J Obstet Gynecol 137:136–137, 1980

253. Shevchuk MM, Fenoglio CM, Lattes R et al: Malignant mixed tumor of the vagina probably arising in mesonephric rests. Cancer 42:214–223, 1978

254. Marchetti DL, Piver MS, Tsukada Y, Reese P: Prevention of vaginal recurrence of stage I endometrial adenocarcinoma with postoperative vaginal radiation. Obstet Gynecol 67:399, 1986

255. Lifshitz S, Newland WH, Dolan TE et al: Ovarian carcinoma presenting as a vaginal lesion. JAMA 239:1788–1789, 1978

256. Sogani PC, Whitmore WF Jr: Solitary vaginal metastasis from unsuspected renal cell carcinoma. J Urol 121:95–97, 1979

257. Pineda A, Sall S: Metastasis to the vagina from carcinoma of the breast. J Reprod Med 20:243–245, 1978

258. Weitzner S, Dressner SA: Vaginal metastasis from adenocarcinoma of the pancreas. Ann Surg 40:256–258, 1974

259. Raider L: Remote vaginal metastases from carcinoma of the colon. Am J Roentgen Rad Ther Nucl Med 97:944–950, 1966

260. Mazur MT, Hsueh S, Gersell DJ: Metastases to the female genital tract: Analysis of 325 cases. Cancer 53:1978–1984, 1984

Pathology in Gynecology and Obstetrics, Fourth Edition, edited by Claude Gompel and Steven G. Silverberg. J. B. Lippincott Company, Philadelphia © 1994.

3 | *The Cervix*

The frequent morphologic alterations of inflammatory, hormonal, or tumorous origin in the uterine cervix constitute a vast field of clinicopathologic investigation that has been greatly exploited since the beginning of this century. These studies are of value to us notably with respect to the early diagnosis of cancer, knowledge of the extremely varied pictures of cervical infections, and discovery of new histologic and clinical concepts such as the entities of dysplasia and in situ carcinoma. The study of the uterine cervix has been of general interest and has led, for example, to the investigation of intraepithelial cancers of other organs, such as the bronchus, the larynx, and the stomach. The role of viruses in the early stages of carcinogenesis of solid tumors has been studied in greatest detail in the cervix. These few remarks serve to illuminate the important position of the cervix in pathologic anatomy.

EMBRYOLOGY

The uterine cervix is of mesodermal origin. It arises from the fusion of the middle portions of the müllerian ducts; the adjacent mesenchyme gives rise to the connective tissue stroma and muscle fibers. The stratified squamous epithelium of the ectocervix originates from the epithelium of the primitive uterine canal derived from the urogenital sinus.[1] The glandular epithelium becomes mucus-producing by metaplasia from the primitive cuboidal epithelium derived from the müllerian ducts. During the late fetal and neonatal period, the junction between the two epithelia is located on the ectocervix; this ectropion may be the result of maternal hormonal stimulation.[2] The cervical stroma is invaded by straight glands issuing from the surface epithelium; these glands ramify secondarily.

ANATOMY

The cervix has a more or less cylindrical shape and forms the inferior third of the uterus. Its lowest part, known as the *portio vaginalis*, projects into the vagina. The external os represents the junction between the portio and the endocervical canal, which itself communicates with the endometrial cavity at the internal os.[3] The average length of the cervix is about 3 cm, its diameter at the base is 3 cm, and its inferior diameter is from 2.5 to 3 cm. It represents a fibromuscular structure covered by a mucosa. The internal surface is covered by rugae directed obliquely toward the upper portion, originating from an anterior and a posterior longitudinal fold. The vascularization issues from branches of the uterovaginal artery and the vaginal artery (a branch of the hypogastric artery).[4] The cervix is innervated by the uterine plexus and contains sensory fibers.[5] The lymphatics from the superficial and deep stroma collect into different channels, which run to the iliac, hypogastric, obturator, and sacral nodes.

HISTOLOGY

The cervix comprises two distinct parts. The *ectocervix* is covered by a stratified squamous epithelium that overlies a dense fibrous stroma.[6–9] The *endocervix* is covered by an unistratified columnar mucosa resting on a stroma rich in mucus-secreting glands. Fluhmann[10] has demonstrated that these glands are actually clefts issuing from the surface mucosa.

The *squamous ectocervical epithelium* is composed of basal, intermediate, and superficial cell layers identical to those of the vaginal mucosa. Five layers are recognizable (Fig. 3-1).

The *basal layer (C1)* is in contact with the basement membrane; this is the reserve cell layer. The cells are oriented perpendicular to the basal lamina and normally exhibit mitotic figures because they constitute the reproductive cells of the epithelium. The enzymes phosphorylase and amylo-1,6-glucosidase, required for glycogen synthesis, are localized in these cells.

Layer C2 consists of two or three rows of parabasal cells; this is the most rapidly proliferative layer. *Layer C3* is characterized by the presence of glycogen[11] (manifested by clear cytoplasm) and the development of intercellular bridges (desmosomes). *Layer C4* is rich in glycogen, and the intercellular bridges begin to disappear; it does not contain eleidin granules like its cutaneous equivalent.

The *superficial layer (C5)* contains large cells with pyknotic nuclei. Eosinophilia of the cytoplasm is related to the presence of keratin microfilaments.[12] Immunohistochemistry reveals the existence of 19 different cytokeratins.[13,14]

The *endocervical muciparous columnar epithelium* is composed of tall cells with elongated basal nuclei and occasional ciliated cells (Figs. 3-2 and 3-3 and Color Fig. 3-1). This mucosa penetrates into the stroma, where it gives rise to glands lined by columnar cells with abundant clear cytoplasm and basal nuclei.[15]

The cervical stroma is dense and comprises fascicles of fusiform connective tissue cells, collagenous and elastic fibers, and scattered smooth muscle fibers. The latter are more numerous in the superior part of the cervix, where they constitute about 15% of the stromal elements. A narrow subepithelial myxoid zone may be present. The stroma does not undergo cyclic histologic modifications such as those of the endometrial stroma.

The junction of the two epithelia occurs normally at the level of the external os by direct contact or more frequently by a transformation zone of metaplastic squamous epithelium (squamocolumnar junction or transformation zone).[16]

The schema adapted from Ober[17] indicates the different modes of junction encountered (Fig. 3-4). During the period of genital activity, the endocervical mucosa tends to extend toward the external cervical orifice (ectopy or ectropion). Before puberty and after ovarian activity ceases, the glandular epithelium is pushed back into the endocervical canal by the squamous ectocervical epithelium (entropion,

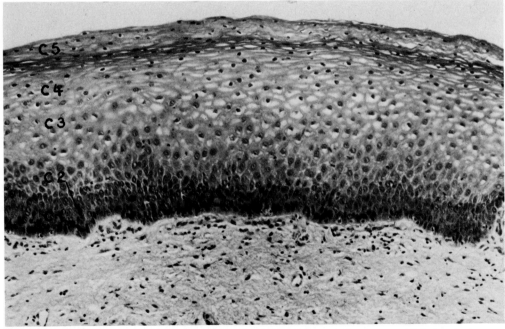

FIGURE 3-1 Normal squamous mucosa of ectocervix: C1, deep layer in contact with basement membrane; C2, parabasal layer constituted by two or three rows of cells; C3, intermediate layer rich in glycogen; C4, layer rich in glycogen and showing beginning disappearance of intercellular bridges; and C5, superficial layer with pyknotic nuclei.

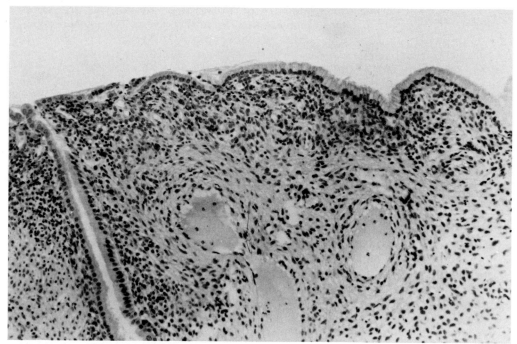

FIGURE 3-2 Endocervical columnar mucosa.

Fig. 3-5).[18,19] The clinical significance is that in post-menopausal women, intraepithelial and invasive squamous carcinomas are seen in the endocervical canal.

The squamous mucosa presents the same hormonal modifications as the vaginal mucosa and undergoes cyclic keratinization in relation to estrogenic activity. It contains glycogen, particularly in the intermediate cell layers (navicular cells). The maturation cycle of the squamous cell takes about 4 days.

With regard to the endocervical glandular mucosa, cyclic modifications are discrete. Wollner[20] has described in the estrogenic phase of the cycle an augmentation of cellular proliferation and of the number of papillary projections of the mucosa. It must be admitted that the endocervical mucosa, although of müllerian origin like the vaginal and endometrial mucosae, reacts only discretely to genital hormonal stimulation. On the contrary, the secretion of glandular cells constitutes the cervical mucous gel and exhibits cyclic variations. The secretion is abundant and alkaline, and it facilitates the penetration of spermatozoa during the estrogenic phase; it is scant, acid, and thick after ovulation, thus hindering sperm migration. Biochemical and electron microscopic studies have revealed the complex structure of the mucous gel.[8] It is composed of a micellar network of glycoproteins in which the intermicellar spaces are occupied by cervical plasma. Crystallization of the mucus is favored by the presence of potassium and sodium chloride ions. The parallel orientation of the glycoprotein micelles during the estrogenic phase fa-

vors sperm migration. This orientation disappears during the progestational phase.

Electron microscopy shows that the endocervical cell cytoplasm contains numerous clear vacuoles related to mucous secretion, as well as filamentous structures of still unknown function (see Fig. 3-3).

The squamocolumnar junction or transformation zone shows the presence of Langerhans cells dispersed among the squamous cells.[21–23] These cells have a vesicular nucleus surrounded by a clear cytoplasm. Their presence can be demonstrated immunohistochemically by the use of monoclonal antibodies to S-100 protein. Langerhans cells are of bone marrow origin and are involved in local immune mechanisms.[24] They form part of the system of mucosal-associated lymphoid tissue similar to that found in other mucosae exposed to the external environment. Their activity is influenced by clinical circumstances such as the presence of human papillomavirus or the existence of cervical intraepithelial neoplasia.[25]

Atypical Ectodermal and Mesodermal Structures

On rare occasions, ectodermal and mesodermal structures have been described in the cervix. Ectodermal structures include hair follicles, sweat glands, and sebaceous glands. Two explanations are proposed: (1) under appropriate stimuli, adult mesodermal tissue is able to form epidermis and epidermal appendages, or (2) misplaced ectodermal embryonal precursors after an abnormal cephalic

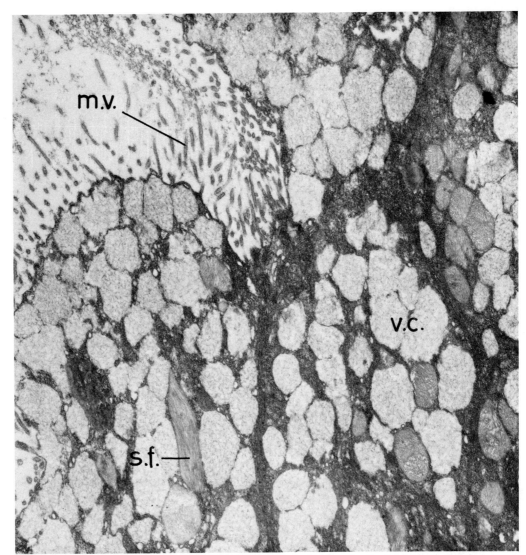

FIGURE 3-3 Electron micrograph (×22,050) of endocervical mucosal cells showing cytoplasmic clear vacuoles of mucin secretion (*v.c.*) and filamentous structures (*s.f.*), with microvilli bordering the apical poles of the cells (*m.v.*).

migration remain in the cervical region. The former theory seems more probable and may represent a metaplastic phenomenon.[26] Atypical localization of mesodermal tissue such as cartilage has been reported in the cervix.[27] This has no clinical significance.

Mesonephric Remnants

Mesonephric remnants representing the distal end of the mesonephric ducts are present in about 1% of cervices.[28] They consist of small tubules or cysts lined by a cuboidal or flattened nonciliated epithe-

FIGURE 3-4 Schematic drawing of the different modes of junction between the squamous and columnar epithelia of the cervix. (Adapted from Ober KG: Les variations morphologiques du col durant la vie de la femme. Bull Soc Belge Gynécol Obstét 28:203–213, 1958).

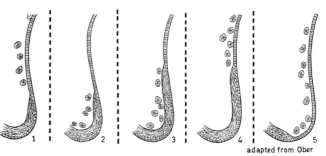

adapted from Ober

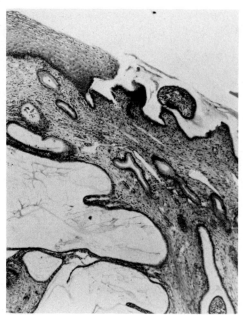

FIGURE 3-5 Zone of squamocolumnar junction and nabothian cysts.

lium and are located in the lateral cervical walls.[28–30] The absence of mucin or glycogen is characteristic of the mesonephric epithelium. Rare cases of adenocarcinoma arising in the lateral wall and consisting of nonmucinous structures have been considered to be related to a mesonephric origin.[28,31]

Histologic Appearance During Pregnancy

The histologic appearance of the cervix is modified during pregnancy.[32,33] The squamous epithelium shows an increase in thickness and hyperactivity of the basal cells manifested by the appearance of supplementary basal cell layers. This hyperplasia only partially involves the epithelium, leaving intact rows of differentiated cells at the surface. When dyspolarity, cellular atypia, and full-thickness epithelial immaturity are seen, these changes should not be attributed to pregnancy but rather to a dysplastic or neoplastic condition.

The endocervical glands also manifest hyperplastic phenomena, accompanied sometimes by squamous metaplasia (Fig. 3-6A). According to Fluhmann,[10] these glands, which actually represent infoldings of endocervical mucosa, will present new and more pronounced invaginations in the course of pregnancy (tunnel clusters). Secretory activity of the cells is augmented, and the apical pole, filled with mucin, presents a bulging appearance. This important proliferation of endocervical mucin-secreting cells results in eversion of the endocervical mucosa into the exocervix, pushing the squamous epithelium away from the external os. This ectropion is a common feature in the primigravida, with eventual secondary erosion of the fragile epithelium. Healing

by replacement with squamous epithelium is the rule after pregnancy. Positive immunoreactivity with S-100 protein has been found in cervical glands during pregnancy.[34]

More marked *microglandular* endocervical hyperplasia (see below) may also occur. It is also observed in patients using oral contraceptives[35] and rarely after menopause.[36] Correlation with a high level of progesterone activity is postulated.

Decidual Change

In pregnancy, there may be a decidual transformation of the cervical stroma (Fig. 3-6B).[37,38] With the extended use of colposcopy, it is more frequently seen both in the endocervix and the ectocervix.[39,40] *Macroscopically*, one observes a small structure that is raised, nodular, and highly vascularized. *Microscopically*, the decidual cells are large, with round nuclei containing conspicuous nucleoli, surrounded by abundant glycogen-rich cytoplasm. If degenerative changes occur, these cells may be irregular with hyperchromatic nuclei. They should not be mistaken for neoplastic cells. Very marked decidual reaction may present as a submucosal tumor or an endocervical polyp composed largely of decidual cells. Regression is observed after the pregnancy.

Arias-Stella Reaction

Gestational Arias-Stella reaction may be observed in endocervical glands (Fig. 3-7).[41] These cellular atypias should not be confused with adenocarcinoma.

MALFORMATIONS

Congenital malformations of the cervix generally accompany those of the corpus uteri. In this form, bicervical uterus, coupled and partitioned cervices, and cervical hypoplasia and aplasia may be encountered.[42] Cervical hoods and "cockscomb" malformations are seen in young women who were exposed in utero to diethylstilbestrol (DES), and they may be associated with infertility or habitual abortion.[43]

INFLAMMATORY DISEASES

Acute Cervicitis

Inflammatory diseases are discussed at length in Chapter 2. The same causal agents may involve the cervix and cause acute and chronic lesions. The infection may be the result of direct invasion of the cervix, spread of an infection from other parts of the genital tract and adjoining organs, or blood-borne contamination. Routine bacteriologic studies often

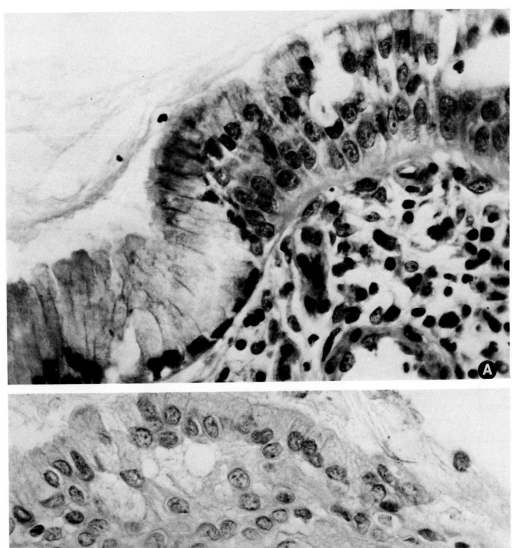

FIGURE 3-6 Photomicrograph of cervix uteri during pregnancy. **(A)** Hyperplasia of glandular epithelium. **(B)** Decidual reaction of stroma.

demonstrate the presence of pathogenic organisms not accompanied by clinical symptoms.

Acute cervicitis may result from primary infection by different organisms such as bacteria, fungi, parasites, or viruses. Table 3-1 indicates the various agents that can cause cervicitis.

Clinically, acute infection is manifested by a purulent, leukorrheal, malodorous discharge. *Macroscopically,* the cervix is edematous, congested, and exhibits an intense red color; the causative organism may be identified in the purulent leukorrheal discharge. The *histologic appearance* is that of a predom-

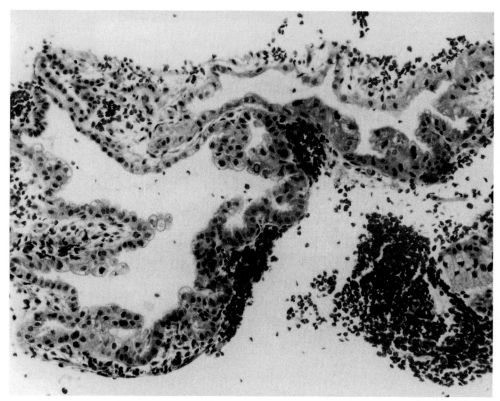

FIGURE 3-7 Arias-Stella reaction of endocervical glands seen in curettage specimen. The angular, hyperchromatic but uniformly dense nuclei are typical.

inantly polymorphonuclear leukocytic inflammatory infiltrate, with marked vascularization and edema of the submucosa (Fig. 3-8). When the squamous epithelium is infiltrated by neutrophils, it may exhibit spongiosis, acanthosis, and nuclear and cytoplasmic vacuolization.

Vaginal smears show an abundant inflammatory exudate rich in neutrophils, histiocytes, and mucus, with the squamous cells presenting diverse nuclear (anisonucleosis, pyknosis, karyorrhexis) and cytoplasmic changes (precocious eosinophilia, vacuolization, and alteration of the cell membrane with cytolysis; Color Fig. 3-2). The intensity of these cytologic alterations is a function of the gravity of the

cervical lesions and permits the observer to follow the evolution of the disease. Columnar endocervical cells may also reveal morphologic alterations such as hypertrophic nuclei and vacuolated cytoplasm.

Repair phenomena appear if the inflammation subsides. Granulation tissue is replaced by regenerating epithelial cells, which exhibit large, hyperchromatic nuclei with frequent mitoses. In smears, these regenerating cells should not be misinterpreted as dysplastic or neoplastic. The absence of definite criteria of malignancy, the recognition of the inflammatory event, and amelioration after treatment of the inflammation may help to solve the problem. These alterations are particularly difficult to interpret when they occur in endocervical columnar cells.[44]

TABLE 3-1.
Causal Agents of Cervicitis

Bacterial agents: Various cocci (streptococci, staphylococci, enterococci), lactobacilli (?), *Gardnerella, Corynebacterium diphtheriae, Neisseria gonorrhoeae, Chlamydia trachomatis, Treponema, Mycobacterium tuberculosis, Leptothrix*
Fungal agents: *Candida albicans, Torulopsis glabrata, Coccidioides immitis, Aspergillus, Toxoplasma, Blastomyces*
Parasitic agents: *Trichomonas vaginalis*
Viral agents: Herpes genitalis, cytomegalovirus, human papillomavirus
Protozoal agents: *Entamoeba histolytica, Balantidium coli, Vorticella*
Helminthic agents: *Schistosoma haematobium/mansoni/japonicum*

Chronic Cervicitis

The existence of chronic infection of the uterine cervix has been recognized for about a century. Before then, the clinical signs of cervicitis such as leukorrhea were attributed to "chronic inflammation of the matrix," the etiology of which was poorly defined. Chronic cervicitis is the most common gynecologic disease and the most common cause of leukorrhea, being discovered in about one third of women examined by gynecologists. Several factors explain its frequency:

1. The cervix is exposed to diverse traumata of genital life.
2. The multiple folds of the cervical mucosa favor microbial pollution.
3. The constant presence of cervical and endometrial secretions constitutes an environment favorable to the development of pathogenic organisms.
4. The rich lymphatic drainage in the region facilitates the dissemination of infections, originating most commonly in the urinary tract.
5. Modifications of the hormonal milieu create morphologic alterations in the mucosa.

The causal organisms are the same as for acute cervicitis (see Table 3-1). The gonococcus, one of the most common, has decreased in frequency since the beginning of the antibiotic era. *Mycoplasma, Chlamydia,* and *Gardnerella vaginalis* have been recognized recently as playing a frequent role.

Macroscopic Appearance. The macroscopic pictures seen in chronic cervicitis are varied. The ectocervix may appear normal, the infection being localized to the endocervical canal, or it may display profound alterations. In the latter case, it is deformed, budding, granular, congested, and edematous, or it may contain more or less extensive zones

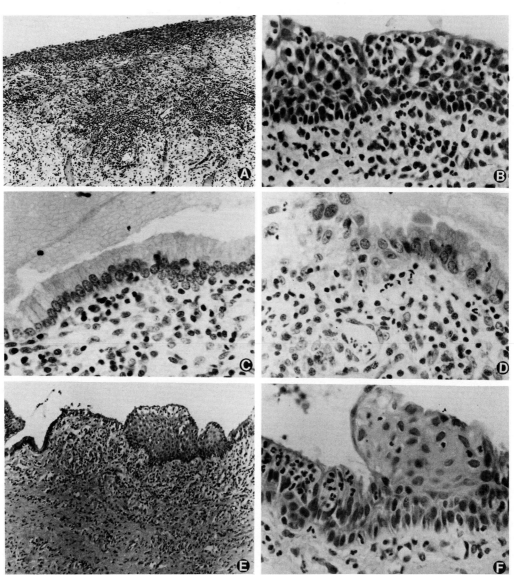

FIGURE 3-8 Acute and chronic cervicitis: microscopic appearances. **(A)** Leukocytic infiltration of epithelium and subjacent stroma, vascular congestion. **(B)** Acute inflammatory infiltrate rich in polymorphonuclear leukocytes invading epithelium and stroma. **(C)** The stroma shows a discrete chronic inflammatory infiltrate rich in lymphocytes and plasma cells, with no alteration of the glandular epithelium. **(D)** Polymorphonuclear leukocytic stromal infiltrate and alterations of the glandular epithelium. **(E)** Focus of squamous metaplasia and leukocytic infiltration. **(F)** Detail of the focus of squamous metaplasia seen in **E**.

of red granular surface erosion. Glandular cysts project under the mucosa, and lacerations are sometimes visible. The extent and severity of these lesions determine the macroscopic appearance and the clinical manifestations. With time, progressive fibrosis takes place occasionally resulting in a cicatricial stenosis of the cervical canal.

Colposcopic examination facilitates the identification of these lesions.[45,46] The best known findings by this technique are (1) true erosion of the mucosa, (2) leukoplakic foci due to mucosal hyperkeratosis, (3) hyperemia and infiltration of the submucosa in the zones of erosion, and (4) ectropion, or the presence of glandular epithelium covering the ectocervix.

Certain chronic infections cause specific anatomic modifications. The most notable of these are condylomata acuminata and the mucous plaques of secondary syphilis.

Microscopic Appearance. The histologic lesions provoked by chronic inflammatory phenomena are varied, and their intensity depends on local and systemic factors (Figs. 3-8 and 3-9). The most discrete consist of lymphoplasmacytic infiltration and vascular congestion of the submucosa without alteration of the squamous or glandular mucosa. This type of lesion is extremely frequent and often is of little clinical significance. When the inflammatory infiltrate is more extensive, it reaches the basal layers of the epi-

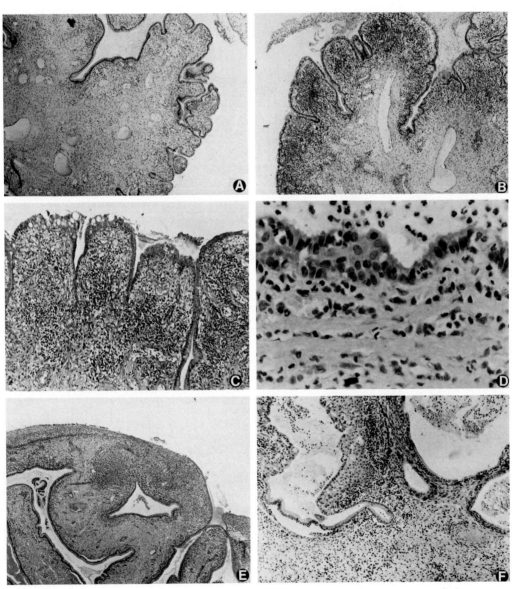

FIGURE 3-9 Chronic cerviticis: microscopic appearances. **(A,B)** Papillary structure of the endocervical mucosa with leukocytic infiltration. **(C)** Degenerative alterations of surface epithelium. **(D)** Leukocytic inflammatory infiltrate and discrete squamous metaplasia at left. **(E)** Papillary structure of endocervical mucosa, leukocytic stromal infiltrate. **(F)** Focus of squamous metaplasia.

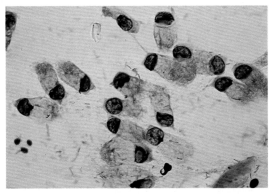

Color Figure 3-1

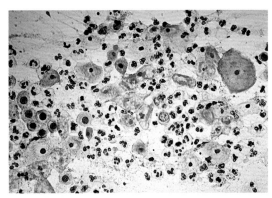

Color Figure 3-2

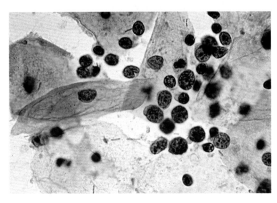

Color Figure 3-3

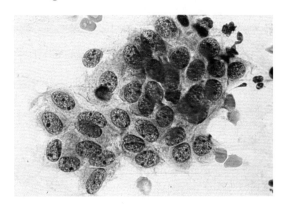

Color Figure 3-4

Color Figure 3-1   Cervical smear: normal endocervical cells. The presence of endocervical cells such as these or of metaplastic cells (see Color Figs. 3-7 and 3-8) should be noted as an indication that the smear has attained the squamous–columnar junction.

Color Figure 3-2   Cervical smear: atypia due to *Trichomonas vaginalis* infection. Note aniso-nucleosis, nuclear hyperchromasia, and perinuclear haloes. The inflammatory background and the presence of the parasite (see Color Fig. 3-5) aid in the distinction from condyloma (Color Figs. 3-10 through 3-12) and dysplasia (Color Figs. 3-22 through 3-25).

Color Figure 3-3   Cervical smear: follicular cervicitis. Numerous benign lymphocytes must not be mistaken for endometrial cells or cells exfoliated from a small cell carcinoma or malignant lymphoma.

Color Figure 3-4   Cervical smear: endocervical cells showing hyperplasia with nuclear atypia in biopsy-proven severe acute and chronic endocervicitis with microglandular hyperplasia. (Compare with Color Figs. 3-6, 3-31, and 3-32.)

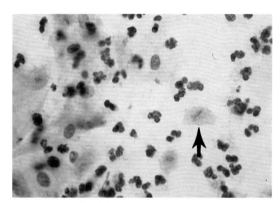

Color Figure 3-5

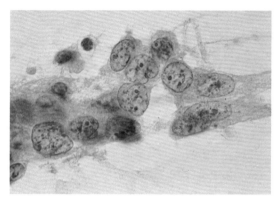

Color Figure 3-6

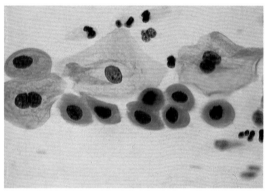

Color Figure 3-7

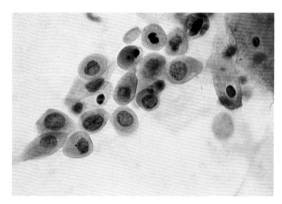

Color Figure 3-8

Color Figure 3-5 Cervical smear: trichomoniasis. Several organisms with distinct nuclei are present in an inflammatory background *(arrow)*.

Color Figure 3-6 Cervical smear: atypia due to endocervical repair phenomenon. Note variability in cell size and enlarged nuclei with prominent nucleoli and granular chromatin. (Compare with Color Figs. 3-4, 3-31, and 3-32.)

Color Figure 3-7 Cervical smear: squamous metaplasia. Group of parabasal-type cells in a row with cytoplasmic molding and flattening at one surface.

Color Figure 3-8 Cervical smear: atypical metaplasia. Small cells similar in shape and orientation to those seen in Color Figure 3-7 but with moderate nuclear atypia. Abnormal chromatin clumping of dysplasia in parabasal or metaplastic cells is absent. (Compare with Color Figs. 3-23 through 3-25.)

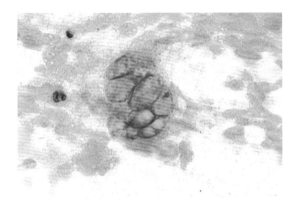

Color Figure 3-9

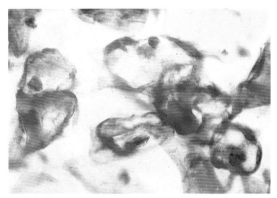

Color Figure 3-10

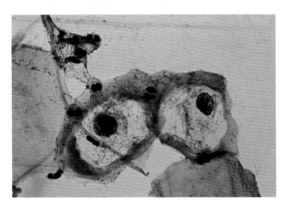

Color Figure 3-11

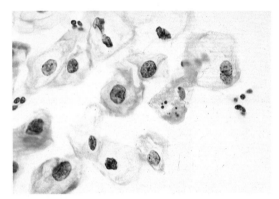

Color Figure 3-12

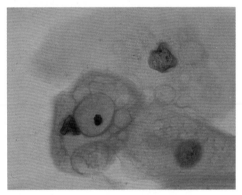

Color Figure 3-13

Color Figure 3-9 Cervical smear: *Herpesvirus hominis* type 2 infection. Multinucleated cells with "ground-glass" nuclei can be seen.

Color Figure 3-10 Cervical smear: flat condyloma or wart virus infection. Typical cytoplasmic haloes and peripheral cytoplasmic thickening of squamous cells with orangeophilic or fuchsia red staining. Nuclei are small, dense, and irregular.

Color Figure 3-11 Cervical smear: flat condyloma or wart virus infection. Koilocytotic cells with cytoplasmic haloes, peripherally dense cytoplasm, and "raisinoid" nuclei.

Color Figure 3-12 Cervical smear: flat condyloma or wart virus infection. Pronounced cytoplasmic vacuolation and moderate nuclear atypia including binucleation. This should be reported as "mild dysplasia of probable viral origin."

Color Figure 3-13 Cervical smear: chlamydial cervicitis. Cell with typical cytoplasmic inclusion with distinct borders.

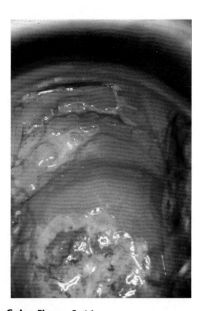

Color Figure 3-14

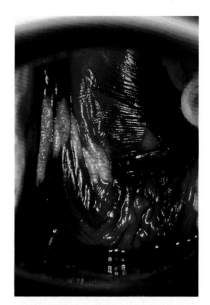

Color Figure 3-15

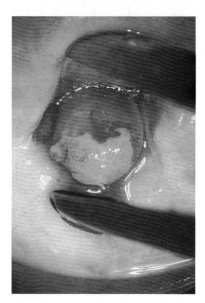

Color Figure 3-16

Color Figure 3-17

Color Figure 3-14   Positive Schiller test in extensive cervicitis. Squamous epithelium is only slightly stained by iodine. No dysplasia was present (Courtesy of Dr. R. Cartier)

Color Figure 3-15   Positive Schiller test in vaginal condyloma. Cervix is normal and is deeply stained by iodine. (Courtesy of Dr. R. Cartier)

Color Figure 3-16   Colposcopic view of herpetic ulcers of anterior vaginal fornix and cervix. (Courtesy of Dr. R. Cartier)

Color Figure 3-17   Colposcopic picture of endocervical polyp. The polyp protrudes through the external os and shows squamous metaplasia (white) on its surface. (Courtesy of Dr. R. Cartier)

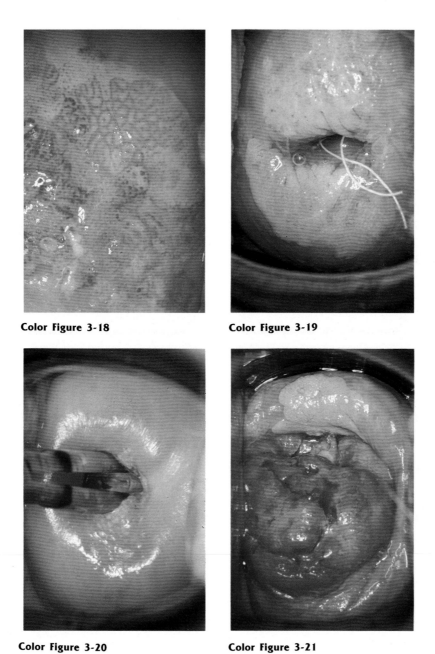

Color Figure 3-18

Color Figure 3-19

Color Figure 3-20

Color Figure 3-21

Color Figure 3-18 Colposcopic picture of severe dysplasia (CIN III). After application of acetic acid, the cervix shows a polymorphous appearance, with mosaic punctation, marked congestion, and a white cuffed gland opening at the lower left of the figure. (Courtesy of Dr. R. Cartier)

Color Figure 3-19 Colposcopic picture of severe dysplasia (CIN III). Acetowhite epithelium indicates a large ectocervical lesion. The squamocolumnar junction is visible at the external os. An IUD string protrudes from the endocervical canal. (Courtesy of Dr. R. Cartier)

Color Figure 3-20 Colposcopic picture of severe dysplasia (CIN III). Examination using a Palmer polyp forceps as endocervical speculum demonstrates that the endocervical mucosa is white and smooth, with no squamocolumnar junction visible (compare with Color Fig. 3-19). (Courtesy of Dr. R. Cartier)

Color Figure 3-21 Colposcopic picture of invasive squamous cell carcinoma. This large fungating tumor extends to the posterior vaginal wall. Note atypical pattern of surface blood vessels. (Courtesy of Dr. R. Cartier)

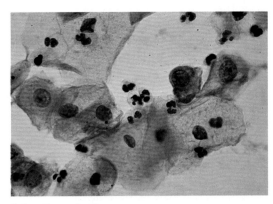

Color Figure 3-22

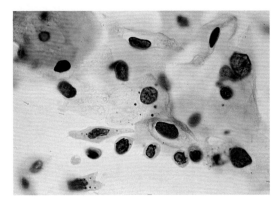

Color Figure 3-23

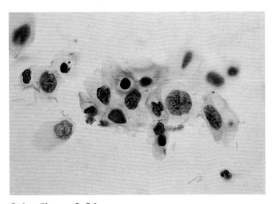

Color Figure 3-24

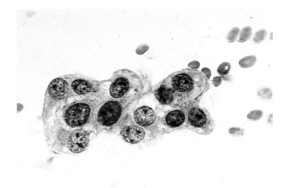

Color Figure 3-25

Color Figure 3-22 Cervical smear: mild dysplasia (CIN I). Dyskaryosis and slight nuclear atypia of superficial and intermediate squamous cells.

Color Figure 3-23 Cervical smear: moderate dysplasia (CIN II). Intermediate and parabasal squamous cells show anisonucleosis, nuclear hyperchromasia, and fine chromatin clumping.

Color Figure 3-24 Cervical smear: moderate dysplasia (CIN II). Intermediate and parabasal squamous cells show anisonucleosis, nuclear hyperchromasia, and fine chromatin clumping.

Color Figure 3-25 Cervical smear: severe dysplasia (CIN III). Parabasal dyskaryosis of small squamous cells with basophilic cytoplasm and marked nuclear atypia.

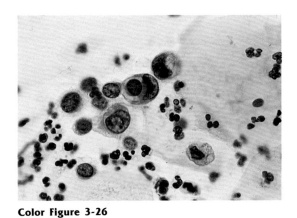

Color Figure 3-26

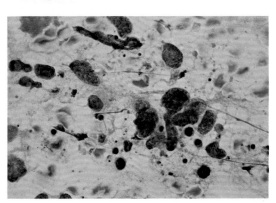

Color Figure 3-27

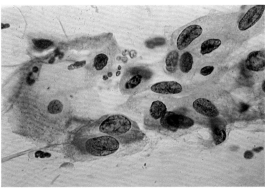

Color Figure 3-28

Color Figure 3-29

Color Figure 3-26 Cervical smear: squamous carcinoma in situ (CIN III or CIS). Findings are similar to those in Color Figure 3-25, but less cytoplasm is present. The similarity of these two cases argues in favor of the CIN classification.

Color Figure 3-27 Cervical smear: squamous carcinoma in situ (CIN III or CIS), large cell type. This smear is similar to that depicted in Color Figure 3-26, but the neoplastic cells are considerably larger (figures taken at same magnification). The uniformity of the neoplastic cells and the absence of a "tumor diathesis" are factors against the diagnosis of invasive large cell carcinoma (compare with Color Fig. 3-29).

Color Figure 3-28 Cervical smear: invasive keratinizing squamous cell carcinoma. Cells with malignant nuclei and voluminous cytoplasm showing keratinization.

Color Figure 3-29 Cervical smear: invasive squamous cell carcinoma, large cell nonkeratinizing type. In addition to nuclear criteria of malignancy, cells are pleomorphic and there is a necrotic background ("tumor diathesis"). (Compare with Color Fig. 3-27).

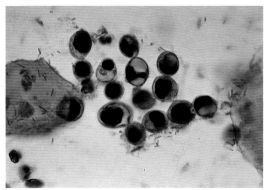

Color Figure 3-30

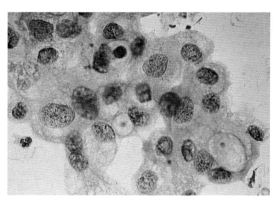

Color Figure 3-31

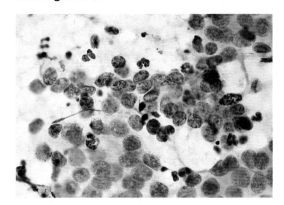

Color Figure 3-32

Color Figure 3-30 Cervical smear: invasive small cell carcinoma. Cells are small, round, and fairly uniform. "Tumor diathesis" was present elsewhere in the smear.

Color Figure 3-31 Cervical smear: adenocarcinoma of endocervix. The neoplastic cells are in a papillary cluster and show the usual nuclear criteria of malignancy. Compared with adeno-carcinoma of the endometrium (Color Figs. 3-32 and 4-6), the cells of endocervical adeno-carcinoma are larger and have large cytoplasmic vacuoles; they are also more likely to contain macronucleoli (not seen in this figure). Also compare with benign endocervical atypias in Color Figures 3-4, 3-6, and 3-8.

Color Figure 3-32 Cervical smear: adenocarcinoma of endometrium extending to cervix (direct scrape and smear of tumor). Compare with Color Figure 3-31.

thelium, spreads within the stroma, and surrounds the endocervical glands. This infiltrate is composed of lymphocytes, neutrophils, plasma cells, and histiocytes. If lymphoid follicles are prominent, the designation *follicular cervicitis* is applied (Fig. 3-10 and Color Fig. 3-3). *Cervical smears* may reveal the presence of a characteristic rich pleomorphic infiltrate composed of lymphoid cells and macrophages. *Follicular cervicitis* is frequently associated with chlamydial infection.[47] It is more frequent in postmenopausal women and should not be confused microscopically with a leukemic or lymphomatous lesion.[48] The endocervical mucosa reacts by proliferating and developing superficial papillary formations that may project at the external orifice of the cervix (ectropion). The endocervical mucosa, congestive and proliferating, forms a visible collar around the cervical os.

The squamous epithelium is more resistant, and the lesions are limited at this stage to the basal cell layers. These cells show discrete nuclear and cytoplasmic atypias, and leukocytes infiltrate the epithelium.

In more severe cervicitis, all the histologic structures are altered or destroyed by the inflammatory infiltrate. Either the epithelia are replaced by inflammatory infiltrates or they present cytologic alterations of reactive type (Fig. 3-11). The squamous epithelium shows hyperkeratosis, acanthosis, and anomalies of size and shape of cells and of nuclei. Intracellular glycogen is diminished or absent. This disappearance of glycogen is demonstrated clinically by the Schiller test (the cervical mucosa is stained brown by iodine except in areas in which glycogen is deficient). These cellular anomalies should not be confused with cervical intraepithelial neoplasia (CIN). The stroma is congested, edematous, and contains numerous leukocytes and histiocytes concentrated around blood vessels. The glands are dilated, cystic (*nabothian cysts*; Fig. 3-12), or destroyed by the inflammation. Nabothian cysts result from blockage of the endocervical gland necks by inflammation or subsequent squamous metaplasia. Vascular congestion favors the appearance of hemorrhages, especially during pregnancy.

Repair phenomena appearing in longstanding cervicitis are characterized by considerable cellular alterations of squamous and columnar cells which should not be confused with CIN.[49] They correspond to an epithelial proliferation replacing the destroyed epithelium. The presence of enlarged nucleoli is the expression of active repair protein synthesis (cell regeneration). The nuclei, though enlarged, irregular, and hyperchromatic, lack the very marked anomalies of neoplastic cells. The columnar cells have large clear, hypochromatic nuclei, conspicuous nucleoli, and dense eosinophilic cytoplasm. Mitoses are normal. The nuclear–cytoplasmic ratio is within normal limits. These repair anomalies are well illustrated in postconization smears and biopsies and after radiation therapy.

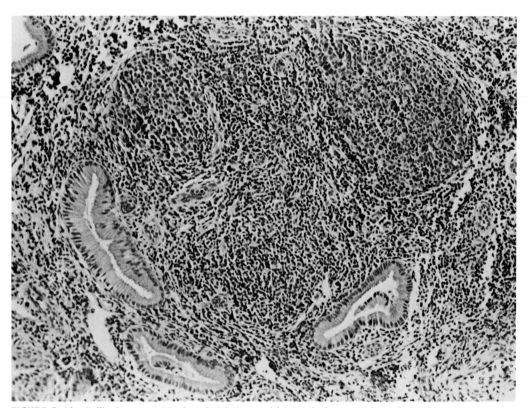

FIGURE 3-10 Follicular cervicitis: lymphoid tissue with germinal centers in endocervix.

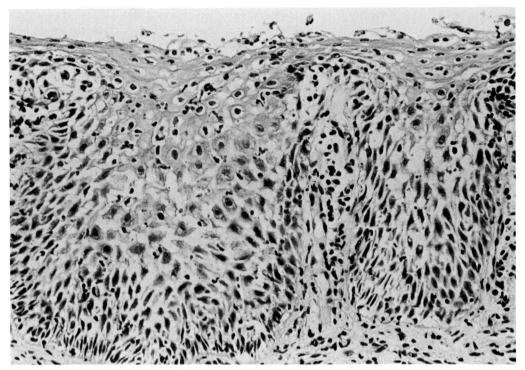

FIGURE 3-11 Cervicitis with mild reactive atypia of squamous mucosa.

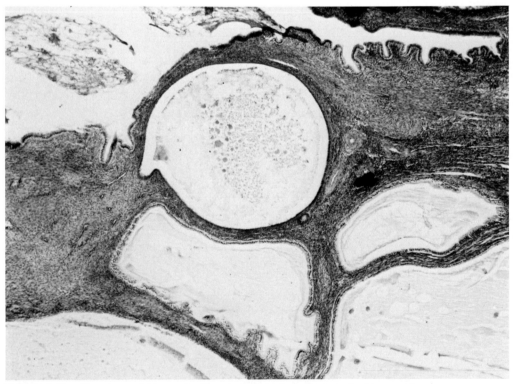

FIGURE 3-12 Chronic cervicitis: cystic dilatation of cervical glands (nabothian cysts).

Erosion and Squamous Metaplasia

The term *erosion* has been used in several different senses, but because the early description by Meyer[50] emphasized its relation to inflammatory processes, it will be considered at this point. Most important is that the common usage of the term does not denote an erosion in the histopathologic sense (ie, mucosal denudation or ulceration), but rather an outgrowth of endocervical columnar epithelium onto the portio (ectropion), where, because the thinner mucosa is relatively transparent, the underlying blood vessels give the area involved (often a ring-like zone around the external os) a red or eroded appearance. To understand its development, it is necessary to recall that the external os of the cervix represents the normal boundary between mucus-secreting glandular epithelium and stratified squamous epithelium (transformation zone).

Modifications in pH, under the influence of bacterial or hormonal factors, bring about disturbances in the equilibrium between the two epithelia. In the first stage, the glandular epithelium proliferates onto the squamous territory by the following mechanism: an elevation of pH provokes maceration of the squamous epithelium, which becomes infiltrated by polymorphonuclear leukocytes, degenerates, disappears, and is replaced by glandular epithelium. When the pH is lowered, the glandular epithelium this time recedes before the squamous lining. The latter creeps under the columnar cells, pushes them back, invades the necks of the glands, and produces the picture of *squamous metaplasia* (Figs. 3-13 through 3-16). Thus, the localization of the borderline or transformation zone varies according to the factors mentioned previously and is better visualized with the use of the colposcope, which can also determine the location and extent of cervical lesions. These lesions are so common that they can be considered as physiologic changes expressing the search for a constant equilibrium between the two epithelia.

Although the inflammatory etiology of cervical erosion represents the classic theory, many authors agree with Fluhmann[51] that the lesion is more often either congenital or acquired from an ectropion secondary to trauma. Biopsies often show papillary projections of columnar epithelium overlying a stroma devoid of inflammatory cells. The classic explanation of squamous metaplasia is also not accepted by all authors. According to the historic work of Meyer,[50] the image of metaplasia is produced when the squamous epithelium becomes dominant and insinuates itself under the glandular epithelium; it therefore becomes evident that the term *metaplasia* is inexact because it is not a case of epithelial transformation but rather of squamous epithelialization. The term *epidermization* has been used for this phenomenon—although incorrectly, because true epidermis does

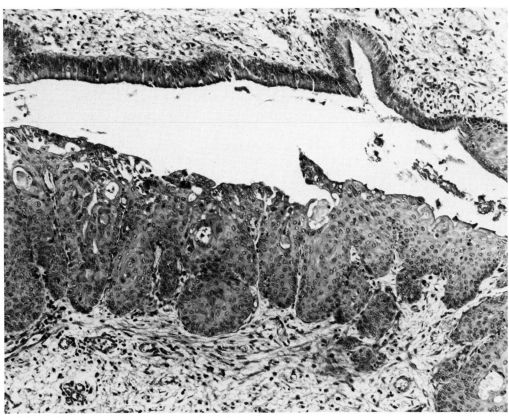

FIGURE 3-13 Squamous metaplasia at the level of a cervical gland neck.

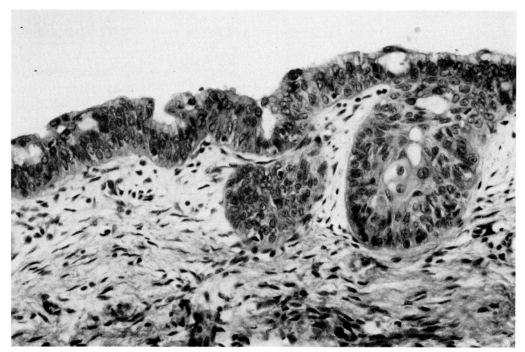

FIGURE 3-14 Squamous metaplasia (*right*), arising in reserve cell hyperplasia (*left*).

not participate. Usage and numerous works, however, have consecrated these terms.

The second hypothesis postulates the existence of a true metaplasia (squamous prosoplasia of Fluhmann) arising from the pluripotential subcolumnar reserve cell (Fig. 3-17). These cells, also called *basal cells,* are capable of undergoing, under the influence of diverse stimuli, various transformations such as simple proliferation, hyperplasia, metaplasia, and anaplasia. Numerous authors have shown convincing pictures in favor of the hypothesis.[49,52–55] According to them, these cells have a potential for differentiation into either muciparous glandular epithelium or squamous epithelium. The presence of mucus in squamous cell plaques illustrates this double potential.

The immature squamous metaplasia resulting from the proliferation of reserve cells pushes the overlying endocervical epithelium toward the surface (see Figs. 3-15 and 3-16). The immature metaplastic cells are rather small, contain no abundant glycogen, and often have an eosinophilic cytoplasm. When these cells differentiate, they become similar to normal squamous cells constituting a mature squamous epithelium.

Supporters of the true metaplasia theory reject the idea of epithelial migration because of pictures in which the border between the normal and the atypical metaplastic zones is sharp. Another argument in favor of the metaplasia hypothesis is the existence of foci of metaplasia distant and isolated from the squamocolumnar junction. Our own experience indicates

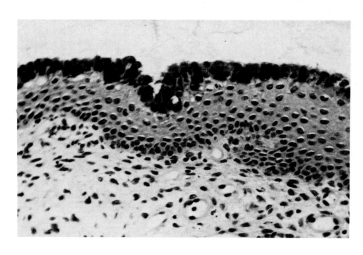

FIGURE 3-15 Squamous metaplasia: mucin stain demonstrating the columnar superficial layer.

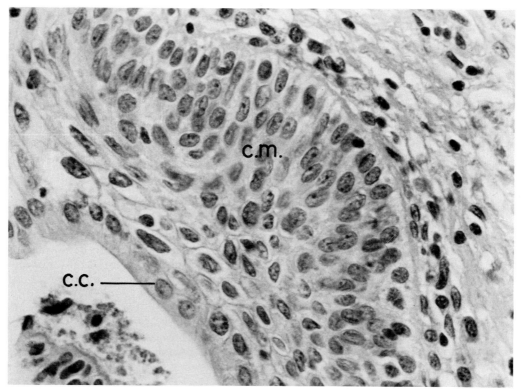

FIGURE 3-16 Squamous metaplasia: columnar (*c.c.*) and squamous (*c.m.*) cells.

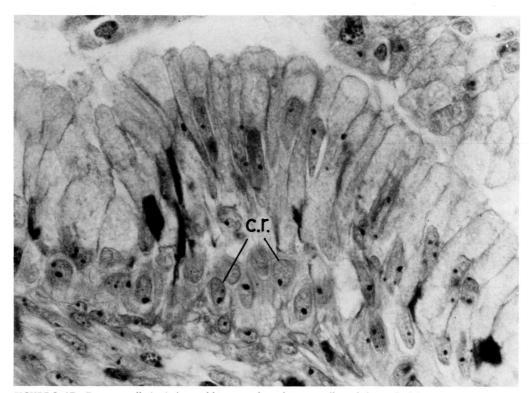

FIGURE 3-17 Reserve cells (*c.r.*) situated between the columnar cells and the underlying stroma.

that both mechanisms exist, but the one mediated by subcolumnar reserve cells is far more common. Interestingly, the origin of these reserve cells itself remains a mystery.[53,56–58] They may originate from multipotential basal cells, from endocervical columnar cells, from stromal cells, or from embryonic endodermal cells. Hormonal stimuli and local factors may play a role in this proliferation.

It is important to know these histologic pictures to avoid confusion with cancer, because of the immaturity of metaplastic epithelium. The absence of cellular atypia and of bizarre mitoses and the presence of normal stratification of the squamous epithelium are morphologic supports for the benign character of these lesions.

Cytology in Cervicitis and Squamous Metaplasia

The great majority of abnormal cervicovaginal smears exhibit atypia on the basis of cervical inflammation or metaplasia. These pictures, although themselves not of great clinical significance, are important to recognize to avoid the false diagnosis of a dysplastic or neoplastic process. Although the changes of inflammatory and metaplastic lesions will be described separately, in most cases they occur together and are frequent.[59] Normal and abnormal cervical cells are illustrated in Figure 3-18.

Cervicitis

In chronic cervicitis, the background of the smear is generally normal, although in rare cases of follicular cervicitis (see above), numerous lymphocytes and larger germinal center cells may be exfoliated, raising the differential diagnosis with a malignant lymphoma (see Color Fig. 3-3). In acute cervicitis, the smears are usually rich in neutrophils, with many large clumps of necrotic debris. The neutrophils may cluster around epithelial cells, and in endocervicitis may be found within the cytoplasm of large, often markedly atypical endocervical cells. The offending organisms, particularly *Trichomonas vaginalis,* may be identified in the smears as well (Color Figs. 3-2, 3-4, and 3-5). Reserve cells, easily observed in biopsies, are not frequently identifiable in the smears. Only in marked reserve cell hyperplasia may one notice the presence of small, round, regular cells with round normochromatic nuclei surrounded by a slim rim of cyanophilic cytoplasm. They desquamate in syncytial aggregates.

More important is the cellular atypia that may be encountered in these smears (see Color Fig. 3-2). These are seen predominantly in acute cervicitis, and chronic cervicitis exhibits few cytologic changes. Parabasal cells are often increased in number and show degenerative phenomena such as karyorrhexis, nuclear pyknosis, and cytoplasmic vacuolization.

Some variation in size and shape of epithelial cells may be seen, and nuclei may be slightly to moderately enlarged, with a uniform "ground glass" appearance. Endocervical cells (see Color Fig. 3-4) and their nuclei may be markedly enlarged, and the nuclei may contain one or more large, prominent nucleoli. The endocervical cells may be multinucleate, show mitotic figures, and contain intracytoplasmic vacuoles and neutrophils. Naked nuclei are frequently seen. These changes may be extremely difficult to differentiate from those of endocervical or endometrial adenocarcinoma (see text below and Color Figs. 3-31 and 3-32).

Some additional changes resulting from specific organisms may also be encountered. The pictures in herpesvirus and papillomavirus infections are discussed later. In *Trichomonas* infection, atypical cellular changes may be prominent (see Color Fig. 3-2). The nuclear anomalies include enlargement, blurring of nuclear structure, irregularity of form, multinucleation, finely granular hyperchromatism, and clumping of chromatin along the nuclear membrane. These worrisome nuclear atypias are usually combined with characteristic cytoplasmic findings, which aid in the differential diagnosis from dysplasia: the presence of clear perinuclear haloes and of marked cytoplasmic eosinophilia. The organisms usually can be identified as well. However, there is no reason that trichomoniasis and dysplasia or even cancer cannot coexist, and therefore if the diagnosis of atypia secondary to *Trichomonas* infection is made, a repeat smear should always be obtained after treatment of the infection to be sure that the cellular anomalies do not persist.

Marked inflammatory changes affecting both squamous and glandular cells may be attributed to the presence of an intrauterine device (IUD). The cellular atypias (see Chapter 4) are accompanied by a severe inflammatory reaction. The age of the patient and the presence of an IUD may help to make the correct diagnosis.[60–62]

Immunodeficiencies or immunodepressive drugs can favor the development of infections, particularly herpes simplex and human papillomavirus.[63]

Repair and Regeneration

Although not related to typical cervicitis, the cytologic changes encountered in repair and regeneration (Color Fig. 3-6) should be mentioned here. These changes are similar to those described earlier as typical of inflammatory changes in endocervical cells, and similarly may be difficult to differentiate from carcinoma. These cells vary in size, and their enlarged, irregular, slightly hyperchromatic nuclei reveal nucleolar hypertrophy. The vacuolated cytoplasm may be infiltrated with polymorphonuclear leukocytes. The absence of marked hyperchromatism and the persistence of cohesiveness between cells are in favor of the benign and metaplastic origin of the lesion. The etiology is a recent surgical proce-

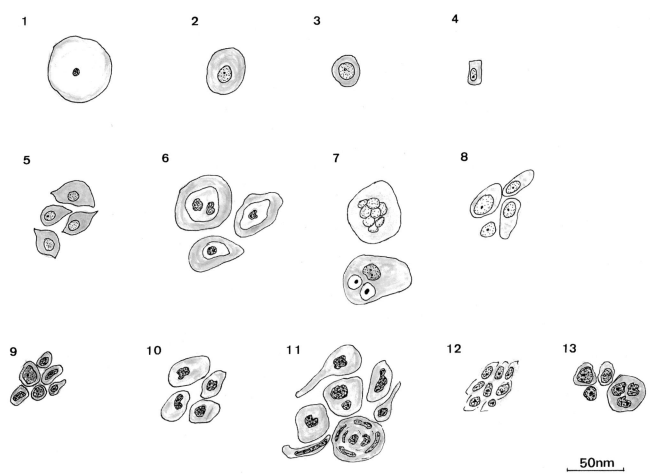

FIGURE 3-18 Schematic representation of cervicovaginal cytology: (1) superficial squamous cell; (2) intermediate squamous cell; (3) parabasal squamous cell; (4) columnar endocervical cell; (5) mature squamous metaplasia; (6) cytologic alterations compatible with human papillomavirus (koilocytes); (7) cytologic alterations compatible with *Herpesvirus* (multinucleate cell) and *Chlamydia* infection (cytoplasmic inclusions); (8) inflammatory benign changes of columnar endocervical cells; (9) CIN, small cell type; (10) CIN, intermediate cell type; (11) CIN, differentiated superficial type; (12) differentiated adenocarcinoma of endocervix; and (13) undifferentiated adenocarcinoma of endocervix.

dure rather than infection, although cautery, cryocoagulation diathermy, radiation therapy, and past infection may represent causal agents. Because of the diagnostic problems that these changes may pose, the history of prior surgery or irradiation should always be supplied by the clinician submitting a smear in such a case.

Squamous Metaplasia

In *squamous metaplasia,* parabasal-type cells are numerous in the smear. Many of these form clusters that are contiguous with endocervical cells, mimicking the close relation between these two cell types encountered in biopsy specimens. The metaplastic cells (Color Fig. 3-7) are larger than adjacent endocervical cells and have slightly enlarged nuclei and, frequently, well-developed intercellular bridges. One surface of the cluster of metaplastic cells is frequently flattened, suggesting that it arose in the en-

docervical canal. The cytoplasm may contain fine mucin vacuoles. Clusters of altered endocervical cells with marked vacuolated cytoplasm overlie the metaplastic zones, which contributes to their desquamation. The metaplastic cells occasionally show nuclear atypia that may range in degree from mild to severe (Fig. 3-19 and Color Fig. 3-8). The hyperchromatism, chromatin clumping, and nuclear irregularity of dysplasia are not present, however. If they are, and if the atypical metaplasia is severe, the diagnosis of a dysplasia arising in metaplastic epithelium should be suggested. Clusters of altered endocervical cells are often present; they have a vacuolated cytoplasm that pushes the nucleus to the periphery. The nuclei are regular, normochromatic, and moderately enlarged. Leukocytes infiltrate the cytoplasm and contribute to the existence of lytic phenomena. To summarize, all these cytologic anomalies can be classified into three main categories: immature, mature, and atypical metaplasia.

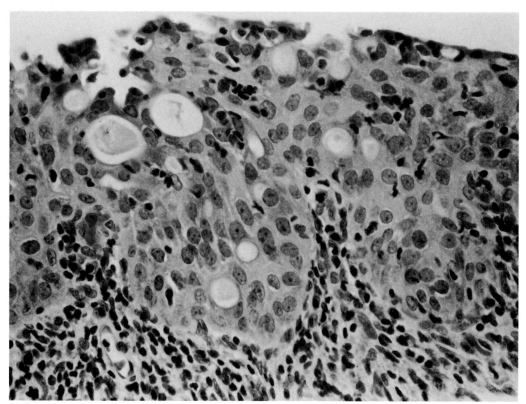

FIGURE 3-19 Squamous metaplasia with nuclear enlargement and moderate atypia.

Immature squamous metaplasia is characterized by the presence of elongated streaks of round, oval, or elongated cells with large, regular nuclei and a dense, predominantly cyanophilic cytoplasm. Nucleoli may be prominent. They have the size of parabasal or intermediate cells.

Mature squamous metaplasia is represented by larger cells, usually isolated, round, or elongated, with a lower nuclear–cytoplasmic ratio than that observed in immature metaplasia. The nuclei have a finely dispersed chromatin. The density of the cytoplasm is usually higher than in normal squamous cells and varies from one cell to another and in different areas of the same cell. One may note the presence of bipolar cells with a finely elongated cytoplasm at both ends of the cell.

Atypical metaplasia is characterized by the appearance of moderate cellular anomalies such as binucleation, nuclear enlargement, moderate hyperchromatism, and prominent nucleoli. Some disorder in the cellular arrangement is observable when large clusters are present.[64]

Specific Infections

Herpes Genitalis

This common viral infection is due to a DNA-containing poxvirus with a diameter of 150 nm, which is surrounded by a protein capsid. Viruses are located in the host cell nucleus and modify the cellular metabolism by inducing the synthesis of proteins necessary for the replication of viral DNA. Two types, herpes simplex viruses 1 and 2 (HSV-1 and HSV-2), are described; the distinction is based on serologic studies because they are morphologically identical. HSV-1 is responsible for lesions appearing in infancy and adolescence, and HSV-2 occurs predominantly after puberty. In pregnant women, the risk of transmitting the virus to the fetus is great, resulting in major fetal abnormalities and specific infections such as conjunctivitis.[65] It is also responsible for fetal mortality and abortion.

Cervicitis due to infection with herpes genitalis has acquired added importance because of the suggestion by different authors that this virus may play a role in the development of cervical carcinoma.[66-68]

Seroepidemiologic studies have demonstrated that patients with cervical cancer have a significantly higher incidence of neutralizing antibodies against HSV-2 and that patients with antibodies to HSV-2 are more susceptible to invasive cancer than women without such antibodies.[69,70] Prospective studies have confirmed these data; in patients with herpes genitalis, dysplasia is statistically more frequent than in control groups of patients.[71] These studies suggest that the viral infection precedes the development of dysplasia and carcinoma. In addition, cervical cancers have been induced in mice by local application of inactivated herpesvirus,[72] and the virus has been observed by electron microscopy in cervical carcinoma cells in tissue culture.[73] These data were challenged by other studies; Adam and colleagues[69] did not demonstrate an increase of HSV-2 antibody titers in cervical cancer patients. Vonka and associates[74] showed that the incidence of antibodies correlates with sexual behavior and socioeconomic status of patients rather than with the existence of neoplasia. Furthermore, in several studies cervical atypias preceded the herpetic infection more often than they followed it.[75,76] Thus, the data supporting the role of HSV-2 as a cervical carcinogen or cocarcinogen are intriguing but by no means conclusive.

Diagnosis. The diagnosis relies on cervical cultures, antibody serology, and clinical cytology. Herpetic cervicitis may be seen clinically as multiple, superficial, painful ulcers of the mucosa resulting from the transformation of papules and vesicles. The clinical lesions usually are more severe in the primary manifestation of the disease. In recurrent, even clinically silent, episodes, cellular alterations are observed in the biopsy or smear. The virus isolation is difficult and has to be done during the acute phase of the disease. After the first infection, the virus remains dormant in the sacral root ganglia of the spinal cord. *Histologically,* it is an ulcerative lesion with typical epithelial cell alterations. If a biopsy is obtained during the vesiculopapular phase, one may observe suprabasal intraepithelial vesicles. Some cells present in the vesicles exhibit intranuclear eosinophilic inclusions. The morphologic alterations caused by the virus are observed in squamous, endocervical columnar, and metaplastic cells.

Cytology. More frequently the disease is recognized by these same alterations in cytologic material if the smears are taken during the acute stage of the disease (2 to 3 weeks). The smears should be taken from the edge and bed of ulceration because the vesicular content is inflammatory and does not reveal typical cells. The cellular changes include (1) enlarged nuclei with homogenized, opaque, basophilic content ("ground glass" nuclei) corresponding to the massive presence of the virus; (2) large multinucleated cells characterized by internuclear molding and the existence of intranuclear eosinophilic inclusions surrounded by a clear halo; and (3) late degenerative phenomena expressed by hyperchromatic, large nuclear debris. The cytoplasm is dense, and degenerative vacuoles are often present.[49] Nucleoli are conspicuous and moderately enlarged. Ng and associates[77] have emphasized that the classic large eosinophilic nuclear viral inclusions are seen predominantly in recurrent infections, whereas primary infections are characterized by "ground glass" nuclei with unusually clear nucleoplasm (Fig. 3-20 and Color Fig. 3-9). These data were not confirmed by Vesterinen and colleagues.[78]

Multinucleation is not a specific image of HSV; it is also encountered in trophoblastic cells, in nonspecific giant cells observed in postmenopausal smears or in cervicitis, and in postsurgical foreign-body multinucleated giant cells. A case of measles cervicitis in a 20-year-old pregnant woman revealed in the Papanicolaou smear the presence of innumerable multinucleate superficial and intermediate cells and metaplastic elements.[79]

Human Papillomavirus

Molecular biology techniques have established that human papillomaviruses (HPV) are associated with a spectrum of genital lesions including condyloma acuminatum, flat condyloma, CIN, and invasive carcinoma.[80–84]

HPV is a heterogeneous group of DNA viruses, and at least 68 different types have been isolated using molecular hybridization and restriction enzymes analyses.[85,86] Among these, about 30 types have been identified in the lower female genital tract.[87,89]

Different data favor the role of HPV in the etiology of cervical neoplasia, but many aspects of this re-

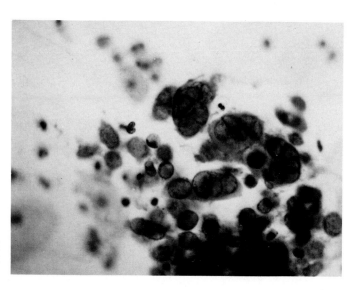

FIGURE 3-20 Herpetic cervicitis: appearance of cervical smear in primary infection, showing multinucleated cells with "ground glass" nuclei.

lation remain to be clarified. HPV antigens have been identified in tissue sections of CIN,[90–92] and HPV particles have been observed ultrastructurally in koilocytotic cells (Fig. 3-21).[92]

Human cervical cancer lines such as HeLa cells may contain HPV DNA.[93] Metastatic cervical cancer and the primary tumor may harbor the same HPV type.[94] HPV DNA can be integrated in the cell nuclear DNA in high-grade dysplasia and carcinoma. It is also frequently reported in immunodeficient patients (eg, patients with lymphomas, AIDS, or immunosuppressed organ transplants).

Condylomatous lesions seem to be a frequent disease of the cervix and may be detected frequently in adult women screened by cytology. Meisels and coworkers[95] estimate in retrospect that about 70% of their cervical dysplasias are related to condylomatous lesions, and condylomas may progress to dysplasia and carcinoma in situ. Different authors[85,96–100] have shown that high-grade intraepithelial neoplasms and invasive carcinoma of the cervix are mostly related to papillomavirus types 16, 18, 31, 33 and 35, whereas types 6 and 11 are associated with flat condyloma and low-grade intraepithelial neoplasia. This correlation is not constant, because high-risk types of viruses do not necessarily correspond to high-grade lesions and, on the contrary, lesions with HPV-6 and -11 occasionally may progress to carcinoma. This finding confirms the existence of at least two biologic subsets, one with a greater risk of progression to more severe forms of intraepithelial neoplasia and invasive carcinoma.[101,102]

Different findings should be mentioned to emphasize the need for additional studies before reaching a definite conclusion on the role of HPV in lower female genital tract oncogenesis.

1. About 10% of the female population harbors HPV, and more than 60% of this population has a normal Pap spear and no clinical lesion. The wide distribution of the HPV does not militate against its role in cervical oncogenesis, but it must be confirmed by more prospective epidemiologic studies.[103,104]
2. The correlation between the type of cervical lesion and the type of HPV present is not always as expected (see above).
3. The unpredictable evolution of CIN may be linked with the diversity of genital HPV types associated with the lesion.[84]
4. In a small percentage of case, HPV may have no role in the development of CIN.[105]
5. The correlation between the morphologic image and the presence of HPV is not constant; typical CIN images are not accompanied by HPV and vice versa.
6. Strict cytologic and histologic criteria should be used for the diagnosis of HPV infection to avoid overdiagnosis and subsequent overtreatment.

Colposcopy. The colposcope identifies four types of condylomatous lesions[45,46]:

1. The florid condyloma acuminatum is charac-

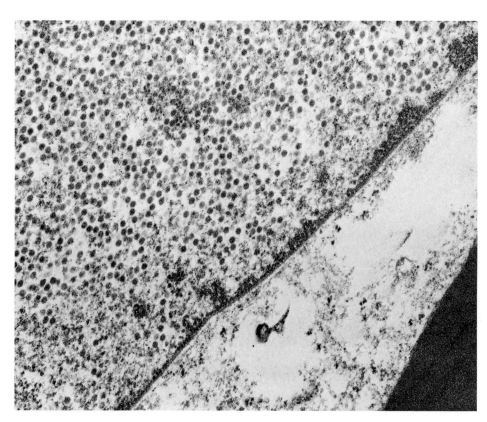

FIGURE 3-21 Electron micrograph of intranuclear papillomavirus particles in condyloma. (Courtesy of Drs. Bennett A. Jenson and Robert J. Kurman, Georgetown University Medical Center, Washington, DC)

terized by a white thickened epithelium with finger-like projections.

2. The spiked condyloma shows a white area with roughened peaks.
3. The flat condyloma reveals a flat, white lesion with a mosaic pattern, in which vessels are not apparent.
4. Condylomatous cervicitis or vaginitis shows a red epithelium with raised white dots and can be found alone or in association with flat condyloma.

Histopathology.   Histologically, condyloma presents three main structural variations:

1. A papillary growth (*condyloma acuminatum*) is characterized by a papillomatous exophytic proliferation (Fig. 3-22). This type is more commonly seen on the external genitalia. The epithelium shows acanthosis, hyperkeratosis, parakeratosis, and cellular atypia.
2. A rare type, the *inverted condyloma*, shows a downward proliferation into the stroma (involving endocervical glands) and has often been confused with carcinoma (Fig. 3-23).
3. The most common type is the *flat condyloma*, which exhibits the same cellular atypias but lacks the papillomatous or inverting proliferation (Figs. 3-24 and 3-25). The terminology is actually contradictory, because condyloma means a focal raised lesion and not a flat structure. The term *noncondylomatous cervical HPV infection* is more correct, but it is difficult to change a denomination consecrated by daily usage.

The characteristic *cellular changes* present in all types of condyloma (see Figs. 3-24 and 3-25) are the existence of superficial and intermediate cells with (1) voluminous clear, glycogen-poor cytoplasm and (2) an irregular, hyperchromatic or pyknotic nucleus. The localization of the cytoplasmic organelles at the periphery of the cell creates the impression of a thickened cell membrane surrounding a perinuclear halo (*koilocytosis*). Ireland* has referred to the nuclei as "raisinoid," emphasizing their irregularly wrinkled appearance. Binucleate cells are common.[106] Parakeratosis is constant, and small peaks of superficial epithelium (perhaps abortive papillae) are seen even in the flat lesions.

The presence of HPV alterations in the intermediate and superficial cells and not in the parabasal layers can be explained by the fact that viral structural antigens are not synthesized in proliferating basal cells but occur in the differentiated cells, which are permissive for the synthesis of the structural proteins of the virus.

The simultaneous presence of condylomatous lesions in the superficial layers of the epithelium and dysplasia in the basal layers may shed some light on

*Ireland: Personal communication.

the development of *intraepithelial neoplasia* (see Figs. 3-48, 3-49 and 3-50). Hyperplasia of parabasal cells occurs beneath the areas of virus-induced atypias; this induced proliferation of the parabasal layers is susceptible to neoplastic transformation through the potentiating action of the viral agent. The morphologic manifestation of the viral infestation is not apparent in the parabasal cells that contain the viral genome; on the contrary, when the cells differentiate, they become permissive for synthesis of the viral structural proteins and their manifestations become apparent.

The failure to detect HPV antigens in more severe forms of dysplasia and carcinoma in situ can be interpreted as a disturbance in virus production when the neoplastic transformation has taken place or as a suppression of virus protein synthesis in cells that already show evidence of HPV infestation.[96]

Cytology.   Cytologic examination is the routine technique for the detection of HPV infection in the genital tract: it is economical, convenient and rapid (Color Figs. 3-10 through 3-12).[106,107] Papanicolaou-stained smears reveal the presence of koilocytes. These elements are intermediate or superficial squamous cells and metaplastic-type cells from the transformation zone. Their nuclei are eccentrically located, hyperchromatic, enlarged, irregular, and wrinkled, or small and dense, and surrounded by a clear cytoplasmic halo, which is itself surrounded by peripheral dense blue-green or fuchsia-red cytoplasm. This staining is very different from the normal orangeophilia. This zone corresponds to cytoplasmic necrosis. Binucleation or multinucleation is common. The degree of nuclear abnormality varies from mild to marked. Phagocytosed material may be present in the clear space. These cells constitute small aggregates or are isolated. In early stages of the viral infection, one may observe clumps of rounded and blunt cells with dense and opaque cytoplasm representing the first morphologic alterations. Dyskaryotic cells are present and characterized by a yellow or orangeophilic cytoplasm and a small, dense nucleus without prominent nucleoli. Metaplastic-type immature cells from the transformation zone reveal the same alteration: nuclear enlargement, moderate hyperchromatism, bi- or multinucleation, and peripherally condensed cyanophilic cytoplasm. Columnar endocervical cells do not reveal specific changes. According to these descriptions, the koilocyte is a dyskaryotic cell with a very typical perinuclear halo. These various cellular alterations, described by Koss and Durfee[108] under the term *koilocytosis*, had been called *nearo-carcinoma* by Ayre[109] and *balloon cells* by Meisels and Fortin.[106] These authors had guessed the viral origin of the cellular alterations.

Natural History and Prognosis.   The natural history and prognosis of cervical HPV infection are still

(*Text continued on page 94.*)

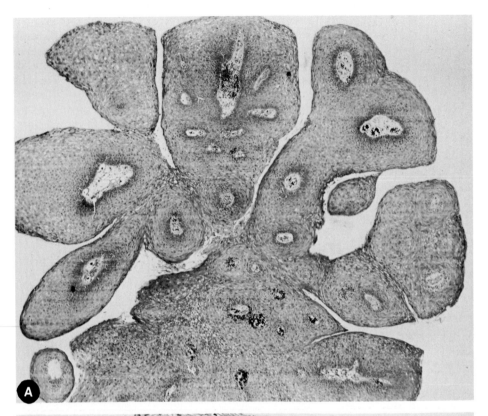

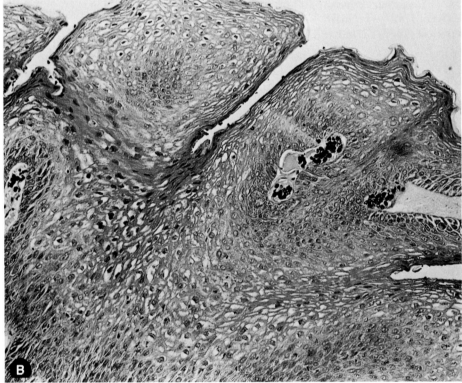

FIGURE 3-22 Condyloma acuminatum of cervix. **(A)** Low-power view of papillary growth pattern. **(B)** Detail showing koilocytotic atypia.

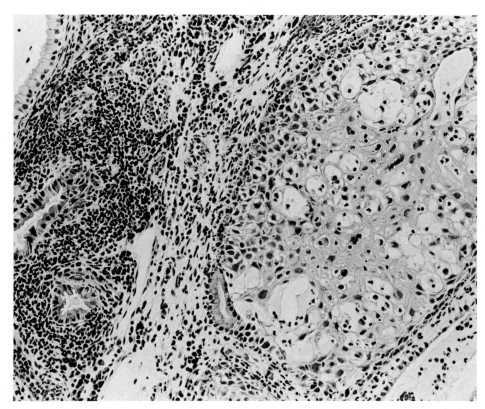

FIGURE 3-23 Inverted condyloma involving endocervical gland.

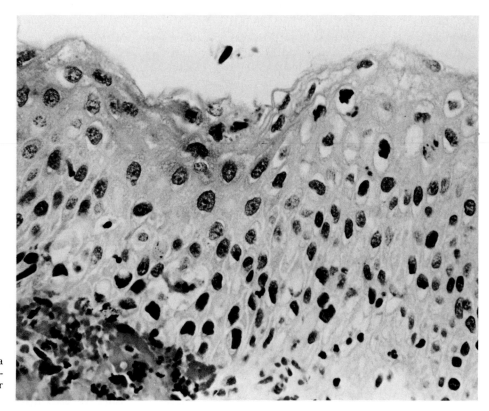

FIGURE 3-24 Flat condyloma showing peaks of surface epithelium and typical cellular manifestations.

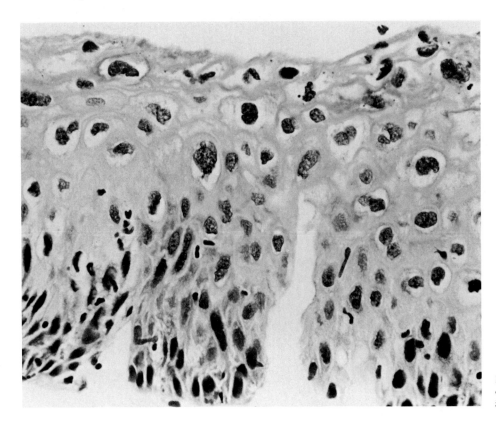

FIGURE 3-25 Flat condyloma demonstrating "raisinoid" nuclei and perinuclear haloes.

poorly understood. One would expect condylomatous lesions unassociated with classic dysplasia or carcinoma in situ to be less likely to progress to cancer if untreated, but this has not been demonstrated adequately. The specific antigenic type of HPV (particularly types 16 and 18) and the presence of aneuploid cells may portend progression, but most laboratories cannot routinely perform the studies necessary to yield these data. Dysplasia may be seen directly beneath the superficial layers showing condylomatous manifestations, immediately adjacent to the condylomatous lesion, or at some distance from it in the same or a different biopsy specimen. Because the clinical significance of these different patterns is not clearly understood, it is recommended that the treatment and follow-up of the "pure" cervical condyloma be the same as for cervical dysplasia at the present time.[110,111]

This story is not at all complete, and more correlative histologic and virologic analysis, further characterization of HPV types, and prospective studies of low-grade CIN lesions are needed before the exact role of HPV will be determined. At present, cytology is the most practical method to detect virus-associated cellular abnormalities.

Trichomonas Cervicitis

It has been estimated that as many as 20% to 25% of adult women harbor the parasite *Trichomonas vaginalis* in the lower genital tract, although many of these women are asymptomatic. Inflammatory reactions due to *Trichomonas* are characteristically intermittent and difficult to treat.

Histologically, cervical vascular congestion is followed by edema, cellular inflammatory infiltrates, and ulceration of the squamous mucosa (Fig. 3-26). This picture is nonspecific unless the parasite is identified, usually in cervicovaginal smears (see discussion above and in Chap. 2). When the infection is severe, one may observe reserve cell hyperplasia, squamous metaplasia, and superficial papillomatosis of columnar cells. Patients with *Trichomonas* infections often have notable epithelial atypia in cytologic material, which should regress after treatment of the infection (see Chap. 2). Cervical cancer and precancerous states are also more frequent in women with trichomoniasis, probably coincidentally rather than causally.[112-115]

Chlamydial Cervicitis

Chlamydial cervicitis is a common sexually transmitted disease often restricted to the cervix and the urethra.[116-118] The organism may be responsible for other infections such as endometritis, salpingitis, trachoma, and lymphogranuloma venereum. Contamination of the neonate during delivery may cause conjunctivitis and pneumonia.

The cervical infection is asymptomatic or clinically associated with a mucopurulent endocervical discharge.[119] It has been reported that *Chlamydia trachomatis* infection may produce follicular cervicitis.[47,120]

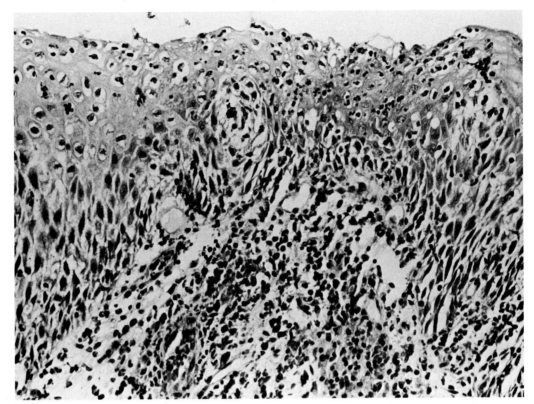

FIGURE 3-26 *Trichomonas* cervicitis, with acute and chronic inflammation and reactive atypia of squamous mucosa.

The organisms, which measure about 300 nm, enter squamous metaplastic and endocervical columnar cells, multiply, and constitute intracytoplasmic inclusions. After lysis of the cell, the elementary bodies are free and enter new cells.

Electron microscopy has confirmed that the cytoplasmic vesicles contain several morphologic forms (elementary bodies, reticulate bodies, and intermediate forms) typical of *Chlamydia*.[121] These obligate intracellular organisms are classified as bacteria. *Histologically,* chlamydial cervicitis consists of a chronic inflammatory infiltrate with macrophages, plasma cells, lymphocytes, neutrophils, and eosinophils.

Cytology. The elementary bodies cannot be identified in Papanicolaou-stained smears, but the presence of intracytoplasmic aggregates of elementary bodies produces cellular changes that can be observed microscopically.[122–128] First, numerous, small vacuolated structures are present in the cytoplasm, suggesting a "moth-eaten" appearance. Dot-like structures occupy these vacuoles. Later, these aggregates condense and develop the distinct intracytoplasmic inclusion underlined by a well-defined wall (Color Fig. 3-13). Multinucleation is common. The typical cytoplasmic inclusions are not always present, and therefore the diagnosis is based on tissue culture and immunodiagnosis.[129]

Cervical Tuberculosis

Cervical tuberculosis represents only 1% of cases of genital tuberculosis and is secondary to tuberculous endometritis and salpingitis. Several observations have revealed the simultaneous presence of cervical tuberculosis and epidermoid carcinoma, although no etiologic relation has been established.[130–132]

Macroscopic Appearance. The cervix is proliferative, irregular, and sometimes ulcerated, and suggests the existence of a malignant tumor. Examination of the biopsy makes the diagnosis, but it should be confirmed by culture of *Mycobacterium tuberculosis.*

Histology. The lesion is a typical tuberculous granuloma; epithelioid cells and Langhans' giant cells surrounded by lymphocytes, with little or much central caseation.

Cytology. Cytology of tuberculosis includes the presence of clusters of epithelioid cells, lymphocytes, and huge multinucleated giant cells. If all these components are present, the diagnosis of tuberculosis can be suspected. This eventuality is rare, especially in the regions of the world where tuberculosis has been treated effectively. The epithelioid cells form aggregates of large, pale, cyanophilic, irregular cells with oval, vesicular nuclei. The multinucleated giant cells have numerous, peripherally located small nuclei.[133-135]

Other Granulomatous Lesions

Other granulomatous lesions that can involve the cervix are the *foreign body giant cell granuloma* secondary to a previous surgical procedure and *schistosomiasis* (bilharziasis). Schistosomiasis is characterized microscopically by multinucleate giant cell granulomas surrounding the eggs with their characteristic spines.[136,137]

A case of *ceroid granuloma* been described in the cervix.[138] The cervical biopsy revealed an ulcerated granulomatous lesion of the epithelium with macrophages containing ceroid pigment. A tampon-related etiology has been suggested. Protozoa uncommonly observed in cervical smears are *Entamoeba histolytica* and *Vorticella*.[139,140]

Langerhans cell histiocytosis of the lower genital tract is a rare disease thought to represent a disorder of immune regulation; a few cases have been described involving the cervix.[141] Microscopy reveals a cellular granulomatous infiltrate composed almost exclusively of proliferating Langerhans cells with associated inflammatory cells. Immunohistochemically, these cells express S-100 protein. Elongated Birbeck granules are visible at the electron microscopic level.

Cervical Syphilis

Next to vulvar chancre, cervical chancre is most frequent in the female genital tract.[142] The lesion may be confused with a simple cervical erosion. In the great majority of cases, it is situated at the circumference of the external os. The chancre presents in one of two forms: (1) an ulcer with indurated base and elevated borders, surrounded by a zone of edema, or (2) a simple nonindurated erosion covered by a gray membranous exudate. Search for the treponeme is mandatory in all doubtful lesions; its demonstration permits the differential diagnosis from granuloma inguinale, acute gonorrhea, chancroid, and carcinoma.

Secondary papular lesions of the cervix have been described rarely, and tertiary lesions are very rare. Chapter 1 provides a microscopic description of these lesions.

Other Specific Infections

Other rare specific infections are occasionally seen. *Cytomegalovirus*,[143-146] which belongs to the herpesvirus group, is serologically common, but clinical manifestations are rare. It may be associated with herpesvirus and HPV. In cervical smears, columnar cells are more frequently affected and contain round, large intranuclear inclusions surrounded by a clear halo (Fig. 3-27). Cervical *actinomycosis* has been

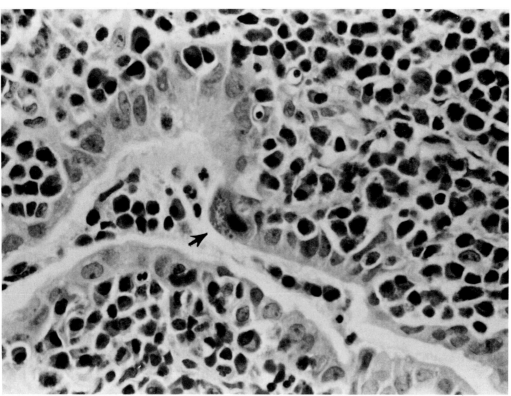

FIGURE 3-27 Cytomegalovirus cervicitis: endocervical cell with nuclear and cytoplasmic inclusions (*arrow*).

reported.[147] The typical filaments and peripheral palisading clubs are easily recognized. Some cases have been associated with use of intrauterine contraceptive devices.[148,149] Rare cases of *giant cell arteritis* limited to the cervix have been described.[150–152] These seem to be incidental findings of no clinical importance. The nematode *Ascaris lumbricoides* has been mentioned in cervicovaginal smears,[139,153] as have microfilariae.[154]

BENIGN TUMORS AND TUMOR-LIKE LESIONS

Endocervical Polyp

The cervical polyp is a pedunculated tumorous formation developing at the surface of the cervix. It is considered a hyperplastic phenomenon of the epithelium and stroma rather than a true neoplasm. It is sometimes accompanied by small hemorrhages, either spontaneous or on contact, and by leukorrhea, but most often it is asymptomatic. It is more common in middle-aged women and multigravidas.

Macroscopic Appearance. The cervical polyp presents as a single small spherical mass that herniates at the level of the cervical orifice and usually measures several millimeters in diameter. It is usually attached to the cervical wall by a short stalk but is occasionally sessile. The surface is smooth, shiny, and pale pink, or granular, lobulated, and dark red (Fig. 3-28). Signs of secondary infection are frequent. More rarely, the lesion actually may be an endometrial polyp attached by a long stalk to the isthmus or to the corporeal mucosa and exteriorized at the cervical orifice.

Microscopic Appearance. The cervical polyp is covered by a glandular epithelium showing frequent foci of squamous metaplasia (Fig. 3-29). It contains a loose, edematous, richly vascularized connective tissue stroma, infiltrated by inflammatory cells of predominantly lymphoplasmacytic type. This inflammatory infiltrate is found in 80% of cases; it is more marked in the presence of ulceration of the surface epithelium. Highly vascularized polyps are occasionally encountered. The development of dysplasia and in situ or invasive carcinoma in a polyp occurs in less than 1% of cases.[155] In a case with malignant change, it is important to verify the integrity of the base of the stalk at the implantation site. Another possibility is the secondary invasion of the polyp by an adjacent carcinoma. A small number of polyps contain in their stroma large, clear cells with foamy cytoplasm containing lipids; their significance is not known.[156] Bizarre stromal cells with hyperchromatic nuclei may be encountered rarely in pseudosarcomatous

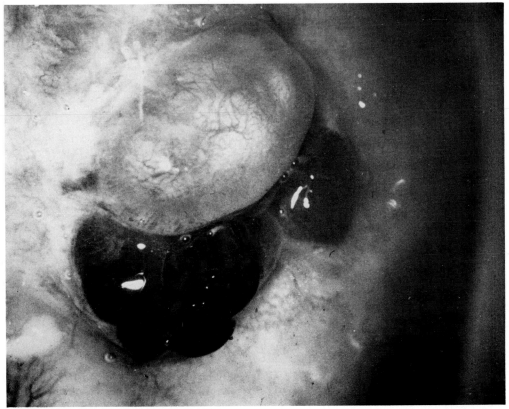

FIGURE 3-28 Endocervical polyp: clinical appearance.

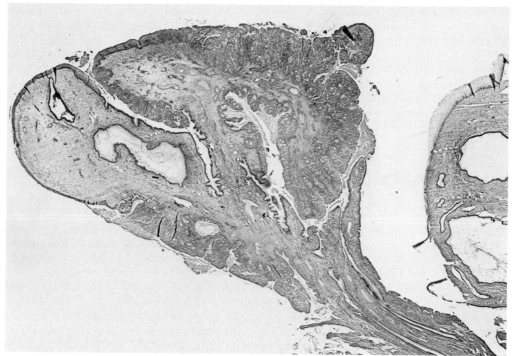

FIGURE 3-29 Endocervical polyp with zones of squamous metaplasia.

botryoid polyp of the cervix. Decidual reaction is encountered in some pregnancies (decidual polyp).[37–40,157]

Cytology. The cervical smear may reveal inflammatory or dysplastic lesions of the epithelium lining the polyp. Eroded areas are the origin of repair changes (see above). Abundant aggregates of columnar cells are present when a direct scraping of the polyp is obtained. Numerous endocervical columnar cells showing no cellular atypia and accompanied by abundant inflammatory cells may suggest the existence of a polyp.

Squamous Papilloma

The squamous papilloma is a polypoid formation covered by a papillomatous squamous epithelium beneath which is a richly vascularized stroma.[158,159] It is a rare tumor, usually encountered during pregnancy, which represents less than 1% of the benign tumors of the cervix. Chronic inflammatory conditions such as gonorrhea, tuberculosis, and viral infections are said to favor its appearance, but this notion demands confirmation. The evolution of these lesions is benign, and excision is curative.

Macroscopic Appearance. The tumor has the form of an ectocervical polyp and is several millimeters in diameter.

Microscopic Appearance. The covering squamous epithelium shows papillomatosis, hyperkeratosis, ac-

anthosis, and parakeratosis. Mitoses are infrequent. The stroma is richly vascularized and contains a chronic inflammatory infiltrate. Benign epithelial atypia or (rarely) in situ or invasive carcinoma may develop in the epithelium.[160,161] *Condyloma acuminatum* is a particular, usually multiple, very exuberant type of squamous papilloma. This and other papillomavirus-induced lesions are discussed earlier in the chapter.

Leiomyoma

The leiomyoma is a single spherical or nodular tumor consisting of smooth muscle fibers and fibrous connective tissue (Fig. 3-30). It is a relatively infrequent tumor in the cervix and represents less than 10% of all uterine myomas.[162] It may be immense and either encapsulated or diffuse. It is often associated with leiomyomata of the corpus uteri and resembles them histologically. Different forms of degeneration identical to those observed in leiomyomas of the corpus may occur. Malignant transformation is rare.[51] The vascular leiomyoma is an association of a leiomyomatous growth with abundant, disseminated, thick-walled vessels.

Glandular Hyperplasias and Metaplasias

A number of benign endocervical glandular proliferative lesions lacking cytologic atypia or premalignant significance have been described. Their main clinical

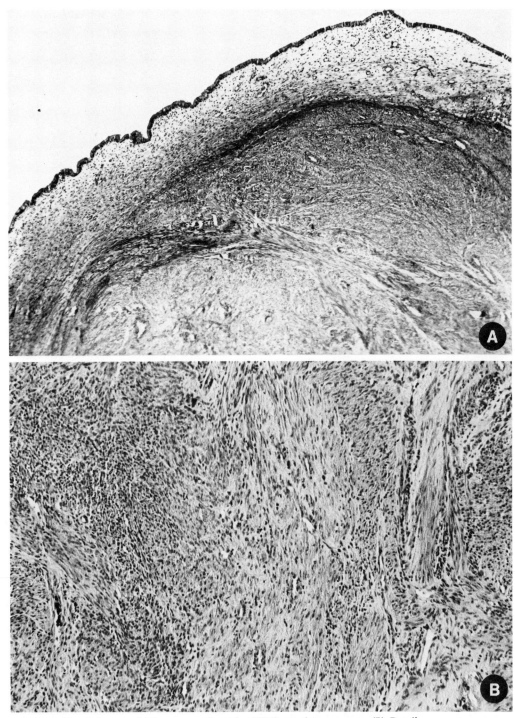

FIGURE 3-30 Submucosal leiomyoma of cervix. **(A)** General appearance. **(B)** Detail.

importance lies in the occasional tendency of the inexperienced pathologist to misinterpret them as adenocarcinoma.

Tunnel Clusters

Tunnel clusters,[51,163] sometimes referred to as *adenomatous hyperplasia*,[163,164] are characterized by the presence of groups of endocervical glands, often cystic, with columnar, cuboidal, or flattened epithelium (Fig. 3-31). These glands contain mucus and are surrounded by a fibrous stroma disposed in concentric layers. The lesions are situated in the endocervix and may extend the entire length of this portion but rarely involve the ectocervix. They lack glandular angularity and a surrounding inflammatory stromal response, differentiating them from minimal deviation adenocarcinoma.

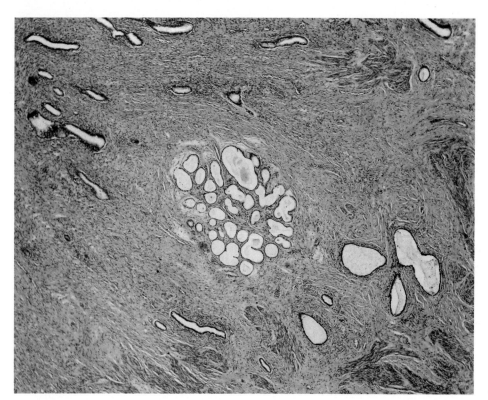

FIGURE 3-31 Tunnel cluster of endocervix.

Microglandular Hyperplasia

Frequently seen in women taking oral progestational agents for contraception and in pregnant and postpartum women is a lesion known as *microglandular hyperplasia* (MGH; Fig. 3-32).[165–167] *Clinically*, it may simulate an endocervical polyp or occur in the endocervical clefts and present no evident macroscopic lesion.

Microscopically, MGH shows numerous irregular glandular structures disposed in a dense or reticulated pattern and lined by hyperplastic cuboidal cells. Small glands containing intraluminal mucin and neutrophils fuse to form larger cystic spaces. The glands often appear continuous with the surrounding stroma, and two or more adjacent glands share "party walls," being lined by the same single layer of cells. The presence of subcolumnar reserve cells and squamous metaplasia is often observed. Mitoses are very rare. The stroma is loose and edematous and shows vascular congestion, multiplication of vessels, and leukocytic infiltration that is predominantly lymphoplasmacytic.

The benign character of the lesion is emphasized by the uniformity of the cells (which often contain subnuclear vacuoles), the absence of stromal invasion, the generally absent mitotic activity, and the clinical history. Immunohistochemically, there is no reaction for carcinoembryonic antigen (CEA), which helps in the differential diagnosis with adenocarcinoma.[168,169] Leslie and Silverberg[166] have emphasized that rare atypical cases may be encountered, by virtue of cytologic atypia (Fig. 3-33) or an unusual clin-ical presentation (eg, in a postmenopausal woman or in the endometrium). Their schema for differential diagnosis from adenocarcinoma of endocervix and endometrium is reproduced in Table 3-2. Rare cases of endometrial or endocervical adenocarcinoma may present with an MGH-like picture in a curettage or biopsy specimen.[166,170] Thus, the differential diagnosis may be confusing in both directions.

Deep Nabothian Cysts

Nabothian cysts (see Fig. 3-12) have been described above as part of the picture of chronic cervicitis. These generally are located immediately beneath the endocervical or metaplastic surface epithelium, but occasionally they can be found deep in the cervical wall, where they may be confused with a type of adenocarcinoma known as *minimal deviation adenocarcinoma*.[171] The uniform round contours and cystic dilatation of the nabothian cysts and the absence of a stromal reaction around them should prevent this error.

Diffuse Laminar Endocervical Glandular Hyperplasia

Jones and colleagues[172] have described this lesion as an incidental finding in specimens from hysterectomies performed for other indications. It consists of a glandular proliferation confined to the inner third of the cervical wall and sharply demarcated from the underlying stroma. The glands are of moderate size, evenly and closely spaced, and highly differentiated.

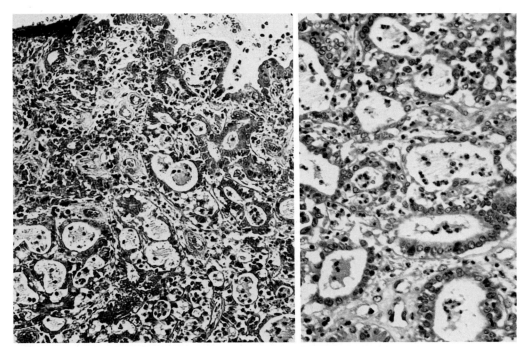

FIGURE 3-32 Microglandular hyperplasia in woman receiving oral contraceptives: general appearance (*left*) and detail (*right*).

Marked inflammation and reactive atypia may be present. The absence of irregular and deep stromal infiltration and of a desmoplastic stromal response help in the differential diagnosis from minimal deviation adenocarcinoma.

Glandular Metaplasias

In addition to the ubiquitous squamous metaplasia, endocervical glands can also undergo *intestinal, endometrial,* and *tubal metaplasia.* Intestinal metaplasia is predominantly encountered in neoplastic (in situ or invasive) glandular epithelia. Endometrial metaplasia is uncommon, and by definition must be located distal to the endometrial-endocervical junction and be unassociated with endometrial stroma (endometriosis). Tubal metaplasia[173,174] is the most common of these conditions, occurring in 31% of hysterectomy specimens in one recent series, and even more frequently in cases from which many tissue blocks were submitted for microscopic examination.[174] In this lesion, the surface epithelium, glands, or both are lined focally by a pseudostratified epithelium containing all three cell types (ciliated, secretory, and in-

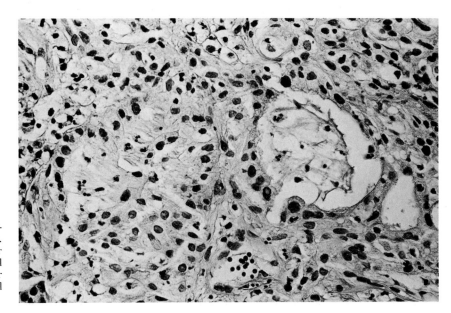

FIGURE 3-33 Microglandular hyperplasia of cervix with focal nuclear atypia. (Leslie KO, Silverberg SG: Microglandular hyperplasia of the cervix: Unusual clinical and pathological presentations and their differential diagnosis. Prog Surg Pathol 5:95–114, 1984)

TABLE 3-2.
Differential Diagnosis of Microglandular Hyperplasia from Endocervical and Endometrial Adenocarcinoma

	Microglandular Hyperplasia	Endocervical Adenocarcinoma	Endometrial Adenocarcinoma
Age	Predominantly young	Usually over 40	Usually over 40
Menstrual status	Predominantly premenopausal, frequently pregnant	40% premenopausal	Predominantly postmenopausal
Constitution	No special characteristics	No special characteristics	Obese, hypertensive, diabetic, nulliparous
Hormone usage	Oral contraceptive therapy (predominantly progestational effect)	Oral contraceptive therapy?	Estrogen effect
Atypia	Rare (inflammatory)	Characteristically present	Characteristically present
Mitoses	Extremely rare	Characteristically present	Characteristically present (numerous)
Architecture	Central core of glands with peripheral stromal pseudoinfiltration. Glands share "party walls." No true cribriform areas	Usually little cribriform pattern. Glands separated by scirrhous or edematous stroma	Diffuse stromal infiltration by glands. Solid sheets of cells may be central (morules), peripheral, or both. Glands "independent" except in cribriform areas
Inflammatory cells	Always present; within glands, glandular epithelium, and stroma	May be absent or inconspicuous without necrosis	May be absent or inconspicuous without necrosis
Mucin	Present in gland lumina, not in cells or stroma	Voluminous mucin in cells and gland lumina	Generally not prominent; when present, mainly apical and intraluminal
Squamous metaplasia	Characteristically present	Uncommon	Present in up to 50% of cases—squamous element frequently histologically malignant
Tissue CEA	Uniformly negative	Usually positive	Usually negative

Leslie KO, Silverberg SG: Microglandular hyperplasia of the cervix: Unusual clinical and pathological presentations and their differential diagnosis. Prog Surg Pathol 5:95–114, 1984

tercalated) seen in the normal fallopian tube. The main significance of this lesion is its potential confusion with adenocarcinoma in situ histologically or with any glandular neoplasia cytologically. The observation of ciliated cells should lead to the correct diagnosis. Tubal metaplasia is illustrated in this chapter in the section on adenocarcinoma in situ (see Fig. 3-80).

Mesonephric Remnants, Cysts, and Hyperplasias

Mesonephric remnants or rests in the cervix are a common incidental finding.[175] They are situated deep in the substance of the lateral walls of the endocervix and are lined by cuboidal epithelium. There is no secretion of mucus or glycogen and no ciliation. The histologic distinction between deep endocervical glands, especially malignant ones, and mesonephric rests is important to make.[28,176] Most important is the nonciliated and nonmuciparous nature of the mesonephric epithelium and the usual presence of a central slit-like duct from which the small glands radiate (Fig. 3-34). Dense eosinophilic material in the gland lumina is also characteristic. Ferry and Scully[28] have proposed a classification and a definition of the mesonephric lesions that should avert misdiagnosis (Table 3-3). These lesions, with the exception of mesonephric remnants, are rare, with mesonephric carcinoma being the rarest.

Papillary Adenofibroma

Papillary adenofibroma is a rare lesion. First delineated by Abell,[177] it is characterized by a lobulated and papillary configuration, with flattened endocervical epithelium covering a compact or loose solid growth of small, uniform fibroblasts (Fig. 3-35). No

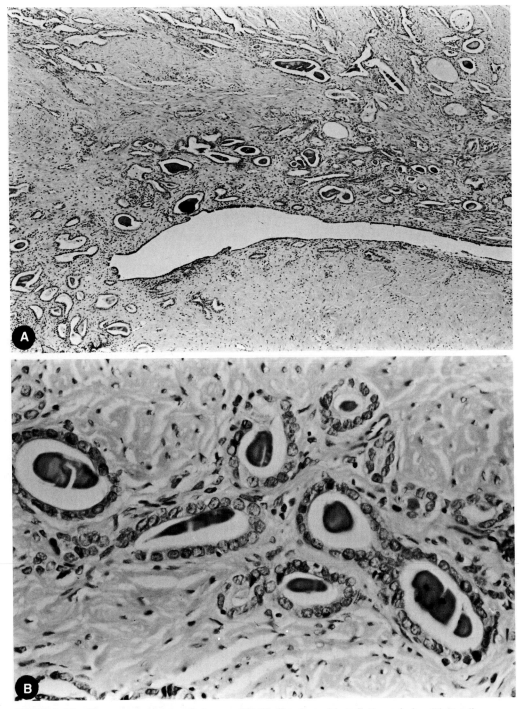

FIGURE 3-34 Hyperplastic mesonephric rests. **(A)** Slit-like duct with radiating tubules. **(B)** Detail of tubules lined by nonciliated, nonmuciparous cuboidal cells, with dense eosinophilic material in lumina.

smooth muscle cells and no mitoses are observed. Microscopically, it resembles adenofibromas arising in the ovary and the endometrium.[178] Most of the cases are described in postmenopausal women. The evolution is benign, but the lesion must be differentiated from the closely related müllerian adenosarcoma (see Chap. 4).

Rare Benign Tumors

Let us also note briefly a few rare cases of *hemangioma,*[179] *blue nevus,*[180] *traumatic neuroma,*[181] *ganglioneuroma,*[182] *neurilemmoma,*[183] and *granular cell tumor.*[184] *Glial polyps* of the cervix are probably sequelae of a previous occult abortion.[185] A few authors have

TABLE 3-3.
Mesonephric Lesions of the Cervix

Mesonephric remnants
Mesonephric cysts
Lobular mesonephric hyperplasia
Diffuse mesonephric hyperplasia
Mesonephric ductal hyperplasia
Mesonephric carcinoma

Adapted from Ferry JA, Scully RE: Mesonephric remnants, hyperplasia, and neoplasia in the uterine cervix: A study of 49 cases. Am J Surg Pathol 14:1100–1111, 1990.

noted the presence in the cervix of *sebaceous glands,* which are products of metaplastic phenomena from squamous epithelium or represent misplaced embryonic tissue.[186–188]

The *müllerian papilloma* (previously called *mesonephric papilloma*) is a rare cervical or vaginal benign tumor of infancy.[189–191] It is characterized by papillary structures lined by a cuboidal epithelium and underlain by a loose fibrovascular stroma. The presence of mucin-filled cells and the ultrastructural appearance have confirmed the müllerian origin.[192]

Cervical Endometriosis

More than 100 cases of cervical endometriosis have been published,[193–195] but our experience suggests that the lesion is far more common. The most rea-

sonable pathogenic mechanism is post-traumatic implantation of fragments of endometrium.[196] The clinical history frequently reveals the existence of prior gynecologic trauma during a delivery or a curettage. Why is this implantation rare, considering the frequency of passage of endometrial debris into and through the cervix with each menstrual period? One may explain this rarity by the resistance of the untraumatized intact squamous epithelium to the implantation of endometrial fragments. Thus, the lesion is seen most frequently after combined cervical conization and endometrial curettage.

The lesion is asymptomatic or may cause premenstrual hemorrhages. More rarely, they are inter- or postmenstrual. It develops in the adult women between 20 and 50 years of age.

Macroscopic Appearance. Cervical endometriosis does not always present a typical appearance. The presence of a slightly elevated, dark red or brown cystic structure suggests a focus of endometriosis. Endometriosis may also present as a zone of erosion, a granular-surfaced nodule, or a proliferating lesion; these may arouse suspicion of malignancy, and only microscopic examination permits the assessment of their true nature.

Histologic examination shows endometrial glands (proliferative or secretory) surrounded by endometrial stroma. To be labeled *endometriosis,* this lesion should have no connection with the adjacent endometrium. Stromal endometriosis that emphasizes the stromal proliferation has been described.[197] A case

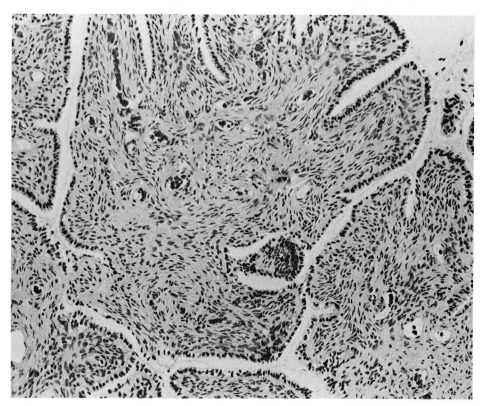

FIGURE 3-35 Papillary adenofibroma of cervix.

of adenocarcinoma has been reported within a focus of cervical endometriosis.[198]

Cytology may reveal the presence of well-preserved endometrial cells of epithelial and stromal origin. The visual or colposcopic observation of a cervical lesion must be correlated with the abundance of endometrial cells and suggests the diagnosis.[199]

CERVICAL INTRAEPITHELIAL NEOPLASIA (DYSPLASIA AND IN SITU CARCINOMA, LOW- AND HIGH-GRADE SQUAMOUS INTRAEPITHELIAL LESIONS)

Although many descriptions of the precancerous lesions are found in the literature of the late 19th century and early 20th century (Cullen[200] illustrated changes of carcinoma in situ as early as 1900), the first attempt to classify the precancerous lesions can be attributed to Broders[201] in 1932. The term *cervical dysplasia* was mentioned by Papanicolaou[202] in 1949, and Reagan[203] in 1953 defined the lesion as an atypical hyperplasia of the cervical squamous epithelium. The important contribution of Reagan pointed out that the clinical prognosis cannot be determined from the morphologic appearance of the lesion, and he introduced the notion that two categories of lesions are present in the cervical epithelium : an ill-defined category that includes various benign alterations (dysplasia), and carcinoma in situ, which represents the precursor of invasive carcinoma. Because dysplasia is considered to comprise epithelial atypical changes below the level of carcinoma in situ, the crucial definition is that of the latter lesion.

The definition established in 1961 by the International Committee for Histological Definitions[204] was strictly histologic:

> Only those cases should be classified as carcinoma in situ which, in the absence of invasion, show a surface epithelium in which, throughout its whole thickness, no differentiation takes place. The process may involve the lining of the cervical glands without thereby creating a new group. It is recognized that the cells of the uppermost layers may show some slight flattening. The very rare case of an otherwise characteristic carcinoma in situ which shows a greater degree of differentiation belongs to the exceptions for which no classification can provide.

Koss[205,206] has suggested a broader functional definition of carcinoma in situ as "a lesion confined to the epithelium of the uterine cervix, morphologically resembling invasive cancer."

The disadvantage of this dual terminology was to tend to represent dysplasia and carcinoma in situ as two different diseases. We know that the epithelial changes of the cervix form a continuous spectrum of the same disease. To meet this major objection, the term *cervical intraepithelial neoplasia (CIN)* was pro-

posed by Richart[207-210] to indicate the spectrum of epithelial changes constituting various forms of dysplasia and in situ squamous cell carcinoma. This nomenclature recognizes the concept of a single disease, considers dysplasia as a neoplastic entity, and correlates histologic images with adequate treatment. When the CIN terminology is used, we prefer that the lesions not be subclassified as CIN I, II, and III, although most systems now do this; the reason is that the entire philosophic basis of CIN terminology is to emphasize the continuous spectrum of these lesions.

More recently, a new classification for cytologic diagnosis has been proposed by a committee convened under the auspices of the National Cancer Institute in Bethesda in 1988,[211] with further modification in 1991.[212] This Bethesda system suggests the use of only two grades to qualify these morphologic anomalies: *low-grade* and *high-grade squamous intraepithelial lesions*. Richart has proposed to modify the CIN classification accordingly into two groups,[213] although some arguments exist to maintain the subdivision of CIN into three grades.[214] Table 3-4 summarizes the three current classifications and their relation to one another.

Difficulties in Studying Cervical Intraepithelial Neoplasia

The difficulties involved in attempting to study the natural history of cervical dysplasia and in situ carcinoma result largely from the following almost insurmountable obstacles.

Lack of Universally Accepted Definitions

We have just mentioned the different classifications proposed in the last decades. Unanimity has not been reached, although the tendency is to adopt a uniform simple terminology that would communicate the necessary information to the physician. More biologic, epidemiologic, and pathologic infor-

TABLE 3-4.
Classifications of Cervical Intraepithelial Neoplasia

CIN	Classical	Bethesda
CIN I ———— Mild dysplasia		Low-grade SIL*
CIN II ———— Moderate dysplasia		
CIN III ⟨ Severe dysplasia / Carcinoma in situ		High-grade SIL

SIL, squamous intraepithelial lesion

*Low-grade SIL also encompasses HPV-related cellular changes (condyloma, koilocytotic atypia). This is designed as a cytopathologic reporting system, whereas the other two are histopathologic.

mation is needed to clarify the pathogenesis of the different steps of cervical cancerization, for example, to be able to separate benign and potentially malignant lesions that reveal similar cytohistologic images.

Observer Disagreement in Histopathologic Diagnosis

Numerous authors[215–218] have demonstrated a remarkable variability in the interpretation of identical lesions by different pathologists (or even by the same pathologist on different days). Although these different interpretations usually vary only slightly (eg, mild versus moderate dysplasia, *not* moderate dysplasia versus invasive cancer), they indicate that any population study based on biopsy diagnosis is subject to considerable observer bias.

Possible Differences in Natural History Based on Etiologic Agents

The demonstration that most lesions classified as CIN are related to HPV infection[80–84,87–89,99,102,110,219–222] has raised a new caveat in the study of these atypias. We now need to differentiate "pure" condyloma, dysplasia or carcinoma in situ without evidence of condyloma, and various patterns of coexistence of the two processes, before we can attempt follow-up studies. The suggestion that particular viral subtypes may be more likely to be associated with lesions that progress indicates that morphologic interpretations alone may be inadequate in the study of these lesions.[82,84,85,87,89,99,100,223–226] It is generally accepted that types 16 and 18 belong in this "high-risk" group; some investigators also include types 31, 33, 45, and 56, whereas others assign these types (as well as 30, 34, 40, and 47) to an intermediate risk category; types 6, 11, and 42 are universally considered low risk.[222–226] Finally, because none of these distinctions was made in the classic studies of earlier years, all their conclusions must be reexamined.

Effect of the Investigative Procedure on the Process Being Studied

Several investigators[206,208] have shown that even small punch biopsies that do not remove all of the abnormal epithelium can induce subsequent replacement of dysplastic or in situ carcinomatous epithelium by benign mucosa. Because the interpretation of colposcopic and cytologic observations is even more variable than that of biopsy material, we must conclude that no method of study will give us a definitive, quantitative picture of the natural history of CIN. Similarly, although we will continue to use the terms *dysplasia* and *carcinoma in situ* in the classic sense to delineate certain cytologic and histopathologic pictures, we must remember that no studies— whether cytogenetic,[223,227] electron microscopic,[228] chromosomal,[229,230] immunohistochemical,[231,232] or tissue cultural[210,233]—have succeeded in delineating

the exact stage at which dysplastic changes become irreversible and malignant.

Possible Progression to Invasive Cancer

Nevertheless, an impressive body of evidence has been assembled to support the concept of an origin of invasive cancer from these lesions:

1. These lesions occur in the same population groups, and groups with low prevalence rates for one lesion have low prevalence rates for all.[234]
2. The prevalences of dysplasia, in situ carcinoma, and invasive carcinoma are similar in women examined for the first time.[49,235,236]
3. Studies of untreated women with dysplasia and carcinoma in situ have shown subsequent development of invasive carcinoma.[237–239]
4. Women with invasive carcinoma have been found, on review of previous biopsy specimens, to have had prior dysplasia, in situ carcinoma, or both.[240]
5. Coexistence of these lesions frequently can be demonstrated by serial sections of cervices.[237,241]
6. There is a constant spatial relationship, in that all of these lesions arise most frequently in the region of the squamocolumnar junction or the transformation zone; when lesions of varying severity (eg, dysplasia and in situ carcinoma) coexist, the least severe pattern is usually seen in the most exterior site. Similar histologic patterns are seen in similar sites (eg, keratinizing dysplasia and keratinizing invasive carcinoma both involve the portio with greater frequency).[49,237,242]
7. There is a constant temporal relationship; the median age for dysplasia is 5 to 10 years younger than that for invasive carcinoma— the actual ages vary with the population studied, but this progression always applies.[49,206,235,243]
8. Studies of populations previously screened by cytologic examination have demonstrated up to 1200 times higher incidence of in situ carcinoma, and 100 times higher incidence of invasive carcinoma, in women initially found to have dysplasia.[235]
9. Incidence rates of, and death rates from, invasive cervical carcinoma have been lowered substantially in populations of women subjected to mass cytologic screening in whom dysplasia and in situ carcinoma were efficiently detected and treated.[244–250]

The exact rates of progression to invasive cancer of dysplasia and carcinoma in situ are not known, for reasons previously explained, but most authors believe that mild dysplasias are more likely to regress than progress, in situ carcinomas are much more likely to become invasive if untreated, and moderate and severe dysplasias fall somewhere in between. In a series of 49 cases of severe dysplasia reported by Westergaard and Norgaard,[251] 57.1 % progressed to in situ and microinvasive carcinoma. Similar data, accumulated from many studies predominantly in the Anglo-American and European literature, have been summarized by various authors.[203,206,236,238,252,253]

Methods of Identification and Diagnosis

Macroscopic Appearance. CIN does not have a characteristic macroscopic appearance. The cervix often appears entirely normal, and occasionally shows nonspecific pictures of leukoplakia, erosion, or cervicitis. The most suspicious of these is a zone of *leukoplakia* (by definition, a white plaque), but one study demonstrated that only 10% of patients with clinical leukoplakia had dysplasia or in situ carcinoma.[254]

Schiller Test. As a supplement to clinical inspection of the cervix, Lugol's solution may be applied to its surface. A positive stain is given when the iodine reacts with glycogen-rich normal squamous epithelium (Color Figs. 3-14 and 3-15). When glycogen is depleted, as in absence (erosion, inflammatory ulcer) or abnormality (metaplasia, dysplasia, carcinoma in situ) of the squamous epithelium, the stain will be negative (interestingly, this is considered a positive test). Thus, the test can locate abnormalities to be biopsied but cannot define the type of lesion present.

Colposcopy. It was in 1923 that Hinselmann,[255] aware of the imperfection of then extant methods for the diagnosis of cervical cancer, devised a system of a stereoscopic microscope with direct lighting of the cervix for improvement of the quality of visual examination. The colposcope was born, enabling the observer to describe with great precision the physiologic and pathologic variations in the cervical mucosa and to establish the relationship between these macroscopic modifications and the corresponding histologic pictures (Color Figs. 3-16 through 3-21). The usual magnification factor is 16, and the main features examined are the vascular patterns, surface patterns, interpapillary distances, and color relationships. Particularly important are zones of white epithelium, foci showing a punctate vascular pattern, and zones of mosaicism (polygonal areas of white epithelium separated by red borders of highly vascularized connective tissue papillae). These elementary solitary or multiple lesions at times represent inflammatory conditions, at times benign atypias, and at times lesions of CIN.

The advantages of colposcopy may be summarized as follows: it precludes the necessity of conization biopsy for visible benign lesions and localizes the best biopsy site when biopsy is deemed necessary.[256-261] As far as invasive carcinoma is concerned, visual examination alone is most often sufficient to suspect the diagnosis, whereas colposcopy facilitates the diagnosis of minuscule lesions. The method does not permit the visualization of subepithelial lesions or of lesions within the endocervical canal.

Cytology. Cytologic examination has contributed greatly to the early diagnosis of dysplasia and in situ carcinoma, and it possesses the advantage over the Schiller test and colposcopy of demonstrating lesions originating in the endocervical canal. This technique has been shown to be of great value as a mass population screening device, and some authors have predicted that widespread use of exfoliative cytology could completely eradicate invasive cervical carcinoma within a population, by detecting epithelial atypias at an earlier, curable stage (CIN, dysplasia, or in situ carcinoma).[244,245,248,262-265]

The other major advantage of this method is that it can be practiced by the gynecologist and by the physician untrained in this specialty, with a cytotechnologist and a cytopathologist being required at a later time to interpret the smears obtained. If the cervical scraping includes a good sampling of the endocervical canal, the chances of missing an intraepithelial lesion are slight. However, the true *false-negative* rate of cytology is not negligible and may represent 10% of cases.[266,267] These cases are by definition identified retrospectively; if the clinical examination and the cytology report are both negative, there is no adequate prospective clinical follow-up. False-negative reports are engendered both by the absence of suspicious cells in the smears (which may be otherwise adequate or inadequate) and by a wrong interpretation of the cellular atypias present. Different endocervical sampling instruments have been introduced to increase the chance of obtaining a smear from the squamocolumnar junction (transformation zone). Although some authors[268,269] are enthusiastic, others are reluctant to use them[206] because of the poor quality of the smears. In addition, it has been recommended that the false-negative rate could be reduced substantially by taking two smears rather than one at the time of pelvic examination.[249] Vaginal pool aspiration increases the chances of detecting endometrial lesions as well.

Is the presence of endocervical columnar cells necessary to consider a smear adequate? This rule should not be strictly applied in our experience. If the smears are richly provided with well-preserved and fixed cells, and if endocervical mucus is present with inflammatory and metaplastic cells trapped in it, one should consider these smears technically adequate. Mitchell and Medley[270] have suggested that the endocervical component of the cervical smear be defined on the basis of metaplastic cells alone or in combination with columnar cells. Their study tends to show that metaplastic cells are a more important marker than columnar cells.

The optimal interim period between screening examinations has been debated recently, and this period can influence the clinical impact of a false-negative report. We agree with the guideline proposed by the American Cancer Society[271] that "all women who are or have been sexually active, or have reached age 18 years, have an annual Pap test and pelvic examination. After a woman has had three or more consecutive satisfactory normal annual examinations, the Pap test may be performed less frequently at the discretion of her physician." This opinion is not shared by all authors in view of the medical cost of yearly tests. With the exception of women with positive herpes II antibodies or with previously diagnosed HPV infection or CIN, triennial screening can be proposed.[246,249] Some investigators still think that periods longer than 1 year will demotivate the women.

The cytologic picture of in situ carcinoma differs only in degree from that of invasive carcinoma on the one hand and severe dysplasia on the other. Although many authors claim a high degree of accuracy in differentiating these lesions cytologically, we believe that tissue examination (biopsy or conization) is required for a definitive diagnosis. Cytologic interpretations should always be expressed in histologic terminology so that the cytologic and biopsy diagnoses are comparable. The Bethesda system[212] is summarized in Table 3-5 as an advisable terminology.

Histology. The final diagnosis of any malignant or suspicious cervical lesion should be made by biopsy. Much has been written arguing the relative merits of multiple punch biopsies and conization biopsy, the latter being the technique that samples the entire circumference of the squamocolumnar junction. There is no doubt that the conization specimen, when totally sectioned, embedded, and examined in detail by the pathologist by a technique such as that of Foote and Stewart,[272,273] will reveal lesions that may not have been sampled by prior punch biopsies;[266] but many have questioned whether the additional information is often of enough significance to justify the occasional morbidity of the procedure. Colposcopically directed biopsies combined with endocervical curettage can provide the same information with less morbidity.[259,260,274,275] Conization (by cold knife, laser, or loop excision) is advised when the entire lesion cannot be located or visualized by colposcopy (positive or inadequate endocervical curettage specimen). Some workers also recommend conization for in situ carcinoma.[276]

The pathologist working with conization specimens must be sure to section and examine the entire specimen. Usually 15 to 25 tissue pieces are submitted for histologic preparation if the specimen permits, and at least three or four levels of each should be examined. Some authors have recommended routine serial step sectioning of all tissue blocks,[277] but we believe that the imposition of this task on a busy laboratory is simply not practical; certainly, any block with a suspicious lesion should be subjected to step sectioning. Another question that is often raised

TABLE 3-5.
The 1991 Bethesda System

Adequacy of the specimen
  Satisfactory for evaluation
  Satisfactory for evaluation but limited by . . . (specify reason)
  Unsatisfactory for evaluation . . . (specify reason)
General categorization (optional)
  Within normal limits
  Benign cellular changes: See descriptive diagnosis
  Epithelial cell abnormality: See descriptive diagnosis
Descriptive diagnoses
  Benign cellular changes
    Infection
      Trichomonas vaginalis
      Fungal organisms morphologically consistent with *Candida* spp
      Predominance of coccobacilli consistent with shift in vaginal flora
      Bacteria morphologically consistent with *Actinomyces* spp
      Cellular changes associated with herpes simplex virus
      Other
    Reactive changes
      Reactive cellular changes associated with
        Inflammation (includes typical repair)
        Atrophy with inflammation ("atrophic vaginitis")
        Radiation
        Intrauterine contraceptive device (IUD)
        Other
  Epithelial cell abnormalities
    Squamous cell
      Atypical squamous cells of undetermined significance: Qualify*
      Low-grade squamous intraepithelial lesion encompassing: HPV,** mild dysplasia/CIN I
      High-grade squamous intraepithelial lesion encompassing: Moderate and severe dysplasia/CIS, CIN II and CIN III
    Squamous cell carcinoma
    Glandular cell
      Endometrial cells, cytologically benign, in a postmenopausal woman
      Atypical glandular cells of undetermined significance: Qualify*
      Endocervical adenocarcinoma
      Endometrial adenocarcinoma
      Extrauterine adenocarcinoma
      Adenocarcinoma: not otherwise specified
  Other malignant neoplasms: Specify
  Hormonal evaluation (applies to vaginal smears only)
    Hormonal pattern compatible with age and history
    Hormonal pattern incompatible with age and history: Specify
    Hormonal evaluation not possible due to: Specify

*Atypical squamous or glandular cells of undetermined significance should be further qualified as to whether a reactive or a premalignant/malignant process is favored.

**Cellular changes of human papillomavirus (HPV)—previously termed koilocytosis, koilocytotic atypia, or condylomatous atypia—are included in the category of low-grade squamous intraepithelial lesion.

is that of performing frozen section on conization specimens; again, we believe that the advantages are offset by the difficulty of the procedure, the lack of immediately important therapeutic information to be gained (most microinvasive carcinomas will not be treated differently from CIN), and the inherent risk of error involved (an average of 12.6% incorrect diagnoses in one literature review[278]). In reporting the final results of a conization biopsy for carcinoma in situ, the pathologist should always mention the adequacy of the upper and lower resection margins, particularly if the uterus may be retained. A recent study showed a 12% incidence of residual tumor in postconization uteri with adequate margins, compared with 82% when margins were inadequate. Margin involvement was a better predictor of residual disease at repeat surgery than was abnormal follow-up cytology.[279]

Diagnosis of Cervical Intraepithelial Neoplasia (Dysplasia and Carcinoma In Situ, Low-Grade and High-Grade Squamous Intraepithelial Lesions)

Histologic Appearance

The great majority of intraepithelial lesions originate at the squamocolumnar junction or transformation zone and may involve the epithelium of the adjacent endocervical gland necks. Reserve cells differentiate into squamous epithelium through the steps of squamous metaplasia. We are all familiar with the common picture of biopsies from the junction: the coexistence of areas of normal squamous epithelium, columnar glands and foci of basal hyperplasia, and squamous metaplasia combined with inflammatory infiltrates.

CIN is characterized by the combination of the following elementary lesions (Figs. 3-36 through 3-47):

(*Text continued on page 113.*)

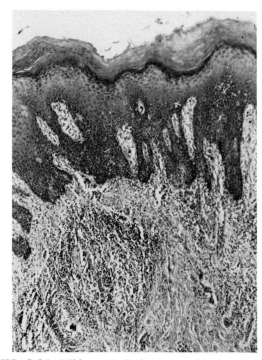

FIGURE 3-36 Mild cervical dysplasia with hyperkeratosis (leukoplakia).

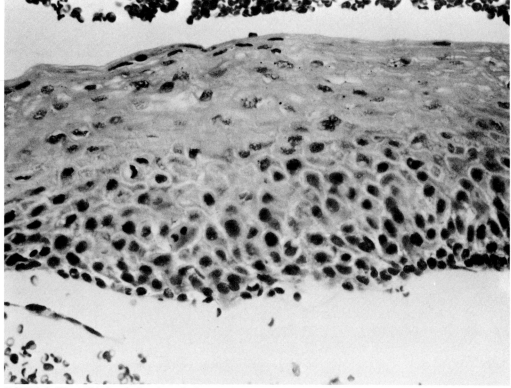

FIGURE 3-37 Mild dysplasia: dyspolarity, nuclear atypia, and mitotic figures in lower half of mucosa only.

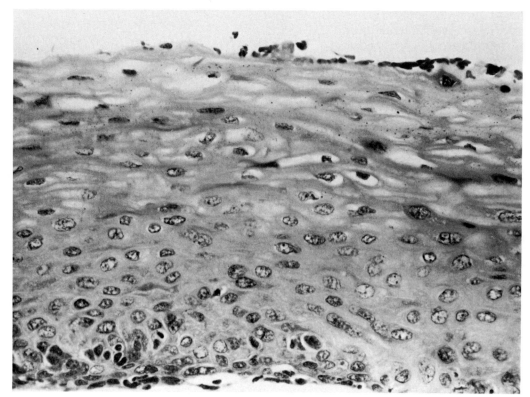

FIGURE 3-38 Mild dysplasia: slightly more atypia but fewer mitoses than in Figure 3-37.

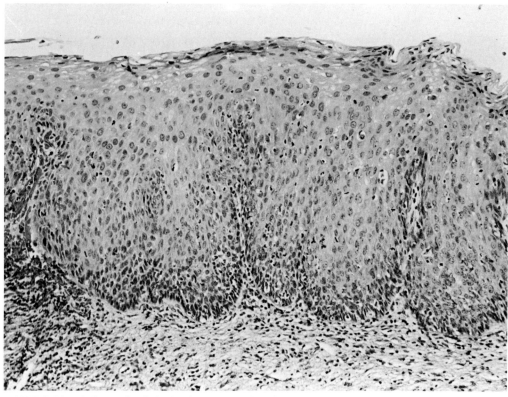

FIGURE 3-39 Moderate dysplasia: focal parakeratosis and epithelial peaking suggest origin in flat condyloma.

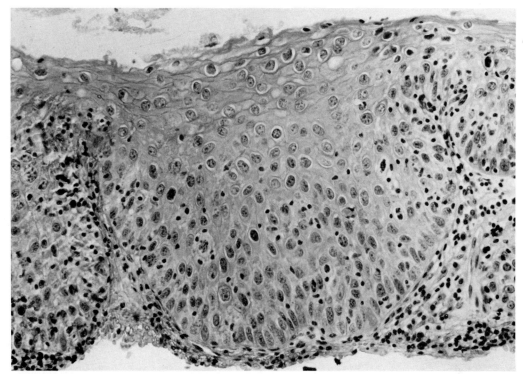

FIGURE 3-40 Moderate dysplasia: detail.

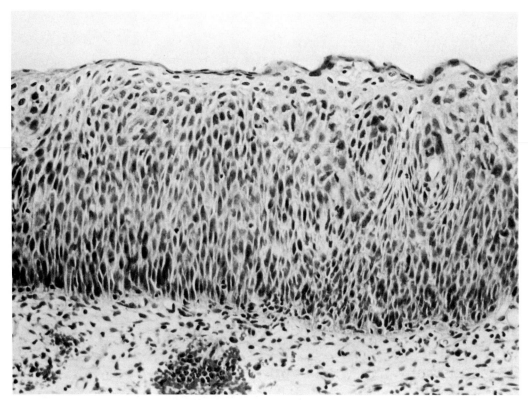

FIGURE 3-41 Severe dysplasia: flattening and maturation limited to upper fifth of mucosa.

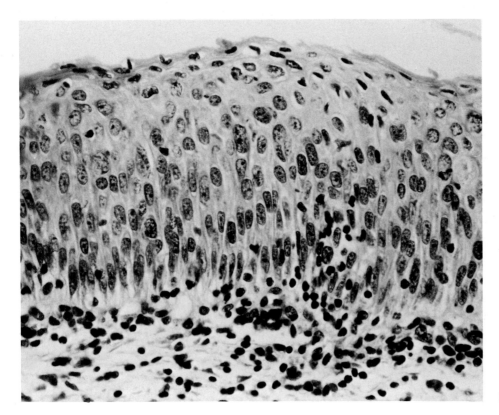

FIGURE 3-42 Severe dysplasia.

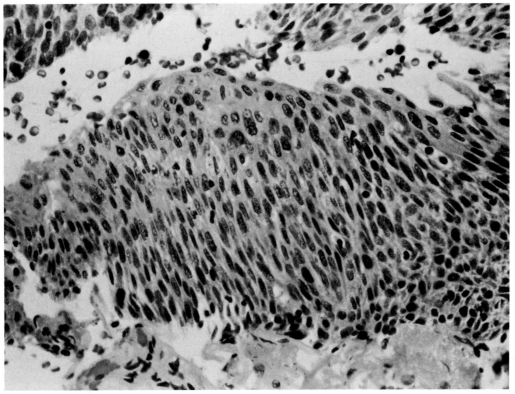

FIGURE 3-43 Borderline lesion of high-grade CIN. Iatrogenic loss of some surface epithelium in this endocervical curettage specimen makes it difficult to distinguish between severe dysplasia and in situ carcinoma.

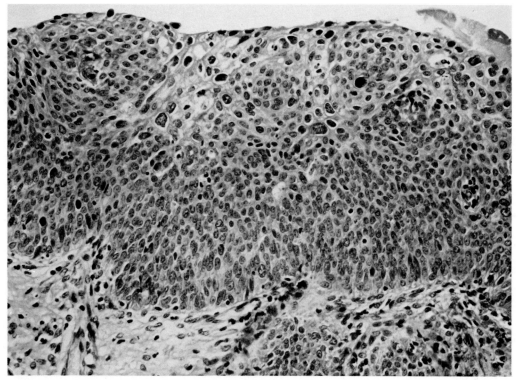

FIGURE 3-44 In situ carcinoma: microscopic appearance.

Hyperplasia of the basal cell layers, particularly layers C1 and C2, occurs with or without cellular anomalies. The basal layer is augmented in thickness and encroaches on the intermediate layers. The basal cells are normal in appearance or may show discrete cytologic modifications (increase in size of cells or of nuclei, irregularities of shape). In high-grade CIN (carcinoma in situ) there is a total lack of maturation toward the surface with uniform proliferation of immature cells. Minor degrees of flattening may be seen but the cells at the surface are as immature as those at the base, and do not show such features of

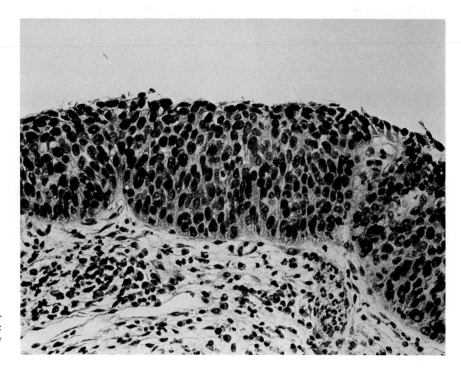

FIGURE 3-45 In situ carcinoma composed of basal-type cells. (Silverberg SG: Surgical pathology of the uterus. New York, John Wiley & Sons, 1977)

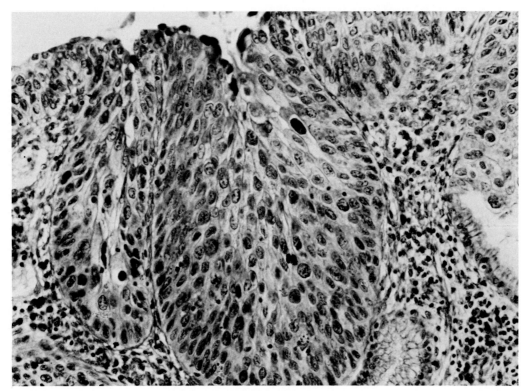

FIGURE 3-46 Carcinoma in situ with gland neck extension: detail of cells.

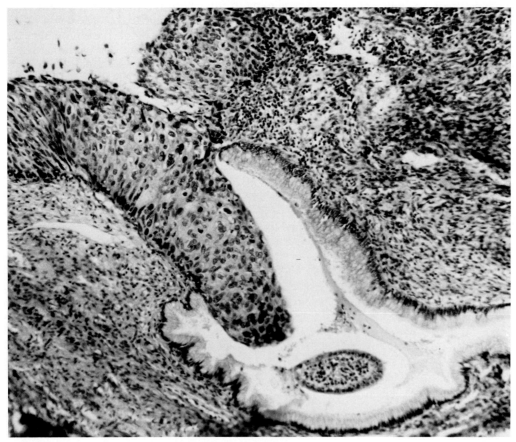

FIGURE 3-47 In situ carcinoma: extension into endocervical glands.

squamous differentiation as increased cytoplasm, cytoplasmic glycogen, and sharp intercellular borders.

Anomalies of size and shape are found in cells and nuclei, principally in the intermediate and deep epithelial layers. Premature keratinization may be present. *Nuclear hyperchromatism* is present, often with relatively normal cytoplasm. *Quantitative and qualitative abnormalities of mitoses* include increased mitotic rate, with abnormal mitoses usually confined to the lower half of the epithelium in low-grade CIN (mild and moderate dysplasia) and distributed in all levels in severe dysplasia and carcinoma in situ. The presence of three-part mitoses or three-group metaphase multipolar spindles and multinucleate cells is a good indicator of the severity of the lesion.[281-284] DNA ploidy is another expression of these anomalies.[285]

The *nuclear–cytoplasmic ratio* (expression of nuclear area to cytoplasmic area) increases with the severity of the lesion. *Acanthosis* occurs with accentuation of the papillary structure. *Dyspolarity* is present, with disturbance of the normal orderly maturation toward the surface. *Leukocytic and histiocytic infiltration* of the subjacent stroma is accompanied by anarchic angiogenesis.

Decrease of surface maturation is a variable criterion, largely based on the epithelium of origin. Thus, dysplasias arising in native squamous epithelium (ie, distally) tend to show extensive surface maturation, frequent isolated cell keratinizations, and prominent parakeratosis, and tend to be considered mild or moderate (keratinizing dysplasia). On the other hand, dysplasias arising in metaplastic epithelium possess few of these characteristics, appear immature, and often are labeled *severe dysplasia*. Severe dysplasia may be difficult to differentiate from carcinoma in situ and both are encompassed by the term *CIN III*.

There is *extension of the abnormal epithelium* into underlying cervical gland necks, generally more extensive in CIN III (see Figs. 3-46 and 3-47). Fluhmann clearly showed many years ago that this histologic picture does not indicate invasion[51] because the deep-seated nests of tumors are rounded, with intact basement membranes and no surrounding stromal response. Residual glandular epithelium often facilitates the diagnosis.

Different combinations of these elementary lesions will explain the highly various aspects of CIN.

Mild Dysplasia (CIN I).

The morphologic alterations are limited to the basal and parabasal layers of the native squamous epithelium or to the area of squamous metaplasia. Nuclear anomalies are minimal, with mild hyperchromasia and anisonucleosis. Dyspolarity is moderate. The nuclear–cytoplasmic ratio can be slightly increased. Stratification and differentiation of intermediate and superficial squamous layers are preserved. Few mitoses are observed.

Moderate Dysplasia (CIN II).

The cell polarity is disturbed in the lower two thirds of the epithelium,

and stratification is maintained in the upper third. Cellular atypia is present throughout the epithelium but is less evident in superficial cells. The nuclear–cytoplasmic ratio is increased. Surface maturation persists even if some abnormal nuclei are observed. Mitoses, some abnormal, are present.

Severe Dysplasia and In Situ Carcinoma (CIN III).

Dyspolarity is present in all layers of the epithelium. Nuclear atypias are severe and abundant. Anomalies of cellular size and shape are constant. Nuclear hyperchromasia is pronounced, and the nuclear–cytoplasmic ratio is notably increased, particularly in parabasal and intermediate cells. Superficial maturation is absent or minimal. Stratification may persist superficially or may be absent in CIN III of metaplastic type. Mitoses are present in all layers, and abnormal figures are evident. The more severe lesions correspond to carcinoma in situ. Then maturation is totally absent, but parallel arrangement of the most superficial cells may persist, probably for mechanical reasons. Extension into the cervical gland necks is frequent.

Study of the different cytokeratins elaborated by cervical cells and revealed by immunocytochemistry allows the distinction between normal ecto- and endocervical cells, reserve cells, squamous metaplasia, and CIN.[231,232] These determinations probably add little to routine histopathology for diagnostic purposes.

Different classifications of CIN III have been proposed, which recognize three major types based on the predominant pattern:

1. *The small cell type* (poorly differentiated or anaplastic carcinoma), composed of small cells with sometimes elongated nuclei and no sign of keratinization, suggesting the structure of basal cells
2. *The large cell type*, also referred to as *nonkeratinizing* or *moderately well differentiated*
3. *The keratinizing type*, which reveals differentiation and keratin formation. Surface keratinization is prominent and nuclear abnormalities are present even in these keratinized cells. As mentioned earlier, in some classification systems these keratinizing lesions are all considered dysplasias.

The differential diagnosis of dysplasia from *condyloma* (HPV infection-related atypia) is based on the observation that routinely visible condylomatous atypias involve predominantly the superficial and intermediate cell layers of the mucosa, whereas dysplasias begin in the basal and parabasal cell layers and grow toward the surface with increasing severity. Findings such as peaking of the surface epithelium, koilocytotic perinuclear haloes, and irregularly wrinkled, "raisinoid," often bizarre nuclei are characteristic of condyloma, whereas dysplastic cells are usually more uniform, contain hyperchromatic but not wrinkled or pyknotic nuclei, and demonstrate more frequent mitotic figures. Abnormal mitoses should not be seen in condyloma without coexisting dysplasia. Classic dysplasia may coexist with condyloma (Figs. 3-48 through 3-50) in one or more of three fashions: (1) involving the basal and parabasal cell layers beneath a superficial condylomatous atypia; (2) immediately adjacent to a condylomatous lesion; or (3) synchronous with but spatially distant from a condyloma.

Dysplasia may also be difficult to differentiate from *atypical squamous metaplasia* or *reactive (repair) atypia* of the squamous mucosa secondary to inflammation. The disorderly dyspolarity of dysplasia is absent in both of these situations, mitotic figures are rare, and nuclei, although they may be large, are generally normochromatic or less hyperchromatic than in dysplasia. In inflammatory atypias, the inflammatory cells usually extend into the altered epithelium, whereas the inflammation associated with dysplasia is generally limited to the stroma. Immunoperoxidase staining for involucrin is said to be negative in most dysplasias and positive in 95% of normal, metaplastic, and condylomatous epithelia.[286] At the other end of the spectrum, the distinction of severe dysplasia from in situ carcinoma may pose problems, as discussed above. The inclusion of both severe dysplasia and in situ carcinoma in the CIN III grouping, however, indicates that the treatment and prognosis of these lesions depend more on their distribution (eradicable or not by conservative therapy) than on their exact histologic pattern.

Cytologic Appearance

The number of exfoliated cells depends on the method of collection, the skill of the sample taker, the extension and the location of the lesion, and the severity of atypia (Figs. 3-51 and 3-52 and Color Figs. 3-22 through 3-25).

Low-Grade Squamous Intraepithelial Lesion (Mild Dysplasia, CIN I). Superficial and intermediate squamous cells or metaplastic cells reveal mild atypia characterized by enlarged and irregular nuclei with a finely granular chromatin. Hyperchromasia is discrete. Anisonucleosis is not prominent. Nucleoli are inconspicuous. The nuclear–cytoplasmic ratio is slightly increased.

High-Grade Squamous Intraepithelial Lesion. This classification in the Bethesda system includes both moderate dysplasia (CIN II) and severe dysplasia and carcinoma in situ (CIN III). Because there are usually cytologic differences between these lesions, we will discuss them here separately. In *moderate dysplasia (CIN II)*, squamous cells of all cellular layers (parabasal, intermediate, and superficial) or metaplastic cells reveal moderate nuclear abnormalities. One observes anisonucleosis, nuclear enlargement, and folding of the nuclear membrane. Nucleoli are inconspicuous. The nuclear–cytoplasmic ratio is increased by enlargement of the nucleus or decrease in size of the cytoplasm. Cytoplasmic staining is cyano-

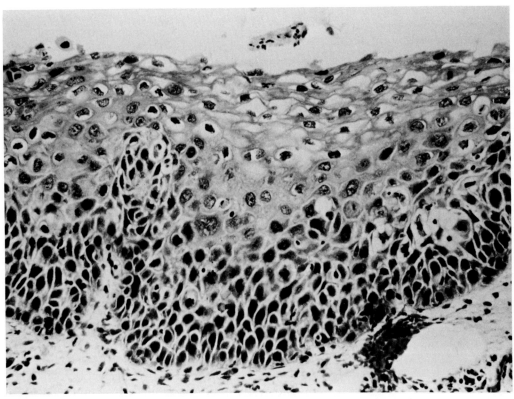

FIGURE 3-48 Flat condyloma with underlying mild dysplasia.

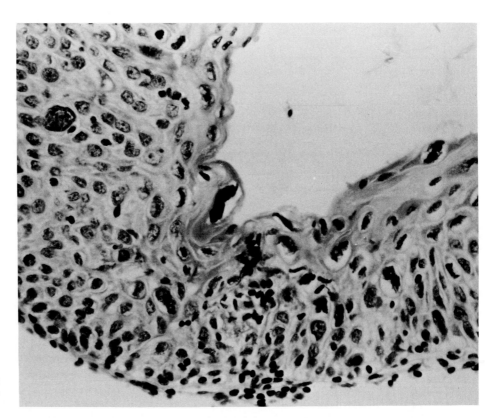

FIGURE 3-49 Flat condyloma with underlying mild to moderate dysplasia.

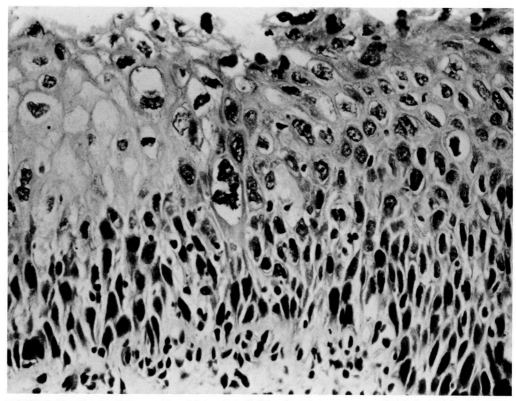

FIGURE 3-50 Flat condyloma with mild dysplasia (*left*), and moderate to severe dysplasia (*right*).

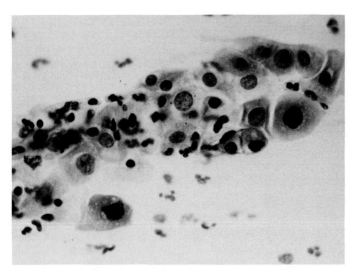

FIGURE 3-51 Moderate dysplasia: appearance of cervical smear.

philic or eosinophilic when cellular maturation is precocious.

Severe dysplasia/carcinoma in situ (CIN III) exhibits the most atypical lesions. Depending on the histologic type, the cells are small or large with or without cytoplasmic keratotic differentiation. The smears are rich in atypical cells and form aggregates of disorderly arranged elements. Nuclei are large, irregular, and hyperchromatic with scanty surrounding cytoplasm. Enlarged eosinophilic nucleoli are visible in the dense coarse chromatin. Bizarre-shaped cells may be present. The nuclear–cytoplasmic ratio is significantly increased, particularly in undifferenti-

ated cells. Indistinct cell borders create pseudosyncytial structures.

The three histologic types of carcinoma in situ can be differentiated cytologically (Color Figs. 3-26 and 3-27). According to the cell type, the smears will show predominantly (1) small cells with large nuclei and basophilic cytoplasm occurring singly or in clusters; (2) large cells with basophilic or, less often, acidophilic orange cytoplasm; or (3) keratinized cells with abundant homogeneous eosinophilic cytoplasm and dark, often dense, irregular or pyknotic nuclei; the tadpole cell is commonly present in this type. A clear-cut distinction between the different types is

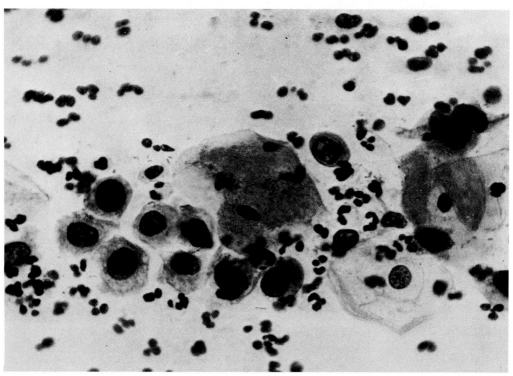

FIGURE 3-52 In situ carcinoma: appearance of cervical smear.

not always possible and mixed forms occur. Cells exfoliated from in situ carcinoma are usually more numerous, more uniform, and smaller than those seen in dysplasia, often grow in syncytia, and are round, with little cytoplasm surrounding their large, hyperchromatic, coarsely granular nuclei (see Fig. 3-52). The general background, as in dysplasia, is usually "clean" (lacking cell debris), but an inflammatory diathesis can be present, although this characteristic is classically attributed to invasive carcinoma.

The cytologic *differential diagnosis* with inflammatory, regenerative and metaplastic atypias has been discussed previously, and that with invasive squamous cell carcinoma will be discussed below.

INVASIVE MALIGNANT TUMORS

Cervical cancer represents about 10% of all cancers in women and 25% to 45% of female genital cancers. It was estimated that in the United States in 1991, 13,000 women would develop invasive cervical cancer and 7,000 women would die of the disease. It is found with the same frequency among almost all populations except Jews and certain other people such as the Fiji Islanders and with higher frequency among populations in which routine cytologic screening has not been adopted. Low socioeconomic status and poor sexual hygiene represent important factors in the increase of carcinoma in certain populations.

Invasive malignant cervical tumors consist of about 85% squamous carcinomas, 15% adenocarcinomas and adenosquamous carcinomas, and rare cases of sarcomas and metastatic tumors. Table 3-6 summarizes the International Society of Gynecological Pathologists (ISGP) classification of invasive cervical squamous carcinomas.[226]

Carcinoma of the cervix is a rapidly fatal disease; 95% of untreated patients are dead at the end of the fifth year after diagnosis. We should emphasize, at the beginning of the discussion, the social importance of cancer of the cervix uteri, which strikes about 2% of all women who attain the age of 80 years. More than 50% of the patients whose tumors are detected and treated early may hope for a survival of 5 or more years. This figure approaches

TABLE 3-6.
International Society of Gynecological Pathologists Classification of Invasive Squamous Cell Carcinomas

Keratinizing
Nonkeratinizing
Verrucous
Warty (condylomatous)
Papillary (transitional)
Lymphoepithelioma-like

100% when the diagnosis of cancer is made in the noninvasive stage. These figures show the importance of diagnosing this disease in its early stages and, toward that end, of persuading the female population to have regular gynecologic examinations, which should always include cytologic smears.

Clinically, the easy access to the lesion, the slow growth of the tumor, and the efficacy of therapeutic modalities should increase the frequency of cure. If they are neglected by the patient, the first symptoms may escape a cursory examination, and too often the tumor evolves to a stage in which therapy is hazardous and palliative.

Squamous Cell Carcinoma

Epidemiology and Etiology. The etiology of cervical squamous cancer is unknown, but certain factors influence the frequency of its appearance. The rarity of this lesion among Jewish women has led some workers to suppose a genetic factor, but a more widely held notion is that of a protective role of male circumcision. This latter hypothesis is confirmed by some studies that found that, among those natives of the Fiji islands who practice circumcision, the cervical cancer incidence was only one eighth as high as among those who abstain from this practice. Similar data have been obtained from the Moslem and Hindu populations of India, the former of whom practice circumcision, whereas the latter do not. The definite role of circumcision is not settled, even if its protective effect has been confirmed in different epidemiologic studies. Smegma appears to be a causal factor. The carcinogenic properties of smegma may be due to the transformation of its cholesterol by a bacterium (*Mycobacterium smegmatis*) into a unknown carcinogen. Another hypothesis has been proposed by Reid,[287] who emphasized the carcinogenic role of the nuclear DNA of spermatozoa, which could act in the same way as DNA of carcinogenic viruses when penetrating into the nuclei of host cells of the epithelium. As no objective evidence has been offered, these theories still need confirmation.[288]

Some studies support the concept that smoking may represent a risk factor. Nicotine may lower the immunologic defense of the cervix or make it more susceptible to viral infection.[289] A significant decrease in the Langerhans cell population, producing local immunodepression, has been observed in both normal cervical epithelium and CIN among cigarette smokers.[290]

The influence of the type of sexual life appears equally evident. Cervical cancer is statistically more frequent in the multiparous women than in the nulliparous; this frequency does not seem rigorously proportional to the number of pregnancies. It is equally more frequent in the group of married women without children than among virgins, and women with cervical cancer also seem to have begun to have sexual relations at an earlier age than women in a control population. The works of Gagnon[291] and of Schömig[292] have noted the relative frequency of cancer of the cervix among Danish prostitutes, and attribute this in part to sexual hyperactivity. The anatomic modifications, traumata, and inflammatory lesions that are the result of genital activity and multiparity provoke important histologic alterations, but we must also remember the infections (particularly viral) and hormonal stimuli to which these women are exposed (the roles of herpesvirus and HPV have been discussed in detail earlier). Age also appears to play a role, because the condition is found with greatest frequency in women between 45 and 55 years of age. The frequency curve, very low below 20 years, rises slowly between 20 and 30 years, and then rapidly until age 50, and finally descends progressively beyond 55 years of age. At the Institut Bordet, 11% of the patients with cervical cancer were under 40 years of age (Fig. 3-53). With more precocious sexual habits, these lesions appear at an earlier age, and it is now common to detect dysplasias in patients as young as 15 years. Consequently, cytologic screening should be recommended with the beginning of sexual intercourse. It is interesting to note that the most frequent age of appearance of carcinoma in situ is between 30 and 40 years, that is, about 10 years earlier than invasive carcinoma. The rôle played by estrogens in the genesis of

these tumors is not established with certitude. Although cervical cancers have been produced in mice by administering high doses of estrogens, there is no clinical evidence that the situation is the same in the human female.

Jones and colleagues,[293] in a intensive study of the epidemiologic factors that we have just cited briefly, have cast doubt on the validity of these as isolated factors. They think that precocious sexual maturity, a reflection of varied socioeconomic factors, constitutes a background favoring the appearance of cancer.

Finally, in recent years, the evidence for induction or promotion of cervical neoplasia by different transmissible agents has become more persuasive. Among these agents are HPV[80–105,294,295] and, with considerably weaker evidence, HSV-2,[66–74] cytomegalovirus,[296] and chlamydia.[47] *Trichomonas vaginalis,* once regarded as a potential promoting agent, is no longer considered as such.[113–115,117]

Extensive recent studies tend to show that the development of intraepithelial and invasive cervical neoplasia may be favored by sexually transmitted agents. These findings suggest that there may be different forms of dysplasia due to different causes and with subsequently different natural histories. Although the natural history of the various forms of CIN (dysplasia and carcinoma in situ) cannot be predicted on morphologic grounds alone, it is important that these lesions continue to be reported according to the degree of morphologic abnormality.[110]

The mention of the virus-associated alterations should not modify the clinical and therapeutic approach to the lesion until more information is available on the differing relations (if any) of the transmissible agents to the natural history of the disease.

Development and Detection. The advanced stages of squamous cell carcinoma are comparatively more frequent in elderly women, in whom stage 0 (carcinoma in situ) represents only a small fraction of the total number of cases. After an intensive cytologic screening program in a community, these figures in all women will change to indicate a considerably higher frequency of stage 0 and I cases and, a few years later, a much lower frequency of stage III and IV cases, suggesting that many potential advanced cases have been detected at an earlier stage by this method.[244–248,297] An important conclusion should be drawn from these statements: *the absolute necessity of early detection.* For this reason, better education of the public and of the practicing physician and the organization of this detection survey on a population-wide level should be actively encouraged.

The tumor develops most frequently at the level of the squamocolumnar epithelial junction. The localization of the tumor therefore depends on the location of this junction in the cervix. This explains why about 20% of cases originate within the cervical

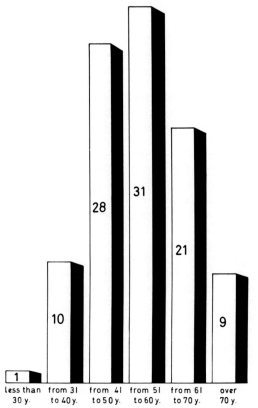

FIGURE 3-53 Percentage of incidence of cervical carcinoma as a function of age (4147 cases).

canal, a location in which clinical detection is more difficult.

At first invisible to the naked eye, the early structural changes are limited to a small region and consist of lesions of intraepithelial or early invasive type. The Schiller test visualizes them as pale iodonegative plaques. It is at this submacroscopic stage that methods of detection (cytology and colposcopy) have their major value. The method of transformation of a normal cell into a cancer cell is unknown, but several facts define the manner of appearance of early cancer:

1. The tumor passes through a first intraepithelial or noninvasive stage, and in the course of a second stage invades the underlying tissues. The first stage may be prolonged for months or years or, on the contrary, may represent only a first brief step in the development of the tumor.
2. Certain carcinomas appear to invade the stroma from their onset, without an earlier intraepithelial stage.
3. The tumor may originate in a single focus or as multicentric cancerous zones. It is not rare to find separate foci of in situ carcinoma separated by intervening normal mucosa. The multicentric character demonstrates that the etiologic agent acts at several foci in the cervix.
4. The transformation of benign into malignant cells should take place in young immature cells, that is, among the basal cells of the squamous epithelium or the reserve cells of the columnar epithelium.

Macroscopic Appearance. The tumor grows progressively and becomes visible to the naked eye. It presents as an elevated granular zone, darker red than the normal mucosa, which bleeds easily on contact. Two macroscopic forms are encountered:

1. The proliferative, papillary, or exophytic form. The tumor projects from the surface and forms multiple budding masses that are hemorrhagic and very friable, often with surface necrosis.
2. The infiltrating or endophytic form burrows into the cervical canal and forms a hard submucosal mass that causes augmentation of the volume of the cervix while, in the early stages, leaving the surface intact. At a later stage than in the proliferative form, the mucosa shows necrotic ulcers.

These two forms are distinguishable when the tumor is small. At a more advanced stage, the tumor involves the entire cervix and the adjacent vaginal wall and presents as a large necrotic ulcer crater (Fig. 3-54).

The international classification adopted in 1950 and modified in 1974 and 1985 subdivides cervical

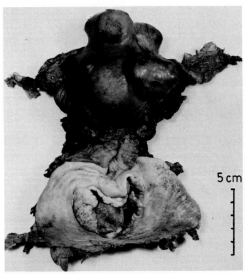

FIGURE 3-54 Squamous cell carcinoma: macroscopic appearance.

cancer into five macroscopic stages (Table 3-7).[226,298] The classification of a tumor should be made as a result of clinical examination before the institution of therapy. In the case of hesitation between two stages, the less advanced must be chosen.

The use of this classification permits comparison of therapeutic results from any medical institutions in the world. This staging is done on the basis of clinical examination; pathologic examination of a re-

TABLE 3-7.
Clinical Staging of Invasive Squamous Carcinoma (FIGO)

Stage 0. Intraepithelial (in situ) carcinoma
Stage I. Invasive carcinoma strictly limited to the cervix
  Stage Ia. Preclinical carcinoma—can only be diagnosed microscopically
    Stage Ia1. Minimal microscopic invasion
    Stage Ia2. Microscopic stromal invasion not exceeding 7 mm horizontally and 5 mm vertically, as measured from the base of the epithelium, either surface or glandular, from which the lesion originates
  Stage Ib. The lesion is larger than in stage Ia2, whether clinically apparent or not
Stage II. Carcinoma extending beyond the cervix proper but not reaching the pelvic wall: cancer involving the vagina, but not its lower third
  Stage IIa. No obvious involvement of the parametrium (involvement of upper two thirds of vagina only)
  Stage IIb. Obvious involvement of parametrium
Stage III. Cancer extending to the pelvic wall and/or involving the inferior third of the vagina and/or causing hydronephrosis or nonfunctioning kidney
  Stage IIIa. No extension to the pelvic wall
  Stage IIIb. Extension to the pelvic wall or hydronephrosis or renal nonfunction
Stage IV: Cancer extends beyond the true pelvis or involves the mucosa of the bladder or rectum
  Stage IVa. Spread to adjacent organs
  Stage IVb. Spread to distant organs

sected, biopsied, or postmortem specimen often changes the stage of a tumor, but for the sake of comparison of therapeutic modalities only the clinical staging should be used.[299,300] This point of view is open to criticism, because it enables the staging to be based on nonobjective criteria. However, although a classification based on gross and microscopic pathologic data would be more objective and precise, in practice this would eliminate most cases of advanced disease from analysis, because surgery is seldom performed in these instances. Therefore, this method unjustly weighs all reports with an unbalanced number of stage 0 and I cases.

Histologic Classification. Squamous carcinomas of the cervix have been the object of numerous histologic classifications elaborated with the intent of finding a relationship between the histologic type, the clinical prognosis, and the efficacy of surgical and radiotherapeutic modalities.

Martzloff[301] divided these tumors into three groups according to the dominant cell type: superficial keratinized, intermediate, and basal types. This classification has the merit of being simple and easily reproducible. A slightly modified approach simply distinguishes differentiated or spinocellular and undifferentiated or basocellular epitheliomas.

Broders[302] proposed four groups of epidermoid carcinomas, depending on the percentage of undifferentiated cells: group I is the most highly differentiated, containing only 0 to 25% undifferentiated cells, whereas group IV is the undifferentiated form (75% to 100%), with groups II and III in intermediate positions. Pendl[303] used no fewer than 5 groups and 16 subgroups to classify the cervical epithelial tumors, although this long classification does include the adenocarcinomas. It is, in our opinion, too involved and subjective.

Recent workers have used three groupings originally suggested by Wentz and Reagan[304] and revised in 1973 by Reagan and Ng:[305]

Group I: keratinizing type
Group II: large cell nonkeratinizing type
Group III: small cell type (small cell nonkeratinizing type)

This classification has two advantages. First, it conforms to modern theories of histogenesis, in which keratinizing cancers arise from ectocervical mucosa by way of dysplasia, large cell nonkeratinizing cancer arises from endocervical squamous metaplasia by way of dysplasia and large cell in situ carcinoma, and small cell carcinoma arises from endocervical reserve cell hyperplasia by way of small cell carcinoma in situ. Second, it appears to convey useful prognostic information (group II tumors showing the best survival and group III the worst in many series, particularly in cases treated by radiation therapy).[304–308] However, equal numbers of more recent studies have failed to confirm the histogenetic relation,[309–312] and some of these same studies have failed to confirm the prognostic utility of tumor grading.

In addition, the utility of the Wentz and Reagan classification is compromised by the fact that it is now known that most small cell carcinomas of the cervix are not of squamous type but actually represent neuroendocrine carcinomas.[313–316] The ISGP classification[226] (see Table 3-6) does not include a small cell variant of squamous cell carcinoma, and classifies small cell carcinomas separately on the assumption that they are all neuroendocrine. This classification also adds to the classical keratinizing and nonkeratinizing types four other patterns: verrucous, warty or condylomatous, papillary or transitional, and lymphoepithelioma-like. We recommend including the warty type (more common in the vulva—see Chapter 1) with the keratinizing group and classifying the three others—all rare in the cervix—separately from squamous carcinoma.

In addition to the classifications discussed so far, the prognostic significance of which is questionable, other authors have favored a "malignancy grading system" that evaluates eight different factors: structure, cell type, nuclear atypia, mitotic activity, pattern of invasion, type of tumor margin, vascular invasion, and host inflammatory response.[317,318] Although these investigators have found this system useful in providing prognostic information, it is complex and is not widely used.

Another observation that has provided useful information in several reports is the presence of stainable mucin within tumor cells in tumors diagnosed without special stains as squamous cell carcinomas.[319–323] Most studies have demonstrated either a greater likelihood of lymph node metastases or a poorer prognosis or both in these *squamous carcinomas with mucin secretion,*[320,323] which Thelmo and colleagues referred to as *mucoepidermoid carcinoma.*[322]

The histologic appearance represents only one prognostic element. Other factors are significant, most notably the degree of extension of the tumor at the time of diagnosis (see Table 3-7). For example, a clinical stage III cervical carcinoma has a poorer prognosis for long survival than a stage I or II lesion, regardless of the histologic appearances of the two tumors being compared. A small biopsy may reveal a local histologic appearance different from that which predominates in the entire tumor.

Microscopic Appearance. Squamous cell carcinoma is composed of epithelial cell cords and nests, the size and shape of which vary greatly from one case to the next. The point of origin of the tumor from the epithelium may be definite and easily seen when the tumor is small, if the biopsy happens by chance to include this region. More often, a large tumor shows surface ulceration and necrosis, with no evidence of its exact point of origin. The cell cords are disposed in random fashion and form multiple arborescences of all sizes.

In the *keratinizing type*, the cells are large, well differentiated, and show foci of keratinization with cornified pearls. A few mitotic figures are present. The cell cords are arranged in an infiltrative pattern (Fig. 3-55). By convention, a single pearl characterizes a squamous carcinoma as keratinizing, but even multiple single keratinized cells do not. If the tumor surface is papillary and hyperkeratotic, the term *warty carcinoma* can be used.

The *large cell nonkeratinizing type* is characterized by large and moderately differentiated cells, with a large, round nucleus, prominent nucleolus, and voluminous cytoplasm but no cornified pearls. Typically the tumor-stromal border is well demarcated (Figs. 3-56 and 3-57). In a few of these tumors, the cells are smaller and may be spindled, resembling the basaloid type of carcinoma described more fully in Chapter 1.

From the cytologic point of view, the cells are of variable size and irregular in shape; these variations are often independent of the cell type, because the presence of even one cornified pearl classifies an otherwise poorly differentiated tumor as a keratinizing (group I) carcinoma. The cytoplasm is basophilic (except in foci of keratinization) and its glycogen content is slight or none. The nuclei are enlarged, with an increased ratio of nucleus to cytoplasm. They present diverse anomalies of form (anisonucleosis) and size, the chromatin is abundant and irregularly disposed, and multinucleation is frequent.

The nucleolus is also enlarged, and multiple nucleoli are encountered in a single nucleus. The presence of these nucleolar anomalies is one of the most certain cytologic indications of the neoplastic nature of the cells. Staining with methylpyronine and microspectrophotometry permit study of the DNA content of the nuclei and evaluation of the volumetric variations of the nucleoli. Mitoses are more abundant than in benign lesions, and they show quantitative alterations such as pluripolar mitoses and disorderly distribution of chromosomes.

Several histochemical methods have been applied to the study of the uterine cervix, but none has established absolute criteria of malignancy.[324,325] Immunohistochemistry brings some valuable information but also no specific diagnostic data. CEA and cytokeratins are expressed in most squamous carcinomas. The blood group isoantigens A, B and H, normally present in the cervical epithelium, have not been detected in squamous carcinomas.[326,327]

Results of *electron microscopic* study of invasive squamous carcinomas have not disclosed specific characteristics of malignancy.[328] We know, however, that even in very anaplastic tumors, ultrastructural evidence of squamous differentiation is usually present.[329]

Cytologic Appearance. Invasive squamous cell carcinomas differ from their in situ counterparts primarily by greater pleomorphism and the presence of a "tumor diathesis" (an amorphous precipitate composed of debris from breakdown of tumor cells and erythrocytes). Most of the tumor cells are smaller than normal squamous cells, and the nuclear–cytoplasmic ratio is increased. The usual nuclear features of malignancy are present, and the size, shape, and cytoplasmic appearance of the tumor cells vary with

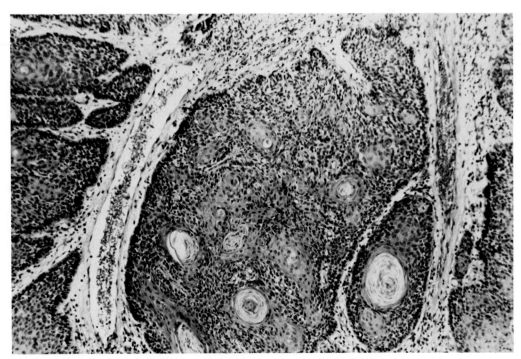

FIGURE 3-55 Keratinizing squamous cell carcinoma: microscopic appearance.

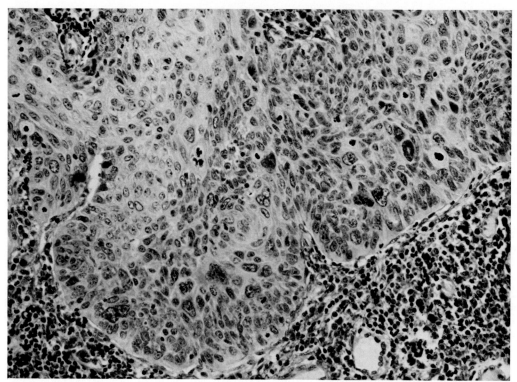

FIGURE 3-56 Large cell nonkeratinizing squamous carcinoma: microscopic appearance.

the histologic type of the tumor. Keratinizing tumors generally exfoliate the fewest, the largest, and the most pleomorphic cells, whereas large cell nonkeratinizing cancers exfoliate greater numbers of more uniform cells with less cytoplasm, no keratinization, and prominent nucleoli (Figs. 3-58 and 3-59 and Color Figs. 3-28 and 3-29). Small cell carcinoma (Color Fig. 3-30) differs from the large cell nonkeratinizing type predominantly in size.

Invasive carcinomas are more frequently missed cytologically than are in situ cancers, because the former are often covered by a surface layer of inflammatory and necrotic debris that may mask the underlying cancer; therefore, *grossly visible cervical lesions should always be biopsied*. Punch biopsy of an invasive carcinoma eliminates the necessity for conization, the main purpose of which is to *rule out* the presence of invasive carcinoma.

Evolution, Metastatic Dissemination, Prognosis, and Treatment. After extending along the surface and into the wall of the cervix, the tumor surpasses the anatomic limits of the cervix and invades the paracervical regions and, more rarely, the corpus uteri. Extension to the corpus does not change the clinical stage.

The parametria are invaded rather early, with an apparent predilection for the left parametrium. Lymphography of the normal genital system shows that the lymph flow is more rapid on the right than on the left for reasons of anatomic disposition. The relative torpor of the left-sided lymphatic circulation favors the implantation of neoplastic cells.

The lymphatic dissemination of cancer cells is generally early, and lymphatic metastases may be present when the primary tumor is still small,[330] although in one series[331] the parametrium, or at least the parametrial border of the cervix, was always involved in cases in which lymph node metastases were present. The percentage of lymph node metastases in lesions of all clinical stages combined ranges from 20% to 50% in various series.[332–334] There appears to be a definite increase in the proportion of cases with positive lymph nodes as the clinical stage advances and the tumor size increases. There may be a difference in frequency of lymph node involvement that depends on the histologic type of the primary tumor; Nogales and Botella-Llusia[335] have reported only 8% involvement in "basal cell" squamous cancers, as compared with 51.8% in "spindle cell" squamous and 84.8% in adenocarcinomas. Chung and coworkers[336] claim that, regardless of clinical stage, poorly differentiated tumors are more likely than well-differentiated ones to metastasize to pelvic or paraortic lymph nodes, and Boyce and associates[337] note more lymph node metastases in cases with primary tumors exceeding 10 mm in depth. Stendahl and coworkers[318] have developed a multiparameter grading system that they also claim exceeds clinical staging alone in prognostic value. The prognostic significance of vascular or lymphatic invasion is debatable; different studies have claimed that this histologic finding is[338] and is not[339] associated with a poorer survival rate. The depth of invasion of the tumor is a significant prognostic factor; tumor invasion exceeding 10 mm in depth is a poor prognostic

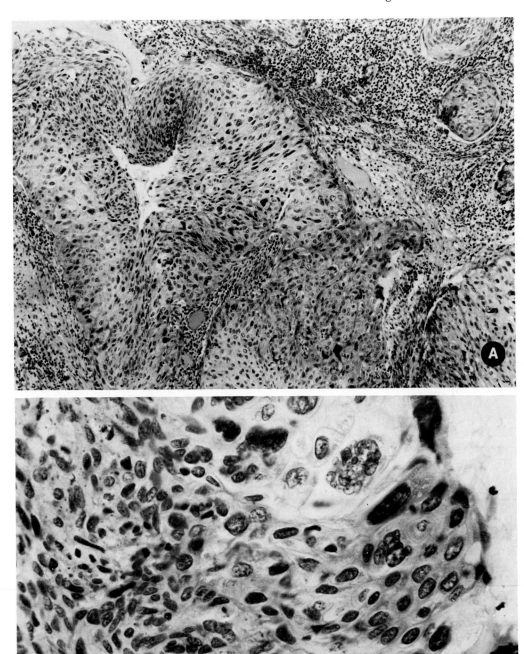

FIGURE 3-57 Large cell nonkeratinizing squamous carcinoma. **(A)** General appearance. **(B)** Detail.

factor and is associated with increased incidence of pelvic node metastases and local extension.[337]

Metastatic lymphadenopathy develops in the following manner (Fig. 3-60). A first nodal group is involved, comprising the highest external iliac and the hypogastric nodes. Among these, the middle node of the internal chain of the external ilial group, named the *obturator node,* appears to be most frequently invaded. A second group is subsequently reached, comprising the common iliac, sacral, and aortic nodes. However, a more distant node may be involved when the first order nodes are intact; for ex-

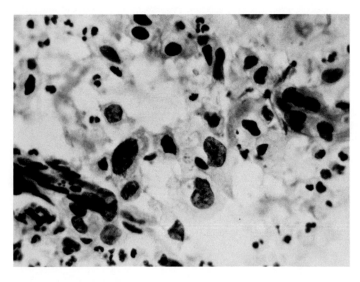

FIGURE 3-58 Keratinizing squamous cell carcinoma: cytologic appearance. Note pleomorphism and "tumor diathesis."

ample, it is not rare to see a supraclavicular node invaded as the first indication of a disseminated tumor.[340] The commonly involved nodes, in descending order of frequency, have been stated to be parametrial, common ilial, paracervical, hypogastric, obturator, external iliac, aortic, sacral, and inguinal.

When the tumor continues its evolution, it involves the vesicovaginal and rectovaginal regions, the bladder, the rectum, and the low ureteral region (Fig. 3-61). In the bladder, the serosa and muscular layers are invaded, but rarely the mucosa. Similarly, the rectal wall is invaded in its submucosal layers by the lymphatic route. The ureters are frequently obstructed (about 80% of autopsied cases), sometimes by external compression, sometimes by radiation fibrosis in the absence of residual tumor (this last event may occur many years after primary therapy). The sequelae of this ureteral involvement consist of alterations of the upper urinary tract (hydronephrosis, pyelographic abnormalities, pyelonephritis, and disorders of renal function). Uremia and sepsis intervene frequently and are the most common causes of

death. Distant metastases may involve any of the viscera; the liver, lungs, bones, adrenals, ovaries, and brain are among the most frequently involved (Fig. 3-62).

Studies of prognostic criteria have often been contradictory, but it is universally accepted that *clinical stage* (see Table 3-7) is the most important prognostic indicator. In most series, clinical stage 0 (in situ) cancers are associated with 5-year survival rates of close to 100%. This figure drops to 75% to 80% in stage I, 50% to 60% in stage II, about 30% in stage III, and 10% in stage IV. Extension to the corpus does not advance the stage but may worsen the prognosis.[341] Within the group of stage I tumors, tumor size and depth of invasion correlate well with survival.[342,343] Five-year survival rates are good indications of the therapeutic results, because more than 90% of deaths caused by cervical cancer occur within the first 5 years after treatment.[317,344]

The prognostic significance of most other indicators remains debatable. We have already discussed such factors as tumor type and grade, presence of

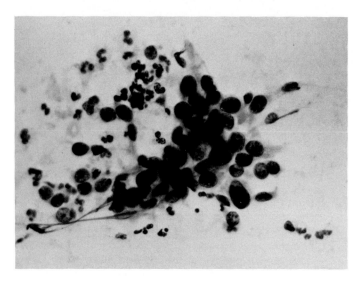

FIGURE 3-59 Large cell nonkeratinizing squamous cell carcinoma: cytologic appearance.

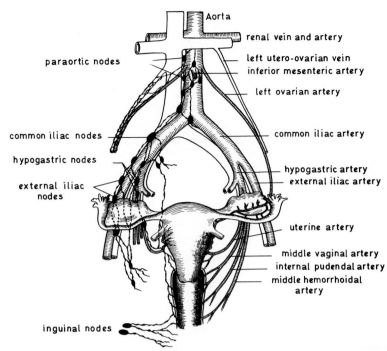

FIGURE 3-60 Lymphatic system of the genital organs.

stainable mucin, and lymphatic or vascular space invasion in the section on classification. Other investigators have been more interested in the host immune response. Both host cellular immunity and tumor-associated antigens have been demonstrated in cervical carcinoma, and this field deserves further exploration. Squamous cell carcinoma antigen (SCC-A) and CA-125 are said to predict and to detect recurrent disease.[345,346] In another series, invasive squamous carcinomas infected with HPV-16 spread to the parametria and pelvic nodes significantly more often than did HPV-16-negative tumors,[347] whereas HPV-18[348,349] or absence of HPV[350] suggested a worse prognosis to other investigators.

Lymphoplasmacytic infiltration of the tumor

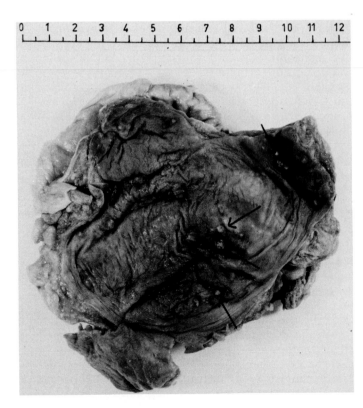

FIGURE 3-61 Squamous cell carcinoma of the cervix: bladder with metastases invading submucosally.

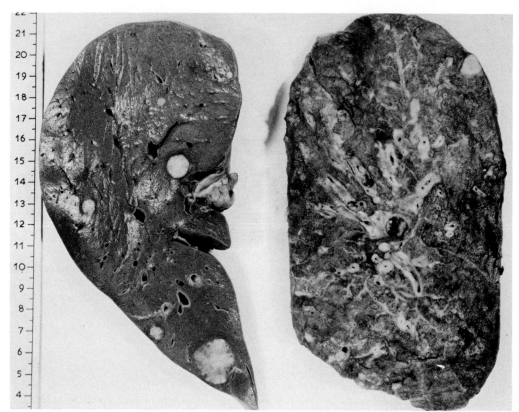

FIGURE 3-62 Squamous cell carcinoma of cervix: hepatic (*left*) and pulmonary (*right*) metastases.

may have a significant value in the prognostic evaluation.[338,351,352] Age 60 or older can be considered a prognostic factor; prognosis of patients in this age category is significantly better than that of patients in younger age groups in some series.[353] A report of Sorensen and colleagues[354] has shown that the nuclear volume is of prognostic value for objective malignancy grading. Such factors as AgNOR counts,[352] flow cytometry,[355] and oncogene overexpression[356,357] have been assigned prognostic significance in recent studies. In summary, the ideal prognostic factors still remain to be defined in this disease.

Studies have shown that therapeutic results—particularly in advanced stages—are improved when patients are treated in large centers by specialists skilled in the treatment of this disease.[358] The longstanding battle between advocates of surgery (Wertheim hysterectomy in stage I or II and exenteration for more advanced cases) and radiation therapy largely has been abandoned, because the therapeutic results are about equal.[359,360] The advent of high-voltage radiation therapy has greatly lowered the incidence of complications of treatment, and most institutions are treating most patients by this modality. Combination chemotherapy in advanced stages is being tested, and induction chemotherapy may potentiate surgery or radiation therapy in earlier stages.[361] An interdepartmental tumor conference or consultation system involving gynecologic and radiation oncologists and patholo-gists usually guarantees optimal and individualized treatment for each patient.

Microinvasive Squamous Carcinoma

The term *microinvasive squamous carcinoma* has been used to define an early stage of invasive squamous carcinoma in which no lesion is visible clinically and the diagnosis is first made histologically.[362–372,374–378] Criteria for diagnosis have varied markedly over the past 30 years, creating some confusion in the definition and treatment of the lesion. The depth of invasion, the configuration of the invasive tongues of neoplastic epithelium, and the evaluation of vascular and lymphatic permeation are among the subjects of contention. According to different proposed classifications, the maximal stromal invasion varies from 1 mm[364] to 9 mm,[365] and some authors include three-dimensional measurements in the definition.[366,368] The ultimate goal is to describe a lesion that can be treated safely by more conservative means than other squamous cancers.

In the clinical staging system of the International Federation of Gynecology and Obstetrics (FIGO; Tables 3-7 and 3-8), microinvasive carcinoma is considered stage Ia, which can be divided into Ia1 (invasive foci confined to a few tongue-like processes) and Ia2 (measurable tumor limited to a depth of less than 5 mm with a horizontal dimension of less than 7 mm).[367,378]

TABLE 3-8.
Criteria for Diagnosis of Microinvasive Squamous Carcinoma of the Cervix

Criteria	International Federation of Gynecology and Obstetrics (FIGO)	Society of Gynecologic Oncologists	Japanese Joint Study Committee
Size	Ia1: tongue-like processes only Ia2: up to 5 mm deep,* 7 mm wide	Up to 3 mm deep*	Up to 3 mm deep*
Lymphatic/vascular space involvement	May be present	No	No
Confluent growth pattern	May be present	May be present	No

*Measured from base of overlying epithelium.

Other studies[368,369,377] have indicated that lesions with a maximal stromal penetration of 3 mm and no lymphatic/vascular space invasion (LVSI) have an excellent prognosis, with virtually no potential for recurrence or metastasis. The definition of the Society of Gynecologic Oncologists (SGO) meets these criteria.[377] It states that "neoplastic epithelium invades the stroma in one or more places to a depth of 3 millimeters or less below the epithelium and lymphatic or vascular involvement is not demonstrated." It is not stated, however, how many serial step sections are needed to rule out deeper invasion or lymphatic or vascular permeation. Finally, the definition of the Japanese Joint Study Committee on Stage Ia Cancer of the Uterine Cervix[376] accepts a depth of 3 mm or less but excludes cases with either LVSI or confluent invasion. We tend to favor this lattermost definition.

Histology. The very early manifestation of microinvasion is the presence of a nidus of well-differentiated cells originating from the basal layers of the epithelium and disrupting the basement membrane. Downward tongue-like processes develop from this initial invasion and expand into the stroma vertically and horizontally. Multiple foci may develop. Confluent growth is characterized by anastomosing tongues of tumor cells with pushing borders.[370] The most common cellular growth patterns are finger-like cords, networks of confluent strands, or small clusters. The histologic types are, with decreasing frequency, large cell nonkeratinizing, keratinizing, and small cell types.[371]

Capillary/lymphatic space invasion should be diagnosed with care. The presence of endothelial cells is mandatory to affirm this invasion. Clear spaces around tumor cells may represent fixation artifacts. Roche and Norris[372] demonstrated that the finding of LVSI is directly proportional to the number of levels examined, and many more cases would be excluded by the SGO and Japanese criteria if dozens of levels were examined routinely.

It is important not to diagnose microinvasion when only endocervical gland extension is present.

In true microinvasion, the invasive tongues of cancer have angular rather than round and smooth contours, lack a surrounding "basement membrane" (as seen with the light microscope), and almost invariably show evidence of increased differentiation (eg, increased volume of eosinophilic cytoplasm, and intercellular bridges) compared with overlying epithelium, which has the appearance of in situ carcinoma or (less frequently) dysplasia (Figs. 3-63 through 3-65 and Table 3-9).

Microinvasive carcinoma can be diagnosed only in an adequate specimen, defined as a cone biopsy or hysterectomy specimen. In punch biopsies, the diagnosis may occasionally be suggested, but conization or hysterectomy remains mandatory for confirmation.

Cytology. The picture is usually that of coexisting in situ and invasive carcinoma. Some authors claim great accuracy in the exact cytologic diagnosis of the lesion, whereas others, like us, experience considerable difficulty. The most frequently reported criteria are (1) the presence of inflammation and necrosis ("tumor diathesis"); (2) abnormal cells in syncytial groupings; (3) abnormal cells whose nuclei have irregular chromatin distribution; and (4) abnormal cells with prominent nucleoli.[373]

Clinical Features. The incidence of microinvasive carcinoma as a proportion of in situ carcinomas has varied from 3% to 50% of in situ carcinoma in reported series,[374] pointing out the need for an adequate definition. The true incidence is probably around 5% to 10%. The *clinical significance* of the lesion is that, despite its invasive nature, it can be treated conservatively (like in situ carcinoma) with great success. We believe that for this statement to be true, all cases with lymphatic or blood vessel invasion and all cases with confluent tumor nests in the stroma must be eliminated from the microinvasive group and treated more vigorously. As discussed above, this concept is still controversial, with some authors (and the FIGO definition) stating that the depth of invasion should be the only significant fac-

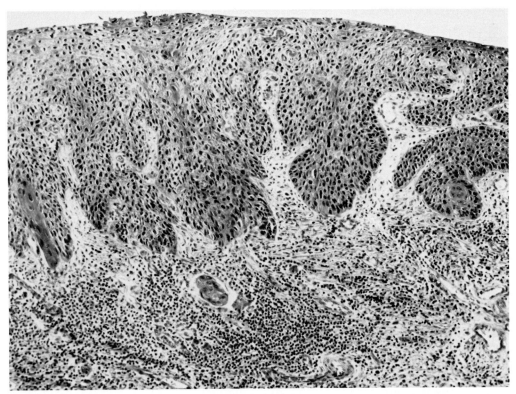

FIGURE 3-63 Microinvasive carcinoma: invasive tongues and one discontinuous nest of differentiated malignant cells.

tor. Boyes and colleagues[375] have suggested the separate term *occult invasive carcinoma* for the confluent tumors and have shown an appreciable incidence of recurrence, metastasis, or both, when this group is treated conservatively. Yamabe[376] has discussed the importance of separating local (eg, vaginal stump) recurrences from true metastases, because it is the lat-

ter which should be used to define the group of cases requiring more aggressive treatment.

Carcinoma of the Cervical Stump

The appearance of a cancer in a cervical stump (ie, that portion remaining after supracervical hysterec-

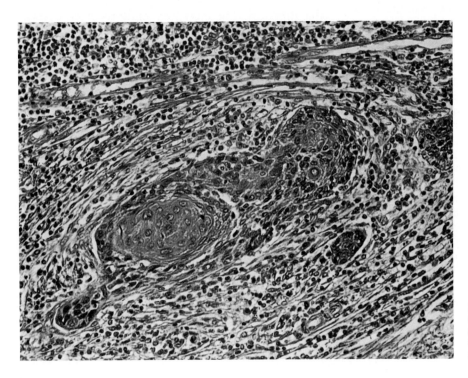

FIGURE 3-64 Microinvasive carcinoma: detail of a nest of tumor cells showing central squamous differentiation, lack of basement membrane, and surrounding stromal reaction.

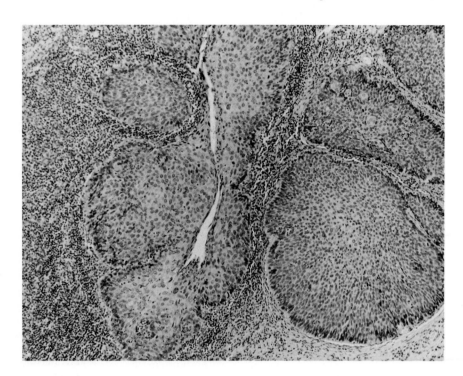

FIGURE 3-65 High-grade CIN extending into and completely replacing endocervical glands. Note roundness of the tumor nests, good circumscription from surrounding stroma, and lack of squamous differentiation.

tomy) poses important clinical problems.[379–381] It represents 4% to 8% of cervical cancers. Of the 183 cases cited by Creadick,[380] 14 were intraepithelial. Among the invasive cancers, the various histologic subtypes are found in about the same proportions as in the intact cervix, and even sarcomas have been reported.[382] Their macroscopic and microscopic appearance do not differ from those of cervical cancers in the intact uterus: only the therapeutic problems are different. It is more difficult, technically speaking, to irradiate or to operate on a cervical stump.

This is why, after a subtotal hysterectomy, it is necessary to verify the state of the cervix and to eliminate the presence of a neoplastic lesion. The complete avoidance of supracervical hysterectomy eliminates the problem entirely. If the tumor is detected less than 2 years after subtotal hysterectomy, it was probably already present at the time of initial surgery.[381]

Verrucous Carcinoma

This rare form of very well-differentiated squamous cell carcinoma may develop in the cervix,[383] but it is more common in the vulva and vagina and has been

TABLE 3-9.
Differential Diagnosis of Cervical Microinvasive Carcinoma Versus CIN With Gland Extension

Criteria	Microinvasion	CIN With Gland Extension
Size of tumor nests	Variable	Uniform
Shape of tumor nests	Angular	Rounded
Basement membrane	Absent	Present
Stromal inflammation	Present	Often absent
Squamous differentiation (eosinophilic cytoplasm) in tumor nests	Present	Absent (tumor cell differentiation $\geqq$ surface epithelium)
Adjacent glands	Variable	Usually present, often focally involved by CIN
Lymphatic/vascular space invasion	Sometimes*	Never
Confluence of tumor nests	Sometimes*	Never

*May be excluded by definition of microinvasion.

discussed in Chapters 1 and 2. Microscopically, it is characterized by marked papillomatosis, normal squamous maturation, and the absence of cellular atypia. The tumor expands into the underlying stroma by pushing, bulky rete pegs with smooth margins. This lesion requires a full-thickness excisional biopsy to be recognized. The differential diagnosis comprises condyloma acuminatum and well-differentiated squamous carcinoma. If treated by adequate local excision, metastases should not occur.

Papillary Squamous Cell Carcinoma

This rare form of carcinoma, reported by Randall and associates,[384] reveals a papillary, wart-like macroscopic appearance corresponding microscopically to fibrovascular cores covered with a dysplastic epithelium showing moderate to severe cellular atypia. The lesion can be in situ or invasive, and a cone biopsy or hysterectomy specimen is necessary to rule out stromal invasion. The ISGP classification (see Table 3-6) uses *papillary transitional cell carcinoma* as a synonym for this lesion because of its resemblance to bladder carcinoma. The cytologic atypia distinguishes it from verrucous carcinoma or benign papilloma. If invasive, the tumor can metastasize, sometimes as a late event.[384]

Lymphoepithelioma-Like Carcinoma

Lymphoepithelioma-like carcinoma is another tumor included in the ISGP classification as a variant of squamous cell carcinoma.[226] It is a rare lesion, usually well circumscribed, consisting of solid nests of undifferentiated cells with indistinct cell borders and an interspersed marked inflammatory infiltrate of lymphocytes, plasma cells, and eosinophils.[385,386] Similar tumors in the nasopharynx and salivary glands have been referred to as *lymphoepitheliomas,* and in the breast as *medullary carcinomas.* The behavior of this lesion in the cervix remains to be defined, but one report has suggested a relatively favorable prognosis.[385] The differential diagnosis includes inflamed squamous cell carcinoma, glassy cell carcinoma, and malignant lymphoma. The first two have larger cells with distinct cell borders; the last may require immunohistochemical evaluation for definitive diagnosis.

Small Cell Neuroendocrine Carcinoma

Small cell neuroendocrine carcinomas[313–316,387–389] exhibit small or intermediate-type cells that arise from argyrophilic cells present in the ectocervical or endocervical epithelium[390,391] or from undifferentiated stem cells. The neoplastic cells are arranged in nests or sheets or are disposed in single files. They have hyperchromatic nuclei with finely dispersed chromatin and an elevated nuclear–cytoplasmic ratio

(Fig. 3-66). Molding, crushing and overlapping modify the disposition of the nuclei. Intermediate-type cells are larger and exhibit a pale, eosinophilic cytoplasm with ill-defined borders. Their nuclei are oval and uniform. In both types mitoses are numerous. Nucleoli are inconspicuous. Necrosis is common, particularly in tumors growing in large nests or sheets. Foci of squamous or glandular differentiation are not rare.[313] A high prevalence of HPV types 16 and particularly 18 has been reported in neuroendocrine carcinomas.[388]

The differential diagnosis includes squamous cell and adenocarcinoma, carcinoid tumor, stromal sarcoma, and malignant lymphoma. Immunohistochemical and ultrastructural studies can establish the diagnosis in problem cases. Argyrophilic granules vary in quantity from one case to another and may require prolonged search at the light microscopic and ultrastructural levels. Positive immunoreaction is observed for cytokeratins, CEA, chromogranin, neuron-specific enolase, synaptophysin, and a variety of polypeptides such as ACTH, serotonin, calcitonin, gastrin, and somatostatin.[315,389,391]

Few cytologic reports are available, and rarely the tumor has been discovered by cytology.[315,316] The aggressive, often voluminous tumor generally is clinically evident. Smears reveal small cells with round or oval hyperchromatic nuclei and scant basophilic cytoplasm. Nucleoli are small and inconspicuous. In some cases, glandular structures coexist with the neuroendocrine cells.[387,392]

The prognosis is poor, and distant metastases are often present at the time of initial diagnosis or soon thereafter. Liver and bones are frequently involved, as in small cell carcinoma of the lung. Chemotherapy may produce a response but rarely a cure.

Carcinoid Tumor

It is not clear whether a better differentiated neuroendocrine tumor that may be classified as pure carcinoid tumor occurs in the uterine cervix. This tumor appears in the ISGP classification as a synonym for

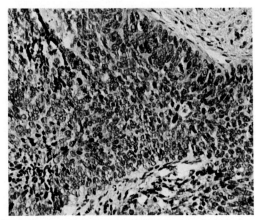

FIGURE 3-66 Small cell carcinoma: microscopic appearance.

adenocarcinoma with features of carcinoid tumor, and Kurman and colleagues question whether a pure carcinoid of the cervix exists.[226] We have seen rare cases (Fig. 3-67) that appear to represent pure carcinoids, usually found as incidental microscopic lesions in cervices removed or biopsied for other indications. More commonly, the typical carcinoid pattern is seen focally in otherwise typical small cell carcinomas or adenocarcinomas.

Adenocarcinoma

Thirty or forty years ago, 95% of all cancers of the uterine cervix were of squamous origin, and adenocarcinomas and their precursor lesions were considered rarities. In subsequent years, the cytologic detection and early treatment of precursors of squamous carcinoma have reduced the frequency of that lesion in many parts of the world, and the proportion of cervical cancers that have an adenocarcinomatous component has increased to 15% or greater in recent reports. Some of these reports have suggested that the absolute as well as the relative incidences of adenocarcinoma may be rising.[393,394]

As these glandular lesions become more common, we are learning more about their clinical and pathologic manifestations, including the recognition of new variants of invasive adenocarcinoma, of precursor lesions, and of benign neoplastic and nonneoplastic lesions that may enter into their differential diagnosis.[395–399] The new ISGP classification of cervical glandular tumors, other nonsquamous epithelial tumors, and glandular tumor-like lesions is presented in Table 3-10.

Adenocarcinoma does not display the same relationship to sexual activity that has been described previously for squamous cell carcinoma, which suggests that different etiologic factors are involved.[400] Nevertheless, the two tumors or their preinvasive variants frequently coexist in the same patient,[401,402] and adenocarcinomas have been associated with HPV, particularly type 18.[82,83,89,402–404] Dallenbach-Hellweg[405] has suggested a link between oral contraceptive usage and the development of cervical adenocarcinomas in young women, but these data have not been confirmed in other series.[406]

Invasive Mucinous Adenocarcinoma

The prototype for adenocarcinoma of the cervix is the mucinous type, particularly its endocervical variant. This is a tumor largely limited to adult women, whose average age is about 50 years. From 80% to 90% of the patients present with abnormal uterine bleeding, although other complaints occur and up to 20% of patients may be asymptomatic. Some of these latter cases are detected by an abnormal Papanicolaou smear, but in most series 50% or more of women with adenocarcinoma of the cervix have a normal smear.[407]

The *gross appearance* of adenocarcinoma of the cervix is variable, some of the tumors presenting as exophytic, polypoid, or papillary processes (Fig. 3-68), whereas others have a grossly normal surface and grow entirely endophytically. In some cases,

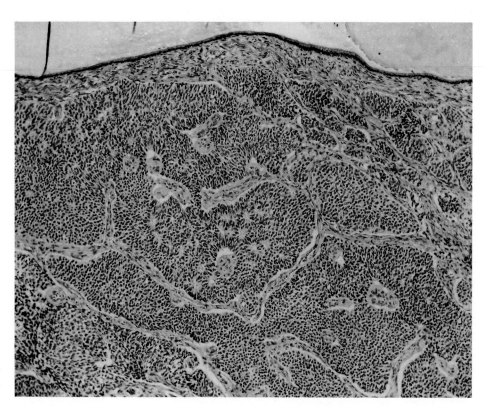

FIGURE 3-67 Carcinoid tumor of the cervix. This tumor was an incidental microscopic finding.

TABLE 3-10.
International Society of Gynecological Pathologists
Classification of Cervical Glandular Tumors and Tumor-Like
Lesions (1991)

Glandular Lesions
  Endocervical polyp
  Müllerian papilloma
  Glandular atypia
  Atypical hyperplasia (glandular dysplasia)
  Adenocarcinoma in situ
  Adenocarcinoma
    Mucinous (endocervical, intestinal, and signet-ring types)
    Endometrioid
    Clear cell
    Minimal deviation (adenoma malignum)
    Papillary villoglandular
    Serous
    Mesonephric
Glandular Tumor-Like Lesions
  Microglandular hyperplasia
  Mesonephric remnants
  Mesonephric hyperplasia
  Arias-Stella reaction
  Endometriosis
  Cysts
  Intestinal metaplasia
  Tubal metaplasia
  Tunnel clusters
Other Epithelial Tumors
  Adenosquamous carcinoma
  Glassy cell carcinoma
  Adenoid cystic carcinoma
  Adenoid basal carcinoma
  Carcinoid tumor (adenocarcinoma with features of carcinoid tumor)
  Small cell carcinoma
  Undifferentiated carcinoma

gross examination of the cervix may even reveal only benign changes.

Microscopically, as mentioned above, the most common type is adenocarcinoma of endocervical type, which is said to account for about 70% of all cervical adenocarcinomas.[395] By definition, these tumors must contain at least some cells in which cytoplasmic mucin can be demonstrated. In most of these tumors, glands of variable size and shape infiltrate through the wall of the cervix, with a variable amount of stromal reaction around them. There is at least some cellular stratification, loss of mucin, nuclear enlargement, hyperchromasia, and mitotic activity, and the severity of these changes varies with the differentiation of the tumor (Figs. 3-69 through 3-72).

Unlike *endometrioid adenocarcinomas*—whether of endocervical or endometrial origin—the glands generally do not grow together in a cribriform pattern and usually are unassociated with a prominent squamous component. Mucin can be demonstrated in the cytoplasm of at least some of the cells of endocervical-type adenocarcinomas, whereas mucin usually is present only at the apical borders of the tumor cells and in tumor lumina in endometrioid adenocarcinomas. This difference is reflected in differences in immunohistochemical reactivity. For example, CEA is said by some authors to be much more common in endocervical than in endometrial adenocarcinoma,[408,409] although others deny this difference.[410] Some authors claim that vimentin immunoreactivity is much more common in endometrial than in endocervical adenocarcinoma, and 1C-5, a

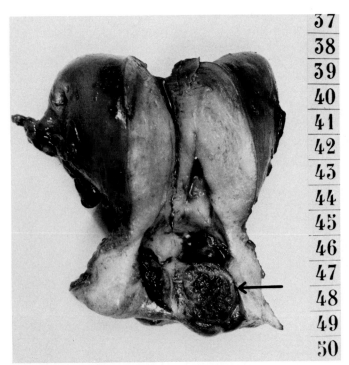

FIGURE 3-68 Adenocarcinoma of the cervix: macroscopic appearance.

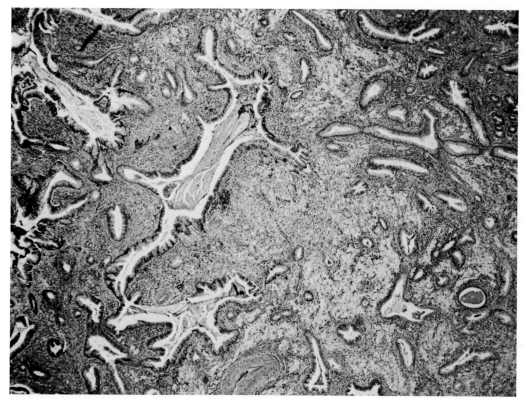

FIGURE 3-69 Well-differentiated adenocarcinoma of endocervical type: low-power photomicrograph of angular glands infiltrating stroma.

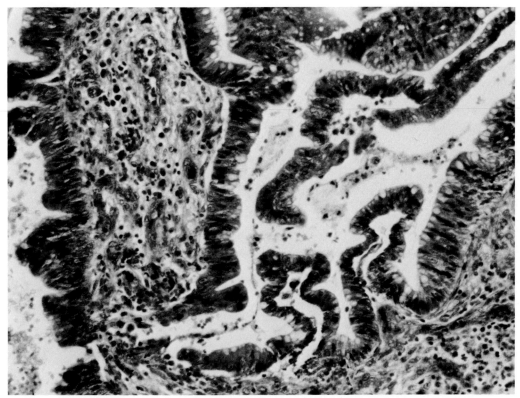

FIGURE 3-70 Well-differentiated endocervical adenocarcinoma: detail of invasive malignant glands.

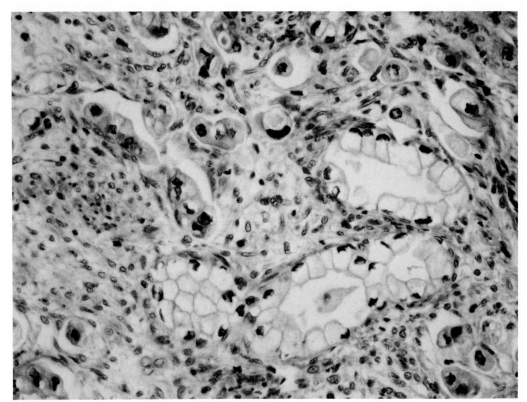

FIGURE 3-71 Moderately differentiated (grade II) adenocarcinoma of the cervix with intracytoplasmic mucin globules within malignant glands and in single signet-ring cells.

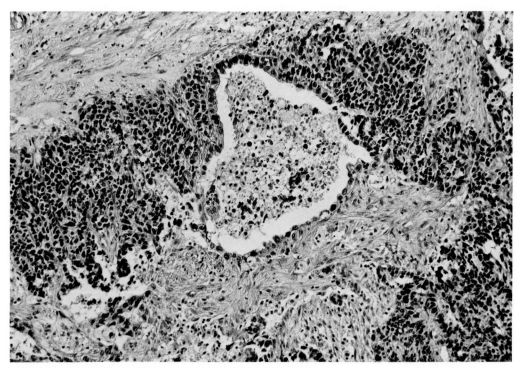

FIGURE 3-72 Largely undifferentiated adenocarcinoma of the cervix.

new monoclonal antibody, has also proved useful in one published report.[411] These stains and histologic appearances differentiate between adenocarcinomas of endometrioid and endocervicoid *types,* rather than of endometrial and endocervical *origin.*[412] Because as many as 15% to 20% of primary adenocarcinomas of the endocervix are of endometrioid type, and about 5% of adenocarcinomas of the endometrium are of mucinous (generally endocervicoid) type, the site of origin of these tumors will always be stated incorrectly by any test relying on histologic appearance or markers of differentiation. The presence of a typical endometrial or endocervical stroma identifies the involved tissue site but may not indicate tumor origin, because carcinoma of the endometrium may extend downward to involve the endocervix and vice versa. The differential diagnosis of endocervical versus endometrial adenocarcinoma is summarized in Table 3-2.

As endocervical adenocarcinomas become more undifferentiated, they may contain solid areas that cannot be differentiated from poorly differentiated squamous carcinoma or even small cell carcinoma (see Fig. 3-72). Even the presence of cervical squamous dysplasia or in situ carcinoma does not resolve the differential diagnosis between poorly differentiated adenocarcinoma and poorly differentiated squamous carcinoma, because these lesions accompany about 40% of cases of well-documented cervical adenocarcinoma.[401,413]

The level of differentiation of cervical adenocarcinoma is important, because it has been shown in numerous studies to be associated with prognosis, well-differentiated tumors having better survival rates than poorly differentiated ones.[407,414,415] Poorly differentiated tumors also tend to present in higher clinical stages, and sometimes it is difficult to separate the prognostic effects of grade and stage. This is also a problem when comparing the outcomes of adenocarcinomas and squamous carcinomas of the cervix. Most studies have suggested that adenocarcinoma is associated with a poorer prognosis, but this is not always true when tumors of the same clinical stage are compared.[393,416,417] The routes of local and distant metastatic spread are the same as for squamous cell carcinoma.

Cytologic Findings. Although the cytologic characteristics of endocervical adenocarcinoma are well established, as many as half of the cases in some series have been missed by cytologic examination.[407,418] The reason for this high false-negative rate is that adenocarcinomas frequently arise high in the endocervical canal and beneath an intact surface mucosa, so that the cells may easily be missed unless vigorous direct endocervical sampling is performed. In endocervical adenocarcinoma, the tumor cells in cytologic material occur most frequently in clusters, often with a papillary arrangement (Color Fig. 3-31). The papillary or glandular arrangement is less apparent in more poorly differentiated tumors.

The cells are generally elongated, with an apparent apical pole and peripheral nucleus; this polarity is a useful distinguishing feature from the more common cervical squamous cell cancers. The cytoplasm is often vacuolated and lacks evidence of keratinization. The nucleus is round to oval and shows considerable enlargement and variation in size and shape from one cell to the next. There is prominent clumping of chromatin within the nuclear substance and along the nuclear membrane, and one or more large prominent nucleoli. The background often shows the same necrotic debris or "tumor diathesis" seen in squamous cell carcinoma.

The cytologic differential diagnosis is with benign reactive endocervical and metaplastic conditions (see Color Figs. 3-4 through 3-8), with large cell nonkeratinizing squamous cell carcinoma of the cervix (see Color Fig. 3-29), and with adenocarcinoma of the endometrium (Color Fig. 3-32). This last distinction is the most difficult; even histologically it may be a problem to differentiate these two entities (see above). The cells of an endocervical adenocarcinoma are generally larger, with larger nuclei and nucleoli and greater cytoplasmic vacuolization, than those of endometrial cancer (compare Color Figs. 3-31 and 3-32). Adenocarcinoma cells arising from the ovary, the fallopian tube, or an extragenital primary cancer metastatic to the genital tract are usually unaccompanied by a tumor diathesis.

Other Types of Invasive Adenocarcinomas

In addition to the most common mucinous tumor of endocervical type, rarer invasive mucinous tumors may show intestinal or signet-ring differentiation.[407,419,420] Any of the other types of differentiation seen elsewhere in the female genital tract may be encountered, including endometrioid (as discussed above), clear cell, and serous adenocarcinomas. *Endometrioid adenocarcinoma* is the most common of these, comprising 15% to 20% of endocervical adenocarcinomas in most reports.[395] As mentioned above, this tumor needs to be differentiated both from the endocervical type of tumor and from adenocarcinoma arising in the endometrium.

Clear Cell Adenocarcinoma. Clear cell adenocarcinoma is seen most frequently in young women who have been exposed to DES in utero, but it is also encountered in all age groups in DES-unexposed patients.[421,422] The DES-related tumors invariably involve the ectocervix, often extending upward into the endocervix or downward into the vagina; indeed, many of these may have originated in the vagina and extended upward to involve the cervix. Microscopically, the tumors grow in varying mixtures of tubulocystic, solid, and papillary patterns, and are characteristically composed of clear or hobnail cells, with some tumors containing many flattened cells as well. The clear cells are characteristically rich in glycogen and poor in mucin. The appearance of these tumors is illustrated in Chapters 2 and 4. The differential diagnosis of these tumors includes other types of adenocarcinoma, as well as the Arias-Stella reaction (see Fig. 3-7) and yolk sac carcinoma—the former seen predominantly in pregnancy and the latter almost exclusively in infancy.

Serous Adenocarcinoma. Also important in the differential diagnosis of clear cell adenocarcinoma is primary serous adenocarcinoma of the cervix. This is an extremely rare tumor, only a few cases of which are described in the literature.[423] Its histologic appearance is similar to that of serous carcinomas in more common sites, such as the ovary, fallopian tube, and endometrium.

Minimal Deviation Adenocarcinoma. Another uncommon type of cervical adenocarcinoma is minimal deviation adenocarcinoma, also known as *adenoma malignum*.[424–431] The controversy over this lesion extends to its classification; Young and Scully[395] characterize it as a variant of endocervical-type adenocarcinoma, whereas the ISGP classification (see Table 3-10) lists it as a separate and independent variant. This is because Kaminski and Norris[426] included an endometrioid type in their report, whereas most others have limited the diagnosis of minimal deviation adenocarcinoma to tumors of endocervical type. In any event, the defining feature is that the glands comprising the tumor lack significant nuclear strati-

fication, pleomorphism, or mitotic activity, although the glands are usually of bizarre shape, with numerous angular outpouchings, and deeply infiltrate the cervical wall (Figs. 3-73 and 3-74). These tumors can be confused with usual endocervical adenocarcinomas but are even more likely to be confused with benign lesions, such as tunnel clusters[51,164] (see Fig. 3-31), deep nabothian cysts,[171] and mesonephric hyperplasias (see Fig. 3-34).[28,175,176] Among the distinctive features of minimal deviation adenocarcinoma are the irregular and angular appearance of the glands, the presence of a stromal reaction around at least some of them as they infiltrate the cervical wall, the presence of large amounts of mucin in the cytoplasm of the neoplastic cells (a distinction from mesonephric hyperplasia), and the presence of CEA demonstrated immunohistochemically in the tumor cells (not seen in benign glandular lesions of the cervix, although certainly it is present in many adenocarcinomas).[428,429,432] The tumors are often large and clinically apparent, but small biopsies may yield a false-negative diagnosis. The tumor is seen in some women in association with the Peutz-Jeghers syndrome.[399,427,430]

Cytologic diagnosis is difficult. The exfoliated cells resemble normal columnar endocervical cells, and cellular atypias are scarce. Only the crowding of the columnar elements may suggest the existence of some cervical pathology.[431]

Controversy surrounds the *prognosis* of minimal deviation adenocarcinoma. The tumor initially was thought to have an extremely poor prognosis, but Silverberg and Hurt[424] subsequently suggested that this might be related to misdiagnosis and consequent delayed treatment. Kaminski and Norris[426] also re-

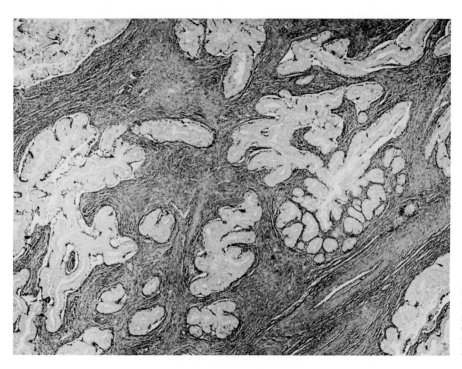

FIGURE 3-73 Minimal deviation adenocarcinoma of cervix: infiltrating glands with angular pointed contours. (Silverberg SG: Surgical pathology of the uterus. New York, John Wiley & Sons, 1977)

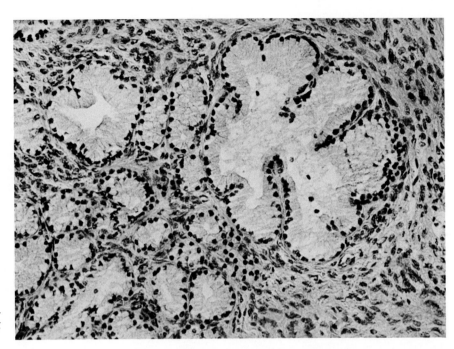

FIGURE 3-74 Minimal deviation adenocarcinoma of the cervix: detail showing lack of cellular atypia.

ported a relatively favorable prognosis, but both Kaku and Enjoji[425] and Gilks and colleagues[427] have noted unfavorable results even in patients who appeared to be adequately treated. Larger series need to be analyzed, but it appears that the tumor has a poor prognosis and needs to be treated vigorously.

Well-Differentiated Villoglandular Adenocarcinoma. Another type of tumor whose pathology and natural history are still being characterized is well-differentiated villoglandular adenocarcinoma.[433,434] The results of two published series of 13 and 24

cases, respectively, suggest that this tumor occurs preferentially in young women (average age in the lower thirties) and has an extremely favorable prognosis. The tumor grows predominantly exophytically, with a prominent papillary component. The papillae typically have a fibrous stroma and are lined by stratified cells showing only modest cytologic atypia (Figs. 3-75 and 3-76). The tumor may show endocervical, endometrial, or intestinal differentiation, and frequently has an admixture of these types. Superficial invasion into the cervical wall is usually seen, but deep invasion is uncommon and distant metastases

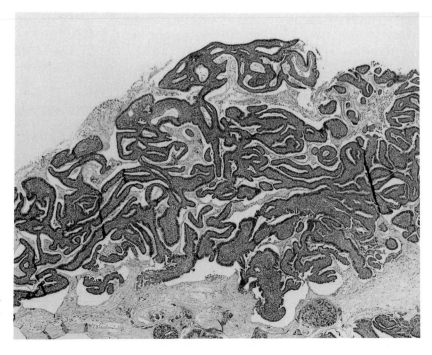

FIGURE 3-75 Well-differentiated villoglandular adenocarcinoma: typical architectural picture at low magnification. (Courtesy of Dr. Mirka Jones, Washington, DC)

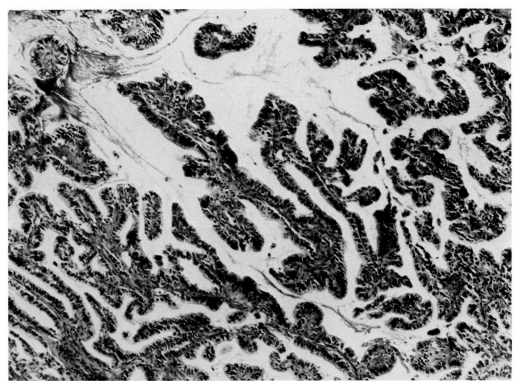

FIGURE 3-76 Well-differentiated villoglandular adenocarcinoma: villoglandular architecture and low cytologic grade are characteristic of the invasive component of this tumor.

have not been seen in any of the 37 cases reported. A few patients treated by less than hysterectomy (predominantly cone biopsy) have shown long-term survival, as have all of the other patients with adequate follow-up. These data seem to suggest that radical surgery and adjuvant therapy are not necessary for the successful treatment of the great majority of these tumors. In our case material, a relation to the use of oral contraceptives was suggested, although the data are not conclusive.[434] The cytologic appearance of these tumors has not been characterized.

Mesonephric Adenocarcinoma. The final subtype of invasive adenocarcinoma listed in the ISGP classification is mesonephric adenocarcinoma. This is probably the rarest subtype, with only 7 well-documented cases in the literature, including 4 in one recent report.[28] Despite early reports equating mesonephric origin with clear cell carcinoma (see above), it is now recognized that clear cell carcinomas are of müllerian type. True mesonephric carcinomas are best recognized by their location deep in the cervical wall, their tubular pattern (reminiscent of benign mesonephric remnants but more atypical and more haphazardly arranged), and the lack of involvement of endocervical mucosa.[28,226,399]

In Situ Adenocarcinoma

With the recent increase in the relative—if not the absolute—frequency of invasive adenocarcinoma of the cervix, it is not surprising that adenocarcinoma in situ (AIS) has been encountered more frequently as well, leading to a better understanding of its pathologic appearance and natural history. This term was first introduced in 1953,[435] and the true population-based frequency is still not known, in part because AIS is thought to be frequently underdiagnosed.[396,436–439] It is diagnosed far less frequently than the corresponding squamous CIN, but 50% or more of cases of AIS show coexisting squamous CIN.[440,441]

As with well-differentiated villoglandular adenocarcinomas, AIS lesions are generally divided into endocervical, endometrioid, and intestinal types. Both in the literature[396,440] and in our own experience, the vast majority of cases have been predominantly of endocervical type, although occasional glands showing endometrioid or intestinal differentiation may be encountered. We prefer to consider this lesion as the exact opposite of minimal deviation adenocarcinoma of the cervix; whereas minimal deviation adenocarcinoma is characterized by glands that are architecturally malignant and cytologically benign, AIS consists of architecturally unremarkable glands showing cytologic evidence of malignancy.

Thus, the glands are normally situated in the cervix and are of normal size and shape, but they reveal cellular stratification, loss of polarity, increased nuclear size, hyperchromasia, loss of cytoplasmic mucin, and mitotic activity (Figs. 3-77 and 3-78). A cribriform glandular pattern has been reported by some authors in AIS, but others might consider this

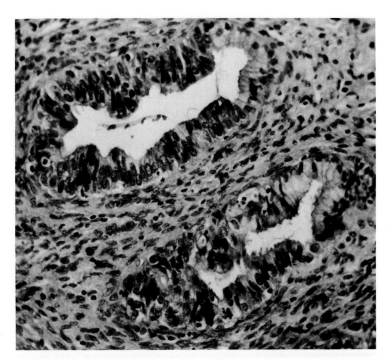

FIGURE 3-77 Adenocarcinoma in situ of the cervix. These two glands are only partially filled by malignant epithelium, are of normal size and shape, and show no stromal reaction around them.

a manifestation of microinvasion (Fig. 3-79). AIS is seen most frequently in the region of the transformation zone of the cervix, and most cases involve both glandular and surface epithelium. It is not completely understood whether the lesion is invariably unicentric or frequently multicentric.

Several studies[402,403] have indicated that HPV is frequently associated with AIS (as it is with invasive cervical adenocarcinoma), and that the type most frequently seen is HPV-18. Ploidy studies are only beginning to be reported, and their diagnostic or prognostic significance remains to be determined.[442] Immunohistochemistry is not diagnostically useful.[443]

The *differential diagnosis* of AIS is predominately with tubal metaplasia, glandular atypias—both reactive and preneoplastic—of lesser degree, and microinvasive adenocarcinoma. Microglandular hyperplasia, cervical endometriosis, and Arias-Stella reaction

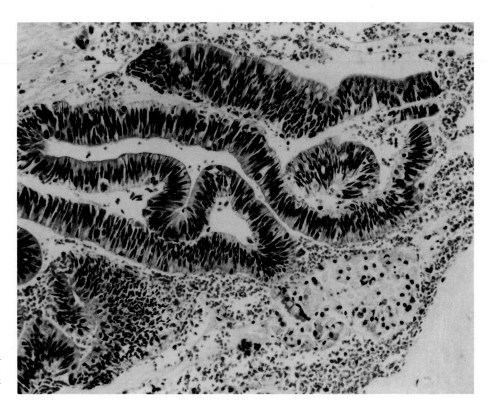

FIGURE 3-78 Adenocarcinoma in situ in curettage specimen. Conization is necessary to rule out stromal invasion.

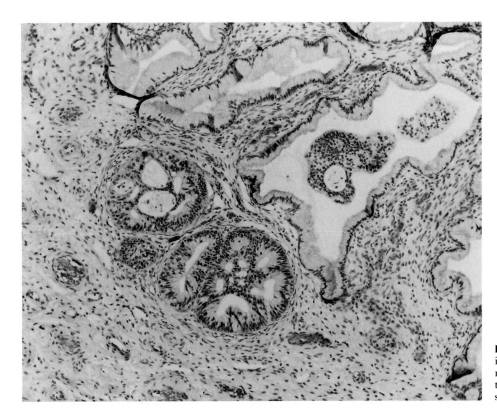

FIGURE 3-79 Adenocarcinoma in situ versus microinvasive adenocarcinoma. The cribriform pattern probably signifies early stromal invasion.

have been mentioned.[396] In cases that we see in consultation, the most frequent misdiagnosis is that of tubal metaplasia.[173,174] The absence of nuclear atypia and mitotic activity and the presence of ciliated cells in this lesion should serve to differentiate it from AIS (Fig. 3-80).

Cytologically, AIS resembles invasive adenocarci-

noma but usually lacks a tumor diathesis.[444–446] The definitive diagnosis, in which stromal invasion is ruled out, must be made in a conization or hysterectomy specimen. If the conization resection margins are negative, this procedure is usually therapeutic as well. In one recent study, only 1 of 7 patients reported and only 1 of 25 reviewed in the literature had residual

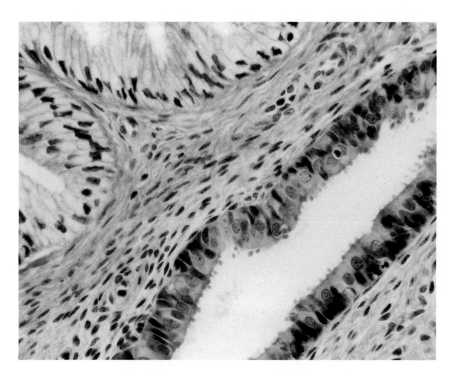

FIGURE 3-80 Tubal metaplasia of endocervical gland (*lower right*). Compare with normal glands at upper left and with adenocarcinoma in situ in Figures 3-77 and 3-78.

disease at hysterectomy when the cone biopsy margins were uninvolved.[447] Evaluation of an endocervical curettage performed after the cone biopsy may be useful. Although the lesion is inferred to have the potential to progress to invasive adenocarcinoma if inadequately treated, only rare cases have been reported as showing such progression.[439,448]

Endocervical Glandular Dysplasia

Much more difficult differential diagnostic problems involve the distinction of AIS from endocervical glandular dysplasia (EGD) at the lower end of the spectrum and microinvasive adenocarcinoma at the upper end. We believe that the diagnostic criteria for both of these lesions have been poorly defined in the literature, and it is not clear that the natural history of either of them differs significantly from that of AIS. The natural history of AIS itself is very poorly established despite the large number of reported cases. The best attempts at definitions of EGD have been made by Jaworski[396] and Brown and Wells,[449] but they are still difficult to understand. Jaworski states that "it should be realized that EGD and AIS form a spectrum and that a sharp division between the two is not possible." When one adds to this confusion the problem of distinguishing glandular dysplasia from reactive glandular atypia secondary to inflammatory lesions, we find that we rarely make the diagnosis of glandular dysplasia in our own practice. When we do, it defines a lesion in which glands in an uninflamed region of the cervix (to rule out reactive atypias) are architecturally unremarkable but

display moderate nuclear enlargement, hyperchromatism, and atypia, with less stratification, mitotic activity, and severe atypia than seen in AIS (Fig. 3-81).

The *cytologic appearance* is characterized by strips of columnar cells showing nuclear pseudostratification and different degrees of atypia.[446] Rosettes indicate the glandular origin of the lesion. Numerous tightly crowded clumps of atypical cells confirm without doubt the existence of an endocervical lesion that requires further investigation. Isolated cells are of little diagnostic value because inflammatory changes may mimic dysplastic anomalies. Differential diagnostic difficulties are posed by inflammatory and repair changes. For example, postconization smears may reveal numerous densely cellular clumps with pseudostratified nuclei that puzzle the cytopathologist.

Microinvasive Adenocarcinoma

Equally confusing as the distinction between AIS and EGD is that between AIS and microinvasive adenocarcinoma. Some investigators have defined microinvasive or "early invasive" adenocarcinoma as a tumor that invades into the underlying cervical stroma to a depth of less than 5 mm as measured from the mucosal surface of the endocervical canal.[436,450] Others use different measurements, whereas yet others (including ourselves) do not measure at all, but merely try to distinguish lesions characterized by invasion of only a few cells or a few glands. Still other authors recommend against using the diagnosis of microinva-

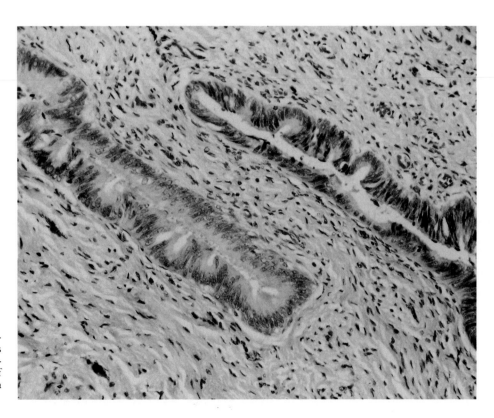

FIGURE 3-81 Endocervical glandular dysplasia. The atypia seen is less than that encountered in adenocarcinoma in situ. The lack of inflammation in adjacent stroma rules out a reactive atypia.

sive adenocarcinoma at all, and Jaworski[396] summarizes the confusion by stating that "the existence of microinvasive adenocarcinoma as an entity remains in dispute."

Given this confusion, it hardly seems appropriate to pontificate at length on the diagnostic criteria for this questionable lesion, but we have made the diagnosis in our laboratories when we encounter a lesion reminiscent of AIS but showing: (1) individual cells, often of apparent squamous type, dropping off into the stroma; (2) a higher concentration of cytologically malignant glands, often with small sizes and variable shapes, than would be expected in normal endocervix or endocervix involved by AIS; (3) glands that have grown together in a confluent pattern (see Fig. 3-79); or (4) glands that are irregular in orientation and have elicited a stromal response (Fig. 3-82). In our experience, this has always been an extremely focal change, and we have not found it necessary to measure these lesions. Invasive adenocarcinomas that are measurable—even if only 2 or 3 mm in greatest dimension—should be diagnosed as invasive adenocarcinoma, although the pathologist may wish to specify their dimensions.

As mentioned above, the *natural history* of all these lesions (EGD, AIS, and microinvasive adenocarcinoma) is poorly understood. It appears that many patients can be managed by cone biopsy alone, but that it is important for the pathologist to check and report the adequacy of the cone biopsy margins. We believe that—until extensive data to the contrary are available—measurable small invasive adenocarcinomas should be treated more aggressively.

Adenosquamous Carcinoma

Adenosquamous carcinoma of the cervix is a difficult lesion to define, because there are several candidates for this designation. First, it has become increasingly apparent over the past few years that the presence of stainable mucin in otherwise typical squamous carcinomas of the cervix portends a poorer prognosis; different authors have used the terms *adenosquamous carcinoma, mucoepidermoid carcinoma,* and *mixed carcinoma* to define tumors identified by positive mucin staining.[319-323] Some authors have also used the term *adenosquamous carcinoma* to characterize "collision" tumors, in which two different tumors—a squamous cell carcinoma and an adenocarcinoma—coexist in the same cervix. Third, certain endometrioid carcinomas of the cervix with squamous differentiation (Fig. 3-83) may logically be referred to as *adenosquamous carcinomas.* In our opinion, only the fourth type—a single carcinoma of endocervical type in which both squamous and glandular differentiation are identifiable without special stains—should be designated as adenosquamous carcinoma (Figs. 3-84 and 3-85).

Defined in this manner, adenosquamous carcinoma is a relatively uncommon tumor, although there is a possibility that it is increasing in frequency, and the question of a relation to oral contraception and to pregnancy has been raised. Most epidemiologic features are closer to those of squamous cell carcinoma than those of adenocarcinoma.[451] Adenosquamous carcinoma has been said by some authors to have a particularly unfavorable prognosis,

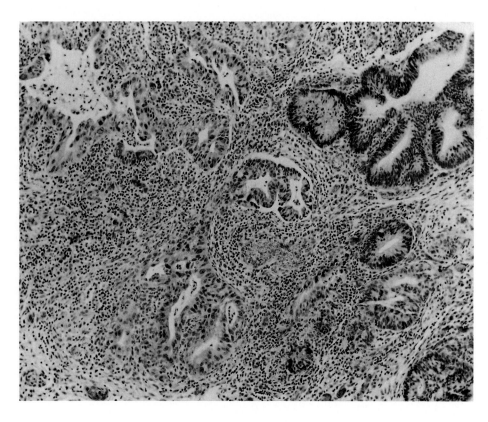

FIGURE 3-82 Microinvasive adenocarcinoma. Glands with in situ adenocarcinoma are seen on the right. The focus of invasion is seen almost in its entirety in this photomicrograph.

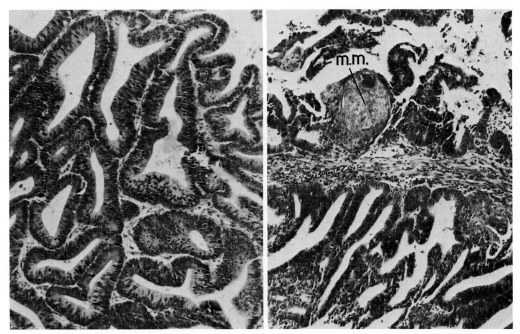

FIGURE 3-83 Adenoacanthoma type of mixed carcinoma of the cervix. *m.m,* squamous metaplasia.

but it is not always clear which of the definitions referred to above is being quoted in this situation.[416,452] Other studies have suggested that the prognosis is no worse than that for comparably staged squamous cell carcinoma.[453,454] The cytologic diagnosis is unreliable.

Glassy Cell Carcinoma

Controversy surrounds the diagnosis and clinical significance of glassy cell carcinoma, which is considered by most authors to be a variant of adenosquamous carcinoma. The tumor is generally easy to

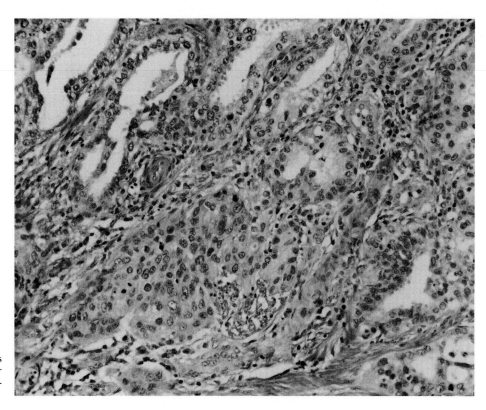

FIGURE 3-84 Adenosquamous carcinoma. This invasive cancer shows both glandular and squamous differentiation.

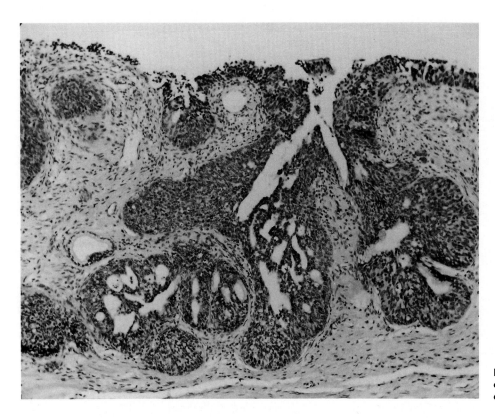

FIGURE 3-85 Adenosquamous carcinoma in situ. Biphasic differentiation in a noninvasive tumor.

diagnose microscopically, because it is composed of characteristic sheets of large cells with abundant eosinophilic or amphophilic, ground-glass or finely granular cytoplasm, prominent cell borders, large nuclei with prominent solitary nucleoli, and a notable stromal inflammatory infiltrate of eosinophils and plasma cells, which divides the tumor into neoplastic cell islands (Fig. 3-86). By the usual definition, an easily recognizable component of classical squamous cell or adenocarcinoma should not be present. Although this tumor is said by some authors to be associated with a typical clinical history, including an appearance in younger, often pregnant patients, and a particularly poor prognosis,[455] other authors who have studied the same subject have denied that it is a distinct entity and believe that the glassy cell morphologic pattern occurs focally in other types of cervical carcinoma.[456,457] Thus, although the diagnosis can usually be made easily, it remains questionable whether it should be made.

Adenoid Basal Carcinoma and Adenoid Cystic Carcinoma

Adenoid basal carcinoma and adenoid cystic carcinoma were once regarded as a single entity, but further studies have shown that they are clinically and pathologically distinct. Adenoid basal carcinoma has an excellent prognosis, whereas adenoid cystic carcinoma is frequently fatal. Different features suggest that these tumors are closely related: (1) they both

contain basaloid, squamous, and glandular elements; (2) adenoid cystic carcinoma may reveal the presence of basaloid nests of cells or exhibit foci of squamous differentiation; and (3) they both appear preferentially in elderly women.

Adenoid basal carcinoma usually does not reveal any palpable mass. An abnormal smear (usually indicative of an overlying CIN) is the most common clinical finding. *Microscopically,* one observes small, regular, round or oval nests of cells suggesting those of basal cell carcinoma (Fig. 3-87).[458–460] These cells are small, with oval, hyperchromatic nuclei surrounded by a thin rim of cytoplasm. Mitoses are rare. The cells nests may contain small lumina. Foci of squamous differentiation are commonly observed, and association with squamous dysplasia, carcinoma in situ or early invasive squamous cell carcinoma has been reported. The tumor cells are immunoreactive for cytokeratins but not for CEA, epithelial membrane antigen, or S-100 protein.[460] The prognosis is good.

Adenoid cystic carcinoma presents as a polypoid or infiltrating cervical mass often accompanied by bleeding. Some of the patients have synchronous mucinous or other epithelial ovarian tumors.

Microscopically, small basal cells form cords, sheets and cellular nests which infiltrate a stroma modified by fibroblastic proliferation, hyalinization and myxoid change (Fig. 3-88). Mitoses are frequent. Cylindromatous structures and palisading arrangements of cells are similar to those observed in the more common salivary gland location of adenoid

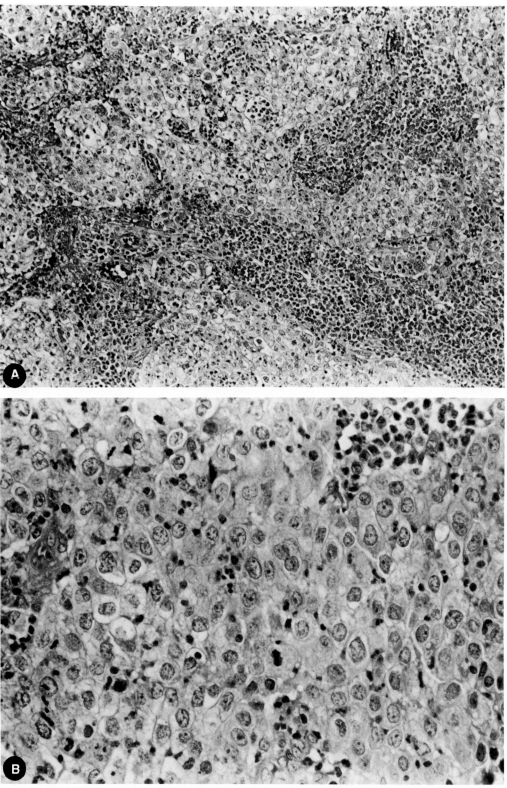

FIGURE 3-86 Glassy cell carcinoma. **(A)** Low-power photomicrograph showing prominent in-flammatory reaction. **(B)** Detail of malignant cells.

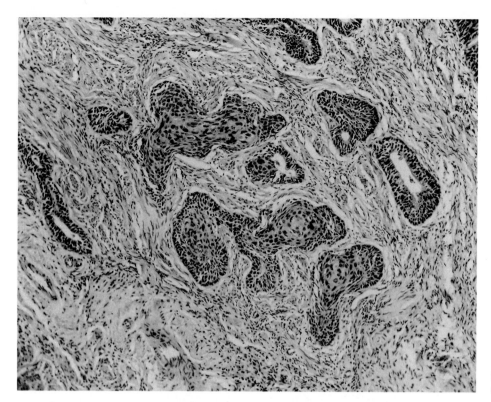

FIGURE 3-87 Adenoid basal cell carcinoma.

cystic carcinoma. Immunohistochemically, the tumor cells express cytokeratins, CEA and epithelial membrane antigen, and, less frequently, S-100 protein.[461] Myoepithelial differentiation is rare in the cervical tumor, although it is expressed in almost all the similar salivary gland tumors. The clinical prognosis is very poor.[459-461]

Invasive Carcinoma of the Cervix and Pregnancy

The appearance of an invasive cervical carcinoma during pregnancy is an uncommon event (0.05% of pregnancies).[462] However, this combination represented 3.6% and 4.5% of all cervical carcinomas in

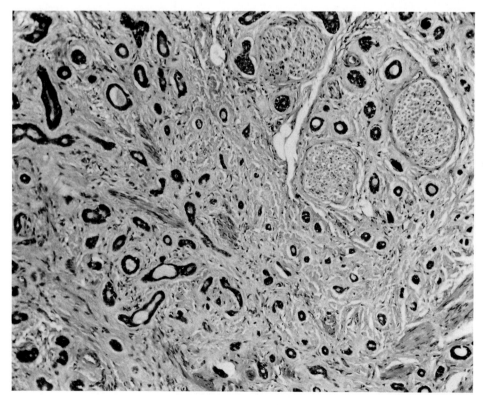

FIGURE 3-88 Adenoid cystic carcinoma.

two series.[463,464] Does pregnancy exert an influence on the evolution of the tumor? Contrary to widespread belief, there is no significant evidence that CIN and invasive carcinoma behave differently during pregnancy; the former should be managed conservatively[465,466] and the latter managed as in the non-pregnant patient.[464,467,468]

In the great majority of cases, these tumors are in situ or invasive squamous cell carcinomas. Some adenocarcinomas and mixed adenosquamous carcinomas have been described. Glücksmann[469] reported that mixed carcinomas are proportionately more frequent in pregnant than non-pregnant women. This finding has not been confirmed by all authors.[467]

Cancer of the Cervix and Radiation Therapy

The question of radiation therapy and cervical cancer may be considered from two different viewpoints: that of the action of radiation on the tumor cells, and that of the clinicopathologic sequelae of irradiation.

Radiation therapy (x-rays and interstitial radium or cesium) acts on tumors and their beds by three mechanisms:

1. Destruction of cancer cells by arrest of cellular divisions, alterations of mitoses, cytolysis, and pyknosis; development of bizarre cells from among the cells injured but not killed by radiation (Fig. 3-89)
2. Appearance of endarteritis with destruction of the vascular architecture, and tissue necrosis with inflammatory granulomata containing foreign body giant cells
3. Tissue fibrosis (often showing many atypical and even bizarre fibroblastic cells).

The sequelae of radiation therapy may be found in the tumor or in the adjacent organs (Fig. 3-90). The injured organs show endarteritis, telangiectasis, cellular necrosis, leukohistiocytic infiltrates, secondary fibrosis, and swelling and degeneration of collagen fibers. These lesions may appear many years after the cessation of radiation therapy. Rarely, new tumors may be induced by radiation.[470,471] The cytologic or histologic diagnosis of cervical dysplasia after radiation therapy (usually within 3 years) is often a sign of subsequent recurrence of cervical cancer with poor survival.[472]

Attempts have been made, with variable degrees of success, to predict the success or failure of radiation therapy in an individual case by biopsy or cytologic evaluation. The biopsy method[473,474] consists of pre- and post-treatment tumor biopsies to evaluate the degree of alteration in the tumor cells brought about by the course of irradiation. The cytologic technique,[475–478] on the other hand, calls for the evaluation of radiation-induced changes in *benign* cells. Each of these methods has been claimed by its proponents to have a high degree of accuracy in predicting within a short while (usually 1 week) after the beginning of treatment which patients are likely to survive 5 years if treated by irradiation alone (radiation responsive) and which are likely to succumb to their disease unless surgical therapy is added (radiation resistant). However, the values of these methods have been much disputed by other workers in the field. The biopsy method, in particular, is often impractical because of the difficulties encountered in biopsying a necrotic, friable, hemorrhagic tissue. Some types of cancer, such as keratinizing squamous carcinoma, have been said to be usually radioresistant,[304–306] but newer studies do not confirm this finding.[311,312]

Sarcomas and Other Rare Tumors

Primary sarcomas of the cervix are rare. *Sarcoma botryoides* or *embryonal rhabdomyosarcoma* is encountered at a later age in the cervix (mean age about 18 years) than in the vagina.[479,480] *Macroscopically*, the tumor has the form of a polypoid mass with a smooth irregular surface protruding through the external os and measuring a few centimeters in diameter. *Microscopically*, it is characterized by a loose and vascular stroma containing large elongated and small round undifferentiated cells. The rhabdomyoblasts have a dense eosinophilic cytoplasm in which cross striations may be observed. These cells are immunoreactive for myoglobulin or desmin. A condensed zone of small round cells with hyperchromatic nuclei is often present under the columnar mucosa (cambium layer). The mitotic rate can be moderately elevated (up to about 10 mitotic figures per 10 high-power fields). Foci of heterologous tissue such as cartilage may be present. This tumor should be distinguished from adenosarcoma, which usually contains more glandular structures, and from endocervical stromal sarcoma, which occurs at a later age, does not reveal a typical cambium layer, and does not exhibit rhabdomyoblasts. Cervical embryonal rhabdomyosarcomas have a better prognosis than the vaginal tumors.[480,481]

Stromal sarcoma, described by Abell and Ramirez,[482] has been reported rarely in the cervix (endocervical stromal sarcoma).[483,484] It appears late in the reproductive period or after menopause. This rare tumor is analogous with endometrial stromal sarcoma. *Macroscopically*, it consists of a polypoid or an infiltrating mass arising in the cervix. *Microscopically*, ovoid, spindled, or stellate cells with enlarged, hyperchromatic nuclei are arranged in a fascicular pattern infiltrating the stroma, with persisting normal endocervical glands (Fig. 3-91). Mitoses are abundant, and foci of edema, necrosis, and hemorrhage with inflammatory infiltrates are observed. This tumor must be differentiated from a *spindle cell* or *sarcomatoid carcinoma*, often only with the aid of ultrastructural or immunohistochemical (intermediate filaments) studies, and from an endometrial

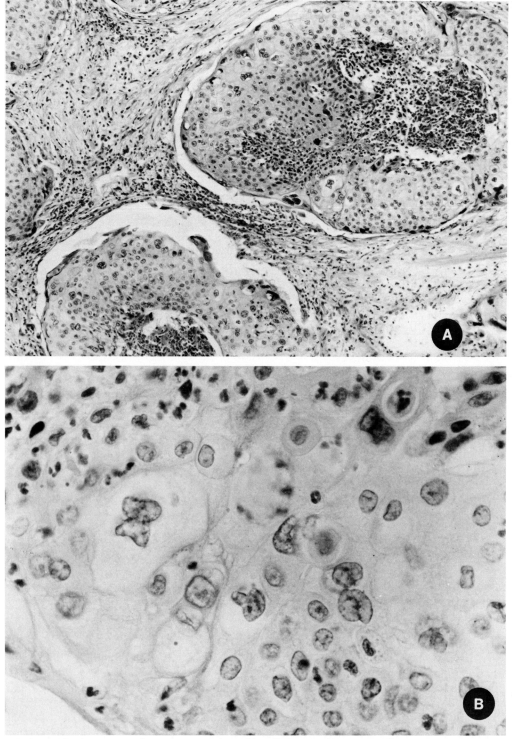

FIGURE 3-89 Squamous cell carcinoma: action of irradiation on the tumor cells.

stromal sarcoma extending to the cervix. Also reported are rare cases of *leiomyosarcoma*,[485] *Wilms' tumor*,[486] *osteosarcoma*,[487] *fibroxanthosarcoma*,[488] *liposarcoma*,[489] *malignant schwannoma*,[490] *germ cell tumor*,[491] *choriocarcinoma*,[492,493] and *malignant melanoma*.[494–496] *Carcinosarcomas*[382,497] and *adenosarcomas* similar in appearance to those seen more frequently in the endometrium are occasionally primary tumors of the cervix, but more often represent extensions from an endometrial primary source.

Lymphomas

Although lymphomas frequently infiltrate the cervix in cases of advanced disease, primary localizations

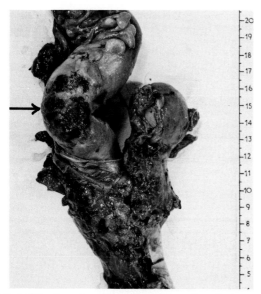

FIGURE 3-90 Sequela of an overdose of radiation: tissue necrosis in the colon.

are rarely reported (Fig. 3-92).[498–503] The main clinical symptom is vaginal bleeding.

Macroscopically, the cervix is diffusely enlarged and may present nodular polypoid deformations. Tissue sections show the typical aspect of malignant lymphoma: a diffuse or nodular, white to tan, homogeneous, granular dense structure. The vagina and uterine corpus may be involved.

Microscopically, the cervical stroma is infiltrated by nodules of different size. The overlying epithelium is rarely infiltrated. The various histologic types of non-Hodgkin's malignant lymphoma have been described. Diffuse "histiocytic" lymphoma was diagnosed more frequently in the series of Harris and Scully.[503] Hodgkin's disease and Burkitt's lymphoma have been mentioned in rare cases.[504,505]

If there is no evidence of dissemination beyond the uterus, cervix, or vagina, the prognosis is excellent, in contradiction to primary ovarian lymphoma, which is almost always a manifestation of known or occult disease outside the genital tract.[503]

Granulocytic sarcoma of the cervix is a mass of granulocytic leukemic cells. The patient may or may not be known to have leukemia when the cervical mass develops;[503,506] if the leukemia is not already manifest clinically, the diagnosis can easily be missed unless the possibility is kept in mind and a chloracetate esterase stain and immunochemical stain for lysozyme are performed. Prognosis is poor, because most patients develop acute leukemia.[507] Decidualized stroma should not be confused with lymphoma.[508]

METASTATIC TUMORS

Metastases to the cervix uteri are very rare; only the fallopian tube is a less frequent site of metastatic disease in the female genital tract.[509] Wallach and Edberg[510] attempt to explain this rarity by invoking the small volume of the cervix, its poor supply of vessels and lymphatics, and the absence of studies involving careful searches for metastases to this organ. These metastases arise, in most reported cases, from ovarian and endometrial primaries (the latter often by direct extension). Of extragenital primary sites, the most common are mammary,[511] gastric,[512,513] pulmonary,[514] and intestinal.[515] A few cases of secondary cervical involvement by tumors of the liver, pancreas, kidney, and gallbladder have been reported. Because almost all these tumors are adenocarcinomas, the differential diagnosis from primary cervical adenocarcinoma must be kept in mind.[516,517] The problem of the distinction between endometrial and endocervical primary adenocarcinomas is discussed earlier in this chapter and in Chapter 4. Metastatic malignant melanoma, usually from a primary tumor of the vulva, has been reported. It is best differentiated from primary cervical melanoma by the absence of junctional activity.[494–496]

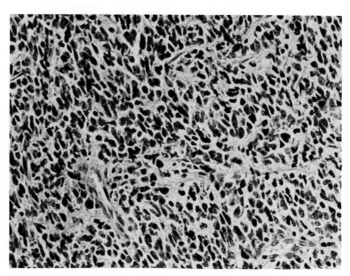

FIGURE 3-91 Endocervical stromal sarcoma: microscopic appearance.

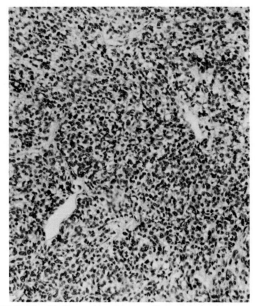

FIGURE 3-92 Maligant lymphoma of the cervix.

The cytologic diagnosis of metastatic cancer to the cervix is a rare eventuality. The presence in the cervical smear of malignant cells that do not resemble the usual patterns of genital cancer and lack a tumor diathesis of necrotic debris may orient the diagnosis to a metastatic tumor. We have observed in cervicovaginal smears malignant cells originating from the breast, the gastrointestinal tract, and the skin (malignant melanoma).

References

1. Rosenthal AH, Hellman LM: The epithelial changes in the fetal cervix including the role of reserve cells. Am J Obstet Gynecol 64:260–270, 1950
2. Forsberg JG: Cervicovaginal epithelium: Its origin and development. Am J Obstet Gynecol 115:1025–1043, 1973
3. Krantz KE: The anatomy of the human cervix, gross and microscopic. In Blandau RJ, Mossighi K, eds. Biology of the cervix, pp 57–69. Chicago, University of Chicago Press, 1973
4. Fanger H, Barker BE: Capillaries and arterioles of cervix. Obstet Gynecol 22:419–421, 1963
5. Duperroy G: L'innervation du col utérin chez la femme: Quelques particularités morphologiques. Gynécol Obstét 52:506–517, 1953
6. Madile BM: The cervical epithelium from fetal age to adolescence. Obstet Gynecol 47:536–539, 1976
7. Rubio CA, Soderberg G, Grant CA et al: The normal squamous epithelium of the human uterine cervix: A histological study. Pathol Eur 11:157–162, 1976
8. Ferenczy A, Richart RM: Female reproductive system: Dynamics of scan and transmission electron microscopy. New York, John Wiley & Sons, 1974
9. Feldman D, Romney SL, Edgcomb J, Valentine T: Ultrastructure of normal, metaplastic, and abnormal human uterine cervix: Use of montages to study the topographical relationship of epithelial cells. Am J Obstet Gynecol 150:573–588, 1984
10. Fluhmann CF, Dickmann Z: The basic pattern of the glandular structures of the cervix uteri. Obstet Gynecol 11:543–555, 1958
11. Henry JS, Latour JPA: Glycogen in the squamous epithelium of the cervix uteri. Am J Obstet Gynecol 74:610–615, 1957
12. Hackermann M, Grubb C, Hill KR: The ultrastructure of normal squamous epithelium of the human cervix uteri. J Ultrastruct Res 22:443–457, 1968
13. Moll R, Franke WW, Schiller DL et al: The catalog of human cytokeratins: Patterns of expression in normal epithelia, tumors, and cultured cells. Cell 31:11–24, 1982
14. Fetissof F, de Muret A, Serres G et al: Cytokératines et épithélium malpighien de l'exocol. Arch Pathol (Paris) :10:262–267, 1990
15. Topkins P: Histologic appearance of endocervix during menstrual cycle. Am J Obstet Gynecol 58:654–663, 1949
16. Syrjänen KJ: The normal cervix: Concept of the transformation zone. The Cervix and the Lower Female Genital Tract 10:83–88, 1992
17. Ober KG: Les variations morphologiques du col durant la vie de la femme. Bull Soc Belge Gynécol Obstét 28:203–213, 1958
18. Pixley E: Basic morphology of the prepubertal and youthful cervix: Topographic and histologic features. J Reprod Med 16:221–230, 1976
19. Crompton AC: The cervical epithelium during the menopause. In Jordan JA, Singer A, eds. The cervix. London, Saunders, 1976
20. Wollner A: The menstrual cycle in the human cervical mucosa and its clinical significance. Am J Surg 57:331–335, 1942
21. Morris HHB, Gatter KC, Stein H, Mason DY: Langerhans' cells in human cervical epithelium: An immunohistological study. Br J Obstet Gynaecol 90:400–411, 1983
22. Figueroa CD, Caorsi I: Ultrastructural and morphometric study of the Langerhans cell in the normal human cervix. J Anat 90:669–682, 1980
23. Fox H, Kazzaz B, Langley FA: Argyrophil and argentaffin cells in the female genital tract and in ovarian mucinous cysts. J Pathol 88:479–488, 1964
24. Edwards JN, Morris HHB: Langerhans' cells and lymphocyte subsets in the female genital tract. Br J Obstet Gynaecol 92:974–982, 1985
25. McArdle JP, Muller HK: Quantitative assessment of Langerhans' cells in human cervical intraepithelial neoplasia and wart virus infection. Am J Obstet Gynecol 154:509–515, 1986
26. Robledo MC, Vazquez JJ, Contreras-Mejuto F, Lopez-Garcia G: Sebaceous glands and hair follicles in the cervix uteri. Histopathology 21:278–280, 1992
27. Roth E, Taylor HB: Heterotopic cartilage in the uterus. Obstet Gynecol 27:838–844, 1966
28. Ferry JA, Scully RE: Mesonephric remnants, hyperplasia, and neoplasia in the uterine cervix: A study of 49 cases. Am J Surg Pathol 14:1100–1111, 1990
29. Scherrick JC, Vega JG: Congenital intramural cysts of the uterus. Obstet Gynecol 19:486–493, 1962
30. Wolfe SA: Gartner's duct lesions of the cervix. Am J Obstet Gynecol 39:312–322, 1940
31. Hart WR, Norris HJ: Mesonephric adenocarcinomas of the cervix. Cancer 29:106–113, 1972
32. Chapman GB, Mann EC, Wegryn R, Hull C: The ultrastructure of human cervical epithelial cells during pregnancy. Am J Obstet Gynecol 88:3–16, 1964
33. Singer A: The cervical epithelium during pregnancy and the puerperium. In Jordan JA, Singer A, eds. The cervix. London, Saunders, 1976
34. Nakamura Y, Moritsuka Y, Ohta Y et al: S-100 protein in glands within decidua and cervical glands during early pregnancy. Hum Pathol 20:1204–1209, 1989
35. Taylor HB, Irey NS, Norris HJ: Atypical endocervical hyperplasia in women taking oral contraceptives. JAMA 202:637–639, 1967

36. Chumas JC, Nelson B, Mann WJ et al: Microglandular hyperplasia of the uterine cervix. Obstet Gynecol 66:406–409, 1985

37. De Brux J, Dupré-Froment J, Bret J: Déciduose du col utérin: Aspects histologiques et cytologiques. Gynécol Obstét 58:304–317, 1959

38. Lepage F, Schramm B: La déciduose du col de l'utérus. Gynécol Obstét 54:550–563, 1955

39. Danos M, Holmquist ND: Cytologic evaluation of decidual cells: A report of two cases with false abnormal cytology. Acta Cytol 11:325–330, 1967

40. Schneider V, Barnes LA: Ectopic decidual reaction of the uterine cervix. Acta Cytol 25:616–622, 1981

41. Schneider V: Arias-Stella reaction of the endocervix. Acta Cytol 25:224–228, 1981

42. Geary WL, Weed JC: Congenital atresia of the uterine cervix. Obstet Gynecol 42:213–217, 1943

43. Jefferies JA, Robboy SJ, O'Brien PC et al: Structural anomalies of the cervix and vagina in women enrolled in the diethylstilbestrol adenosis (DESAD) project. Am J Obstet Gynecol 148:59–66, 1984

44. Bibbo M, Keebler CM, Wied GL: The cytologic diagnosis of tumor repair in the female genital tract. Acta Cytol 15:133–137, 1971

45. Cartier R: Colposcopie pratique, 2nd ed. Paris, Laboratoire Cartier, 1984

46. Kolstad P, Stafl A: Atlas of colposcopy, 2nd ed. Baltimore, University Park Press, 1977

47. Gupta PK, Lee EF, Erozan YS et al: Cytologic investigations of *Chlamydia* infection. Acta Cytol 23:315–320, 1979

48. Roberts TH, Ng ABP: Chronic lymphocytic cervicitis: Cytologic and histopathologic manifestations. Acta Cytol 19:235–243, 1975

49. Patten SF: Diagnostic cytology of the uterine cervix, 2nd ed. Baltimore, Williams & Wilkins, 1978

50. Meyer R: Über Epidermoidalisierung (Ersatz des Schleimepithels durch Plattenepithel) an der Portio Vaginalis Uteri nach Erosion, an Cervicalpolypen und in der Cervicalschleimhaut; ein Betrag zur Frage der Stückendiagnose und des Precancertösen Stadiums. Zentralbl Gynakol 47:946–960, 1923

51. Fluhmann CF: The cervix uteri and its diseases. Philadelphia, WB Saunders, 1961

52. Burghardt E: Early histological diagnosis of cervical cancer. Philadelphia, WB Saunders, 1973

53. Johnson LD: The histopathological approach to early cervical neoplasia. Obstet Gynecol Surv 24:735–767, 1969

54. Philippe E: Elektronmikroskopische Untersuchungen über die sogennanten Reservezelle am Zylinderepithel der menschlichen cervix uteri. Arch Gynäk 218:295–311, 1975

55. Lawrence DW, Shingleton HM: Early physiologic squamous metaplasia of the cervix: Light and electron microscopic observations. Am J Obstet Gynecol 137:661–671, 1980

56. Rosenthal AH, Hellman LM: The epithelial changes in the fetal cervix including the role of "reserve cells." Am J Obstet Gynecol 64:260–270, 1950

57. Gould RR, Barter RA, Papadimitriou JM: An ultrastructural, cytochemical and autoradiographic study of the mucous membrane of the human cervical canal with reference to subcolumnar basal cells. Am J Pathol 95:1–16, 1979

58. Song J: The human uterus: Morphogenesis and embryological basis for cancer. Springfield, IL, Charles C. Thomas, 1964

59. Howard L Jr, Erickson CC, Stoddard LD: A study of the incidence and histogenesis of endocervical metaplasia and intraepithelial carcinoma: Observation on 400 uteri removed for noncervical disease. Cancer 4:1210–1233, 1951

60. Gupta PK: Intrauterine contraceptive devices: Vaginal cytology, pathologic changes, and clinical implications. Acta Cytol 26:571–613, 1982

61. Gupta PK, Burroughs F, Luff RD et al: Epithelial atypia associated with intrauterine contraceptive devices (IUD). Acta Cytol 22:286–291, 1978

62. Risse EKJ, Beerthuizen RJCM, Vooijs GP: Cytologic and histologic findings in women using an IUD. Obstet Gynecol 58:569–573, 1981

63. Matas AJ, Simmons RL, Najarian JS: Chronic antigenic stimulation, herpesvirus infection, and cancer in transplant recipients. Lancet 1:1277–1279, 1975

64. Crum CP, Egawa K, Fu YS et al: Atypical immature metaplasia (AIM): A subset of human papillomavirus infection of the cervix. Cancer 51:2214–2219, 1983

65. Florman AL, Gershon AA, Blacket PR, Nahmias AJ: Intrauterine infection with herpes simplex virus. JAMA 225:129–132, 1973

66. Kessler II: Perspective on the epidemiology of cervical cancer with special reference to the herpes virus hypothesis. Cancer Res 34:1091–1110, 1974

67. Aurelian L: Persistence and expression of the herpes simplex virus type 2 genome in cervical tumor cells. Cancer Res 34:1126–1135, 1974

68. Gilman SC, Dockerty JJ, Clarke A, Rawls WE: Reaction patterns of herpes simplex virus type 1 and type 2 proteins with sera of patients with uterine cervical carcinoma and matched controls. Cancer Res 40:4640–4647, 1980

69. Adam E, Levy AH, Rawls WE, Melnick JL: Seroepidemiologic studies of herpesvirus type 2 and carcinoma of cervix. I. Case-control matching. J Natl Cancer Inst 47:941–952, 1971

70. Poste G, Hawkins DG, Thomlinson J: Herpesvirus hominis infection of the female genital tract. Obstet Gynecol 40:871–890, 1972

71. Fenoglio CM, Galloway DA, Crum CP et al: Herpes simplex virus and cervical neoplasia. Prog Surg Pathol 4:45–82, 1982

72. Wentz WB, Reagan JW, Heggie AD et al: Induction of uterine cancer with inactivated herpes simplex virus, type 1 and type 2. Cancer 48:1783–1790, 1981

73. Takeda M: Virus identification in cytologic and histologic material by electron microscopy. Acta Cytol 13:206–209, 1969

74. Vonka V, Kanka J, Hirsch I et al: Prospective study on the relationship between cervical neoplasia and herpes simplex type-2 virus. II. Herpes simplex type-2 antibody presence in sera taken at enrollment. Int J Cancer 33:61–66, 1984

75. Amstey MS: Current concepts of herpesvirus infection in the woman. Am J Obstet Gynecol 117:717–725, 1973

76. Ng ABP, Reagan JW, Lindner E: The cellular manifestations of primary and recurrent herpes genitalis. Acta Cytol 14:124–129, 1970

77. Ng ABP, Reagan JW, Yen SSC: Herpes genitalis: Clinical and cytopathologic experience with 256 patients. Obstet Gynecol 36:645–651, 1970

78. Vesterinen E, Purola E, Saksela E, Leinikki P: Clinical and virological findings in patients with cytologically diagnosed gynecologic herpes simplex infections. Acta Cytol 21:199–205, 1977

79. Heimann A, Scanlon R, Gentile J et al: Measles cervicitis: Report of a case with cytologic and molecular biologic analysis. Acta Cytol 36:727–730, 1992

80. Syrjanen KJ: Condylomatous lesions in dysplastic and neoplastic epithelium of uterine cervix. Surg Gynecol Obstet 150:372–376, 1980

81. Fletcher S: Histopathology of papilloma virus infection of the cervix uteri: The history, taxonomy, nomenclature and reporting of koilocytotic dysplasia. J Clin Pathol 36:616–624, 1983

82. Wilczynski SP, Bergen S, Walker J et al: Human papillomaviruses and cervical cancer: Analysis of histopathologic features associated with different viral types. Hum Pathol 19:697–704, 1988

83. Arends MJ, Wyllie AH, Bird CC: Papillomavirus and human cancer. Hum Pathol 21:686–698, 1990

84. Bergeron C, Barasso R, Beaudenon S et al: Human papillomavirus associated with cervical intraepithelial neoplasia: Great diversity and distinct distribution in low- and high-grade lesions. Am J Surg Pathol 16:641–649, 1992

85. Lorincz AT, Quinn AP, Lancaster WD, Temple GF: A new

type of papillomavirus associated with cancer of the uterine cervix. Virology 159:187–190, 1987

86. Tawheed A, Beaudenon S, Favre M, Orth G: Characterization of human papillomavirus type 66 from an invasive carcinoma of uterine cervix. J Clin Microbiol 29:2656–2660, 1991

87. Kadish AS, Burk RD, Kress Y et al: Human papillomavirus of different types in precancerous lesions of the uterine cervix: Histologic, immunocytochemical and ultrastructural studies. Hum Pathol 17:384–392, 1986

88. Carmichael JA, Maskens PD: Cervical dysplasia and human papillomavirus. Am J Obstet Gynecol 160:916–918, 1989

89. Nuovo GJ, Darfler MM, Imprain CC, Bromley SE: Occurrence of types of human papillomavirus in genital tract lesions. Am J Pathol 138:53–58, 1991

90. Woodruff JD, Braun L, Cavalieri R et al: Immunological identification of papillomavirus antigen in condyloma tissues from the female genital tract. Obstet Gynecol 56:727–732, 1980

91. Morin C, Braun L, Casa-Cordero et al: Confirmation of the papillomavirus etiology of condylomatous lesions of the cervix by the peroxidase-antiperoxidase technique. J Natl Cancer Inst 66:831–835, 1981

92. Meisels A, Morin C: Human papillomavirus and cancer of the uterine cervix. Gynecol Oncol 12:S111–S123, 1981

93. Popescu N, DiPaolo J, Amsbaugh S: Integration of human papillomavirus 18 DNA sequences on HeLa cell chromosomes. Cytogenet Cell Genet 44:58–62, 1987

94. Lancaster WD, Castellano C, Santos C et al: Human papillomavirus deoxyribonucleic acid in cervical carcinoma from primary and metastatic sites. Am J Obstet Gynecol 154:115–119, 1986

95. Meisels A, Fortin R, Roy M: Condylomatous lesions of the cervix. II. Cytologic, colposcopic and histopathologic study. Acta Cytol 21:379–390, 1977

96. Kurman RJ, Sanz LE, Jenson AB et al: Papillomavirus infection of the uterine cervix. I. Correlation of histology with specific structural antigens and DNA sequences. Int J Gynecol Pathol 1:17–28, 1982

97. Kurman RJ, Jenson AB, Lancaster WD: Papillomavirus infection of the cervix. II. Relationship to intraepithelial neoplasia based on the presence of specific viral structural proteins. Am J Surg Pathol 7:39–52, 1983

98. Dürst M, Gissmann L, Ikenberg H, zur Hausen H: A papillomavirus DNA from a cervical carcinoma and its prevalence in cancer biopsy samples from different geographic regions. Proc Natl Acad Sci U S A 80:3812–3815, 1983

99. Willett GD, Kurman RJ, Reid R et al: Correlation of the histologic appearance of intraepithelial neoplasia of the cervix with human papillomavirus types. Int J Gynecol Pathol 8:18–25, 1989

100. Kurman RJ, Schiffman MH, Lancaster WD et al: Analysis of individual human papillomavirus types in cervical neoplasia: A possible role for type 18 in rapid progression. Am J Obstet Gynecol 159:293–296, 1988

101. Reid R, Stanhope CR, Herschman BR et al: Genital warts and cervical cancer. I. Evidence of an association between subclinical papillomavirus infection and cervical malignancy. Cancer 50:377–387, 1982

102. Reid R, Crum CP, Herschman BR et al: Genital warts and cervical cancer. III. Subclinical papilloma viral infection and cervical neoplasia are linked by a spectrum of continuous morphologic and biologic change. Cancer 53:943–953, 1984

103. Zur Hausen H: Papillomaviruses in anogenital cancer as a model to understand the role of viruses in human cancer. Cancer Res 49:4677–4681, 1989

104. Bauer HM, Ting Y, Greer CE et al: Genital human papillomavirus infection in female university students as determined by a PCR-based method. JAMA 265:472–477, 1991

105. Riou G, Favre M, Jeannel D et al: Association between poor prognosis in early-stage invasive cervical carcinomas and non-detection of HPV DNA. Lancet 335:1171–1174, 1990

106. Meisels A, Fortin R: Condylomatous lesions of the cervix. I. Cytologic patterns. Acta Cytol 20:505–509, 1976

107. Purola E, Savia E: Cytology of gynecologic condyloma acuminatum. Acta Cytol 21:26–31, 1977

108. Koss LG, Durfee GR: Unusual patterns of squamous epithelium of the uterine cervix: Cytologic and pathologic study of koilocytotic atypia. Cancer 12:1171–1193, 1959

109. Ayre JE: Role of the halo cell in cervical carcinogenesis: A virus manifestation in premalignancy? Obstet Gynecol 15:481–491, 1960

110. Kaufman R, Koss LG, Kurman RJ, et al: Letter to the editor. Statement of caution in the interpretation of papillomavirus-associated lesions of the epithelium of the uterine cervix. Int J Gynecol Pathol 2:100, 1983

111. Crum C, Fu YS, Kurman RJ, Okagaki T, Twiggs LB, Silverberg SG: Editorial Board Symposium: Practical approach to cervical human papillomavirus related intraepithelial lesions. Int J Gynecol Pathol 8:388–399, 1989

112. Bechtold E, Reicher NB: The relationship of *Trichomonas* infestations to false diagnoses of squamous carcinoma of the cervix. Cancer 5:442–457, 1952

113. Koss LG, Wolinska WH: Trichomonas vaginalis cervicitis and its relationship to cervical cancer: A histocytochemical study. Cancer 12:1171–1193, 1959

114. Bertini B, Hornstein M: The epidemiology of trichomoniasis and role of this infection in the development of carcinoma of the cervix. Acta Cytol 14:325–332, 1970

115. La Vecchia C, Franceschi S, Decarli A et al: Sexual factors, venereal disease and the risk of intraepithelial and invasive neoplasia. Cancer 58:935–941, 1986

116. Forsey T, Darougar S, Dines RJ et al: Chlamydial genital infection in Addis Ababa, Ethiopia: A seroepidemiologic survey. Br J Vener Dis 58:370–373, 1982

117. Schlachter J, Hill EC, King EB et al: *Chlamydia trachomatis* and cervical neoplasia. JAMA 248:2134–2138, 1982

118. Harrison HR, Phil D, Costin M et al: Cervical *Chlamydia trachomatis* infection in university women: Relationship to history, contraception, ectopy, and cervicitis. Am J Obstet Gynecol 153:224–251, 1985

119. Paavonen J, Vesterinen E, Meyer B et al: Colposcopic and histologic findings of cervical chlamydia infection. Obstet Gynecol 59:712–715, 1982

120. Swanson J, David A, Eschenbach E et al: Light and electron microscopic study of *Chlamydia trachomatis* infection of the uterine cervix. J Infect Dis 131:678–687, 1975

121. Gupta PK, Shurbazi MS, Mintor LF et al: Cytopathologic detection of *Chlamydia trachomatis* in vaginopancervical (fast) smears. Diagn Cytopathol 4:224–229, 1988

122. Bibbo M, Wied GL: Cytology of inflammatory reactions, tissue repair, effects of IUD, contaminants and microbiologic classification including chlamydial organisms. Chicago Tutorials of Cytology, 3rd ed, 1982

123. Lindner E, Geerling S, Nettum JA et al: The cytologic features of *Chlamydia* cervicitis. Acta Cytol 29:676–682, 1985

124. Shafer MA, Chew KL, Kromhout LK et al: Chlamydial endocervical infections and cytologic findings in sexually active female adolescents. Am J Obstet Gynecol 151:765–771, 1985

125. Bernal JN, Martinez MA, Dabancens A: Evaluation of proposed cytomorphologic criteria for the diagnosis of *Chlamydia trachomatis* in Papanicolaou smears. Acta Cytol 33:309–313, 1988

126. Dunlop EMC, Garner A, Darougar S et al: Colposcopy, biopsy, and cytology results in women with chlamydial cervicitis. Genitourin Med 65:22–31, 1989

127. Kiviat NB, Paavonen JA, Wolner-Hanssen P et al: Histopathology of endocervical infection caused by *Chlamydia trachomatis*, herpes simplex virus, *Trichomonas vaginalis*, and *Neisseria gonorrhoeae*. Hum Pathol 21:831–837, 1990

128. Dorman SA, Danos LM, Wilson DJ et al: Detection of chlamydial cervicitis by Papanicolaou stained smears and culture. Am J Clin Pathol 79:421–425, 1983

129. Shiina Y: Cytomorphologic and immunocytochemical

studies of chlamydial infections in cervical smears. Acta Cytol 29:683–691, 1985

130. Nogales F, Vilar E: Etude clinique et thérapeutique de la tuberculose du col utérin: Travail basé sur 102 cas. Rev Fr Gynecol Obstet 52:275–283, 1957

131. Chalmers JA: Coincident carcinoma and tuberculosis of the uterine cervix. Br J Obstet Gynaecol 65:438–439, 1958

132. Schaefer C: Tuberculosis of female genital tract. Clin Obstet Gynecol 13:965–998, 1970

133. Meisels A, Fortin R: Genital tuberculosis cytologic detection. Acta Cytol 19:79–81, 1975

134. Misch KA, Smithies A, Twomey D et al: Tuberculosis of the cervix: Cytology as an aid to diagnosis. J Clin Pathol 29:313–316, 1976

135. Angrish K, Verma K: Cytologic detection of tuberculosis of the uterine cervix. Acta Cytol 25:160–162, 1981

136. Berry A: A cytopathological and histopathological study of bilharziasis of the female genital tract. J Pathol Bacteriol 91:325–338, 1966

137. Youssef AF, Fayad MM, Shafeck MA: Bilharziasis of the cervix uteri. Br J Obstet Gynaecol 77:847–851, 1970

138. Al-Nafussi AI, Hughes D, Rebello G: Ceroid granuloma of the uterine cervix. Histopathology 21:282–284, 1992

139. DeTorres EF, Benitez-Bribiesca L: Cytologic detection of vaginal parasitosis. Acta Cytol 17:252–257, 1973

140. Hermann GI, Deininger JT: Vorticella, an usual protozoa [sic!] found on endocervical smear (Letter). Acta Cytol 7:129–130, 1963

141. Axiotis CA, Merino MJ, Duray PH: Langerhans cell histiocytosis of the female genital tract. Cancer 67:1650–1660, 1991

142. Tcherktoff V, Ober WB: Primary chancre of the cervix uteri. N Y State J Med 66:1921–1924, 1966

143. Morse AR, Coleman DV, Gardner SD: An evaluation of cytology in the diagnosis of herpes simplex virus infection and cytomegalovirus infection of the cervix uteri. Br J Obstet Gynaecol 81:393–398, 1974

144. Griffiths PD, Campbell-Benzie A, Heath RB: A prospective study of primary cytomegalovirus infection in pregnant women. Br J Obstet Gynaecol 87:308–314, 1980

145. Kumar ML, Gold E, Jacob IB et al: Primary cytomegalovirus infection in adolescent pregnancy. Pediatrics 74:493–500, 1984

146. Naib ZM: Exfoliative cytology, 3rd ed. Boston, Little, Brown & Co, 1985

147. Richter GA, Pratt JH, Nichols DR, Coulam CB: Actinomycosis of the female genital tract organs. Minn Med 55:1003–1006, 1972

148. Gupta PK, Hollander DH, Frost JK: Actinomycetes in cervicovaginal smears: An association with IUD usage. Acta Cytol 20:295–297, 1976

149. Bhagavan BS, Gupta PK: Genital actinomycosis and intrauterine contraceptive devices. Hum Pathol 9:567–578, 1978

150. Crow J, McWhinney N: Isolated arteritis of the cervix uteri. Br J Obstet Gynaecol 86:393–398, 1979

151. Gloor E, Schaller MD, Dubois PY: Artérite à cellules géantes à localisation gynécologique: Présentation de deux cas. J Gynécol Obstét Biol Reprod 11:785–788, 1982

152. Marrogi AJ, Gersell DJ, Kraus FT: Localized asymptomatic giant cell arteritis of the female genital tract. Int J Gynecol Pathol 10:51–58, 1991

153. Bhambhani S: Egg of *Ascaris lumbricoides* in cervicovaginal smear. Acta Cytol 28:92, 1984

154. Pandit AA, Khilnani PH, Powar AS: Detection of microfilariae in cervical cytology (Letter). Acta Cytol 36:451–452, 1992

155. Aaro LH, Jacobson LJ, Soule EH: Endocervical polyps. Obstet Gynecol 21:659–665, 1963

156. Harris HR: Foam cells in the stroma of carcinoma of the body of the uterus and uterine cervical polyps. J Clin Pathol 11:19–22, 1958

157. Bory R, de Brux J, Curtz J: Les polypes muqueux du col. Rev Fr Gynécol Obstét 54:687–702, 1959

158. Gilbert EF, Palladino A: Squamous papillomas of the uterine cervix: Review of the literature and report of a giant papillary carcinoma. Am J Clin Pathol 46:115–121, 1966

159. Kazal HL, Long JP: Squamous cell papillomas of the uterine cervix: A report of 20 cases. Cancer 11:1049–1059, 1958

160. Goforth JL: Squamous cell papilloma of the cervix uteri. South Med J 49:921–926, 1952

161. Marsh MR: Papilloma of the cervix. Am J Obstet Gynecol 64:281–291, 1952

162. Sites EC, Coury JJ, Barss JA: Cervical myoma simulating an ectopic pregnancy. Am J Obstet Gynecol 71:221–222, 1956

163. Sherrer CW, Parmley T, Woodruff JD: Adenomatous hyperplasia of the endocervix. Obstet Gynecol 49:65–68, 1977

164. Segal GH, Hart WR: Cystic endocervical tunnel clusters: A clinicopathologic study of 29 cases of so-called "adenomatous hyperplasia." Am J Surg Pathol 14:895–903, 1990

165. Taylor HB, Irey NS, Norris HJ: Atypical endocervical hyperplasia in women taking oral contraceptives. JAMA 202:637–639, 1967

166. Leslie KO, Silverberg SG: Microglandular hyperplasia of the cervix: Unusual clinical and pathological presentations and their differential diagnosis. Prog Surg Pathol 5:95–114, 1984

167. Chumas JC, Nelson B, Mann WJ et al: Microglandular hyperplasia of the uterine cervix. Obstet Gynecol 66:406–409, 1985

168. Speers WC, Picaso LC, Silverberg SG: Immunohistochemical localization of carcinoembryonic antigen in microglandular hyperplasia and adenocarcinoma of the endocervix. Am J Clin Pathol 79:105–107, 1983

169. Steeper TA, Wick MR: Minimal deviation adenocarcinoma of the uterine cervix ("adenoma malignum"). Cancer 58:1131–1138, 1986

170. Young RH, Scully RE: Uterine carcinomas simulating microglandular hyperplasia: A report of six cases. Am J Surg Pathol 16:1092–1097, 1992

171. Clement PB, Young RH: Deep Nabothian cysts of the uterine cervix: A possible source of confusion with minimal deviation adenocarcinoma ("adenoma malignum"). Int J Gynecol Pathol 8:340–348, 1989

172. Jones MA, Young RH, Scully RE: Diffuse laminar endocervical glandular hyperplasia: A benign lesion often confused with adenoma malignum (minimal deviation adenocarcinoma). Am J Surg Pathol 15:1123–1129, 1991

173. Suh K-S, Silverberg SG: Tubal metaplasia of the uterine cervix. Int J Gynecol Pathol 9:122–128, 1990

174. Jonasson JG, Wang HH, Antonioli DA, Ducatman DS: Tubal metaplasia of the uterine cervix: A prevalence study in patients with gynecologic pathologic findings. Int J Gynecol Pathol 11:89–95, 1992

175. Huffman JW: Mesonephric remnants in cervix. Am J Obstet Gynecol 56:23–40, 1948

176. Ayroud Y, Gelfand MM, Ferenczy A: Florid mesonephric hyperplasia of the cervix: A report of a case with review of the literature. Int J Gynecol Pathol 4:245–254, 1985

177. Abell MR: Papillary adenofibroma of the uterine cervix. Am J Obstet Gynecol 110:990–993, 1971

178. Vellios F, Ng ABP, Reagan JW: Papillary adenofibroma of the uterus: A benign mesodermal mixed tumor of Müllerian origin. Am J Clin Pathol 60:543–551, 1973

179. Ahern JK, Allen NH: Cervical hemangiomas: A case report and review of the literature. J Reprod Med 21:228–231, 1978

180. Patel DS, Bhagavan BS: Blue nevus of the uterine cervix. Hum Pathol 16:79–86, 1985

181. Barua R: Post-cone biopsy traumatic neuroma of the uterine cervix. Arch Pathol Lab Med 113:945–947, 1989

182. Fingerland A, Sikl H: Ganglioneuroma of the cervix uteri. J Pathol 47:631–634, 1938

183. Gwavava NJ, Traub AI: A neurilemmoma of the cervix. Br J Obstet Gynaecol 87:444–446, 1980

184. Copas P, Dyer M, Hall DJ, Diddle AW: Granular cell myoblastoma of the uterine cervix: A case report. Diagn Gynecol Obstet 3:251–254, 1981

185. Grönross M, Meurman L, Kahra K: Proliferating glia and other heterotopic tissues in the uterus: Fetal homografts? Obstet Gynecol 61:261–266, 1983

186. Ehrmann RL: Sebaceous metaplasia of the human cervix. Am J Obstet Gynecol 105:1284–1286, 1969

187. Bonilla Musoles F, Monmeneu RM, Simon C, Serra V: Can the uterine cervix grow a moustache? Eur J Gynaecol Oncol 10:145–146, 1989

188. Fichera G, Santanocito A: Pilosebaceous cystic ectopy of the uterine cervix. Clin Exp Obstet Gynecol 16:21–25, 1989

189. Selzer I, Nelson HM: Benign papilloma (polypoid tumor) of the cervix uteri in children: Report of 2 cases. Am J Obstet Gynecol 84:165–169, 1962

190. Janovski MS, Kasdon EJ; Benign mesonephric papillary and polypoid tumors of the cervix in childhood. J Pediatr 63:211–216, 1963

191. Andrews CF, Jourdain L, Damjanov I: Benign cervical mesonephric papilloma of childhood: Report of a case studied by light and electron microscopy. Diagn Gynecol Obstet 3:39–43, 1981

192. Ulbright TM, Alexander RW, Kraus FT: Intramural papilloma of the vagina: Evidence for müllerian histogenesis. Cancer 48:2260–2266, 1981

193. Gardner HL: Cervical and vaginal endometriosis. Clin Obstet Gynecol 9:358–372, 1966

194. Wolfe SA, Mackles A, Greene HJ: Endometriosis of the cervix: Classification and analysis of 17 cases. Am J Obstet Gynecol 81:111–123, 1961

195. Richmond HG: Endometriosis of the cervix. J Pathol 106:viii, 1972

196. Ridley JH: The histogenesis of endometriosis: A review of facts and fancies. Obstet Gynecol Surv 23:1–35, 1968

197. Clement PB, Young RH, Scully RE: Stromal endometriosis of the uterine cervix: A variant of endometriosis that may simulate a sarcoma. Am J Surg Pathol 14:449–455, 1990

198. Chang SH, Maddox WA: Adenocarcinoma arising within cervical endometriosis and invading the adjacent vagina. Am J Obstet Gynecol 110:1015–1017, 1971

199. Veiga-Ferreira MM, Leiman G, Dunbar F, Margolius KA: Cervical endometriosis: facilitated diagnosis by fine needle aspiration cytologic testing. Am J Obstet Gynecol 157:849–856, 1987

200. Cullen TS: Cancer of the uterus. Philadelphia, WB Saunders, 1909

201. Broders AC: Carcinoma in situ contrasted with benign penetrating epithelium. JAMA 99:1670–1674, 1932

202. Papanicolaou GN: Survey of actualities and potentialities of exfoliative cytology in cancer diagnosis. Ann Intern Med 31:661–674, 1949

203. Reagan JW, Seideman IL, Saracusa Y: Cellular morphology of carcinoma in situ and dysplasia or atypical hyperplasia of uterine cervix. Cancer 6:224–235, 1953

204. Editorial: International agreement of histological terminology for the lesions of the uterine cervix. Acta Cytol 6:235–236, 1962

205. Koss LG: Dysplasia: A real concept or a misnomer? Obstet Gynecol 51:374–379, 1978

206. Koss LG: Diagnostic cytology and its histopathologic bases, 4th ed. Philadelphia, JB Lippincott, 1992

207. Richart RM: Colpomicroscopic studies of the distribution of dysplasia and carcinoma in situ on the exposed portion of the human uterine cervix. Cancer 18:950–954, 1965

208. Richart RM: Influence of diagnostic and therapeutic procedures on distribution of cervical intraepithelial neoplasia. Cancer 19:1635–1638, 1966

209. Richart RM: The natural history of cervical intraepithelial neoplasia. Clin Obstet Gynecol 10:748–784, 1967

210. Richart RM, Lerch VV, Barron BA: A time-lapse cinematographic study in vitro of mitosis of normal human cervical epithelium, dysplasia, and carcinoma in situ. J Natl Cancer Inst 39:571–577, 1967

211. The Bethesda system for reporting cervical/vaginal cytologic diagnoses: Developed and approved at the National Cancer Institute workshop in Bethesda, Maryland, December 12–13, 1988. Hum Pathol 21:704–708, 1990

212. The revised Bethesda system for reporting cervical/vaginal cytologic diagnoses: Report of the 1991 Bethesda workshop. Acta Cytol 36:273–276, 1992

213. Richart RM: A modified terminology for cervical intraepithelial neoplasia. Obstet Gynecol 75:131–133, 1990

214. Anderson MC, Brown CL, Buckley CH et al: Current views on cervical intraepithelial neoplasia. J Clin Pathol 44:969–978, 1991

215. Cocker J, Fox H, Langley FA: Consistency in the histological diagnosis in epithelial abnormalities of the cervix uteri. J Clin Pathol 21:67–70, 1968

216. Holmquist ND, McMahan CA, Williams OD: Variability in classification of carcinoma in situ of the uterine cervix. Arch Pathol 84:334–345, 1967

217. Ismail SM, Colclough AB, Dinnen JS et al: Observer variation in histopathological diagnosis and grading of cervical intraepithelial neoplasia. Br Med J 298:707–710, 1989

218. Robertson AJ, Anderson JM, Swanson Beck J et al: Observer variability in histopathological reporting of cervical biopsy specimen. J Clin Pathol 42:231–238, 1989

219. Crum CP, Mitao M, Levine TRV, Silverstein SJ: Cervical papilloma viruses segregate within morphologically distinct precancerous lesions. J Virol 54:675–681, 1985

220. Syrjänen S, Syrjänen K, Mäntyjävi R et al: Human papilloma virus (HPV) DNA sequence demonstrated by in situ DNA hybridization in serial paraffin-embedded cervical biopsies. Arch Pathol Lab Med 239:39–48, 1986

221. Reid R, Greenberg M, Jenson AB et al: Sexually transmitted papillomavirus infection. I. The anatomic distribution and pathologic grade of neoplastic lesions associated with different viral types. Am J Obstet Gynecol 156:212–222, 1987

222. Arends MJ, Wyllie AH, Bird CC: Papillomaviruses and human cancer. Hum Pathol 21:686–698, 1990

223. Clavel C, Zerat L, Binninger I et al: DNA content measurement and in situ hybridization in condylomatous cervical lesions. Diagn Molec Pathol 1:180–184, 1992

224. DePalo G, Stefanon B, Bandieramonte G: Treatment of genital human papillomavirus infection. The Cervix and the Lower Female Genital Tract 10:119–124, 1992

225. Kiviat NB, Koutsky LA, Critchlow CW et al: Prevalence and cytologic manifestations of human papilloma virus (HPV) types 6, 11, 16, 18, 31, 33, 35, 42, 43, 44, 45, 51, 52, and 56 among 500 consecutive women. Int J Gynecol Pathol 11:197–203, 1992

226. Kurman RJ, Norris HJ, Wilkinson E: Tumors of the cervix, vagina, and vulva. Atlas of tumor pathology, 3rd series, fascicle 4. Washington, DC, Armed Forces Institute of Pathology, 1992

227. Hanselaar AG, Vooijs GP, Oud PS et al: DNA ploidy patterns in cervical intraepithelial neoplasia grade III, with and without synchronous invasive squamous cell carcinoma: Measurements in nuclei isolated from paraffin-embedded tissue. Cancer 62:2537–2545, 1988

228. Shingleton HM, Richart RM, Weiner J, Spireo D: Human cervical intraepithelial neoplasia: Fine structure of dysplasia and carcinoma in situ. Cancer Res 28:695–706, 1968

229. Stanley MA, Kirkland JA: Chromosome and histologic patterns in preinvasive lesions of the cervix. Acta Cytol 19:142–147, 1975

230. Nishiya I, Ishizaki Y, Sasaki M: Nuclear DNA content and the number of Barr bodies in premalignant and malignant lesions of the uterine cervix. Acta Cytol 25:407–411, 1981

231. Dabbs DJ, Geisinger KR: Selective applications of immunohistochemistry in gynecological neoplasms. Pathol Annu 28(1):329–353, 1993

232. Mittal KR, Demopoulos RI, Goswami S: Patterns of keratin

19 expression in normal, metaplastic, condylomatous, atrophic, dysplastic, and malignant cervical squamous epithelium. Am J Clin Pathol 98:419–423, 1992

233. Wilbanks GD: Tissue culture in early cervical neoplasia. Obstet Gynecol Surv 24:804–837, 1969

234. Wynder EL: Epidemiology of carcinoma in situ. Obstet Gynecol Surv 24:697–711, 1969

235. Stern E: Epidemiology of dysplasia. Obstet Gynecol Surv 24:711–723, 1969

236. Davesa SS: Descriptive epidemiology of cancer of the uterine cervix. Obstet Gynecol 63:605–612, 1984

237. Burghardt E, Östör AG: Colposcopy: cervical pathology, 2nd ed. New York, G. Thieme Verlag, 1991

238. Hall JE, Walton L: Dysplasia of the cervix: A prospective study of 206 cases. Am J Obstet Gynecol 100:667–671, 1968

239. Spriggs Al: Natural history of cervical dysplasia. Clin Obstet Gynecol 8:65–79, 1981

240. Jones HW Jr, Galvin GA, Te Linde RW: Re-examination of biopsies taken prior to the development of invasive carcinoma of the cervix. In Proceedings of the Third National Cancer Conference, p 678. Philadelphia, JB Lippincott, 1957

241. Carson RP, Gall EA: Preinvasive carcinoma and precancerous metaplasia of cervix: Serial block survey. Am J Pathol 30:15–29, 1954

242. Hulka BS, Redmond CK: Factors related to progression of cervical atypias. Am J Epidemiol 93:23–32, 1971

243. Gottardi G, Marzi MM, Zaninetti P et al: Cervical intraepithelial neoplasia (CIN) in 648 teenagers. Ann Ostet Ginecol Med Perinat 101:391–396, 1980

244. Christopherson WM, Parker JE, Mendez WM, Lundin FE Jr: Cervix cancer death rates and mass cytologic screening. Cancer 26:808–811, 1970

245. Johanesson G, Geirson G, Day N: The effect of mass screening of cancer in Iceland 1965–1974 on the incidence and mortality of cervical carcinoma. Cancer 21:418–425, 1978

246. Boon ME, De Graaff Guilloud JC: Cost effectiveness of population screening and rescreening for cervical cancer in the Netherlands. Acta Cytol 25:539–542, 1981

247. Eddy DM: Appropriateness of cervical cancer screening. Gynecol Oncol 12:S168–S187, 1981

248. Benedet JL, Anderson GH: Cervical intraepithelial neoplasia in British Columbia: A comprehensive program for detection, diagnosis and treatment. Gynecol Oncol 12: S280–S291, 1981

249. Beilby JOW, Guillebaud J, Steele ST: Paired cervical smears: A method of reducing the false-negative rate in population screening. Obstet Gynecol 60:46–48, 1982

250. Parkin DM, Collins W, Clayden AD: Cervical cytology screening in two Yorkshire areas: Pattern of service. Public Health 95:311–321, 1981

251. Westergaard L, Norgaard M: Severe cervical dysplasia. Control by biopsies or primary conization? A comparative study. Acta Obstet Gynecol Scand 60:549–554, 1981

252. Östör A: Natural history of cervical intraepithelial neoplasia: A critical review. Int J Gynecol Pathol 12:186–192, 1993.

253. Spriggs AL, Boddington MM: Progression and regression of cervical lesions: Review of smears from women followed without initial biopsy or treatment. J Clin Pathol 33:517–522, 1980

254. Brown D Jr, Kaufman RH, Gardner HL: Leukoplakia of the cervix. Am J Obstet Gynecol 116:214–221, 1973

255. Hinselmann H: Einführung in die Kolposcopie. Hamburg, P. Hartung Verlag, 1933

256. Cartier R. Colposcopie pratique. Basel, S. Karger, 1977

257. Coppleson M, Pixley E, Reid BL: Colposcopy: A scientific and practical approach to the cervix in health and disease, 3rd ed. Springfield IL, Charles C. Thomas, 1986

258. Kolstad P, Stafl A: Atlas of colposcopy, 3rd ed. Baltimore, University Park Press, 1982

259. Singer A, Walker P: What is the optimum treatment of cervical premalignancy? Br J Obstet Gynaecol 89:335–337, 1982

260. Helmerhorst ThJM: Clinical significance of endocervical curettage as part of colposcopic evaluation: A review. Int J Gynecol Cancer 2:256–262, 1992

261. Stafl A, Wilbanks GD: An international terminology of colposcopy: Report of the Nomenclature Committee of the International Federation of Cervical Pathology and Colposcopy. Obstet Gynecol 77:313–314, 1991

262. Laara E, Day NE, Hakama E: Trends in mortality from cervical cancer in the Nordic countries: Association with organized screening programmes. Lancet 1:1247–1249, 1987

263. Macgregor JE, Teper S: Mortality from carcinoma of cervix uteri in Britain. Lancet 2:774–776, 1978

264. Marsan NC, Jacquemier J, Sabatier P, Seradour B: Enquête épidémiologique sur les lésions virales et CIN du col: Etude multicentrique rétrospective dans les centres publics et privés. Arch Anat Cytol Pathol 38:215–225, 1990

265. Dickinson LE: Control of cancer of the uterine cervix. Gynecol Oncol 3:1–9, 1975

266. Carmichael JA, Jeffrey JF, Steele HD, Ohlke ID: The cytologic history of 245 patients developing invasive cervical carcinoma. Am J Obstet Gynecol 148:685–690, 1984

267. Van der Graaf Y, Vooijs GP, Gaillard HLJ, Go DMDS: Screening errors in cervical cytology smears. Acta Cytol 31:434–438, 1987

268. Boon ME, De Graaff Guilloud JC, Rietveld WJ: Analysis of five sampling methods for the preparation of cervical smears. Acta Cytol 33:843–848, 1989

269. Vooijs GP, Elias A, Van der Graaf Y, Velig S: Relationship between the diagnosis of epithelial abnormalities and the composition of cervical smears. Acta Cytol 29:323–328, 1985

270. Mitchell H, Medley G: Influence of endocervical status on the cytologic prediction of cervical intraepithelial neoplasia. Acta Cytol 36:875–880, 1992

271. Fink DJ: Change in American Cancer Society guidelines for detection of cervical cancer. Cancer 38:127–128, 1988

272. Matseoane S, Williams SB, Navarro C et al: Diagnostic value of conization of the uterine cervix in the management of cervical neoplasia: A review of 756 consecutive patients. Gynecol Oncol 47:287–291, 1992

273. Foote FW Jr, Stewart FW: The anatomical distribution of intraepithelial epidermoid carcinoma of the cervix. Cancer 1:431–440, 1948

274. Chanen W, Rome RM: Electrocoagulation diathermy for cervical dysplasia and carcinoma in situ: A 15 year survey. Obstet Gynecol 61:673–679, 1983

275. Drescher CW, Peters WA Jr, Roberts JA: Contribution of endocervical curettage in evaluating abnormal cervical cytology. Obstet Gynecol 62:343–347, 1983

276. Andersch B, Moinian M: Diagnostic and therapeutic viewpoints on cervical intraepithelial neoplasia: 10 year follow-up of a conization material. Gynecol Obstet Invest 13:193–205, 1982

277. Nichols TM, Boyes DA, Fidler HK: Advantages of routine step serial sectioning of cervical cone biopsies. Am J Clin Pathol 49:342–346, 1968

278. Powell JM, Jones FS, Dougherty RE, Diddle AW: Cervical carcinoma: Correlation of microtome cryostat, cytologic and histologic diagnoses. Obstet Gynecol 33:476–481, 1969

279. Paterson-Brown S, Chappatte OA, Clark SK et al: The significance of cone biopsy resection margins. Gynecol Oncol 46:182–185, 1992

280. Baak JPA: Mitosis counting in tumors (Editorial). Hum Pathol 21:683–685, 1990

281. Dustin P, Parmentier R: Données expérimentales sur la nature des mitoses anormales observées dans certains épithéliomas du col utérin. Gynécol Obstét 52:258–265, 1953

282. Koller PS: The role of chromosomes in cancer biology. New York, Springer Verlag, 1972

283. Winkler B, Crum CP, Fujii T et al: Koilocytotic lesions of the cervix: The relationship of mitotic abnormalities to the

presence of papillomavirus antigens and DNA nuclear content. Cancer 53:1081–1087, 1984

284. Mourits MJE, Pieters WJLM, Hollema H, Burger MPM: Three group metaphase as a morphologic criterion of progressive cervical intraepithelial neoplasia. Am J Obstet Gynecol 167:591–595, 1992

285. Bibbo M, Dytch HE, Alenghat E et al: DNA ploidy profiles as prognostic indicators in CIN lesions. Am J Clin Pathol 92:261–265, 1989

286. Warhol MJ, Antonioli DA, Pinkus GS et al: Immunoperoxidase staining for involucrin: A potential diagnostic aid in cervicovaginal pathology. Hum Pathol 13:1095–1099, 1982

287. Reid BL: Cancer of the cervix uteri: Review of causal factors with an hypothesis as to its origin. Med J Aust 1:375–383, 1965

288. Tenis M, Wilson F, Nelson JH Jr: Relation of circumcision to cancer of the cervix. Am J Obstet Gynecol 117:1056–1066, 1973

289. Hellberg D, Nilsson S, Haley NJ et al: Smoking and cervical intraepithelial neoplasia: Nicotine and cotinine in serum and cervical mucus in smokers and non smokers. Am J Obstet Gynecol 158:910–913, 1988

290. Barton SE, Maddox PH, Jenkins D et al: Effect of cigarette smoking on cervical epithelial immunity: A mechanism for neoplastic change? Lancet 2:652–654, 1988

291. Gagnon F: Contribution to the study of the etiology and prevention of cancer of the cervix of the uterus. Am J Obstet Gynecol 60:516–522, 1950

292. Schömig G: Die weiblichen Genitalkarzinom bei sexueller Enthaltsamkeit. Strahlentherapie 92:156–158, 1953

293. Jones EG, MacDonald I, Breslow L: A study of epidemiologic factors in carcinoma of the uterine cervix. Am J Obstet Gynecol 76:1–10, 1958

294. Schneider A, Meinhardt G, Kirchmayor R, Schneider V: Prevalence of human papillomavirus genome in tissues from lower genital tract as detected by molecular in situ hybridization. Int J Gynecol Pathol 10:1–14, 1991

295. Bonfiglio TA, Stoler MH: Human papilloma virus and cancer of the uterine cervix. Hum Pathol 19:621–622, 1988

296. Melnick JL, Lewis R, Wimberly I et al: Association of cytomegalovirus (CMV) infection with cervical cancer: Isolation of CMV from cell culture derived from cervical biopsy. Intervirology 10:115–119, 1978

297. Starreveld AA, Hill GB, Brown LB et al: Effect of screening on the incidence of cervical cancer in Alberta. Can Med Assoc J 125:1105–1109, 1981

298. Lanciano RM, Won M, Hanks GE: A reappraisal of the International Federation of Gynecology and Obstetrics staging system for cervical cancer: A study of patterns of care. Cancer 69:482–487, 1992

299. Shingleton HM, Fowler WC Jr, Koch GG: Pretreatment evaluation in cervical cancer. Am J Obstet Gynecol 110:385–389, 1971

300. Van Nagell JR Jr, Roddick JW Jr, Lowin DM: The staging of cervical cancer: Inevitable discrepancies between clinical staging and pathologic findings. Am J Obstet Gynecol 110:973–978, 1971

301. Martzloff HK: Carcinoma of the cervix uteri: A pathological and clinical study with particular reference to the relative malignancy of the neoplastic process as indicated by the predominant type of cancer. Bull Johns Hopkins Hosp 34:141–149, 1923

302. Broders AC: Carcinoma, grading and practical application. Arch Pathol 2:376–381, 1926

303. Pendl O: Histologische Klassifizierung und Ergebnisse der Strahlenbehandlung des Carcinome Colli Uteri. Radiol Austriaca 4:95–126, 1951

304. Wentz WB, Reagan JW: Survival in cervical cancer with respect to cell type. Cancer 12:384–388, 1959

305. Reagan JW, Ng ABP: The cellular manifestations of uterine carcinogenesis. In Norris HJ, Hertig AT, Abell MR, eds. The uterus. Baltimore, Williams & Wilkins, 1973

306. Finck FM, Denk M: Cervical carcinoma: Relationship between histology and survival following radiation therapy. Obstet Gynecol 35:339–343, 1970

307. Sidhu GS, Koss LG, Barber HRK: Relation of histologic factors to response of stage I epidermoid carcinoma of cervix to surgical treatment. Obstet Gynecol 35:329–338, 1970

308. Swan DS, Roddick JW: A clinical-pathological correlation of cell type classification for cervical cancer. Am J Obstet Gynecol 116:666–670, 1973

309. Chung CK, Stryker JA, Ward SP et al: Histologic grade and prognosis of carcinoma of the cervix. Obstet Gynecol 57:636–642, 1981

310. Crissman JD. Makuch R, Budhraja M: Histopathologic grading of squamous cell carcinoma of the uterine cervix: An evaluation of 70 stage Ib patients. Cancer 55:1590–1596, 1985

311. Crissman JD, Budhraja M, Aron BS, Cummings G: Histopathologic prognostic factors in stage II and III squamous cell carcinoma of the uterine cervix: An evaluation of 91 patients treated primarily with radiation therapy. Int J Gynecol Pathol 6:97–103, 1987

312. Zaino R, Ward S, Frauenhoffer E: Histopathologic predictors of behavior of squamous carcinoma of the cervix (Abstract). Lab Invest 60:108A, 1989

313. Groben P, Reddick R, Askin F: The pathologic spectrum of small cell carcinoma of the cervix. Int J Gynecol Pathol 4:42–57, 1985

314. Barrett RJ II, Davos I, Leuchter RS et al: Neuroendocrine features in poorly differentiated and undifferentiated carcinomas of the cervix. Cancer 60:2325–2330, 1987

315. Gersell DJ, Mazoujian G, Mutch DG, Rudloff MA: Small cell undifferentiated carcinoma of the cervix: A clinicopathologic, ultrastructural, and immunocytochemical study of 25 cases. Am J Surg Pathol 12:684–698, 1988

316. Walker J, Mills SE, Taylor PT: Cervical neuroendocrine carcinoma: A clinical and light microscopic study of 14 cases. Int J Gynecol Pathol 7:64–74, 1988

317. Bichel P, Jakobsen A: Histopathologic grading and prognosis of uterine cervical carcinoma. Am J Clin Oncol 8:247–254, 1985

318. Stendahl Y, Eklund G, Willen R: Prognosis of invasive squamous cell carcinoma of the uterine cervix: A comparative study of the predictive values of clinical staging IB–III and a histopathologic malignancy grading system. Int J Gynecol Pathol 2:42–54, 1983

319. Benda JA, Platz CE, Bushsbaum H, Lifshitz S: Mucin production in defining mixed carcinoma of the uterine cervix: A clinicopathologic study. Int J Gynecol Pathol 4:314–27, 1985

320. Buckley CH, Beards CS, Fox H: Pathological prognostic indicators in cervical cancer with particular reference to patients under the age of 40 years. Br J Obstet Gynaecol 95:47–56, 1988

321. Ireland D, Cole S, Kelly P, Monaghan JM: Mucin production in cervical intraepithelial neoplasia and in stage Ib carcinoma of cervix with pelvic lymph node metastases. Br J Obstet Gynaecol 94:467–472, 1987

322. Thelmo WL, Nicastri AD, Fruchter R, Spring H, DiMaio T, Boyce J: Mucoepidermoid carcinoma of the uterine cervix stage IB. Int J Gynecol Pathol 9:316–324, 1990

323. Colgan TJ, Auger M, McLaughlin JR: Histopathologic classification of cervical carcinomas and recognition of mucin-secreting squamous carcinomas. Int J Gynecol Pathol 12:64–69, 1993

324. Hopman BC: Histochemical methods applied to benign and malignant squamous epithelium of the cervix uteri. Am J Obstet Gynecol 79:346–369, 1960

325. Thiery M, Willighagen RJG: Enzyme histochemistry of squamous cell carcinoma of the uterine cervix. Am J Obstet Gynecol 95:1059–1067, 1966

326. Davidsohn I, Kovarik S: Isoantigens A, B, and H in benign and malignant lesions of the cervix. Arch Pathol 87:306–314, 1969

327. Bonfiglio TA, Feinberg MR: Isoantigen loss in cervical neoplasia. Arch Pathol Lab Med 100:307–310, 1976

328. Hinglais Guillard N, Moricard R, Bernhard W: Ultrastructure des cancers pavimenteux invasifs du col utérin chez la femme. Bull Cancer (Paris) 48:283–316, 1961

329. Auersperg N, Erber H, Worth A: Histologic variation among poorly differentiated invasive carcinomas of the uterine cervix. J Natl Cancer Inst 51:1461–1478, 1973

330. Heller PB, Lee RB, Leman MH et al: Lymph node positivity in cervical cancer. Gynecol Oncol 12:328–335, 1981

331. Beyer FD Jr, Murphy A: Patterns of spread of invasive cancer of the human cervix. Cancer 18:34–40, 1965

332. White CD, Morley GW, Kumar NB: The prognostic significance of tumor emboli in lymphatic or vascular spaces of the cervical stroma in stage IB squamous cell carcinoma of the cervix. Am J Obstet Gynecol 149:342–349, 1984

333. Henriksen E: The lymphatic spread of carcinoma of the cervix and of the body of the uterus: A study of 420 necropsies. Am J Obstet Gynecol 58:924–942, 1949

334. Matsuyama T, Inoue I, Tsukamoto N et al: Stage IB, IIa, and IIb cervix cancer, postsurgical staging, and prognosis. Cancer 54:3072–3077, 1984

335. Nogales F, Botella-Llusia J: The frequency of invasion of the lymph nodes in cancer of the uterine cervix: A study of the degree of extension in relation to the histological type of tumor. Am J Obstet Gynecol 93:91–94, 1965

336. Chung CK, Nahnas WA, Zaino R et al: Histologic grade and lymph node metastasis in squamous cell carcinoma of the cervix. Gynecol Oncol 12:348–354, 1981

337. Boyce J, Fruchter RG, Nicastri AD et al: Prognostic factors in stage I carcinoma of the cervix. Gynecol Oncol 12:154–165, 1981

338. Baltzer J, Lohe KJ, Koepcke W et al: Histological criteria for the prognosis in patients with operated squamous cell carcinoma of the cervix. Gynecol Oncol 13:184–194, 1982

339. White CD, Morley GW, Kumar NB: The prognostic significance of tumor emboli in lymphatic or vascular spaces of the cervical stroma in stage IB squamous cell carcinoma of the cervix. Am J Obstet Gynecol 149:342–349, 1984

340. Ketcham AS, Chretien PB, Hoye RC et al: Occult metastases to the scalene lymph nodes in patients with clinically operable carcinoma of the cervix. Cancer 31:180–183, 1973

341. Perez CA, Camel HM, Askin F, Breaux S: Endometrial extension of carcinoma of the uterine cervix: A prognostic factor that may modify staging. Cancer 48:170–180, 1981

342. Burghardt E, Pickel H, Haas J, Lahousen M: Prognostic factors and operative treatment of stage IB to IIB cervical cancer. Am J Obstet Gynecol 156:988–996, 1987

343. Gauthier P, Gore H, Shingleton HM et al: Identification of histopathologic risk groups in stage IB squamous cell carcinoma of the cervix. Obstet Gynecol 66:569–574, 1985

344. Paunier JP, Declos L, Fletcher GH: Causes, time of death and sites of failure in squamous-cell carcinoma of the uterine cervix on intact uterus. Radiology 88:555–562, 1967

345. Yazigi R, Munoz AK, Richardson B, Risser R: Correlation of squamous cell carcinoma antigen levels and treatment response in cervical cancer. Gynecol Oncol 41:135–138, 1991

346. Goldberg S, Sklar A, O'Hanlan KA et al: CA-125: A potential prognostic indicator in patients with cervical cancer. Gynecol Oncol 40:222–224, 1991

347. Girardi F, Fuchs P, Haas J: Prognostic significance of human papillomavirus type 16 DNA in cervical cancer. Cancer 69:2502–2504, 1992

348. Walker J, Bloss JD, Liao S, Berman M, Bergen S, Wilczynski SP: Human papillomavirus genotype as a prognostic indicator in carcinoma of the uterine cervix. Obstet Gynecol 74:781–785, 1989

349. Burnett AF, Barnes WA, Johnson JC et al: Prognostic significance of polymerase chain reaction detected human papillomavirus of tumors and lymph nodes in surgically treated Stage IB cervical cancer. Gynecol Oncol 47:343–347, 1992

350. Riou G, Faure M, Jeannel D et al: Association between poor prognosis in early stage invasive cervical carcinomas and nondetection of HPV DNA. Lancet 335:1171–1174, 1990

351. Minucci D, Cinel A, Arslan Pagnini C et al: Prognostic evaluation in uterine cervix carcinoma in relation to the lymphoplasmacyte infiltrate and to the cyto-histologic type. Clin Exp Obstet Gynecol 7:185–193, 1980

352. Tosi P, Cintorino M, Santopietro R et al: Prognostic factors in invasive cervical carcinomas associated with human papillomavirus (HPV): Quantitative data and cytokeratin expression. Path Res Pract 188:866–873, 1992

353. Kodama S, Kanazawa K, Honna S, Tanaka K: Age as a prognostic factor in patients with squamous cell carcinoma of the uterine cervix. Cancer 68:2481–2485, 1991

354. Sorensen FB, Bichel P, Jakobsen A: DNA level and stereologic estimates of nuclear volume in squamous cell carcinomas of the uterine cervix: A comparative study with analysis of prognostic impact. Cancer 69:187–199, 1992

355. Jakobsen A, Bichel P, Kristensen GB, Nyland M: Prognostic influence of ploidy level and histopathologic differentiation in cervical carcinoma stage IB. Eur J Cancer 24:969–972, 1988

356. Bourhis J, Le MG, Barrois M et al: Prognostic value of c-myc proto-oncogene overexpression in early invasive carcinoma of the cervix. J Clin Oncol 8:1789–1796, 1990

357. Hayashi Y, Hachisuga T, Iwasaka T et al: Expression of the ras oncogene product and EGF receptor in cervical squamous cell carcinoma and its relationship to lymph node involvement. Gynecol Oncol 40:147–151, 1991

358. Graham S, Priore RL, Schueller EF, Burnett W: Epidemiology of survival from cancer of the cervix. J Natl Cancer Inst 49:639–647, 1972

359. Burghardt E, Baltzer J, Tulusan AH, Haas J: Results of surgical treatment of 1028 cervical cancers studied with volumetry. Cancer 70:648–655, 1992

360. Hopkins MP, Morley GW: Radical hysterectomy versus radiation therapy in stage IB squamous cell cancer of the cervix. Cancer 68:272–277, 1991

361. Markham M: Systemic therapy for gynecologic cancer. Curr Opin Oncol 4:939–945, 1992

362. Sedlis A, Sol S, Tsukada Y et al: Microinvasive carcinoma of the uterine cervix: A clinical-pathologic study. Am J Obstet Gynecol 133:64–74, 1979

363. Philippe E, Ritter, Starkova O: Le carcinome microinvasif du col utérin: Diagnostic et indications thérapeutiques. J Gynecol Obstet Biol Reprod (Paris) 11:255–265, 1982

364. Averette HE, Nelson JH, Ng ABP et al: Diagnosis and management of microinvasive (stage IA) carcinoma of the uterine cervix. Cancer 38:414–425, 1976

365. Larsson G, Alm P, Gullberg B et al: Prognostic factors in early invasive carcinoma of the uterine cervix: A clinical, histopathologic, and statistical analysis of 343 cases. Am J Obstet Gynecol 146:145–153, 1983

366. Burghardt E, Holzer E: Diagnosis and treatment of microinvasive carcinoma of the cervix uteri. Obstet Gynecol 49:641–653, 1977

367. Tsukamoto N, Kaku T, Matsukuma K et al: The problem of stage Ia (FIGO, 1985) carcinoma of the uterine cervix. Gynecol Oncol 34:1–6, 1989

368. Lohe KJ: Early squamous carcinoma of the uterine cervix. I. Definition and histology. III. Frequency of lymph node metastases. Gynecol Oncol 6:10–30, 51–59, 1978

369. Creasman WT, Fetter BF, Clark-Pearson DL et al: Management of stage IA carcinoma of the cervix. Am J Obstet Gynecol 153:164–172, 1985

370. Seski JC, Abell MR, Morley GW: Microinvasive squamous carcinoma of the cervix: Definition, histologic analysis, late results of treatment. Obstet Gynecol 50:410–414, 1977

371. van Nagell JR, Greenwell N, Powell DF et al: Microinvasive carcinoma of the cervix. Am J Obstet Gynecol 145:981–991, 1983

372. Roche WD, Norris HJ: Microinvasive squamous carcinoma of the cervix: The significance of lymphatic invasion and confluent patterns of stromal growth. Cancer 36:180–186, 1975

373. Covell JL, Frierson HF Jr: Intraepithelial neoplasia mimicking microinvasive squamous-cell carcinoma in endocervical brushings. Diagn Cytopathol 8:18–22, 1992

374. Savage EW: Microinvasive carcinoma of the cervix. Am J Obstet Gynecol 113:708–717, 1972

375. Boyes DA, Worth AJ, Fidler HK: The results of treatment of 4389 cases of pre-clinical cervical squamous carcinoma. Br J Obstet Gynaecol 77:769–780, 1970

376. Yamabe T: The problem of microinvasive carcinoma of the cervix. In Kurihara S et al, eds. Cervical pathology and colposcopy, pp. 137–142. New York, Elsevier Science Publishers, 1985

377. Sevin B-U, Nadji M, Averette HE et al: Microinvasive carcinoma of the cervix. Cancer 70:2121–2128, 1992

378. Burghardt E, Girardi F, Lahousen M et al: Microinvasive carcinoma of the uterine cervix (International Federation of Gynecology and Obstetrics Stage IA). Cancer 67:1037–1045, 1991

379. Petersen LK, Mamsen A, Jakobsen A: Carcinoma of the cervical stump. Gynecol Oncol 46:199–202, 1992

380. Creadick RN: Carcinoma of the cervical stump. Am J Obstet Gynecol 75:565–574, 1958

381. Wolff JP, Lacour J, Chassagne D, Berend M: Cancer of the cervical stump: A study of 173 patients. Obstet Gynecol 39:10–16, 1972

382. Waxman M, Waxman JS, Alinovi V: Heterologous malignant mixed tumor of the cervical stump. Gynecol Oncol 16:422–428, 1983

383. Bennett JL, Clement PB: Verrucous carcinoma of the uterine cervix and endometrium. Diagn Gynecol Obstet 2:197–203, 1980

384. Randall ME, Andersen WA, Mills SE et al: Papillary squamous cell carcinoma of the uterine cervix: A clinico-pathologic study of nine cases. Int J Gynecol Pathol 5:1–10, 1985

385. Hasumi K, Sugano H, Sakamoto G et al: Circumscribed carcinoma of the uterine cervix with marked lymphocytic infiltration. Cancer 39:2503–2507, 1977

386. Mills SE, Austin SB, Randall ME: Lymphoepithelioma-like carcinoma of the uterine cervix: A distinctive, undifferentiated carcinoma with inflammatory stroma. Am J Surg Pathol 9:883–889, 1985

387. Van Nagell JR, Powell DE, Gallion HH et al: Small cell carcinoma of the uterine cervix. Cancer 62:1586–1593, 1988

388. Stoler MH, Mills ME, Gersell DJ, Walker AN: Small-cell neuroendocrine carcinoma of the cervix. Am J Surg Pathol 15:28–32, 1991

389. Ueda G, Shimizu C, Shimizu H et al: An immunohistochemical study of small-cell and poorly differentiated carcinoma of the cervix using neuroendocrine markers. Gynecol Oncol 34:164–169, 1989

390. Fox H, Kazzaz B, Langley FA: Argyrophil and argentaffin cells in the female genital tract and in ovarian mucinous cysts. J Pathol Bacteriol 88:479–488, 1964

391. Scully RE, Aguirre P, DeLellis RA: Argyrophilia, serotonin, and peptide hormones in the female genital tract and its tumors. Int J Gynecol Pathol 3:51–70, 1984

392. Miles PA, Herrera GA, Mena H et al: Cytologic findings in primary malignant carcinoid tumor of the cervix, including immunohistochemistry and electron microscopy performed on cervical smears. Acta Cytol 29:1003–1008, 1985

393. Vesterinen E, Forss M, Nieminen U: Increase of cervical adenocarcinoma: A report of 520 cases of cervical carcinoma including 112 tumors with glandular elements. Gynecol Oncol 33:49–53, 1989

394. Schwartz SM, Weiss NS: Increased incidence of adenocarcinoma of the cervix in young women in the United States. Am J Epidemiol 124:1045–1047, 1986

395. Young RH, Scully RE: Invasive adenocarcinoma and related tumors of the uterine cervix. Semin Diagn Pathol 7:205–227, 1990

396. Jaworski RC: Endocervical glandular dysplasia, adenocarcinoma in situ, and early invasive (microinvasive) adenocarcinoma of the uterine cervix. Semin Diagn Pathol 7:190–204, 1990

397. Lawrence WD: Advances in the pathology of the uterine cervix. Human Pathol 22:792–806, 1991

398. Yeh I, LiVolsi VA, Noumoff JS: Endocervical carcinoma. Pathol Res Pract 187:129–144, 1991

399. Norris HJ, McCauley KM: Unusual forms of adenocarcinoma of the cervix: An update. Pathol Annu 28(1):73–95, 1993

400. Korhonen MO: Epidemiological differences between adenocarcinoma and squamous cell carcinoma of the uterine cervix. Gynecol Oncol 10:312–317, 1980

401. Maier RC, Norris HJ: Coexistence of cervical intraepithelial neoplasia with primary adenocarcinoma of the endocervix. Obstet Gynecol 56:361–364, 1980

402. Tase T, Okagaki T, Clark BA et al: Human papillomavirus DNA in adenocarcinoma in situ, microinvasive adenocarcinoma of the uterine cervix, and coexisting cervical squamous intraepithelial neoplasia. Int J Gynecol Pathol 8:8–17, 1989

403. Farnsworth A, Laverty C, Stoler MH: Human papillomavirus messenger RNA expression in adenocarcinoma in situ of the uterine cervix. Int J Gynecol Pathol 8:321–330, 1989

404. Smotkin D, Berek JS, Fu YS: Human papillomavirus DNA in adenocarcinoma and adenosquamous carcinoma of the uterine cervix. Obstet Gynecol 68:241–244, 1986

405. Dallenbach-Hellweg G: On the origin and histological structure of adenocarcinoma of the endocervix in women under 50 years of age. Pathol Res Pract 179:38–50, 1984

406. Jones MW, Silverberg SG: Cervical adenocarcinoma in young women: Possible relationship to microglandular hyperplasia and use of oral contraceptives. Obstet Gynecol 73:984–989, 1989

407. Hurt WG, Silverberg SG, Frable WJ et al: Adenocarcinoma of the cervix: Histopathologic and clinical features. Am J Obstet Gynecol 129:304–315, 1977

408. Wahlstrom T, Korhonen M, Lindgren J et al: Distinction between endocervical and endometrial adenocarcinoma with immunoperoxidase staining of carcinoembryonic antigen in routine histologic tissue specimens. Lancet 2:1159–1160, 1979

409. Nanbu Y, Fujii S, Konishi I et al: Immunohistochemical localizations of CA 125, carcinoembryonic antigen, and CA 19-9 in normal and neoplastic glandular cells of the uterine cervix. Cancer 62:2580–2588, 1988

410. Cohen C, Shulman G, Budgeon LR: Endocervical and endometrial adenocarcinoma: An immunoperoxidase and histochemical study. Am J Surg Pathol 6:151–157, 1982

411. Kudo R, Sasano H, Koizumi M, Orenstein JM, Silverberg SG: Immunohistochemical comparison of new monoclonal antibody 1C-5 and carcinoembryonic antigen in the differential diagnosis of adenocarcinoma of the uterine cervix. Int J Gynecol Pathol 9:325–336, 1990

412. Silverberg SG: Histogenetic interpretation of immunohistochemical staining results. In Kindermann G, Lampe B, eds. Immunohistochemische Diagnostik gynäkologischer Tumoren, pp 17–21. New York, George Thieme Verlag, 1992

413. Choo YC, Naylor B: Coexistent squamous cell carcinoma and adenocarcinoma of the uterine cervix. Gynecol Oncol 17:168–174, 1984

414. Berek JS, Hatcher NF, Fu YS et al: Adenocarcinoma of the uterine cervix: Histologic variables associated with lymph node metastasis and survival. Obstet Gynecol 65:46–52, 1985

415. Hopkins MP, Schmidt RW, Roberts JA et al: Gland cell carcinoma (adenocarcinoma) of the cervix. Obstet Gynecol 72:789–795, 1988

416. Hopkins MP, Schmidt RW, Roberts JA et al: The prognosis and treatment of stage I adenocarcinoma of the cervix. Obstet Gynecol 72:915–921, 1988

417. Moberg PJ, Einhorn N, Silfversward C, Soderberg G: Adenocarcinoma of the uterine cervix. Cancer 57:407–410, 1986

418. Saigo PE, Wolinska WH, Kim WS, Hajdu SI: The role of cytology in the diagnosis and follow-up of patients with cervical adenocarcinoma. Acta Cytol 29:785–794, 1985

419. Azzopardi JG, Hou LT: Intestinal metaplasia with argentaffin cells in cervical adenocarcinoma. J Pathol 90:686–690, 1985

420. Fox H, Wells M, Harris M, McWilliam LJ et al: Enteric tumours of the lower female genital tract: A report of three cases. Histopathology 12:167–176, 1988

421. Kaminski PF, Maier RC: Clear cell adenocarcinoma of the cervix unrelated to diethylstilbestrol exposure. Obstet Gynecol 62:720–727, 1983

422. Hanselaar AG, Van Leusen ND, De Wilde PC, Vooijs GP: Clear cell adenocarcinoma of the vagina and cervix: A report of the Central Netherlands Registry with emphasis on early detection and prognosis. Cancer 67:1971–1978, 1991

423. Gilks CB, Clement PB: Papillary serous adenocarcinoma of the uterine cervix: A report of three cases. Mod Pathol 5:426–431, 1992

424. Silverberg SG, Hurt WG: Minimal deviation adenocarcinoma ("adenoma malignum") of the cervix. Am J Obstet Gynecol 123:971–975, 1975

425. Kaku T, Enjoji M: Extremely well-differentiated adenocarcinoma ("adenoma malignum") of the cervix. Int J Gynecol Pathol 2:28–41, 1983

426. Kaminski PF, Norris HJ: Minimal deviation carcinoma (adenoma malignum) of the cervix. Int J Gynecol Pathol 2:141–153, 1983

427. Gilks CB, Young RH, Aguirre P et al: Adenoma malignum (minimal deviation adenocarcinoma) of the uterine cervix: A clinicopathological and immunohistochemical analysis of 26 cases. Am J Surg Pathol 13:717–729, 1989

428. Michael H, Grawe L, Kraus FT: Minimal deviation endocervical adenocarcinoma: Clinical and histologic features, immunohistochemical staining for carcinoembryonic antigen, and differentiation from confusing benign lesions. Int J Gynecol Pathol 3:261–276, 1984

429. Bulmer JN, Griffin NR, Bates C et al: Minimal deviation adenocarcinoma (adenoma malignum) of the endocervix: Histochemical and immunohistochemical study of two cases. Gynecol Oncol 36:139–146, 1990

430. Young RH, Welch WR, Dickersin GR et al: Ovarian sex cord tumor with annular tubules: Review of 74 cases including 27 with Peutz-Jeghers syndrome and four with adenoma malignum of the cervix. Cancer 50:1384–1402, 1982

431. Szyfelbein WM, Young RH, Scully RE: Adenoma malignum of the cervix: Cytologic findings. Acta Cytol 28:691–698, 1984

432. Speers WC, Picaso LG, Silverberg SG: Immunohistochemical localization of carcinoembryonic antigen in microglandular hyperplasia and adenocarcinoma of the endocervix. Am J Clin Pathol 79:105–107, 1983

433. Young RH, Scully RE: Villoglandular papillary adenocarcinoma of the uterine cervix: A clinicopathological analysis of 13 cases. Cancer 63:1773–1779, 1989

434. Jones MW, Silverberg SG, Kurman RJ: Well differentiated villoglandular adenocarcinoma of uterine cervix: A clinicopathological study of 24 cases. Int J Gynecol Pathol 12:1–7, 1993

435. Friedell GH, McKay DG: Adenocarcinoma in situ of the endocervix. Cancer 6:887–897, 1953

436. Quizibash AH: In situ and microinvasive adenocarcinoma of the uterine cervix: A clinical, cytologic and histologic study of 14 cases. Am J Clin Pathol 64:155–170, 1975

437. Anderson ES, Arffmann E: Adenocarcinoma in situ of the uterine cervix: A clinico-pathologic study of 36 cases. Gynecol Oncol 35:1–7, 1989

438. Luesley DM, Jordan JA, Woodman CBJ et al: A retrospective review of adenocarcinoma-in-situ and glandular atypia of the uterine cervix. Br J Obstet Gynaecol 94:699–703, 1987

439. Boon ME, Baak JPA, Kurver PJH et al: Adenocarcinoma in situ of the cervix: An underdiagnosed lesion. Cancer 48:768–773, 1981

440. Jaworski RC, Pacey NF, Greenberg ML et al: The histologic diagnosis of adenocarcinoma in situ and related lesions of the cervix uteri. Cancer 61:1171–1181, 1988

441. Ostör AG, Pagano R, Davoren RAM et al: Adenocarcinoma in situ of the cervix. Int J Gynecol Pathol 3:179–190, 1984

442. Jaworski RC, Jones A: DNA ploidy studies in adenocarcinoma in situ of the uterine cervix. J Clin Pathol 43:435–436, 1990

443. Gloor E, Hurlimann J. Cervical intraepithelial glandular neoplasia (adenocarcinoma in situ and glandular dysplasia): A correlative study of 23 cases with histologic grading, histochemical analysis of mucins, and immunohistochemical determination of the affinity for four lectins. Cancer 58:1272–80, 1986

444. Ayer B, Pacey NF, Greenberg ML et al: The cytologic diagnosis of adenocarcinoma in situ of the cervix uteri and related lesions. I. Adenocarcinoma in situ. Acta Cytol 31:397–411, 1987

445. Ayer B, Pacey NF, Greenberg M: The cytologic diagnosis of adenocarcinoma in situ of the cervix uteri and related lesions. II. Microinvasive adenocarcinoma. Acta Cytol 32:318–324, 1988

446. Pacey F, Ayer B, Greenberg M: The cytologic diagnosis of adenocarcinoma in situ of the cervix uteri and related lesions. III. Pitfalls in diagnosis. Acta Cytol 32:325–330, 1988

447. Hopkins MP, Roberts JA, Schmidt RW: Cervical adenocarcinoma in situ. Obstet Gynecol 71:842–844, 1988

448. Ireland D, Hardiman P, Monaghan JM: Adenocarcinoma of the uterine cervix: A study of 73 cases. Obstet Gynecol 65:82–85, 1985

449. Brown LJR, Wells M: Cervical glandular atypia associated with squamous intraepithelial neoplasia: A premalignant lesion? J Clin Pathol 39:22–28, 1986

450. Teshima S, Shimosato Y, Kishi K et al: Early stage adenocarcinoma of the uterine cervix. Histopathologic analysis with consideration of histogenesis. Cancer 56:167–172, 1985

451. Brinton LA, Tashima KT, Lehman HF et al: Epidemiology of cervical cancer by cell type. Cancer Res 47:1706–1711, 1987

452. Gallup DG, Harper RH, Stock RJ: Poor prognosis in patients with adenosquamous cell carcinoma of the cervix. Obstet Gynecol 65:416–422, 1985

453. Shingleton HM, Gore H, Bradley DH, Soong SJ: Adenocarcinoma of the cervix. I. Clinical evaluation and pathologic features. Am J Obstet Gynecol 139:799–814, 1981

454. Yazigi R, Sandstad J, Muñoz AK et al: Adenosquamous carcinoma of the cervix: Prognosis in stage IB. Obstet Gynecol 75:1012–1015, 1990

455. Littman P, Clement PB, Henriksen B et al: Glassy cell carcinoma of the cervix. Cancer 37:2238–2246, 1976

456. Maier RC, Norris HJ: Glassy cell carcinoma of the cervix. Obstet Gynecol 60:219–224, 1982

457. Costa MJ, Kenny MB, Hewan-Lowe K, Judd R: Glassy cell features in adenosquamous carcinoma of the uterine cervix: Histologic, ultrastructural, immunohistochemical, and clinical findings. Am J Clin Pathol 96:520–528, 1991

458. Daroca PJ, Dhurandhar HN: Basaloid carcinoma of the uterine cervix. Am J Surg Pathol 4:235–239, 1980

459. Van Dinh T, Woodruff JD: Adenoid cystic and adenoid basal carcinomas of the cervix. Obstet Gynecol 65:705–708, 1985

460. Ferry JA, Scully RE: "Adenoid cystic" carcinoma and adenoid basal carcinoma of the uterine cervix: A study of 28 cases. Am J Surg Pathol 12:134–144, 1988

461. Mazur MT, Battifora HA: Adenoid cystic carcinoma of the uterine cervix: Ultrastructure, immunofluorescence and criteria for diagnosis. Am J Clin Pathol 77:494–500, 1982

462. Stone ML, Weingold AB, Sall S: Cervical carcinoma in pregnancy. Am J Obstet Gynecol 93:479–485, 1965

463. Williams TJ, Brack CB: Carcinoma of the cervix in pregnancy. Cancer 17:1486–1491, 1964

464. Sivanesaratram V, Jayalakshmi P, Loo C: Surgical management of early invasive cancer of the cervix associated with pregnancy. Gynecol Oncol 48:68–75, 1993

465. Hellberg D, Axelson O, Gad A, Nilsson S: Conservative

management of the abnormal smear during pregnancy. Acta Obstet Gynecol Scand 66:195–199, 1987

466. Ostergard DR, Nieberg RK: Evaluation of abnormal cervical cytology during pregnancy with colposcopy. Am J Obstet Gynecol 134:756–758, 1979

467. Hacker NF, Berek JS, Lagasse LD et al: Carcinoma of the cervix associated with pregnancy. Obstet Gynecol 59:735–746, 1982

468. Nisker JA, Shubat M: Stage IB cervical carcinoma and pregnancy: Report of 49 cases. Am J Obstet Gynecol 145:203–206, 1983

469. Glücksmann A: Relationship between hormonal changes in pregnancy and the development of "mixed carcinoma" of the uterine cervix. Cancer 10:831–837, 1957

470. Hoffman M, Roberts WS, Cavanagh D: Second pelvic malignancies following radiation therapy for cervical cancer. Obstet Gynecol Surv 40:611–617, 1985

471. Parkash V, Carcangiu ML: Uterine papillary serous carcinoma after radiation therapy for carcinoma of the cervix. Cancer 69:496–501, 1992

472. Fujimora M, Ostrow RS, Okagaki T: Implication of human papillomavirus in postirradiation dysplasia. Cancer 68:2181–2185, 1991

473. Glücksmann A: Can radiosensivity and histopathology of cervical cancer be correlated? JAMA 193:823–824, 1965

474. Sugimori H, Taki I: Radiosensivity test for cervical cancer. Acta Cytol 16:331–335, 1972

475. Gompel C: Possibilités d'appréciation de l'évolution d'un cancer génital par la cytologie exfoliatrice après radiothérapie. Bull Soc Belge Gynéc Obstét 28:71–76, 1958

476. Graham RM, Graham JB: Cytological prognosis in cancer of the uterine cervix treated radiologically. Cancer 8:59–70, 1955

477. Green TH Jr: Further trial of a cytologic method for selecting either radiation or radical operation in the primary treatment of cervical cancer. Am J Obstet Gynecol 112:544–555, 1972

478. Gupta S, Mukherjee K, Gupta YN, Kumar M: Sequential radiation changes in cytology of vaginal smears in carcinoma of cervix uteri during radiotherapy. Int J Gynaecol Obstet 25:303–308, 1987

479. Ortner A, Weiser G, Haas H et al: Embryonal rhabdomyosarcoma (botryoid type) of the cervix: A case report and review. Gynecol Oncol 13:115–119, 1982

480. Daya DA, Scully RE: Sarcoma botryoides of the uterine cervix in young women: A clinicopathological study of 13 cases. Gynecol Oncol 29:290–304, 1988

481. Brand E, Berek JS, Nieberg RK et al: Rhabdomyosarcoma of the uterine cervix: Sarcoma botryoides. Cancer 60:1552–1560, 1987

482. Abell MR, Ramirez JA: Sarcomas and carcinosarcomas of the uterine cervix. Cancer 31:1176–1192, 1973

483. Jaffe R, Altaras M, Berheim J et al: Endocervical stromal sarcoma: A case report. Gynecol Oncol 22:105–108, 1985

484. Abdul-Karim FW, Bazi TM, Sorensen K et al: Sarcoma of the uterine cervix: Clinicopathologic findings in three cases. Gynecol Oncol 26:103–111, 1987

485. Jawalelar KS, Zacharopoulou M, McCaffrey RM: Leiomyosarcoma of the cervix uteri. South Med J 74:510–511, 1981

486. Bell DA, Shimm DS, Gang DL: Wilms' tumor of the endocervix. Arch Pathol Lab Med 109:371–373, 1985

487. Crum CP, Rogers BH, Andersen W: Osteosarcoma of uterus: Case report and review of the literature. Gynecol Oncol 9:256–268, 1989

488. Bonfiglio TA, Patten SF Jr, Woodworth FE: Fibroxanthosarcoma of the uterine cervix. Cytopathologic and histologic manifestations. Acta Cytol 20:501–504, 1986

489. Veliath AJ, Hannah P, Ratnakar C et al: Primary liposarcoma of the cervix: A case report. Int J Gynaecol Obstet 16:75–79, 1978

490. Junge J, Horn T, Bock J: Primary malignant schwannoma of the uterine cervix: Case report. Br J Obstet Gynaecol 96:111–116, 1989

491. Pyrah RD, Redman TF: Teratoma of the uterus with an associated congenital anomaly. J Pathol 95:291–295, 1968

492. Tsukamoto N, Nakamura M, Kashimura M et al: Primary cervical choriocarcinoma. Gynecol Oncol 9:99–107, 1980

493. Tripathi R, Pratap VK: Choriocarcinoma of cervix: Case report. Br J Obstet Gynaecol 89:267–269, 1982

494. Kristiansen SB, Anderson R, Cohen DM: Primary malignant melanoma of the cervix and review of the literature. Gynecol Oncol 47:398–403, 1992

495. Yu HC, Ketabchi M: Detection of malignant melanoma of the uterine cervix from Papanicolaou smears: A case report. Acta Cytol 31:73–76, 1987

496. Mordel N, Mor-Yosef S, Ben-Baruch N et al: Malignant melanoma of the uterine cervix: Case report and review of the literature. Gynecol Oncol 32:375–380, 1989

497. Hall-Craggs M, Toker G, Nedwich A: Carcinosarcoma of the uterine cervix: A light and electron microscopic study. Cancer 48:151–169, 1981

498. Komaki R, Cox J, Hansen R et al: Malignant lymphoma of the uterine cervix. Cancer 54:1699–1704, 1984

499. Taki I, Aozasa K, Kurokawa K: Malignant lymphoma of the uterine cervix: Cytologic diagnosis of a case with immunocytochemical corroboration. Acta Cytol 29:607–611, 1985

500. Mann R, Roberts WS, Gunasakeran S et al: Primary lymphoma of the uterine cervix. Gynecol Oncol 26:127–134, 1987

501. Khoury G, Robinson A: Lymphoma of uterine cervix. Eur J Surg Oncol 15:65–67, 1989

502. Matsuyama T, Tsukamoto N, Kaku T et al: Primary malignant lymphoma of the uterine corpus and cervix. Acta Cytol 33:228–232, 1989

503. Harris NL, Scully RE: Malignant lymphoma and granulocytic sarcoma of the uterus and vagina: A clinicopathologic analysis of 27 cases. Cancer 53:2530–2545, 1984

504. Nasiell M: Hodgkin's disease limited to the uterine cervix: A case report including cytologic findings in the cervical and vaginal smears. Acta Cytol 8:16–18, 1964

505. Andrews SJ, Hernandez E, Woods J et al: Burkitt's like lymphoma presenting as a gynecologic tumor. Gynecol Oncol 30:131–136, 1988

506. Spahr J, Behm FG, Schneider V: Preleukemic granulocytic sarcoma of cervix and vagina: Initial manifestation by cytology. Acta Cytol 25:55–60, 1982

507. Abeler V, Kjorstad KE, Langholm R et al: Granulocytic sarcoma (chloroma) of the uterine cervix: Report of two cases. Int J Gynecol Pathol 2:88–92, 1983

508. Armenia CS, Shaver DN, Moddesher MW: Decidual transformation of the cervical stroma simulating reticulum cell sarcoma. Am J Obstet Gynecol 89:808–816, 1964

509. Mazur MT, Hsueh S, Gersell DJ: Metastases to the female genital tract: Analysis of 325 cases. Cancer 53:1978–1984, 1984

510. Wallach JB, Edberg S: Carcinoma metastatic to the uterine cervix. Am J Obstet Gynecol 77:990–995, 1959

511. Yazigi R, Sandstad J, Munoz AK: Breast cancer metastasizing to the uterine cervix. Cancer 61:2558–2560, 1988

512. McGill F, Adachi A, Karimi N et al: Abnormal cervical cytology leading to the diagnosis of gastric cancer. Gynecol Oncol 36:101–105, 1990

513. Atobe Y, Yoshimura T, Kako H et al: Gastric cancer diagnosed by biopsy of the uterine cervix. Gynecol Oncol 26:135–139, 1987

514. Takeda M, King DE, McHenry MJ et al: Lung cancer metastatic to the uterine cervix. Acta Cytol 25:442, 1981

515. Zhang Y, Zhang P, Wei Y: Metastatic carcinoma of the cervix uteri from the gastrointestinal tract. Gynecol Oncol 15:287–290, 1983

516. Way S: Carcinoma metastatic in the cervix. Gynecol Oncol 9:298–302, 1980

517. Lemoine NR, Hall PA: Epithelial tumors metastatic to the uterine cervix: A study of 33 cases and review of the literature. Cancer 57:2002–2005, 1986

Pathology in Gynecology and Obstetrics, Fourth Edition, edited by Claude Gompel and Steven G. Silverberg. J. B. Lippincott Company, Philadelphia © 1994.

4 | *The Corpus Uteri*

EMBRYOLOGY

The corpus uteri arises as a result of the fusion of the caudal portions of the müllerian ducts, which themselves arise as invaginations of coelomic epithelium. From the beginning of its formation, the lumen of this canal is lined by a columnar epithelium, from which the endometrial glands later proliferate.[1] Whether these glands induce the formation of endometrial stroma or vice versa is still being debated, but certainly these two structures—as well as the smooth muscle fibers, which arise during the fourth month of fetal life—are intimately related during the course of their development. This intimate relationship is reproduced pathologically in the development of endometriosis and of certain tumors, in each of which two or three of these elements may coexist.[2,3] All three are ultimately of coelomic, and thus of mesodermal, origin. The corpus is well formed by the 21st week of gestation; its subsequent development is limited to an increase in size, although it remains smaller than the cervix well into childhood.[4]

ANATOMY

The corpus uteri has the form of a pyramid, the apex of which is bent toward the base. It presents two surfaces and three borders and measures, in the adult, 45 to 50 mm in height, 50 mm in width, and 25 mm in thickness. The weight under normal conditions ranges from 40 to 70 g, the higher weights prevailing in the multipara and the lower weights after the menopause.[5] Uterine size measured in vivo by new radiographic techniques probably reflects physiologic conditions better than the classic autopsy studies.[6,7] Considerable symmetrical enlargement may occur in the absence of demonstrable pathology; the mechanism of this change is unknown because it may occur in nulliparous and parous women.[8]

MALFORMATIONS

When the development and fusion of the müllerian ducts and the disappearance of the septum do not take place normally, a series of malformations that depends on several mechanisms ensues (Fig. 4-1).[9–11] The most reduced malformation is the *uterus arcuatus*, which presents a heart-shaped appearance and often an outline of a median partition at the base. These anomalies are frequently associated with vaginal, tubal, or urinary tract (single kidney, double ureter, pelvic kidney) anomalies.

Recently, a series of anomalies has been described in women who were exposed in utero to diethylstilbestrol (DES), including hypoplasia, a

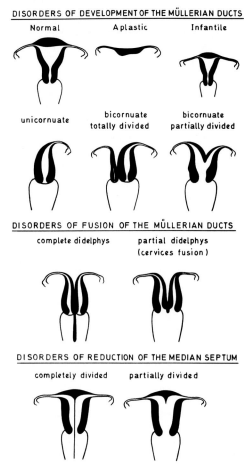

DISORDERS OF DEVELOPMENT OF THE MÜLLERIAN DUCTS

Normal   Aplastic   Infantile

unicornuate   bicornuate totally divided   bicornuate partially divided

DISORDERS OF FUSION OF THE MÜLLERIAN DUCTS

complete didelphys   partial didelphys (cervices fusion)

DISORDERS OF REDUCTION OF THE MEDIAN SEPTUM

completely divided   partially divided

FIGURE 4-1 Congenital malformations of the uterus.

T-shaped uterus, and constriction bands in the endometrial cavity;[12,13] more is known of their hysterographic than of their morphologic appearances. These and other anomalies in these women may result in fertility disorders.

A rare malformation not related to müllerian maldevelopment is uterine arteriovenous fistula.[14] This lesion is more commonly acquired than congenital.

HISTOLOGY

From the histologic point of view, the uterus consists of three layers: the serosa, myometrium, and endometrium. The *serosa* or *visceral peritoneum* is composed of mesothelial cells.

The *muscular layer* or *myometrium* is composed of smooth muscle fibers separated by collagen and elastic fibers; this muscular layer is divided into an external zone of longitudinal fibers, a middle zone of interdigitating fibers coursing in all directions, and an internal zone of circular fibers.[1,15] The in-

ternal zone is particularly well developed in the inferior portion of the uterine corpus (isthmic zone). A lateral muscle bundle has been described as extending from the cornua to the cervix;[16] this has been designated the *fasciculus cervicoangularis* and may play a role in conduction.

The role of the *mucosa* or *endometrium* is to provide a site of implantation and nutrition for the fertilized egg. The endometrial surface is covered by a columnar epithelium, into which the glands open. The glands are distributed in a stroma formed of round to ovoid cells. Around the glands is a fibrillar network and a characteristic vascular apparatus. Three successive layers in the endometrium can be distinguished.[1,17] The *deep layer* or *basalis* comprises the depths of the glandular cul-de-sacs, which during the menstrual cycle respond only feebly to estrogenic stimulation and never to progesteronal stimulation. Some of these cul-de-sacs have a tendency to penetrate into the adjacent myometrium. When this phenomenon is pronounced, it is interpreted as adenomyosis. The stroma of the deep layer is dense and composed of small rounded cells with little cytoplasm. Some authors have denied the existence of a functionally distinct basalis.[18]

The *middle layer* or *spongiosa* occupies the greatest part of the thickness of the endometrium and reacts intensely to hormonal stimulation. The vascular apparatus is well developed.

The *superficial layer* or *compacta* includes the necks of the glands and the surface epithelium. During the luteal phase, the glandular convolutions in this layer are less accentuated than in the spongiosa. The surface epithelium does not show the same cyclical variations as the rest of the mucosa.

Endometrial *vascularization* involves a distribution that is unique to this organ.[19–21] Two types of arteries, basal and spiral, arise from the myometrial arteries to supply the endometrium.

The *basal arteries*, whose territory is confined to the deep part of the endometrium, do not vary in structure during the course of the menstrual cycle. Their independence of the ovarian hormones is confirmed experimentally by the fact that, in the rhesus monkey, they are not involved by the hyalinization that is found in the spiral and myometrial arteries.

The spiral arteries penetrate to the surface of the mucosa and undergo evident cyclical modifications (Figs. 4-2 and 4-3). During the proliferative phase, they are less numerous, moderately spiral, and localized to the deep part of the functional zone. Progressively during the course of the secretory phase, their digitations increase and their spiral structure becomes more accentuated. They reach the superficial part of the functional zone and attain their maximum growth at the premenstrual period. They feed into the capillary and venous lakes situated under the endometrial surface. At the end of the cycle, their walls show lesions consisting of hyalinization and alterations of the elastic fibers.

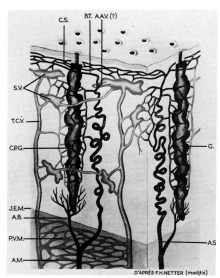

FIGURE 4-2 Schematic representation of the spiral arteries. *A.M.,* myometrial artery; *A.S.,* spiral artery; *A,B.,* basal artery; *A.A.V.,* arteriovenous anastomosis.

Cellular Components of the Endometrium

The Epithelium of the Glandular System

The *glandular cell* is a columnar element whose height varies from 6 to 20 μm according to the phase of the cycle. The nucleus is elongated but becomes round and vesicular during the secretory phase. The cytoplasm is the site of synthesis of RNA, proteins, mucopolysaccharides, glycogen, lipids, and various enzymes. The massive production of glycogen after ovulation justifies the term *secretory phase.*

The ultrastructure of the glandular cells reveals the typical organelles of epithelial cells.[22] The chromatin structure is finely distributed and bordered by the double-layered nuclear envelope; the nucleolus is rich in RNA and has a maximal volume at the time of ovulation. The endoplasmic reticulum, a ramified system of tubules and cisternae, is covered with numerous small granules rich in RNA (ribosomes). Some of the ribosomes are free in the cytoplasmic matrix. The Golgi apparatus or zone is a group of vacuoles and cisternae situated in the juxtanuclear region; it is concerned with synthesis and concentration of secretory products. Lysosomes are more abundant during the late secretory phase.

Mitochondria are numerous and are bordered by a double membrane that sends numerous digitations or cristae through the thickness of the matrix. The mitochondria play an essential role in the cellular mechanisms of oxidation because of their richness in enzymes.

Intensely osmophilic lipid inclusions are found disseminated in the cytoplasm. The significance of their variations in size and shape is not precisely defined. Rounded granular formations of the size of a mitochondrion may be connected with the lysosomes; these are known as *microbodies.*

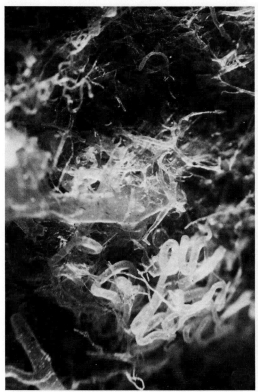
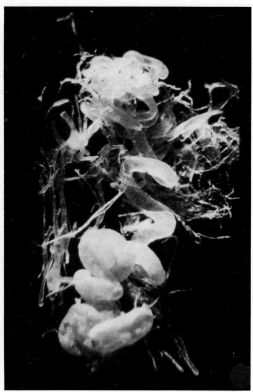

FIGURE 4-3 Casts of spiral arteris.

The ciliated cell appears as a clear cell dispersed among the glandular cells; the former are most numerous during the late proliferative phase and in endometrial hyperplasia, suggesting an estrogen-dependent mechanism. The cilia possess a complex structure consisting of nine double filaments grouped around an axial double filament (Fig. 4-4). The whole structure is surrounded by a thin casing of cytoplasm.

The other (nonciliated) cells show an apical pole covered with simple cytoplasmic prolongations (microvilli) that give a hairy appearance to the cells (Fig. 4-5). Other cells are found at the bases of the glands and have central small round nuclei and clear cyto-

plasm. These ciliated cells have not yet reached the luminal surface, where they can extrude their cilia.

The Superficial Epithelium

The superficial epithelium is composed of a layer of columnar cells that are rich in RNA and glycogen (Fig. 4-6).

Endometrial Stroma

Stromal cells arise from pluripotential mesenchymal cells. They are elongated elements with irregular nuclei that will become predecidual cells during the

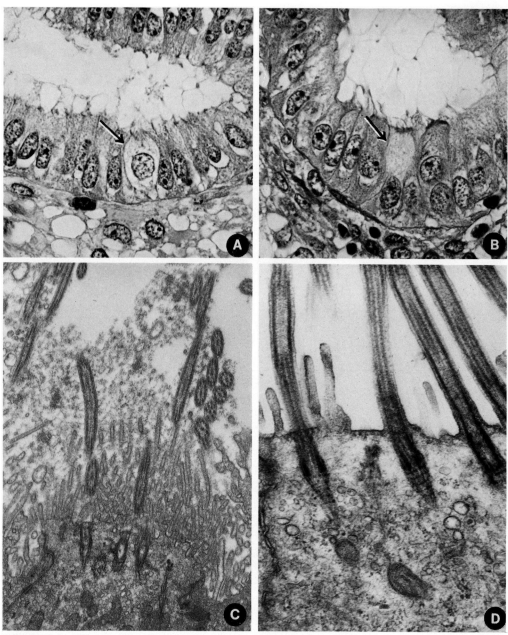

FIGURE 4-4 Ciliated cells of the endometrium. **(A,B)** Optical microscopy. **(C,D)** Electron micrographs (×23,400 and ×34,500).

late secretory phase. Glycogen and lipids are found in the abundant cytoplasm of predecidual cells. Other stromal cells have been thought to transform to endometrial granulocytes, the cytoplasmic phloxinophilic granules of which contain relaxin, which dissolves the reticulin fibers surrounding individual stromal cells immediately before menstruation.[23] More recent studies have identified these cells as lymphoid in nature.[24–26]

The *basal lamina* underlies the epithelial elements and separates them from the subjacent stroma (Fig. 4-7). Its structure varies depending on whether it is examined by optical or electron microscopy. Under the electron microscope, it appears as a dark band, about 250 nm thick, rich in reticulin fibers that run parallel to the cellular membranes of the glandular cells. It is separated from this cell membrane by a clearer zone of the same thickness. The deep surface of the membrane is in direct contact with the stromal cells and collagen fibers.

Examined with the optical microscope after silver impregnation, it appears thicker and measures about 2500 nm. This indicates that in addition to the structures that we have just described, ordinary histologic methods also stain fibrillar elements that make up part of the underlying stroma. The periodic acid-Schiff (PAS) stain is positive and reveals the presence of mucopolysaccharides.

MECHANISM OF HORMONAL INFLUENCES ON THE ENDOMETRIUM

Different portions of the endometrium respond differently to hormonal stimuli. It has been shown that estrogen- and progesterone-binding proteins (receptors) are present in normal human endometrium and mediate the effects of these hormones on the endometrial cycle.[27–30] These receptors appear to be

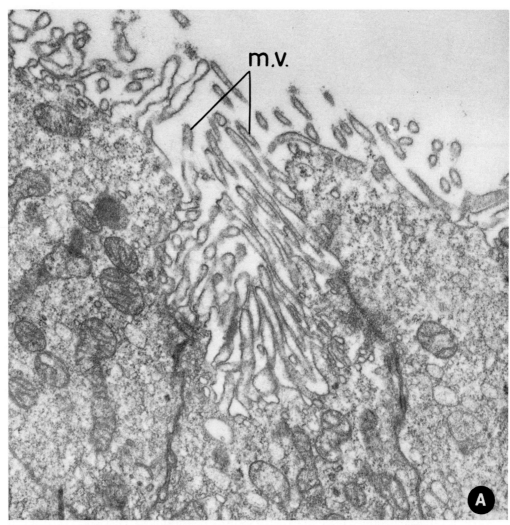

FIGURE 4-5 **(A)** Early proliferative phase (electron micrograph): cytoplasmic microvilli (*m.v.*) bordering the apical pole (×27,300). **(B)** Early proliferative phase (electron micrograph): endometrial stromal cells: nuclei (*n.*) and collagen fibers (*f.c.;* ×10,800).

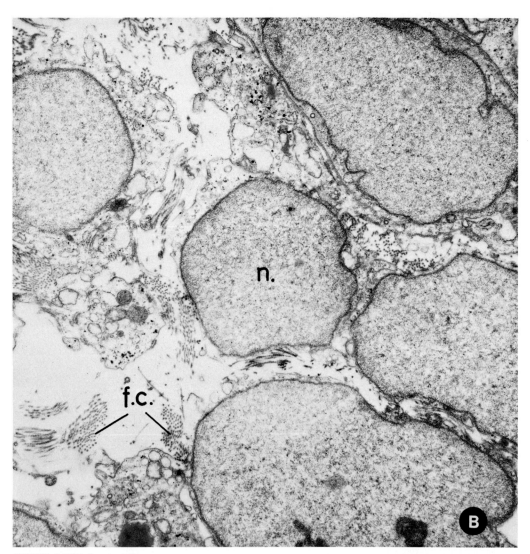

FIGURE 4-5(B) *(continued)*

more numerous in glandular than in stromal cells and in endometrium of the fundus than of the isthmus or lower uterine segment. Estrogen increases the concentration of these receptors, whereas progesterone decreases them.[31] Steroid hormone molecules combine with their cytoplasmic receptors, and the complex moves to the nucleus, where it affects DNA-dependent RNA transcription and, ultimately, the appearance of the endometrium.

The production of different enzymes within the endometrium is influenced by the ovarian hormones that act on these receptors. For example, alkaline phosphatase is found in greatest concentration in glandular epithelial cells during the estrogenic phase, whereas estradiol dehydrogenase (which converts estradiol to estrone) is increased by progesterone and thus is found mostly in the luteal phase.[32,33] The endometrium can also produce hormones, such as prostaglandins and prolactin.[34,35]

CYTOLOGY OF NORMAL ENDOMETRIUM

The cytologic appearance of normal endometrial cells depends on their source. Endometrial glandular cells generally are seen in vaginal pool smears during the first 10 days of each menstrual cycle, in which situation they present as compact balls of uniform small cells with dark nuclei showing varying degrees of degeneration and very little preserved cytoplasm (Color Fig. 4-1). In vaginal material, the presence of endometrial cells after the tenth day of a cycle or in a postmenopausal woman who is not cycling because of exogenous hormones should suggest the possible presence of an endometrial hyperplasia or (particularly if the cells are atypical) carcinoma.

In material obtained by direct aspiration of the endometrial cavity, on the other hand, endometrial cells should be seen at all times, even in the absence of pathology, and should be better preserved. The glandular columnar cells are smaller than those of the endocervix and may appear as clusters with well-defined borders ("honeycomb" pattern; Color Fig. 4-2), as an elongated palisade, or as single cells. The nuclei are rounded or ovoid and exhibit finely granular chromatin and a nucleolus that may be prominent. In the luteal phase, the nuclei are rounder and paler and the cytoplasm more abundant and frequently vacuolated. Occasional ciliated cells may be encountered; if they are numerous, a hyperestrogenic state is suggested.

Endometrial stromal cells are also seen, and they are particularly numerous at the end of the menstrual phase. These cells resemble the glandular cells but may have less well-defined cell borders (Color Fig. 4-3). Like glandular epithelial cells, they become loaded with glycogen during the luteal phase.

PHYSIOLOGIC MECHANISMS OF MENSTRUATION

The intimate mechanisms of menstruation still are not entirely elucidated. One may appreciate the long road followed since the earliest studies by reading the first chapter of the "Traité des maladies des femmes," written in Paris in 1761 by J. Astruc,[36] Royal Professor of Medicine and consultant physician to King Louis XV. We have extracted and translated the following passage:

> The understanding of the structure of the matrix and of the distribution of its vessels is sufficient to state that it is from the venous appendages that this blood must flow. These are all venous ramifications; those which advance the farthest in the cavity of the matrix are the only ones which pene-

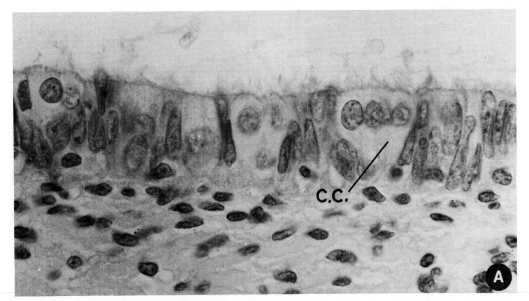

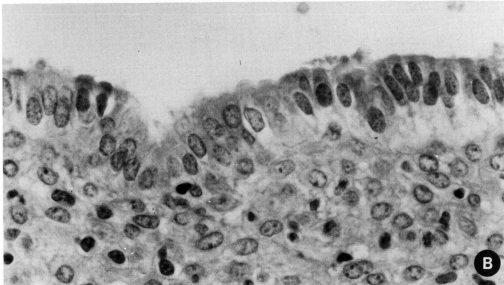

FIGURE 4-6   Covering epithelium of endometrium; ciliated cells (*c.c.*).

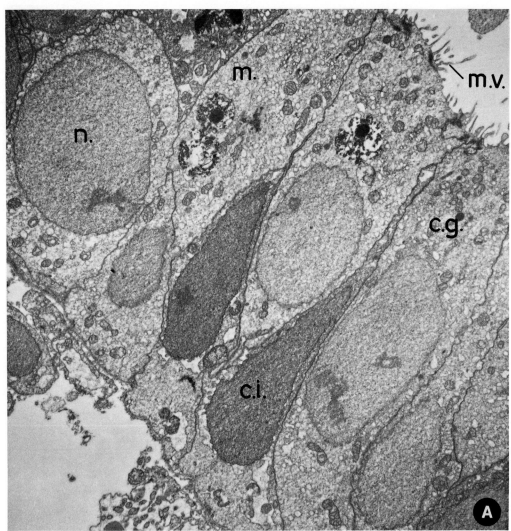

FIGURE 4-7 **(A)** Endometrial glands in early proliferative phase (electron micrograph): glandular cells (*c.g.*): intercalated cells (*c.i.*); nuclei (*n.*); mitochondria (*m.*); microvilli (*m.v.*; ×7500). **(B)** Early proliferative phase (electron micrograph); mitochondrion (*m.*); basement membrane (*m.b.*); collagen fibers (*f.c.*). The structure of the basement membrane is easily visible here. It is constituted, from top to bottom, by the basal membrane of the cell, a clear space, and a dark band. The entire structure is about 250 nm thick and rich in reticulin.

trate the full thickness of the tunica interior. These are kinds of venous endings which should be destined for some usage in the design of nature, but, however, have none in the ordinary order of the circulation. Finally, these are vein endings simply wrinkled at their extremities and therefore capable of extending, folding, opening without tearing. All these facts form so many presumptions that should make one conjecture that it is from these appendages that bleeding takes place into the cavity of the matrix during menstruation.

The theory proposed in 1761 by Astruc (Fig. 4-8), based essentially on visual observation and good sense, as the author himself said, permitted the prediction with remarkable prescience of the existence of the spiral arteries and of their mechanism of action in the process of menstruation.

The endometrial vessels were described for the first time in 1754 by Hunter, who compared their convolutions to the undulations of a snake.[21] It was not until 1847 that the existence of a true mucosa was recognized by Coste. It was described histologically for the first time in 1873 by Kundrat and Engelmann; in 1877, Leopold described the spiral arteries; and in 1908, Hitschmann and Adler[37] recognized the cyclical nature of the histologic modifications of the endometrium. Schröder[38,39] was the first to synthesize these diverse observations; he recognized the relationship existing between maturation of the ovarian follicle and the proliferative phase of the endometrium and between the corpus luteum and the secretory phase.

Subsequent studies over the next three quarters of a century have served to increase our knowledge

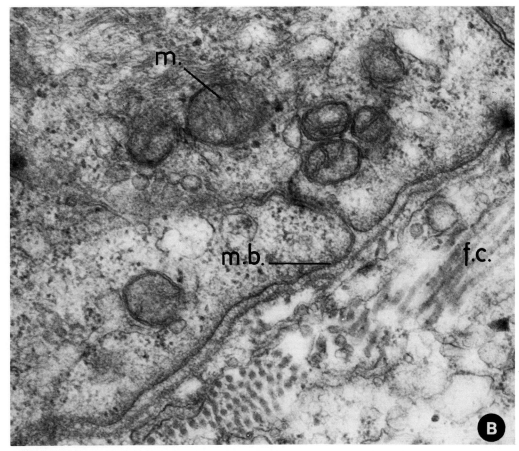

FIGURE 4-7(B) *(continued)*

greatly but still have not provided a universal explanation for the phenomenon of menstruation. For the purposes of the diagnostic pathologist who is seeking to correlate structure with function, much has been learned about the normal cyclical variations of the endometrium. The information provided by these studies is summarized in the following section.

CYCLICAL VARIATIONS OF THE ENDOMETRIUM

Histologic Modifications of the Endometrium

An essential role of the histologic modifications of the endometrium under the influence of ovarian hormonal stimulations is the preparation of the mucosa for the implantation of the fertilized ovum. The morphologic conditions necessary for this implantation are reproduced with a remarkable regularity and constancy in the absence of fertilization.

These modifications are under the influence of the estrogenic hormones during the first half of the cycle and of progesterone and estrogens during the second half. The combination of these two hormonal activities conditions the appearance of the endometrium. Their production is under the influence of the anterior pituitary through the mediation of the hormones of follicular maturation or stimulation (follicle-stimulating hormone [FSH]) and of luteinization (luteinizing hormone [LH]). The anterior pituitary is itself under the influence of the central nervous system through the hypothalamus.

The aspects of the uterine mucosa are classified schematically in eight phases. If we consider the duration of the "normal" (ie, average) cycle to be 28 days, the phases are as follows:

1. The early proliferative (estrogenic) phase (days 4–9)
2. The late proliferative (estrogenic) phase (days 10–14)
3. The phase of ovulation (interval phase) (days 14 and 15)
4. The early secretory (luteal, progestational) phase (days 16–18)
5. The mid-secretory (luteal, progestational) phase (days 19 and 20)
6. The late secretory (luteal, progestational) phase (days 21–25)
7. The immediately premenstrual phase (days 26–28)
8. The menstrual phase (days 1–3).

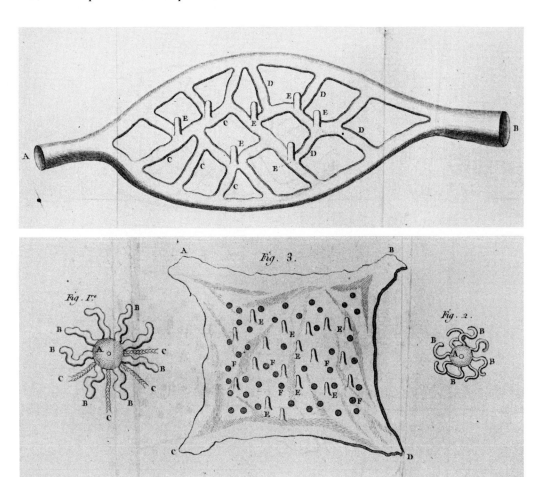

FIGURE 4-8 Representation of the vascularization of the endometrium (Astruc J: Traité des maladies des femmes. Paris, PG Cavelier, 1761).

This system is useful diagnostically as well as descriptively, because it has been shown that about 75% to 80% of endometrial biopsies can be dated histologically within 2 days in either direction.[40–42] Exact dating with reference to circulating hormone levels or the onset of the next menses is much less accurate. Because it is easier to demonstrate day-to-day variations in postovulatory endometria, it has been suggested that the designation of day 1 should be assigned to the first day after ovulation (day 15 in the schema presented here), rather than the first day of menstrual bleeding.[41] We have no objection to this system but emphasize that all clinicians and pathologists within a given institution should use and understand the same system.

Although the lengths of the proliferative and secretory portions of the cycle both average 14 days, the former may vary in presumably "normal" women from 9 to 21 days and the latter from 9 to 17 days,[40] thus pointing out again the imprecision of the comments presented below.

Because of these variations, particularly in the secretory phase, correlation between histologic dating and chronologic dating is considerably better if the LH peak rather than the date of the next menstrual period is used as the chronologic standard.[43,44]

Endometrial morphology also has been shown to correlate well with corpus luteum morphology[44] and the date of ovulation determined by ultrasonography.[45] Morphometric analysis of the endometrium may be even more reliable than standard histopathology,[46,47] but it is considerably more time and labor intensive.

Early Proliferative Phase (Days 4–9)

General Appearance of the Mucosa. The thickness of the endometrium at the beginning of the cycle is about 1 to 2 mm. The glands have regular contours, are of small diameter, and are dispersed in a relatively dense stroma (Fig. 4-9). The middle part of the endometrium may contain a few clumps of lymphocytes, which have no pathologic significance (Fig. 4-10). This appearance characterizes the mucosa, which, after having reconstituted its anatomic integrity, undergoes a phase of growth of its glands, stroma, and vessels. The covering superficial epithelium, now completely regenerated, is cylindrical and contains ATPase and alkaline phosphatase. It is rich in ciliated and mucus-secreting cells.

Glandular Epithelium. The glandular columnar cell shows a basal elongated nucleus and abundant

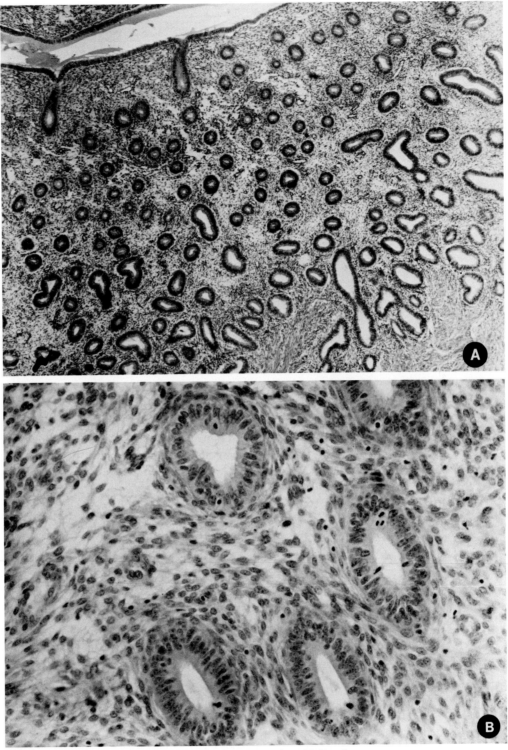

FIGURE 4-9 Early proliferative phase. **(A)** Low-power view. **(B)** Detail.

apical cytoplasm bordered by microvilli (see Fig. 4-5A). The nuclei are not all situated at the same level, and this variation creates a pseudostratified appearance that must not be confused with the picture of hyperplasia. Mitoses are frequent; they are found at the apical pole of the cell and in the middle if the gland is sectioned transversely. The cytoplasm of the glandular cells contains small elongated mitochondria. RNA synthesis is very active, as indicated by the abundance of free ribosomes and granular endoplasmic reticulum. Ciliated cells are dispersed in the glandular epithelium (see Figs. 4-4 and 4-6).

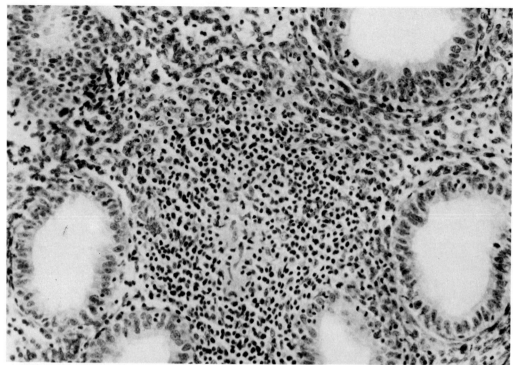

FIGURE 4-10 Early proliferative phase: lymphocytic infiltrate.

Stroma. The stroma is dense and richly populated with small cells containing rounded or elongated nuclei (see Fig. 4-9*B*). Ultrastructurally, they resemble fibroblasts and produce numerous collagen fibers (see Fig. 4-5*B*). Mitoses are present. Between the cells, there is a well-developed collagenous network formed of bundles of fibers anastomosing in all directions. Here and there, one may find rare leukocytes in the concentration of about one per square millimeter of endometrium. Thin-walled spiral arteries are situated in the deep layers; they give rise to a few collaterals that irrigate the periglandular capillary plexus. The moderately dilated venous networks empty into the venous plexus, which form lakes in regions of anastomoses of venous trunks. These reassemble into collecting trunks that enter the myometrium.

Late Proliferative Phase (Days 10–14)

General Appearance of the Mucosa. The thickness of the endometrium increases to about 2 to 3 mm. The gland contours become more sinuous, and their diameters increase as well. At this time, numerous glands have convoluted contours, and the surface epithelium forms large undulations (Fig. 4-11). The stroma is abundant. Edema appears between the cells at the onset of this phase and tends to regress before ovulation. The spiral arteries continue their development and reach the superficial part of the endometrium. The arteriolar walls thicken and become enriched in elastic fibers. The capillaries, lymphatics, and veins grow and dilate. Sometimes in the deep layers there exist a few small lymphoid follicles, the presence of which has no pathologic significance.

Glandular Epithelium. Proliferation of the glandular cells is evidenced by the number of mitoses present. Their nuclei are elongated and enlarged and are always found at the base of the cell (see Fig. 4-11). Ultrastructurally, RNA synthesis is still very active. The Golgi apparatus is well developed, and lipid droplets are present in the apical part of the cytoplasm. The number of ciliated cells increases proportionately, but they remain in the minority. Clear cells appear as isolated and dispersed elements at the base of the glandular epithelium.[48] Their abundant clear cytoplasm stands out against the darker appearance of the neighboring cells. These cells appear to be precursors of fully ciliated cells and are useful markers of estrogenic activity because they are rarely seen in inactive or atrophic endometria.

Toward the 14th day of the cycle, fine glycogen inclusions appear ultrastructurally at the basal pole of the glandular cell. They accompany the presence of voluminous mitochondria in intimate relation with the endoplasmic reticulum. This morphologic connection suggests that these two organelles play collaborative roles in the synthesis of glycogen. A microtubular system distinct from the endoplasmic reticulum has been described by Cavazos;[49] these structures are said to be spatially and temporally related to glycogen. Clyman[50] has more recently denied their existence and believes that they are tonofilaments. The cytoplasm of the glandular cells shows three distinct zones when examined by electron microscopy: the basal zone, in which the glycogen appears (Fig. 4-12*A*), the juxtanuclear zone, in which the mitochondria are elongated and less numerous, and the apical zone. The apical zone con-

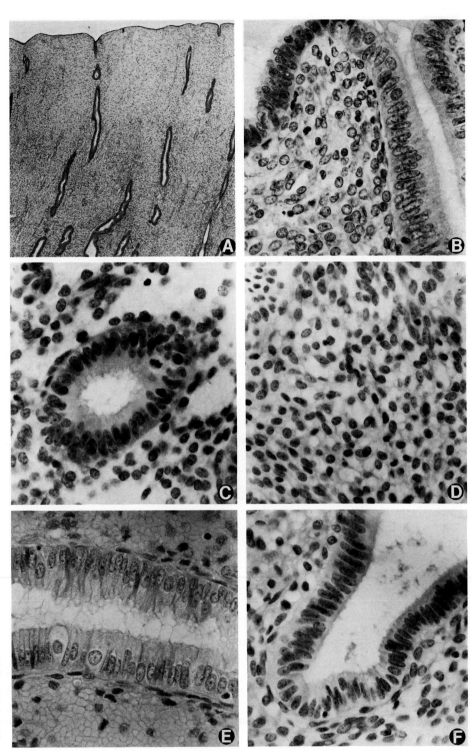

FIGURE 4-11 Late proliferative phase. **(A)** General appearance. **(B)** Surface epithelium and gland neck. **(C)** Mitosis in gland. **(D)** Stroma. **(E)** Gland showing a ciliated cell and a small clear cell (*at right*). **(F)** Proliferative gland showing a clear cell toward the bottom.

tains numerous mitochondria, well-developed endoplasmic reticulum, lipid inclusions, and vacuoles that are either simple or filled with microvesicles. The Golgi apparatus, situated immediately above the nucleus, comprises a series of longitudinal fissures and rounded vacuoles. These submicroscopic modifications are connected with the secretory activities of the cell.[51]

The basement membrane loses its rectilinear disposition and presents more and more numerous and accentuated invaginations toward the glandular epithelium; these are the precursors of the connective tissue spines of the secretory phase.

Stroma. The stroma increases in volume and is composed of stellate cells anastomosed to one another (see Fig. 4-11). It forms a loose network containing more or less abundant edema fluid, which

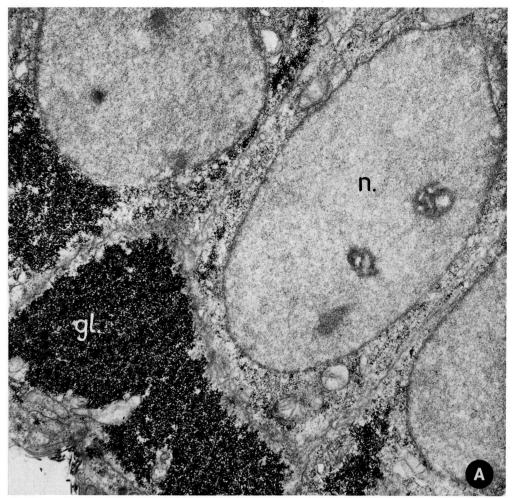

FIGURE 4-12 **(A)** Early secretory phase (electron micrograph ×10,800). *n.,* nuclei; *gl.,* glycogenic vacuoles. **(B)** Intranuclear tubular structures.

tends to diminish immediately after ovulation. A few leukocytes are found here and there. Mitoses are numerous.

Ovulatory (Interval) Phase (Days 14–15)

The combined influence of estrogens and progesterone characterizes the ovulatory phase. Edema of the compact layer begins to develop. Transient focal hemorrhagic phenomena may appear, limited to the superficial portion of the endometrium (Fig. 4-13); this is manifested clinically by a small loss of blood in about 5% of women. Microscopic examination shows tiny hemorrhagic foci situated below the surface epithelium.

Early and Mid-Secretory Phases (Days 16–20)

General Appearance of the Mucosa. The thickness of the endometrium is at its maximum (3 to 5 mm). The glands are numerous, and their caliber has increased in comparison with the preceding phase. The "sawtooth" appearance of their contours is caused by invaginations of the membrane and of the adjacent stroma, which form small connective tissue axes on which are implanted the glandular cells. However, their presence is not indispensable for the diagnosis of a secretory endometrium. Their number and height increase during the course of this phase. The surface epithelium is markedly convoluted. The stroma is abundant and of loose consistency. The vessels continue their growth, the walls of the spiral arteries thicken and their spiralization increases, and the foci of edema in the spongiosa (which tend to regress somewhat between days 12 and 18) again become more numerous. The basal endometrium continues to show a discrete proliferative appearance and is not affected by the postovulatory modifications.

Glandular Epithelium. About 24 to 72 hours after ovulation, basal vacuoles appear in the secretory glandular cells;[41,52] they represent the massive glycogen content of the cytoplasm and correspond to the beginning of progestational activity (Figs. 4-14 and 4-15; see Fig. 4-12).

Color Figure 4-1

Color Figure 4-2

Color Figure 4-3

Color Figure 4-4

Color Figure 4-1 Poorly preserved benign endometrial glandular cells in vaginal smear.

Color Figure 4-2 Endometrial glandular cells in "honeycomb" pattern in endometrial aspirate.

Color Figure 4-3 Endometrial stromal cells (*right*) in vaginal smear taken during menses. The large ball of glandular cells (*left*) is markedly degenerated.

Color Figure 4-4 Vaginal smear from an IUD wearer, showing both atypical columnar cells (*right*) and "IUD cells" with a high nuclear–cytoplasmic ratio (*left*). (Courtesy of Dr. Prabodh K. Gupta, Hospital of the University of Pennsylvania, Philadelphia)

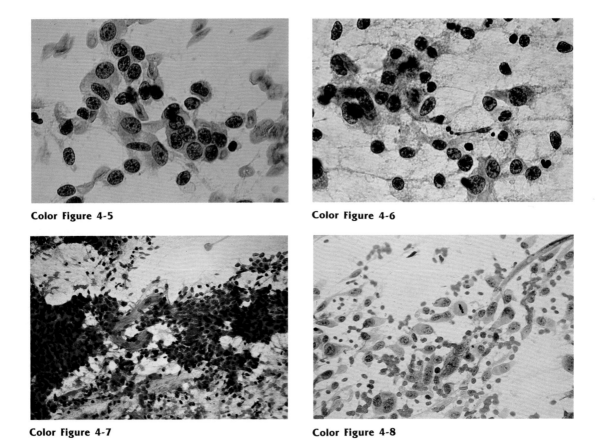

Color Figure 4-5

Color Figure 4-6

Color Figure 4-7

Color Figure 4-8

Color Figure 4-5 Complex hyperplasia (endometrial aspirate).

Color Figure 4-6 Well-differentiated adenocarcinoma (endometrial aspirate). Atypia is increased only slightly from Color Figure 4-5.

Color Figure 4-7 Aspirate of adenoacanthoma: squamous cells in center surrounded by well-differentiated adenocarcinoma cells.

Color Figure 4-8 Leiomyosarcoma: cytologic picture featuring marked pleomorphism, spindled tumor cells, and mitotic figures.

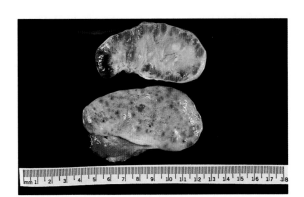

Color Figure 6-1

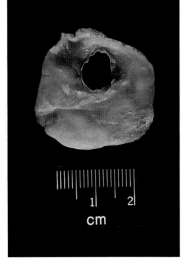

Color Figure 6-2

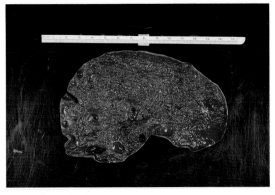

Color Figure 6-3

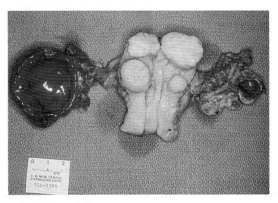

Color Figure 6-4

Color Figure 6-1 Hyperreactio luteinalis. Cortical and cut surfaces of one of two enlarged ovaries in a woman with a twin pregnancy.

Color Figure 6-2 Ovary with hyperthecosis. Tan cortical stromal nodules are present. The benign cyst and the corpus luteum are incidental.

Color Figure 6-3 Massive edema of the ovary. The ovary is enlarged, and clear fluid exudes from the cut surface.

Color Figure 6-4 Endometriosis of the ovary. The bilateral "chocolate cysts" are associated with uterine leiomyomata.

Color Figure 6-5

Color Figure 6-6

Color Figure 6-7

Color Figure 6-8

Color Figure 6-5 Serous tumor of low malignant potential. Coarse polypoid processes project into the cyst lumen.

Color Figure 6-6 Mucinous tumor of low malignant potential. These are generally large, multiloculated cystic neoplasms.

Color Figure 6-7 Carcinosarcoma. The tumor is composed of malignant epithelial and mesenchymal elements.

Color Figure 6-8 Smear from serous cystadenoma showing a broad flat sheet of uniform cohesive cells with small regular nuclei.

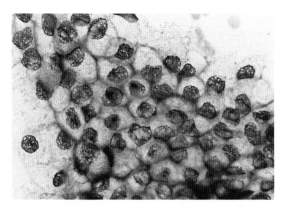

Color Figure 6-9

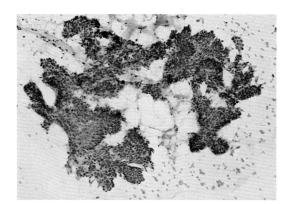

Color Figure 6-10

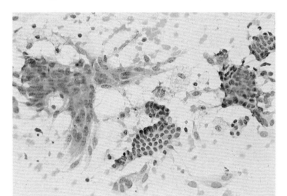

Color Figure 6-11

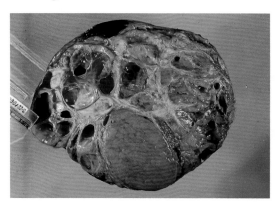

Color Figure 6-12

Color Figure 6-9 Smear from mucinous cystadenoma. Uniform cohesive cells in a honeycomb arrangement.

Color Figure 6-10 Fine needle aspirate of serous cystadenocarcinoma of the ovary. Papillary clusters have frequent branches composed of small, tightly packed cells with high nuclear–cytoplasmic ratio and nuclear hyperchromasia. (Courtesy of M. Nadji, MD, University of Miami, Miami, FL).

Color Figure 6-11 Transabdominal needle aspirate of an endometrioid tumor of low malignant potential. Glandular elements (*right*) contrast with the squamous component (*left*). (Courtesy of M. Nadji, MD, University of Miami, Miami, FL).

Color Figure 6-12 Granulosa cell tumor. Granulosa cell tumors typically are partially cystic. The intervening solid areas are soft and tan or yellow.

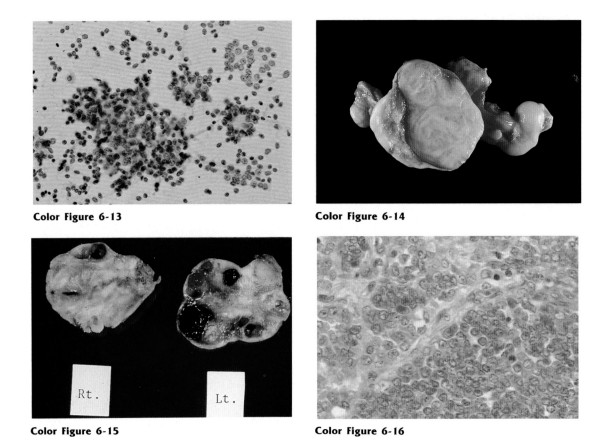

Color Figure 6-13

Color Figure 6-14

Color Figure 6-15

Color Figure 6-16

Color Figure 6-13 Fine-needle aspirate of granulosa cell tumor. Groups of cells with uniform oval nuclei, indistinct cytoplasmic borders, and structures resembling Call-Exner bodies. (Courtesy of M. Nadji, MD, University of Miami, Miami, FL)

Color Figure 6-14 Thecoma. Firm solid tumor with a whorled, yellow and white cut surface.

Color Figure 6-15 Sex cord tumor with annular tubules. Multiple yellow tumor nodules were found in both ovaries in a patient with Peutz-Jeghers syndrome.

Color Figure 6-16 Small cell carcinoma. Small cells with scanty cytoplasm are adjacent to larger cells with more abundant eosinophilic cytoplasm.

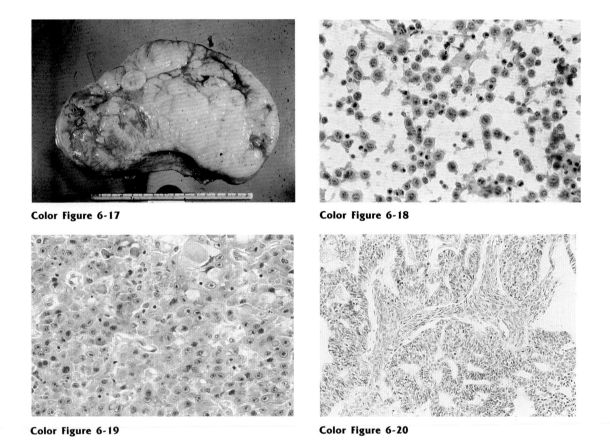

Color Figure 6-17

Color Figure 6-18

Color Figure 6-19

Color Figure 6-20

Color Figure 6-17   Dysgerminoma. The dysgerminoma is a solid neoplasm with a fleshy, white or tan cut surface.

Color Figure 6-18   Dysgerminoma of the ovary. Transvaginal aspirate showing isolated or loosely bound cells with large nuclei and prominent nucleoli. Lymphocytes are intimately associated with tumor cells. (Courtesy of M. Nadji, MD, University of Miami, Miami, FL).

Color Figure 6-19   Hepatoid yolk sac tumor. Other yolk sac patterns were seen elsewhere in this tumor.

Color Figure 6-20   Glandular endometrioid yolk sac tumor resembling endometrioid carcinoma. Other yolk sac patterns were found elsewhere in this tumor.

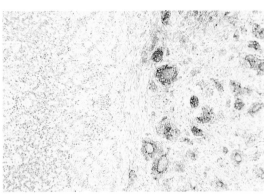

Color Figure 6-21

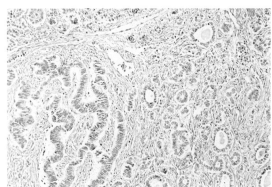

Color Figure 6-22

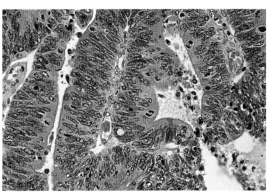

Color Figure 6-23

Color Figure 6-24

Color Figure 6-21   Mature (benign) cystic teratoma with extensive infarction following torsion.

Color Figure 6-22   Strumal carcinoid. The neoplasm contains trabecular arrangements of cells typical of carcinoid (*left*) and follicles resembling thyroid tissue (*right*).

Color Figure 6-23   Strumal carcinoid. Immunoperoxidase stain of the tissue block seen in Color Figure 6-22. Thyroglobulin is present in the cells lining the follicles but not within the cells in the trabeculae.

Color Figure 6-24   Metastatic adenocarcinoma from the large intestine.

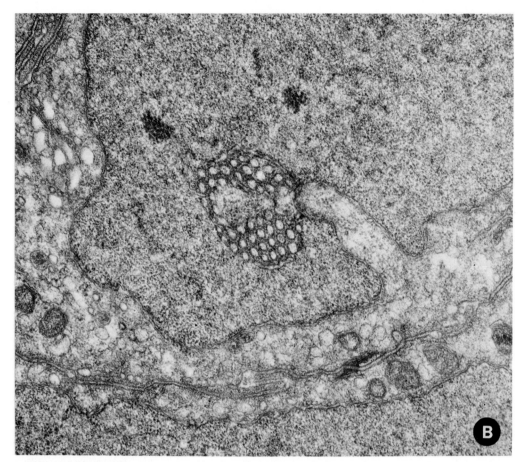

FIGURE 4-12(B) *(continued)*

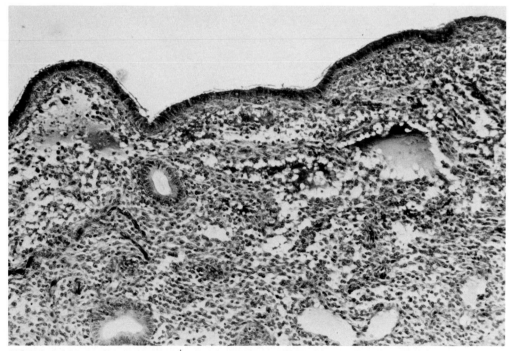

FIGURE 4-13 Ovulatory phase: superficial intermenstrual hemorrhage *(mittelschmerz)*.

Glycogen may appear in the endometrial glands under the action of estrogens alone. It is present in small quantities during anovulatory cycles and may be explained by deficient luteinization of a persistent follicle. However, a combination of estrogenic and progestational activity is necessary for its presence in significant quantities. Therefore, we may consider the presence of basal vacuoles in significant numbers as a sign of the beginning of activity of the corpus luteum. These vacuoles are seen at first in a few cells, and then progressively in all the glands of the functional strata. By day 18, they move into an apical po-

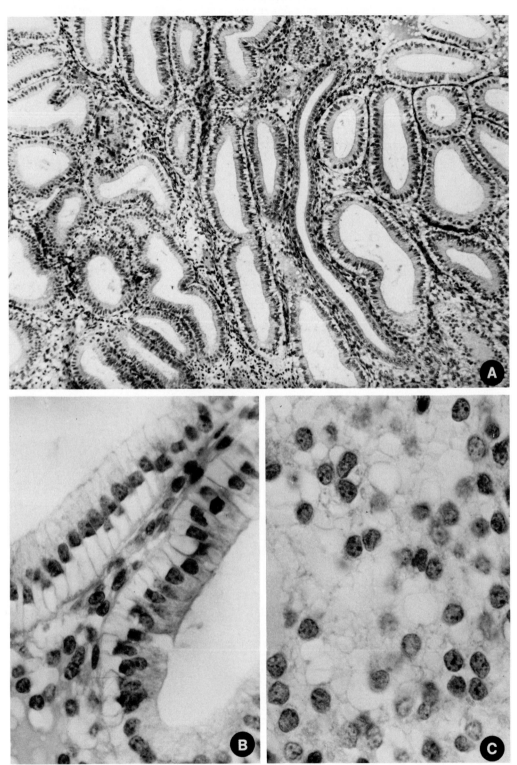

FIGURE 4-14 Early secretory phase: basal vacuoles containing glycogen. **(A)** General appearance. **(B,C)** Details of vacuoles and stroma.

sition (this may be called the *mid-secretory phase*), and by day 20 discrete vacuoles disappear, with glycogen expanding throughout the entire cell (Fig. 4-16).

Toward the end of this stage, an amorphous substance is found in the gland lumina. This substance is stainable with eosin and contains products of secretion and cellular debris in the process of necrosis.

With the electron microscope, intranuclear tu-

bular structures (see Fig. 4-12*B*), formed by tubules or canaliculi in parallel or concentric distribution, have been demonstrated in the secretory phase, apparently related to a strong balanced progesterone effect.[53] In hyperestrogenic states, cytoplasmic annulate lamellae have been seen at this time. These small clusters of paired parallel membranes converge at regular intervals and are found in supranuclear loca-

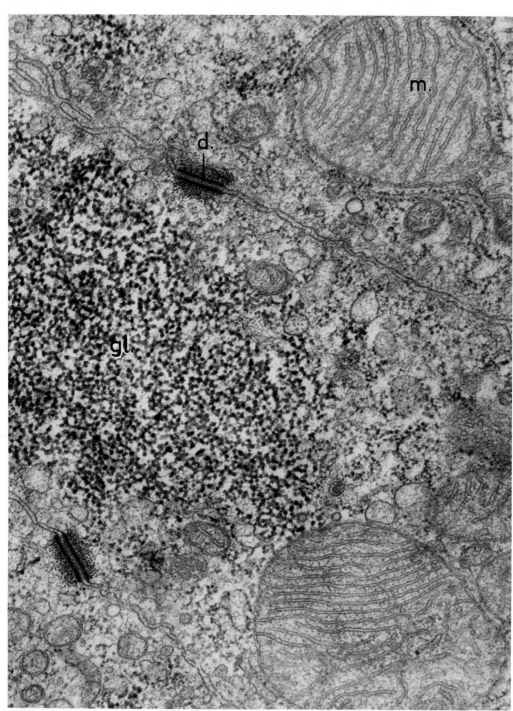

FIGURE 4-15 Early secretory phase (electron micrograph, ×84,000). The glycogen, stained with ferric hydroxide, is seen as round granules grouped in large masses. A large mitochondrion is present in each of the cells. The desmosomes binding two cellular membranes are easily seen. *gl.,* glycogen; *m.,* mitochondria; *d.,* desmosomes.

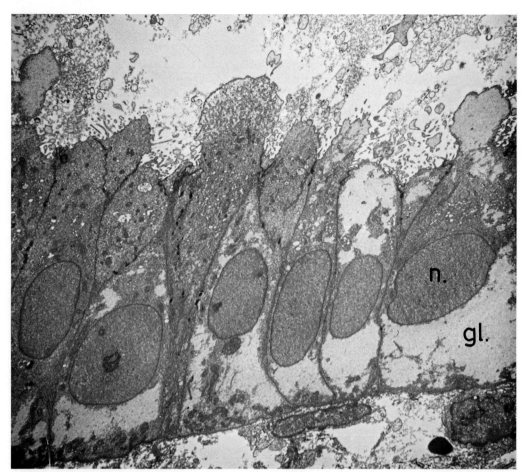

FIGURE 4-16 Endometrium at 22nd day of cycle (electron micrograph, ×4200) showing the distribution of glycogen throughout the cytoplasm.

tions when estrogenic stimulation is marked and in the subnuclear zone when luteal changes are also seen.[54] Their origin may be from the nuclear membrane or from the Golgi apparatus. Their significance is unknown.

Stroma. The stroma presents a looser appearance; edema reappears and attains its maximum intensity around the 22nd day (Fig. 4-17). The cells are always separated and of stellate shape. The rounded or elongated nuclei are only rarely in mitosis.

Late Secretory Phase (Days 21–25)

General Appearance of the Mucosa. The mucosa is edematous and succulent but by the end of this phase begins to show regressive changes. It contains numerous glands with marked sawtooth configurations (Figs. 4-18 and 4-19). The glandular convolutions attain their maximal intensity and may be so well developed that the glands assume a papillary aspect. These modifications involve the strata spongiosa and compacta and leave the basalis intact. The stroma is abundant, loose, and edematous. The predecidual reaction begins around the vessels toward the 24th day and extends to the entire superficial part of the stroma. The spiral arterioles (Fig. 4-20) attain their full development, and their most superficial appendages are situated immediately beneath the surface epithelium. Occasionally they run parallel to this epithelium for as long a distance as 1 mm. They become prominent around day 23.

Glandular Epithelium. The secretory glandular cells contain voluminous round basal nuclei.[52] The chromatin is finely dispersed, and the nucleolus can be seen easily. The cytoplasm bulges and herniates into the gland lumen. It contains pools of glycogen; other cells have lost their glycogen and are evolving toward a resting state. This bulging appearance of the superior pole brings to mind secretion of apocrine type, but electron microscopic observations point toward the diffusion of the glycogen into the glandular lumen. Some of the microvilli contain plaques of glycogen and have the appearance of a club (Fig. 4-21). The mitochondria are small and numerous and are localized principally in the supranuclear region. The rough endoplasmic reticulum is well developed. The Golgi apparatus is voluminous and presents dilated vacuoles and cisterns. Lipid inclusions and vesicles persist in the supranuclear region. The lateral cell membranes show numerous

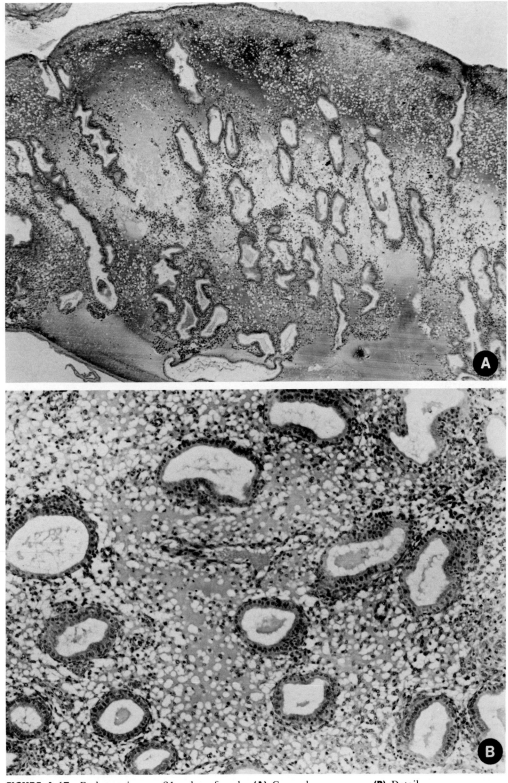

FIGURE 4-17 Endometrium at 21st day of cycle. **(A)** General appearance. **(B)** Detail.

convolutions. The basement membrane forms invaginations that constitute the axes of connective tissue spines (Fig. 4-22). The formation of these spines constitutes one of the criteria of progestational activity. They appear more rapidly than the predecidualization of the stroma but require higher doses of progesterone. Here and there, between the secretory cells, are found intercalated cells with dark, dense cytoplasm and ovoid nuclei, stretched out between two adjacent cells. There are fewer ciliated cells than during the proliferative phase. Small clear cells are also rare.

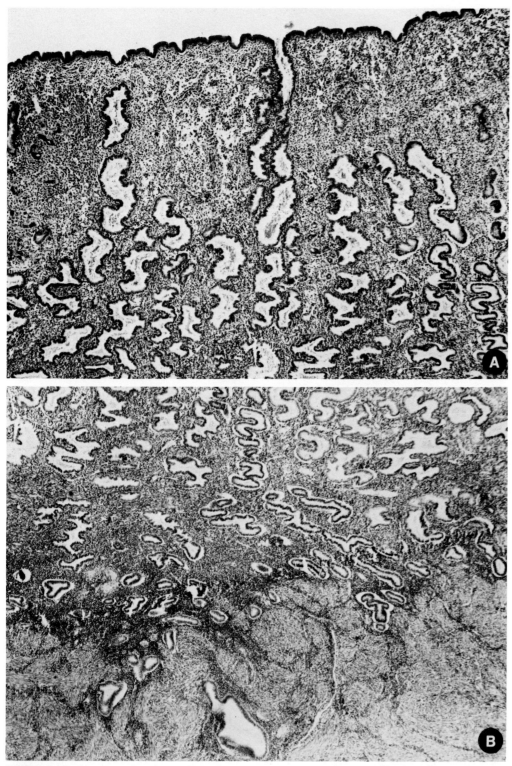

FIGURE 4-18 Late secretory phase. **(A)** Superficial portion of endometrium. **(B)** Deep portion of endometrium.

This characteristic appearance of the secretory gland persists until 3 days before menstruation. Then, the first signs of mucosal involution appear, following the fall of estrogen and progesterone levels.

In some endometria in which histologic examina- tion reveals a very recent implantation of the ovum, typical progestational hyperplasia may be seen. This is manifested at first by more marked edema and congestion of the capillary network of the compact layer. Subsequently, the normal manifestations of lu- teal impregnation are more accentuated, notably de-

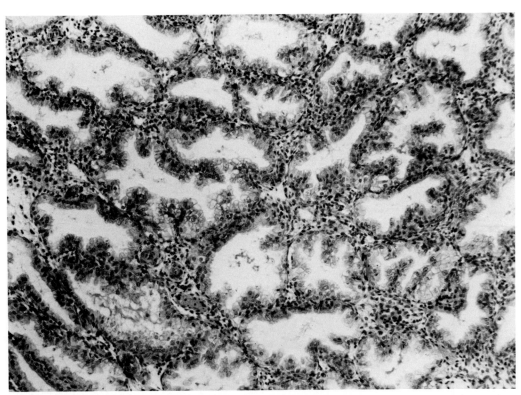

FIGURE 4-19 Late secretory phase: gland with sawtooth contours.

cidual change, edema, glandular secretion, and development of the spiral arteries.

Stroma. Stromal edema is accentuated and the connective tissue network becomes more and more loose. The stroma of the functional layers undergoes predecidual change (Fig. 4-23A), manifested by a major increase in cytoplasmic glycogen. Appearing at first around spiral arterioles (decidual cuffs) around day 24, these cells eventually form large plaques; they are easily recognizable by their size and their clear cytoplasm. Their number decreases in the deeper functional layers.

A particular cell type makes its appearance at this phase (Fig. 4-23B): the granulocyte or metrial cell, characterized by an indented nucleus and by round eosinophilic cytoplasmic granules whose chemical structure differs from that of the granules of eosinophilic polymorphonuclear leukocytes. The granules are stained by the method of Lendrum with tartrazine phloxine and by that of Weigert with methyl violet. Immunohistologic studies have been reported to demonstrate that this polypeptide molecule represents relaxin.[23] These cells are localized with predilection in the compact zone and around blood vessels. They are found only during the secretory phase and in the first 3 months of pregnancy. They were thought for many years to be derived from endometrial stromal cells and to be involved in menstruation and implantation, but more recent studies have indicated that they are either T lymphocytes or macrophages.[24–26]

True polymorphonuclear leukocytes are also found in the stroma, almost exclusively from day 26 on, and reflect the approach of the menses.[55] Ultrastructurally, stromal cell cytoplasmic organelles increase in number and size, and collagen precursors are secreted into the extracellular space, where polymerization occurs.

Premenstrual Phase (Days 26–28)

This brief phase is essentially an accentuation of the late secretory phase. The predecidual stromal reaction has spread to involve the entire compacta, whereas the underlying spongiosa is comprised largely of "sawtooth" glands that show profound shrinkage and diminished secretions. Dilated thin-walled capillaries are prominent near the endometrial surface. Stromal leukocytic infiltrates are marked, and discrete glandular and stromal hemorrhages are present.

Menstrual Phase (Days 1–3)

The mucosa becomes fragmented and desquamates as large or small fragments of debris (Fig. 4-24). The stroma retracts and shows dense foci of cells compressed against each other (Fig. 4-25), adjacent to still edematous or superficial hemorrhagic zones. At this time, the mucosa undergoes marked dehydration. The leukocytic infiltrate reaches its maximal intensity. The glandular cells, some of which are still secretory, whereas others are already in an exhausted state, become necrotic and lose their tinctorial affinity. Desquamation usually involves small fragments but may in the case of *membranous dysmenorrhea* consist of large scraps of mucosa. The spiral arteries are dilated and show gaping apertures. Their walls present signs of degeneration: confluence of endothelial cells, hyalinization of muscular fi-

bers, and disappearance of elastic fibers. The capillaries and venous plexus are also dilated. The absence of thrombi in the vessels broken off by desquamation suggests the existence of a mechanism of control of vasoconstriction in the arteries remaining in place. Fibrils of fibrin are present in small amounts in the capillaries and stroma during the

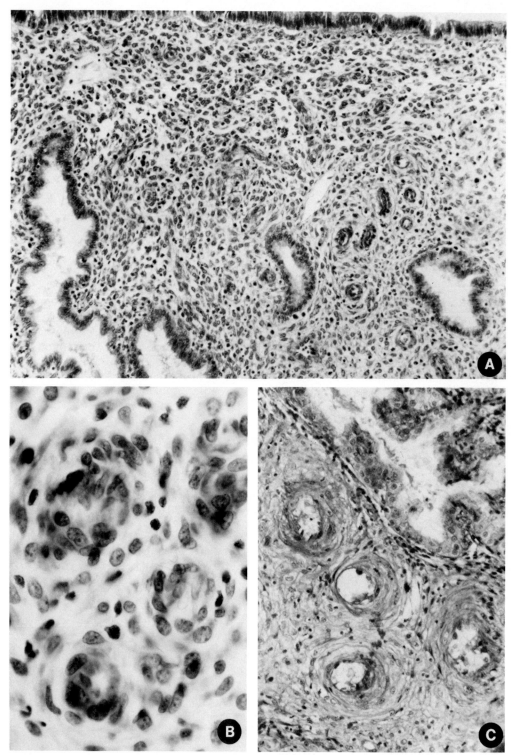

FIGURE 4-20 Late secretory phase: spiral arteries. **(A)** General appearance. **(B,C)** Details.

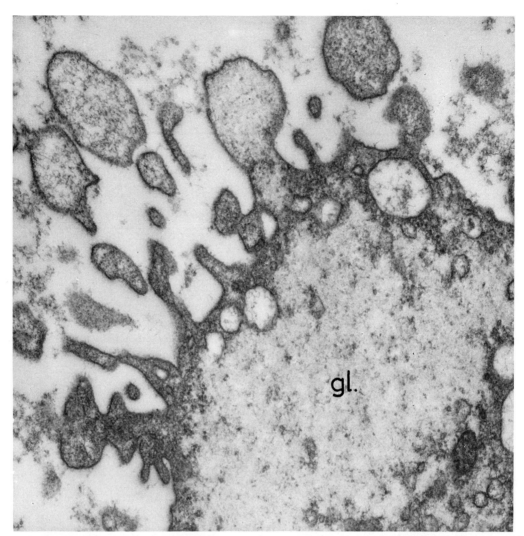

FIGURE 4-21 Late secretory phase (electron micrograph, ×43,350); detail of apical pole of glandular cell showing the presence of glycogen in the microvilli.

premenstrual phase. Subsequent fibrinolytic activity with dissolution of the clots explains the fluidity of the menstrual blood. Desquamation involves the compacta and at least part of the spongiosa; how much spongiosa remains above the basalis is still debated.[18,56] Menstrual shedding generally lasts about 72 hours.

Subsequently, the regenerative phase begins and is accomplished very rapidly, because at the end of menstruation the surface epithelium is already practically reconstituted.[57,58] Reorganization of the stromal components is evident by the fifth day.

Histologic Appearances of the Endometrium Encountered Outside the Menstrual Cycle, and Pathologic Appearances

Modifications in histologic appearance of the endometrium due to physiologic states encountered outside the menstrual cycle and to pathologic states may be separated schematically into three groups:

1. Physiologic states outside the period of functional activity
2. Normal histologic pictures whose moment of appearance is pathologic
3. Histologic pictures invariably of pathologic nature.

This classification points out the importance of clinical data in the interpretation of an endometrial biopsy or curettage. A picture that may be entirely normal at one period during the cycle becomes pathologic at another moment. It is therefore essential that the pathologist be in possession of the pertinent clinical information to interpret the pictures observed.

Physiologic States of the Mucosa Outside the Functional Period

Fetal Endometrium. Differentiation of the uterine mucosa is terminated around 4½ months of fetal life.[1,17] It consists at this time of a cuboidal epithe-

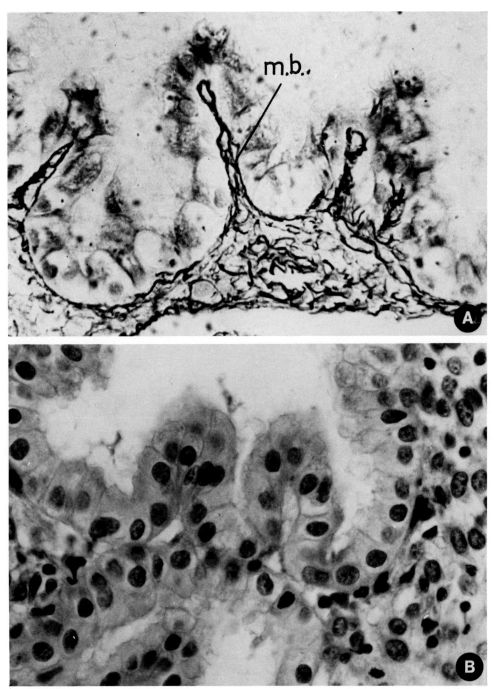

FIGURE 4-22 Late secretory phase: connective tissue spines. **(A)** Reticulin stain showing the basement membrane (*m.b.*). **(B)** Hematoxylin and eosin stain.

lium covering a dense stroma and containing small cells; the glands are practically nonexistent, and the surface epithelium presents a few large undulations (Fig. 4-26). Around the fifth month, estrogenic stimulation begins, and this is prolonged until about 7½ months. A few glands appear, lined by columnar epithelium with elongated nuclei, and the stroma shows an outline of vascularization in its deep layer. Toward the eighth month, the glands develop and are lined by epithelium showing secretory activity, proved by the presence of glycogen in the glandular

cells; the stroma is loose and edematous. This secretory activity persists until birth and then regresses and is succeeded by a state of atrophy about 1 month after delivery. The histologic pictures of the fetal uterus are due to fetal and maternal hormonal stimuli, predominantly estrogens. The fetal hormones are of extraovarian, notably adrenal cortical, origin.

Infantile Endometrium. Infantile endometrium is of atrophic type. The glands are few in number, of

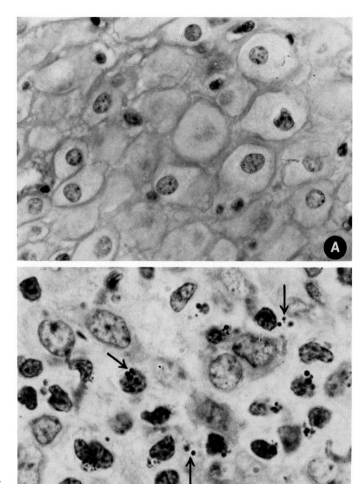

FIGURE 4-23 Late secretory phase. **(A)** Predecidual reaction of the stroma. **(B)** Granular or lymphoreticular cells of the stroma.

small caliber, and lined by columnar or cuboidal epithelium. Mitoses are absent. The stroma is composed of small cells compressed one against the others. The vascularization is rudimentary.

Pubertal Endometrium. At the moment of puberty, the first signs of estrogenic stimulation appear and are soon followed by the first menstrual cycles, of which most are anovulatory.[4]

Postpartum Endometrium. Postpartum regeneration of the endometrium generally is complete within 3 weeks. In women who are not breast-feeding, the first ovulation usually takes place during the seventh postpartum week. During the preceding menstrual period, the endometrium often reveals venous thrombi and hyalinization of arterial walls. In the weeks following delivery, during the first postpartum cycle, there is most frequently moderate or diminished estrogenic stimulation and more rarely signs of secretory activity. The most frequent complication seen in the postpartum endometrium is the presence of retained placental cotyledons or an exaggerated placental site (exuberant proliferated intermediate trophoblast) with secondary inflammatory

changes (endometritis). Thrombosed and secondarily hyalinized vessels may be responsible for the existence of small hyalin masses (hyalin bodies) that may be the cause of hemorrhages. Curettage usually suppresses this type of complication.

Postmenopausal Endometrium. *Atrophy* of the endometrium proceeds progressively after the menopause, and in some cases this transformation may take years.[1,17,31,59,60] This is why it is not rare to find after the menopause signs of proliferative or, more rarely, secretory activity. The existence of extraovarian sources of genital hormones, notably the adrenal cortices, and to a lesser extent persistent ovarian activity, explains the persistence of hormonal response long after menopause. MacBride[61] reported in 1521 cases of curettage in menopausal women that the endometrium was of atrophic type in 31.5% and of cystic atrophic type in 42.7%. Hyperplasia was seen in 12.6% of women, who were usually only a few years postmenopausal. This series is of more than historic interest, because it serves as a baseline before the era of menopausal hormone replacement.

The *macroscopic appearance* of the atrophic mucosa is pale, thin, and smooth. It measures about 0.4

mm in thickness. The *histologic picture* is characterized by the presence of scanty glands of regular contours and small caliber, lined by a single layer of small cylindrical cells (Fig. 4-27). The stroma is dense and composed of small round cells. The vascularization is poorly developed. Arteriosclerotic le-

sions may be found (Fig. 4-28). When atrophy has been present for a long time (ie, in women older than 65 years), it is often of cystic type (Fig. 4-29). The formation of cysts is apparently due to obstruction of the gland necks with secondary subjacent dilatation. This picture of cystic atrophy should not be

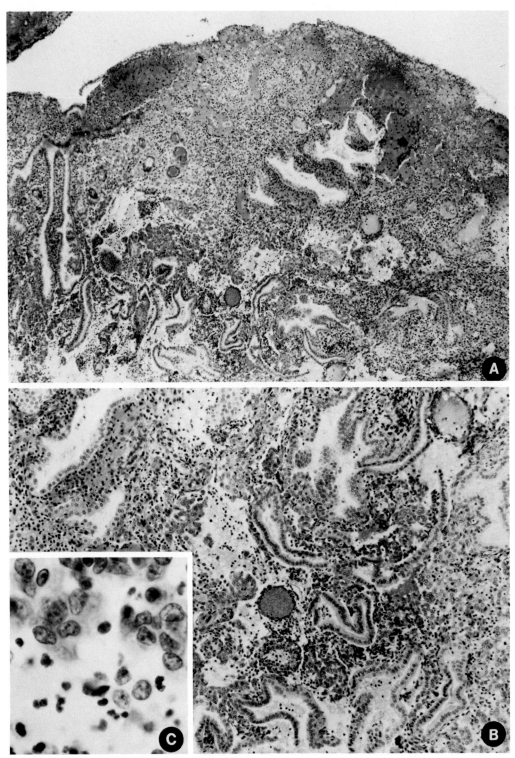

FIGURE 4-24 Menstrual phase. **(A)** General appearance. **(B,C)** Details showing stromal disintegration and leukocytic infiltration.

confused with that of cystic hyperplasia, in which the gland epithelium is stratified and mitotically active. In some atrophic endometria, the small elongated glands take an orientation parallel to the mucosal surface. The reason for this flattening is not understood.

Postmenopausal bleeding in an atrophic endometrium can be explained by myometrial arteriosclerosis, venous congestion in uterine prolapse, and venous bleeding accompanying rupture of atrophic endometrial cysts.

The same pictures of atrophy are encountered after surgical or radiotherapeutic[62] castration, in total ovarian functional insufficiency,[63,64] in certain disease states such as Sheehan's and Schmidt's syndromes, and occasionally after prolonged oral contraception.[65]

Normal Histologic Pictures Whose Moment of Appearance Is Pathologic

Persistent Estrogenic Endometrium (Anovulatory Cycle). Anovulatory cycles are more frequent than previously thought. Many postmenarchal and premenopausal cycles are anovulatory, and during the reproductive years anovulatory cycles are of a sporadic character in some women. Their frequency has been evaluated by Levan and Szanto[66] in a study of 261 biopsies performed in 103 patients: they found 9 patients who presented 14 anovulatory cycles. These were more frequent in women older than 40 years. Since the study was reported in 1944, it did not include any women who had received exogenous hormones.

The anovulatory cycle, defined as a cycle terminating in a menstrual period in the absence of ovulation, is a frequent cause of sterility. Irregular and heavy menstrual periods may also be seen. The intensity and duration of estrogenic activity vary according to the mode of regression of the persistent follicle with subsequent modification of the duration of the cycle. The estrogenic secretion of the persistent follicle may last only a few days or remain at a low level during the entire cycle. Sometimes there is a moderate follicular luteinization due to abnormal gonadotropin activity.

Microscopic examination of the endometrium shows an absence of secretory changes in the second part of the cycle and a pronounced proliferative activity (Fig. 4-30). Glycogen may be present in small amounts when there is follicular luteinization or abnormal hypophyseal activity. Erythrocytes may be seen in the stroma and fibrin thrombi in dilated capillaries.

Ovulation, with the appearance of normal postovulatory endometrial maturation, can be induced by clomiphene citrate, a weak estrogen. The feedback effect of this drug increases the release of gonadotropins with subsequent ovulation.

The differential diagnosis must be made between anovulatory cycle and late ovulation, which can take place during the third week of the cycle. A biopsy to confirm the former condition should be taken during the fourth week.[67,68]

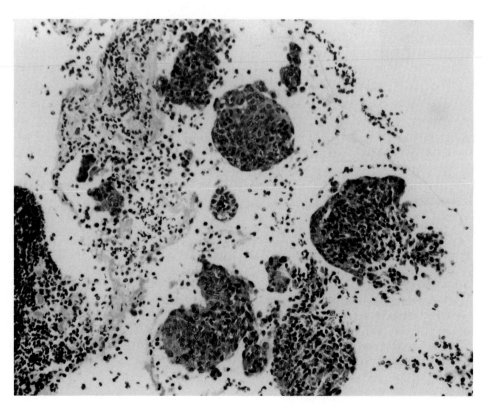

FIGURE 4-25 Menstrual endometrium showing compact aggregates of endometrial stroma.

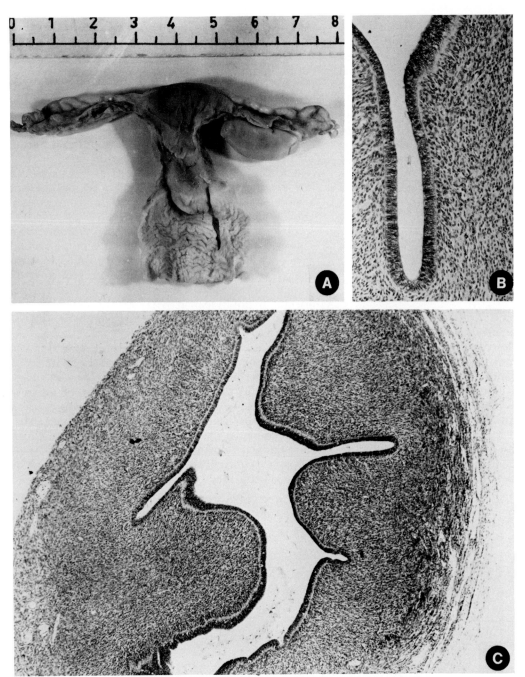

FIGURE 4-26 Fetal endometrium. **(A)** General appearance of the uterus, vagina, tubes, and ovaries. **(B)** Superficial epithelium and precursor of gland. **(C)** General appearance of the endometrium.

Luteal Phase Dysfunction. Luteal phase defects are demonstrable in up to 3% or 5% of infertile women and up to 35% of habitual aborters.[69–74] However, they are also encountered in women with a completely normal reproductive history.[75] These defects may be divided into the short luteal phase,[76] in which the interval between ovulation and menstruation is 10 days or less, and the inadequate luteal phase, in which the interval is normal but progesterone output is low. Hyperprolactinemia may be demonstrated in both disorders, whereas low FSH levels are seen only in the short luteal phase.[77] In the latter circumstance, the usual etiology is a defect in the pituitary–hypophyseal axis, and treatment consists of clomiphene or gonadotropin. The inadequate luteal phase may be due to corpus luteum deficiency, relative estrogenic hypersecretion, or local disturbances of the receptivity of the endometrium to progestational hormones.

In either situation, endometrial biopsy shows evidence of ovulation, but the histologic appearance is inappropriate for the date at which the biopsy was

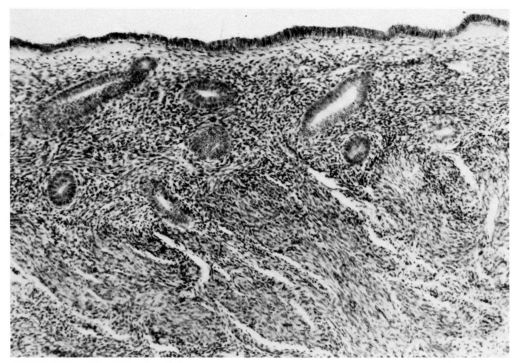

FIGURE 4-27 Atrophic endometrium.

taken. A discrepancy of 3 days or more must be seen (Fig. 4-31), because 2 days is within the normal range of error of endometrial biopsy interpretation. The picture may be entirely normal except for the retardation (coordinated pattern), or there may be an intrinsic abnormality (dissociated pattern). In the latter type, which is seen with increased estrogenic activity or decreased responsiveness to progesterone, proliferative and secretory endometrium may coexist or there may be glandular-stromal dissociation, with one of these elements appearing more advanced in the cycle than the other.

For the diagnosis of this dissociated pattern (which also has been called *irregular maturation*), the

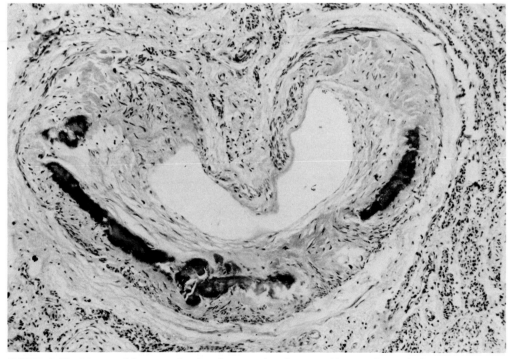

FIGURE 4-28 Myometrial artery showing degenerative changes with secondary calcification.

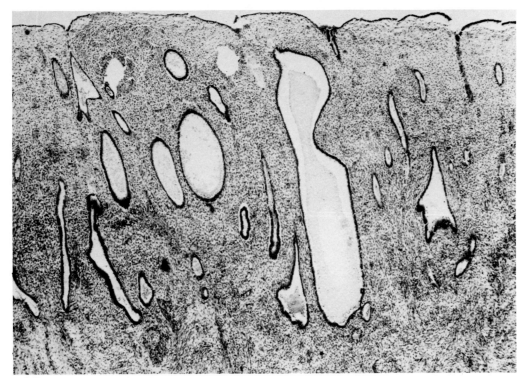

FIGURE 4-29 Cystic atrophic endometrium.

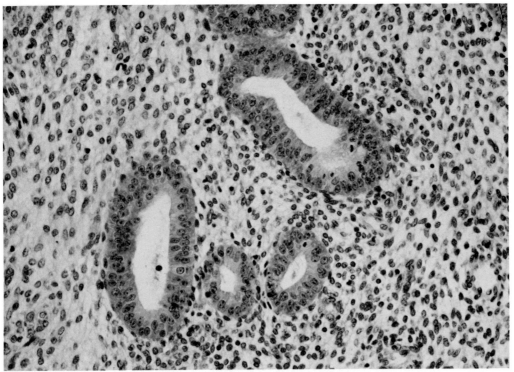

FIGURE 4-30 Endometrium at 22nd day of cycle; anovulatory cycle with relative hyperestrogenism.

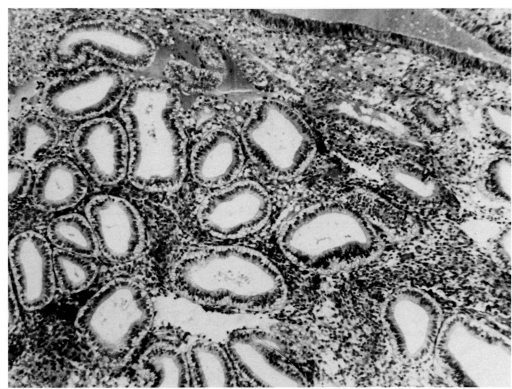

FIGURE 4-31 Endometrium at 26th day of cycle: coordinated type of luteal phase defect (basal vacuoles).

contrasting pictures must be found totally within the functional layer of the endometrium (Fig. 4-32). The presence of an endometrial polyp must be excluded, because in this latter lesion it is common to find endometrium that is totally or partially nonreactive to hormonal stimuli. It is also essential to ensure that the biopsy does not come from the isthmic region (lower uterine segment), which does not manifest distinct cyclic modifications. Endometritis must also be excluded, as should treatment with exogenous hormones (Fig. 4-33).

Although luteal phase deficiency is thought by many to be an important cause of infertility, this has been questioned by a recent study in which this was never the only factor in an infertile patient and in which clomiphene citrate therapy was equally effective in inducing pregnancy in the presence or absence of luteal phase defects.[78] Clement has summarized some of the controversy over this entity in a recent symposium.[79]

Histologic Pictures of Pathologic Nature

Endometrial Hypoplasia. Endometrial hypoplasia (inactive endometrium) secondary to ovarian hypofunction is characterized by a thin mucosa containing resting glands of regular contours and small caliber (Fig. 4-34).

The epithelium is constituted by cuboidal cells with flattened or ovoid nuclei situated in the basal part of the cytoplasm. Ciliated cells are rare. Mitoses are not seen. The stromal cells are small and take a fibroblastic appearance. The vascular apparatus is poorly developed.

Ovarian hypofunction, often resulting from hypophyseal gonadotropic insufficiency or autoimmune oophoritis, is ordinarily encountered in young girls or in women around the age of 40 (precocious menopause).[63,64,79] Hypomenorrhea or amenorrhea is the rule. Hypoplastic endometrium can rarely be seen in the presence of histologically normal ovaries containing follicles and corpora lutea. The defect has been characterized as a deficient ovarian aromatizing enzyme system.

Endometrial Hyperplasia. The clinical and pathologic significance of endometrial hyperplasia is in many respects analogous to that of dysplasia of the cervix uteri. As in this latter lesion, the pictures of endometrial hyperplasia vary from an image only slightly distorted from normal to a picture indistinguishable from that of a lesion that has been designated carcinoma in situ. Also, as in the case of cervical dysplasia, it appears that the changes seen in endometrial hyperplasia may be reversible (either spontaneously or with treatment), may persist unchanged for many years, or may follow a relentless progression over a period of time, perhaps through an in situ phase, into clinically apparent invasive carcinoma. The final analogy that we may draw be-

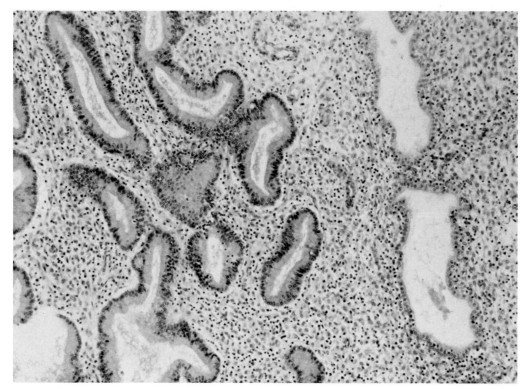

FIGURE 4-32 Irregular maturation (dissociated pattern of luteal phase defect) of endometrium: simultaneous presence of secretory and proliferative glands.

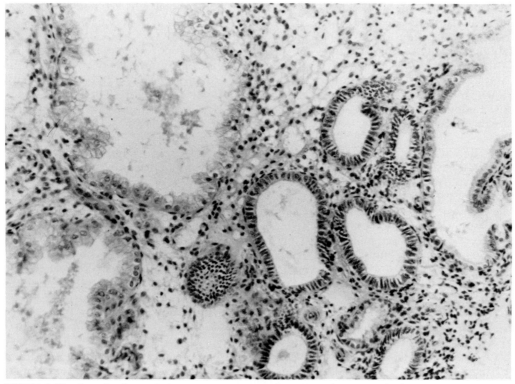

FIGURE 4-33 Complex hyperplasia treated by progestogens (irregular maturation).

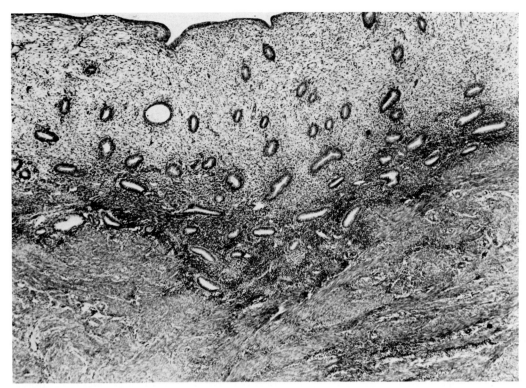

FIGURE 4-34 Hypoplastic endometrium.

tween these two lesions is that the diagnosis of both, and of the early malignant changes associated with them, is clouded by the profusion of different terminologies that have been proposed in the past and by the often highly subjective factors in distinguishing histopathologic pictures.

Because of the premalignant significance of this lesion, it will be discussed in greater detail in the section on endometrial carcinoma.

Endometrium of Irregular Shedding. Synonyms are *irregular desquamation* and *endometrium of prolonged luteal activity.* Examination of the endometrium in certain cases of profuse and prolonged menstruation shows glands in all stages of involution intimately associated with other glands of secretory type; the stroma is retracted and abundant[80] (Figs. 4-35 and 4-36). This picture becomes pathologic when it is found 5 days or more after the onset of the men-

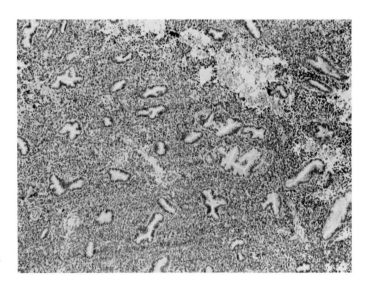

FIGURE 4-35 Irregular shedding: shrunken star-shaped glands in compact stroma.

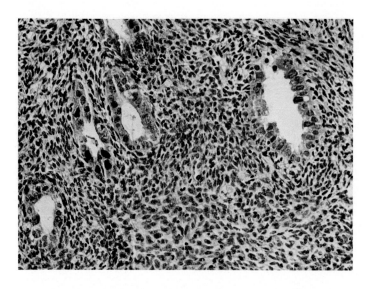

FIGURE 4-36 Irregular shedding (detail). Contracted glands show focal secretory activity and Arias-Stella changes (case of tubal ectopic pregnancy).

strual period. A small biopsy will not suffice; only a complete curettage of the mucosa can furnish the pathologist with the necessary elements for diagnosis. The existence of an organic disease should be eliminated before the diagnosis is made, because anomalies of desquamation and regeneration may be provoked by an endometrial polyp, uterine leiomyoma, or placental retention.

The retraction of the endometrium by resorption of the stromal edema, the fragmentation and separation of the mucosal debris, and the subsequent regeneration of the endometrium—phenomena that take place normally in the course of 36 to 72 hours—have their evolution prolonged beyond this time. The histologic picture is a consequence of slowing of the menstruation process. Retraction of the stroma by loss of extra- and intracellular fluid following the fall of progesterone levels does not take place completely. This causes retention of functional endometrium and of fragments of secretory mucosa adjacent to mucosa in involution. The arteries have thick hyalinized walls and are increased in diameter.

Endometrial Pattern With Oral Contraceptive Agents. The use of certain progestational agents as inhibitors of ovulation produces an increasingly more common histologic appearance of the endometrium, which we may conveniently classify among the prolonged luteal activities. These changes have been described frequently in the literature.

The administration of synthetic progestational agents (19 nor-testosterone and 17 α-hydroxyprogesterone derivatives) in association with ethinyl estradiol or mestranol from the 5th to the 24th day of the cycle provokes the appearance of precocious signs of luteinization around days 12 to 14. The histologic picture varies according to the drug dosage, the number of cycles of therapy, and other individual factors.[23,81,82] It is characterized by diminution of glandular proliferation and minimal secretion,

stromal decidualization, and the absence of mitoses (Fig. 4-37). At the 24th day, we find an atypical secretory state in which are seen glands of small caliber that are inactive and without mitoses or connective tissue spines. The stroma is very congested and shows venous lacunae and decidualization. Another characteristic finding is suppression of the spiral arterioles with development of thin-walled sinusoids.

After a few cycles, the glands are small, secretion is minimal or absent, and the epithelium is devoid of mitoses. Large doses produce earlier and more intense changes. A rare complication after many cycles is amenorrhea with persistent and irremediable endometrial atrophy.[65,83] Decidual necrosis and Arias-Stella changes have been described in rare cases.

The regimen described here is the one most commonly prescribed for oral contraception and is known as *combined therapy*. Other agents are known as *sequentials* and are characterized by an estrogen given alone from the 5th to the 19th day of the cycle, followed by 5 days of estrogen combined with a progestogen. Cycles with these agents are characterized histologically by prolonged proliferative activity preceding a shortened and less intense secretory phase.[84] Cases of endometrial hyperplasia and carcinoma have been reported after prolonged sequential therapy (Fig. 4-38). The vast majority of these cases occurred after the administration of a sequential agent (Oracon) that combined a strong estrogen with a particularly weak progestin.[85] It was subsequently shown that Oracon was the only oral contraceptive associated with an increased risk of endometrial carcinoma and that other oral contraceptives appear to be associated with a decreased risk.[86,87] In any event, all sequential agents were removed from the American and Canadian markets in 1976.

Intramuscular Administration of Long-Acting Progestogens. Long-acting progestogens (eg, Provera) administered intramuscularly produce characteristic endometrial changes that may persist for several

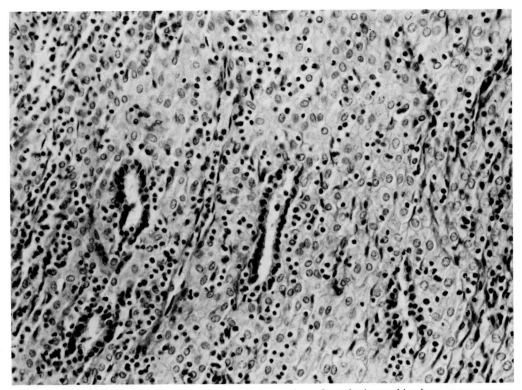

FIGURE 4-37 Endometrial biopsy after the administration of synthetic combined-type progestational agents.

months. These changes consist of decidualization of the compacta and a functional layer composed of small inactive glands, spindle cell stroma, and widely dilated venules (Fig. 4-39). Other changes reported with pure progestogens include discrete stromal cell atypias and scanning electron microscopic findings of defective cilioneogenesis.[88]

Other Progestins and the Endometrium. Progestins, alone or in combination with estrogenic agents, are

administered in other situations and dosages. One of the most common patterns of administration is in the form of combined or sequential estrogen/progestin therapy in postmenopausal women, for the main purpose of decreasing the severity of osteoporosis and cardiovascular disease without the increased risk of endometrial carcinoma noted in women who receive estrogen alone.[86,87] The sequential regimens are generally associated with endometrial histologic appearances similar to those seen in

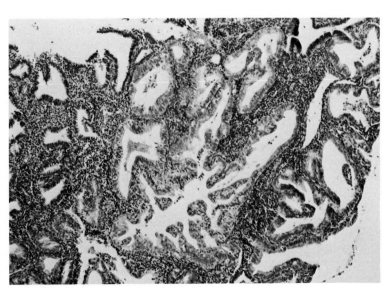

FIGURE 4-38 Focus of early adenocarcinoma of endometrium in a 34-year-old woman after 4 years of sequential oral contraceptive medication. No residual tumor was found at hysterectomy.

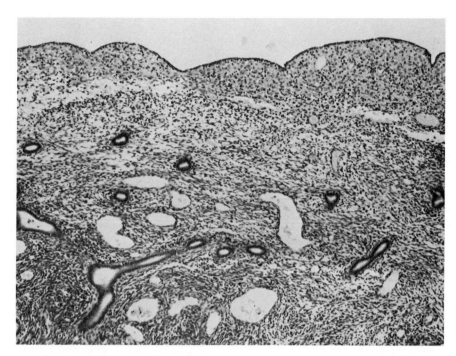

FIGURE 4-39 Endometrium at hysterectomy in a woman who received intramuscular progestogen (Provera) 1 month previously.

cycling premenopausal women, depending on when in the artificial cycle the biopsy is performed, and varying with the relative doses of estrogen and progestin. The combined continuous regimens, which are preferred by many women because of the absence of monthly withdrawal bleeding, are associated with an unpredictable endometrial response for the first 3 to 6 months, followed by an inactive or atrophic endometrium.[89,90] Patients who experience breakthrough bleeding after achieving amenorrhea for some time have in some instances been found to have polyps or carcinomas.[89]

Progestational agents can also be administered for contraceptive purposes in other than oral forms. Among the pathways of administration encountered in experimental or—in some parts of the world—clinical situations are progestin-releasing intrauterine or intracervical devices, subcutaneous implants, nasal sprays, and others. These seem to share a final common pathway of effect on the endometrium similar to those discussed above for oral or intramuscular progestogens.[91] The progestin-releasing devices may lead to endometrial stromal calcification, small polyps, and thick-walled fibrotic blood vessels after several years.[91,92]

Endometrial Pattern With Intrauterine Contraceptive Devices. Intrauterine contraceptive devices (IUDs) consist of diverse metal and plastic loops, bows, and other structures that are retained within the uterus and exert a contraceptive effect by a mechanism that is not clearly established. One of the two most widely accepted hypotheses assumes that the ovum arrives in the uterus when the endometrium is out of phase for implantation (endometrial asynchronism), whereas the other favors a primary

retardation of the biochemical maturation of the endometrium.[93]

Several studies have investigated endometrial histology after prolonged retention of the IUD. However, both IUDs and studies related to them have become less popular in the Western world in recent years. Although Rozin and his colleagues[94] noted no significant histologic abnormality except for chronic endometritis in 17% of cases, other workers have described minor but consistent focal changes.[93,95,96] The most common of these is superficial stromal edema beneath the IUD, often with some fibrosis and increased superficial vascularity consisting of large thin-walled vascular channels. A precocious decidual reaction around the vessels, sometimes accompanied by discrete hyalinization, also has been noted. Endometrial dating is often, but by no means always, behind the expected pattern. Significant changes in the glands have not been described. True endometritis can be diagnosed only by finding inflammation away from the immediate vicinity of the IUD. Copper-containing IUDs may influence various biochemical mechanisms and have a spermotoxic effect. The findings associated with progestin-impregnated devices have been discussed above.[91] A rare complication of the shield-type IUD has been fatal sepsis during pregnancy.[97]

The *cytologic findings* in IUD wearers have been reviewed by Risse and associates[98] and by Gupta.[99] Prominent among these is the finding of *Actinomyces* organisms (see Fig. 4-57) in the cervicovaginal smears of about 10% of women with an IUD in place and in about 25% of IUD wearers with symptoms of infection (eg, brown, foul-smelling vaginal discharge).[99,100] Some of these women may develop clinically significant, often unilateral, salpingitis and tubo-ovarian abscesses due to these organisms. See Chapter 5 for a more complete discussion of this problem.

Another worrisome cytologic complication of the IUD is the appearance of atypical cells in Pap smears. The most commonly encountered atypias are represented by vacuolated columnar cells (Fig. 4-40*A* and Color Fig. 4-4), which probably are derived from atypical endocervical hyperplasia, endometrial tubal metaplasia, or both, and by *IUD cells* of indeterminate type with a high nuclear–cytoplasmic ratio (Fig. 4-40*B* and Color Fig. 4-4), which are thought to be of histiocytic or endometrial origin. The differential diagnosis of the former cell type must include various adenocarcinomas, but the age of the patient, small number of atypical cells, and absence of a "tumor diathesis" all militate against a malignant diagnosis, as does the prompt disappearance of these cells after removal of the IUD. The IUD cells bear a strong resemblance to the "third-type

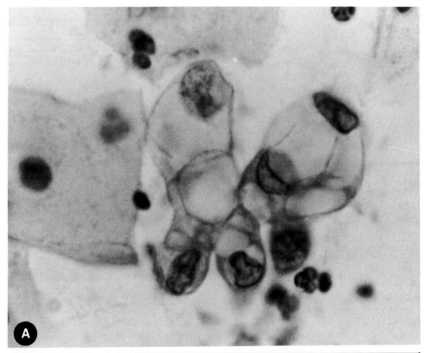

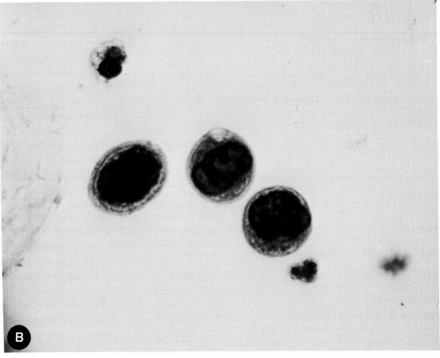

FIGURE 4-40 Atypical cells seen in cervicovaginal Papanicolaou smears of IUD wearers. **(A)** Vacuolated columnar cells. **(B)** Cells of probable histiocytic or endometrial origin resembling "third-type" cells of cervical in situ squamous carcinoma. (Gupta PK: Intrauterine contraceptive devices: Vaginal cytology, pathologic changes and clinical implications. Acta Cytol 26:571–613, 1982)

cells" of squamous cell carcinoma in situ, and this differential diagnosis is summarized in Table 4-1. The most helpful single feature is the absence of dysplastic cells of a lesser degree of atypia in smears with IUD cells. Dysplasias and carcinomas can, of course, occur in IUD wearers, but there is no good evidence to suggest an increased frequency of these lesions in this population.

Other Iatrogenic Stimuli. Premenopausal infertile women in whom some form of in vitro fertilization is being considered may be subjected to *mock cycles*, in which their endogenous menstrual cycle is suppressed with an agent such as leuprolide (Lupron) and an exogenous cycle stimulated with estrogen and progesterone. Biopsies are performed during these cycles to determine how closely the iatrogenic cycle simulates a natural one; thus, a biopsy performed on day 18 or day 26 should be evaluated to determine whether it conforms to the corresponding date of a natural idealized 28-day cycle or one with a shortened or lengthened proliferative phase.[101]

Clomiphene citrate is an agent that is thought to bind estrogen receptors in the hypothalamus (antiestrogenic effect), promoting secretion of FSH with subsequent increased estrogen production followed by an LH surge. Clomiphene is used as an inducer of

ovulation in certain infertile women and has been shown to have estrogenic and antiestrogenic effects in various organs. In a recent study, Benda noted that secretory-phase endometrial biopsies from infertility patients receiving clomiphene showed a characteristic hypoestrogenic effect (less tortuous glands than normal, scant secretions, inspissated luminal secretions, low cuboidal late secretory glandular epithelium, and sometimes smaller than normal decidualized stromal cells).[102]

Postcoital contraception (also known as *morning after pills*) is available in many parts of the world.[103] Several different types of agents are used, and their effects on the endometrium are variable and in some instances poorly described. RU 486, an antiprogesteronal steroid, has been noted to cause degenerative changes in endometrial stroma and endothelial cells.[103]

Endometrium of Traumatic Amenorrhea (Asherman's Syndrome). Another iatrogenic condition is the rare Asherman's syndrome, which is characterized clinically by secondary amenorrhea or hypomenorrhea and pathologically by destruction of the endometrium with subsequent synechial (and rarely calcific) obliteration of the uterine cavity.[104,105] More than 25% of all the cases in the literature have been reported from Israel, the site of the first description of the entity. The etiology generally involves a vulnerable endometrium affected by inflammation and trauma. The great majority of all cases follow curettage related to pregnancy, usually postpartum or postabortal. Other operative procedures may also be represented, and a small proportion of cases are unrelated to surgical trauma; these latter cases are usually the result of tuberculous endometritis.[104] A new cause is laser ablation of the endometrium, which is performed under hysteroscopic control for the conservative management of dysfunctional uterine bleeding.[106,107]

The underlying endometrium in this condition is often functional, and the presence of adenomyosis is common. Treatment (if desired) is by repeat dilatation and curettage, usually followed by insertion of an IUD and administration of estrogenic hormones.[104,108]

Histologic Modifications of the Endometrium in the Presence of Trophoblast. Characteristic endometrial histologic modifications occur in the presence of ectopic pregnancy, hydatidiform mole, and choriocarcinoma. Pictures of endometrial regression have been described in cases of extrauterine pregnancy with fetal death. According to Baniecki,[109] these histologic modifications are divided into three stages. First, the decidual reaction regresses but persists around convoluted and hyalinized arterioles. Subsequently, the decidual reaction disappears, the stroma retracts, and arteriolar hyalinization is aggravated. In the third stage, stromal retraction continues, and the glands are small and round and still show signs of discrete secretory activity (Fig. 4-41; see Fig. 4-36).

TABLE 4-1.
Differentiating Features of IUD Cells versus Carcinoma In Situ Cells

	IUD cells	Carcinoma In Situ Cells
Tissue fragments	Present	Absent
Cell quantity	Scant	Generally abundant
Dysplastic cells	Absent	Present
Inflammation	Generally present	Generally absent
Bizarre forms	Present	Absent
Preservation	Poor	Good
Nuclear envelope	Wrinkled	Wavy
Chromatin	Clumped and fuzzy	Granular and uniform
Nucleoli	Present	Absent
Multinucleation	Present	Absent
Crisp cytoplasm (squamoid, metaplastic)	Present	Absent

Adapted from Gupta PK: Intrauterine contraceptive devices. Vaginal cytology, pathologic changes, and clinical implications. Acta Cytol 26:571–613, 1982.

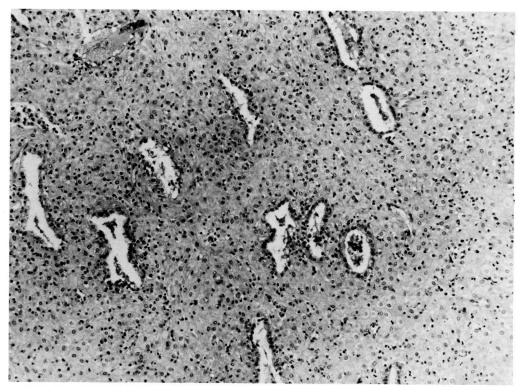

FIGURE 4-41 Regressive transformation of endometrium in the presence of an extrauterine pregnancy.

This regressive transformation of the endometrium permits suspicion of the existence of an extrauterine pregnancy in the process of degeneration. This picture is not specific and is found in irregular shedding, in certain intrauterine abortions, during oral contraceptive administration, and even in the normal mucosa in its resting phase.

Arias-Stella[110,111] studied specifically the endometrial glands in curettings from women carrying ectopic pregnancies and found the characteristic nuclear and cytoplasmic atypical changes (Fig. 4-42A) that have come to bear his name (*Arias-Stella phenomenon*). He attributes these cellular alterations to the presence of chorionic tissue. The mechanism of appearance of these changes has not been definitely elucidated, although they appear in most instances to represent a response to elevated levels of chorionic gonadotropin. Although some authors have considered them to be regressive changes,[112] Silverberg[113] has shown that they are present with presumably normal intrauterine gestations, and Wagner and Richart[114] have demonstrated that the constituent glandular cells are polyploid. These two observations and others like them suggest that the phenomenon is proliferative and secretory rather than regressive.

These changes are encountered in all of the following conditions: normal pregnancy, postabortal and postpartum metropathies, ectopic pregnancy, and chorionic tumors. We have seen them on rare occasions in the absence of any known source of gonadotropic hormonal stimulation. Although Arias-

Stella himself emphasized their significance in the diagnosis of ectopic pregnancy (particularly when neither decidua nor chorionic villi are seen in an endometrial curettage specimen), Kjer and Eldon[115] have noted that ectopic pregnancy was present in only 16% of cases in which endometrial Arias-Stella phenomenon was observed. In cases of intrauterine pregnancy, the changes may be seen as early as the 12th day of gestation and may persist for up to 8 weeks following the expulsion of the placental tissue.

Histologic examination shows large, irregular, hyperchromatic glandular nuclei surrounded by abundant vacuolated cytoplasm. The nuclei are disposed in all directions, not necessarily following the greatest axis of the cell. The epithelium of the glands is stratified and sometimes assumes a pseudopapillary disposition. In some cases, particularly when associated with an abnormal gestation or a tumor, secretory vacuolation may be minimal. Hobnail and clear cell epithelial changes, described predominantly in gestational endometria, probably represent limited variants of Arias-Stella phenomenon.

The diagnostic value of these endometrial changes is relative, as seen previously, because they lack specificity. Nonetheless, they at least permit the strong suspicion of an ectopic pregnancy or a chorionic tumor when they are found on endometrial biopsy in the absence of other findings diagnostic of intrauterine pregnancy. Ultrastructural studies have shown that these cells have high metabolic activity, expressed by a well-developed endoplasmic retic-

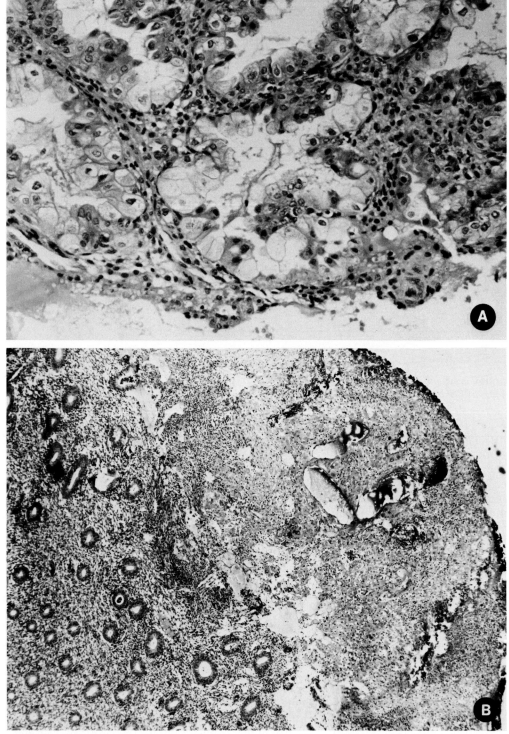

FIGURE 4-42 **(A)** Atypical cellular changes in association with pregnancy described by Arias-Stella. **(B)** Superficial retained placental tissue in the process of necrosis.

ulum and the presence of numerous glycogen granules.[116]

Differential Diagnosis. Differential diagnosis of these alterations must be made with clear cell carcinoma of the endometrium. In the latter condition, although the cytology is similar, the architectural features of stromal invasion are present. The Arias-Stella phenomenon may be seen in intrauterine endometrial glands, in foci of endometriosis, in endocervical glands, in the glands of vaginal adenosis, and in the mucosa of the fallopian tube. Finally, nuclear pseudoinclusions occasionally seen within the glandular cells should not lead to confusion with a herpetic or cytomegaloviral endometritis.[117]

Postabortal Endometrium. Surface re-epithelialization is completed by 1 week postabortion, and signs of active proliferation are present around 10 days postabortion. Ovulation, which occurs around day 44 after a normal delivery, appears earlier after abortion. Decidual fragments have been found during the first 3 weeks postabortum (Fig. 4-42*B*). The inflammatory reaction that is often present (poly-

morphonuclear leukocytes and plasma cells) is not accompanied by clinical signs of endometritis. This foreign body reaction follows the necrosis of degenerating decidua and trophoblast.

Mucus- or Lipid-Laden Macrophages in the Endometrial Stroma. Large macrophages with abundant foamy cytoplasm (Fig. 4-43) are occasionally encoun-

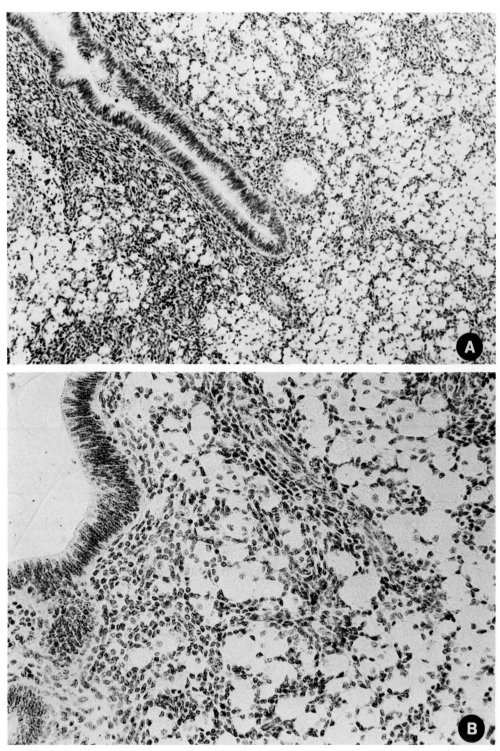

FIGURE 4-43 Fatty degeneration of stromal cells. **(A)** General appearance. **(B)** Detail. (Courtesy of Dr. R. Cordier)

tered in banal mucosae, polyps, hyperplasias, and carcinomas and low-grade stromal tumors of the endometrium. Their pathologic significance is not clear. Macrophages containing mucicarminophilic and PAS-positive substances probably represent phagocytosis of material coming from the glands. Cells rich in lipids (neutral fats) are seen with greater frequency in cases of carcinoma and may arouse a suspicion of malignancy even when seen in an otherwise benign curettage; however, in a late secretory endometrium, these probably represent merely a regressive phenomenon.[118] The mechanism of appearance of these cells is unknown. Ultrastructural studies have shown them to be of stromal origin.[119] When seen in association with carcinoma, they are of no prognostic or other clinical significance.[120] This picture is different from that observed after the injection of contrast media, in which case a true foreign-body granulomatous reaction is seen.

Glandular Invaginations or Double Contours.

Invaginations of the glandular epithelium sometimes appear in endometrial glands. On occasion, the base of invagination is visible and forms a papillary digitation. More often, the plane of section does not pass through the region of implantation, and the image formed is that of several concentric epithelial walls or glands within glands (Fig. 4-44). This image does not necessarily result from poor fixation or the trauma of the biopsy technique, because it is also found in hysterectomy specimens fixed in toto with no manipulation of the endometrium before fixation. Plastic reconstitutions have been carried out by Hampson and Gerlis,[121] who attribute the origin of these invaginations to the disposition of the endometrial vessels. They appear especially in the deep parts of the glands, which are irrigated by the basal arteries. This vascularization, more abundant than that of the spiral arteries, causes a difference in the development of the gland and the appearance of these epithelial invaginations.

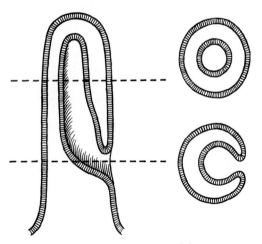

FIGURE 4-44 Endometrium: double glandular contours.

"Cracking" Artifact of the Glands.

The glands are separated from the stroma by an empty space (Fig. 4-45). This artifact is caused by tardy fixation.

Hemorrhage.

Diffuse recent hemorrhages may be due to the manipulations of the biopsy procedure. A method of eliminating them is to wash the curettings rapidly in physiologic liquid (normal saline) before placing them in the fixative.

Postradiotherapeutic and Postcurettage Lesions.

Irradiation of the normal uterine mucosa,[122] as in the course of radiation therapy of cervical cancer, produces atrophy of the mucosa with bizarre glandular cells, nuclear pyknosis, and loss of the tinctorial affinities of the cells (Fig. 4-46). Similar pictures may occur as *regenerative atypias* after previous curettage. Flattened surface epithelial cells may be present within 3 days after curettage, but it takes 7 to 9 days or more for complete restoration of the endometrium; regeneration is even slower if the curettage was performed in the secretory phase[123] and may take 3 months or more after total endometrial ablation by laser.[106]

If the curettage or radiation therapy was administered for endometrial carcinoma, it is important not to misinterpret these reactive glandular changes as residual carcinoma. A false impression of myometrial invasion by carcinoma may be given, particularly if these changes are seen in glands participating in adenomyosis. As in the differential diagnosis of the Arias-Stella phenomenon (see above), the absence of architectural features of stromal invasion is of primary importance.

After radiation therapy, the stroma shows cytologic alterations of atypical nature and is infiltrated with leukocytes. If the dose of radiation is very high, phenomena of necrosis dominate. Depending on the modalities of irradiation, the atrophy may be complete or followed by partial regeneration. Appearance of malignant endometrial tumors several years after pelvic irradiation has been reported.[124]

Foci of Dense Stromal Cellularity.

The appearance of nodular aggregates of closely packed but otherwise cytologically normal stromal cells was noted by Picoff and Luginbuhl[125] in 10.7% of the endometria that they examined. This finding was almost always associated with bleeding for 24 hours or longer, either physiologic (menstruation) or pathologic, and was not specific for any one diagnostic entity. The researchers ascribed the origin of these foci to compaction of stromal cells rather than to hyperplasia. We have seen these "stromal balls" misinterpreted as carcinoma, but they are totally lacking in cytologic atypia (see Fig. 4-25).

Fibrin in the Endometrial Stroma.

Clumps of material identifiable as fibrin are not infrequently seen in

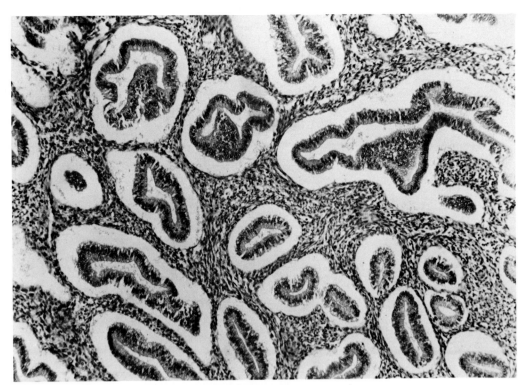

FIGURE 4-45 Glandular retraction with "cracking" artifact.

curetted endometria and seem to be associated with the presence of abnormal bleeding. Picoff and Luginbuhl[126] have proposed that these fibrin clumps may be the histologic evidence of an underlying defect in the fibrinolytic mechanism in these states.

ENDOMETRIAL METAPLASIAS

A great number of metaplastic phenomena can occur in the endometrium, some appearing after known etiologic stimuli and others occurring without known antecedents. The metaplasias can be grouped into epithelial and stromal types and will be discussed in that order. Hendrickson and Kempson[127] have classified the epithelial metaplasias into seven categories:

1. morules and squamous metaplasia
2. papillary metaplasia
3. ciliated cell or tubal metaplasia
4. eosinophilic metaplasia
5. mucinous metaplasia
6. hobnail metaplasia
7. clear cell metaplasia.

The newer classification of the International Society of Gynecological Pathologists (ISGP; Table 4-2) expands these seven to nine, notes that most of them are not truly metaplastic phenomena, and includes nonepithelial metaplastic and related changes.[128]

Squamous Metaplasia

Squamous metaplasia of slight or considerable proportion is seen in endometria under a large variety of circumstances (Fig. 4-47). Among these are excessive hormonal stimulation, intrauterine administration of chemicals, presence of an IUD, vitamin A deficiency, senility, polyps, tumors, chronic inversion, chronic endometritis (including tuberculous and luetic endometritis), and pyometra.[129] Very extensive squamous metaplasia is sometimes designated as *ichthyosis uteri*, especially if it largely covers the surface of the endometrium. Foci that are epidermoid in appearance but lack intercellular bridges are known as *morules* (Fig. 4-48).[130]

The main significance of these proliferations is that, like many of the other epithelial metaplasias, they are frequently confused with cancer. It is important to remember that carcinoma of the endometrium is diagnosed primarily from the glandular component. If the glands appear benign and do not invade their own stroma, and if the squamous or morular elements are also histologically benign, it is safe to assume that the overall lesion is benign.[131] If the glands show malignant characteristics, the diagnosis is adenocarcinoma with squamous differentiation (see below).

It has been hypothesized that squamous metaplasia may be a precursor of squamous cell carcinoma of the endometrium, but this malignant transformation, if it occurs at all, is extremely rare, because only about 30 cases of pure squamous cell carcinoma of the endometrium have been reported.

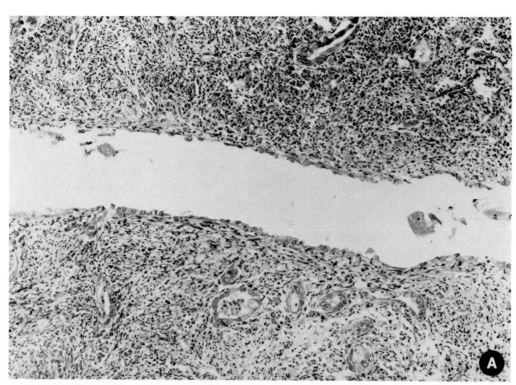

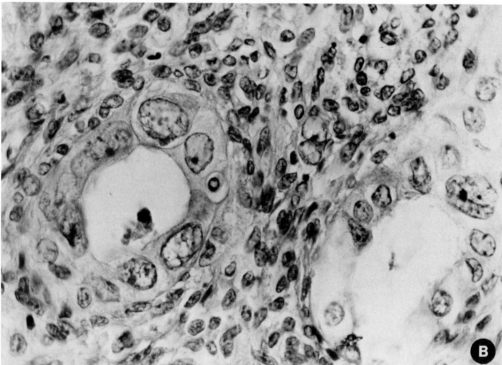

FIGURE 4-46 Postradiotherapeutic lesions in a previously normal endometrium. **(A)** General appearance. **(B)** Detail.

Papillary Proliferation and Surface Syncytial Change

It is often difficult to differentiate papillary proliferation from surface syncytial change. They tend to occur together, although the latter is more common.

Both usually are found at or near the endometrial surface. Surface syncytial change is characterized by cells that appear to form a syncytium (Fig. 4-49) but may contain papillary projections as well (Fig. 4-50). When the papillae contain fibrovascular stromal cores, the designation of papillary proliferation is

TABLE 4-2.
Endometrial Metaplasias and Related Changes

Epithelial metaplastic and related changes
   Squamous metaplasia and morules
   Mucinous metaplasia (including intestinal)
   Ciliary change
   Hobnail change
   Clear cell change
   Eosinophilic cell change (including oncocytic)
   Surface syncytial change
   Papillary proliferation
   Arias-Stella change

Nonepithelial metaplastic and related changes
   Smooth muscle metaplasia
   Osseous metaplasia
   Cartilaginous metaplasia
   Fatty change
   Glial tissue
   Foam cell change
   Retained fetal products

Silverberg SG, Kurman RJ: Tumors of the uterine corpus and gestational trophoblastic disease. In Atlas of tumor pathology, 3rd series, fascicle 3. Washington, DC, Armed Forces Institute of Pathology, 1992

preferable. The overall appearance is often reminiscent of microglandular hyperplasia of the endocervix, but this endometrial lesion is usually seen in patients under estrogenic stimulation rather than progestational stimulation. The surface location of the lesion, the cytologically bland nuclei, the indistinct cytoplasmic margins, and the frequent penetra-

tion of the lesion by neutrophils all help make the differential diagnosis from papillary serous or endometrioid adenocarcinoma. Although surface syncytial change appears to be benign, we have now seen several cases in which it was associated with an underlying carcinoma, so this possibility should always be kept in mind.

Ciliary Change

Ciliary change is commonly known as *tubal metaplasia*, but it may or may not include the full spectrum of cell types seen in adult fallopian tubal mucosa. The characteristic feature is the presence of glands lined by cells with bland nuclei, brightly eosinophilic cytoplasm, and numerous cilia (Fig. 4-51). In some instances, intercalated and muciparous cells may also be present, intensifying the resemblance to tubal epithelium. This change also seems to be more common in endometria in hyperestrogenic states.[132]

As in most of the epithelial metaplasias, the main significance of this lesion lies in its frequent confusion with more worrisome lesions, particularly atypical hyperplasia, which is also often recognized at low power by the presence of cytoplasmic eosinophilia. The main distinction is the presence of ciliated cells and the absence of nuclear stratification and atypia in ciliary change. However, carcinomas containing many ciliated cells do occur in the endometrium, and these are best diagnosed by architectural evidence of stromal invasion.[133]

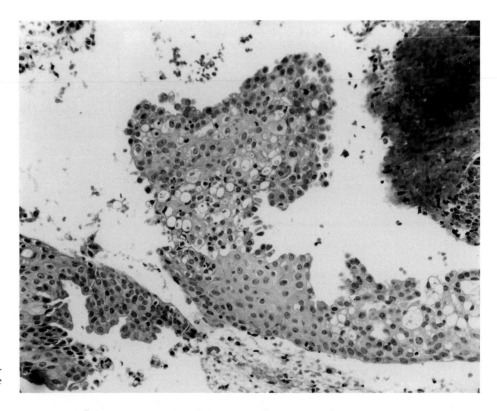

FIGURE 4-47 Squamous metaplasia in endometrial curettage specimen.

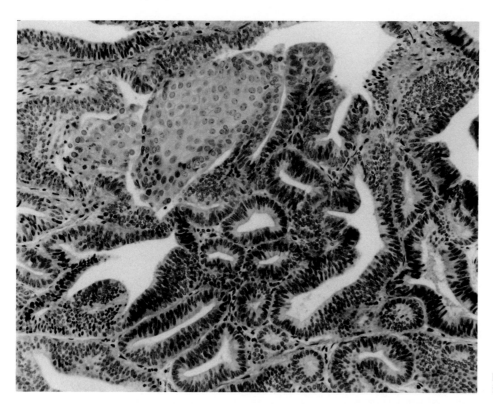

FIGURE 4-48 Morular metaplasia in hyperplastic endometrium.

Eosinophilic Cell Change

Eosinophilic cell change includes cells with the brightly eosinophilic cytoplasm of ciliary change but without the cilia (see Fig. 4-49). Occasionally these cells may demonstrate the typical features of oncocytes, in which case some nuclear atypia may also be present.[134] In most instances, however, the absence of atypia helps in the differential diagnosis from atypical hyperplasia.

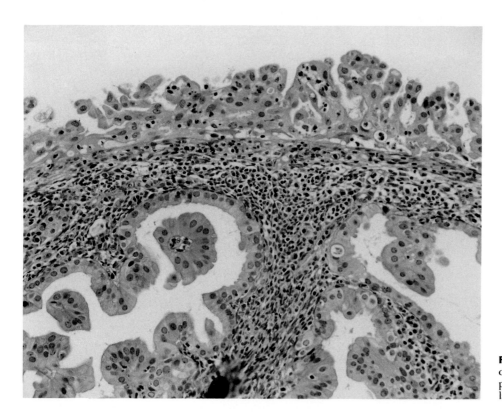

FIGURE 4-49 Surface syncytial change and underlying eosinophilic cell change with focal papillary proliferation.

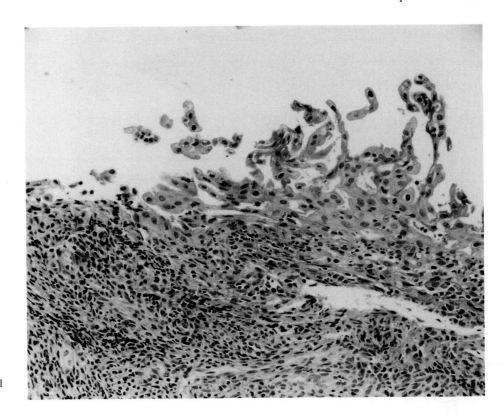

FIGURE 4-50 Surface syncytial change with papillary features.

Mucinous Metaplasia

Mucinous metaplasia is usually a true endocervical metaplasia because, as in the case of full tubal metaplasia, the lesion seems to represent an example of cells in the endometrium differentiating along another müllerian pathway. Demopoulos and Greco[135] have shown that the endometrial epithelial cells in mucinous metaplasia are identical to endocervical epithelial cells both ultrastructurally and histochemically. Occasionally, an intestinal type of mucinous metaplasia is encountered.

Although the usual appearance of this uncommon metaplasia consists of glands lined by tall columnar mucin-secreting cells (Fig. 4-52), we have seen examples in which this metaplastic endocervical-type epithelium developed a secondary microglandular hyperplasia (Fig. 4-53).

As with the other types of metaplasia, the main significance of this lesion is its distinction from the uncommon endocervical-type mucinous carcinoma arising in the endometrium.[136,137] When mucinous metaplasia is seen in a curettage or biopsy specimen, it may be difficult to appreciate that the source of

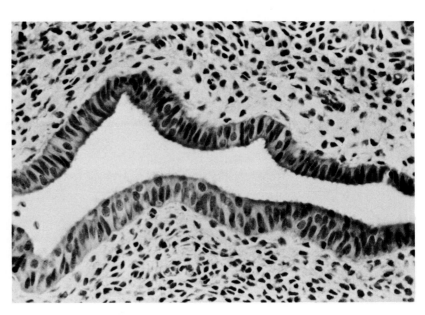

FIGURE 4-51 Tubal metaplasia. Ciliated and intercalated cells are present.

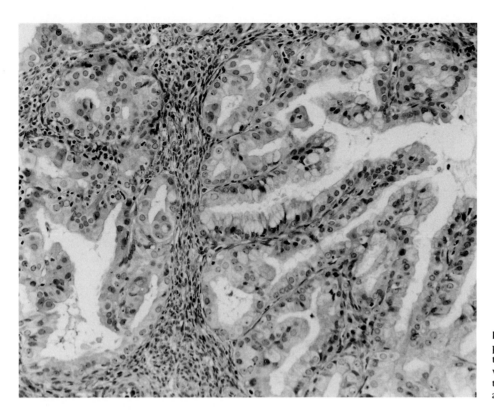

FIGURE 4-52 Mucinous metaplasia of endometrium. Although the cells are mostly of endocervical type, a few goblet cells (intestinal-type mucinous metaplasia) are present.

the specimen was indeed the endometrium rather than the endocervix.

Hobnail and Clear Cell Changes

Two other epithelial changes described by Hendrickson and Kempson[127] are the hobnail and clear cell types. These are both rare and, as would be expected, their differential diagnosis lies mainly with clear cell carcinoma and Arias-Stella phenomenon.

Like the latter, they are both encountered mainly in gestational endometria. We have observed hobnail cells in the endometrium not infrequently as a response to trauma.

Frequency of Epithelial Metaplastic and Related Changes

Careful searches for these lesions have not been performed in large series of consecutive otherwise

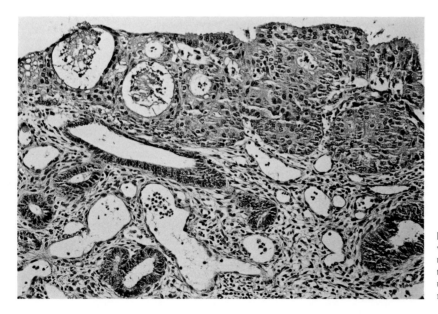

FIGURE 4-53 Microglandular hyperplasia with squamous metaplasia in endocervical-type surface epithelium overlying endometrial basalis. Section is from high in the uterine corpus and is not contiguous with mucosa of endocervical canal.

normal endometrial specimens, so we do not know their population-based prevalences. Many of them, as mentioned above, seem to be related to specific hormonal stimuli (including Arias-Stella change, which is discussed earlier in this chapter). In our own anecdotal experience, the most commonly seen forms other than Arias-Stella change have been (in descending order of frequency) ciliary change, surface syncytial change, and squamous metaplasia and morules. Because these pictures often occur together, it is not unusual to see two or three of them in the same specimen (see Fig. 4-49). There are no known clinical signs or symptoms associated with these lesions, so that they are basically incidental findings in endometrial specimens seen by the pathologist for other reasons.

One of these reasons may be endometrial hyperplasia or carcinoma, and one or more of the metaplastic and related changes may be noted either within the hyperplastic or neoplastic epithelium or in the nonlesional endometrium accompanying it.[138-140] This phenomenon seems to be more common in the United States than in Japan, and in well-differentiated than in poorly differentiated carcinomas, and is probably a favorable prognostic marker when seen in association with carcinoma.

Mesenchymal Metaplasias and Related Changes

In addition to epithelial changes, certain rare types of metaplastic and related changes occur in the endometrial stroma (see Table 4-2). These involve the formation of islands of benign cartilage, bone, smooth muscle, and adipose and perhaps glial tissue. Also encountered are foam cell change (discussed above) and retained fetal products (listed in this classification because they enter into the differential diagnosis of most of the other changes).

Smooth muscle metaplasia is the most common of these mesenchymal metaplasias, as would be expected from the well-known ability of endometrial stroma to differentiate into smooth muscle.[141] These are usually small foci of typical benign smooth muscle, which have sometimes been referred to as *intraendometrial leiomyomas*. Smooth muscle, apart from blood vessel walls, is also seen in about 1% of endometrial polyps (adenomyomatous polyps). Its main differential diagnosis is with epithelial morules.

Foci of *osseous*[142] and *cartilaginous*[143] *metaplasia* are encountered rarely in the endometrium, usually in the postabortal state. These lesions occasionally may represent fetal parts from a previous abortion, but more often they represent a true metaplasia, because their origin from endometrial stromal cells may be demonstrable. These benign metaplasias occasionally can be seen within the stroma of an endometrial carcinoma or sarcoma and should not lead to the erroneous diagnosis of a carcinosarcoma (malignant mixed mesodermal tumor), in which the heterologous stromal elements are histologically malignant.[144]

Glial tissues in the uterus represent the most controversial of these lesions,[145-147] because only mesodermal-derived tissues would be expected to be within the metaplastic capabilities of the endometrial stroma. Most observers of these lesions have postulated an origin from a previous abortion. Although the glial tissues may present in the endometrium per se, they are most frequently found in a cervical polyp. They may be associated with foci of cartilage, bone, and squamous epithelium. Occasionally they may resemble a true glioma.[147]

INFLAMMATORY DISEASES OF THE ENDOMETRIUM

Discussion of the inflammatory pathology of the endometrium formerly occupied a major position in tracts of anatomic pathology. Its importance has been reduced considerably since the discovery of the genital hormones, because most of these histologic alterations are in reality due to modifications of the hormonal equilibrium. Furthermore, the use of antibiotics has reduced the frequency of infections.

Endometritis is encountered in acute or chronic form. In the past it was most often of bacterial origin, and in most cases the causative organism was a streptococcus, staphylococcus, colibacillus, enterococcus (principally in puerperal infection), gonococcus, or tubercle bacillus.

More recent reports[148-151] have stressed the importance of anaerobic infections of the endometrium and of using appropriate culture techniques to identify these infections. Specific organisms that have been identified with increasing frequency include *Chlamydia trachomatis*,[148,151,152] which is sometimes identified in the endometrium of salpingitis patients with irregular bleeding; *Ureaplasma urealyticum*,[153] which has been mentioned as a possible cause of infertility; *Mycoplasma* organisms,[154] which have been mentioned as a cause of infertility; *Toxoplasma gondii*,[155] which has been associated with repeated spontaneous abortions; and *Actinomyces* species,[99,100] which have been seen notably in women using IUDs.

Acute Endometritis

Acute Puerperal Infection

Postpartum endometritis, the frequency and severity of which have diminished considerably since the discovery of antibiotics, represented a major scourge in maternities a half century ago. The pathologic anatomy of this infection was the object of a very complete study by Halban and Koehler,[156] based on 163 autopsied cases. The bacteria isolated include group A hemolytic streptococci, hemolytic *Staphylococcus aureus*, and various anaerobes. Mixed infections are common, and *Chlamydia* are seen frequently in late infections.[148,151]

The *etiology* should be looked for in surgical interventions, minor daily traumata to the genital organs, perineal and cervical lacerations, or curettages. The internal surface of the uterus is edematous and congested, dark in color, covered with petechiae, and involved by ulcers of diverse sizes. When the infection is aggravated, there is necrosis of the decidua with gray shreds of tissue eliminated spontaneously, among which are found vestiges of chorionic villi. Necrotic decidua can be seen, however, in the absence of significant endometritis. The ulcerated surfaces are covered with a purulent necrotic exudate. The infection extends to the myometrium, which is soft and edematous and may, in certain cases, undergo partial or even total necrosis. In these most severe but fortunately rare cases, greatly feared complications include uterine necrosis, propagation of the infection into the fallopian tubes, and extension into lymphatics and veins. Notable sequelae include thrombophlebitis with pulmonary emboli, parietal or intraligamentous abscesses, peritonitis, and episodes of septicemia.

Microscopically, the endometrial mucosa is invaded or even replaced by an acute inflammatory infiltrate that extends into the myometrium. Zones of tissue necrosis and microabscesses are more or less extensive and bacterial colonies are found in them. Thrombi with periarterial inflammatory infiltrates are also seen.

Gonococcal Endometritis

Contamination of the endometrium takes place by the ascending route. The endometrium presents the classic signs of an acute infection: stromal and intraglandular infiltration with neutrophils, marked vascular congestion, edema, and necrotic alteration of the glands and stroma by the inflammatory process.

Uteroadnexal Infarction

The uteroadnexal infarct is a rare and ominous lesion. It consists of gangrenous phenomena of toxic origin appearing at the beginning or end of pregnancy. At the beginning of pregnancy, the infarct is in general a complication of abortion; at the end of pregnancy, it is related to toxemia.[157]

The *etiology* may be of autonomic neural reflex origin (vascular spasm) or may involve bacterial toxicity when there is a secondary infection. The organisms responsible are predominantly anaerobes (*Clostridium perfringens*) and streptococci. *Clinical manifestations* are a state of shock, signs of septicemia, and an acute painful abdominal syndrome, with eventual complications of oliguria or anuria, myocarditis, and hypofibrinogenemia.

Macroscopically, the uterus is dark red with black or gray zones corresponding to hemorrhagic or necrotic foci. The vessels are all thrombosed. Sections reveal a largely necrotic myometrium. Perforation is occasionally seen. Infarction may extend to the adnexa and the parametria, which also appear dark red or black.

Histologically, there is infarction with massive hemorrhage and secondary necrosis, the cause of which is found more often in reflex arterial spasm than in venous thrombosis.

The evolution is always grave and necessitates rapid intervention with resection of the involved structures. Infarction of the uterus may also occur rarely as a complication of arteriosclerosis, thromboembolism, or dissecting aneurysm.

Chronic Endometritis

Bacterial Endometritis

The origin of a chronic endometritis should be searched for in inflammatory lesions of other portions of the genital system, particularly the fallopian tubes, which secondarily involve the endometrium.[151] These lesions are often secondary to minor traumata of the cervix, vagina, and perineum during delivery. The periodic desquamation of the endometrium explains why these lesions rarely attain the intensity and chronicity of those of the cervix. They are characterized by lymphoplasmacytic infiltrates of the stroma and glands. Because lymphocytes and even lymphoid follicles may be found in normal endometria,[1,24–26] most authors require the presence of plasma cells for the diagnosis of chronic endometritis.[158,159] Although these may be difficult to find, their presence (and that of endometritis) is suggested when an endometrium shows a phase discrepancy in the absence of another cause or shows pronounced spindle cell alteration of the stroma (Fig. 4-54).

Cases of chronic endometritis frequently show proliferative responses of the endometrial glands that may be characterized by architectural (Fig. 4-55) or, less frequently, cytologic atypia (see Fig. 4-54B). Pathologists should realize that this proliferative response precludes dating the endometrium, and they should not fall into the trap of overdiagnosing a chronic endometritis as an endometrial hyperplasia.

A frequent cause of chronic endometritis is placental retention (see Fig. 4-42B). This etiology is easily recognized by the presence of placental villi that may be well preserved, in the process of hyalinization, or reduced to hyaline and fibrous masses. In other cases, islands of decidual cells surrounded by leukocytic and histiocytic infiltrates persist in the depths of the endometrium and maintain chronic inflammatory foci. These cells should not be confused with the groups of stromal foam cells found in zones of tumor necrosis.

Endometrial Tuberculosis

The development of endometrial tuberculosis is related to that of pulmonary tuberculosis. Dissemina-

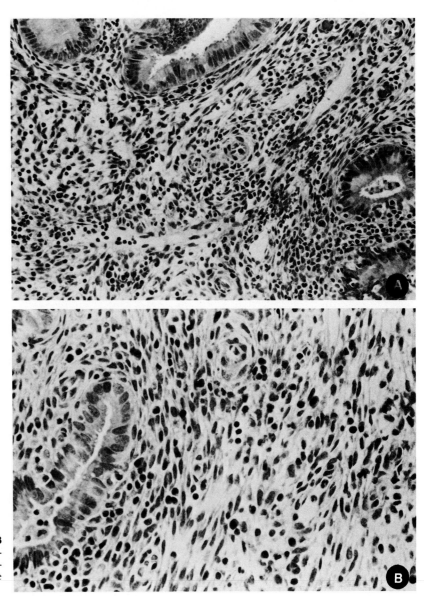

FIGURE 4-54 Chronic endometritis. **A** and **B** are from different cases, but both show spindled and edematous stroma infiltrated by lymphocytes and plasma cells. **B** also shows some reactive atypia of an endometrial gland.

tion takes place by the hematogenous route. Endometrial localization is, in the great majority of cases, secondary to a tubal lesion and represents the second most frequent genital site of this infection. It is found most commonly in young women between 15 and 40 years of age and is very rare after the menopause.[160]

Endometrial tuberculosis is often asymptomatic and may be discovered in the course of a routine gynecologic examination, often performed because of sterility.

Sharman[161] detected 216 cases of endometrial tuberculosis among 3804 cases of sterility, an incidence of 5.6%. Sutherland[162] found the incidence of tuberculosis to be 1.1% among 5521 curettages and 1.4% among 864 hysterectomy specimens. However, the incidence is considerably lower today in most Western countries.

The most readily observed *symptoms* are amenor-rhea, menorrhagia, and rarely metrorrhagia. Sterility is the rule, with only rare exceptions. Peritoneal dissemination should be searched for, because this is a possible complication.

The *macroscopic appearance* of the mucosa is not always typical and may not be particularly suspicious. Occasionally, small yellow miliary granulomata are visible grossly on the mucosal surface. At an advanced stage of the disease, caseous abscesses may be seen in the mucosa and the myometrium.

The *microscopic appearance* is characterized by the presence of a granuloma rich in epithelioid cells surrounded by lymphocytes and containing Langhans-type giant cells in variable number (Fig. 4-56). Caseation is rare. These tubercles are found throughout the mucosa. In many cases, all the classic elements of the granuloma may not be present; there may be epithelioid cells without giant cells or without the surrounding crown of lymphocytes, or per-

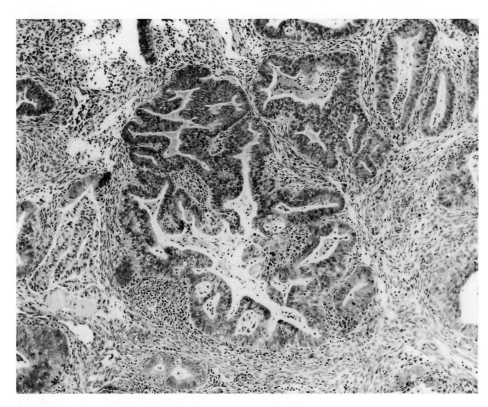

FIGURE 4-55 Chronic endometritis with marked reactive architectural atypia of endometrial glands.

haps even just diffuse lymphoplasmacytic infiltrates in the stroma and in dilated gland lumina.[163,164] In cases of sterility, these latter lesions should incite a careful search for typical granulomata, either in new sections of the original pathologic material or in a repeat biopsy. The demonstration of acid-fast bacilli by histologic means is usually impossible, and culture of the endometrium and its inoculation into the guinea pig remain indispensable for confirmation of the tuberculous nature of the lesion. Accordingly, when this diagnosis is a likely possibility, a portion of the curettings should be sent for these cultural studies rather than fixed in toto in formalin or similar material for microscopic study. Because the granulomata take up to 2 weeks to develop and are most frequently seen in the spongiosa and compacta, which are shed every 4 weeks, curettage should be performed during the premenstrual or menstrual phase.[164]

In any case of endometritis, but particularly those of tuberculous etiology, marked atypical proliferation of endometrial glands may be present. This should not be confused with a true hyperplasia or even carcinoma of the endometrium.

Viral Endometritis

Rare cases of intranuclear inclusions associated with chronic or acute endometritis have been reported in cases of herpes simplex[165] and cytomegalovirus.[166] These may be important as causes of abortion or perinatal infection. Dardi and colleagues[117] have pointed out that nuclear pseudoinclusions similar to

viral inclusions may be seen in some cases of Arias-Stella phenomenon and should not lead to confusion with viral endometritis.

Endometritis Associated with Intrauterine Contraceptive Devices

IUDs may induce a focal acute or chronic inflammatory response, which may be diffuse or limited to the endometrium immediately beneath the device. Of considerably more importance is pelvic infection in some IUD users by *Actinomyces* species, particularly *Actinomyces israelii*.[99,100] The organisms typically present as isolated, irregular, spidery, dark brown to black bodies (Fig. 4-57). Also encountered are filamentous forms and "sulfur granules" consisting of a dense central mass of tangled hyphae surrounded by peripheral, radiating, club-shaped filaments. Because other organisms and even debris from the IUD surface may simulate this morphology, Gupta[99] has recommended that the diagnosis be confirmed by a fluorescent antibody technique.

In about 10% of IUD users, *Actinomyces* organisms are seen on vaginal smears.[99] Some of these women develop significant pelvic infections, particularly salpingitis, which is often unilateral. This complication is discussed in more detail in Chapter 5.

Other Causes of Endometritis

Virtually every organism has at one time or another been reported as a cause of at least a single case of endometritis. In addition to the organisms already mentioned, these include *parasites*,[155,167,168] the most important of which worldwide are schistosomal, and various *fungi*,[169] the endometrial localization of which is generally an incidental finding in a case of widely disseminated infection. These organisms all produce granulomatous endometritis, as does *sarcoidosis*.[170] Granulomatous endometritis may also be caused by foreign bodies, particularly talc.

Malacoplakia[171] has been reported in the endometrium, although it is more frequently seen in the urinary or intestinal tract. It presents as a xanthogranulomatous inflammatory process, in which Michaelis-Gutmann bodies (intracellular and extracellular calcific spherules) are found. The etiology is thought to be bacterial. Cases of xanthogranulomatous or histiocytic endometritis without

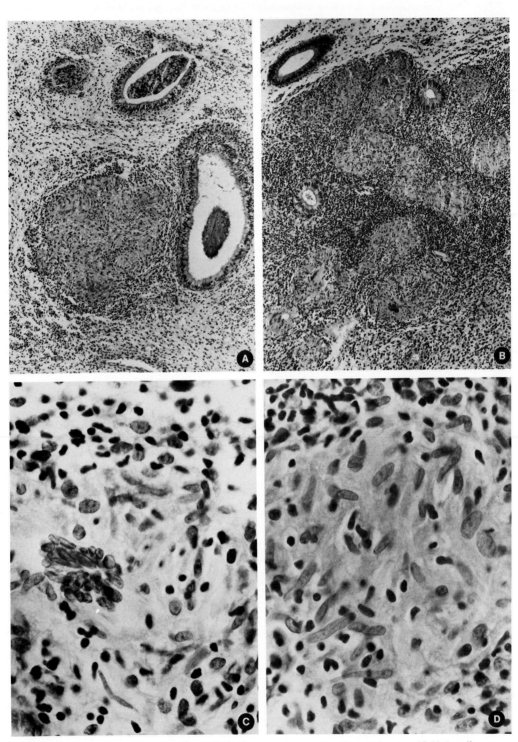

FIGURE 4-56 Endometrial tuberculosis. **(A,B)** Noncaseating giant cell granulomata. **(C,D)** Detail of epithelioid cells and giant cells.

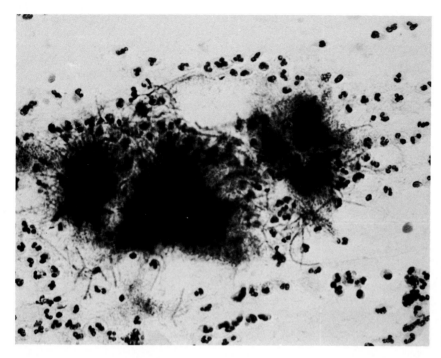

FIGURE 4-57 *Actinomyces* organisms in Papanicolaou-stained cervicovaginal smear from an IUD wearer. These dense "spidery" bodies are the most common pattern in which the organisms are encountered. (Gupta PK: Intrauterine contraceptive devices: Vaginal cytology, pathologic changes and clinical implications. Acta Cytol 26:571–613, 1982)

Michaelis-Gutmann bodies are probably of similar origin.[172]

Vasculitis

A rare inflammatory lesion of the uterus, as well as other portions of the female genital tract, is arteritis, which is usually diagnosed incidentally in specimens received for other clinical indications.[173,174] These lesions may represent an isolated finding of no clinical significance or be part of a generalized vasculitis, which is often previously undiagnosed. Based on a literature review of 35 cases in addition to their 2 cases, Bruch and colleagues[174] suggest that granulomatous arteritis is usually a systemic disease requiring corticosteroid therapy, whereas necrotizing arteritis of polyarteritis type (Fig. 4-58) is most often an isolated finding requiring no treatment. Bell and colleagues, however, report 3 cases of extensive giant cell arteritis of the female genital tract, of which one required systemic treatment and one was asymptomatic for 17 years after surgery without any intervening treatment.[173]

ADENOMYOSIS

Adenomyosis consists of endometrial glands and stroma within the myometrium. It is frequently called *endometriosis interna* to differentiate it from endometriosis externa, which is characterized by the presence of extrauterine localizations of similar benign endometrial glands and stroma. Because the latter is an extrauterine disease, the most frequent localizations of which are related to peritoneal mesothelium, it is discussed in Chapter 7 on the female peritoneum. However, the uterine serosa and immediately subserosal myometrium may be involved by endometriosis externa, so not every case of deeply situated endometrium in the uterine corpus represents adenomyosis.

Definition

Because the junction of endometrium and myometrium in a normal uterus is often irregular, multiple sections of most uteri show endometrial glands and stroma penetrating at least superficially into the myometrium. Therefore, the definition of adenomyosis is arbitrary, and the depth of penetration required for the diagnosis determines such factors as the frequency of the condition and its clinical significance. We generally use the dividing line of one medium-power ($\times$ 100) microscopic field below the endometrial–myometrial junction as the distinction between "physiologic" penetration of endometrium into the myometrium and the "disease" of adenomyosis. Others have accepted either shallower or deeper penetration. In the former case, adenomyosis is seen in most hysterectomy specimens and is of little clinical significance, whereas in the latter it is a relatively rare diagnosis usually associated with characteristic clinical findings and gross uterine enlargement.[175–180]

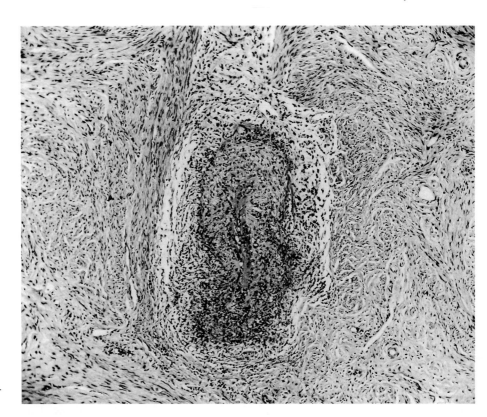

FIGURE 4-58 Isolated necrotizing angiitis in myometrium.

Frequency and Clinical Presentation

Reported frequencies of adenomyosis in hysterectomy specimens vary from less than 10% to greater than 50%. In our own material, because of the diagnostic criteria that we apply, the figure is probably closer to but slightly above the lowest reported.

If one accepts such a low prevalence figure, adenomyosis will frequently be a symptomatic disease. It occurs primarily in women in the reproductive years, and it is most commonly associated with abnormal menstrual bleeding, dysmenorrhea, uterine enlargement, and occasionally infertility. However, because adenomyosis is associated with endometriosis externa in about 15% of cases, and with uterine myomata in more than 50%,[179] it is often difficult to know to which lesion to ascribe the symptoms. Because of the nonspecificity of these symptoms, and because many women with adenomyosis have no symptoms whatsoever, the diagnosis usually is not made preoperatively.[178]

Pathogenesis

In most instances, adenomyosis appears to represent a diverticulosis of endometrium into the myometrium. Thus, serial sections of the uterus frequently show that the islands of endometrium that appear to be isolated deep in the myometrium are actually in contact with the overlying endometrium. Some cases, however, may arise by metaplasia from multipotential mesenchymal cells located around blood vessels within the myometrium.

Macroscopic Appearance

The uterus is of normal size in 20% to 25% of cases, and in many of the others the enlargement is at least partly due to associated myomata. However, some cases may show massive enlargement without any other disease. In these instances, the enlargement is symmetrical and occurs primarily as a result of smooth muscle hypertrophy around the deep-seated islands of endometrium.

In some cases, the lesions may be grossly visible as small pink or gray-white zones that are less dense and less firm than the surrounding myometrium. In rare cases, these foci are dark red as a result of hemorrhage. Small cysts are occasionally seen. If the lesion is solitary and focal, it is sometimes called an *adenomyoma*.

Microscopic Appearance

The endometrium seen within the myometrium is generally inactive or proliferative and only rarely shows functional changes consonant with the ovarian hormonal cycle and with the appearance of the overlying normal endometrium. This histologic appearance correlates with the observation by Tamaya and associates that estrogen receptors are always present in foci of adenomyosis but progesterone receptor levels are low or absent.[181] In pregnancy, foci of adenomyosis may show glandular secretions and decidual stroma.[182]

Because of the lack of hormonal response, neither fresh hemorrhage nor deposits of hemosiderin pigment are generally seen in adenomyosis, as they usually are in endometriosis externa. Hyperplastic smooth muscle fibers are usually seen around the ectopic endometrial glands and stroma. The ultrastructural appearance of adenomyotic glandular epithelium is said to be less differentiated than that of normal proliferative endometrium.[183]

Malignant Transformation

Ectopic endometrium, whether in adenomyosis or endometriosis externa, shares with normally situated endometrium the ability to undergo hyperplastic or malignant change. To accept a carcinoma as having arisen within adenomyosis, the overlying endometrium must be thoroughly sampled to prove that it is not involved, and such cases are rare.[184]

Much more frequent is the extension of a carcinoma arising in the overlying endometrium into the islands of adenomyosis. In these instances, the nests of carcinoma within the myometrium have rounded rather than irregular contours, and residual benign endometrial stroma may be seen at their periphery. The poor prognosis generally associated with true deep myometrial invasion is not present.[184,185]

The term *stromal endometriosis* has been used in the past to describe intramyometrial lesions composed of benign-appearing endometrial stromal cells without glands. Although it was once assumed that these represented a variant of adenomyosis that might demonstrate malignant behavior, it is now generally accepted that these lesions represent low-grade endometrial stromal sarcoma, which is discussed later in this chapter.

BENIGN TUMORS

Leiomyoma

The leiomyoma is a very common benign uterine tumor found in about 40% of women after the age of 35 years.[186] Synonyms are *fibroma, myoma,* and *fibroid.* This tumor is often called *fibroma,* and usage has consecrated this false term. In reality, the tumor takes its origin in the smooth muscle fibers of the myometrium.

The *pathogenesis* is not clear. There does not seem to be any hereditary factor, but its demonstration would be difficult because of the great frequency of the tumor.[187] Certain clinical facts suggest the existence of a hormonal factor: the tumor appears during the period of genital activity and stabilizes or regresses after the menopause. It sometimes increases in size and demonstrates atypias during pregnancy or administration of oral contraceptives.[188,189] Serum growth hormone and estradiol levels are elevated in women with myomata,[190] and estrogen and progesterone receptors have been demonstrated in the tumors.[191,192] Attempts to reproduce the tumor experimentally using hormones have met with partial failure. The appearance of disseminated fibromatous tumors in the abdominal cavity of the guinea pig and the rabbit has been provoked by the administration of estrogens.[193] However, these experimental tumors have not been morphologically identical to human uterine leiomyomata; they are fibromas rather than myomas. The regression of the tumor after the menopause and after the administration of a gonadotropin-releasing hormone agonist (Lupron)[194,195] may not be a hormonal phenomenon but rather may be explicable by vascular involution; the shrinkage of leiomyomas after radiation therapy is at least in part the result of the same mechanism. Additional evidence of at least partial hormone dependence of these tumors is provided by studies showing increased mitotic activity during the secretory phase of the menstrual cycle[196,197] and ultrastructural evidence of increased differentiation (myofilaments, dense bodies) in leiomyoma cells cultured with estrogen and progesterone added to the media.[198] To conclude, we may say that sex steroid hormones influence the growth of the leiomyoma but that we can not conclusively affirm that they bring about its original appearance.

Other substances such as growth factors have been suggested to play a role in tumorigenesis.[187] Cytogenetic studies have demonstrated clonal chromosomal abnormalities in one-third to one-half of leiomyomas, but numerous different abnormalities are found.[199,200] The demonstration that uterine leiomyomas are less commonly found in the cervix and more commonly in the fundus than would be expected based on the intrauterine distribution of normal smooth muscle has been presented as a possible clue to histogenesis.[192] Nevertheless, the origin of this common tumor is still in doubt.

Clinical Signs. Many asymptomatic myomata are discovered during a routine gynecologic examination. Others are manifested by the following symptoms: pain, menorrhagia or metrorrhagia, dysmenorrhea, urinary disturbances, and constipation. The most frequent complications are compression of neighboring organs, torsion, and necrosis. Fetal death as a result of compression has been described (Fig. 4-59). Spontaneous abortion and infertility are frequent associations,[186] and abruptio placentae, intrapartum increased pain, and premature labor have been reported as clinically significant complications during pregnancy.[201]

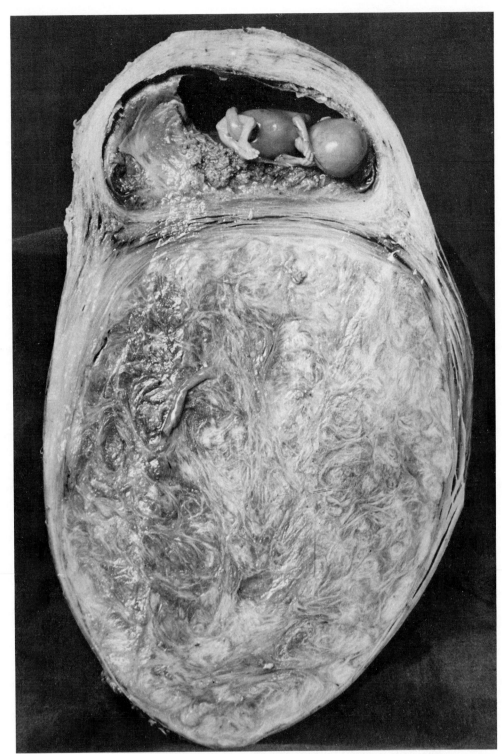

FIGURE 4-59 Leiomyoma and dead fetus.

Macroscopic Appearance. The uterine myoma is spherical, firm and elastic in consistency, and white. Sections through it show pearly tissue, with the typical appearance of whorled bundles of smooth muscle fibers (Fig. 4-60). These are separated by a connective tissue stroma that varies in quantity. Hemorrhagic and necrotic foci are identified by their dark red or yellow color and their softer consistency. Hyalinized or calcified nodules are frequently seen; their number and size vary greatly from one case to another. Myomata sometimes attain a size of 20 cm or more in diameter. They are usually multiple but may be solitary.

Submucous leiomyomata are the least frequent.

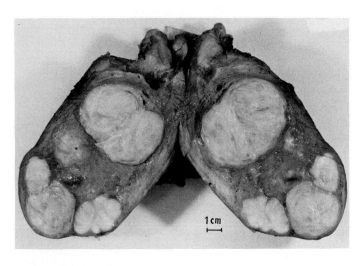

FIGURE 4-60 Intramural leiomyomata.

They often cause significant uterine hemorrhages. They are occasionally pedunculated and may prolapse into the cervical orifice of the vagina. Their mass causes phenomena of compression, and they often become superficially ulcerated, necrotic, and inflamed.

Intramural myomata are not detected when they are small; when large, they bulge under the mucosa or the serosa. They are the most frequent leiomyomata (see Fig. 4-60).

Subserous myomata herniate beneath the peritoneal serosa and are frequently pedunculated. If the pedicle is long, the tumor floats in the peritoneal cavity. It may undergo torsion or rupture, and in the latter case the tumor becomes migratory or aberrant and may adhere to other intra-abdominal organs, from which it receives a new vascular supply (*parasitic myoma*). Also seen are leiomyomas of the broad ligament, which are difficult to distinguish clinically from an ovarian mass (Fig. 4-61).

Microscopic Appearance. The leiomyoma consists of anastomosed and whorled fascicles of fusiform cells of uniform size. The nuclei are elongated and

their extremities rounded (Figs. 4-62 and 4-63). Mitoses are not frequent. Blood vessels are small and not numerous. Between the bundles of smooth muscle fibers are found variable amounts of fibrous connective tissue. When the tumor is richly cellular, it must not be confused with leiomyosarcoma; the absence of bizarre cellular atypia, infiltrative borders, and numerous mitoses facilitates the identification of the lesion as benign.

Leiomyomas may present several types of degenerative histologic transformation: hemorrhage, necrosis, hyalinization, fibrosis, and calcification. Hyaline degeneration appears grossly as a smooth, homogeneous, translucent zone; if it is located interstitially, it is difficult to recognize grossly. Histologically, it consists of eosinophilic bands infiltrating the muscle bundles or of homogeneous plaques in which all cellular structure has disappeared. When the hyalinized zones present liquefaction and edema, there appear gelatinous and myxoid plaques or even cystic cavities measuring up to several millimeters in diameter. Calcification is particularly frequent after liquefaction, hemorrhage, or necrosis.

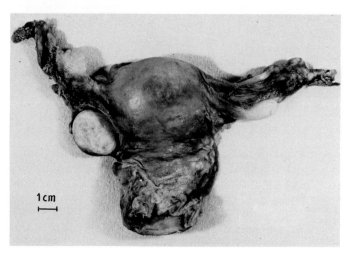

FIGURE 4-61 Leiomyoma of broad ligament.

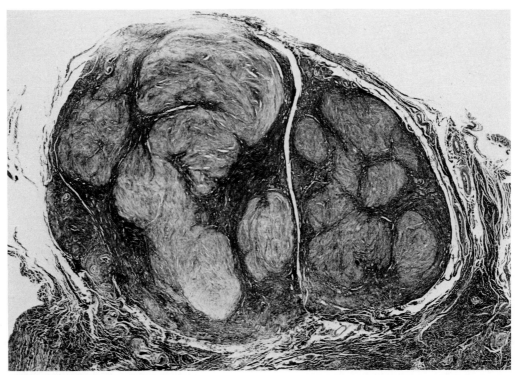

FIGURE 4-62   Intramural leiomyoma.

Often seen in association with these degenerative changes are symplastic giant cells (*bizarre, symplastic,* or *pleomorphic leiomyoma*; Fig. 4-64). These may be mono- or multinucleate and are characterized by large, often monstrous, hyperchromatic nuclei that appear degenerative rather than malignant. The invariable absence or paucity of mitotic figures, the absence of tumor necrosis, the usual youth of the patient, and the frequent history of pregnancy or oral contraceptive usage all help in the differential diagnosis from leiomyosarcoma.

Certain other histologic changes occasionally seen in leiomyomata may represent manifestations of the metaplastic capabilities of the cell of origin. These include foci that, at the light microscopic level, resemble neurilemoma[202] or hemangiopericytoma.[203] Also seen are smooth muscle tumors containing foci of adipose tissue (*lipoleiomyoma*)[204–206] of endometrial stroma, or of tubular or cord-like structures that may be reminiscent of ovarian sex cord elements (Fig. 4-65).[207,208] Sex cord–like structures may also be seen in endometrial stromal tumors or may form tumors with no obvious muscular or stromal differentiation, so a classic leiomyomatous component must be observed for the diagnosis of leiomyoma with sex cord–like foci. Devaney and

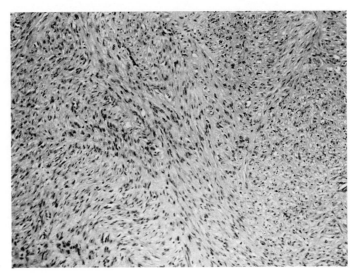

FIGURE 4-63   Leiomyoma: detail of histologic structure.

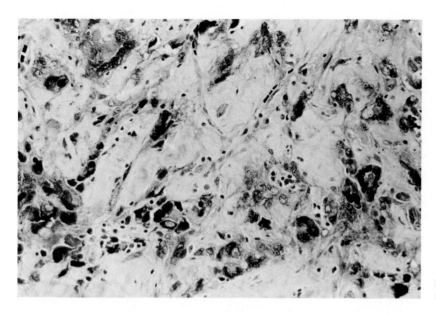

FIGURE 4-64 Symplastic giant cells in leiomyoma with edema and hyalinization.

Tavassoli[209] have claimed on the basis of immunohistochemical studies that all sex cord–like tumors are combined smooth muscle and endometrial stromal tumors.

Endometrial Changes in the Presence of a Leiomyoma. The mechanical compression exerted by a submucous leiomyoma causes atrophy of the overlying endometrium. The glands are flattened and lined by cuboidal and flat epithelium. There is no secretory activity. The stroma is dense and formed of small round cells. Dilated venous spaces are present throughout the endometrium. The picture of irreg-

ular shedding (see above) has been described in these cases.

Evolution and Treatment. Sarcomatous transformation is rare but should be systematically searched for in any smooth muscle tumor that increases rapidly in volume, particularly after the menopause, or that grossly shows softening, hemorrhage, or cystic degeneration. Liebsohn and colleagues found unsuspected leiomyosarcoma in 1% of a series of hysterectomies performed for presumed leiomyomas.[210] Symptomatic leiomyomata are classically treated by myomectomy (if uterine preservation is desired)[211] or

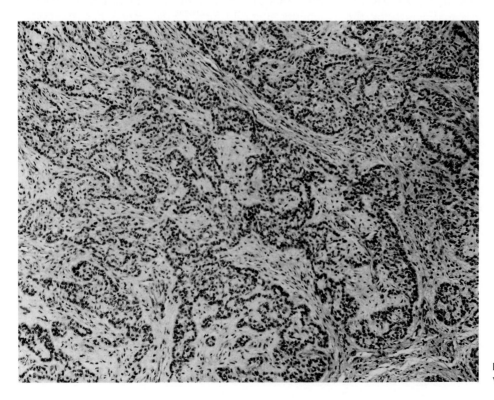

FIGURE 4-65 Uterine leiomyoma with sex cord–like differentiation.

hysterectomy, but recent therapeutic alternatives include medical treatment with a gonadotropin-releasing hormone agonist (Lupron),[194,195] hysteroscopic resection,[212] and Lupron followed by hysteroscopic laser devascularization of the tumor.[213] Recurrences have been reported in 15% of cases treated by myomectomy.[214]

Variants of Leiomyoma

The ISGP classification of uterine smooth muscle tumors (Table 4-3) includes several histologic variants (lipoleiomyoma and cellular, epithelioid, and bizarre leiomyomas) and variants characterized by an unusual growth pattern (metastasizing leiomyoma, intravenous leiomyomatosis, and diffuse leiomyomatosis).[215,216] *Lipoleiomyoma* and *bizarre (symplastic) leiomyoma* have been discussed above. *Cellular leiomyoma* is defined as a benign smooth muscle tumor that is significantly more cellular than the surrounding myometrium. Because the interpretation of "significantly" varies from one pathologist to another, the relative frequency of these tumors varies. The important fact to remember is that these tumors are differentiated from leiomyosarcoma by their bland nuclear appearance and lack of notable mitotic activity. The remaining variants will be discussed in the following paragraphs.

Epithelioid Leiomyoma. Muscle fibers may undergo modifications that cause them to resemble epithelial elements,[217] sometimes during pregnancy. In the *leiomyoblastoma* variant, the cells may be nested in a hyalinized stroma, the nuclei are voluminous and round, and the cytoplasm becomes strongly eosinophilic and homogeneous (Fig. 4-66).[218,219] A *clear cell* type is characterized by cells with voluminous clear cytoplasm (Fig. 4-67).[217,220]

These epithelioid leiomyomas are probably analogous to similar tumors described originally in the stomach and, like their gastric counterparts, may occasionally behave malignantly.[216,217] Because the tumors by definition are virtually all markedly atypical histologically, it is difficult to predict which will metastasize; however, frequent mitotic figures and evidence of local aggressiveness are helpful features. The origin of the clear vacuoles seen in the cytoplasm of the clear cell leiomyomas is controversial, but one ultrastructural study has suggested that they are derived from swollen mitochondria.[219]

The third category of epithelioid leiomyoma is the plexiform type, usually called *plexiform tumorlet*. These small lesions, usually incidental findings in uteri removed for other reasons, were first reported by Borghard-Erdle and Hirsch[221] and were subsequently reported under a variety of names, reflecting the lack of unanimity on their histogenesis. Ultrastructural studies have subsequently shown them to be of smooth muscle origin,[222] and indeed plexiform foci may be found within otherwise typical smooth muscle tumors of the uterus. When they occur as separate lesions, they are small, usually solitary but occasionally multiple, well localized but unencapsulated, and usually found in the myometrium near its junction with the endometrium. Histologically, they are composed of randomly oriented rows or plexiform masses of uniform small cells with clear vesicular nuclei, separated by abundant connective tissue stroma (Fig. 4-68). All plexiform tumorlets reported have been benign.[215,223]

Intravenous Leiomyomatosis. Intravenous leiomyomatosis has as a typical feature worm-like masses within the veins of the uterus and broad ligaments.[224-226] This gross picture resembles that of low-grade endometrial stromal sarcoma. However, these masses are not composed of endometrial stromal tissue but rather of intermingled smooth muscle and fibrous tissue containing very prominent small blood vessels. The masses are often lobulated by the presence of small clefts and show none of the whorled pattern that is so common in the "usual" leiomyoma. No significant cellular atypia is seen in the usual case, and mitoses are rare. The cases reported have almost all been associated with "typical" myomas, but controversy rages over whether the intravenous myomatous tissue arises from invasive uterine myomas or from the vein walls themselves. Only 25% of the cases have shown extension beyond the broad ligaments, and only rare deaths have been reported, resulting from direct extension of tumor into the inferior vena cava and the right atrium. Metastases do not occur, and even when resection has been incomplete, patients usually have shown no further evidence of disease. Any of the leiomyoma variants (eg, cellular, epithelioid, bizarre) may show this intravascular growth pattern.[226,227] If mitoses are

---

TABLE 4-3.
Uterine Smooth Muscle Tumors

Leiomyoma
    Variants:
        Cellular
        Epithelioid
        Bizarre (symplastic, pleomorphic)
        Lipoleoimyoma

Smooth muscle tumor of uncertain malignant potential

Leiomyosarcoma
    Variants
        Epithelioid
        Myxoid

Other smooth muscle tumors
    Metastasizing leiomyoma
    Intravenous leiomyomatosis
    Diffuse leiomyomatosis

Mixed endometrial stromal and smooth muscle tumors

Silverberg SG, Kurman RJ: Tumors of the uterine corpus and gestational trophoblastic disease. In Atlas of tumor pathology, 3rd series, fascicle 3. Washington, DC, Armed Forces Institute of Pathology, 1992

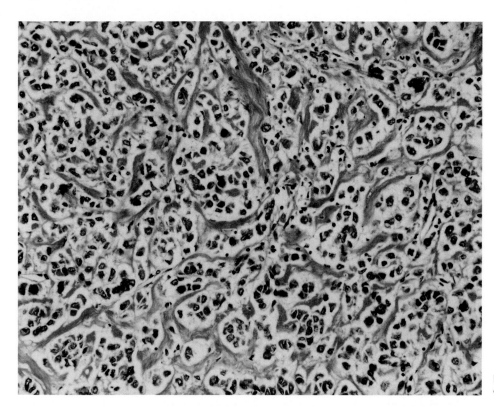

FIGURE 4-66 Epithelioid leiomyoma, leiomyoblastoma type.

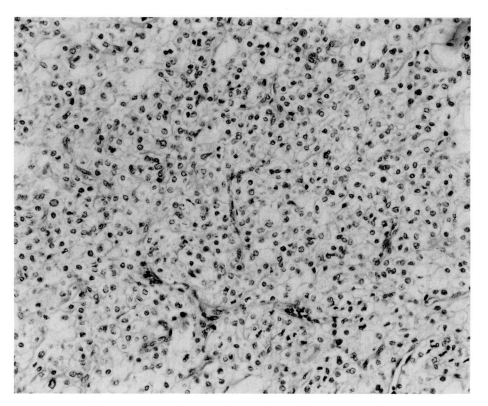

FIGURE 4-67 Epithelioid leiomyoma, clear cell type.

sparse and myometrial (rather than vascular) invasion is absent, leiomyosarcoma usually can be ruled out.

Metastasizing Leiomyoma. Metastasizing leiomyoma is equally rare, with only about two dozen cases documented.[228–230] The usual clinical history in these cases has been the appearance of pulmonary metastases several years after hysterectomy for "benign" leiomyomata. Histologic examination of both the pulmonary and uterine tumors has in each case (when both were available) demonstrated the typical cellular pattern of benign leiomyoma. The burden of proof in these cases is on the author making the assertion, and we believe that in the absence of serial sections of the entire uterus, it cannot be definitively stated that a leiomyosarcoma was not originally present; nevertheless, the published photomicrographs of the pulmonary tumors do indeed look benign, as do our cases. An alternative explanation is that the pulmonary lesions may be primary pulmonary leiomyomas. However, lymph node metastases have been reported.[228] Finally, the almost invariable history of surgery suggests iatrogenic dissemination of biologically benign tumors.

Endometrial Polyp

The endometrial polyp consists of a mass of endometrial tissue appended to the mucosa by a pedicle. Polyps are of diverse sizes, may be single or multiple, and are located in all parts of the uterine cavity. Usually they measure from 0.5 to 3 cm in diameter. They may appear long after the menopause or during active genital life.

Clinical Manifestations. Frequently, the polyp is asymptomatic and represents a fortuitous discovery during the course of a clinical examination or in the dissection of a surgical specimen. In some cases, its presence is manifested by hemorrhages. When voluminous, it may herniate at the cervical orifice, and in some cases it becomes ulcerated. Large polyps have been reported to develop in postmenopausal breast cancer patients receiving tamoxifen.[231,232]

Macroscopic Appearance. The polyp presents as a small, gray or pink, smooth-surfaced, firm mass (Fig. 4-69). It is attached to the mucosa by a stalk of variable length or may be sessile. In some cases, polyps are numerous and disseminated throughout the entire endometrial cavity.

Microscopic Appearance. The polyp is covered by a cuboidal or flattened epithelium, which is sometimes eroded. The endometrial tissue may undergo cyclic modifications, but more commonly it shows a nonfunctional appearance of discrete proliferative or atrophic type.[233,234]

Hyperplasia may be present. About 1% of polyps contain smooth muscle (*adenomyomatous polyp*). The presence of cystic glands is common, dilated thick-walled vessels are prominent, and the stroma is fibrotic, permitting the diagnosis of a polyp in material obtained by curettage, in which the stalk is not

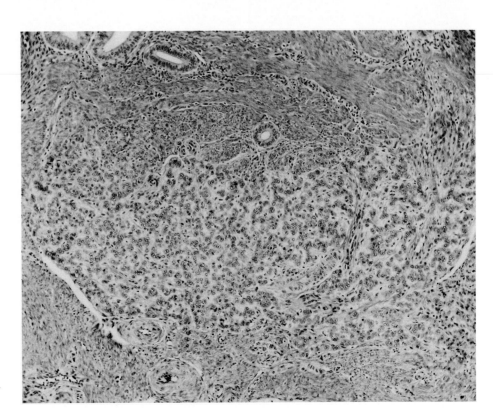

FIGURE 4-68 Epithelioid leiomyoma, plexiform tumorlet type.

visible (Figs. 4-70 and 4-71). Similar changes may be seen in a nonpolypoid configuration within the endometrium, often related to the basalis, suggesting that polyps arise as localized proliferations or hyperplasias of basalis-type endometrium. Indeed, Dallenbach-Hellweg[23] includes polyps in her discussion of endometrial hyperplasia, although many polyps, particularly in postmenopausal women, are composed of atrophic endometrium.

Prognosis, Evolution, and Treatment. The great majority of endometrial polyps are benign. Their evolution may be asymptomatic or accompanied by hemorrhagic manifestations. Focal (Fig. 4-72) or diffuse hyperplasia within the polyp is not uncommon. A small number show malignant transformation, which may or may not be limited to the polypoid mass itself. In these cases, it is difficult to determine whether one is dealing with a carcinoma that has

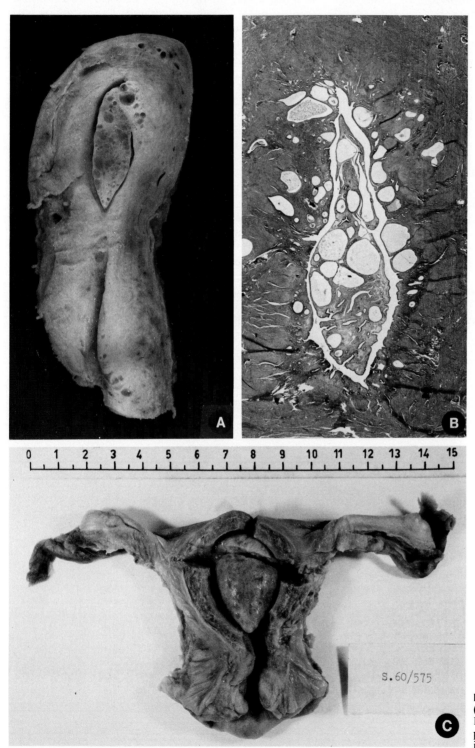

FIGURE 4-69 Endometrial polyp. **(A)** Macroscopic appearance. **(B)** Microscopic appearance of same polyp. **(C)** Macroscopic appearance in another case.

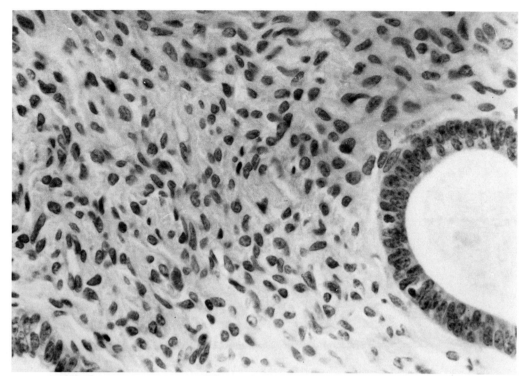

FIGURE 4-70 Endometrial polyp: fibroblastic appearance of stroma.

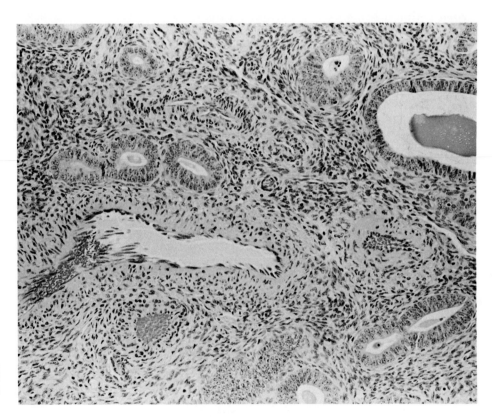

FIGURE 4-71 Endometrial polyp: detail showing thick-walled blood vessels, fibrotic stroma, and glands of proliferative phase type.

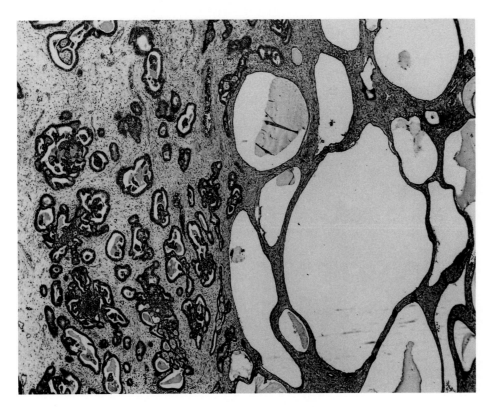

FIGURE 4-72 Complex hyperplasia (*left*) in an endometrial polyp.

arisen within a benign polyp or with a carcinoma, malignant from its onset, of polypoid type. When the carcinoma is limited to the polyp and is of endometrioid type, the prognosis is excellent; however, serous and clear cell adenocarcinomas[235,236] and carcinosarcomas[237] can disseminate even when confined to a polyp. Surgical excision with adequate pathologic examination is the treatment of choice for all polyps.

Vascular Tumors

The benign vascular tumors comprise *hemangiomas* and *lymphangiomas*. In 1955, Pedowitz and coworkers[238] found 128 published cases in the literature, to which they added 10 personal cases, but some of these were probably cases of low-grade endometrial stromal sarcoma. They are congenital but are discovered most frequently between the ages of 40 and 60 years, usually producing menstrual disturbances or some other form of hemorrhage.[239] They rarely attain sufficient size to be palpable. In a few cases, observation of the pulsatile character of the tumor during laparotomy has led to the correct diagnosis.

Hemangiomas may be subserous and pedunculated or intramural. They are less commonly found within the endometrium. They vary in size from a few millimeters to several centimeters (Fig. 4-73). *Histologically*, they are composed of small interwoven capillaries (capillary hemangioma), large dilated capillaries (cavernous hemangioma), or vessels surrounded by cuffs of smooth muscle fibers (angiomyo-

ma). Cavernous hemangioma of the uterus may be associated with angiomatous lesions of other sites.

Lymphangiomas are rare. They are composed of lymphatic vessels, recognizable by the absence of erythrocytes in their lumina. Their differential diagnosis is with the adenomatoid tumor (see below).

The treatment of choice for these tumors is surgical excision. Radiation therapy appears to bring about regressions that are temporary at best.

Lipoma

More than 100 cases of lipomatous tumors of the uterus have been reported.[206,240,241] Most of these have been associated with vascular and leiomyomatous elements and have been designated *lipoleiomyomas, angiomyolipomas,* or *benign mixed mesodermal tumors.*[242] Although related to myomata, 90% of uterine lipomatous tumors have occurred in women older than 40 years. The origin of these tumors may be from multipotential mesenchymal tissue or from the adipose tissue in the adventitia of uterine blood vessels.

Adenomatoid Tumor

Of the 76 reported cases of adenomatoid tumors in women found in a review of the literature by Teel,[243] 35 were situated in the uterus, 33 in the fallopian tube, 5 in the ovary, 1 in the broad ligament, and 1 in parovarian connective tissue. Regardless of the location, they are usually asymptomatic, classically discovered during an operation for an unrelated condition. In the uterus, they are usually found in a subserosal location, reflecting their now generally accepted mesothelial histogenesis.[244–247] Multiple sections of routine hysterectomy specimens reveal adenomatoid tumors in 0.6% to 1.2% of cases.[244,246]

Macroscopic Appearance. The lesions generally are small and usually are located at or near the serosal surface. They may resemble leiomyomata. However, they are generally softer and may have infiltrating borders. Occasional tumors that are large and extend to the endometrium have been reported.[248]

Microscopic Appearance. The most common pattern is the adenoid[245] or tubular one, consisting of anastomosing tubules lined by flattened to cuboidal cells (Fig. 4-74). In many instances, these tubules may assume an angiomatoid configuration; for this reason, these tumors were frequently confused with lymphangiomas in the past. Less common are solid and cystic growth patterns.[245,247]

Infiltration of the myometrium is frequently seen, and cases submitted to us in consultation are often thought to represent adenocarcinomas. Important distinguishing features include the subserosal location of the adenomatoid tumor, its lack of cellular atypia and mitotic activity, and the absence of myometrial destruction or a stromal response suggestive of invasion by a malignant tumor. The differential diagnosis with lymphangioma is aided by the presence of immunohistochemically detected epithelial antigens in the adenomatoid tumor. The *evolution* of the uterine adenomatoid tumor is benign.

Other Benign Tumors

Rare cases of *nonchromaffin paraganglioma* have been referred to briefly in the literature.[249] Somewhat less rare are *papillary adenofibroma, atypical polypoid adenomyoma,* and *adenomyomatosis.* Because these three benign lesions seem to be part of a spectrum including the low-grade malignant tumor known as *müllerian adenosarcoma,* they will be discussed in the later section on malignant neoplasms. *Stromal nodule* is also discussed later with endometrial stromal sarcomas. Such rare uterine benign lesions as *neurofibroma,*[209] *melanotic schwannoma,*[209] *fetal rhabdomyoma,*[250] *postoperative spindle cell nodule,*[251] and *inflammatory pseudotumor*[252] have been reported.

ENDOMETRIAL HYPERPLASIA

Endometrial hyperplasia embraces a spectrum of histologic appearances that have been compared with those of cervical dysplasia. As in the latter, the milder forms of endometrial hyperplasia tend to occur in younger patients and in the great majority of cases to regress, either spontaneously or after treatment. The more severe forms, occurring pre-

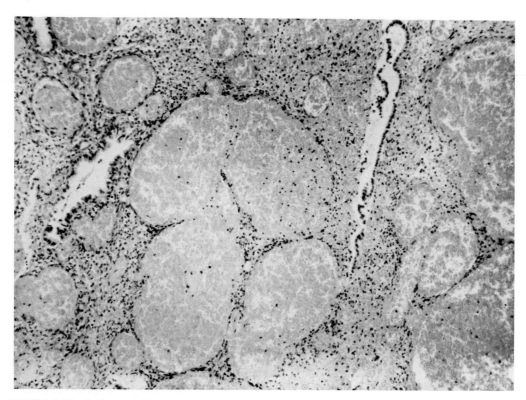

FIGURE 4-73 Endometrial hemangioma.

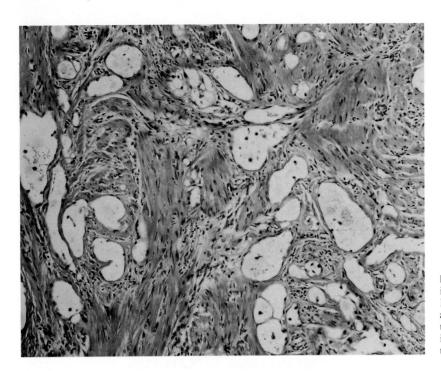

FIGURE 4-74 Adenomatoid tumor infiltrating the myometrium. (Silverberg SG, Kurman RJ: Tumors of the uterine corpus and gestational trophoblastic disease. Atlas of tumor pathology, 3rd series, fascicle 3. Washington, D.C., Armed Forces Institute of Pathology, 1992)

dominantly in peri- and postmenopausal women, appear to have a significant premalignant potential, the evidence for which will be discussed below.

Clinically, the hyperplasia is manifested principally by abnormal uterine bleeding, whose severity is not necessarily proportional to that of the histologic changes.[253] Endometrial hyperplasias are uncommon in asymptomatic women, with a reported prevalence of slightly more than 8 cases per 1000 screened postmenopausal women.[254] There is an association with obesity (and a Western diet), nulliparity, diabetes mellitus, hypertension, and endogenous and exogenous hyperestrinism.[253-255]

Macroscopic Appearance. The *macroscopic appearance* of endometrial hyperplasia may not vary significantly from the normal, or it may show considerable thickening of either the entire mucosa or focal regions. When focal thickening occurs, the lesion may acquire a polypoid aspect. The consistency is usually soft and the color pale pink. Curettage usually yields increased amounts of tissue.

Microscopic Appearance. The *microscopic appearance* depends on the degree of hyperplasia. Lesions of different degrees of severity have been given diverse names by different authors. The current ISGP nomenclature[128] uses the terms *hyperplasia* and *atypical hyperplasia* to refer to processes without and with cytologic (nuclear) atypia respectively, and each of these is divided into a *simple* and a *complex* (adenomatous) type, reflecting the degree of architectural complexity.[256-261] In all patterns, by definition the volume of endometrium is increased, although this may not be apparent in a small biopsy specimen.

Simple Hyperplasia

Simple hyperplasia is the least distressing form histologically. In this form, there is an increase in both the glandular and stromal compartments, and although the ratio of glands to stroma is somewhat increased, the glands are not markedly crowded (Figs. 4-75 and 4-76). The numerous glands usually include many that are dilated or cystic, the height of the epithelium varying inversely with the degree of dilatation. The slightly dilated glands are lined by stratified proliferative type epithelium, whereas the markedly dilated ones may show stratified, cuboidal, or, rarely, flattened epithelium (see Fig. 4-75). Rarely, in this or one of the other types of hyperplasia, some or all of the glands show secretory changes (*secretory hyperplasia*). The general appearance of the endometrium has been likened to the small and large holes of Swiss cheese, and this pattern is often referred to as "Swiss cheese hyperplasia." It is frequently polypoid. Ciliated cells are numerous; mitoses are present but are not numerous, and no atypical mitoses are seen. No dyspolarity or nuclear atypia is present. The gland lumina may contain cellular debris. The stromal cells are densely packed and have small nuclei and scanty cytoplasm; mitoses are present.[262] The spiral arteries are poorly developed, but the superficial capillaries are numerous and uniformly distributed. Hyaline deposits in the stroma are frequent and may represent residual products of incomplete fibrinolysis caused by local enzymatic deficiencies. This lesion should not be confused with the pattern of cystic atrophy seen predominantly in postmenopausal women, in which the epithelium of all the glands is flattened and inactive. Similarly, the presence of a few cysts is common in

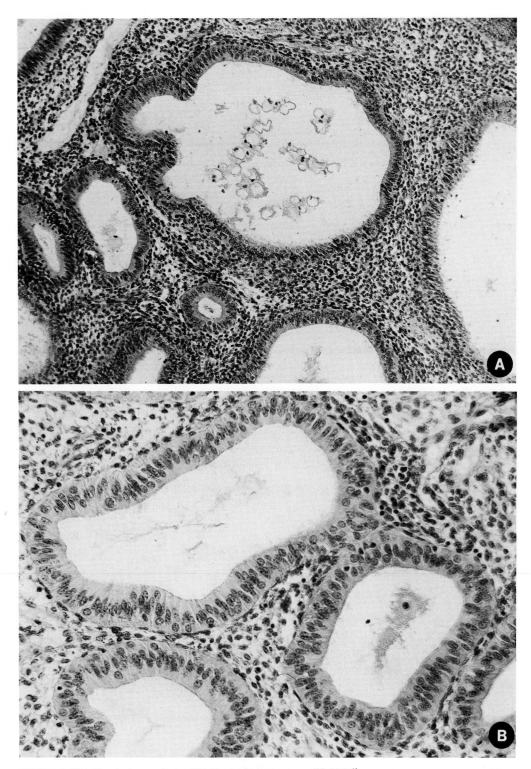

FIGURE 4-75 Simple hyperplasia. **(A)** General appearance. **(B)** Detail.

endometritis, in endometria overlying submucous myomata, and even in normal endometria. Therefore, the mere presence of dilated glands or cysts does not establish the diagnosis of simple hyperplasia. Opinions concerning the premalignant potentialities of this lesion are unanimous in assigning it a very low risk of progression to cancer (probably in the range of 1% to 5%).[256,257,259,260,263]

Complex Hyperplasia

Complex hyperplasia (Figs. 4-77 and 4-78; see Fig. 4-76B) may involve the entire endometrium or may be found in foci intermingled with normal or simple hyperplastic endometrium . The glands are closely packed and distributed irregularly in a cellular compact stroma. The glandular to stromal ratio is mark-

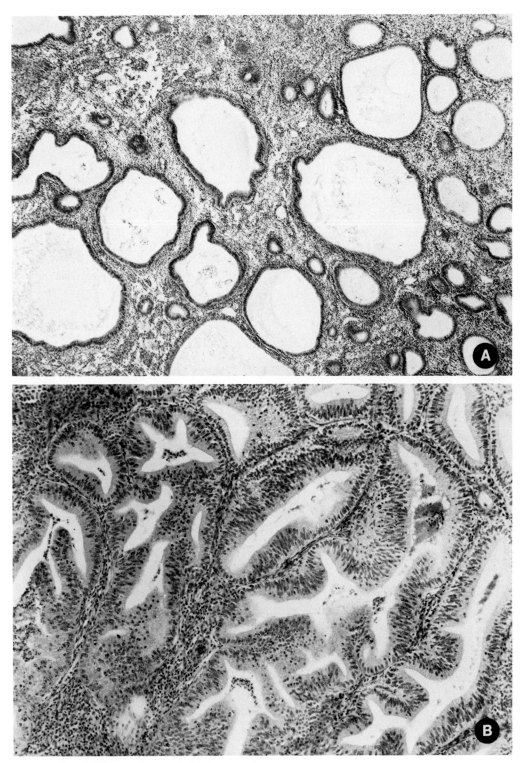

FIGURE 4-76 Endometrial hyperplasia. **(A)** Simple. **(B)** Complex.

edly increased. The glands are often irregular in size and shape. Outpouching or branching of these glands is a common feature (see Fig. 4-78); small bud-like projections may be pinched off to form small nests of closely packed glands in a microfollicular pattern. The epithelium is usually stratified and proliferative in appearance; mitoses are frequent. Cellular atypia is not present. Lipid-laden stromal cells (foam cells) may be noted.

The overall frequency of transformation of this lesion to carcinoma is not entirely clear. It is around 25% according to Sherman and Brown[264] and

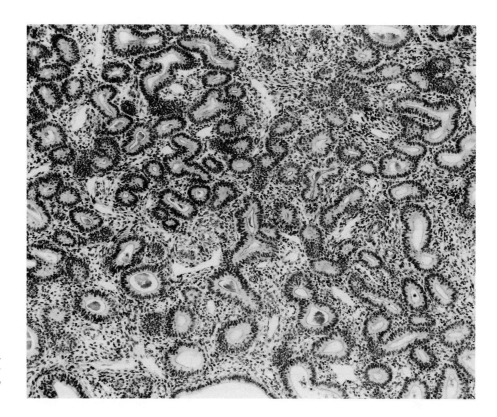

FIGURE 4-77 Complex hyperplasia. Glands are crowded and show some architectural atypia but no nuclear atypia.

Wentz[265] and less than 10% for most other investigators.[256,257,261,263,266] Curettage of this lesion usually yields more voluminous material than in the case of simple hyperplasia, and the patients tend to be somewhat older.

Atypical Hyperplasia

Atypical hyperplasia appears to be the same lesion that is alternately called *marked adenomatous hyperplasia,*[267] *anaplasia,*[268] or *carcinoma in situ*[269–271] in

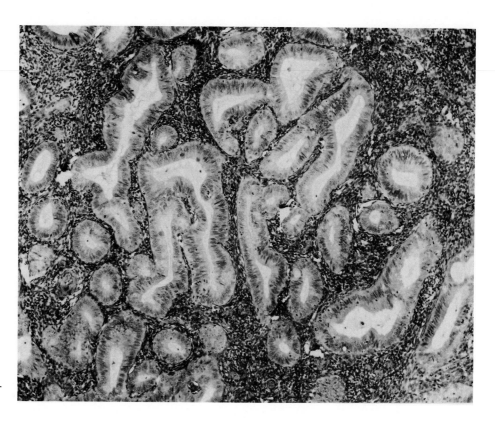

FIGURE 4-78 Complex hyperplasia. Nuclear atypia is absent.

the older literature. This lesion is usually focal and may be of simple or (more commonly) complex architectural type, but in addition the glandular epithelium demonstrates cellular atypia. Cellular disorientation, anisocytosis, and stratification are common (Figs. 4-79 through 4-81). Papillary projections and syncytial formations are often seen projecting into gland lumina (see Fig. 4-81). Mitoses are present but are no different in number or appearance from those in other hyperplastic lesions. Nuclear hyperchromatism, clumping of chromatin, and enlarged nucleoli are present. The nuclei tend to be round rather than columnar. Some cases are also characterized by marked cytoplasmic eosinophilia (see Figs. 4-80 and 4-81); these have been designated carcinoma in situ by some authors, but there is little evidence that this is a more advanced lesion than the more common noneosinophilic variant. Whatever term is chosen by the individual pathologist, the clinical significance of the lesion should be fully understood by both the clinician and the pathologist. If untreated, a large proportion of these lesions will probably progress to cancer,[256,257,261,263–266] although the exact figure in different reports ranges from 25% to 80%. In some of these studies, the complex type has had a higher progression rate than the simple type.

Premalignant Potential

What is the evidence for considering endometrial hyperplasia as a lesion with a significant premalignant potential? As in cervical lesions of this nature, the major studies along these lines may be divided into those of prospective, retrospective, and concurrent nature.

The earliest observation of the concurrent existence of endometrial hyperplasia in uteri examined because of the known presence of endometrial adenocarcinoma was that of Cullen[272] in 1900; he believed that this atypical change was not pathognomonic of carcinoma but rather an early change suggestive of a nearby cancer. Subsequently, many case reports and systematized studies have accumulated that show the simultaneous presence of endometrial hyperplasia and carcinoma; these studies are summarized in the review of Scully.[273]

Retrospective studies of previous biopsies in patients seen with endometrial carcinoma have suggested a significant relationship between these two lesions. These studies have been summarized by Foster and Montgomery,[268] who state that in 88 case reports of endometrial carcinoma extracted from the literature in which prior material was also reviewed, 61 of the 88 previous biopsies were reported as abnormal, most having shown varying degrees of hyperplasia. In the series in which this information is available, the degree of these changes seems to vary inversely with the amount of time that elapsed between the early biopsy and the subsequent demonstration of carcinoma.[265,274]

The other main avenue of approach to the natural history of endometrial hyperplasia has been the prospective follow-up of patients demonstrated to have this lesion on endometrial biopsy who are sub-

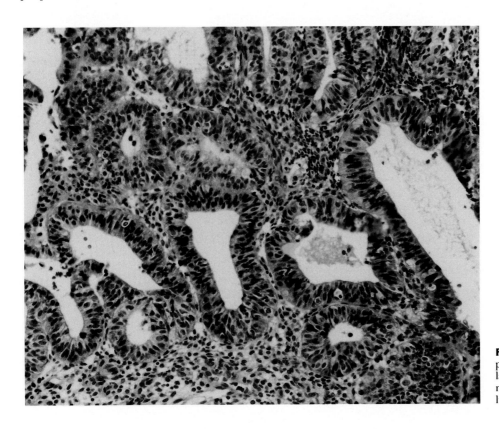

FIGURE 4-79 Atypical hyperplasia (complex). Note the irregular stratification and the roundness of nuclei. Debris in the gland lumina is a common feature.

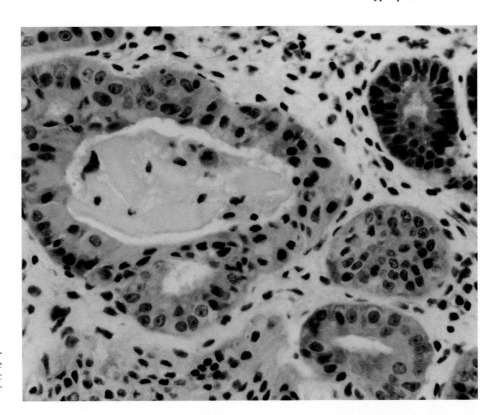

FIGURE 4-80 Atypical hyperplasia. These atypical glands have eosinophilic cytoplasm, dyspolaric cell stratification, and nuclear atypia.

sequently either treated conservatively or untreated and observed clinically and biopsied at intervals thereafter. Of 23 patients with atypical hyperplasia followed pathologically by Copenhaver,[275] 8 subsequently developed invasive carcinoma. TeLinde and colleagues[276] report the same progression in all of their 14 patients who had a second curettage from 10 months to 23 years later. Gusberg and Kaplan[267] report 191 patients with a pathologic diagnosis of "adenomatous hyperplasia" of variable severity (probably including all types in the current nomenclature). Of the 90 treated by immediate hysterectomy, 20% had coexistent carcinoma; of those untreated in this fashion, 68 patients were followed for 1 year or more, and 8 developed carcinoma from 1½ to 9 years later.

In more recent studies, Wentz[265] reported subsequent carcinoma within 2 to 8 years in 27% of women with adenomatous (here probably meaning complex) hyperplasia, 82% with atypical hyperplasia, and 100% with "adenocarcinoma in situ." Sherman and Brown[264] found carcinoma developing within 2 to 18 years in 22% of women with adenomatous (also comparable to complex) hyperplasia, 57% with atypical hyperplasia, and an almost identical 59% with adenocarcinoma in situ. In contrast to this latter series, in which all the patients were older than 50 years, Chamlian and Taylor[277] reported the development of adenocarcinoma in only 14% of women 35 years or younger with adenomatous or atypical hyperplasia who were followed for 1 to 14 years. Thus, the age of the patient seems to influence the risk of progression to carcinoma, and we would an-

ticipate that the mediation of exogenous estrogens would do so as well (hyperplasias developing in the estrogen-treated women should be more likely to regress and less likely to progress if the source of exogenous hormone is withdrawn). Few studies have critically analyzed the relation of exogenous estrogens to endometrial hyperplasias,[255] although the magnitude of this problem in recent years is demonstrated by the fact that, of 48 consecutive patients who underwent hysterectomy for atypical hyperplasia in the series of Tavassoli and Kraus,[278] 39 had previously received exogenous hormones. In this series, in which hysterectomy was performed more or less immediately after the diagnosis of atypical hyperplasia, 25% of the uteri contained at least a single focus of well-differentiated carcinoma, but another 15% had neither hyperplasia nor carcinoma despite the absence of intervening treatment with progestational agents.

More recent studies have tended to use more modern terminology for the lesions analyzed, but they still have involved relatively limited numbers of cases with varying follow-up periods and intervening treatment. Kurman and colleagues[263] found progression rates to carcinoma of 1% in cases of simple hyperplasia, 3% in complex hyperplasia, and 23% in atypical hyperplasia (8% of those with the simple architectural pattern and 29% of those with complex atypical hyperplasia). The follow-up ranged from 1 to 26.7 years after the diagnosis of hyperplasia. Many of the patients received hormones in the intervening period, but this treatment had little influence on the progression rate. In addition to those cases

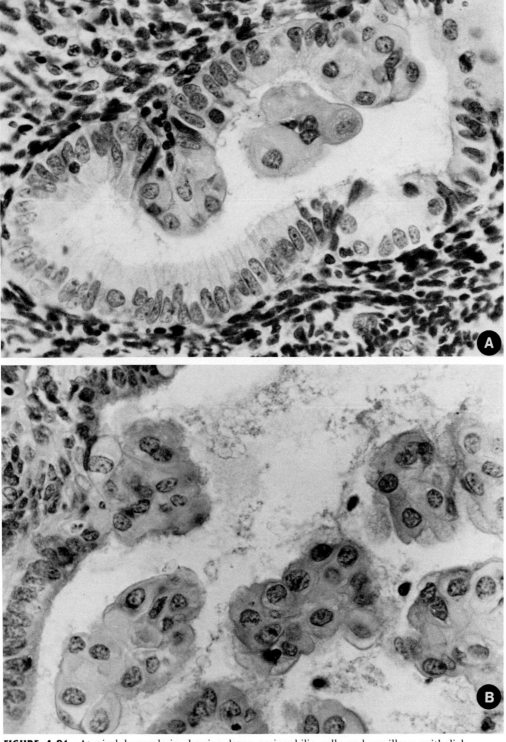

FIGURE 4-81 Atypical hyperplasia showing large eosinophilic cells and papillary epithelial infoldings.

that progressed to carcinoma, another 19% of both atypical and typical hyperplasias persisted.

Huang and associates[257] studied a somewhat smaller group of patients with hyperplasia, who had a subsequent endometrial specimen from 1 to 13 years later. Some patients received hormones and some were untreated. Twenty-four percent of patients with hyperplasia with nuclear atypia showed progression to carcinoma, versus 2.9% of hyperplasias without atypia. This study also included 38 patients originally diagnosed with hyperplasia whose specimens were interpreted on review as persistent proliferative endometrium; none of these progressed to either atypical hyperplasia or carcinoma. Schwartz and colleagues[288] reviewed a subset of the same cases reported by Huang and colleagues and confirmed their findings. Immunohistochemical staining of the original blocks with monoclonal antibodies B72.3 and MSN-1 proved that neither was better than cytologic atypia in predicting the behavior of endometrial hyperplasia, although MSN-1 showed some promise.

Ferenczy and Gelfand,[261] in the latest of a series of reports, studied 85 peri- and postmenopausal women with endometrial hyperplasia without (65 patients) and with (20 patients) cytologic atypia. In this prospective study, all women were treated with a uniform regimen of medroxyprogesterone acetate and followed from 2 to 12 years (mean 7 years). In the group without atypia, 20% had persistence or recurrence of hyperplasia and none developed carcinoma. Of the 20 patients with atypical hyperplasia, 15 (75%) had persistence or recurrence and 5 (25%) developed adenocarcinoma at 2 to 7 years (mean 5.5 years).

Baak and associates[279] compared morphometric analysis with standard morphologic criteria in a series of 39 patients. They estimated that in their population the ratio of hyperplasia to carcinoma was about 4.5 to 1, and about 2% of all hyperplasias were atypical. On follow-up, none of 8 patients with simple hyperplasia developed carcinoma, versus 2 of 20 (10%) with either complex hyperplasia or atypical simple hyperplasia and 5 of 11 (45%) with atypical complex hyperplasia. The specificity of prediction was better with these criteria, but the sensitivity was higher with morphometry.

To summarize these and other studies in this complex field, we can say, first, that the perfect study still has probably not been done. For one thing, the different terminologies that have been used for this group of lesions make different studies in the literature extremely difficult to compare. For another, the diagnosis of hyperplasia made on a biopsy or a curettage specimen usually has provoked hormonal, radiotherapeutic, or definitive surgical (hysterectomy) treatment and will no doubt continue to do so in the future, making it virtually impossible to obtain follow-up on a large series of untreated patients. Despite formal data, it seems prudent to accept the thesis that atypical hyperplasia, as previously defined, carries a significant risk of progression to carcinoma, particularly in the postmenopausal woman. Additional evidence for the separation of atypical hyperplasia comes from cytologic,[280] microspectrophotometric,[281,282] flow cytometric,[283] immunohistochemical,[284-288] morphometric,[279,289,290] and chromosomal[291] studies that all show a close relation of this form of hyperplasia to adenocarcinoma. Some studies of proliferation markers have shown a wider separation between all the hyperplasias and adenocarcinomas (Sasano H, personal communication).[292] Ultrastructural studies are somewhat contradictory;

in some studies, atypical hyperplasias look more like milder hyperplasias, whereas in others they more closely resemble carcinomas.[293,294] Of the hyperplasias without atypia, simple hyperplasia clearly has no significant premalignant potential, whereas that of complex hyperplasia is probably small but possibly real.

Differential Diagnosis. The *differential diagnosis* of these hyperplastic lesions depends on the type of hyperplasia being considered (Table 4-4). Simple hyperplasia has its differential diagnosis primarily with cystic atrophy and with polyps containing cystically dilated glands.[295] Because simple hyperplasia is frequently polypoid, this latter distinction may be more apparent than real. The main features to look for in simple hyperplasia are the proliferative rather than atrophic appearance of all or nearly all the glands and the participation of the stroma in the hyperplastic process. Polyps are identifiable by their fibrotic stroma and thick-walled blood vessels. Complex hyperplasia may be difficult to distinguish from a normal endometrium in late proliferative phase, a polyp or polyps, a chronic endometritis, or a *disordered proliferative endometrium* (Fig. 4-82). The latter appearance may be associated with anovulatory cycles and has irregularly distributed, sometimes architecturally abnormal glands. However, the volume of endometrium is not increased, and the stromal compartment is neither increased (as in simple hyperplasia) nor decreased (as in complex hyperplasia), thus leaving the glandular–stromal ratio normal for a proliferative-phase endometrium. In normal prolifer-

---

TABLE 4-4.
Differential Diagnosis of Endometrial Hyperplasia

Simple
  Cystic atrophy
  Polyp(s)
  Disordered proliferative phase
  Normal cycling endometrium with compression artifact

Complex
  Polyp(s)
  Chronic endometritis
  Disordered proliferative phase
  Normal cycling endometrium with compression artifact
  Atypical polypoid adenomyoma
  Simple hyperplasia
  Complex atypical hyperplasia
  Adenocarcinoma (rarely)

Atypical
  Ciliary change
  Surface syncytial change
  Papillary proliferation
  Eosinophilic cell change
  Arias-Stella change
  Chronic endometritis (rarely)
  Other hyperplasias
  Adenocarcinoma

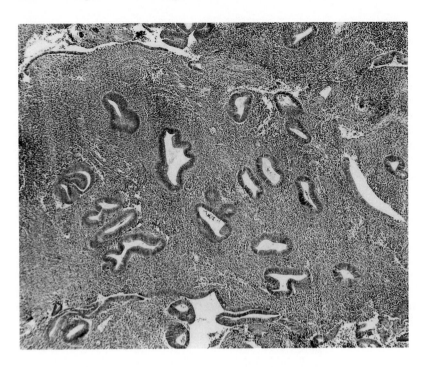

FIGURE 4-82 Disordered proliferative endometrium. The glands are irregularly distributed and somewhat irregular in shape, but the gland-to-stromal ratio is unchanged.

ative endometrium, the regularity of the glandular distribution should prevent confusion. In chronic endometritis, it is important to identify the inflammatory infiltrate; stromal edema, spindle cells, or both are commonly seen as well.

Finally, atypical hyperplasia must be distinguished from ciliary, eosinophilic, papillary and surface syncytial changes on the one hand, and focal adenocarcinoma on the other. The former distinction is based largely on the absence of cytologic and nuclear atypias in the metaplasias and related changes (see above), whereas we believe that the distinction from carcinoma is best made on the basis of the presence or absence of stromal invasion (see below).[128,260,296] Other authors who have dealt with the problem of the differentiation between atypical hyperplasia and well-differentiated carcinoma have proposed criteria that seem markedly different on first reading,[258,278,279,296–299] but in fact will yield similar results if applied to a series of practical rather than theoretical cases. Metaplastic changes, particularly squamous metaplasia or morules, in a complex hyperplasia (Fig. 4-83) should not lead to a diagnosis of adenocarcinoma unless the glands show the appropriate features.

Computer-aided diagnosis may prove to be of value in the future,[289,290,300,301] or we may fall back on the concept of endometrial intraepithelial neoplasia (EIN)[264,266] for those focal lesions in which treatment should be the same regardless of whether the lesion is called *severe atypical hyperplasia* or *focal well-differentiated adenocarcinoma*.

Additional differential diagnoses of all of the hyperplasias are with each other. Clues to avoid pitfalls in this area have been presented in the earlier section on microscopic appearance.

Cytologic Detection and Diagnosis. Cytologic detection and diagnosis of endometrial hyperplasias are still controversial; some authors claim excellent results for purely cytologic techniques,[280,302,303] whereas most[304–309] find histologic specimens far better than cytologic specimens for making the diagnosis. Our experience supports the latter viewpoint, although we certainly have been able to suggest the diagnosis of hyperplasia in some situations. With vaginal or cervical material, the only way that the suspicion of hyperplasia can be raised is by finding endometrial cells at an abnormal time (after the tenth day of a menstrual cycle or after the menopause), often in association with an abnormal hormonal background (numerous superficial cells in a scrape from the lateral vaginal wall suggesting estrogenic stimulation in a postmenopausal woman). In material obtained directly from the endometrial cavity, and less frequently in an endocervical aspirate, the presence of endometrial hyperplasia is suggested by abundant cellular material in which cell clusters show increased cell volume, anisonucleosis, and stratification or piling up of cells, without the more severe abnormalities seen in adenocarcinoma (Color Fig. 4-5). In Vuopala's literature survey,[309] however, even direct endometrial aspiration was able to detect only 20% to 70% of hyperplasias in various series, and false-positive diagnoses of carcinoma were not infrequent. We agree with Vuopala, Bibbo and coworkers,[304] Gusberg and Milano,[306] and others that sampling techniques that obtain material suitable for histologic study are preferable for the detection and diagnosis of these hyperplastic lesions.

Treatment. The *treatment* of these lesions is of interest both to the clinician and the pathologist. In

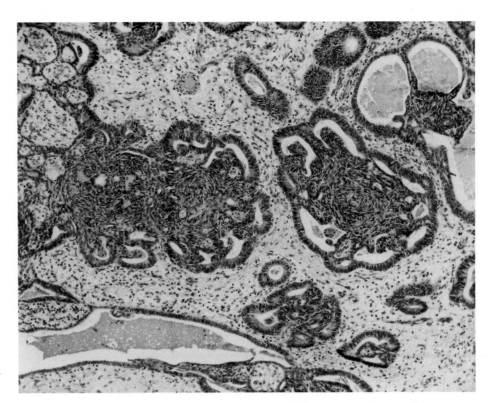

FIGURE 4-83 Complex hyperplasia with morular metaplasia. The glands do not satisfy the criteria for the diagnosis of adenocarcinoma.

postmenopausal women, the wisest course to follow is probably hysterectomy, which will be permanently curative for all noninvasive lesions. In younger women, therapy may profitably be directed along endocrine lines. Any underlying source of abnormal estrogenic stimuli (eg, polycystic ovarian syndrome, ovarian cyst or tumor, hyperthecosis, exogenous estrogen administration) should be uncovered and treated. Specific therapy for the endometrial lesion consists of the administration of progestational agents; in most cases of hyperplasia without atypia, the hyperplastic changes regress considerably, and usually completely, and progression to invasive carcinoma after this treatment is rare.[261,265,310] The endometrium after treatment may take on a completely normal histologic appearance, show glandular atrophy with stromal decidual reaction, or show persistent hyperplasia of lesser severity than in the pretreatment biopsy. Atypical hyperplasias, on the other hand, frequently persist or progress despite treatment and must be monitored carefully. A new alternative to progestin treatment is the oral administration of danazol; more studies on this agent must be reported.[311]

MALIGNANT TUMORS

Malignant tumors of the uterus can be classified as epithelial (carcinomas, the most common), nonepithelial, and mixed epithelial-nonepithelial (Table 4-5). There are also a few other rare tumors such as

sex cord–like tumors, tumors of germ cell type, neuroectodermal tumors, and malignant lymphomas. In addition to these primary tumors, there are metastatic tumors, more commonly epithelial than sarcomatous. Cancers of the corpus uteri represent about 10% to 15% of the malignant tumors seen in women. They appear with greatest frequency between 50 and 70 years of age.

Primary Tumors

Carcinoma

Carcinoma of the endometrium accounts for about 90% of malignant tumors of the uterine corpus. It is the fourth most common cancer in Western women and the most frequent invasive gynecologic cancer. Its frequency tends to increase with the increased longevity of the population, because 75% of cases appear after the age of 50 years (Fig. 4-84). This increasing frequency, combined with the decreasing incidence of invasive cervical cancer, has greatly modified the formerly quoted proportion of 10 cervical cancers to 1 endometrial cancer in favor of the latter. The most recent epidemiologic surveys, however, have noted a decline in endometrial cancer incidence in the United States since 1975, generally attributed to decreasing estrogen usage.[312,313] Endometrial carcinoma is rare before the age of 40 years.[85,314,315] Classically, 95% of endometrial carcinomas have been adenocarcinomas, and 95% have occurred after the menopause. In more recent series, as many as 50% of the tumors have contained

TABLE 4-5.
Malignant Tumors of the Uterine Corpus

Epithelial
Endometrial carcinoma
  Endometrioid
    Adenocarcinoma
      Variants:
        Secretory
        Ciliated cell
    Adenocarcinoma with squamous differentiation
      Adenocarcinoma with squamous metaplasia
        (adenoacanthoma)
      Adenosquamous carcinoma
  Serous adenocarcinoma
  Clear cell adenocarcinoma
  Mucinous adenocarcinoma
  Squamous cell carcinoma
  Mixed carcinoma
  Undifferentiated carcinoma

Nonepithelial
Endometrial stromal tumors
  Low-grade stromal sarcoma
  High-grade stromal sarcoma
Leiomyosarcoma (see Table 4-3)
Other soft-tissue tumors
  Homologous
  Heterologous

Mixed Epithelial-Nonepithelial
Adenosarcoma
  Homologous
  Heterologous
Carcinosarcoma (malignant mixed mesodermal tumor;
  malignant mixed müllerian tumor)
  Homologous
  Heterologous

Silverberg SG, Kurman RJ: Tumors of the uterine corpus and gestational trophoblastic disease. Atlas of tumor pathology, 3rd series, fascicle 3. Washington, DC, Armed Forces Institute of Pathology, 1992

squamous elements, and many tumors have affected premenopausal women.[316,317]

Etiology. The etiology is not known, but several favorable factors have been demonstrated. In general, these are the same as for endometrial hyperplasia, reinforcing the concept of the premalignant potential of this lesion. Many of these factors have been related to prolonged or exaggerated estrogenic stimulation,[318–320] including nulliparity, failure of ovulation (eg, polycystic ovary syndrome),[321] late menopause, obesity (adipose tissue increases estrone formation),[322] feminizing mesenchymal ovarian tumors,[323] ovarian stromal hyperplasia and hyperthecosis,[324] and exogenous estrogen (including tamoxifen) administration.[325–328]

Factors that have not been related to the estrogen hypothesis of carcinogenesis include diabetes, hypertension, prior pelvic irradiation,[124] and familial predisposition.[329,330] Animal experiments have produced conflicting data on estrogen carcinogenicity; a neoplastic response has been demonstrated in ani-

mals such as rats, mice, and rabbits but not in subhuman primates. Numerous studies have indicated that estrone is the most important estrogen in endometrial carcinogenesis and that this hormone is produced primarily by extraglandular aromatization of plasma androstenedione.[320,331,332] Estrogen receptors have been demonstrated in normal and neoplastic endometrium,[332–336] adding to the evidence for specific responsiveness of this tissue. Some authors[336–339] have postulated that endometrial carcinomas that develop in this hormonal milieu have a more favorable prognosis than those that do not. Finally, the role of oncogene alterations in the development and natural history of endometrial hyperplasia is just beginning to be defined.[340,341]

Clinical Signs. The dominant clinical sign of carcinoma is painless vaginal bleeding, at first slight and at intervals, later continuous and profuse. Pain appears only late in the course of the disease. Postmenopausal bleeding should be emphasized as an important sign. In one study, endometrial carcinoma was found in 107 (13.7%) of 782 patients with this complaint.[342]

Diagnosis. The methods of diagnosis of endometrial carcinoma include study of the clinical signs (metrorrhagia, white blood-tinged discharge, pain), hysterography,[343] hysteroscopy,[344] sonoangiogra-

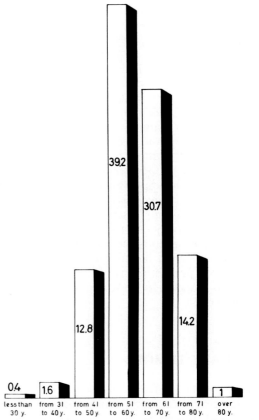

FIGURE 4-84 Adenocarcinoma of endometrium: frequency (percentage) of appearance as a function of age (879 cases).

phy,[345] ultrasonography,[346] exfoliative cytology, and (ultimately) histologic examination. Early diagnosis is often the result of the practice of exfoliative cytology;[254,306,307,347,348] the finding of neoplastic cells in vaginal, cervical, or endometrial secretions brings about the discovery of some asymptomatic cases. Endometrial aspiration is the technique of choice,[304,306,309,349] because it produces fewer false-negative results than cervical scrapings (the poorest technique) or vaginal pool or endocervical aspiration (intermediate in value). Despite these technical precautions, the percentage of false-negative reports remains in the range of 10% or greater, pointing out the need for adequate endometrial biopsy in clinically worrisome cases.[304,309,347,348]

In recent years, new instruments and techniques have permitted direct histologic sampling of the endometrium as an outpatient procedure.[304–306,309] Although dilatation and curettage under anesthesia is generally considered the most reliable procedure, it does not sample the entire endometrium in most cases,[350] and it is far more expensive and prone to complications than the outpatient procedures.[351]

Macroscopic Appearance.

With the exception of a few tumors that arise in deep-seated foci of adenomyosis, endometrial carcinoma begins on the surface of the uterus, most frequently on the posterior wall. It develops slowly and presents in one of two macroscopic forms: localized or diffuse.

Localized carcinoma consists of a round, polypoid, or exophytic mass that is friable and often shows surface ulceration. The uterine cavity is progressively encroached on by soft, easily detachable neoplastic masses, which are embedded superficially in the myometrium (Fig. 4-85).

Diffuse carcinoma extensively infiltrates the thickened and indurated mucosa (Fig. 4-86). The volume of the uterus is increased but rarely surpasses that of a 3-month pregnancy. In advanced cases, the uterine cavity is filled with tumor, which may block the cervical canal and cause hematometra or pyometra.

Microscopic Appearance and Histologic Grading of Endometrioid Adenocarcinoma.

Endometrioid adenocarcinoma is the most common type of carcinoma seen in the endometrium (see Table 4-5). It is characterized by numerous rounded glands of generally small and uniform size disposed in random fashion. They are lined by stratified epithelium, the cells of which show nuclear atypia and mitoses, the number and character of which vary according to the degree of differentiation of the tumor. The cells usually are oriented with their axes perpendicular to the basement membrane. In many cases, the degree of differentiation varies from one region to another.

The abundance of the connective tissue stroma also varies. It is in general well vascularized and contains prominent leukocytic and histiocytic infiltrates. Stromal foam cells are often seen.[120] Reactive fibrosis may be prominent. Foci of benign cartilaginous or osseous metaplasia are rarely present, but they must be differentiated from their malignant counterparts in mixed mesodermal tumors.[144]

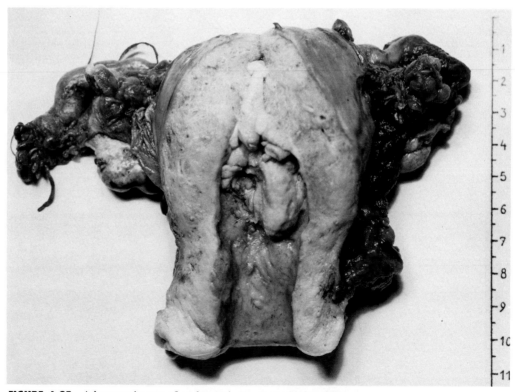

FIGURE 4-85 Adenocarcinoma of endometrium: macroscopic appearance.

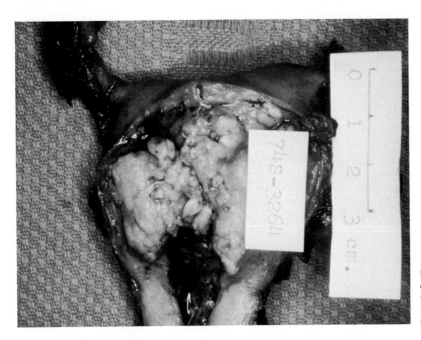

FIGURE 4-86 Diffuse macroscopic pattern of endometrial carcinoma with deep myometrial invasion despite small size of uterus (compare with Fig. 4-85, in which a much larger uterus shows a more limited tumor).

The International Federation of Gynecology and Obstetrics (FIGO) and ISGP grading system for endometrioid adenocarcinoma is based primarily on the concept that these tumors become less differentiated by deviating from a glandular or papillary pattern to form solid sheets.[128,352]

Well-differentiated (grade I) adenocarcinoma is characterized by 5% or less of a nonsquamous and nonmorular solid growth pattern. The glands are of regular contour and little cellular atypia. The only histologic finding suggesting malignancy is the overabundance of glands, which are crowded against each other with either no stroma separating them or separated by a reactive fibrous stroma or necrotic debris (Figs. 4-87 through 4-90). Pluristratification is present in most of the glands (Fig. 4-91). Mitoses may be numerous. The nuclei are larger than in normal cells, and their contours are indented. The nucleoli are enlarged, and the nuclear–cytoplasmic ratio is moderately augmented. If marked nuclear

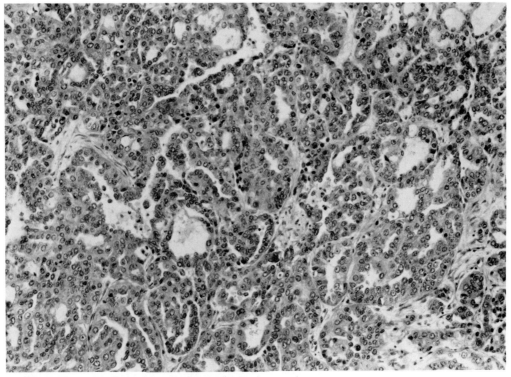

FIGURE 4-87 Well-differentiated (FIGO grade I) adenocarcinoma.

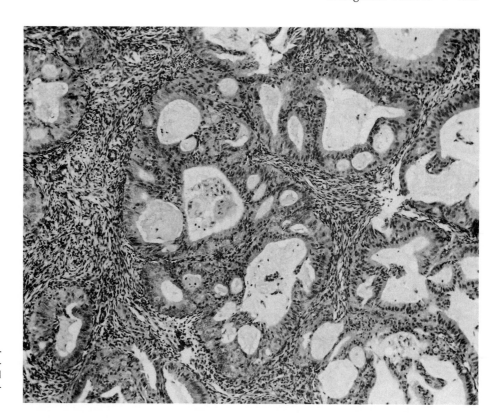

FIGURE 4-88 Focal well-differentiated (FIGO grade I) endometrioid adenocarcinoma in atypical hyperplasia. Note cribriform (confluent) pattern of glands.

atypia is present, the FIGO grade is elevated to grade II.

Papillary structures may be prominent in some tumors (*papillary* or *villoglandular endometrioid adenocarcinomas*). These tumors must be distinguished from papillary clear cell or serous carcinomas (see below). The main diagnostic feature is that the cells are similar to those of the classic glandular endometrioid pattern (Figs. 4-92 and 4-93).[353]

Electron micrographs have not demonstrated morphologic characteristics specific for the cancer cell. The modifications of fine structure of the malignant

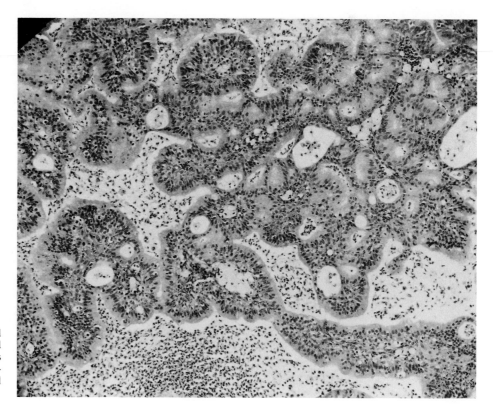

FIGURE 4-89 Well-differentiated (FIGO grade I) endometrioid adenocarcinoma showing necrosis of stroma between glands, identified by replacement of stromal cells by neutrophils.

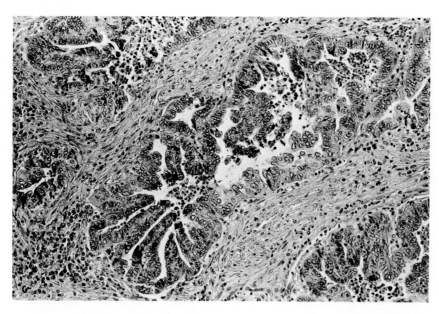

FIGURE 4-90 Adenocarcinoma of endometrium with stromal fibrosis.

cell are more of a quantitative than a qualitative nature.[293,294,354,355]

The nuclei are multilobate and show more or less deep invaginations of the membranes. They have a dense homogeneous structure, in which is found a voluminous nucleolus (Fig. 4-94). Enlargements of about 50,000 times permit recognition of the filamentous and granular structure of this organelle, as has been described in phase-contrast microscopy. Its contours are poorly defined, but its components appear in parallel rows of round parti-

cles measuring about 15 nm in diameter each. The nucleolus contains principally RNA (Feulgen-negative and ribonuclease-positive).

The cytoplasm contains numerous mitochondria of similar size and appearance as those in normal endometrial cells. The lysosomes or dense bodies are found in greater number than in normal cells and their size is variable; most, however, are of the same size as mitochondria. They contain catabolic enzymes such as urease, phosphatases, and desoxyribonucleases.

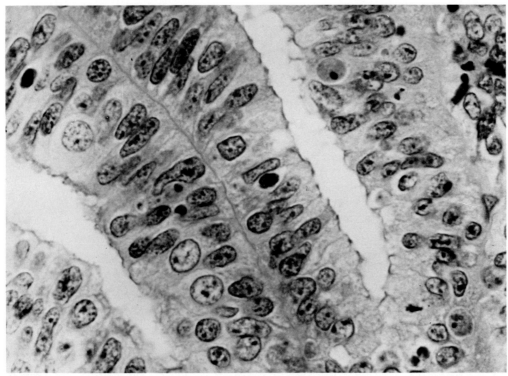

FIGURE 4-91 Well-differentiated adenocarcinoma: detail of a gland.

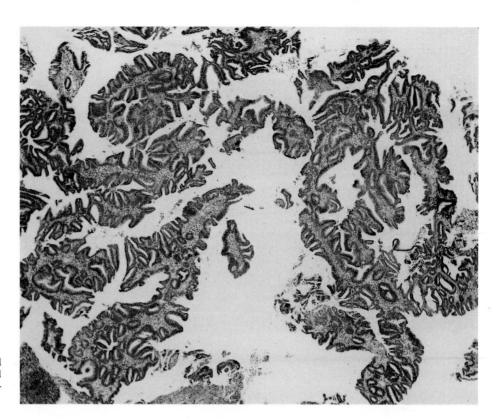

FIGURE 4-92 Well-differentiated (FIGO grade I) endometrioid adenocarcinoma of papillary (villoglandular) type.

The Golgi apparatus is well developed and sometimes shows dilatation of its vacuolar structures (Fig. 4-95). The appearance of the endoplasmic reticulum does not differ significantly from that of the normal cell; rarely, the membranes separate to form vacuoles of varied shapes.

Pools of lipid with irregular contours are found disseminated in the cytoplasm, and many cells contain variable amounts of glycogen (see Fig. 4-95). The cell membranes are sinuous and here and there reveal desmosomes. Bundles of fine filaments of about 10 nm in diameter, frequently related to des-

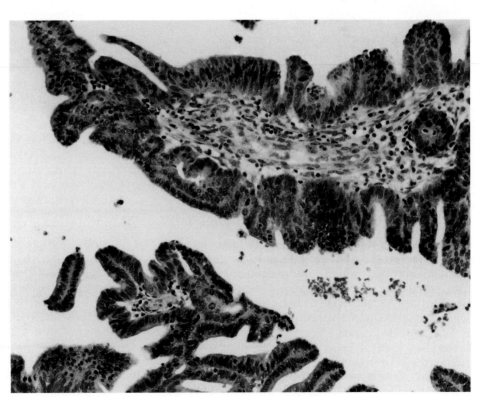

FIGURE 4-93 Well-differentiated (FIGO grade I) endometrioid adenocarcinoma of papillary (villoglandular) type. Note the low-grade cytologic features (compare with Fig. 4-103).

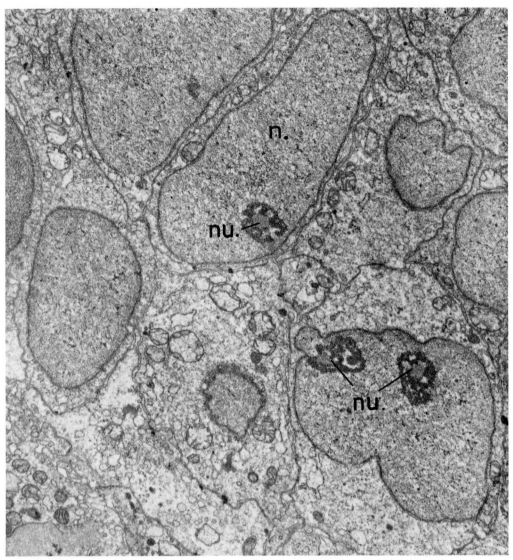

FIGURE 4-94 Adenocarcinoma of endometrium (electron micrograph, ×12,000): indented nuclei (*n.*), voluminous nucleoli (*nu.*), and convoluted cell membranes. The irregular nuclear contours, the volume of the nucleoli, and the anarchic distribution of the cells characterize the neoplastic nature of the cells.

mosomes, are more numerous than in normal endometrial cells. Basement membranes such as we have described in the normal endometrium are found around the neoplastic cell masses and constitute the junction between the epithelial elements and the stroma. This fact casts doubt on the classic description of rupture of the basement membrane as one of the cardinal manifestations of cancer. The stromal cells show irregularity of their nuclear and cytoplasmic contours. Bundles of collagen fibers insinuate among them in all directions.

The *differential diagnosis* between well-differentiated adenocarcinoma and certain atypical hyperplasias is difficult, and the pathologist must call on his or her fund of experience in distinguishing between the two lesions.[128,258,260,295-299] Haphazardly arranged glands, polystratification, and moderate nuclear atypia are typically found in cancer but are

seen in some cases of hyperplasia as well. The absence of myometrial invasion cannot be considered proof of benignity, because many carcinomas become invasive only as a late event. The most important single criterion of carcinoma is the presence of stromal invasion, which may present as diminution or loss of stroma between glands (see Figs. 4-87, 4-88, and 4-96), as stromal necrosis (see Fig. 4-89), or as stromal fibrosis (see Fig. 4-90). The absence of this criterion is also important for distinguishing benign postradiotherapy atypias in hysterectomy specimens from persistent tumor.[356]

Moderately differentiated (grade II) adenocarcinoma is a predominantly glandular lesion, but it contains a significant minority (6% to 50%) of solid cell nests, often composed of anaplastic cells (Fig. 4-97). Even the glandular component usually shows more atypia than is seen in grade I adenocarcinomas.

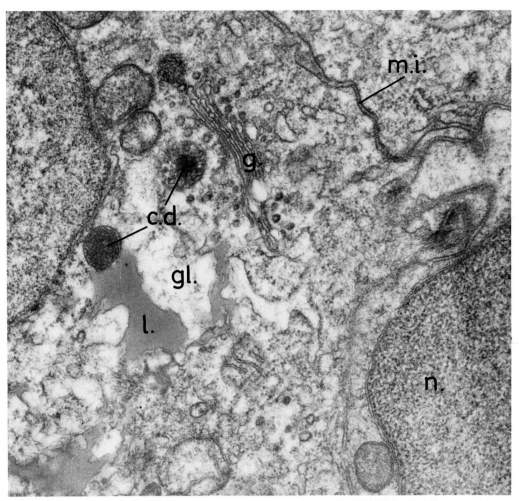

FIGURE 4-95 Adenocarcinoma of endometrium (electron micrograph, ×42,000), *n.*, nucleus; *g.*, Golgi apparatus; *c.d.*, lysosomes or dense bodies; *gl.*, glycogen; *l.*, lipids; *m.i.*, cell membranes.

Poorly differentiated (grade III) adenocarcinoma consists predominantly of solid cell nests (Fig. 4-98), with glandular elements seen in less than 50% of the tumor or perhaps not at all. Differential diagnosis of this lesion from a carcinosarcoma (if malignant glands are present) or endometrial stromal sarcoma (if no glands are seen) may be extremely difficult. In some instances, a residual nesting of epithelial type may be seen (see Fig. 4-98) and may be accentuated with a reticulin stain. In others, electron microscopic evidence of epithelial differentiation or immunohistochemical demonstration of keratin filaments[357] may be the only evidence that the tumor is, indeed, a pure carcinoma. As we shall see, these markers of epithelial differentiation may also be present in tumors that are classically considered to be of stromal origin.

Adenocarcinoma in situ. Adenocarcinoma in situ is a term that has been used in different ways by different observers. Some researchers[269–271] have used it to describe the lesion that we call atypical hyperplasia (see above), associated with a particular cytoplasmic eosinophilia, whereas others[299] have suggested that it

be used to describe a particularly small focus of what we would designate as invasive adenocarcinoma. Because the endometrium is the epithelium of the uterine corpus, this term could also be used to describe any adenocarcinoma that has not yet invaded the myometrium. With this wide discrepancy in its definition, we agree with such authors as Tavassoli and Kraus[278] and Fox and Buckley[266] that it is best not to use this term at all. Certainly, if only a small focus of adenocarcinoma invading its own stroma is seen in a curettage or a hysterectomy specimen, it should be so described and treatment should be discussed with the clinician.

Secretory Carcinoma. A variant of endometrioid adenocarcinoma has been designated secretory carcinoma; it consists of very well-differentiated cells forming glands that differ slightly if at all from those of normal secretory endometrium (Fig. 4-99). These tumors are rare in pure form but occur more frequently as foci within other endometrioid carcinomas.[358] They appear to be associated with a favorable prognosis.

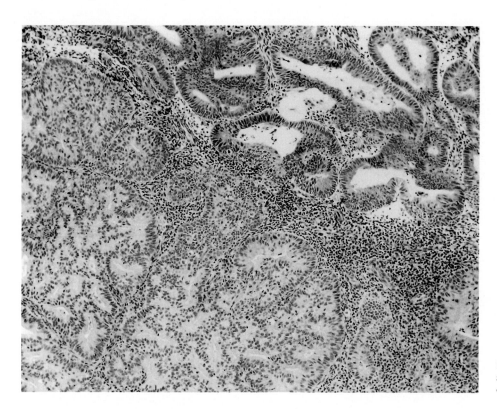

FIGURE 4-96 Well-differentiated adenocarcinoma (*bottom left*) and complex hyperplasia (*top right*).

Ciliated cell adenocarcinoma. Ciliated cell adenocarcinoma is another uncommon variant of endometrioid adenocarcinoma. In this form, the neoplastic glands are composed predominantly or exclusively of ciliated cells.[359] The outcome of the few cases reported has been relatively favorable. The differential diagnosis is with the much more common benign ciliary change, in which stromal invasion is obviously not present.

Adenocarcinoma with Squamous Differentiation (Adeno-acanthoma [Adenocarcinoma with Squamous Metaplasia] and Adenosquamous Carcinoma). In the past decades, concepts of these tumors have changed considerably. They originally were thought to be rare tumors, characterized by foci of benign squamous metaplasia within an adenocarcinoma, and carrying a better prognosis than that of adenocarcinoma without this additional finding.[360] In the past quarter century,[316,317,361–365] these tumors became recognized as fairly common (up to 50% of endometrial carcinomas in some series). Although it was originally thought that this reflected a true increase in incidence in recent years,[361] most subsequent studies have not revealed such an increase.[316,363,366] The separation of adenocarcinomas with squamous elements into adenoacanthomas and mixed adenosquamous carcinomas resulted from the work of Ng and colleagues.[361] The former lesion is characterized by squamous or morular elements that appear histologically benign and generally grow either on the surface of the endometrial tumor or within gland lumina (Figs. 4-100 and 4-101). The glandular ele-

ments are almost always of histologic grade I; the prognosis is at least as favorable as for similar-grade adenocarcinomas and in our hands is probably even more favorable. On the other hand, in adenosquamous carcinomas, the squamous elements possess cellular characteristics of malignancy and usually invade the stroma (Fig. 4-102). The glandular elements are usually moderately or poorly differentiated, and indeed sometimes it is difficult to distinguish the undifferentiated portion of a grade II or III adenocarcinoma from poorly differentiated squamous elements. In such a case, unless squamous differentiation can be demonstrated clearly, the diagnosis of adenosquamous carcinoma should not be made. The criteria for squamous differentiation adopted by ISGP[128] are as follows:

1. keratinization demonstrated with standard staining techniques
2. intercellular bridges
3. three or more of the following four criteria:
   sheet-like growth without gland formation or palisading
   sharp cell margins
   eosinophilic and thick or glassy cytoplasm
   a decreased nuclear–cytoplasmic ratio (compared with foci elsewhere in the same tumor).

Although the criteria discussed above for benignity versus malignancy of the squamous elements can then be applied, the ISGP and several recent reports[317,364,365] have recommended the use of the more inclusive term *adenocarcinoma with squamous*

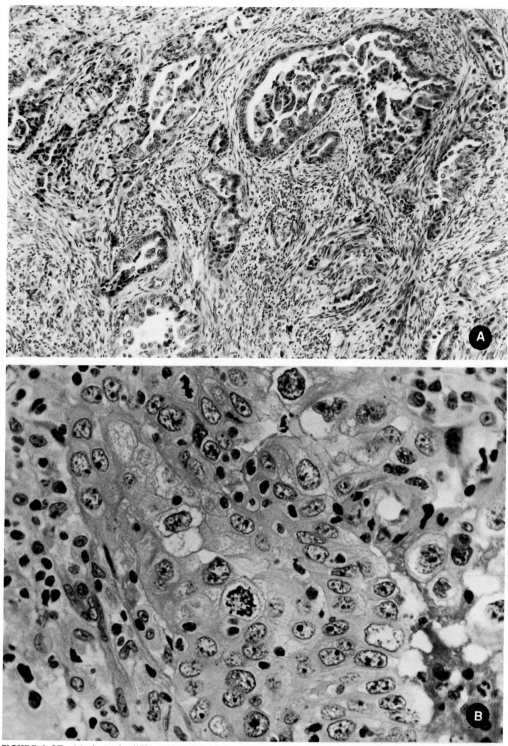

FIGURE 4-97 Moderately differentiated (FIGO grade II) adenocarcinoma. **(A)** Glandular components. **(B)** Detail of solid component.

differentiation for both adenoacanthoma and adenosquamous carcinoma, on the basis of the demonstration that the grade of the glandular component rather than the appearance of the squamous elements is most important prognostically.

The differential diagnosis of adenoacanthoma is with extensive squamous or morular metaplasia (see above) associated with benign glandular elements, frequently in the form of endometrial hyperplasia (see Figs. 4-48 and 4-83). The diagnosis of this type of carcinoma is made from the glandular elements, which must show the features previously described for grade I or II adenocarcinoma. In adenoacanthoma, the glandular elements almost always domi-

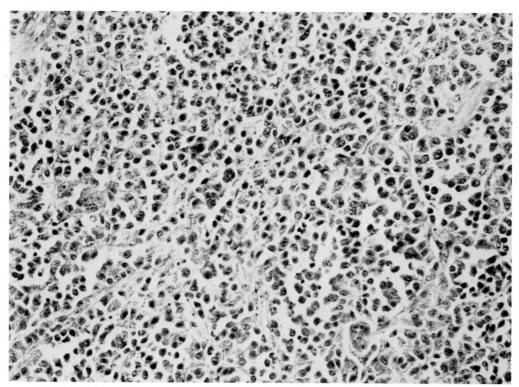

FIGURE 4-98 Poorly differentiated (FIGO grade III) adenocarcinoma.

nate the squamous or morular ones. In adenosquamous carcinoma, although the glandular elements most often dominate, the squamous component may be equally prominent or even dominate the picture. Indeed, we have seen adenosquamous carcinomas that we thought were pure squamous cell carcinomas of the endometrium until multiple sections were taken. Similarly, adenosquamous carcinoma may metastasize as an adenocarcinoma, a pure squamous cell carcinoma, or in a mixed pattern. As mentioned above, the usual poor survival figures reported for

adenosquamous carcinoma are thought to be due largely to the generally poor differentiation of the glandular elements. The squamous elements in this tumor are said to be aneuploid, as opposed to those in adenoacanthoma.[366]

Squamous Cell Carcinoma or Epidermoid Carcinoma. Squamous cell carcinoma or epidermoid carcinoma of the endometrium is rare, with about 30 cases reported.[367] It originates in a focus of benign

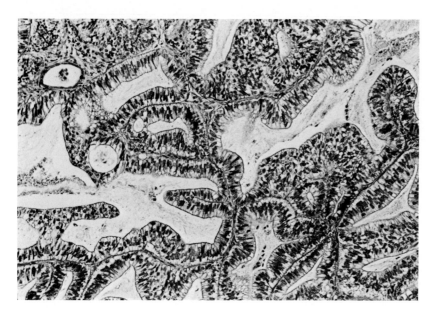

FIGURE 4-99 Secretory carcinoma: back-to-back glands cytologically resembling normal early secretory endometrium.

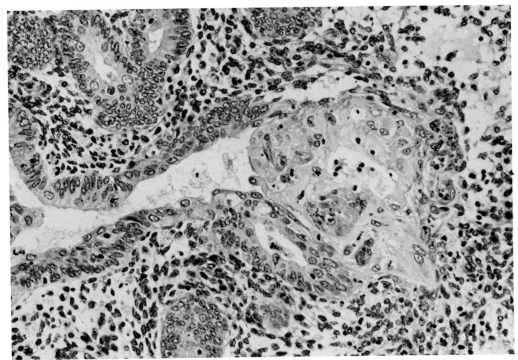

FIGURE 4-100 Adenoacanthoma (adenocarcinoma with squamous metaplasia) of endometrium: histologically benign squamous epithelium within gland lumen.

squamous metaplasia or as an overgrowth of an adenosquamous carcinoma. To establish a corporeal epidermoid carcinoma as definitely of endometrial origin, one must prove the absence of foci of adenocarcinoma in the endometrium, of coexistent invasive epidermoid carcinoma of the cervix, and of any continuity between the tumor and the cervical squamous mucosa.[368,369] These rare cases are composed of cords and nests of poorly differentiated squamous cells, among which are outlines of pearls and other foci of keratinization. Nuclear anomalies and mitoses are of variable prominence.

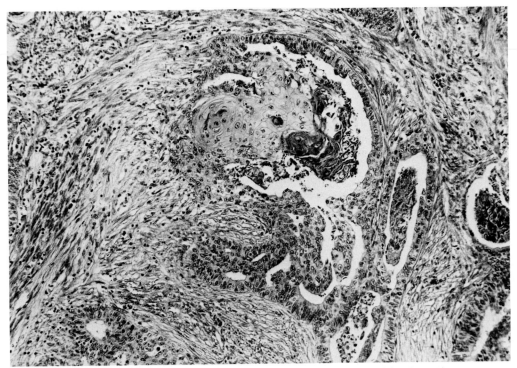

FIGURE 4-101 Adenoacanthoma (adenocarcinoma with squamous metaplasia) of endometrium.

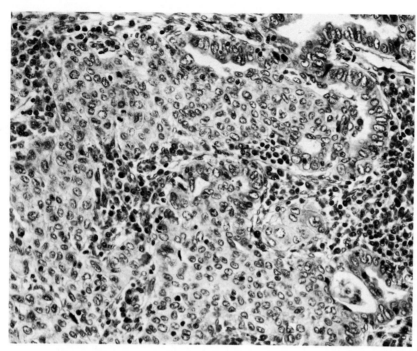

FIGURE 4-102 Adenosquamous carcinoma: detail of neoplastic glands and invasive, histologically malignant, squamous elements.

Serous Carcinoma. *Serous carcinoma* is probably the most important of the nonendometrioid adenocarcinomas, both because of its frequency (5% to 10% of all endometrial carcinomas) and its distinctive natural history. It is defined as a primary carcinoma of the endometrium that is histologically identical to its more common counterpart seen in the ovary.[235,236,370–376] This type of tumor is generally seen in older women and is usually moderately to poorly differentiated (Fig. 4-103). Characteristic histologic findings include broad papillae with fibrovascular cores, lined by secondary papillae with tufting and exfoliation of small clusters of cells. Psammoma bodies are a frequent but not universal finding. The cells and their nuclei are generally smaller and rounder than those of most endometrioid adenocarcinomas. The differential diagnosis includes papillary variants of both classic endometrioid and clear cell carcinoma, as well as the papillary metaplasia usually seen at or near the endometrial surface (see above). Although they frequently occur in small uteri, serous carcinomas generally extensively invade the myometrium within lymphatics or blood vessels (Fig. 4-104), are usually disseminated beyond the uterus at the time of diagnosis, and have a very poor prognosis. It has recently been shown that dissemination (perhaps really multifocal peritoneal neoplasia) is a major threat even when serous carcinoma in the uterus is limited to the endometrium or an endometrial polyp.[235,236,375,376]

Clear Cell Adenocarcinoma. This tumor, like serous carcinoma, is associated with a poor prognosis even when apparently confined to the uterine corpus or to the endometrium itself.[236] It comprises about 4% of endometrial carcinomas.[373,377–380] It occurs predominantly in postmenopausal women and is often in an advanced stage when first detected. Microscopically, the characteristic feature is the presence of large tumor cells with voluminous clear cytoplasm containing glycogen. A second population of cells projecting individually into lumina (hobnail cells) may be as numerous or even more so than the clear cells. Mucin may be present in lumina but rarely in tumor cell cytoplasm. The stroma is often focally hyalinized. The tumor cells grow in tubular (Fig. 4-105), papillary (Fig. 4-106), solid (Fig. 4-107), or mixed architectural patterns. The nuclei are usually pleomorphic and, if these tumors are to be graded at all, nuclear grading should be used exclusively. The differential diagnosis is with benign clear cell, hobnail cell, and Arias-Stella changes, and with serous carcinoma. The latter may frequently coexist with clear cell carcinoma.[376]

Mucinous Adenocarcinoma. *Mucinous adenocarcinoma* comprised 9% of all stage I endometrial carcinomas in one series[381] but is much less common in our experience. It is defined as an adenocarcinoma in which most of the tumor cells contain prominent intracytoplasmic mucin (Fig. 4-108). The tumor is usually well differentiated and the prognosis is favorable.[381,382] The differential diagnosis includes mucinous metaplasia (distinguishable on architectural features), primary endocervical adenocarcinoma, and otherwise typical endometrioid endometrial adenocarcinomas with minor foci of mucinous differentiation or abundant luminal rather than intracytoplasmic mucin.

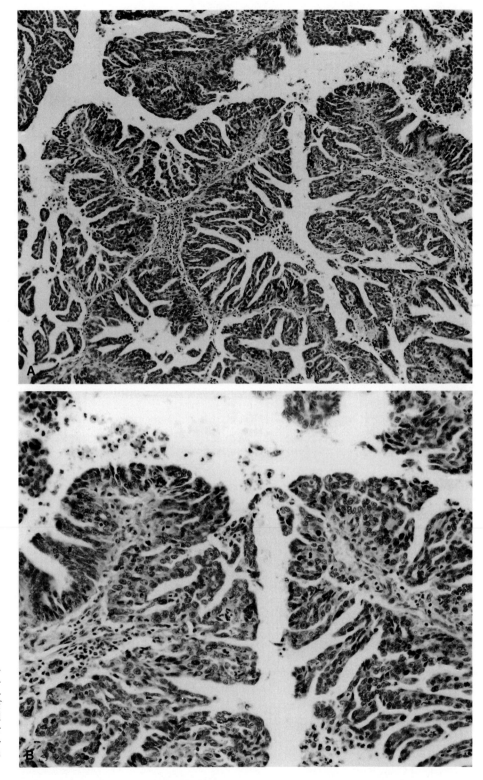

FIGURE 4-103 Serous adenocarcinoma. **(A)** Low-power photomicrograph showing complex papillary architecture. **(B)** Detail of small cells with round nuclei and frequent mitotic figures; tumor cells and necrotic debris are exfoliated into lumina. Compare with Figures 4-92 and 4-93.

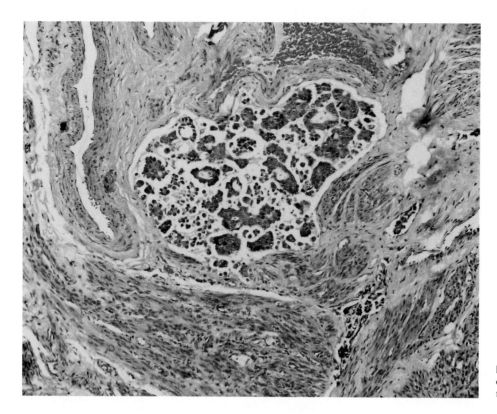

FIGURE 4-104 Serous adenocarcinoma of endometrium invading myometrial lymphatics.

Other Forms of Carcinoma. In addition to these histologic types of carcinoma, certain other patterns have been reported in the endometrium. Some cases of adenocarcinoma indistinguishable from the more common types described here may be shown, with appropriate stains, to contain argyrophil cells.[383]

This demonstration is probably not of prognostic significance. Much more rare is a true *small cell carcinoma* of the endometrium resembling similar tumors seen in the bronchial tree.[384,385] These and other *undifferentiated carcinomas*[385] have a very poor prognosis.

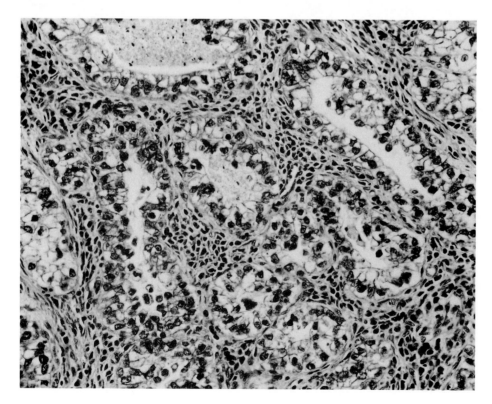

FIGURE 4-105 Clear cell adenocarcinoma, tubular pattern.

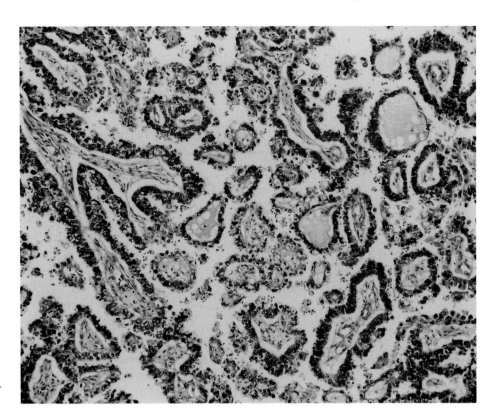

FIGURE 4-106 Clear cell adeno-carcinoma, papillary pattern.

Other tumor types that occur more frequently in the cervix, but have been reported in the endometrium, include *glassy cell carcinoma,*[386] *verrucous carcinoma,*[387] and adenocarcinomas with *giant cell carcinoma*[388] and with *trophoblastic differentiation.*[389]

Mixed Carcinomas. *Mixed carcinoma of the endometrium* is a carcinoma containing more than one of the cell types described above. For the tumor to be characterized as mixed, the second type must comprise at least 10% of the total volume of the tumor,

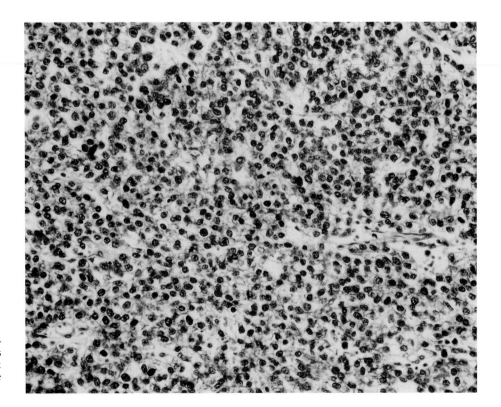

FIGURE 4-107 Clear cell adeno-carcinoma, solid pattern. Figures 4-105 through 4-107 represent different fields within the same tumor.

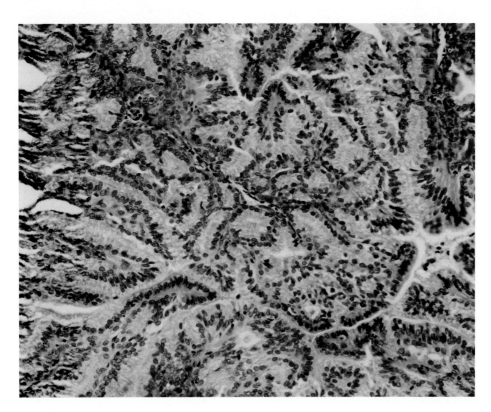

FIGURE 4-108 Mucinous adenocarcinoma of endometrium.

as estimated from the examination of multiple sections. The types of tumor encountered and their relative proportions should be specified in the pathology report. The prognostic implications of mixed carcinomas in which the subordinate type is less favorable have been poorly characterized, but Sherman and colleagues have suggested that tumors with 25% or more of a serous pattern display the unfavorable prognostic characteristics of pure serous carcinoma.[376]

Cytology. We prefer techniques that provide histologic rather than cytologic material for the definitive diagnosis of endometrial carcinoma, and techniques are available that provide such material on an outpatient basis in most cases. In a summary of the literature, Vuopala[309] noted an accuracy rate of 97% in the diagnosis of endometrial carcinoma with the Vabra aspiration technique, as compared with 42% to 70% in techniques relying predominantly on cytologic interpretation of vaginal or cervical material, 73% for endocervical aspiration, and 75% to 88% for techniques using cytologic interpretation of material obtained directly from the endometrial cavity. The criteria for diagnosis of endometrial carcinoma from vaginal or cervical material are similar to those described for endometrial hyperplasia and often merely involve finding endometrial cells at the wrong time (late in the menstrual cycle or in a postmenopausal woman). In the case of carcinoma, these cells usually show greater cytologic atypia than is encountered in most hyperplasias.

Although poorly differentiated endometrial carcinomas usually do not pose any problems in cytologic diagnosis, a well-differentiated or grade I lesion may be difficult to distinguish from hyperplasia or even normal endometrium. The major distinguishing characteristic is cell size, which is generally larger than that of any benign endometrial cell, although smaller than the malignant endocervical cell. The cell size in endometrial carcinoma increases as the differentiation decreases. In addition to size, the nuclear chromatin is irregularly distributed and varying degrees of hyperchromasia are present (Color Fig. 4-6). The nucleus is generally round to oval, as is the cell itself. Although isolated cells may be seen, small groups are the rule. Enlarged solitary nucleoli are the general rule, although occasionally multiple nucleoli may be seen in a single nucleus. The cytoplasmic borders are usually indistinct, and one, several, or many vacuoles may be present in the cytoplasm. The cells often contain leukocytes or cellular debris. Relatively few tumor cells may be seen, particularly in material obtained distant from the endometrial cavity itself and in well-differentiated carcinomas. In these cases, an inflammatory diathesis consisting of cellular debris, leukocytes, erythrocytes, histiocytes, and fibrin may provide the first clue to the diagnosis of a carcinoma.

Although this discussion is largely relevant to adenocarcinoma of the endometrioid type, other histologic types may be diagnosed by finding the appropriate cells in cytologic material: benign squamous cells coexisting with malignant glandular ones in adenoacanthoma (Color Fig. 4-7), malignant glandular and squamous cells in adenosquamous carcinoma, abundant well-preserved cytoplasm (occasionally optically clear) in clear cell carcinoma, and papillary structures with occasional psammoma bodies in serous carcinoma.

Staging of Endometrial Carcinoma. The FIGO clinical staging system in use for many years was superseded in 1988 by a surgical staging system (Table 4-6).[352] Clinical staging is now supposed to be used only for patients who are not candidates for staging by laparotomy, usually for medical reasons (eg, marked obesity and severe diabetes). The extent of surgical staging in an individual patient—for example, whether lymph node dissection will be performed—is often based on an estimate of risk versus benefit, which in turn is based on an assessment of tumor type and grade, extension to involve the cervix, and depth of myometrial invasion. Most studies have shown the intraoperative evaluation of these factors to be more reliable by frozen section than by gross evaluation only of the hysterectomy specimen.[390-392]

One effect of surgical staging is to eliminate the confusion formerly caused by the use of fractional (endometrial and endocervical) curettage to identify carcinomas that have extended to the cervix (stage II). If such a procedure is performed, the pathologist should remember that the presence of carcinoma in the specimen submitted as "endocervix" does not confirm stage II disease unless cancerous invasion of endocervical stroma can be demonstrated histologically.[390,393,394] The value of separating new surgical stages IIA and IIB has been confirmed in one recent report in which the recurrence rates in these two stages were 0 and 63% respectively.[395]

Another problem encountered in staging endometrial carcinomas involves the best definition of stage III disease. It has been shown in several series[396-399] that some patients with carcinoma involving the endometrium and one or both ovaries probably have separate primaries rather than metastatic disease. In these cases, the patients are usually young, the tumors well-differentiated, and the prognosis excellent, in contrast to other patients with true stage III disease.

Despite these problems, several studies have already confirmed the value of surgical staging of endometrial carcinoma.[395,400,401] Because grading is included in the new staging system, the advisability of raising the architectural grade for "inappropriate" nuclear atypia has been questioned by some investigators.[402,403]

Evolution, Prognosis, and Treatment. The degree of differentiation in adenocarcinoma shows good correlation with the clinical prognosis. As a general rule, the better differentiated the tumor, the longer the median survival (all other factors, such as size, myometrial invasion, clinical stage, patient age, and adequacy of initial therapy, being equal).[390,400,401,404-406] Only endometrioid adenocarcinoma and its variants can be graded reproducibly and meaningfully by the usual criteria.

Adenocarcinoma of the endometrium remains localized for a long time and, for this reason, has a more favorable evolution than carcinoma of the cervix. Metastatic dissemination by the lymphatic route involves the hypogastric, iliac, aortic, and lumbar nodes, but rarely occurs in the absence of myometrial or cervical invasion.[400,407,408] It is common to find intralymphatic tumor infiltrates beneath the vaginal mucosa as the first sign of recurrence after surgical or radiation therapy;[409] modifications of the lymphatic circulation brought about by postradiotherapeutic secondary fibrosis may be invoked to explain these retrograde localizations. The occurrence of ovarian and pelvic peritoneal metastases by means of the intratubal route,[410] by a mechanism identical to that advanced to explain these localizations of endometriosis, may not be of great importance.[411] Peritoneal dissemination in cases of serous carcinoma may represent multifocal carcinomatosis.[235,236,375,376] Hematogenous metastases generally appear late in the course of the disease and localize with greatest frequency in the lungs, liver, and bones. In extensive cases, the tumor breaks through the uterine serosal surface and involves the peritoneum. Considering all clinical and histologic groupings together, endometrial adenocarcinoma shows a 5-year survival rate in the range of 70%, somewhat more favorable than that of cervical carcinoma.[412] By clinical stage, the 5-year survival rate is about 75% to 80% in stage I, 50% to 60% in stage II, 30% in stage III (but better if the only extrauterine tumor is in the ovaries),[396-399] and 10% in stage IV. These survival rates are better in the corresponding surgical stages.[412] They are generally worse for serous, clear cell, pure squamous cell, and undifferentiated carcinomas.

TABLE 4-6.
The 1988 FIGO Surgical Staging System for Uterine Corpus Carcinoma

Stage I: Confined to the uterine corpus
   IA Tumor limited to endometrium
   IB Invasion of less than half of the myometrium
   IC Invasion of more than half of the myometrium

Stage II: Uterine cervix involved
   IIA Endocervical glandular involvement only
   IIB Cervical stromal invasion

Stage III: Pelvic extension
   IIIA Tumor invades serosa and/or adnexa and/or positive
       peritoneal cytology
   IIIB Vaginal metastasis
   IIIC Metastases to pelvic and/or paraaortic lymph nodes

Stage IV: Extrapelvic extension
   IVA Tumor invasion of bladder and/or bowel mucosa
   IVB Distant metastases including intra-abdominal and/or
       inguinal lymph nodes

Regardless of the histologic type, the presence and extent of myometrial invasion are important prognostic features. Most important is the observation that endometrioid tumors without any myometrial invasion have a negligible risk of metastasis.[390,400,401] The extent of myometrial invasion, when present, definitely relates to the likelihood of metastasis and death. Different authors have proposed different ways of measuring the extent of myometrial involvement,[413,414] although the classic expression of invasion into the inner, middle, or outer third of the myometrium is the system that we have usually used, and the inner or outer half is now mandated by FIGO. It is important not to overinterpret as myometrial invasion the extension of carcinoma into "tongues" of endometrium penetrating shallowly into the myometrium or extension into foci of adenomyosis.[184,185] Rounded rather than angular tumor borders, as well as residual nests of benign endometrial stromal cells, are helpful in both of these circumstances.

In addition to these tumor-related factors, host-related factors are of prognostic importance. The favorable prognosis of endometrial carcinoma in young women, particularly in association with the Stein-Leventhal syndrome, has long been noted, and observations have indicated that elderly patients with endometrial carcinoma have a particularly poor prognosis.[415] The significance of a host immunologic response is probably also considerable.[338]

Other factors of unfavorable prognostic significance include the presence of myometrial lymphatic/vascular space invasion,[416–419] involvement of the lower uterine segment by cancers limited to the corpus,[420,421] and positive peritoneal cytology.[422–424] It is hotly debated whether the latter finding is an independent indicator of poor prognosis, with most studies claiming that it is not independent of other factors such as stage and grade. The last major histologic factor associated with prognosis is the presence in nonneoplastic endometrium accompanying the tumor of hyperplastic[425,426] or metaplastic changes,[139,140] which appears to convey a more favorable prognosis. This goes along with the observation that carcinomas developing in a background of endogenous or exogenous hyperestrinism tend to be of a more favorable type.[326,337,339,427]

Other nonmorphologic factors may also be important in prognosis. These include the presence of estrogen and progesterone receptors in the tumor[333,334,336] (although a primary carcinoma and its metastases may not show the same pattern[428]), the finding of specific oncogene alterations,[340,341] and quantitative features including those analyzed by flow cytometry.[429–431]

Treatment is determined in large measure by the surgical staging findings and usually is limited to surgery in favorable cases. Vaginal or external irradiation may be added (formerly often before surgery, now usually postoperatively).[432–434] Some medically inoperable patients may be treated by radiation therapy alone.[435] Chemotherapy[436] or hormonal therapy[437] can be used for advanced or recurrent disease. The presence of hormone receptors in the tumor augurs a favorable response to treatment with progestins.[437] Recurrences in endometrial carcinoma are detectable within 2 years in 70% of the cases destined to recur.[438]

Uterine Sarcomas and Mixed Epithelial-Nonepithelial Tumors

Malignant connective tissue and mixed tumors are more common in the corpus than in the cervix uteri and characteristically appear in mature women. They represent 5% or fewer of malignant uterine corporeal tumors, although they constitute a higher percentage in black women. Their clinical presentation is essentially identical to that of endometrial carcinoma: serosanguineous or frankly hemorrhagic discharge; presence of a palpable mass; pain when the tumor is extensive; cachexia, anemia, and metastatic generalization at the terminal stage. The background of hyperestrogenism and the clinical triad of obesity, hypertension, and diabetes often seen in women with endometrial carcinoma are of less significance in relation to sarcomas. Epidemiologic factors are difficult to analyze in this heterogeneous group of tumors, because factors favoring the development of, for example, leiomyosarcoma may be entirely different from those related to carcinosarcoma. Unfortunately, most studies tend to consider all of these tumors as a single group.[439] We do know that pelvic irradiation seems to play a role in the development of carcinosarcomas but probably not of the other tumors in this group.[440] Hyperestrinism may also contribute to the development of carcinosarcomas.[441]

The classification of uterine sarcomas and mixed tumors is presented in Table 4-5, with the exception of the malignant smooth muscle tumors (leiomyosarcomas), which are included in Table 4-3. The discussion here will focus first on pure endometrial stromal tumors, then the mixed tumors (including some benign variants) of endometrial origin, and finally on leiomyosarcoma and rare malignant tumors of the uterine corpus.

Any classification, no matter how complete, must still leave room for an occasional undifferentiated or unclassifiable sarcoma, as well as for malignant tumors the epithelial or nonepithelial nature of which is not apparent. We hope that future studies will resolve continuing problems about the nature, treatment, and natural history of such lesions.

Endometrial Stromal Tumors. Although the uterine tumors of pure endometrial stromal type were first described in 1908,[442] they were not well characterized until the classic study of Norris and Taylor in 1966.[443] This latter publication divided the endometrial stromal tumors into three types with very different clinical implications:

1. Stromal nodule, a benign tumor
2. Low-grade endometrial stromal sarcoma, formerly known as *endolymphatic stromal myosis*, a malignant tumor of generally indolent aggressive behavior
3. High-grade endometrial stromal sarcoma, a fully malignant tumor with a generally unfavorable prognosis.

The pathologic criteria for distinguishing these three lesions have become somewhat controversial in recent years, with the proposed addition of a fourth diagnostic entity—poorly differentiated endometrial sarcoma.[444]

Despite the controversy at the higher end of the spectrum of malignancy in this group of neoplasms, the criteria for the diagnosis of the benign *stromal nodule* have remained constant. This lesion is defined as a well-circumscribed tumoral proliferation of uniform cells resembling the stromal cells of normal proliferative-phase endometrium. The key term in this definition is *well-circumscribed,* because the pushing margins of this lesion are essentially the only feature by which it may be distinguished from low-grade endometrial stromal sarcoma. *Nodule* is probably a misleading term, because these lesions can measure up to 15 cm in diameter, with median diameters of 4.0 cm[445] and 5.7 cm[446] in the two largest series reported. In any event, there is complete agreement that stromal nodules—regardless of their size—are completely benign, with no known recurrences or deaths in any published series.

As indicated above, *low-grade endometrial stromal sarcoma* is composed of cells that are essentially identical to those of the benign stromal nodule, the only difference between the tumors being the infiltrative margins of low-grade stromal sarcoma, compared with the virtually total circumscription of the stromal nodule. Low-grade stromal sarcomas may appear grossly well circumscribed, but at least half of these tumors are described as demonstrating diffuse myometrial permeation by worm-like masses or multiple nodules, with gross extrauterine extension in as many as one-third of cases.[444-447] At the microscopic level, these tumors are by definition infiltrating. They are always seen in the myometrium and frequently involve the endometrium as well. Plugs of tumor are commonly identified within lymphatic or venous channels, leading to the frequent designation of this tumor in the older literature as *endolymphatic stromal myosis.* Despite this extensive invasion, these tumors are cytologically no more malignant in appearance than the stromal nodule. The component cells are small and uniform in size and shape, with minimal cytologic atypia and generally few mitotic figures (Figs. 4-109 and 4-110). More than 10 mitotic figures per 10 high-power microscopic fields are occasionally seen, but increased mitotic activity alone, in the absence of other criteria of high-grade malignancy, does not appear to influence the behavior of the tumor. Atypical mitoses are not seen in

the low-grade tumors, and large foci of necrosis are usually absent.

A characteristic feature is the vascular pattern, with many of the numerous vessels in the tumor resembling the spiral arterioles of normal endometrium, with tumor cells arranged in a whorling pattern around them. Additional features occasionally encountered focally or diffusely include epithelioid differentiation, characterized by a glandular or sex cord–like pattern,[446-448] and foci of smooth (and rarely skeletal) muscle differentiation.[449]

Immunohistochemical studies have shown a highly variable pattern, with virtually all tumors positive for vimentin, many for both desmin and smooth muscle actin, and some for epithelial markers.[450,451] Flow cytometric analysis reveals a diploid or near diploid pattern.[452,453] The tumors usually contain estrogen and progesterone receptors and are responsive to progestin therapy.[452,454-456]

Low-grade stromal sarcoma is a malignant tumor, but the initial local recurrence or distant metastasis may take place many years after the initial surgery was performed, especially in the case of tumors that were initially limited to the uterine corpus. It is not at all unusual in our experience to see a patient who presents with a pelvic, abdominal, or even pulmonary tumor with the histologic features of low-grade endometrial stromal sarcoma and a history of hysterectomy for supposed leiomyomata or adenomyosis 10 or 15 years earlier. On histologic review of the hysterectomy specimen, the primary sarcoma generally is identified. These tumors may also be primary in the ovary or in extrauterine and extraovarian foci of endometriosis—a fact that is also true for the other sarcomas and mixed tumors and (as is well known) for endometrioid carcinoma as well.

The differential diagnosis between endometrial sarcomas of low and high grade has become somewhat controversial within the past decade. In the classic article of Norris and Taylor,[443] the distinction between low-grade and high-grade sarcomas of endometrial stromal type was made solely on the basis of mitotic counting, with more than 10 mitotic figures per 10 high-power fields considered diagnostic of the high-grade tumor. More recent studies have suggested that increased mitotic activity alone does not alter the behavior of a low-grade sarcoma, and more than 10 mitoses per 10 high-power fields are even reported in occasional stromal nodules, which still behave benignly if otherwise well differentiated and well circumscribed.[445,446] In 1982, Evans[444] suggested that there were really two fundamental types of sarcoma derived from the endometrial stroma: a tumor for which he retained the name *endometrial stromal sarcoma,* which could be more or less mitotically active but still resembled endometrial stroma histologically, and a tumor that he designated *poorly differentiated endometrial sarcoma,* characterized by its anaplastic appearance, lack of resemblance to normal endometrial stroma, and frequent resemblance to the stromal component of carcinosar-

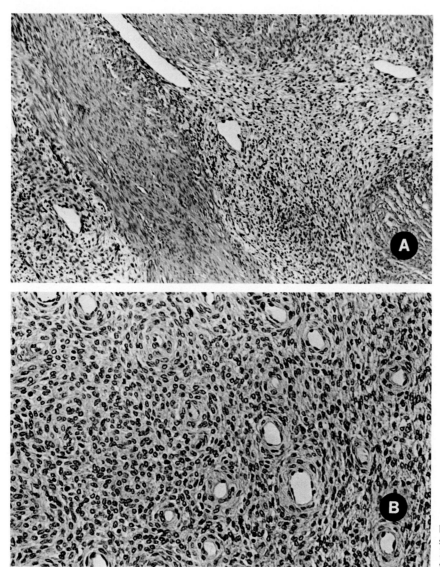

FIGURE 4-109 Low-grade endometrial stromal sarcoma. **(A)** Low-power view. **(B)** Detail. Note prominent vascularity and absence of atypia.

comas. Chang and colleagues[447] have recently endorsed this view. In their large series, neither mitotic activity nor cytologic atypia was predictive of tumor recurrence for patients with stage I sarcomas showing typical endometrial stromal differentiation.

The main question that remains to be answered is whether the complete body of endometrial stromal sarcomas should be divided into two groups with the nomenclature suggested by Norris and Taylor, two groups as defined by Evans, or three groups, as we would prefer—*low-grade stromal sarcoma, high-grade stromal sarcoma,* and *undifferentiated sarcoma.* In an unpublished study of Gynecologic Oncology Group (GOG) cases, we recently used this tripartite classification, accepting as high-grade endometrial stromal sarcomas those tumors that still showed to some extent the vascular pattern and cytologic features of endometrial stromal differentiation, but with considerably more cellular pleomorphism, often accompanied by necrosis, increased mitotic activity, and

atypical mitotic figures as well (Fig. 4-111). Undifferentiated sarcoma was defined as a nonepithelial malignant neoplasm originating in the endometrium but showing no histologic features suggestive of endometrial stromal differentiation, and no features of any of the other common sarcomas (eg, leiomyosarcoma or rhabdomyosarcoma). Using these definitions, both of these tumor types were associated with a high probability of both initial extrauterine spread and subsequent recurrence, with a mortality rate in the range of 50% at a mean 2½-year follow-up. There were no deaths among the patients with low-grade stromal sarcomas in this series, although a few patients had already demonstrated local or distant recurrences. We anticipate that some of the low-grade tumors will prove to be lethal in the future, but probably for the most part more than 5 years after initial treatment.

The highly aggressive behavior of the high-grade and undifferentiated sarcomas is in agreement with

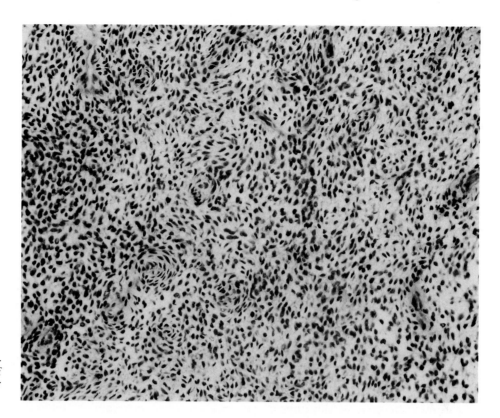

FIGURE 4-110 Low-grade endometrial stromal sarcoma: detail of bland cells and uniform vascular pattern.

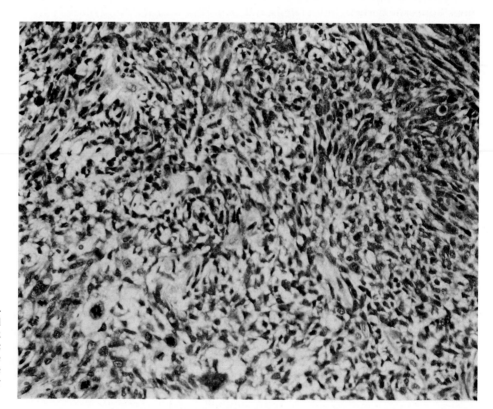

FIGURE 4-111 High-grade endometrial stromal sarcoma. General stromal pattern is retained, but the tumor cells are pleomorphic (compare with Fig. 4-110 at the same magnification). Note the atypical mitotic figure at lower left.

the studies reported in the literature.[444,446,456,457] However, the reported experience with these tumors is limited and perhaps not reliable, in part because they are considerably less common than the low-grade stromal sarcomas, and in part because diagnostic criteria and nomenclature have varied so widely, as discussed above. High-grade stromal sarcomas, in contrast to the low-grade type, tend to be receptor-negative and may be aneuploid.[458,459] Ploidy studies do not predict behavior better than classic histologic analysis.[459]

The primary *differential diagnosis* of the three tumors in this group is with each other. Low-grade stromal tumors must also be distinguished from intravenous leiomyomatosis and the extremely rare uterine *hemangiopericytoma*, which has a similar vascular pattern.[460] The high-grade and undifferentiated sarcomas have their differential diagnosis with poorly differentiated and undifferentiated endometrial carcinomas and other high-grade sarcomas of specific types (eg, malignant fibrous histiocytoma and leiomyosarcoma).

Mixed Epithelial-Nonepithelial Tumors. This group of tumors is one in which both an epithelial and a stromal component contribute to the architecture of the tumor. Because of the unusual composition of this group of tumors, they have always raised questions concerning their histogenesis and pathways of differentiation, as well as the relative contributions of the different elements in determining the natural history, prognosis, and treatment of each tumor in the group.

The nomenclature for the group of tumors presented in Table 4-5 provides a prefix (*adeno-* or *carcino-*) that conveys the benign or malignant appearance of the epithelial component, and a suffix (*-fibroma*, *-myoma*, or *-sarcoma*) that indicates the benign or malignant appearance of the nonepithelial component. Therefore, of the common mixed tumors of malignant type, carcinosarcoma contains both epithelial and nonepithelial elements that are histologically malignant, whereas adenosarcoma is characterized by a benign epithelial component and a malignant stroma.

In the current classification, carcinosarcoma is synonymous with the terms *malignant mixed mesodermal tumor* and *malignant mixed müllerian tumor*. Although we and others have sometimes used the term *carcinosarcoma* to denote a homologous tumor and *malignant mixed mesodermal tumor* to indicate one with heterologous elements, the current terminology uses a single term for both and then specifies whether the tumor is homologous or heterologous.

By definition, any lesion placed in the mixed tumor category must contain separate epithelial and nonepithelial components, both of which are integral parts of the lesion. Therefore, among the lesions that are excluded from this category but may be confused with it are pure endometrial stromal tumors (usually of low grade) in which the stromal cells differentiate focally into tubular, gland-like, or sex cord–like structures, and endometrial carcinomas with spindle cell (sarcomatoid) metaplasia which are identifiable as such with routine histologic staining.

Carcinosarcoma. Carcinosarcoma is the most common of the neoplasms in the uterine mixed tumor group, and the most common endometrial cancer after carcinoma. Many clinical and epidemiologic discussions of "uterine sarcomas" in the literature refer primarily to this tumor. Although common within this group, carcinosarcoma is still a rare tumor, comprising only 2% to 3% of all uterine cancers.[461]

Carcinosarcoma is predominantly a tumor of elderly women, but well-documented cases have occurred in younger patients. They are generally large, bulky, solitary, polypoid masses. The tumors present clinically with abnormal vaginal bleeding, often fill the uterine cavity, and may protrude through the external cervical os. The diagnosis is usually made by endometrial curettage, but sometimes only the epithelial or the stromal component is recognized in the initial specimen. Cervicovaginal smears are often also initially interpreted as adenocarcinoma.[462,463]

The cut surface of a carcinosarcoma of the endometrium is generally fleshy and variegated, with grossly recognizable areas of hemorrhage and necrosis (Fig. 4-112). The tumor usually invades into the myometrium and often has spread beyond the uterine corpus at the time of initial surgery.

Microscopically, carcinosarcomas are characterized by an intimate admixture of malignant epithelial and nonepithelial elements (Figs. 4-112, 4-113 and 4-114). The epithelial component is generally an adenocarcinoma showing one or more of the patterns of differentiation (eg, endometrioid, serous, clear cell) usually encountered in pure endometrial carcinoma. A squamous component is frequently present. There is a tendency for the carcinomatous component to be moderately to poorly differentiated.[464]

The stromal component is usually a high-grade sarcoma of indeterminate type, but may occasionally be well differentiated and may be recognizable as endometrial stromal sarcoma, fibrosarcoma, or leiomyosarcoma. In about half of the cases, there is a heterologous stromal component, meaning that the tumor contains foci of sarcoma differentiating toward elements not normally found in the uterine corpus. The most common type is rhabdomyosarcoma, characterized by a malignant striated muscle component (see Fig. 4-112). Less common elements, in decreasing order of frequency, are chondrosarcoma (see Fig. 4-113), osteosarcoma, and liposarcoma. More than one heterologous element may be present.

The *pathogenesis* and pathway of differentiation of these tumors have been of interest to many investigators. Speculation has centered on whether they represent collision tumors (a mixture of two histogenetically distinct malignant cell populations), com-

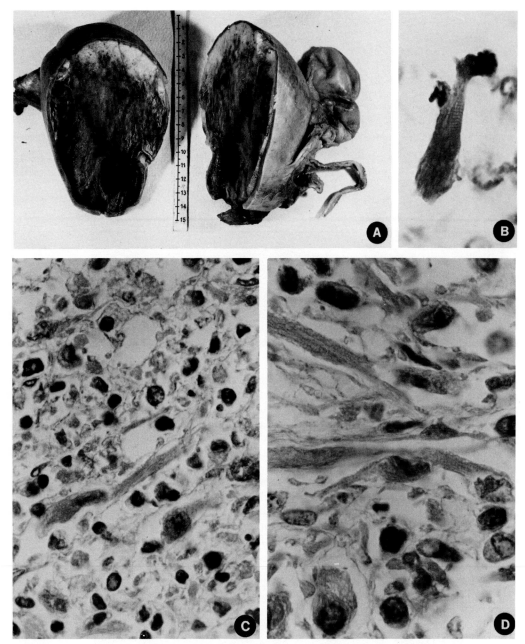

FIGURE 4-112 Carcinosarcoma of corpus uteri. **(A)** Macroscopic appearance. **(B,C,D)** Cytologic and histologic appearances, showing the presence of striated muscle cells.

bination tumors (representing an origin of both elements from a common stem cell), or composition tumors (pure carcinomas with reactive, atypical, but benign stromal elements). These possibilities have been investigated by numerous studies using electron microscopy, tissue culture, heterotransplantation, and immunohistochemistry. Most of the recent studies have been interpreted as supporting the "combination tumor" theory.[464] Of particular interest are immunohistochemical studies[465-467] that have confirmed that epithelial markers such as cytokeratins and epithelial membrane antigen are

frequently displayed by the sarcomatous-appearing cells.

Additional evidence in favor of the combination tumor theory comes from observations that the initial metastases of uterine carcinosarcomas are usually of pure carcinomatous type, less frequently mixed and only rarely of pure sarcomatous appearance.[464,466] Silverberg and colleagues,[464] in a GOG series of 203 cases, noted that metastases to lymph nodes occurred with about the same frequency as in poorly differentiated endometrial carcinomas, and that the presence or absence of metastases at initial

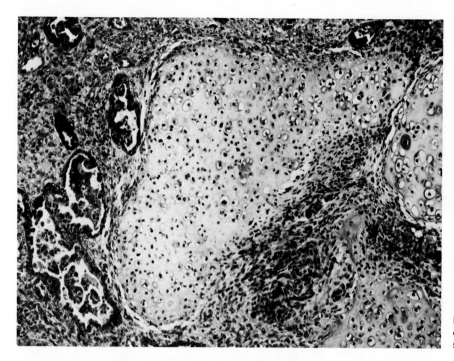

FIGURE 4-113 Carcinosarcoma: adenocarcinoma, stromal sarcoma, and chondrosarcoma.

exploratory laparotomy correlated more closely with the appearance of the epithelial component than that of the stromal component of the primary tumor. All these observations suggest that (1) both the epithelial and nonepithelial elements within these tumors are derived from a single precursor cell type; (2) the carcinomatous component ultimately drives the behavior of the tumor; and (3) perhaps most of the carcinosarcomas are truly metaplastic carcinomas, as encountered in most other organs of the body.

Because of the complex histologic appearance of these tumors, the relationship of the different elements within them to *prognosis* has been investigated in numerous studies over the years, often with variable results. The surgical stage and depth of myometrial invasion have been shown to be important prognostic indicators in almost every large published series, although other pathologic factors have been more controversial.[464] Although early studies suggested that heterologous tumors—particularly those containing rhabdomyosarcoma—had a poorer prognosis than homologous ones, more recent studies generally have not confirmed this observation.[464,468–470]

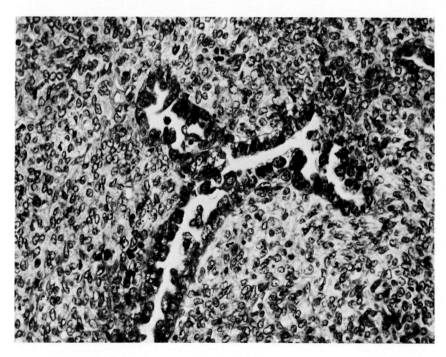

FIGURE 4-114 Carcinosarcoma of endometrium: malignant gland and stroma.

Features related to the frequency of metastases detected at staging laparotomy in the large series of Silverberg and colleagues[464] included the following: a carcinomatous component that was high-grade endometrioid, serous, or clear cell; deep myometrial invasion; lymphatic or vascular space invasion; and involvement of the isthmus or cervix. On the other hand, most features of the stromal component of the primary tumor, including grade, mitotic index, and the presence or absence and types of heterologous elements, showed no relation to the presence of metastases at operation. Longer follow-up is required to determine whether these factors may eventually prove to be of some prognostic significance. Other factors that have not been investigated adequately include the relative proportions of epithelial and nonepithelial elements and the immunophenotype of the tumor (ie, whether or not the stromal component is immunohistochemically positive for epithelial markers).

Initial metastases of these tumors appear to be predominantly of the epithelial component. Thus, metastatic endometrioid, serous, or clear cell carcinoma is typical of early spread from an endometrial carcinosarcoma. Deligdisch and colleagues[471] have noted that subsequent recurrences, on the other hand, were composed largely of sarcomatous elements.

Adenosarcoma. Unlike carcinosarcoma, which has been recognized for many decades, adenosarcoma was first described in 1974.[472] Thus, there are still large gaps in our knowledge of the epidemiology, histogenesis, and clinical and pathologic features of this tumor. Several hundred cases have, however, been reported, with the largest series comprising 100,[473] 31,[474] and 25[475] cases.

Adenosarcoma is defined as a tumor composed of a benign epithelial and a malignant nonepithelial component. It fills the gap between the completely benign (adenofibroma, adenomyoma) and high-grade malignant (carcinosarcoma) neoplasms in the endometrial mixed tumor group.

Adenosarcomas are usually diagnosed in a somewhat younger population than that which is characteristic of carcinosarcoma. The mean age in most series has been between 55 and 60 years, but cases have been seen in younger women and even in children. Like other endometrial malignant tumors, adenosarcomas usually present with abnormal vaginal bleeding. They are usually solitary lesions arising in the uterine fundus and projecting into the endometrial cavity, and average about 5 cm in diameter. They are occasionally associated with prior pelvic radiation or with exogenous or endogenous hyperestrinism.[473]

Microscopically, adenosarcoma is characterized by benign epithelial elements intimately admixed with a malignant stromal component (Fig. 4-115). Many histologic features of the tumor are reminiscent of those of cystosarcoma phyllodes of the breast.[476] Broad, leaf-like, papillary processes are usually present on the surface, and the deeper epithelial component is almost always cuffed by bands of hypercellular stroma. The tumor is usually limited to the endometrium, with a generally sharp

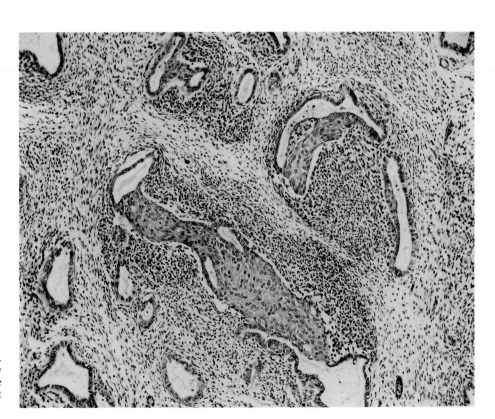

FIGURE 4-115 Adenosarcoma. Benign-appearing glands show squamous metaplasia and are cuffed by hypercellular malignant stroma.

junction between its base and the underlying myometrium. In a proportion of cases that varies from one series to the next, myometrial invasion is present. The myometrial invasion may be deep and may include involvement of vascular and lymphatic spaces. Extrauterine spread was present in the GOG series of Kaku and colleagues in 6 of 31 cases subjected to hysterectomy and staging laparotomy.[474]

The benign epithelial component of the tumor is generally characterized by papillary processes, cystically dilated glands, and compressed slit-like glands. Metaplastic changes and some degree of glandular atypia may be present, but by definition malignant change is absent. If even focal carcinomatous elements are encountered, the diagnosis becomes carcinosarcoma.

The stromal component by definition is cytologically malignant, but it is usually of lower grade than that which is characteristically seen in carcinosarcoma. In most adenosarcomas, the stroma is of homologous type and is composed of spindled or round cells resembling fibroblasts, endometrial stromal cells, or both. Focally dense cuffs of hypercellular stroma surrounding glands are almost always seen. Stromal mitoses are present but, as in the case of atypia, usually do not reach the levels seen in carcinosarcoma. They generally range in number between 3 and 20 mitotic figures per 10 high-power fields. Tumors with fewer than this number of mitoses are generally found to be adenofibromas, which behave in a completely benign manner.

Foci of hemorrhage, necrosis, foam cells, smooth muscle cells, stromal fibrosis, and stromal hyaliniza-tion may be present in varying proportions. A heterologous stromal component—usually rhabdomyosarcoma or chondrosarcoma—may be present. As with carcinosarcoma, it is debatable whether the presence of a heterologous component alters tumor behavior. Sex cord–like elements, consisting of solid nests, trabeculae, and solid or hollow tubules composed of benign-appearing epithelial-type cells, may occasionally be present in the stromal component of the tumor and do not appear to alter its behavior.[477]

The most important histopathologic variant of adenosarcoma is the pattern that has been designated *adenosarcoma with sarcomatous overgrowth*.[474,478] This is defined by the presence of a pure sarcoma—usually of a higher grade and mitotic index than encountered elsewhere in the tumor—that overgrows the typical adenosarcoma to account for at least 25% of total tumor volume (Fig. 4-116). The true frequency of this phenomenon is not known, because it represented 10 of 125 cases of adenosarcoma in one series[478] and 17 of 31 in another.[474] Because the former series was composed largely of consultation cases, and the latter of GOG cases subjected to staging laparotomy, we suspect that the true prevalence of this tumor type is probably intermediate between the two extremes reported.

In both series, nevertheless, sarcomatous overgrowth was an ominous *prognostic* feature, with tumor recurrences developing in 44% to 70% of cases, compared with 14% to 25% of those without sarcomatous overgrowth. Thus, adenosarcoma can in general be considered a relatively favorable malignant tumor unless stromal overgrowth is present.

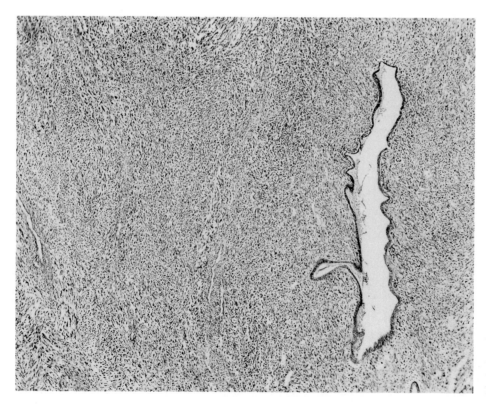

FIGURE 4-116 Adenosarcoma with sarcomatous overgrowth. Pure high-grade sarcoma occupies most of this field and accounts for more than 25% of the tumor sampled for microscopic examination.

Initial recurrences are usually vaginal, pelvic, or abdominal, and often appear at an interval of 5 years or more after hysterectomy. Vaginal recurrences may resemble the primary tumor or be composed of pure sarcoma, whereas distant metastases are almost always composed of the sarcomatous component alone.

As emphasized above, this relatively favorable prognosis is altered dramatically by the presence of sarcomatous overgrowth. An increased risk of recurrence is also noted with myometrial invasion. Other features that have been reported in some series as unfavorable prognostic factors include the presence of extrauterine spread at the time of diagnosis, necrosis in the primary tumor, the presence of heterologous elements (particularly rhabdomyosarcoma), high sarcoma grade, and high mitotic index of the stromal component.[473–476] In the GOG series of Kaku and colleagues,[474] the triad of stromal overgrowth, rhabdomyosarcoma, and lymphatic/vascular space invasion predicted both of the two cases (of a total of 31) in which lymph node metastases were present at the time of exploratory laparotomy. Because these two cases were the only ones in the series with these three findings in the hysterectomy specimen itself, it was suggested that lymphadenectomy might be reserved in the future for similar cases.

Atypical Polypoid Adenomyoma and Papillary Adenofibroma. These two uncommon lesions are grouped together here because they seem to form a continuous clinical and pathologic spectrum with the malignant mixed tumors discussed above and because they are a major part of the differential diagnosis with these tumors. Both lesions have been characterized within the past two decades, although there is some question whether this represents a real increase in frequency. The lesions resemble carcinosarcomas and adenosarcomas in that they consist of both epithelial and stromal elements; they differ, however, in that the epithelial and stromal components are always histologically benign and the lesions are benign in their clinical behavior.[479,480]

Clinically, adenofibromas usually occur in middle-aged to elderly women and atypical polypoid adenomyomas in premenopausal women. They both present most frequently with abnormal vaginal bleeding.

Macroscopically, they present as endometrial polyps of variable size, sometimes large and occasionally occupying the entire endometrial cavity and prolapsing down into the cervix, with atypical polypoid adenomyoma frequently originating in the lower uterine segment. There is a strong tendency for these polyps to be sessile. Foci of hemorrhage and necrosis are generally absent.

Microscopically, the lesions consist of intimate admixtures of epithelial and stromal elements. In the *papillary adenofibroma,*[475,476,481] the basic architecture is papillary, both the epithelial and stromal elements appear benign, and the latter is predominantly fibroblastic (Fig. 4-117). The benign histologic appearance correlates well with the clinical behavior, although adenofibromas can invade the myometrium and pelvic veins[482] and recur locally[483] on rare occasions.

Atypical polypoid adenomyoma is characterized by an intimate admixture of benign endometrial glands and a stroma consisting predominantly or exclusively of equally benign-appearing smooth muscle (Fig.

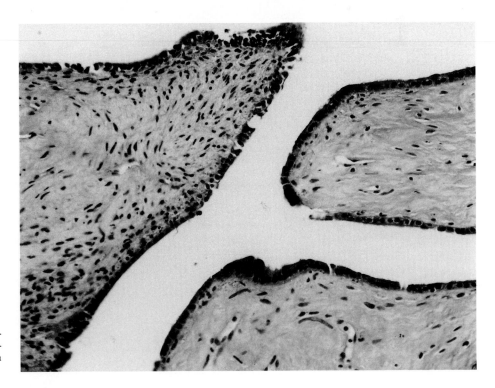

FIGURE 4-117 Papillary adenofibroma. In contrast to adenosarcoma (see Fig. 4-115), the stroma is histologically benign.

4-118). The glands invariably exhibit architectural atypia and may show cytologic atypia (usually slight but occasionally marked) as well. Squamous or morular metaplasia is found in most cases and is often extensive. Although central necrosis may be present in these large metaplastic foci, their cytologic appearance is benign. The stromal component consists of swirling and interlacing fascicles of smooth muscle cells that appear cytologically benign. Mitotic activity in this compartment is usually less than 2 mitotic figures per 10 high-power fields.

Adenocarcinoma has been noted within and associated with this tumor.[484,485] The most important differential diagnosis of atypical polypoid adenomyoma, particularly in a curettage specimen, is with endometrial carcinoma invading the myometrium. It is unusual for myometrial invasion to be demonstrated in a curettage specimen; the glands of atypical polypoid adenomyoma lack cytologic and architectural features of malignancy, and the smooth muscle component exhibits a cellularity and fascicular pattern that would be unusual for myometrium invaded by carcinoma and lacks the usual stromal response to invasive cancer.

Leiomyosarcoma. Leiomyosarcoma represents the most frequent type of pure uterine sarcoma. It may arise in a previously existing benign leiomyoma or de novo from the smooth muscle fibers of the myometrium. Different authors report various frequencies of each of these modes of origin. Stearns and Sneeden[486] believed that 49 of 54 leiomyosarcomas in their series arose in benign myomas, whereas Aaro and colleagues[487] demonstrated this origin in only 22 of their 105 cases, and Taylor and Norris[488] denied it completely. Feulgen microspectrophotometric observations by Herbold and associates[489] seem to confirm that such transitions can take place, although their frequency is still unknown. The 105 leiomyosarcomas in Aaro's series were found in a total of 177 uterine sarcomas and malignant mixed tumors; most other series have also indicated that leiomyosarcomas comprise half or slightly more of all uterine nonepithelial malignant tumors, with most of the others being carcinosarcomas.[490–492] They are predominantly tumors of older women, but cases have been described in young patients. Rapid increase in the size of an apparent leiomyoma after the menopause should arouse suspicion of sarcoma. However, the diagnosis is often first suspected by the pathologist during the examination of a uterus removed for supposedly benign myomata.[210]

Macroscopically, the tumor is found within a leiomyomatous nodule or forms an isolated intramural mass (Fig. 4-119). It presents as a soft or fleshy zone of gray-yellow or pink color, with poorly defined borders. This appearance contrasts with that of benign leiomyomatous tissue, which is firm, white, and shows a prominent whorled pattern on section. Zones of necrosis and hemorrhage are frequent (in one series,[488] necrosis was seen grossly in 74% of leiomyosarcomas versus only 12% of benign cellular myomas). The tumor may be solitary or associated

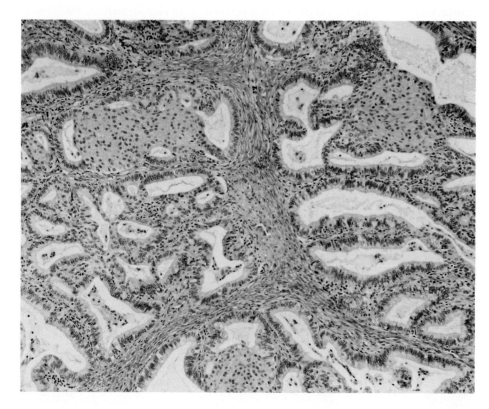

FIGURE 4-118 Atypical polypoid adenomyoma. Architecturally irregular and crowded glands with morular metaplasia are separated by interlacing fascicles of smooth muscle.

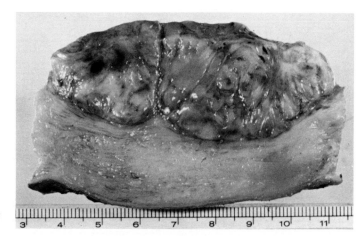

FIGURE 4-119 Leiomyosarcoma: macroscopic appearance of cut surface.

with multiple benign myomata, with different authors disagreeing about which pattern is more frequent.

Occasionally, the tumor grows out of the confines of the uterine wall and forms a nodular, budding, or grape-like mass within the uterine cavity. In advanced stages, the tumor grows inward to involve the endometrial cavity or outward to the peritoneal serosa, at times with distant peritoneal spread.

Microscopically, the tumor is composed of whorled and interwoven bundles of fusiform cells with elongated hyperchromatic nuclei, which may be enormous and bizarre (Fig. 4-120). Mitoses are usually numerous. Some authors have attached a major prognostic significance to the number of mitoses present,[488,491,493] whereas others believe that the macroscopic extent of the tumor and its overall differentiation are equally valuable in this respect.[486,494-497] When the tumor attains a certain volume, it is common to find zones of necrosis, hemorrhage, and edema.

There is considerable confusion in the literature between the diagnosis of leiomyosarcoma and that of cellular or bizarre but benign leiomyoma (Table 4-7 summarizes our criteria). Certain authors believe that a quantitative estimation of mitotic activity will always solve this problem, the figure of 5 mitoses per 10 high-power fields being most often quoted as the dividing line. However, we believe that individual variations, both in tumors and in observers, make this approach untenable.[498-500] The entity of *mitotically active leiomyoma,* a benign tumor generally occurring in young women, in which many normal mitotic figures but no atypia or tumor necrosis is seen, also demonstrates the inutility of using mitotic activity as the single criterion to separate benign from malignant.[501-503] The absence of bizarre nuclei and of atypical mitoses points to a benign tumor; a few giant cells, however, may be found in benign leiomyomas of "symplastic" type (see above). Tumor necrosis is an important additional criterion of leiomyosarcoma, as is obvious invasion of the myometrium.[504,505] The problem of the "benign metastasizing

leiomyoma" has already been discussed; these cases are so rare that they seldom pose a significant problem. Myxoid smooth muscle tumors must be viewed with alarm even in the absence of prominent mitotic activity,[506] because they have been stated to have a high malignant potential. Other lesions to be considered in the differential diagnosis include intravenous leiomyomatosis, spindle cell carcinoma, endometrial stromal sarcoma, rare rhabdomyosarcomas, and other soft-tissue sarcomas.

In recent years, a category of *smooth muscle tumor of uncertain malignant potential* has been added to the classification of smooth muscle tumors (see Table 4-3), to encompass "borderline" lesions with some criteria of malignancy. This is a valuable addition, because it recognizes that we do not know with certainty the true clinical potential of every tumor encountered. This is especially true of some of the variants (such as epithelioid smooth muscle tumors) of which too few cases have been reported. Nevertheless, the prudent pathologist must be wary of overuse of this diagnosis to avoid being labeled by clinical colleagues as a "pathologist of uncertain malignant potential."

Several clinical and pathologic features should be considered in evaluating the *prognosis* of leiomyosarcoma. Poor prognostic factors are marked anaplasia of the tumor cells, high mitotic rate, evidence of blood vessel invasion, obvious malignant tumor on gross inspection, and (perhaps most ominous of all) the postmenopausal state of the patient.[495,497] Published 5-year survival rates have been as variable as the diagnostic criteria, but they probably average 40% or less. The *treatment* of choice is surgical. Irradiation seems to be of little value, but chemotherapy is beginning to show some promise.[507] When metastases occur, they most frequently involve intrapelvic structures, the lungs, and the liver.

Cytologic Appearance of Uterine Sarcomas. Because of the rarity of uterine sarcomas, coupled with the fact that they are almost always symptomatic and

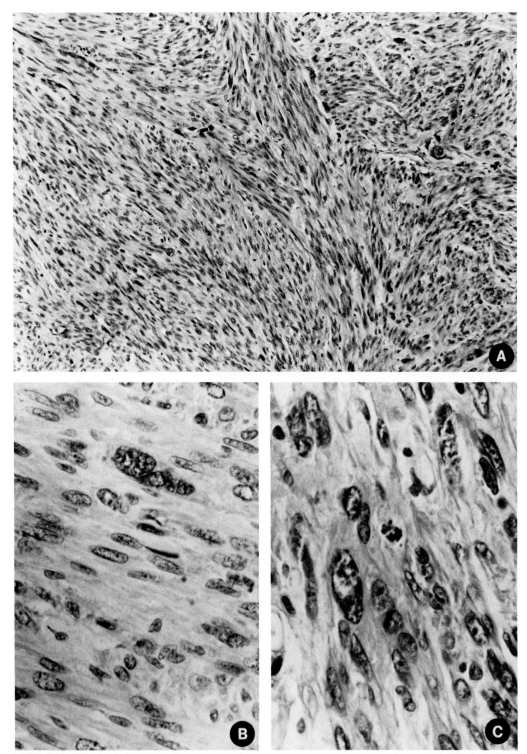

FIGURE 4-120 Leiomyosarcoma of uterus: microscopic appearance. **(A)** General view. **(B,C)** Cytologic details.

therefore not detected by screening procedures, the cytologic appearance of most of these tumors is poorly characterized. In general terms, most of the sarcomas exfoliate highly disorganized clusters of huge polymorphous cells, which lack the grouping into rounded cell balls or papillary structures fre-

quently seen in endometrial carcinoma. Leiomyosarcomas exfoliate the most characteristic cells, with a spindled shape and large markedly irregular nuclei (Color Fig. 4-8). However, because these tumors frequently occur beneath an intact endometrium, malignant cells may not be seen, even with direct

TABLE 4-7.
Differential Diagnosis of Uterine Smooth Muscle Tumors

Hypercellularity	−	+	+	−	−	+	+	−
Atypia	−	+	−	+	−	+	−	+
Prominent mitotic activity	−	+	−	−	+	−	+	+
Diagnosis	M	S	CM	AM	AM	S	S	T

M, benign myoma; *CM,* cellular myoma; *AM,* atypical myoma; *S,* sarcoma; *T,* theoretical combination only.

sampling of the endometrial cavity. Equally distinctive cytologically are the malignant heterologous elements seen in some carcinosarcomas—particularly rhabdomyoblasts with prominent cross-striations (see Fig. 4-112)—but these are even more rarely encountered in cytologic material, because even histologic examination frequently reveals only very small foci of these cells in otherwise homologous tumors.

Other Malignant Tumors of the Corpus Uteri

Among the malignant tumors that have been reported to show rare uterine primary localizations are rhabdomyosarcoma,[508,509] osteogenic sarcoma,[510] chondrosarcoma,[511] liposarcoma,[512] malignant fibrous histiocytoma,[513] angiosarcoma,[514,515] alveolar soft part sarcoma,[516] endodermal sinus tumor,[517,518] primitive neuroectodermal tumor,[519] immature teratoma,[520] malignant rhabdoid tumor,[521] and Wilms' tumor.[522] Malignant lymphomas[523] are usually a manifestation of disseminated disease. They should not be confused with lymphoma-like benign lesions, including leiomyomas with marked lymphoid infiltration.[524,525]

METASTATIC TUMORS OF THE CORPUS UTERI

The corpus uteri may be involved by distant metastases from primary tumors of diverse organs or by local extensions of tumors of other parts of the female genital tract or other pelvic organs. Most frequently, metastases are from ovarian cancers, and it is sometimes difficult to determine whether the primary tumor is ovarian or uterine (or, as is frequently the case, both).[396–399] Of extrapelvic tumors metastasizing to the uterus, by far the most frequent are mammary and gastrointestinal carcinomas (Fig. 4-121).[526,527] Carcinomas of other organs, leukemias and lymphomas, and carcinoid tumors have been reported as rare sources of uterine metastases. Carcinomas of the cervix,[528] ovary, sigmoid, and urinary bladder extend to the corpus uteri directly or by the lymphatic route (Fig. 4-122).

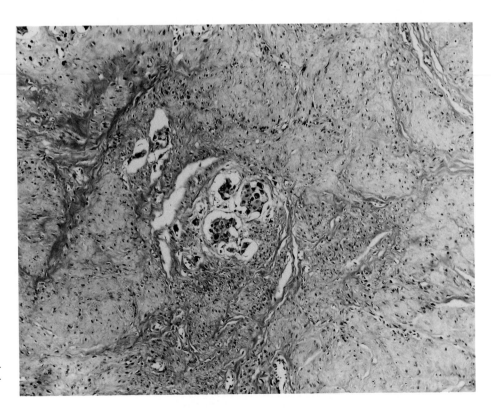

FIGURE 4-121 Metastatic mammary carcinoma in uterine leiomyoma.

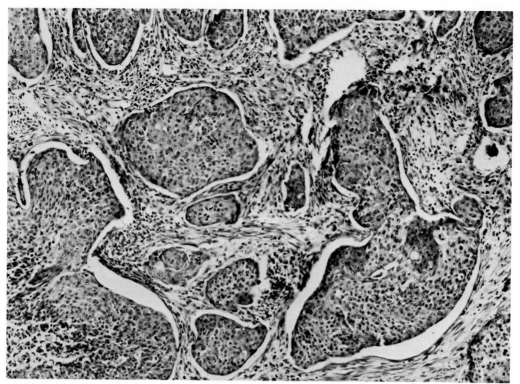

FIGURE 4-122 Squamous cell carcinoma of the cervix extending to the corpus uteri: microscopic appearance.

REFERENCES

1. Hendrickson M, Kempson R: Uterus and fallopian tubes. In Sternberg S, ed. Histology for pathologists, pp 797–834. New York, Raven Press, 1992
2. Kuo TT, London SN, Dinh TV: Endometriosis occurring in leiomyomatosis peritonealis disseminata: Ultrastructural study and histogenetic consideration. Am J Surg Pathol 4:197–204, 1980
3. Mazur MT, Kraus FT: Histogenesis of morphologic variations in tumors of the uterine wall. Am J Surg Pathol 4:59–74, 1980
4. Porcu E, Venturoli S, Fabbri R et al: Uterine development and endocrine relationships after menarche. Am J Obstet Gynecol 161:174–177, 1989
5. Langlois PL: The size of the normal uterus. J Reprod Med 4:220–228, 1970
6. Kurz KH, Tadesse E, Haspels AA: In vivo measurements of uterine cavities in 795 women of fertile age. Contraception 29:495–510, 1984
7. Hricak H: MRI of the female pelvis: A review. AJR 146:1115–1122, 1986
8. Honoré LH: Menorrhagia, diffuse myometrial hypertrophy and the intrauterine contraceptive device: A report of fourteen cases. Acta Obstet Gynecol Scand 58:283–285, 1979
9. Allen N, Cowan LE: Uterus didelphys with unilateral imperforate vagina: Report of 4 cases. Obstet Gynecol 22:422–426, 1963
10. Andrews MC, Jones HW Jr: Impaired reproductive performance of the unicornuate uterus: Intrauterine growth retardation, infertility, and recurrent abortion in five cases. Am J Obstet Gynecol 144:173–176, 1982
11. Buttram VC Jr, Gibbons WE: Müllerian anomalies: A proposed classification. Fertil Steril 32:40–46, 1979
12. Ben-Baruch G, Menczer J, Mashiach S, Serr DM: Uterine anomalies in diethylstilbestrol-exposed women with fertil-ity disorders. Acta Obstet Gynecol Scand 60:395–397, 1981
13. Stillman RJ: In utero exposure to diethylstilbestrol: Adverse effects on the reproductive tract and reproductive performance in male and female offspring. Am J Obstet Gynecol 142:905–921, 1982
14. Forssman L, Lundberg J, Scherstén T: Conservative treatment of uterine arteriovenous fistula. Acta Obstet Gynecol Scand 61:85–87, 1982
15. Schwalm H, Dubrausky V: The structure of the human uterus: Muscles and connective tissue. Am J Obstet Gynecol 94:391–404, 1966
16. Toth S, Toth A: Undescribed muscle bundle of the human uterus: Fasciculus cervicoangularis. Am J Obstet Gynecol 118:979–984, 1974
17. Ferenczy A: Histology of the human endometrium: From birth to senescence. Ann N Y Acad Sci 622:6–27, 1991
18. Nogales-Ortiz F, Puerta J, Nogales FF Jr: The normal menstrual cycle: Chronology and mechanism of endometrial desquamation. Obstet Gynecol 51:259–264, 1978
19. Fanger H, Barker BE: Capillaries and arterioles in normal endometrium. Obstet Gynecol 17:543–550, 1961
20. Farrer-Brown G, Beilby JOW, Tarbit MH: The blood supply of the uterus: 1. Arterial vasculature; 2. Venous pattern. Br J Obstet Gynaecol 77:673–689, 1970
21. Ramsey EM: The story of the spiral arteries. J Reprod Med 6:393–399, 1981
22. Wynn RM: Histology and ultrastructure of the human endometrium. In Wynn RM, ed. Biology of the uterus, pp 341–376. New York, Plenum Press, 1977
23. Dallenbach-Hellweg G: Histopathology of the endometrium, 4th ed. New York, Springer, 1987
24. Bulmer J, Lunny D, Hagin S: Immunohistochemical characterization of stromal leucocytes in nonpregnant human endometrium. Am J Reprod Immunol Microbiol 17:83–90, 1988
25. Kamat B, Isaacson P: The immunocytochemical distribution of leukocytic subpopulations in human endometrium. Am J Pathol 127:66–73, 1987

26. Marshall R, Jones D: An immunohistochemical study of lymphoid tissue in human endometrium. Int J Gynecol Pathol 7:225–235, 1988

27. Senekjian EK, Press MF, Blough RR et al: Comparison of the quantity of estrogen receptors in human endometrium and myometrium by steroid-binding assay and enzyme immunoassay based on monoclonal antibodies to human estrophilin. Am J Obstet Gynecol 160:592–597, 1989

28. Gehring U: Steroid hormone receptors: Biochemistry, genetics, and molecular biology. Trends Biochem Sci 12:399–402, 1987

29. Bergeron C, Ferenczy A, Shyamala G: Distribution of estrogen receptors in various cell types of normal, hyperplastic, and neoplastic human endometrial tissues. Lab Invest 58:338–345, 1988

30. Bergeron C, Ferenczy A, Toft DO et al: Immunocytochemical study of progesterone receptors in the human endometrium during the menstrual cycle. Lab Invest 59:862–869, 1988

31. Whitehead MI, Townsend PT, Pryse-Davies J, Ryder T et al: Actions of progestins on the morphology and biochemistry of the endometrium of postmenopausal women receiving low-dose estrogen therapy. Am J Obstet Gynecol 142:791–795, 1982

32. Holinka CF, Gurpide E: Hormone-related enzymatic activities in normal and cancer cells of human endometrium. J Steroid Biochem 15:183–192, 1981

33. King RJB, Townsend PT, Whitehead MI, Young O, Taylor RW: Biochemical analysis of separated epithelium and stroma from endometria of premenopausal and postmenopausal women receiving estrogen and progestins. J Steroid Biochem 14:979–987, 1981

34. Healy DL, Hodgen GD: The endocrinology of human endometrium. Obstet Gynecol Surv 38:509–530, 1983

35. Riddick DH, Daly DC, Walters CA: The uterus as an endocrine compartment. Clin Perinatol 10:627–639, 1983

36. Astruc J: Traité des maladies des femmes. Paris, PG Cavelier, 1761

37. Hitschmann F, Adler L: Der Bau der Uterusschleimhaut des geschlechtsreifen Weibes mit besonderer Berucksichtigung der Menstruation. Mschr Geburtshilfe Gynaekol 27:1–82, 1908

38. Schröder R: Anatomische Studien zur normalen und pathologischen Physiologie des menstruation-zyklus. Arch Gynaekol 104:27–102, 1915

39. Schröder R: Der anatomische und klinische Begriff des metropathia haemorrhagica. Zentralbl Gynaekol 44:1401–1404, 1920

40. Johannisson E, Parker RA, Landgren B-M, Diczfalusy E: Morphometric analysis of the human endometrium in relation to peripheral hormone levels. Fertil Steril 38:564–571, 1982

41. Noyes RW: Normal phases of the endometrium. In HJ Norris, AT Hertig, MR Abell, eds. The uterus. International Academy of Pathology Monograph 14, pp 110–135. Baltimore, Williams & Wilkins, 1973

42. Trevoux R, De Brux J, Scholler R et al: L'endomètre est-il le fidèle reflet de la sécrétion ovariene? Gynecologie 42:272–277, 1991

43. Li T, Rogers A, Lenton E, Dockery P, Cooke I: A comparison between two methods of chronological dating of human endometrial biopsies during the luteal phase, and their correlation with histologic dating. Fertil Steril 48:928–932, 1987

44. Kim-Björklund T, Landgren BM, Hamberger L, Johannisson E: Comparative morphometric study of the endometrium, the fallopian tube, and the corpus luteum during the postovulatory phase in normally menstruating women. Fertil Steril 56:842–850, 1991

45. Shoupe D, Mishell DJ, Lacarra M et al: Correlation of endometrial maturation with four methods of estimating day of ovulation. Obstet Gynecol 73:88–92, 1989

46. Li T, Dockery P, Rogers A, Cooke I: How precise is histologic dating of endometrium using the standard dating criteria? Fertil Steril 51:759–763, 1989

47. Artacho-Pérula, Roldán-Villalobos R, Roldán-Villalobos A et al: Morphometry and discriminant analysis of the endometrium. Anal Quant Cytol Histol 14:320–329, 1992

48. Vásquez JJ, Dominguez A: The "clear cells" of human endometrium. Virchows Arch A Pathol Anat Histopathol 362:107–114, 1974

49. Cavazos F, Lucas FV: Ultrastructure of the endometrium. In HJ Norris, AT Hertig, MR Abell, eds. The uterus. International Academy of Pathology Monograph 14, pp 136–174. Baltimore, Williams & Wilkins, 1973

50. Clyman MJ, Spiegelman I, Ross T: Appearance of tonofilaments and absence of microtubules in human endometrial glandular epithelium: A function of estrogenic activity. Diagn Gynecol Obstet 4:173–181, 1982

51. Gompel C: The ultrastructure of the human endometrial cell studied by electron microscopy. Am J Obstet Gynecol 84:1000–1009, 1962

52. Roberts DK, Lavia LA, Horbelt DV, Walker NJ: Changes in nuclear and nucleolar areas of endometrial glandular cells throughout the menstrual cycle. Int J Gynecol Pathol 8:36–45, 1989

53. Ancla M, De Brux J: Occurrence of intranuclear tubular structures in the human endometrium during the secretory phase, and of annulate lamellae in hyperestrogenic states. Obstet Gynecol 26:23–33, 1965

54. Armstrong EM, More IAR, McSeveney D, Chatfield WR: Reappraisal of the ultrastructure of the human endometrial glandular cell. Br J Obstet Gynaecol 80:446–460, 1973

55. Poropatich C, Rojas M, Silverberg SG: Polymorphonuclear leukocytes in the endometrium during the normal menstrual cycle. Int J Gynecol Pathol 6:230–234, 1987

56. McLennan CE, Rydell A: Extent of endometrial shedding during normal menstruation. Obstet Gynecol 26:605–621, 1965

57. Christiaens GCML, Sixma JJ, Haspels AA: Hemostasis in menstrual endometrium: A review. Obstet Gynecol Surv 37:281–303, 1982

58. Ferenczy A: Regeneration of the human endometrium. In CM Fenoglio, M Wolff, eds. Progress in surgical pathology, vol 1, pp 157–173. New York, Masson, 1980

59. Hodgen GD, Goodman AL, O'Connor A, Johnson DK: Menopause in Rhesus monkeys: Model for study of disorders in the human climacteric. Am J Obstet Gynecol 127:581–584, 1977

60. Gambrell RD Jr: The menopause: Benefits and risks of estrogen-progestogen replacement therapy. Fertil Steril 37:457–474, 1982

61. MacBride JM: The normal post-menopausal endometrium. Br J Obstet Gynaecol 61:691–697, 1954

62. Kraus FT: Irradiation changes in the uterus. In AT Hertig, HJ Norris, MR Abell, eds. The uterus, pp 457–488. Baltimore, Williams & Wilkins, 1973

63. Board JA, Redwine FO, Moncure CW, Frable WJ, Taylor JR: Identification of differing etiologies of clinically diagnosed premature menopause. Am J Obstet Gynecol 134:936–944, 1979

64. Coulam CB, Ryan RJ: Premature menopause. I. Etiology. Am J Obstet Gynecol 133:639–643, 1978

65. Evrard JR, Buxton BH Jr, Erickson D: Amenorrhea following oral contraception. Am J Obstet Gynecol 124:88–91, 1976

66. Levan AB, Szanto PB: The frequency of anovulatory menstruation as determined by endometrial biopsy. Am J Obstet Gynecol 48:75–80, 1944

67. Chambers JT, Chambers SK: Endometrial sampling: When? Where? Why? With what? Clin Obstet Gynecol 35(1):28–39 1992

68. Collins J: Diagnostic assessment of the ovulatory process. Semin Reprod Endocrinol 8(3):145–155, 1990

69. Balasch J, Vanrell JA: Corpus luteum insufficiency and fertility: A matter of controversy. Hum Reprod 2:557–567, 1987

70. Brodie B, Wentz A: An update on the clinical relevance of luteal phase inadequacy. Semin Reprod Endocrinol 7(2):138–154, 1989

71. McNeely M, Soules M: The diagnosis of luteal phase deficiency: A critical review. Fertil Steril 50:1–15, 1988

72. Olive DL: The prevalence and epidemiology of luteal-phase deficiency in normal and infertile women. Clin Obstet Gynecol 34(1):157–166, 1991

73. Soules M, McLachlar R, Ek M et al: Luteal phase deficiency: Characterization of reproductive hormones over the menstrual cycle. J Clin Endocrinol Metab 69:804–812, 1989

74. Ginsburg KA: Luteal phase defect: Etiology, diagnosis, and management. Endocrinol Metab Clin North Am 21(1):85–104, 1992

75. Davis O, Berkeley A, Naus G et al: The incidence of luteal phase detect in normal, fertile women, determined by serial endometrial biopsies. Fertil Steril 51:582–586, 1989

76. Smith S, Lenton E, Landgren B, Cooke I: The short luteal phase and infertility. Br J Obstet Gynaecol 91:1120–1122, 1984

77. St Michel P, Dizerega J: Hyperprolactinemia and luteal phase dysfunction infertility. Obstet Gynecol Surv 38:248–254, 1983

78. Wentz JC, Kossoy LR, Parker RA: The impact of luteal phase inadequacy in an infertile population. Am J Obstet Gynecol 162:937–945, 1990

79. Clement P: Pathology of gamete and zygote transport: Cervical, endometrial, myometrial, and tubal factors in infertility. In Kraus F, Damjanov I, Kaufman N, eds. Pathology of reproductive failure, pp 140–194. Baltimore, Williams & Wilkins, 1991

80. McKelvey JL, Samuel LT: Irregular shedding of the endometrium. Obstet Gynecol 53:627–636, 1947

81. Ober WB: Effects of oral and intrauterine administration of contraceptives on the uterus. Hum Pathol 8:513–527, 1977

82. Hesla J, Kurman R, Rock J: Histologic effects of oral contraceptives on the uterine corpus and cervix. Semin Reprod Endocrinol 7(3):213–219, 1989

83. Beaconsfield P, Dick R, Ginsburg J, Lewis P: Amenorrhea and infertility after the use of oral contraceptives. Surg Gynecol Obstet 138:571–575, 1974

84. Maqueo M, Becerra C, Mungua H, Goldzieher JW: Endometrial histology and vaginal cytology during oral contraception with sequential estrogen and progesterone. Am J Obstet Gynecol 90:395–400, 1964

85. Silverberg SG, Makowski EL, Roche WD: Endometrial carcinoma in women under 40 years of age: Comparison of cases in oral contraceptive users and non-users. Cancer 39:592–598, 1977

86. Parazzini F, La Vecchia C, Bocciolone L, Franceschi S: The epidemiology of endometrial cancer. Gynecol Oncol 41:1–16, 1991

87. Rubin GL, Peterson HB, Lee NC et al: Estrogen replacement therapy and the risk of endometrial cancer: Remaining controversies. Am J Obstet Gynecol 162:148–154, 1990

88. Ludwig H: The morphologic response of the human endometrium to long-term treatment with progestational agents. Am J Obstet Gynecol 142:796–808, 1982

89. Leather AT, Savvas M, Studd JWW: Endometrial histology and bleeding patterns after 8 years of continuous combined estrogen and progestogen therapy in postmenopausal women. Obstet Gynecol 78:1008–1010, 1991

90. Spowart KJM, Walsh DJ, Hawthorn RJS, Hart DM: Hysteroscopic assessment of the effects of a continuous combined oestrogen-progestogen regime on the endometrium of postmenopausal women. Gynaecol Endoscopy 1:33–35, 1992

91. Silverberg SG, Haukkamaa M, Arko H et al: Endometrial morphology during long-term use of levonorgestrel-releasing intrauterine devices. Int J Gynecol Pathol 5:235–241, 1986

92. Johannisson G: Effects on the endometrium, endo- and exocervix following the use of local progestogen-releasing delivery systems. Contraception 42:403–421, 1990

93. Bonney WA Jr et al: Endometrial response to the intrauterine device. Am J Obstet Gynecol 96:101–113, 1966

94. Rozin S, Sacks MI, Shenker JG: Endometrial histology and clinical symptoms following retention of uterine contraceptive devices. Am J Obstet Gynecol 97:197–202, 1967

95. Czernobilksy B, Rotenstreich L, Mass N, Lancet M: Effect of intrauterine device on histology of endometrium. Obstet Gynecol 45:64–66, 1975

96. Lane ME, Dacalos E, Sobrero AJ, Ober WB: Squamous metaplasia of the endometrium in women with an intrauterine contraceptive device: Follow up study. Am J Obstet Gynecol 119:693–697, 1974

97. Christian CD: Maternal deaths associated with an intrauterine device. Am J Obstet Gynecol 119:441–444, 1974

98. Risse EKJ, Beerthuizen RJCM, Vooijs GP: Cytologic and histologic findings in women using the IUD. Obstet Gynecol 58:569–573, 1981

99. Gupta PK: Intrauterine contraceptive devices: Vaginal cytology, pathologic changes, and clinical implications. Acta Cytol 26:571–613, 1982

100. Duguid HLD, Parratt D, Traynor R: Actinomyces-like organisms in cervical smears from women using intrauterine contraceptive devices. Br Med J 2:534–536, 1980

101. Navot D, Anderson TL, Droesch K et al: Hormonal manipulation of endometrial maturation. J Clin Endocrinol Metab 68:801–807, 1989

102. Benda JA: Clomiphene's effect on endometrium in infertility. Int J Gynecol Pathol 11:273–282, 1992

103. Serfaty D: Le RU 486 en contraception postcoïtale. Gynecologie 43:350–355, 1992

104. Schenker JG, Margalioth EJ: Intrauterine adhesions: An updated appraisal. Fertil Steril 37:593–610, 1982

105. Untawale VG, Gabriel JB Jr, Chauhan PM: Calcific endometritis. Am J Obstet Gynecol 144:482–483, 1982

106. Reid PC, Thurrell W, Smith JHF et al: Nd:YAG laser endometrial ablation: Histological aspects of uterine healing. Int J Gynecol Pathol 11:174–179, 1992

107. Hill DJ, Maher PJ: Pregnancy following endometrial ablation. Gynaecol Endoscopy 1:47–49, 1992

108. Sanfilippo JS, Fitzgerald MR, Badawy SZA et al: Asherman's syndrome: A comparison of therapeutic methods. J Reprod Med 27:328–330, 1982

109. Baniecki H: Das Schleimhautbild des Uterus bei abgestorbener extrauterin-Graviditat. Zentralbl Gynaekol 73:349–355, 1951

110. Arias-Stella J: Atypical endometrial changes associated with the presence of chorionic tissue. Arch Pathol 58:112–128, 1954

111. Arias-Stella J: Atypical endometrial changes produced by chorionic tissue. Hum Pathol 3:450–453, 1972

112. Fienberg R, Lloyd HED: The Arias-Stella reaction in early normal pregnancy: An involutional phenomenon. Hum Pathol 5:183–189, 1974

113. Silverberg SG: Arias-Stella phenomenon in spontaneous and therapeutic abortion. Am J Obstet Gynecol 112:777–780, 1972

114. Wagner D, Richart RM: Polyploidy in the human endometrium with the Arias-Stella reaction. Arch Pathol 85:475–480, 1968

115. Kjer JJ, Eldon K: The diagnostic value of the Arias-Stella phenomenon. Zentralbl Gynaekol 104:753–756, 1982

116. Thrasher TV, Richart RM: Ultrastructure of the Arias-Stella reaction. Am J Obstet Gynecol 112:113–120, 1972

117. Dardi LE, Ariano L, Ariano MC, Gould VE: Arias-Stella reaction with prominent nuclear pseudoinclusions simulating herpetic endometritis. Diagn Gynecol Obstet 4:127–132, 1982

118. Craig JM, Danziger S: Histological distribution and nature of stainable lipids of the human endometrium. Am J Obstet Gynecol 93:1018–1023, 1965

119. Fechner RE, Bossart MI, Spjut H: Ultrastructure of endometrical stromal foam cells. Am J Clin Pathol 72:628–632, 1979

120. Dawagne MP, Silverberg SG: Foam cells in endometrial carcinoma: A clinico-pathologic study. Gynecol Oncol 13:67–75, 1982

121. Hampson F, Gerlis LM: Some form variations in endometrial tubules. Br J Obstet Gynaecol 61:744–749, 1954

122. Kraus FT: Irradiation changes in the uterus. In AT Hertig, HJ Norris, MR Abell, eds. The uterus, pp 457–488. Baltimore, Williams & Wilkins, 1973

123. Johannisson E, Fournier K, Riotton G: Regeneration of the human endometrium and presence of inflammatory cells following diagnostic curettage. Acta Obstet Gynecol Scand 60:451–457, 1981

124. Gallion HH, van Nagell JR Jr, Donaldson ES, Powell DE: Endometrial cancer following radiation therapy for cervical cancer. Gynecol Oncol 27:76–83, 1987

125. Picoff RC, Luginbuhl W: The significance of foci of dense stromal cellularity in the endometrium. Am J Obstet Gynecol 94:820–823, 1966

126. Picoff RC, Luginbuhl W: Fibrin in the endometrial stroma: Its relation to uterine bleeding. Am J Obstet Gynecol 88:642–646, 1964

127. Hendrickson MR, Kempson RL: Endometrial epithelial metaplasias—proliferations frequently misdiagnosed as adenocarcinoma: Report of 89 cases and proposed classification. Am J Surg Pathol 4:525–542, 1980

128. Silverberg SG, Kurman RJ: Tumors of the uterine corpus and gestational trophoblastic disease. Atlas of tumor pathology, 3rd series, fascicle 3. Washington, DC, Armed Forces Institute of Pathology, 1992

129. Baggish MS, Woodruff JD: The occurrence of squamous epithelium in the endometrium. Obstet Gynecol Surv 22:69–115, 1967

130. Dutra F: Intraglandular morules of the endometrium. Am J Clin Pathol 31:60–65, 1959

131. Crum CP, Richart RM, Fenoglio CM: Adenoacanthosis of the endometrium: A clinicopathologic study in premenopausal women. Am J Surg Pathol 5:15–20, 1981

132. Fruin AH, Tighe JR: Tubal metaplasia of the endometrium. Br J Obstet Gynaecol 74:93–97, 1967

133. Hendrickson MR, Kempson RL: Ciliated carcinoma—A variant of endometrial carcinoma: A report of 10 cases. Int J Gynecol Pathol 2:1–12, 1983

134. Bergeron C, Ferenczy A: Oncocytic metaplasia in endometrial hyperplasia and carcinoma (Letter). Int J Gynecol Pathol 7:93–95, 1988

135. Demopoulos RI, Greco MA: Mucinous metaplasia of the endometrium: Ultrastructural and histochemical characteristics. Int J Gynecol Pathol 1:383–390, 1982

136. Czernobilsky B, Katz Z, Lancet M, Gaton E: Endocervical-type epithelium in endometrial carcinoma: A report of 10 cases with emphasis on histochemical methods for differential diagnosis. Am J Surg Pathol 4:481–490, 1980

137. Melhem MF, Tobon H: Mucinous adenocarcinoma of the endometrium. Int J Gynecol Pathol 6:345–355, 1987

138. Andersen WA, Taylor PT Jr, Fechner RE, Pinkerton JA: Endometrial metaplasia associated with endometrial adenocarcinoma. Am J Obstet Gynecol 157:597–604, 1987

139. Kaku T, Tsukamoto N, Tsuruchi N et al: Endometrial metaplasia associated with endometrial carcinoma. Obstet Gynecol 80:812–816, 1992

140. Kaku T, Silverberg SG, Tsukamoto N et al: Association of endometrial epithelial metaplasias with endometrial carcinoma and hyperplasia in Japanese and American women. Int J Gynecol Pathol 12 (in press), 1993

141. Bird CC, Willis RA: The production of smooth muscle by the endometrial stroma of the adult human uterus. J Pathol Bacteriol 90:75–81, 1965

142. Shatia NN, Hoshika MG: Uterine osseous metaplasia. Obstet Gynecol 60:256–259, 1982

143. Roth E, Taylor MB: Heterotopic cartilage in uterus. Obstet Gynecol 27:838–844, 1966

144. Nogales FF, Gomez-Morales M, Raymundo C, Aguilar D: Benign heterologous tissue components associated with endometrial carcinoma. Int J Gynecol Pathol 1:286–291, 1982

145. Grönroos M, Meurman L, Kahra K: Proliferating glia and other heterotopic tissues in the uterus: Fetal homografts? Obstet Gynecol 61:261–266, 1983

146. Hamperl H, Kaufmann C, Ober KG: Wuchernde Glia im Endometrium. Geburtshilfe Frauenheilkd 19:978–982, 1959

147. Young RH, Kleinman GM, Scully RE: Glioma of the uterus: Report of a case with comments on histogenesis. Am J Surg Pathol 5:695–700, 1981

148. Jones R, Mammel J, Shepard M, Fisher R: Recovery of chlamydia trachomatis from the endometrium of women at risk for chlamydial infection. Am J Obstet Gynecol 155:35–39, 1986

149. Monif GRC, Baer H: Impact of diverging anaerobic technology on cul-de-sac isolates from patients with endometritis-salpingitis-peritonitis. Am J Obstet Gynecol 142:896–900, 1982

150. Platt LD, Yonekura ML, Ledger WJ: The role of anaerobic bacteria in postpartum endometritis. Am J Obstet Gynecol 135:814–817, 1979

151. Kiviat NB, Wølner-Hanssen P, Eschenbach DA et al: Endometrial histopathology in patients with culture-proved upper genital tract infection and laparoscopically diagnosed acute salpingitis. Am J Surg Pathol 14:167–175, 1990

152. Weström L: Gynecological chlamydial infections. Infection 10 (Suppl 1):40–45, 1982

153. Stray-Pedersen B, Bruu A-L, Molne K: Infertility and uterine colonization with Ureaplasma urealyticum. Acta Obstet Gynecol Scand 61:21–24, 1982

154. Taylor-Robinson D, McCormack WM: The genital mycoplasmas. N Engl J Med 302:1003–1010, 1063–1067, 1980

155. Stray-Pedersen B, Lorentzen-Styr AM: Uterine Toxoplasma infections and repeated abortions. Am J Obstet Gynecol 128:716–721, 1977

156. Halban J, Koehler R: Die pathologische Anatomie des puerperal Prozesses und ihre Beziehungen zur Klinik und Therapie. Vienna, Braumuller, 1919

157. Hervet E: Infarctus utéro-annexiel post-abortum. Gynecol Obstet 57:48–59, 1958

158. Crum CP, Egawa K, Fenoglio CM, Richart RM: Chronic endometritis: The role of immunohistochemistry in the detection of plasma cells. Am J Obstet Gynecol 147:812–815, 1983

159. Rotterdam H: Chronic endometritis: A clinicopathologic study. Pathol Annu 13:209–231, 1978

160. Schaefer G, Marcus RS, Kramer EE: Postmenopausal endometrial tuberculosis. Am J Obstet Gynecol 112:681–687, 1972

161. Sharman A: Genital tuberculosis. In V Meigs, SH Sturgis, eds. Progress in gynecology, vol III, pp 397–407. New York, Grune & Stratton, 1957

162. Sutherland AM: Genital tuberculosis in women. Am J Obstet Gynecol 79:486–498, 1960

163. Barua R, Kirkland JA, Petrucco OM: Xanthogranulomatous endometritis: Case report. Pathology 10:161–164, 1978

164. Nogales-Ortiz F, Taranco I, Nogales FF Jr: The pathology of female genital tuberculosis: A 31 year study of 1436 cases. Obstet Gynecol 53:422–428, 1959

165. Duncan DA, Varner RE, Mazur MT: Uterine herpes virus infection with multifocal necrotizing endometritis. Hum Pathol 20:1021–1024, 1989

166. Frank TS, Himebaugh KS, Wilson MD: Granulomatous endometritis associated with histologically occult cytomegalovirus in a healthy patient. Am J Surg Pathol 16:716–720, 1992

167. Schenken JR, Tamisiea J: Enterobius vermicularis (pinworm) infection of the endometrium. Am J Obstet Gynecol 72:913–914, 1956

168. Berry A: A cytopathological and histopathological study of bilharziasis of the female genital tract. J Pathol Bacteriol 91:325–338, 1966

169. Salgia K, Bhatia L, Rajashekaraiah KR, Zangan M et al: Coccidiomycosis of the uterus. South Med J 75:614-616, 1982

170. Ho KL: Sarcoidosis of the uterus. Hum Pathol 10:219–222, 1979

171. Molnar JJ, Poliak A: Recurrent endometrial malakoplakia. Am J Clin Pathol 80:762–764, 1983

172. Buckley CH, Fox H: Histiocytic endometritis. Histopathology 4:105–110, 1980

173. Bell DA, Mondschein M, Scully RE: Giant cell arteritis of the female genital tract: A report of three cases. Am J Surg Pathol 10:696–701, 1986

174. Bruch JF, Fernandez H, Antoine C et al: Angéites utérines: Etude anatomoclinique de deux cas et discussion étiopathologique. Gynecologie 41:207–211, 1990

175. Benson RC, Sneeden VD: Adenomyosis: A reappraisal of symptomatology. Am J Obstet Gynecol 76:1044–1061, 1958

176. Bird CB, McElin TW, Manalo-Estella P: The elusive adenomyosis of the uterus—revisited. Am J Obstet Gynecol 112:583–593, 1972

177. Molitor JJ: Adenomyosis: A clinical and pathologic appraisal. Am J Obstet Gynecol 110:275–284, 1971

178. Owolabi TO, Strickler RC: Adenomyosis: A neglected diagnosis. Obstet Gynecol 50:424–427, 1977

179. Weed JC, Geary WL, Holland JB: Adenomyosis of the uterus. Clin Obstet Gynecol 9:412–421, 1966

180. Weseley AC: The preoperative diagnosis of adenomyosis. Diagn Gynecol Obstet 4:105–106, 1982

181. Tamaya T, Motoyama T, Ohono Y et al: Steroid receptor levels and histology of endometriosis and adenomyosis. Fertil Steril 31:396–400, 1979

182. Sandberg EC, Cohn F: Adenomyosis in the gravid uterus at term. Am J Obstet Gynecol 84:1457–1465, 1962

183. Hayata T: Ultrastructural study of glandular epithelium in adenomyosis in comparison with those of proliferative endometrium and well-differentiated endometrial cancer. Am J Obstet Gynecol 165:225–228, 1991

184. Hernandez E, Woodruff JD: Endometrial adenocarcinoma arising in adenomyosis. Am J Obstet Gynecol 138:827–832, 1980

185. Hall JB, Young RH, Nelson JH Jr: The prognostic significance of adenomyosis in endometrial carcinoma. Gynecol Oncol 17:32–40, 1984

186. Vollenhoven B, Lawrence A, Healy D: Uterine fibroids: A clinical review. Br J Obstet Gynaecol 97:285–298, 1990

187. Belaisch J: Leiomyomes: Epidémiologie et hypothèses physiopathologiques. Gynecologie 40:169–174, 1989

188. Norris HJ, Hilliard GD, Irey NS: Hemorrhagic cellular leiomyomas ("apoplectic leiomyoma") of the uterus associated with pregnancy and oral contraceptives. Int J Gynecol Pathol 7:212–224, 1988

189. Fechner RE: Atypical leiomyomas and synthetic progestin therapy. Am J Clin Pathol 49:697–702, 1968

190. Spellacy WN, Le Maire WJ, Buhl WC et al: Plasma growth hormone and estradiol levels in women with uterine myomas. Obstet Gynecol 40:829–834, 1972

191. Soules MR, McCarty KS Jr: Leiomyomas: Steroid receptor content. Variation within normal menstrual cycles. Am J Obstet Gynecol 143:6–11, 1982

192. Cramer SF, Patel A: The nonrandom regional distribution of uterine leiomyomas: A clue to histogenesis? Hum Pathol 23:635–638, 1992

193. Lacassagne A: Modifications progressives de la structure du conduit tubo-utérin chez les lapines soumises à partir de la naissance à des injections répétées d'oestrone (folliculine). CR Soc Biol 120:685–689, 1935

194. Friedman AJ, Harrison-Atlas D, Barbieri RL et al: A randomized, placebo-controlled, double-blind study evaluating the efficacy of leuprolide acetate depot in the treatment of uterine leiomyomata. Fertil Steril 51:251–256, 1989

195. Letterie GS, Coddington CC, Winkel CA et al: Efficacy of a gonadotropin-releasing hormone agonist in the treatment of uterine leiomyomata: Long-term follow-up. Fertil Steril 51:951–956, 1989

196. Kawaguchi K, Fujii S, Konishi I et al: Mitotic activity in uterine leiomyomas during the menstrual cycle. Am J Obstet Gynecol 160:637–641, 1989

197. Tiltman AJ: The effect of progestins on the mitotic activity of uterine fibromyomas. Int J Gynecol Pathol 4:89–96, 1985

198. Kawaguchi K, Fujii S, Konishi I et al: Ultrastructural study of cultured smooth muscle cells from uterine leiomyoma and myometrium under the influence of sex steroids. Gynecol Oncol 21:32–41, 1985

199. Hu J, Surti U: Subgroups of uterine leiomyomas based on cytogenetic analysis. Hum Pathol 22:1009–1016, 1991

200. Pandis N, Heim S, Willén H et al: Histologic-cytogenetic correlations in uterine leiomyomas. Int J Gynecol Cancer 1:163–168, 1991

201. Rice JP, Kay HH, Mahony BS: The clinical significance of uterine leiomyomas in pregnancy. Am J Obstet Gynecol 160:1212–1216, 1989

202. Gisser SD, Young I: Neurilemoma-like uterine myomas: An ultrastructural reaffirmation of their non-Schwannian nature. Am J Obstet Gynecol 129:389–392, 1977

203. Honoré LH: Uterine leiomyoma with hemangiopericytomatous foci: Histogenetic implications. Am J Obstet Gynecol 127:891–892, 1977

204. Honoré LH: Uterine fibrolipoleiomyoma: Report of a case with discussion of histogenesis. Am J Obstet Gynecol 132:635–636, 1978

205. Pounder DJ: Fatty tumours of the uterus. J Clin Pathol 35:1380–1383, 1982

206. Sieinski W: Lipomatous neometaplasia of the uterus: Report of 11 cases with discussion of histogenesis and pathogenesis. Int J Gynecol Pathol 8:357–363, 1989

207. Clement PB, Scully RE: Uterine tumors resembling ovarian sex-cord tumors: A clinicopathologic analysis of fourteen cases. Am J Clin Pathol 66:512–525, 1976

208. Mazur MT, Kraus FT: Histogenesis of morphologic variations in tumors of the uterine wall. Am J Surg Pathol 4:59–74, 1980

209. Devaney K, Tavassoli FA: Immunohistochemistry as a diagnostic aid in the interpretation of unusual mesenchymal tumors of the uterus. Mod Pathol 4:225–231, 1991

210. Leibsohn S, d'Ablaing G, Mishell DR Jr, Schlaerth JB: Leiomyosarcoma in a series of hysterectomies performed for presumed uterine leiomyomas. Am J Obstet Gynecol 162:968–976, 1990

211. Smith DC, Uhlir JK: Myomectomy as a reproductive procedure. Am J Obstet Gynecol 162:1476–1482, 1990

212. Mergui JL, Salat-Baroux J: Indications et techniques du traitement per hystéroscopique des fibromes utérins. Gynecologie 39:374–378, 1988

213. Lesec G, Manhes H: Myolyse: Réflexions sur la physiopathologie de l'involution myomateuse et étude préliminaire. Gynecologie 40:181–187, 1989

214. Buttram VS Jr, Reiter RC: Uterine leiomyomata: Etiology, symptomatology, and management. Fertil Steril 36:433–445, 1981

215. Evans HL, Chawla SP, Simpson C, Finn KP: Smooth muscle neoplasms of the uterus other than ordinary leiomyoma: A study of 46 cases, with emphasis on diagnostic criteria and prognostic factors. Cancer 62:2239–2247, 1988

216. Kempson RL, Hendrickson MR: Pure mesenchymal neoplasms of the uterine corpus: Selected problems. Semin Diagn Pathol 5:172–198, 1988

217. Kurman RJ, Norris HJ: Mesenchymal tumors of the uterus. VI. Epithelioid smooth muscle tumors including leiomyoblastoma and clear cell leiomyoma: A clinical and pathologic analysis of 26 cases. Cancer 37:1853–1865, 1976

218. De Brux J, Ancla M, Bonnenfant JL: Uterine leiomyoblastomas (Myoid tumours of the uterus). Ann Anat Pathol 14:107–118, 1969

219. Chang V, Aikawa M, Druet R: Uterine leiomyoblastoma: Ultrastructural and cytological studies. Cancer 39:1563–1569, 1977

220. Hyde KE, Geisinger KR, Marshall RB, Jones TL: The clear-cell variant of uterine epithelioid leiomyoma: An immunohistologic and ultrastructural study. Arch Pathol Lab Med 113:551–553, 1989

221. Borghard-Erdle AM, Hirsch EF: Glomus tumor of the uterus. Arch Pathol 65:244–246, 1958

222. Nunez-Alonso C, Battifora HA: Plexiform tumors of the uterus: Ultrastructural study. Cancer 44:1707–1714, 1979

223. Kaminski PF, Tavassoli FA: Plexiform tumorlet: A clinical and pathologic study of 15 cases with ultrastructural observations. Int J Gynecol Pathol 3:124–134, 1984

224. Norris HJ, Parmley T: Mesenchymal tumors of the uterus. V. Intravenous leiomyomatosis: A clinical and pathologic study of 14 cases. Cancer 36:2164–2178, 1975

225. Clement PB: Intravenous leiomyomatosis of the uterus. Pathol Annu 23:(Part 2)153–183, 1988

226. Nogales FF, Navarro N, Martinez de Victoria JM et al: Uterine intravascular leiomyomatosis: An update and report of seven cases. Int J Gynecol Pathol 6:331–339, 1987

227. Clement PB, Young RH, Scully RE: Intravenous leiomyomatosis of the uterus: A clinicopathologic analysis of 16 cases with unusual histologic features. Am J Surg Pathol 12:932–945, 1988

228. Abell MR, Littler ER: Benign metastasizing uterine leiomyoma: Multiple lymph nodal metastases. Cancer 36:2206–2213, 1975

229. Williams LJ Jr, Pavlick FJ: Leiomyomatosis peritonealis disseminata: Two case reports and a review of the medical literature. Cancer 45:1726–1733, 1980

230. Wolff M, Silva F, Kaye G: Pulmonary metastases (with admixed epithelial elements) from smooth muscle neoplasms: Report of nine cases, including three males. Am J Surg Pathol 3:325–342, 1979

231. Nuovo MA, Nuovo GJ, McCaffrey RM et al: Endometrial polyps in postmenopausal patients receiving tamoxifen. Int J Gynecol Pathol 8:125–131, 1989

232. Wolf DM, Jordan VC: Gynecologic complications associated with long-term adjuvant tamoxifen therapy for breast cancer. Gynecol Oncol 45:118–128, 1992

233. Lau H, Stoll P: Das Adenom des Corpus uteri. Dtsch Med Wochenschr 87:1005–1012, 1962

234. Peterson WF, Novak ER: Endometrial polyps. Obstet Gynecol 8:40–49, 1956

235. Silva EG, Jenkins R: Serous carcinoma in endometrial polyps. Mod Pathol 3:120–128, 1990

236. Lee KR, Belinson JL: Recurrence in noninvasive endometrial carcinoma: Relationship to uterine papillary serous carcinoma. Am J Surg Pathol 15:965–973, 1991

237. Silverberg SG, Major FJ, Blessing JA et al: Carcinosarcoma (malignant mixed mesodermal tumor) of the uterus: A Gynecologic Oncology Group pathologic study of 203 cases. Int J Gynecol Pathol 9:1–19, 1990

238. Pedowitz P, Felmus LB, Grayzel DM: Vascular tumors of the uterus. I. Benign vascular tumors. Am J Obstet Gynecol 69:1291–1303, 1955

239. Milton PJD, Thonet RGN: Myometrial hemangioma: A rare cause of severe menorrhagia. Case report. Br J Obstet Gynaecol 88:1054–1055, 1981

240. Pounder DJ: Fatty tumours of the uterus. J Clin Pathol 35:1380–1383, 1982

241. Willén R, Gad A, Willén H: Lipomatous lesions of the uterus. Virchows Arch A Pathol Anat Histopathol 377:351–361, 1978

242. Demopoulos RI, Denarvaez F, Kaji V: Benign mixed mesodermal tumors of the uterus: A histogenetic study. Am J Clin Pathol 60:377–383, 1973

243. Teel P: Adenomatoid tumors of the genital tract with special reference of the female. Am J Obstet Gynecol 75:1347–1353, 1958

244. Honoré LH: Uterine mesothelioma. Am J Obstet Gynecol 135:162, 1979

245. Quigley JC, Hart WR: Adenomatoid tumors of the uterus. Am J Clin Pathol 76:627–635, 1981

246. Tiltman AJ: Adenomatoid tumors of the uterus. Histopathology 4:437–443, 1980

247. Livingston EG, Guis MS, Pearl ML et al: Diffuse adenomatoid tumor of the uterus with a serosal papillary cystic component. Int J Gynecol Pathol 11:288–292, 1992

248. Carlier MT, Dardick I, Lagace AF, Sreeram V: Adenomatoid tumor of the uterus: Presentation in endometrial curettings. Int J Gynecol Pathol 5:69–74, 1986

249. Young TW, Thrasher TV: Nonchromaffin paraganglioma of the uterus: A case report. Arch Pathol Lab Med 106:608–609, 1982

250. Jacques SM, Lawrence WD, Malviya VK: Uterine mixed embryonal rhabdomyosarcoma and fetal rhabdomyoma. Gynecol Oncol 48:272–276, 1993

251. Clement PB: Postoperative spindle-cell nodule of the endometrium. Arch Pathol Lab Med 112:566–568, 1988

252. Gilks CB, Taylor GP, Clement PB: Inflammatory pseudotumor of the uterus. Int J Gynecol Pathol 6:275–286, 1987

253. Nogales-Ortiz F, Nogales-Fernandez F, Herraiz Martinez MA, Ortega I: Hiperplasia glandular atípica del endometrio. Consideraciones anatomicoclínicas. Acta Ginecológica 49:182–195, 1992

254. Koss LG, Schreiber K, Oberlander SG et al: Detection of endometrial carcinoma and hyperplasia in asymptomatic women. Obstet Gynecol 64:1–11, 1984

255. Kelsey JL, Hildreth NG: Breast and gynecologic cancer epidemiology. Boca Raton, CRC Press, 1983

256. Fox H: The endometrial hyperplasias. Obstet Gynecol Annu 13:197–209, 1984

257. Huang SJ, Amparo EG, Fu YS: Endometrial hyperplasia: Histologic classification and behavior. Surg Pathol 1:215–229, 1988

258. Kurman RJ, Norris HJ: Evaluation of criteria for distinguishing atypical endometrial hyperplasia from well-differentiated carcinoma. Cancer 49:2547–2559, 1982

259. Norris HJ, Connor MP, Kurman RJ: Preinvasive lesions of the endometrium. Clin Obstet Gynaecol 13:725–738, 1986

260. Silverberg SG: Hyperplasia and carcinoma of the endometrium. Semin Diagn Pathol 5:135–153, 1988

261. Ferenczy A, Gelfand M: The biologic significance of cytologic atypia in progestogen-treated endometrial hyperplasia. Am J Obstet Gynecol 160:126–131, 1989

262. Hanson DJ: Studies of the endometrial stroma in cystic glandular hyperplasia. Am J Clin Pathol 32:152–158, 1959

263. Kurman RJ, Kaminski PF, Norris HJ: The behavior of endometrial hyperplasia: A long-term study of "untreated" hyperplasia in 170 patients. Cancer 56:403–412, 1985

264. Sherman AI, Brown S: The precursors of endometrial carcinoma. Am J Obstet Gynecol 135:947–956, 1979

265. Wentz WB: Progestin therapy in endometrial hyperplasia. Gynecol Oncol 2:362–368, 1974

266. Fox H, Buckley CH: The endometrial hyperplasias and their relationship to endometrial neoplasias. Histopathology 6:493–510, 1982

267. Gusberg SB, Kaplan AL: Precursors of corpus cancer. IV. Adenomatous hyperplasia as stage 0 carcinoma of the endometrium. Am J Obstet Gynecol 87:662–678, 1963

268. Foster LN, Montgomery R: Endometrial carcinoma: A review of prior biopsies. Am J Clin Pathol 43:26–38, 1965

269. Buehl IA, Vellios F, Carter JE, Huber CP: Carcinoma in situ of the endometrium. Am J Clin Pathol 42:594–601, 1964

270. Gore H, Hertig AT: Carcinoma in situ of the endometrium. Am J Obstet Gynecol 94:134–154, 1966

271. Hertig AT, Sommers SC, Bengloff H: Genesis of endometrial carcinoma. III. Carcinoma in situ. Cancer 2:964–971, 1949

272. Cullen TS: Cancer of the uterus. New York, Appleton, 1900

273. Scully RE: Definition of endometrial carcinoma precursors. Clin Obstet Gynecol 25:39–48, 1982

274. Hertig AT, Sommers SC, Bengloff H: Genesis of endometrial cancer. I. A study of prior biopsies. Cancer 2:946–956, 1949

275. Copenhaver EH: Atypical endometrial hyperplasia. Obstet Gynecol 13: 264–268, 1959

276. TeLinde RW, Jones HW Jr, Galvin GA: What are the earliest endometrial changes to justify a diagnosis of endometrial cancer? Am J Obstet Gynecol 66:953–969, 1953

277. Chamlian DL, Taylor HB: Endometrial hyperplasia in young women. Obstet Gynecol 36:659-666, 1970

278. Tavassoli F, Kraus FT: Endometrial lesions in uteri resected for atypical endometrial hyperplasia. Am J Clin Pathol 70:770–779, 1978

279. Baak JPA, Wisse-Brekelmans ECM, Fleege JC et al: Assessment of the risk on endometrial cancer in hyperplasia, by means of morphological and morphometrical features. Pathol Res Pract 188:856–859, 1992

280. Ng ABP: The cellular detection of endometrial carcinoma and its precursors. Gynecol Oncol 2:162–179, 1974

281. Wagner D, Richart RM, Terner JY: Deoxyribonucleic acid content of presumed precursors of endometrial carcinoma. Cancer 20:2067–2077, 1967

282. Ferenczy A: Cytodynamics of endometrial hyperplasia and neoplasia. II. In vitro DNA histoautoradiography. Hum Pathol 14:77–82, 1983

283. Kysela B et al: Flow cytometry (FCM) analysis of endometrial hyperplasia and carcinoma. Neoplasma 37:489–495, 1990

284. Morris WP, Griffin NR, Wells M: Patterns of reactivity with the monoclonal antibodies HMFG1 and HMFG2 in normal endometrium, endometrial hyperplasia and adenocarcinoma. Histopathology 15:179–186, 1989

285. Söderström KO: Lectin binding to human endometrial hyperplasias and adenocarcinoma. Int J Gynecol Pathol 6:356–365, 1987

286. Thor A, Viglione MJ, Muraro R et al: Monoclonal antibody B72.3 reactivity with human endometrium. Int J Gynecol Pathol 6:235–247, 1987

287. Nakopoulou L, Minaretzis D, Tsionou C, Mastrominas M: Value of immunohistochemical demonstration of several epithelial markers in hyperplastic and neoplastic endometrium. Gynecol Oncol 37:346–353, 1990

288. Schwartz AM, Silverberg SG, Fu YS et al: Use of monoclonal antibodies MSN-1 and B72.3 in the prediction of the natural history of endometrial hyperplasia. Int Gynecol Pathol 12:253–258, 1993

289. Norris HJ, Becker RL, Mikel UV: A comparative morphometric and cytophotometric study of endometrial hyperplasia, atypical hyperplasia, and endometrial carcinoma. Hum Pathol 20:219–223, 1989

290. Baak JPA, Kurver PHJ, Diegenbach PC et al: Discrimination of hyperplasia and carcinoma of the endometrium by quantitative microscopy: A feasibility study. Histopathology 5:61–68, 1981

291. Katayama KP, Jones HW: Chromosomes of atypical (adenomatous) hyperplasia and carcinoma of the endometrium. Am J Obstet Gynecol 97:978–983, 1967

292. Wilkinson N, Buckley CH, Chawner L, Fox H: Nucleolar organizer regions in normal, hyperplastic and neoplastic endometria. Int J Gynecol Pathol 9:55–59, 1990

293. Ferenczy A: The ultrastructural dynamics of endometrial hyperplasia and neoplasia. In LG Koss, DV Coleman, eds. Advances in clinical cytology, pp 1–43. London, Butterworths, 1980

294. Klemi PM, Grönroos M, Rayramo L, Punnonen R: Ultrastructural features of endometrial atypical adenomatous hyperplasia and adenocarcinomas and the plasma level of estrogens. Gynecol Oncol 9:162–169, 1980

295. Winkler B, Alvarez S, Richart RM, Crum CP: Pitfalls in the diagnosis of endometrial neoplasia. Obstet Gynecol 64:185–194, 1984

296. Silverberg SG: Surgical pathology of the uterus. New York, John Wiley & Sons, 1977

297. Hendrickson MR, Kempson RL: Surgical pathology of the uterine corpus. Philadelphia, WB Saunders, 1980

298. Hendrickson MR, Ross JC, Kempson RL: Toward the development of morphologic criteria for well-differentiated adenocarcinoma of the endometrium. Am J Surg Pathol 7:819–838, 1983

299. Welch WR, Scully RE: Precancerous lesions of the endometrium. Hum Pathol 8:503–512, 1977

300. Baak JPA, Kurver PHJ, Overdiep SH et al: Quantitative, microscopical, computer-aided diagnosis of endometrial hyperplasia or carcinoma in individual patients. Histopathology 5:689–695, 1981

301. Colgan HJ, Norris HJ, Foster W, Kurman RJ, Fox CH: Predicting the outcome of endometrial hyperplasia by quantitative analysis of nuclear features using a linear discriminant function. Int J Gynecol Pathol 1:347–352, 1982

302. Morse AR, Ellice RM, Anderson MC, Beard RW: Reliability of endometrial aspiration cytology in the assessment of endometrial status. Obstet Gynecol 59:513–518, 1982

303. Tezuka F, Higashiiwai H, Namiki T: Quantitative analysis of nuclear distribution pattern differentiating carcinoma from hyperplasia in endometrial cytologic studies. Am J Clin Pathol 96:648–653, 1991

304. Bibbo M, Kluskens L, Azizi F, Bartels PH et al: Accuracy of three sampling technics for the diagnosis of endometrial cancer and hyperplasia. J Reprod Med 27:622–626, 1982

305. Ferenczy A, Gelfand MM: Appraisal of techniques for the office diagnosis of corpus carcinoma and its precursors. Am J Diagn Gynecol Obstet 1:49–54, 1979

306. Gusberg SB, Milano C: Detection of endometrial cancer and its precursors. Cancer 47:1173–1175, 1981

307. Koss LG, Schreiber K, Moussouris H, Oberlander SG: Endometrial carcinoma and its precursors: Detection and screening. Clin Obstet Gynecol 25:49–61, 1982

308. Studd JWW, Thom M, Dische F, Driver M et al: Value of cytology for detecting endometrial abnormalities in climacteric women receiving hormone replacement therapy. Br Med J 1:846–848, 1979

309. Vuopala S: Diagnostic accuracy and clinical applicability of cytological and histological methods for investigating endometrial carcinoma. Acta Obstet Gynecol Scand Suppl 70:1–72, 1977

310. Kistner RW: Treatment of hyperplasia and carcinoma in situ of the endometrium. Clin Obstet Gynecol 25:63–74, 1982

311. Soh E, Sato K: Clinical effects of Danazol on endometrial hyperplasia in menopausal and postmenopausal women. Cancer 66:983–988, 1990

312. Austin DF, Roe KM: The decreasing incidence of endometrial cancer: Public health implications. Am J Public Health 72:65–68, 1982

313. Marrett LD, Meigs JW, Flannery JT: Trends in the incidence of cancer of the corpus uteri in Connecticut, 1964–1979, in relation to consumption of exogenous estrogens. Am J Epidemiol 116:57–67, 1982

314. Ostör AG, Adam R, Gutteridge BH, Fortune DW: Endometrial carcinoma in young women. Aust N Z J Obstet Gynaecol 22:38–42, 1982

315. Farhi DC, Nosanchuk J, Silverberg SG: Endometrial adenocarcinoma in women under 25 years of age. Obstet Gynecol 68:741–745, 1986

316. Silverberg SG: Significance of squamous elements in carcinoma of the endometrium: A review. Prog Surg Pathol 4:115–136, 1982

317. Zaino RJ, Kurman RJ: Squamous differentiation in carcinoma of the endometrium: A critical appraisal of adenoacanthoma and adenosquamous carcinoma. Semin Diagn Pathol 5:154–171, 1988

318. MacMahon B: Risk factors for endometrial cancer. Gynecol Oncol 2:122–129, 1974

319. Nisker JA, Hammond GL, Davidson BJ et al: Serum sex hormone-binding globulin capacity and the percentage of free estradiol in postmenopausal women with and without endometrial carcinoma. Am J Obstet Gynecol 138:637–642, 1980

320. Gurpide E: Endometrial cancer: Biochemical and clinical correlates. J Natl Cancer Inst 83:405–416, 1991

321. Fechner RE, Kaufman RH: Endometrial adenocarcinoma in Stein-Leventhal syndrome. Cancer 34:444–452, 1974

322. MacDonald PC, Edman CD, Hemsell DL et al: Effect of obesity on conversion of androstenedione to estrone in postmenopausal women with and without endometrial cancer. Am J Obstet Gynecol 130:448–455, 1978

323. McDonald T, Malkasian G, Gaffey T: Endometrial cancer associated with feminizing ovarian tumor and polycystic ovarian disease. Obstet Gynecol 49:654–658, 1977

324. Sasano H, Fukunaga M, Rojas M, Silverberg SG: Hyperthecosis of the ovary: Clinicopathologic study of 19 cases with immunohistochemical analysis of steroidogenic enzymes. Int J Gynecol Pathol 8:311–320, 1989

325. Ziel HK: Estrogen's role in endometrial cancer. Obstet Gynecol 60:509–515, 1982

326. Silverberg SG, Mullen D, Faraci JA et al: Endometrial carcinoma: Clinical-pathologic comparison of cases in postmenopausal women receiving and not receiving exogenous estrogens. Cancer 45:3018–3026, 1980

327. Harlap S: The benefits and risks of hormone replacement therapy: An epidemiologic overview. Am J Obstet Gynecol 166:1986–1992, 1992

328. Malfetano JH: Tamoxifen-associated endometrial carcinoma in postmenopausal breast cancer patients. Gynecol Oncol 39:82–84, 1990

329. Hakala T, Mecklin JP, Forss M et al: Endometrial carcinoma in the cancer family syndrome. Cancer 68:1656–1659, 1991

330. Sandles LG, Shulman LP, Elias S et al: Endometrial adenocarcinoma: Genetic analysis suggesting heritable site-specific uterine cancer. Gynecol Oncol 47:167–171, 1992

331. Longscope C, Pratt JH, Schneider SH, Fineberg SE: Aromatization of androgens by muscle and adipose tissue in vivo. J Clin Endocrinol Metab 46:146–152, 1978

332. Siiteri PK, Schwarz BE, MacDonald PC: Estrogen receptors and the estrone hypothesis in relation to endometrial and breast cancer. Gynecol Oncol 2:228–238, 1974

333. Ehrlich CE, Young PC, Cleary RE: Cytoplasmic progesterone and estradiol receptors in normal, hyperplastic, and carcinomatous endometria: Therapeutic implications. Am J Obstet Gynecol 141:539–546, 1981

334. Billiet G, DeHertogh R, Bonte J, Ide P, Vlaemynck G: Estrogen receptors in human uterine adenocarcinoma: Correlation with tissue differentiation, vaginal karyopyknotic index, and effect of progestogen or anti-estrogen treatment. Gynecol Oncol 10:33–39, 1982

335. Carcangiu ML, Chambers JT: Sex steroid receptors in gynecologic neoplasms. Pathol Annu 27(Part 2):121–152, 1992

336. Kleine W, Maier T, Geyer H, Pfleiderer A: Estrogen and progesterone receptors in endometrial cancer and their prognostic relevance. Gynecol Oncol 38:59–65, 1990

337. Bokhman JV: Two pathogenetic types of endometrial carcinoma. Gynecol Oncol 15:10–17, 1983

338. Deligdisch L: Morphologic correlates of host response in endometrial carcinoma. Am J Reprod Immunol 2:54–57, 1982

339. LaVecchia C, Franceschi S, Gallus G et al: Prognostic features of endometrial cancer in estrogen users and obese women. Am J Obstet Gynecol 144:387–390, 1982

340. Borst MP, Baker VV, Dixon D et al: Oncogene alterations in endometrial carcinoma. Gynecol Oncol 38:364–366, 1990

341. Hetzel DJ, Wilson TO, Keeney GL et al: HER-2/neu expression: A major prognostic factor in endometrial cancer. Gynecol Oncol 47:179–185, 1992

342. Procope BJ: Aetiology of postmenopausal bleeding. Acta Obstet Gynecol Scand 50:311–313, 1971

343. Tak WK, Anderson B, Vardi JR et al: Myometrial invasion and hysterography in endometrial carcinoma. Obstet Gynecol 50:159–165, 1977

344. Gordon A: The history of gynaecological endoscopy (Editorial). Gynaecol Endoscopy 1:3–5, 1992

345. Hata K, Hata T, Manabe A et al: New pelvic sonoangiography for detection of endometrial carcinoma: A preliminary report. Gynecol Oncol 45:179–184, 1992

346. Sahakian V, Syrop C, Turner D: Endometrial carcinoma: Transvaginal ultrasonography prediction of depth of myometrial invasion. Gynecol Oncol 43:217–219, 1991

347. DuBeshter B, Warshal DP, Angel C et al: Endometrial carcinoma: The relevance of cervical cytology. Obstet Gynecol 77:458–462, 1991

348. Mitchell H, Giles G, Medley G: Accuracy and survival benefit of cytological prediction of endometrial carcinoma on routine cervical smears. Int J Gynecol Pathol 12:34–40, 1993

349. Favre J, Bernard P, Besançon D, Siebert S: A five-year experience with intrauterine washing cytology. Acta Cytol 26:623–629, 1982

350. Stock RJ, Kanbour A: Prehysterectomy curettage. Obstet Gynecol 45:537–541, 1975

351. Grimes DA: Diagnostic dilatation and curettage: A reappraisal. Am J Obstet Gynecol 142:1–6, 1982

352. Shepherd JH: Revised FIGO staging for gynaecological cancer. Br J Obstet Gynaecol 96:889–892, 1989

353. Chen JL, Trost DC, Wilkinson EJ: Endometrial papillary adenocarcinomas: Two clinicopathological types. Int Gynecol Pathol 4:279–288, 1985

354. Fu YS, Parks PJ, Reagan JW et al: The ultrastructure and factors relating to survival of endometrial cancers. Am J Diagn Gynecol Obstet 1:55–72, 1979

355. Genton CY, Büchi KA: Are the histological and ultrastructural features of endometrial carcinomas reliable indicators of their steroid receptor content? Gynecol Obstet Invest 13:213–225, 1982

356. Silverberg SG, DeGiorgi LS: Histopathologic analysis of preoperative radiation therapy in endometrial carcinoma. Am J Obstet Gynecol 119:698–704, 1974

357. Bonazzi del Poggetto C, Virtanen I, Lehto VP, Wahlstrom T, Saksela E: Expression of intermediate filaments in ovarian and uterine tumors. Int J Gynecol Pathol 1:359–366, 1982

358. Tobon H, Watkins GJ: Secretory adenocarcinoma of the endometrium. Int J Gynecol Pathol 4:328–335, 1985

359. Hendrickson MR, Kempson RL: Ciliated carcinoma—a variant of endometrial adenocarcinoma: A report of 10 cases. Int J Gynecol Pathol 2:1–12, 1983

360. Novak ER, Nalley WB: Uterine adenoacanthoma. Obstet Gynecol 9:396–402, 1957

361. Ng AB, Reagan JW, Storaasli JP, Wentz WB: Mixed adenosquamous carcinoma of the endometrium. Am J Clin Pathol 59:765–781, 1973

362. Silverberg SG, Bolin MG, DeGiorgi LS: Adenoacanthoma and mixed adenosquamous carcinoma of the endometrium: A clinicopathologic study. Cancer 30:1307–1314, 1972

363. Silverberg SG, Sasano N. Yajima A: Endometrial carcinoma in Miyagi Prefecture, Japan: Histopathologic analysis of a cancer registry-based series and comparison with cases in American women. Cancer 49:1504–1510, 1982

364. Abeler VM, Kjrstad KE: Endometrial adenocarcinoma with squamous cell differentiation. Cancer 69:488–495, 1992

365. Zaino RJ, Kurman R, Herbold D et al: The significance of squamous differentiation in endometrial carcinoma: Data from a Gynecologic Oncology Group study. Cancer 68:2293–2302, 1991

366. Alberhasky RC, Connelly PJ, Christopherson WM: Carcinoma of the endometrium. IV. Mixed adenosquamous carcinoma: A clinical-pathological study of 68 cases with long-term follow-up. Am J Clin Pathol 77:655–664, 1982

367. Abeler VM, Kjørstad KE: Endometrial squamous cell carcinoma: Report of three cases and review of the literature. Gynecol Oncol 36:321–326, 1990

368. Bibro MC, Kapp DS, LiVolsi VA et al: Squamous carcinoma of the endometrium with ultrastructural observations and review of the literature. Gynecol Oncol 10:217–223, 1980

369. Kay S: Squamous cell carcinomas of the endometrium. Am J Clin Pathol 61:264–269, 1974

370. Hendrickson M, Ross J, Eifel P et al: Uterine papillary serous carcinoma: A highly malignant form of endometrial adenocarcinoma. Am J Surg Pathol 6:93–108, 1982

371. Lauchlan SC: Tubal (serous) carcinoma of the endometrium. Arch Pathol Lab Med 105:615–618, 1981

372. Sato N, Mori T, Orenstein JM, Silverberg SG: Ultrastruc-

ture of papillary serous carcinoma of the endometrium. Int J Gynecol Pathol 2:337–348, 1984

373. Fanning J, Evans MC, Peters AJ et al: Endometrial adenocarcinoma histologic subtypes: Clinical and pathologic profile. Gynecol Oncol 32:288–291, 1989

374. Dunton CJ, Balsara G, McFarland M, Hernandez E: Uterine papillary serous carcinoma: A review. Obstet Gynecol Surv 46:97–102, 1991

375. Carcangiu ML, Chambers JT: Uterine papillary serous carcinoma: A study on 108 cases with emphasis on the prognostic significance of associated endometrioid carcinoma, absence of invasion, and concomitant ovarian carcinoma. Gynecol Oncol 47:298–305, 1992

376. Sherman ME, Bitterman P, Rosenshein NB et al: Uterine serous carcinoma: A morphologically diverse neoplasm with unifying clinicopathologic features. Am J Surg Pathol 16:600–610, 1992

377. Christopherson WM, Alberhasky RC, Connelly PJ: Carcinoma of the endometrium. I. A clinicopathologic study of clear-cell carcinoma and secretory carcinoma. Cancer 49:1511–1523, 1982

378. Silverberg SG, DeGiorgi LS: Clear cell carcinoma of the endometrium: Clinical, pathologic and ultrastructural findings. Cancer 31:1127–1140, 1973

379. Webb GA, Lagios MD: Clear cell carcinoma of the endometrium. Am J Obstet Gynecol 156:82–91, 1984

380. Abeler VM, Kjørstad KE: Clear cell carcinoma of the endometrium: A histopathological and clinical study of 97 cases. Gynecol Oncol 40:207–217, 1991

381. Ross JC, Eifel PJ, Cox RS et al: Primary mucinous adenocarcinoma of the endometrium: A clinicopathologic and histochemical study. Am J Surg Pathol 7:715–729, 1983

382. Melhem MF, Tobon H: Mucinous adenocarcinoma of the endometrium. Int J Gynecol Pathol 6:347–355, 1987

383. Inoue M, Ueda G, Yamasaki M et al: Endometrial argyrophil cell adenocarcinoma with indole- or catecholamine precursor uptake and decarboxylation. Int J Gynecol Pathol 1:47–58, 1982

384. Campo E, Brunier MN, Merino MJ: Small cell carcinoma of the endometrium with associated ocular paraneoplastic syndrome. Cancer 69:2283–2288, 1992

385. Abeler VM, Kjørstad KE, Nesland JM: Undifferentiated carcinoma of the endometrium: A histopathologic and clinical study of 31 cases. Cancer 68:98–105, 1991

386. Hachisuga T, Sugimori H, Kaku T et al: Glassy cell carcinoma of the endometrium. Gynecol Oncol 36:134–138, 1990

387. Ryder DE: Verrucous carcinoma of the endometrium: A unique neoplasm with long survival. Obstet Gynecol 59:78S–80S, 1982

388. Jones MA, Young RH, Scully RE: Endometrial adenocarcinoma with a component of giant cell carcinoma. Int J Gynecol Pathol 10:260–270, 1991

389. Pesce C, Merino MJ, Chambers JT, Nogales F: Endometrial carcinoma with trophoblastic differentiation: An aggressive form of uterine cancer. Cancer 68:1799–1802, 1991

390. Sidawy MK, Silverberg SG: Endometrial carcinoma: Pathologic factors of therapeutic and prognostic significance. Pathol Annu 27(Part 2): 153–186, 1992

391. Goff BA, Rice LW: Assessment of depth of myometrial invasion in endometrial adenocarcinoma. Gynecol Oncol 38:46–48, 1990

392. Malviya VK, Deppe G, Malone JM Jr et al: Reliability of frozen section examination in identifying poor prognostic indicators in Stage I endometrial adenocarcinoma. Gynecol Oncol 34:299–304, 1989

393. Kadar NR, Kohorn EI, LiVolsi VA, Kapp DS: Histologic variants of cervical involvement by endometrial carcinoma. Obstet Gynecol 59:85–92, 1982

394. Frauenhoffer EE, Zaino RJ, Wolff TV, Whitney CE: Value of endocervical curettage in the staging of endometrial carcinoma. Int J Gynecol Pathol 6:195–202, 1987

395. Fanning J, Alvarez PM, Tsukada Y, Piver MS: Prognostic significance of the extent of cervical involvement by endometrial cancer. Gynecol Oncol 40:46–47, 1991

396. Bruckman JE, Bloomer WD, Mack A et al: Stage III adenocarcinoma of the endometrium: Two prognostic groups. Gynecol Oncol 9:12–17, 1980

397. Eifel P, Hendrickson M, Ross R et al: Simultaneous presentation of carcinoma involving the ovary and the uterine corpus. Cancer 50:163–170, 1982

398. Montoya F, Martin M, Schneider J et al: Simultaneous appearance of ovarian and endometrial carcinoma: A therapeutic challenge. Eur J Gynaecol Oncol 10:135–139, 1989

399. Eisner RF, Nieberg RK, Berek JS: Synchronous primary neoplasms of the female reproductive tract. Gynecol Oncol 33:335–339, 1989

400. Morrow CP, Bundy BN, Kurman RJ et al: Relationship between surgical-pathological risk factors and outcome in clinical Stage I and II carcinoma of the endometrium: A Gynecologic Oncology Group study. Gynecol Oncol 40:55–65, 1991

401. Wolfson AH, Sightler SE, Markoe AM et al: The prognostic significance of surgical staging for carcinoma of the endometrium. Gynecol Oncol 45:142–146, 1992

402. Nielsen AL, Thomsen HK, Nyholm HCJ: Evaluation of the reproducibility of the revised 1988 International Federation of Gynecology and Obstetrics grading system of endometrial cancers with special emphasis on nuclear grading. Cancer 68:2303–2309, 1991

403. Zaino RJ, Silverberg SG, Norris HJ et al: The prognostic value of nuclear versus architectural grading in endometrial adenocarcinoma: A Gynecologic Oncology Group study. Int J Gynecol Pathol 12 (in press), 1993

404. Hendrickson M, Ross J, Eifel P et al: Adenocarcinoma of the endometrium: Analysis of 256 cases with carcinoma limited to the uterine corpus. Pathology review and analysis of prognostic variables. Gynecol Oncol 13:373–392, 1982

405. Lotocki RJ, Copeland LJ, DePetrillo AD, Muirhead W: Stage I endometrial adenocarcinoma: Treatment results in 835 patients. Am J Obstet Gynecol 146:141–145, 1983

406. Abeler VM, Kjørstad KE: Endometrial adenocarcinoma in Norway: A study of a total population. Cancer 67:3093–3103, 1991

407. Creasman WT, Boronow RC, Morrow CP et al: Adenocarcinoma of the endometrium: Its metastatic lymph node potential—a preliminary report. Gynecol Oncol 4:239–243, 1976

408. Henriksen E: The lymphatic spread of carcinoma of the cervix and of the body of the uterus: A study of 420 necropsies. Am J Obstet Gynecol 58:924–942, 1949

409. Phillips GL, Prem KA, Adcock LL, Twiggs LB: Vaginal recurrence of adenocarcinoma of the endometrium. Gynecol Oncol 13:323–328, 1982

410. Creasman WT, Lukeman J: Role of the fallopian tube in dissemination of malignant cells in corpus cancer. Cancer 29:456–457, 1972

411. Menczer J, Modan M, Gloor E: The significance of positive tubal cytology in patients with endometrial adenocarcinoma. Gynecol Oncol 10:249–252, 1980

412. Pettersson F, ed: Annual report on the results of treatment in gynecological cancer, vol 21. Int J Gynecol Obstet 36(Suppl):1–315, 1991

413. Lutz H, Underwood B Jr, Kreutner A Jr, Miller M: Endometrial carcinoma: A new method of classification of therapeutic and prognostic significance. Gynecol Oncol 6:83–94, 1978

414. Templeton AC: Reporting of myometrial invasion by endometrial cancer. Histopathology 6:733–738, 1982

415. Connelly PJ, Alberhasky RC, Christopherson WM: Carcinoma of the endometrium. III. Analysis of 865 cases of adenocarcinoma and adenoacanthoma. Obstet Gynecol 59:569–575, 1982

416. Sivridis E, Buckley CH, Fox H: The prognostic significance of lymphatic vascular space invasion in endometrial adenocarcinoma. Br J Obstet Gynaecol 94:991–994, 1987

417. Hanson MB, van Nagell JR Jr, Powell DE et al: The prognostic significance of lymph-vascular space invasion in Stage I endometrial cancer. Cancer 55:1753–1757, 1985

418. Gal D, Recio FO, Zamurovic D, Tancer ML: Lymphvas-

cular space involvement: A prognostic indicator in endometrial adenocarcinoma. Gynecol Oncol 42:142–145, 1991

419. Ambros RA, Kurman RJ: Combined assessment of vascular and myometrial invasion as a model to predict prognosis in Stage I endometrioid adenocarcinoma of the uterine corpus. Cancer 69:1424–1431, 1992

420. Creasman WT, Morrow CP, Bundy BN et al: Surgical pathologic spread patterns of endometrial cancer. A Gynecologic Oncology Group study. Cancer 60:2035–2041, 1987

421. Hachisuga T, Kaku T, Enjoji M: Carcinoma of the lower uterine segment: Clinicopathologic analysis of 12 cases. Int J Gynecol Pathol 8:26–35, 1989

422. Grimshaw RN, Tupper WC, Fraser RC et al: Prognostic value of peritoneal cytology in endometrial carcinoma. Gynecol Oncol 36:97–100, 1990

423. Milosevic MF, Dembo AJ, Thomas GM: The clinical significance of malignant peritoneal cytology in Stage I endometrial carcinoma. Int J Gynecol Cancer 2:225–235, 1992

424. Kadar N, Homesley HD, Malfetano JH: Positive peritoneal cytology is an adverse factor in endometrial carcinoma only if there is other evidence of extrauterine disease. Gynecol Oncol 46:145–149, 1992

425. Beckner ME, Mori T, Silverberg SG: Endometrial carcinoma: Nontumor factors in prognosis. Int J Gynecol Pathol 4:131–145, 1985

426. Ayhan A, Yarali H, Ayhan A: Endometrial carcinoma: A pathologic evaluation of 142 cases with and without associated endometrial hyperplasia. J Surg Oncol 46:182–184, 1991

427. Chu J, Schweid AI, Weiss NS: Survival among women with endometrial cancer: A comparison of estrogen users and nonusers. Am J Obstet Gynecol 143:569–573, 1982

428. Runowicz CD, Nuchtern LM, Braunstein JD, Jones JG: Heterogeneity in hormone receptor status in primary and metastatic endometrial cancer. Gynecol Oncol 38:437–441, 1990

429. van der Putten HW, Baak JP, Koenders TJ et al: Prognostic value of quantitative pathologic features and DNA content in individual patients with Stage I endometrial adenocarcinoma. Cancer 63:1378–1387, 1989

430. Zaino RJ, Laskaris A, Whitney C, Sharkey FE: Morphometric analysis of endometrial adenocarcinoma. 2. A comparison of architectural differentiation determined morphometrically with subjective grading. Int J Gynecol Pathol 6:20–28, 1987

431. Stendahl U, Strang P, Wagenius G et al: Prognostic significance of proliferation in endometrial adenocarcinomas: A multivariate analysis of clinical and flow cytometric variables. Int J Gynecol Pathol 10:271–284, 1991

432. Piver MS, Hempling RE: A prospective trial of postoperative vaginal radium/cesium for grade 1–2 less than 50% myometrial invasion and pelvic radiation therapy for grade 3 or deep myometrial invasion in surgical Stage I endometrial adenocarcinoma. Cancer 66:1133–1138, 1990

433. Aalders J, Abeler V, Kolstad P et al: Postoperative external irradiation and prognostic parameters in Stage I endometrial carcinoma: Clinical and histopathologic study of 540 patients. Obstet Gynecol 56:419–427, 1980

434. Marchetti DL, Caglar H, Driscoll DL et al: Pelvic radiation in Stage I endometrial adenocarcinoma with high-risk attributes. Gynecol Oncol 37:51–54, 1990

435. Grigsby PW, Kuske RR, Perez CA et al: Medically inoperable Stage I adenocarcinoma of the endometrium treated with radiotherapy alone. Int J Rad Oncol Biol Phys 13:483–488, 1987

436. Hancock KC, Freedman RS, Edwards CL et al: Use of cisplatin, doxorubicin, and cyclophosphamide to treat advanced and recurrent adenocarcinoma of the endometrium. Cancer Treatment Reports 70:789–791, 1986

437. Kauppila A: Oestrogen and progestin receptors as prognostic indicators in endometrial cancer: A review of the literature. Acta Oncol 28:561–566, 1989

438. Podczaski E, Kaminski P, Gurski K et al: Detection and patterns of treatment failure in 300 consecutive cases of

439. Schwartz SM, Thomas DB: A case-control study of risk factors for sarcomas of the uterus. Cancer 64:2487–2492, 1989

440. Norris HJ, Taylor HB: Postirradiation sarcomas of the uterus. Obstet Gynecol 26:689–694, 1965

441. Press MF, Scully RE: Endometrial "sarcomas" complicating ovarian thecoma, polycystic ovarian disease and estrogen therapy. Gynecol Oncol 21:135–154, 1985

442. Doran AHG, Lockyer C: Two cases of uterine fibroids showing peritheliomatous change: Long immunity from recurrence after operation. Proc R Soc Med 2:25–39, 1908

443. Norris HJ, Taylor HB: Mesenchymal tumors of the uterus. I. A clinical and pathological study of 53 endometrial stromal tumors. Cancer 19:755–766, 1966

444. Evans HL: Endometrial stromal sarcoma and poorly differentiated endometrial sarcoma. Cancer 50:2170–2181, 1982

445. Tavassoli FA, Norris HJ: Mesenchymal tumors of the uterus. VII. A clinicopathological study of 60 endometrial stromal nodules. Histopathology 5:1–10, 1981

446. Fekete PS, Vellios F: The clinical and histologic spectrum of endometrial stromal neoplasms: A report of 41 cases. Int J Gynecol Pathol 3:198–212, 1984

447. Chang KL, Crabtree GS, Lim-Tan SK et al: Primary uterine endometrial stromal neoplasms: A clinicopathologic study of 117 cases. Am J Surg Pathol 14:415–438, 1990

448. Clement PB, Scully RE: Endometrial stromal sarcomas of the uterus with extensive endometrioid glandular differentiation: A report of three cases that caused problems in differential diagnosis. Int J Gynecol Pathol 11:163–173, 1992

449. Lloreta J, Prat J: Endometrial stromal nodule with smooth and skeletal muscle components simulating stromal sarcoma. Int J Gynecol Pathol 11:293–298, 1992

450. Farhood AI, Abrams J: Immunohistochemistry of endometrial stromal sarcoma. Hum Pathol 22:224–230, 1991

451. Franquemont DW, Frierson HF Jr, Mills SE: An immunohistochemical study of normal endometrial stroma and endometrial stromal neoplasms: Evidence for smooth muscle differentiation. Am J Surg Pathol 15:861–870, 1991

452. Dunton CJ, Kelsten ML, Brooks SE et al: Low-grade stromal sarcoma: DNA flow cytometric analysis and estrogen progesterone receptor data. Gynecol Oncol 37:268–275, 1990

453. El-Naggar AK, Abdul-Karim FW, Silva EG et al: Uterine stromal neoplasms: A clinicopathologic and DNA flow cytometric correlation. Hum Pathol 22:897–903, 1991

454. Katz L, Merino MJ, Sakamoto H, Schwartz PE: Endometrial stromal sarcoma: A clinicopathologic study of 11 cases with determination of estrogen and progestin receptor levels in three tumors. Gynecol Oncol 26:87–97, 1987

455. Tosi P, Sforza V, Santopietro R: Estrogen receptor content, immunohistochemically determined by monoclonal antibodies, in endometrial stromal sarcoma. Obstet Gynecol 73:75–78, 1989

456. Sutton GP, Stehman FB, Michael H et al: Estrogen and progesterone receptors in uterine sarcomas. Obstet Gynecol 68:709–714, 1986

457. De Fusco PA, Gaffey TA, Malkasian GD Jr et al: Endometrial stromal sarcoma: Review of Mayo Clinic experience, 1945–1980. Gynecol Oncol 35:8–14, 1989

458. Sabini G, Chumas JC, Mann WJ: Steroid hormone receptors in endometrial stromal sarcomas: A biochemical and immunohistochemical study. Am J Clin Pathol 97:381–386, 1992

459. Hitchcock CL, Norris HJ: Flow cytometric analysis of endometrial stromal sarcoma. Am J Clin Pathol 97:267–271, 1992

460. Muñoz AK, Berek JS, Fu YS, Heintz PAM: Pelvic hemangiopericytomas: A report of five cases and literature review. Gynecol Oncol 36:380–382, 1990

461. Spanos WJ Jr, Peters LJ, Osward MJ: Patterns of recurrence in malignant mixed müllerian tumor of the uterus. Cancer 57:155–159, 1986

462. Tenti P, Babilonti L, La Fianza A et al: Cytology of malig-

nant mixed mesodermal tumour of the uterus: Experience of 10 cases. Eur J Gynaecol Oncol 10:125–128, 1989

463. Costa MJ, Tidd C, Willis D: Cervicovaginal cytology in carcinosarcoma [malignant mixed müllerian (mesodermal) tumor] of the uterus. Diagn Cytopathol 8:33–40, 1992

464. Silverberg SG, Major FJ, Blessing JA et al: Carcinosarcoma (malignant mixed mesodermal tumor) of the uterus: A Gynecologic Oncology Group pathologic study of 203 cases. Int J Gynecol Pathol 9:1–19, 1990

465. Auerbach HE, LiVolsi VA, Merino MJ: Malignant mixed müllerian tumors of the uterus: An immunohistochemical study. Int J Gynecol Pathol 7:123–130, 1988

466. Bitterman P, Chun BK, Kurman RJ: The significance of epithelial differentiation in mixed mesodermal tumors of the uterus: A clinicopathologic and immunohistochemical study. Am J Surg Pathol 14:317–328, 1990

467. DeBrito PA, Silverberg SG, Orenstein JM: Carcinosarcoma (malignant mixed müllerian [mesodermal] tumor) of the female genital tract: Immunohistochemical and ultrastructural analysis of 28 cases. Hum Pathol 24:132–142, 1993

468. Dinh TV, Slavin RE, Bhagavan BS et al: Mixed müllerian tumors of the uterus: A clinicopathologic study. Obstet Gynecol 74:388–392, 1989

469. Nielsen SC, Podratz KC, Scheithauer BW, O'Brien PC: Clinico-pathologic analysis of uterine malignant mixed müllerian tumors. Gynecol Oncol 34:372–378, 1989

470. Podczaski ES, Woomert CA, Steven CH Jr et al: Management of malignant, mixed mesodermal tumors of the uterus. Gynecol Oncol 32:240–244, 1989

471. Deligdisch L, Plaxe S, Cohen CJ: Extrauterine pelvic malignant mixed mesodermal tumors: A study of 10 cases with immunohistochemistry. Int J Gynecol Pathol 7:361–372, 1988

472. Clement PB, Scully RE: Müllerian adenosarcoma of the uterus: A clinicopathologic analysis of ten cases of a distinctive type of müllerian mixed tumor. Cancer 34:1138–1149, 1974

473. Clement PB, Scully RE: Müllerian adenosarcoma of the uterus: A clinicopathologic analysis of 100 cases with a review of the literature. Hum Pathol 21:363–381, 1990

474. Kaku T, Silverberg SG, Major FJ et al: Adenosarcoma of the uterus: A Gynecologic Oncology Group clinico-pathologic study of 31 cases. Int J Gynecol Pathol 11:75–88, 1992

475. Zaloudek CJ, Norris HJ: Adenofibroma and adenosarcoma of the uterus: A clinicopathologic study of 35 cases. Cancer 48:354–366, 1981

476. Vellios F: Papillary adenofibroma-adenosarcoma: The uterine cystosarcoma phyllodes. Prog Surg Pathol 1:205–219, 1980

477. Clement PB, Scully RE: Müllerian adenosarcomas of the uterus with sex cord-like elements: A clinicopathologic analysis of eight cases. Am J Clin Pathol 91:664–672, 1989

478. Clement PB: Müllerian adenosarcoma of the uterus with sarcomatous overgrowth: A clinicopathological analysis of 10 cases. Am J Surg Pathol 13:28–38, 1989

479. Ostör AG, Fortune DW: Benign and low grade variants of mixed Müllerian tumour of the uterus. Histopathology 4:369–382, 1980

480. Clement PB, Scully RE: Uterine tumors with mixed epithelial and mesenchymal elements. Semin Diagn Pathol 5:199–222, 1988

481. Vellios F, Ng ABP, Reagan JW: Papillary adenofibroma of the uterus: A benign mesenchymal mixed tumor of Müllerian origin. Am J Clin Pathol 60:543–551, 1973

482. Clement PB, Scully RE: Müllerian adenofibroma of the uterus with invasion of myometrium and pelvic veins. Int J Gynecol Pathol 9:363–371, 1990

483. Seltzer VL, Levine A, Spiegel G et al: Adenofibroma of the uterus: Multiple recurrences following wide local excision. Gynecol Oncol 37:427–431, 1990

484. Mazur MT: Atypical polypoid adenomyomas of the endometrium. Am J Surg Pathol 5:473–482, 1981

485. Young RH, Treger T, Scully RE: Atypical polypoid adeno-

myoma of the uterus: A report of 27 cases. Am J Clin Pathol 86:139–145, 1986

486. Stearns HC, Sneeden VD: Leiomyosarcoma of the uterus. Am J Obstet Gynecol 95:374–380, 1966

487. Aaro LA, Symmonds RE, Dockerty MB: Sarcoma of the uterus: A clinical and pathological study of 177 cases. Am J Obstet Gynecol 94:101–109, 1966

488. Taylor HB, Norris HJ: Mesenchymal tumors of the uterus. IV. Diagnosis and prognosis of leiomyosarcoma. Arch Pathol 82:40–44, 1966

489. Herbold DR, Fu YS, Silbert SW: Leiomyosarcoma of the broad ligament: A case report and literature review with follow-up. Am J Surg Pathol 7:285–292, 1983

490. Bard DS, Zuna RE: Sarcomas and related neoplasms of the uterine corpus: A brief review of their natural history, prognostic factors, and management. Obstet Gynecol Annu 10:237–265, 1981

491. Christopherson WM, Richardson M: Uterine mesenchymal tumors. Pathol Annu 16(1):215–246, 1981

492. Zaloudek CJ, Norris HJ: Mesenchymal tumors of the uterus. Prog Surg Pathol 3:1–35, 1981

493. Hart WR, Billman JK Jr: A reassessment of uterine neoplasms originally diagnosed as leiomyosarcomas. Cancer 41:1902–1910, 1978

494. Burns B, Curry RH, Bell MEA: Morphologic features of prognostic significance in uterine smooth muscle tumors: A review of eighty-four cases. Am J Obstet Gynecol 135:109–114, 1979

495. Dinh TV, Woodruff JD: Leiomyosarcoma of the uterus. Am J Obstet Gynecol 144:817–823, 1982

496. Hannigan EV, Gomez LG: Uterine leiomyosarcoma: A review of prognostic clinical and pathologic features. Am J Obstet Gynecol 134:557–564, 1979

497. Silverberg SG: Leiomyosarcoma of the uterus: A clinicopathologic study. Obstet Gynecol 38:613–628, 1971

498. Silverberg SG: Reproducibility of the mitosis count in the histologic diagnosis of uterine smooth muscle tumors. Hum Pathol 7:451–454, 1976

499. Donhuijsen K, Schmidt U, Hirche H et al: Changes in mitotic rate and cell cycle fractions caused by delayed fixation. Hum Pathol 21:709–714, 1990

500. Van Diest P, Baak J, Matze-Cok P et al: Reproducibility of mitosis counting in 2,469 breast cancer specimens: Results from the multicenter morphometric mammary carcinoma project. Hum Pathol 23:603–607, 1992

501. O'Connnor DM, Norris HJ: Mitotically active leiomyomas of the uterus. Hum Pathol 21:223–227, 1990

502. Perrone T, Dehner LP: Prognostically favorable "mitotically active" smooth-muscle tumors of the uterus: A clinicopathologic study of ten cases. Am J Surg Pathol 12:1–8, 1988

503. Prayson RA, Hart WR: Mitotically active leiomyomas of the uterus. Am J Clin Pathol 97:14–20, 1992

504. Bell S, Kempson R, Hendrickson M: Smooth muscle neoplasms of the uterus. I. The leiomyoma-leiomyosarcoma spectrum exhibiting standard differentiation. Am J Surg Pathol (in press), 1993

505. Bell S, Kempson R, Hendrickson M: Uterine smooth muscle neoplasms. Pathol Annu (in press), 1993

506. King ME, Dickersin GR, Scully RE: Myxoid leiomyosarcoma of the uterus: A report of six cases. Am J Surg Pathol 6:589–598, 1982

507. Berchuck A, Rubin SC, Hoskins WJ et al: Treatment of uterine leiomyosarcoma. Obstet Gynecol 71:845–850, 1988

508. Dabbs DJ, Silverman JF, Geisinger KR: Immunohistochemical study of uterine stromal sarcoma and rhabdomyosarcoma. Arch Pathol Lab Med 113:1151–1154, 1989

509. Podczaski E, Sees J, Kaminski P et al: Rhabdomyosarcoma of the uterus in a postmenopausal patient. Gynecol Oncol 37:439–442, 1990

510. Piscioli F, Govoni E, Polla E et al: Primary osteosarcoma of the uterine corpus: Report of a case and critical review of the literature. Int J Gynaecol Obstet 23:377–385, 1985

511. Kofinas AD, Suarez J, Calame RJ, Chipeco Z: Chondrosarcoma of the uterus. Gynecol Oncol 19:231–237, 1984

512. Bapat K, Brustein S: Uterine sarcoma with liposarcomatous differentiation: Report of a case and review of the literature. Int J Gynaecol Obstet 28:71–75, 1989

513. Fujii S, Kanzaki H, Konishi I et al: Malignant fibrous histiocytoma of the uterus. Gynecol Oncol 26:319–330, 1987

514. Witkin GB, Askin FB, Geratz JD, Reddick RL: Angiosarcoma of the uterus: A light microscopic, immunohistochemical, and ultrastructural study. Int J Gynecol Pathol 6:176–184, 1987

515. Quinonez GE: Angiosarcoma of the uterus: A case report. Am J Obstet Gynecol 164:90–92, 1991

516. Gray GF Jr, Glick AD, Kurtin PJ, Jones HW III: Alveolar soft part sarcoma of the uterus. Hum Pathol 17:297–300, 1986

517. Ohta M, Sakakibara K, Mizuno K et al: Successful treatment of primary endodermal sinus tumor of the endometrium. Gynecol Oncol 31:357–364, 1988

518. Joseph MG, Fellows FG, Hearn SA: Primary endodermal sinus tumor of the endometrium: A clinicopathologic, immunocytochemical, and ultrastructural study. Cancer 65:297–302, 1990

519. Daya D, Lukka H, Clement PB: Primitive neuroectodermal tumors of the uterus: A report of four cases. Hum Pathol 23:1120–1129, 1992

520. Ansah-Boateng Y, Wells M, Poole DR: Coexistent immature teratoma of the uterus and endometrial adenocarcinoma complicated by gliomatosis peritonei. Gynecol Oncol 21:106–110, 1985

521. Cho KR, Rosenshein NB, Epstein JI: Malignant rhabdoid tumor of the uterus. Int J Gynecol Pathol 8:381–387, 1989

522. Bittencourt AL, Britto JF, Fonseca LE Jr: Wilms' tumor of the uterus: The first report in the literature. Cancer 47:2496–2499, 1981

523. Ferry JA, Young RH: Malignant lymphoma, pseudolymphoma, and hematopoietic disorders of the female genital tract. Pathol Annu 26(Part 1):227–263, 1991

524. Young RH, Harris NL, Scully RE: Lymphoma-like lesions of the lower female genital tract: A report of 16 cases. Int J Gynecol Pathol 4:289–299, 1985

525. Ferry JA, Harris NL, Scully RE: Uterine leiomyomas with lymphoid infiltration simulating lymphoma. Int J Gynecol Pathol 8:263–270, 1989

526. Kumar NB, Hart WR: Metastases to the uterine corpus from extragenital cancers: A clinicopathologic study of 63 cases. Cancer 50:2163–2169, 1982

527. Kumar A, Schneider V: Metastases to the uterus from extrapelvic primary tumors. Int J Gynecol Pathol 2:134–140, 1983

528. Perez CA, Camel HM, Askin F, Breaux S: Endometrial extension of carcinoma of the uterine cervix: A prognostic factor that may modify staging. Cancer 48:170–180, 1981

Pathology in Gynecology and Obstetrics, Fourth Edition, edited by Claude Gompel and Steven G. Silverberg. J. B. Lippincott Company, Philadelphia © 1994.

5 | *The Fallopian Tube*

EMBRYOLOGY

The fallopian tubes arise from the superior portions of the müllerian ducts. This differentiation takes place in the embryo at the 55-mm stage of development.[1,2] The tubes are in vertical position at first, and then accompany the ovaries in their migration, assuming a nearly horizontal position.

ANATOMY

The fallopian tube or oviduct is a musculomembranous tube situated in the superior wing of the broad ligament.[2,3] Its average length measures 10 to 12 cm, and its diameter ranges from 0.4 to 0.9 cm. The tube consists of four segments (Fig. 5-1), which are, from center to periphery:

1. The *interstitial portion,* situated within the uterine wall
2. The *isthmus, or horizontal portion*
3. The *ampulla,* which embraces the ovary in its concavity and is the site of fertilization
4. The *infundibulum* or fimbriated portion.

The ampulla presents sinuosities that are progressively effaced with age. These sinuosities may constitute an obstacle to the flow of secretions and favor the appearance of partial or complete obstructions.

The tubal wall presents longitudinal folds (mucosal rugae) whose number and dimensions increase from the internal orifice to the infundibulum. The tubal canal opens into the superoexternal angle of the uterine cavity by an orifice (ostium uterinum) of about 0.1 cm in diameter;[4] it terminates in the peritoneal cavity through an orifice (peritoneal ostium) measuring 0.2 to 0.3 cm in diameter. The wall consists of a serosa, a muscularis, and a mucosa in continuity with the uterine mucosa.

The tubal arteries arise from the arcade constituted by the internal tubal artery (a branch of the uterine artery) and the external tubal artery (a branch of the ovarian artery).[5] Spiral arterioles in the tubal mucosa react in the same fashion as those of the endometrium during the menstrual cycle.[6] The veins flow into the uterine and ovarian veins. The lymphatics, richly anastomosed with those of the adjacent organs, drain into the ovarian lymphatics and the paraortic lumbar lymph nodes. These lymphatics course along the folds of the tubal mucosa, where they form a network of intercommunicating lymphatic sinusoids. The nerves innervating the tube come from the intermesenteric and hypogastric plexus. Adrenergic fibers predominate over cholinergic fibers.[7]

HISTOLOGY

The tubal wall consists of the following layers: the serosa, subserosa, muscularis, submucosa, and mucosa.

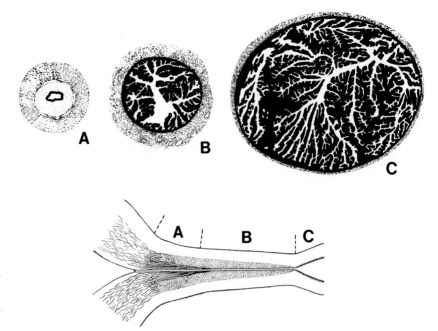

FIGURE 5-1 Normal fallopian tube. Schematic representation of longitudinal and cross sections of the wall. **(A)** Interstitial portion. **(B)** Isthmic portion. **(C)** Ampullary portion. (Adapted from Dubreuil.)

The serosa is the external layer, a peritoneal layer consisting of a mesothelial lining and well-vascularized connective tissue. Cystic or solid (Walthard's cell rests) proliferations of mesothelial cells are often present (see Chap. 6). The subserosa is a loose connective tissue network.

The muscularis is formed by an external plexiform layer thickest at the isthmus; a circular layer, thin in the ampulla and thickening toward the isthmus; and an internal longitudinal layer present in the internal third of the isthmus.

The submucosa is a loose vascularized connective tissue; the mucosa is composed of a cuboidal to columnar unistratified lining. Several cell types are found in the tubal mucosa: secretory, ciliated, interstitial (intercalary or "peg"), and wandering cells (Fig. 5-2). Cyclical changes in the tubal mucosa are not as evident as those of the endometrium. They are manifested by an increase in cell size during the first half of the cycle and by the presence of cytoplasmic glycogen and lipids, especially marked around the 22nd day. Alkaline phosphatase is found in greatest concentration in the apical cytoplasm during the ovulatory phase.

The *secretory cells* are characterized by the presence of an apical border of cytoplasmic microvilli demonstrable by electron microscopy (Fig. 5-3). They have more basophilic cytoplasm than the ciliated cells and possess elongated nuclei with dense chromatin. These elements undergo cyclical modifications.[8-10] They are nearly cuboidal during the early estrogenic phase, become elongated at the time of ovulation, and retain a columnar form until the menstrual phase, at which time they again diminish in height. During the luteal phase, the apical pole herniates into the tubal lumen, and the nucleus comes level with the cell surface, occasionally giving the impression of having been expelled from the epithelium. The increased volume of the cell at this time is responsible for this appearance. These cells possess secretory activity, which is confirmed by the presence of lipids and glycogen in the cytoplasm. Under the electron microscope during the secretory phase, secretory droplets are seen to swell up between the microvilli, which decrease in number and height; the endoplasmic reticulum expands and lysosomes appear during the late portion of this period.

Estradiol and progesterone receptor concentrations can be shown to vary in tubal mucosa during the menstrual cycle.[11] During pregnancy, the secretory cells become filled with glycogen, but the level of lipids is unchanged. They are low and regularly disposed. Increased ergastoplasm, swollen mitochondria, and the presence of secretory granules are seen with the electron microscope. Some tubal mucosae show a true decidual transformation during pregnancy (Fig. 5-4). No specific changes are seen during the postpartum period. *Atrophy* of the tubal mucosa after the menopause takes place slowly, and the functional appearance persists for many years after the cessation of ovarian activity.[12]

The *ciliated cells* are columnar elements of 30 to 35 μm, with clear cytoplasm and a round or oval nucleus situated in the basal part of the cytoplasm. They contrast sharply, by virtue of their pale appearance, with the surrounding secretory cells. The chromatin is gathered in easily visible clumps, and the nucleolus is large. The ciliated cells are often found in groups. They decrease in frequency from the fimbriated end of the tube to its interstitial portion.[3,12,13] They attain their maximal size at the time of ovulation, and thereafter decrease in height until the early estrogenic

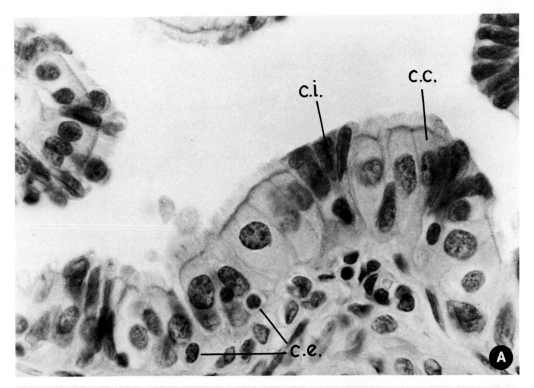

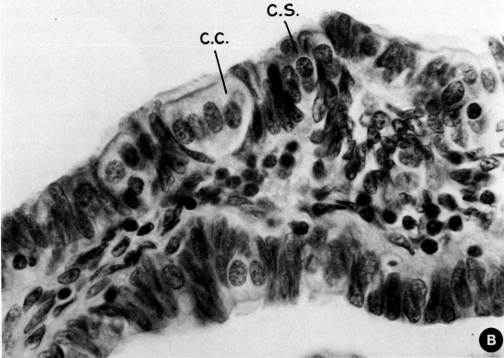

FIGURE 5-2 Fallopian tube: normal histologic appearance showing ciliated cells (*c.c.*), secretory cells (*c.s.*), intercalated cells (*c.i.*), and wandering cells (*c.e.*).

phase. The apical pole is covered with cilia of about 8 μm in length, which reveal the typical structure: nine double filaments disposed around two central filaments, with axes on a parabasal apparatus (see Fig. 5-3). This pattern may be altered in Kartagener's syndrome[14] or after use of an intrauterine contraceptive device (IUD).[15] Cell size increases during the estrogenic phase. Except for these changes, the ciliated cells show no major cyclical variation, although some authors state that about 10% of these cells lose and regenerate their cilia in each menstrual cycle.[10]

The *intercalated cells* or *peg cells,* long and

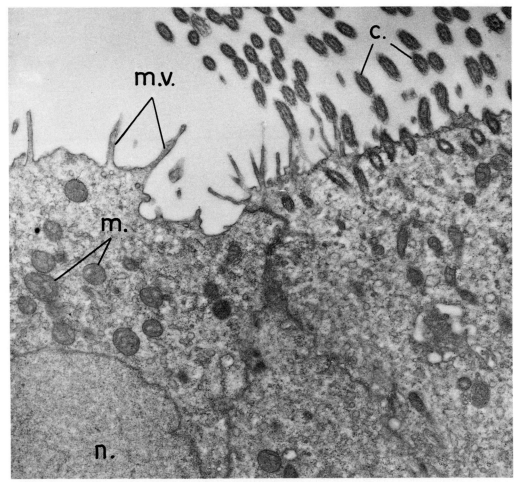

FIGURE 5-3 Electron micrograph of tubal epithelial surface showing microvilli (*m.v.*) and cilia (*c*) in secretory and ciliated cell, respectively. *m.*, mitochondria, *n.*, nucleus.

straight elements, appear crushed between the neighboring elements (see Fig. 5-2). The nucleus, thin and drawn out, is surrounded by a thin, dense, deeply staining rim of cytoplasm. The apical border is composed of cytoplasmic microvilli. This appearance recalls that of an altered secretory cell. Similar elements are encountered in the endometrium during the secretory phase.

The *wandering cells* or *dark cells* described by Andrews are small round cells with a central nucleus and clear cytoplasm situated in the deep part of the epithelium (see Fig. 5-2).[16] They have been shown to be lymphocytes that migrate among the epithelial cells from the subjacent stroma (mucosa-associated lymphoid tissue, or MALT).[17]

MALFORMATIONS

Aplasia of the tube is encountered in unicornuate uterus. Bilateral aplasia is rare. Diverse degrees of *hypoplasia* may be seen, but marked hypoplasia is rare. *Atresia* is generally combined with atresia of a uterine cornu but may be segmental and isolated.[18,19]

The presence of two tubes on one side may be noted, and the existence of multiple external orifices and of diverticula.

Changes have been reported in the tubes of women who had been exposed in utero to diethylstilbestrol (DES). These consist of foreshortened, convoluted tubes with "withered" fimbriae and a pinpoint os, and they seem to be associated with increased frequencies of infertility and ectopic pregnancy.[20] Their prevalence in the DES-exposed population remains unknown.

Although not strictly a malformation, tubal *heterotopia* can follow various forms of pelvic surgery.[21] The most common situation is that of a tube prolapsed into the vaginal vault after vaginal hysterectomy.[22] In this setting, recognition of tubal mucosa and wall (including smooth muscle) avoids confusion with other types of vaginal cysts and tumors (see Chap. 2).

TORSION

Torsion of the fallopian tube usually presents as a painful surgical emergency during the period of ac-

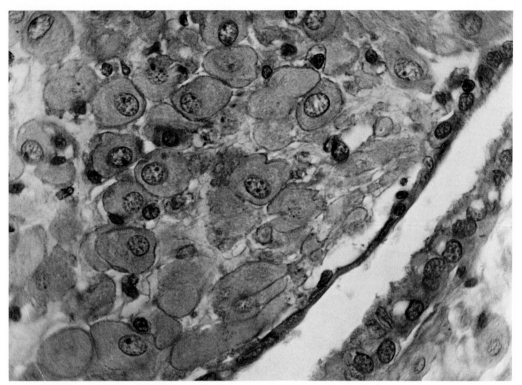

FIGURE 5-4 Tubal mucosa: decidual transformation of stroma.

tive genital life. It is almost always unilateral, but bilateral cases have been reported. Youssef and colleagues divide the etiologic factors into intrinsic and extrinsic conditions.[23] Factors intrinsic to the tube include congenital anomalies, acquired structural defects (hydrosalpinx, tumors, previous surgery), and abnormal peristalsis due to autonomic dysfunction. The extrinsic causes comprise changes in adjacent organs (adhesions, tumors, pregnancy), mechanical factors (trauma, sudden movements), and pelvic congestion. Torsion of an apparently previously normal tube is not rare and has been described on occasion in children and in pregnant women.[24] Isolated torsion of the fimbriated end of the tube is much rarer.[25]

Macroscopic Appearance. The twisted tube may be normal or swollen, and it often contains serous or frankly bloody fluid. Depending on the amount of torsion, which may vary from one half to several twists, severe gangrene may be present. The ovary is involved in the process in about 50% of cases.

Microscopic Appearance. The microscopic appearance is often primarily that of the underlying disease (hydrosalpinx, tumor, or other). The wall of the tube usually shows inflammation, congestion, and edema, and may be completely gangrenous. The prognosis is grave unless surgical measures are instituted rapidly.

INFLAMMATORY DISEASES

Inflammatory disease of the tube, or *salpingitis,* constitutes an important chapter in gynecologic pathology. Although antibiotics have considerably modified the clinical and pathologic aspects of this condition, salpingitis nevertheless remains a severe and relatively common process. It remains responsible for a significant percentage of cases of secondary sterility by occlusion or stenosis. Its frequency varies with the social milieu, and improved hygiene diminishes its incidence.

The most frequently encountered causative organisms in classic studies have been staphylococci, streptococci, *Escherichia coli,* pneumococci, *Proteus, Mycobacterium tuberculosis,* and gonococci. Streptococci and staphylococci that are resistant to antibiotics are common. Gonococcal infection does not account for more than 10% of all cases, although formerly it was far more common. Tubal syphilis has become a great rarity in Europe and North America. A few cases caused by *Enterobius vermicularis* and other parasites have been reported.[26,27]

Recent reports have suggested a possible significance for such organisms as *Chlamydia trachomatis, Mycoplasma hominis, Ureaplasma urealyticum,* and *Bacteroides* and other aerobic species.[28–32] Better documented is the relation between pelvic inflammatory disease (PID), often unilateral, and the IUD. Although certain forms of IUD are frequently associated with minor tubal mucosal structural changes[33] and sterile salpingitis,[34,35] more important statistics are that one third[36] to one half[37] of PID patients in some series have been IUD wearers and that in as many as 87% of patients with PID, *Actinomyces* organisms could be incriminated.[38,39] The presence of the typical "sulfur granules" of *Actinomyces* (see Figs. 5-17 and 4-57) in the vaginal smear of an IUD wearer should raise concern, particularly if signs or symptoms of PID develop. The Dalkon shield IUD has figured most prominently in reports of PID in IUD wearers, and Gram-negative and anaerobic bacteria also have been identified in this situation.[37]

Lukasik compared the flora of the tube and of the cervix in cases of salpingitis and found that these were usually identical when the salpingitis was chronic but that in acute cases they bore no relation to one another.[40] Because the cervix can be easily cultured, this procedure often gives valuable information in cases of chronic salpingitis. More recently, Kiviat and colleagues demonstrated that an endometrial biopsy showing the simultaneous presence of five or more neutrophils per 400× field in surface endometrial epithelium and one or more plasma cell per 120× field in endometrial stroma was highly predictive of the presence of acute salpingitis.[41]

Salpingitis is usually a postpartal or postabortal complication or a tubal extension of a cervicouterine or peritoneal infection. Ascending infections (often chlamydial, less frequently gonococcal) lead to mucosal involvement (*endosalpingitis*) in the earliest stage, whereas postpartal and postabortal infections (usually staphylococcal, streptococcal, and anaerobic) classically spread by means of uterine lymphatics and blood vessels to produce a *perisalpingitis,* with a relative sparing of the tubal lumina.

More rarely, salpingitis may be a complication of a generalized infectious process: typhoid fever, variola, acute colitis with sepsis, or a distant abscess (eg, mastoid, tonsil). The lesions are often bilateral and extend to adjacent organs, principally to the ovaries, pelvic peritoneum, and other pelvic organs. Antibiotic therapy has diminished the frequency and the severity of these extensions. Acute salpingitis may rarely be a complication of tubal ligation.[42]

Acute Salpingitis

The acute pyogenic salpingitides are manifested clinically by fever, pains in the pelvis and iliac fossae, nausea and vomiting, menstrual abnormalities, and pelvic peritonitis. When the infection is not treated correctly, it may pass into a chronic phase, with all the complications discussed below.

Macroscopic Appearance. The tube is enlarged, congested, dark red, and flabby in consistency (Fig.

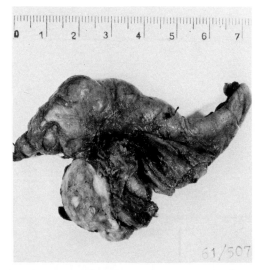

FIGURE 5-5 Acute salpingitis: macroscopic appearance.

5-5). The peritoneum is opacified, and there are loose fibrinous adhesions between the tube and neighboring structures. Section reveals a thick edematous wall with congested mucosal plicae. The lumen contains serous or frankly purulent fluid. The plicae of the infundibulum are thick, turgid, and engorged with blood. The increase in tubal size due to thickening of the wall is much more marked in other pyogenic salpingitides than in gonococcal infection. The increased volume causes accentuation of the tubal angles and favors a superimposed acute obstruction or stenosis.

If obstruction occurs, hydrosalpinx or pyosalpinx ensues, depending on the quality of the exudate. The wall is thick and fibrous, or it may be thin. A possible complication is rupture of the tube.

Microscopic Appearance. When inflammation is discrete, the microscopic lesions may be localized to the mucosa and manifested by stromal edema and infiltration by polymorphonuclear leukocytes and a few plasma cells and lymphocytes. At this stage, the epithelium is not involved. Such infiltration accompanied by vascular congestion may be seen in the normal menstrual cycle during the menstrual phase, and in this circumstance should not be considered to represent an infection. In more severe cases of salpingitis, the epithelium is altered, showing cellular atypia (anisocytosis, anisonucleosis, cytoplasmic vacuolization) and polymorphonuclear leukocytic infiltration (Fig. 5-6). The mucosal rugae are thickened, fill the tubal lumen, and adhere one to another. The surface epithelium may desquamate or become necrotic, leaving a naked submucosa, and microabscesses appear. The vessels are congested, and interstitial hemorrhages take place. Finally, the inflammatory process overflows the mucosa and invades the muscularis, the fibers of which are separated by the leukocytic infiltrates.

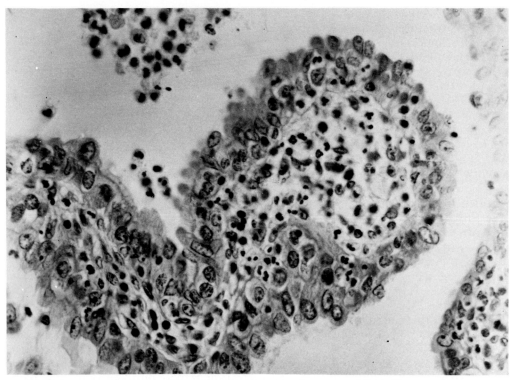

FIGURE 5-6 Acute salpingitis: microscopic appearance, showing neutrophilic infiltrate and mucosal atypia.

When phenomena of necrosis are marked, an abscess is formed that may overflow the tubal wall and invade the ovary (*tubo-ovarian abscess*).[43] The inflammation eventually regresses after one or several acute episodes and is replaced by fibrotic lesions that determine the final anatomic and functional state of the tube. The etiologic microbial agent may be demonstrated by direct microscopic examination or by culture of the secretions or of a tissue fragment.

Several authors have developed clinical staging systems for acute salpingitis.[44,45] These systems may be based on routine clinical examination alone or may be combined with laparoscopic inspection, and they seem to correlate with the eventual clinical outcome. The diagnostic criteria and therapeutic goals in Monif's staging system are summarized in Table 5-1.

Chronic Salpingitis

Salpingitis may be chronic at its onset or it may be a sequel of acute salpingitis. Clinically, it is manifested by pains and menstrual, urinary, and gastrointestinal disturbances. Clinical examination reveals the presence of a tender mass in the vaginal cul-de-sac.

Macroscopic Appearance. Chronic inflammatory lesions of the tube present in two principal forms: hypertrophic or atrophic. In the *hypertrophic form*, the tube is increased in volume and shows accentuated

angles connected by fibrous adhesions (Fig. 5-7). The peritoneal serosa is opacified and gray-yellow, deep red, or brown. There are adhesions to adjacent structures, particularly the ovary, which often participates in the chronic tubal inflammatory processes. Section shows fibrotic thickening of the submucosa and muscularis. The mucosal rugae lose their normal structure and are replaced by thickened mucosal folds that adhere to one another, sometimes forming partitioned cavities of variable size (*follicular salpingitis*). The epithelium is focally ulcerated and necrotic.

TABLE 5-1.
Clinical Staging of Acute Bacterial Salpingitis

Stage	Diagnostic Criteria	Therapeutic Goal
I	Acute endometritis/ salpingitis without peritonitis	Eradication of symptoms and infectivity
II	Salpingitis with peritonitis	Preservation of tubal structure and function
III	Salpingitis with superimposed tubal occlusion or tubo-ovarian complex	Preservation of ovarian function
IV	Ruptured tubo-ovarian abscess	Preservation of life

Monif GRG: Clinical staging of acute bacterial salpingitis and its therapeutic ramifications. Am J Obstet Gynecol 143:489–495, 1982

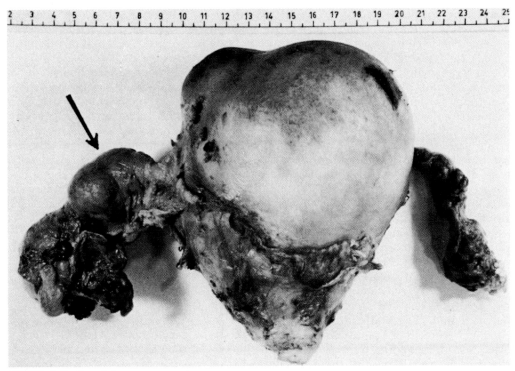

FIGURE 5-7 Pyosalpinx: macroscopic appearance.

In the *atrophic form,* the tube is reduced to a thin, firm cord. Section shows a fibrotic wall with marked diminution of the mucosal rugae.

When the infundibulum and the uterine orifice are obliterated by rugal adhesions, edema, or deformity, a cystic pocket is formed, the contents of which may be purulent (pyosalpinx), serous (hydrosalpinx), or, more rarely, hemorrhagic (hematosalpinx). Chronic *pyosalpinx* shows a thick fibrotic wall, with the internal mucosal surface gray and granular or smooth and shiny. The mucosal folds are atrophic or have disappeared completely. *Hydrosalpinx* forms most frequently by resorption of purulent contents, leaving residual serous or seromucous fluid. This fluid may continue to accumulate as a mucosal secretion or (more important) as a transudate from injured blood vessels.[46,47] The cystic pocket may attain great volume and adhere to adjacent organs. The wall is thin, smooth, and translucent. Section reveals a unilocular or multilocular cavity lined by a flat epithelium and a thin fibrotic muscularis. The multilocular appearance is explained by rugal adhesions with persistent small cavities between them; these cavities later become dilated and filled with fluid. Winston has commented on estrogen and progestin receptor deficiency in the tubal mucosa in hydrosalpinx.[48]

Pyosalpinx and hydrosalpinx may be complicated by hemorrhages that appear in the edematous and congested stroma of the mucosal rugae; this complication is known as *hematosalpinx* (Fig. 5-8). This stroma forms fleshy buds in the zones of epithelial erosion. Hematosalpinx may be confused with an ectopic tubal pregnancy; the absence of fetoplacental debris orients the differential diagnosis toward the inflammatory etiology.

Boer-Meisel and colleagues have suggested that the likelihood of subsequent conception in patients treated for hydrosalpinx could be predicated by a macroscopic analysis of the nature and extent of adhesions, the appearance of the endosalpinx, the thickness of the tubal wall, and the maximal tubal diameter.[49] They were able to combine these observations into scores that resulted in three groups with 77%, 21%, and 3% probabilities of subsequent uterine pregnancy.

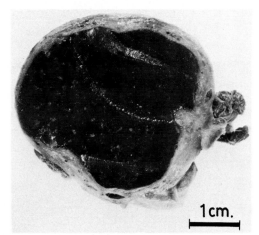

FIGURE 5-8 Hematosalpinx: macroscopic appearance.

Microscopic Appearance. The *hypertrophic form* shows multiplication and enlargement of the mucosal rugae, which become adherent and constitute cystic cavities of variable sizes (Fig. 5-9).The mucosal stroma is edematous, congested, and infiltrated by lymphocytes and plasma cells (Figs. 5-10 and 5-11). There may be small granulomata or microabscesses that destroy the mucosa. The epithelium is atrophic and flattened, and ciliated cells have become rare. In certain cases, mucosal hyperplasia is so pronounced that it is confused with adenocarcinoma. The absence of malignant cytologic abnormalities and the presence of pronounced chronic inflammation permit the recognition of this process as hypertrophic salpingitis. The submucosa and muscularis show lymphoplasmacytic infiltrates and fibrosis. The rugal adhesions with partial or complete tubal obstruction do not prevent the transit of spermatozoa, but they cause abnormal implantations of the egg in the tube.

The *atrophic form* shows effacement of the mucosal folds and marked atrophy of all the layers of the tubal wall. The epithelium is cuboidal or flattened; ciliated cells are as rare as in the hypertrophic form. The inflammatory infiltrates are of the lymphoplasmacytic type. Transit of the egg is disturbed by the slowing of the serous current normally present in the tube.

The microscopic appearance of chronic *pyosalpinx* reveals the tubal wall infiltrated by plasma cells, lymphocytes, neutrophils, and histiocytes. Adhesions between mucosal folds cause the appearance of cystic cavities lined by columnar epithelium or epithelium flattened by the inflammatory process.

The serosa frequently shows fibrous adhesions. The cavity contains a purulent exudate. It is not rare to see foci of acute inflammation complicating a chronic pyosalpinx.

Hydrosalpinx is lined by an atrophic flat epithelium, in which a few mucosal rugae may persist (Fig. 5-12). In the multilocular form, the cystic spaces are lined by an atrophic epithelium overlying a greatly thinned and fibrotic wall. Microscopic evidence of inflammation may be absent but usually is present.

Hematosalpinx reveals stromal hemorrhagic foci and hemorrhages in the mucosal rugae, with rupture of the epithelium and hemorrhagic inundation of the tubal lumen. The mucosa becomes atrophic under the pressure of the hemorrhagic exudate, and it is limited to a single layer of flattened cells. In an ancient hematosalpinx, the wall is reduced to a dense fibrotic layer.

Salpingitis Isthmica Nodosa

Salpingitis isthmica nodosa is a common, usually asymptomatic, lesion. It was described for the first time by Chiari in 1887.[50] It is characterized by muscular hyperplasia with invasion of the muscularis by glandular islands that have usually lost contact with the overlying mucosa. The pathogenesis is still disputed. According to some authors, it is basically a dystrophic lesion of the glandular mucosa accompanied by hyperplasia of smooth muscle fibers (tubal adenomyosis). Because contact with the mucosa can sometimes be demonstrated (Fig. 5-13), other authors prefer the term *diverticulosis*. According to oth-

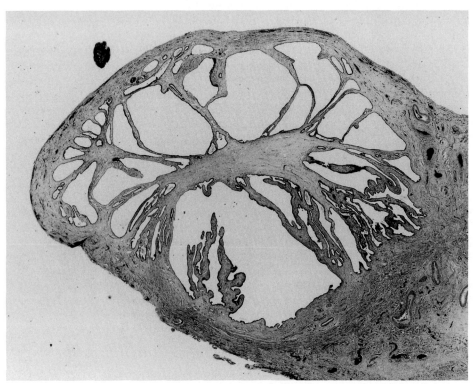

FIGURE 5-9 Follicular salpingitis. Mucosal rugae are adherent and form a network of cystic cavities.

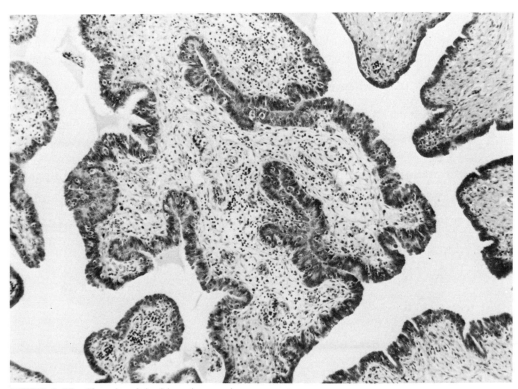

FIGURE 5-10   Chronic salpingitis: microscopic appearance.

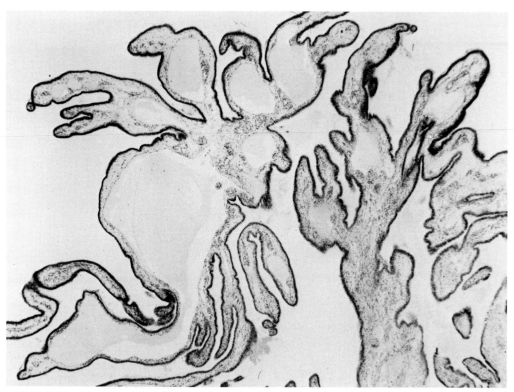

FIGURE 5-11   Chronic salpingitis: marked edema of rugae.

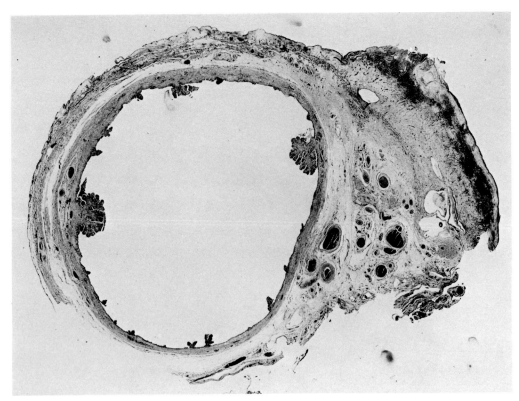

FIGURE 5-12 Hydrosalpinx: microscopic appearance.

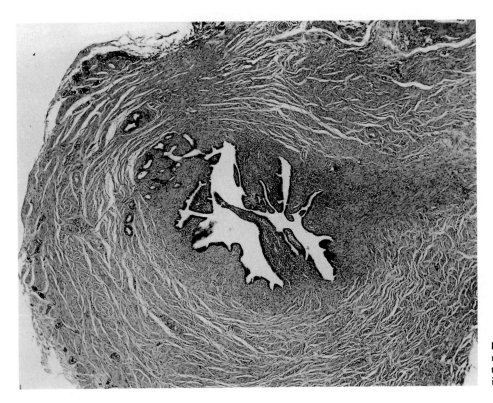

FIGURE 5-13 Salpingitis isthmica nodosa. Early lesion with diverticula extending from the mucosa into the tubal muscular wall.

ers, it is a sequel of chronic salpingitis.[51] It is sometimes considered to be a congenital malformation, although its absence before the menarche militates against this theory. Cioltei and associates have commented on hyperandrogenism in nearly half of their cases of "nodular salpingitis," but the significance of this observation is blunted by their apparent inclusion of salpingitis isthmica nodosa and follicular hydrosalpinx in this grouping.[52]

Macroscopic Appearance. The tubes, principally the isthmic regions, reveal thickened walls in which are noted one or several firm yellow or brown nodules of 1 to 2 cm in diameter.

Microscopic Appearance. In the hypertrophic muscularis, glandular formations not in continuity with the surface epithelium are found, lined by tubal-type epithelium (Fig. 5-14). The smooth muscle fibers surrounding the glands are hyperplastic and hypertrophic. A few discrete lymphoplasmacytic infiltrates are often seen. This lesion should not be confused with true tubal adenomyosis, which consists of invasion of the tubal wall by foci of adenomyosis (endometrial glands and stroma) arising in the uterine cornua.[53]

Tuberculous Salpingitis

About 10% of cases of chronic salpingitis are of tuberculous origin. Its clinical and social importance is great, because about 25% of cases of primary sterility were formerly due to genital tuberculosis. It has recently become a much less common disease, especially in Western countries.[32] Adnexal tuberculosis arises most frequently during adolescence and is accompanied by other manifestations of tuberculosis, notably pleural, peritoneal, pulmonary, nodal, and osseous manifestations. Genital tuberculosis may remain latent for long periods or may manifest itself by discrete clinical signs. Endometrial biopsy undertaken to investigate a case of sterility sometimes uncovers a previously unsuspected gynecologic tuberculous infection.[54]

Tubal contamination takes place by the hematogenous route from the primary pulmonary focus, by lymphatic dissemination after peritoneal or mesenteric lymph nodal involvement, or more rarely by the ascending route from a vaginal infection.

Macroscopic Appearance. The macroscopic appearance of tuberculous salpingitis includes several forms. The least specific form is similar in appearance to any other chronic salpingitis. The *ulcerocaseous* form shows a pale yellow, granular, caseous mass involving a large segment of the tube. The *chronic* form is grossly identical to salpingitis isthmica nodosa. The *miliary* form is characterized by multiple tiny granulomata disseminated on the tubal sur-

face and in the wall. The tube is congested, edematous, and fixed to neighboring organs by numerous adhesions. This miliary form is commonly accompanied by abundant ascitic fluid. These tuberculous granulomata must not be confused with small epithelial inclusion cysts, Walthard's cell rests, or foci of endosalpingiosis. An important characteristic of tuberculous salpingitis is that the infundibulum remains patent, with its fimbriae everted, in about 50% of cases, whereas in gonococcal salpingitis it is almost always obstructed.

Microscopic Appearance. When a caseating granuloma is found, the diagnosis poses no problem: abundant giant cells are seen in the granulomata (Fig. 5-15). In other cases, granulomatous lesions are rare, and serial sections of one or more biopsies are necessary to demonstrate them. The presence of a hyperplastic and adenomatous mucosa, even in the absence of granulomata, should cause suspicion of a tuberculous origin. This hyperplasia should not be confused with adenocarcinoma of the tube, although the latter may coexist with tuberculous salpingitis.

Granulomatous Salpingitis

There are other granulomatous salpingitides besides that of tuberculosis. Their symptomatology is the same as for chronic salpingitis; there may be signs of lesions in other sites. The most frequent complications of these tubal lesions are tubal pregnancy and secondary sterility.

Foreign-Body Granuloma. The causal foreign body often is contrast medium (Lipiodol) introduced during hysterosalpingography (Fig. 5-16). Other foreign bodies are materials deposited during a surgical procedure (eg, talc), silk sutures used for tubal ligation, and lipid or keratin debris from a dermoid cyst. Granulomata rich in epithelioid cells and multinucleated giant cells are found around the foreign material.

Mycotic Inflammatory Granuloma (Actinomycosis). The markedly increased frequency of actinomycotic infection of the tubes in recent years, its often unilateral localization, and its usual relation to the intrauterine device have been commented on earlier.[30] The inflammatory response in these cases is often purulent and granulomatous, although one or the other condition may predominate. Careful search (multiple sections of multiple blocks) may be necessary to demonstrate the typical "sulfur granules" of Gram-positive organisms (Fig. 5-17).

Sarcoidosis
Macroscopic Appearance. The macroscopic appearance, consisting of disseminated miliary nodules, causes the observer to think of tuberculosis.

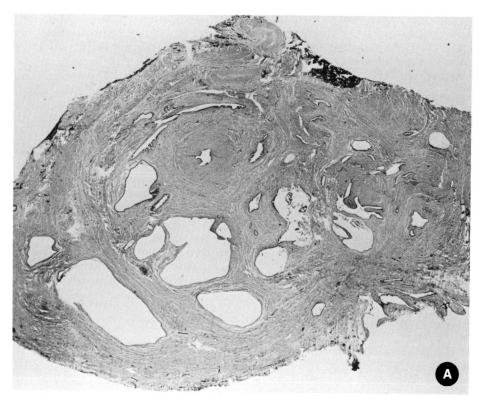

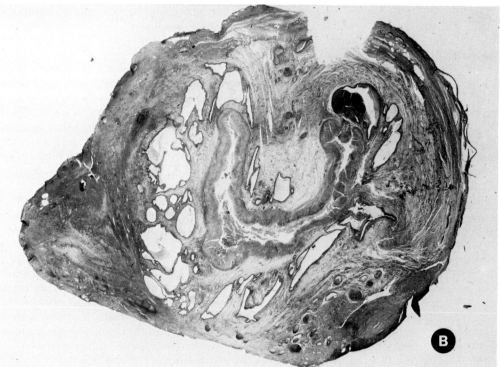

FIGURE 5-14 (A,B) Two cases of salpingitis isthmica nodosa. Both are more advanced than the case shown in Fig. 5-13. (**A** courtesy of Dr. Henry J. Norris and the Armed Forces Institute of Pathology, Washington, DC)

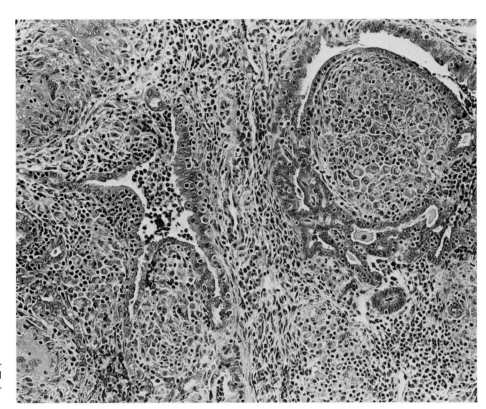

FIGURE 5-15 Tuberculous salpingitis: epithelioid and giant cell granulomata with reactive mucosal hyperplasia.

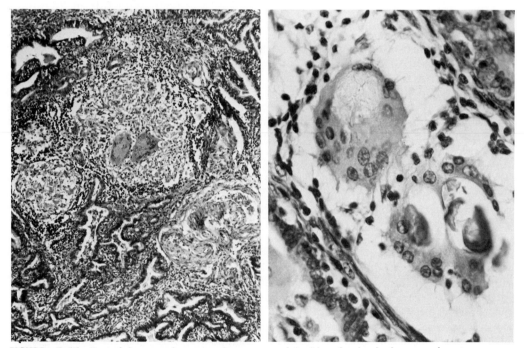

FIGURE 5-16 Postsalpingography granulomatous salpingitis: foreign-body granulomata (Lipiodol).

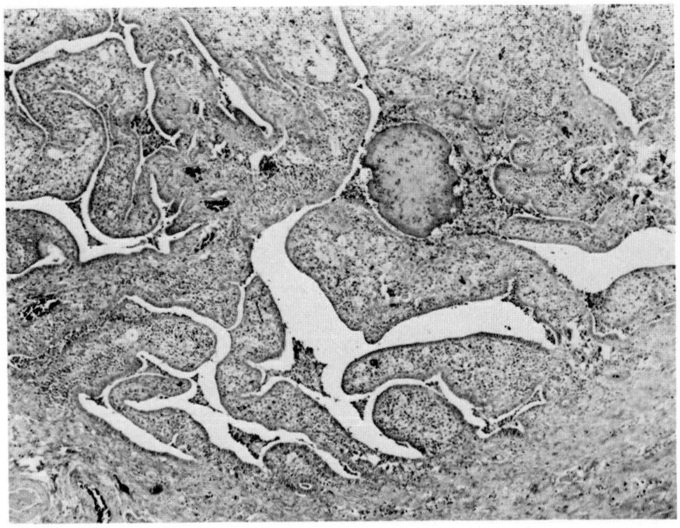

FIGURE 5-17 Actinomycotic salpingitis in an IUD wearer: mixed inflammatory infiltrate, reactive mucosal hyperplasia, and a single "sulfur granule."

Microscopic Appearance. The microscopic picture is that of a giant cell granulomatous process similar to tuberculosis, but without caseation and without tubercle bacilli.

Other Granulomatous Salpingitides. Other conditions associated with granulomatous salpingitis include *parasitic disease* (schistosomiasis, oxyuriasis) and *Crohn's disease* (regional enterocolitis).

Xanthogranulomatous Salpingitis

Xanthogranulomatous salpingitis is a rare lesion that is easily confused with tuberculous salpingitis. It is characterized by the presence of deposits of lipid in the mucosa and submucosa.[55]

Macroscopic Appearance. The macroscopic appearance is that of a chronic salpingitis with pyosalpinx. The mucosa presents a unique appearance of multiple small yellow-white nodules disseminated on the surface (Fig. 5-18A), resembling the surface of a strawberry. This same gross appearance is seen in the gallbladder in cholesterosis (so-called strawberry gallbladder).

Microscopic Appearance. Microscopic examination reveals that these nodules are thickened mucosal rugae filled with numerous lipid-laden macrophages in the stroma (see Fig. 5-18B). This accumulation of macrophages represents a sequel of tissue degeneration or necrosis. In the gallbladder, it is usually explained as a local disturbance in cholesterol metabolism (defect in mucosal resorption or elimination). The reason for this accumulation of lipids in the fallopian tube is not clear. The lesion needs to be differentiated from the collections of histiocytes seen in malacoplakia,[56] in association with endometriosis,[57] and after radiation therapy.[58] The histiocytes contain calcium and iron in the first of the conditions and lipofuscin in the other two.

ENDOMETRIOSIS

Tubal endometriosis develops in the muscularis or beneath the serosa. It is most common in the intramural portion of the tube, but it is occasionally found in the isthmic portion. It may project in polypoid fashion into the tubal lumen and may be associated with infertility.[59] Endometriosis is said to be seen frequently in the proximal tubal segment after partial salpingectomy for sterilization.[60] For a discussion of the pathogenesis of endometriosis, see Chapter 7.[61]

Macroscopic Appearance. Endometriosis presents as small dark blue or black nodules, from a few millimeters to 1 or 2 cm in diameter. These nodules may compress the mucosa and narrow the tubal lumen.

Microscopic Appearance. Microscopically, endometrial glands are surrounded by more or less abundant endometrial stroma, which may undergo decidual transformation during pregnancy or treatment with progestational agents (Fig. 5-19). Endometriosis must not be confused with a well-differentiated adenocarcinoma or an adenofibroma or adenosarcoma.

TUBAL SURGERY IN FERTILITY CONTROL AND STERILITY

The surgical pathologist sees many more normal than abnormal fallopian tubes because of the popularity of tubal surgery as a means of fertility control. Classic abdominal tubal ligation (often at delivery, postpartum, or postabortal) has been supplanted in some institutions by vaginal tubal ligation, laparoscopic tubal electrocoagulation, culdoscopic tubal clipping, or hysteroscopic tubal plugging. Because failure rates of close to 1% have been reported with most of these procedures,[62] the pathologist should be sure that the specimen received represents a complete transection of each tube. Occasionally, multiple sections are necessary to demonstrate the mucosa and lumen. The incidence of histologic salpingitis in puerperal tubal ligation specimens has been quoted as ranging from 7% to 38%, and positive tubal cultures have been obtained in from 0% to 50% of these cases; however, most authors agree that these "infections" are of no clinical significance.[63,64] Stromal decidual change is seen in 3% or more of puerperal tubes and is clinically unimportant.[65]

The reasons for the occasional failure of tubal sterilization procedures are still debated. The type of procedure must play a role, because about half of the pregnancies after failed laparoscopic tubal coagu-

lation are ectopic, whereas almost 90% after failure of other tubal sterilization procedures are intrauterine.[62] Some authors have championed the role of "endosalpingiosis" or "endosalpingoblastosis" (probably in reality salpingitis isthmica nodosa) as evidence of the ability of tubal mucosa to invade and recolonize the poststerilization tubal defect,[62] whereas others have downplayed the significance or even existence of this lesion.[60] Endometriosis and tuboperitoneal fistula are said by others to be common poststerilization tubal lesions. Their clinical significance may be minimal, however, because Rock and coworkers noted no difference in pregnancy rates after tubal reanastomosis in women whose tubes did or did not show these or other less common lesions.[60,66]

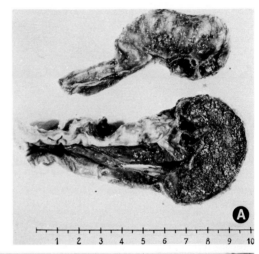

FIGURE 5-18 Xanthogranulomatous salpingitis. **(A)** Macroscopic appearance. **(B)** Microscopic appearance.

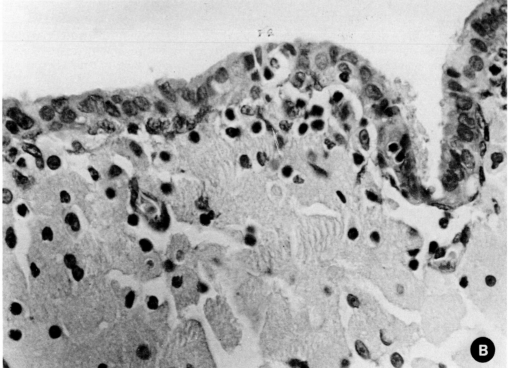

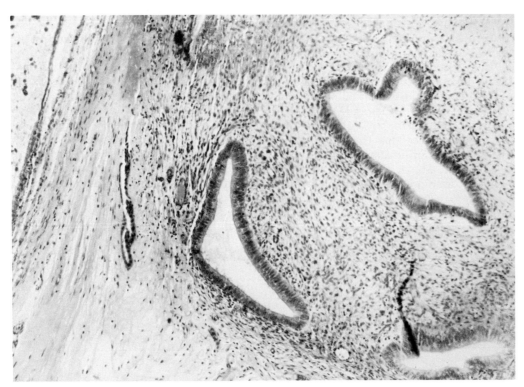

FIGURE 5-19 Tubal endometriosis.

Vasquez and associates have commented on deciliation, polyposis, and loss of mucosal folds as seen by scanning electron microscopy in the tubal isthmus after sterilization.[67] They believe that these lesions increase in severity with time and militate against successful operative reversal of sterilization. Inadequate initial procedures may be blamed for some poststerilization pregnancies, as may spontaneous reanastomosis without initiating pathology, although the latter would seem to be rare.

The pathologist who receives for examination a tube that was ligated at mid-tube years earlier generally encounters some degree of hydrosalpinx in the proximal (uterine) segment and an unremarkable distal (ovarian) segment, each of which ends blindly at a gap measuring 0.5 cm to several centimeters.[68] Mucosal endometriosis may be present at the proximal stump and is thought to result from menstrual reflux followed by implantation in damaged tissues.[60] Polyps projecting into the lumen and a picture resembling salpingitis isthmica nodosa in the wall may be present.[69]

The opposite aspect of tubal surgery consists of operations performed in infertile women in whom tubal pathology is suspected as the cause of the inability to conceive or for reversal of previous tubal sterilization procedures. Microsurgery has been used in these situations since 1959 and is considered by many authors to be the technique of choice.[70-72]

As many as 30% to 40% of cases of female infertility are related to tubal factors.[73] In infertility surgery for tubal disease, one of the most common lesions encountered is a blocked cornu, usually due to postpartal or postabortal inflammation, but also often associated with salpingitis isthmica nodosa, tuberculous salpingitis, tubo-ovarian abscess, polyps, casts of amorphous debris, adenomyosis, or leiomyomata.[48,72-75] After microsurgical treatment of a blocked cornu, 25% to 50% of patients are able to give birth.[72,76] De Brux has determined that the prognosis varies inversely with the severity of disease, and others have confirmed this observation.[72,77,78]

Some idea of the pathology of a blocked tube may be obtained preoperatively or intraoperatively by salpingoscopy.[79] Severe disease is generally evaluated correctly by this method, but histologically proved moderate epithelial or stromal pathology is frequently missed. Ultrastructural examination is even more sensitive for the demonstration of mucosal abnormalities, revealing degenerative changes in ciliated and secretory cells.[79,80]

The other major indication for tubal surgery in infertility occurs when the infertility is iatrogenic, subsequent to one of the tubal sterilization procedures discussed previously.[66,67,76,81] Results in different series are still variable, but Winston reports a 70% to 80% success rate.[76] Vasquez and associates state that results are poorer when the interval after sterilization surgery exceeds 5 years.[67] Siegler, on the other hand, reports that the success rate is independent of this interval, but is poorest with ampullary-isthmic anastomoses and tubes less than 4 cm in length.[81] The tubal specimens from these procedures frequently show pathologic changes, although the prognostic significance of these changes may be minimal (see above). Rock and colleagues report that after unipolar cautery 40% of tubes show endometriosis, 21% show fistulas, and smaller proportions show chronic salpingitis, inclusion cysts, adhesions, or proximal hydrosalpinx.[66] An interesting approach to infertility surgery is the so-called paradoxical oophorectomy, or removal of the normal ovary on the same side as a unilateral diseased tube.[81,82] The rationale here has been described as "putting all the eggs in one (healthy) basket."

BENIGN TUMORS

Leiomyoma

Leiomyoma is also called *fibromyoma or fibroid.* The leiomyoma is a rare tumor in the fallopian tube. It may be solitary or multiple and usually measures from a few millimeters to several centimeters in diameter, although large, clinically significant tumors do occur. It presents macroscopically as a spherical mass protruding under the peritoneal serosa. Microscopically, it appears identical to the uterine leiomyoma: whorled smooth muscle fibers separated by narrow connective tissue bundles.[83,84]

Adenomatoid Tumor

The adenomatoid tumor or mesothelioma is a small, well-demarcated, benign tumor situated in the tubal muscularis or subserosa. It is composed of pseudoglandular formations surrounded by a fibromuscular stroma.[85] Different theories have claimed that the lining cells of these pseudoglandular structures are mesothelial, endothelial, vascular, or epithelial, but ultrastructural and immunohistochemical evidence has established the mesothelial (peritoneal) origin.[86,87] These tumors are rare and are asymptomatic, usually being discovered fortuitously during examination of a surgical or postmortem specimen. They are found during the period of genital activity and are histologically identical to similar tumors of the corpus uteri and the male epididymis.

Macroscopic Appearance. Macroscopic examination reveals a small, well-limited mass visible beneath the peritoneal serosa. Section shows firm, pink-white, homogeneous tissue. Small foci of calcification may be present.

Microscopic Appearance. The microscopic appearance consists of spaces lined by flat or cuboidal cells, surrounded by a stroma rich in collagen fibers and smooth muscle fibers. No cellular atypia or mitotic activity is noted (Fig. 5-20). The flattening of the lining cells, very marked in some cases, has wrongly suggested to some observers a lymphangiomatous origin. In other tumors, the cell nests are massive and contain small cystic spaces. In a few cases, continuity with the peritoneal surface lining has been demonstrated.

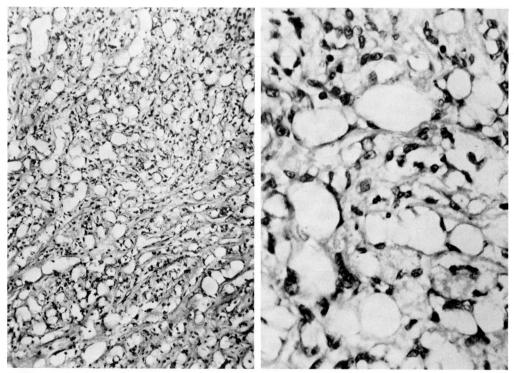

FIGURE 5-20 Adenomatoid tumor of tube. (Hinerman DL, Gould SE: What is your diagnosis? Am J Clin Pathol 37:204, 1962)

Endometrial Polyp and Adenofibroma

These lesions are benign proliferations of epithelium and stroma, which can present as intraluminal masses. The endometrial polyp is common, occurs in the intramural portion of the tube, and is histologically identical to the polyp described in Chapter 4.[59,88] The adenofibroma is rare and consists of tubal epithelium supported by fibrous stroma.[89,90] It also resembles its more common uterine counterpart.

Papillary Tumors

Benign papillomas have been reported rarely in the tube, presenting with hydrosalpinx or with sterility related to tubal occlusion.[91,92] Pathologically, they are composed of papillary processes lined by epithelium resembling normal tubal mucosa, with little stratification, few mitoses, and no atypia.

A lesion that appears to be unique to the fallopian tube and has been reported only in pregnant or postpartum women is the *metaplastic papillary tumor* (Fig. 5-21).[93,94] It was an incidental microscopic finding in all reported cases. The papillae are lined by mucin-secreting cells and cells with eosinophilic cytoplasm, which have been interpreted by some authors as oncocytes,[93] although ultrastructural study of one case[94] did not show the packed mitochondria expected in oncocytes. Mitotic figures are rare, and the tumor does not invade into the wall of the tube. Follow-up findings have been benign in the few cases reported, and it is not known whether the lesion is a hormonally-induced hyperplasia and metaplasia or a true neoplasm.

Teratoma

The fallopian tube is the second most common site (after the ovary) of female genital tract teratoma, with about 50 cases reported.[95] Six of these have been associated with an ectopic pregnancy,[95] and 3 have been malignant (immature).[96] They no doubt arise from germ cells arrested in their maturation toward the genital crest. Their pathologic features are similar to those encountered in the ovary (see Chap. 6).

Other Benign Tumors

Within the tube, rare cases of *hemangioma*,[97] *lipoma*,[98] *fibroma*,[99] *neurilemoma*,[100] and *sex cord tumor with annular tubules*[101] have been reported.

MALIGNANT TUMORS

Primary Tumors

Adenocarcinoma

Adenocarcinoma of the tube arises from the mucosal epithelium. It is an uncommon tumor, but well over 1000 cases have been reported in the literature. It represents about 0.5% of all malignant tumors of the female genital tract,[102] and its incidence in the United States is 3.6 per million women per year, with no recent change in this figure noted.[103] Like epithelial cancers of the ovary and endometrium, tubal carcinoma seems to be less common in Japan.[104] It is encountered in women between 40 and 60 years of age, although patients as young as 18 years have been observed.[105] A high incidence of chronic inflammatory lesions has been noted,[106] but a causal relation has not been established; tuberculosis of the tube is thought by some authors to be frequently associated with carcinoma, but others[107] think that other forms of salpingitis are much more commonly involved. In any event, we must remember that inflammatory lesions of the tube are frequent and that carcinoma is equally rare, and that salpingitis (particularly of tuberculous etiology) may be associated with a hyperplastic mucosal reaction that can be and has been misdiagnosed as carcinoma (see Fig. 5-15). Adenomyosis has been noted in a high percentage of cases by some authors, but again, this is a common lesion.[106]

Other lesions that appear to have a premalignant potential in other portions of the female genital tract have been demonstrated far less frequently in the tube. *Adenomatous hyperplasia* has been discussed in detail by Dougherty and Cotton but has not been shown to be significantly related to carcinoma in the fallopian tube (Fig. 5-22).[108] These authors state that this lesion is often found in conjunction with chronic salpingitis and with estrogen-producing ovarian tumors. Dallenbach-Hellweg found it most commonly associated with endometrial hyperplasia and carcinoma,[109] Stern and coworkers noted it in association with epithelial ovarian tumors and in women receiving exogenous estrogens,[110] and Robey and Silva have commented on a particular association with serous borderline tumors of the ovary.[111] Our experience is similar, but Moore and Enterline doubt the clinical significance of the lesion and believe that careful searching will prove its common occurrence in tubes removed from women with no other disease.[112] In the earliest form, the only abnormalities seen are increased height of the tubal epithelial cells, with crowding and epithelial tufting into the lumen. This is followed by the creation of small glandular spaces within the epithelium. In the most advanced instances, there are numerous small and medium-sized glands crowded together in a greatly thickened epithelium. The cells show hyperchromatism, pseu-

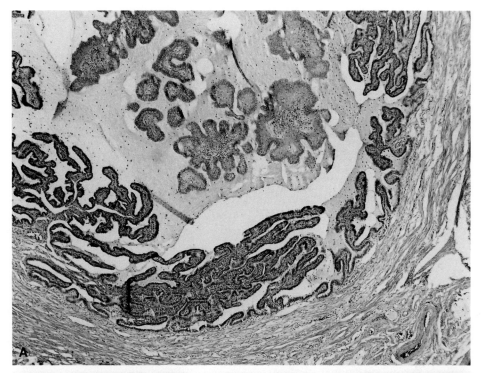

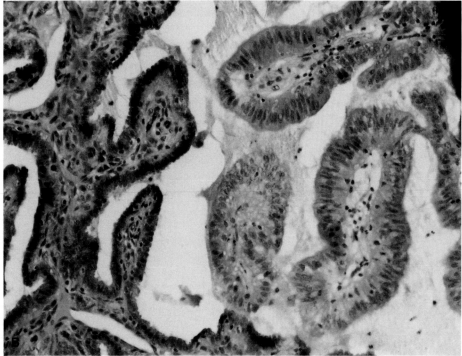

FIGURE 5-21 Metaplastic papillary tumor. **(A)** Low-power view. **(B)** Detail. Compare the normal tubal epithelium (*left*) with the tall columnar cells containing cytoplasm that was eosinophilic in sections stained with hematoxylin-eosin (*right*). Courtesy of Dr. Mirka Jones, Armed Forces Institute of Pathology, Washington, DC)

dostratification, and true stratification; but in contradistinction to carcinoma few mitoses are seen and large abnormal nucleoli are not present. The presence of any mitoses is important, because they are not seen in normal tubal mucosa.

Adenocarcinoma in situ is difficult to differentiate from adenomatous hyperplasia and probably is a more advanced stage of the latter lesion (Fig. 5-23).[110] Bannatyne and Russell stress as important features of in situ carcinoma its focal rather than widespread distribution, frequent and sometimes abnormal mitotic figures, loss of multiple cell types, and marked nu-

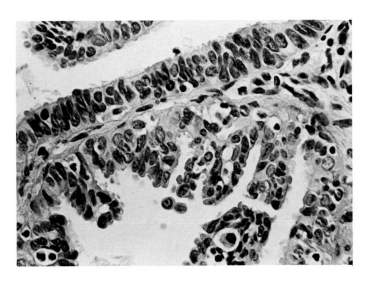

FIGURE 5-22 Adenomatous hyperplasia of tube in a case of ovarian carcinoma. Compare the hyperplastic epithelium (*below*) with the normal tubal mucosa (*above*).

clear pleomorphism with multiple large nucleoli.[113] Because in situ carcinoma is diagnosed after resection, progression to invasive carcinoma can rarely, if ever, be demonstrated. The in situ tubal lesion is usually associated with ovarian or endometrial carcinoma, particularly serous carcinoma of the ovary.[113] *Borderline mucinous and serous tumors* might be considered in situ carcinomas of the tube; two such mucinous lesions, both associated with pseudomyxoma peritonei, have been reported,[114,115] and we have seen a third case that coexisted with an ovarian borderline mucinous tumor (Fig. 5-24).

We must wonder why tubal cancer is so rare, considering that it arises in müllerian-derived epithe-

lium such as that of cervical and endometrial carcinomas, both of which are common lesions, and histologically usually resembles serous carcinoma of the ovary, also a common tumor.[116] This question is one that we are unable to answer at the present time.

Clinical Signs. Clinical signs of invasive carcinoma are not characteristic. They include pain, the presence of an adnexal mass, and serous, purulent, or bloody vaginal discharge. Any of these findings may be absent; the complete triad is seen only rarely. Vaginal discharge is present in about half of the

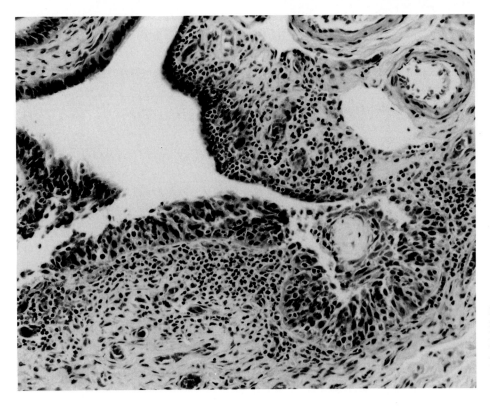

FIGURE 5-23 In situ adenocarcinoma of fallopian tube. Although lymphoid inflammation is present, the mucosal atypia is out of proportion to the infiltrate, and invasive carcinoma was situated nearby.

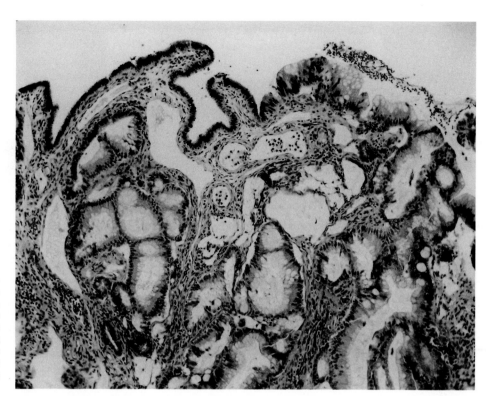

FIGURE 5-24 Borderline mucinous tumor (tumor of low malignant potential) of tubal mucosa. This tumor was an incidental microscopic finding in a patient who also had a borderline mucinous (intestinal-type) tumor of the ipsilateral ovary. Origin of this lesion in the tubal mucosa is seen at top right.

cases. More rarely, intestinal obstruction represents the first sign of the tumor. The diagnosis is made in less than 5% of cases before exploratory laparotomy.[102,107] Clues to the correct diagnosis are furnished by the clinical signs, hysterosalpingography, and vaginal exfoliative cytology. It has been stated that vaginal cytology reveals malignant cells in 60% of cases,[107] but other authors find that this procedure is much more often unrewarding.[105] Endometrial aspiration is probably a more effective cytologic procedure.[117] Carcinomatous cells have been recognized in cul-de-sac washes at the time of vaginal hysterectomy for other indications.[118] Occasionally, the exfoliated malignant cells may be recognized as being of tubal origin, but this is unusual. The cytologic appearance is usually similar to that of serous carcinoma of the endometrium or ovary. Hysterosalpingography is probably the best technique available for making the diagnosis before laparotomy, and ultrasonography is useful.[118]

Even after surgery, definitive diagnosis may be difficult, because tubal origin is difficult to prove in the presence of involvement of the ovary or endometrium, or both. In these situations, the tumor in the tube should look tubal histologically, show a transition from benign epithelium, and perhaps even represent the most bulky tumor mass before a tubal primary is diagnosed with confidence.[119]

Macroscopic Appearance. The tumor may be small or may attain a diameter of several centimeters. In a great number of cases, it is localized to the ampullary portion of the tube and forms an elongated bulge suggestive of chronic salpingitis. When the serosa is not involved, it is smooth and stretched; often fibrous adhesions are present. The tumor involves the right and left tubes with about equal frequency and is bilateral in about 20% of all cases. Coexistent chronic salpingitis is frequently present. On opening the tube, a soft, sometimes encephaloid, tumor mass is seen. It is red or gray and often necrotic, and close inspection often reveals papillary formations (Fig. 5-25). In more advanced cases, the tumor invades completely through the tubal wall and forms papillary nodules on the peritoneal serosal surface; this is usually a late occurrence. The tube frequently becomes obstructed, with the development of a pyosalpinx or hematosalpinx. Isthmic localizations are less frequent, but they show a much more malignant and rapid evolution.

Microscopic Appearance. The most common histologic type is serous papillary adenocarcinoma resembling that more commonly seen in the ovary (Figs. 5-26 and 5-27).[116] In the well-differentiated (grade I) pattern, columnar cells line the connective tissue axes of the papillae and recall the cytologic structure of normal tubal epithelium. Marked cellular atypia is uncommon, but mitoses are frequently seen. Nucleoli are prominent and often multiple.

In the less differentiated tumors, bizarre cellular atypias are numerous and marked; the cells are found in dense nests and sheets, without any morphologic similarity to tubal mucosa. It is not rare to

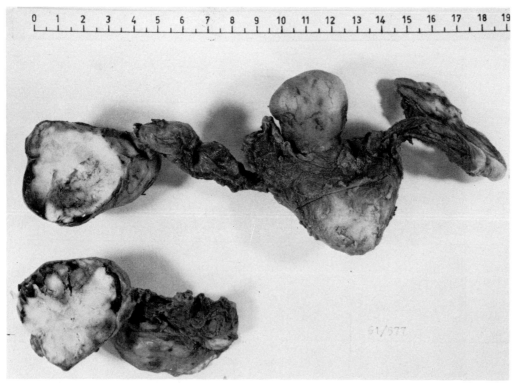

FIGURE 5-25 Well-differentiated adenocarcinoma of tube: macroscopic appearance.

see cystic structures and intracystic papillary formations. Mitoses are numerous.

As elsewhere in the female genital system, other types of carcinoma may be encountered. After serous carcinoma, the most frequent type is *endome-trioid carcinoma*, but only a handful of such cases have been documented.[120,121] A type that may pose a particularly difficult differential diagnostic problem resembles the adnexal tumor of probable wolffian origin (juxta-ovarian tumor).[122] Scattered cases of

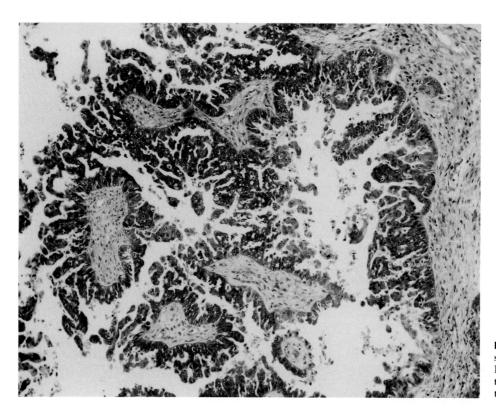

FIGURE 5-26 Well-differentiated serous carcinoma of fallopian tube. Broad papillae are lined by relatively uniform cells with stratification, tufting, and cell exfoliation.

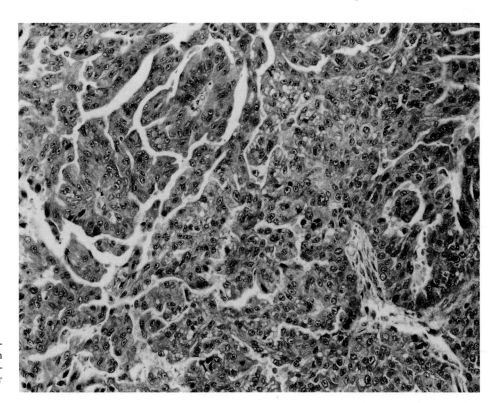

FIGURE 5-27 Poorly differentiated serous carcinoma of fallopian tube. Poorly formed papillae coexist with solid sheets of tumor cells.

clear cell adenocarcinoma,[123] *transitional cell carcinoma,*[124] *glassy cell carcinoma,*[125] and *squamous cell carcinoma*[126] have been reported, as has *mucinous carcinoma of low malignant potential.*[114,115] Endometrial and cervical carcinomas, including *in situ squamous carcinoma of the cervix,* can involve the tubal mucosa by direct extension, but should not be considered primary tubal carcinomas. Primary tubal carcinoma can coexist with primary carcinomas elsewhere in the genital tract, as in the case reported of synchronous papillary mucinous adenocarcinomas of the endocervix and both fallopian tubes.[127]

Prognosis, Evolution, and Treatment. The prognosis of tubal carcinoma is poor, the most favorable results showing only about 40% to 50% 5-year survival.[102,104,128–130] The tumor spreads directly through the fimbriated end of the tube or by penetration through the wall. Lymphatic invasion takes place early and involves the iliac, aortic, and lumbar nodes, the ovaries, the pelvic and abdominal peritoneum, the uterus, the intestine, and the urinary bladder.[127,131,132] Vaginal, ureteral, renal, hepatic, adrenal, pulmonary, splenic, and cutaneous metastases are frequently seen. Survival is better correlated with the gross extent of the tumor at the time of treatment than with histologic differentiation. Most authors[102,128] have advocated the same clinicopathologic staging system as in ovarian cancer, but we prefer a modification of the Dukes system for rectal cancer (Table 5-2).[133] The treatment is primarily surgical; radiation therapy has been used in conjunction

with surgery but has not been demonstrated to improve the therapeutic results. Cisplatin-based combination chemotherapy is promising in localized and advanced-stage cases.[134,135]

Primary Sarcomas

Primary sarcomas of the tube are rare, with only a few dozen cases having been reported. They are predominantly fibrosarcomas and leiomyosarcomas, with even rarer malignant fibrous histiocytomas reported.[136] The clinical evolution is almost always fatal.

TABLE 5-2.
Pathologic Staging of Carcinoma of the Fallopian Tube*

Stage 0	Carcinoma in situ (limited to the tubal mucosa)
Stage 1	Tumor extending into the submucosa and/or muscularis but not penetrating to the serosal surface of the fallopian tube
Stage 2	Tumor extending to the serosa of the fallopian tube
Stage 3	Direct extension of the tumor to the ovary and/or endometrium
Stage 4	Extension of tumor beyond the reproductive organs (eg, other pelvic organs, pelvic soft tissues, peritoneal implants, abdominal viscera)

*The staging of tumor in stages 0, 1, and 2 is not altered by bilateral tubal cancer per se, but the most extensive focus of disease in either tube determines the stage.

Adapted from Schiller HM, Silverberg SG: Staging and prognosis in primary carcinoma of the fallopian tube. Cancer 28:389–395, 1971

Carcinosarcoma

About 40 cases of carcinosarcoma (homologous and heterologous) arising in the fallopian tube have been reported.[137-139] This corresponds to 4% of all such tumors of the female genital tract, the more common localizations being corporeal, ovarian, vaginal, and cervical (in descending order of frequency). These tumors occur predominantly in postmenopausal women, are histologically similar to endometrial carcinosarcomas (see Chap. 4), and share the poor prognosis of uterine carcinosarcoma. A single reported tubal case was bilateral.[139] Anecdotal responses to radiation therapy and chemotherapy have been reported, but the primary treatment is surgical.

Choriocarcinoma

Primary choriocarcinoma of the fallopian tube is a rare lesion; a comprehensive review in 1981 accepted only 76 reported cases.[140] The tubal tumors are gestational in origin and must be differentiated from extensions from the more common intrauterine gestational choriocarcinomas and from choriocarcinomatous components of malignant ovarian germ cell tumors. Symptoms mimic those of a tubal ectopic pregnancy or an ovarian tumor, and the tumor may coexist with an ectopic pregnancy.[141] The gross and microscopic appearance, metastatic pathways, and responsiveness to chemotherapy are similar to those of intrauterine gestational choriocarcinoma.

Metastatic Tumors

Metastatic tumors of the fallopian tube are more frequent than primary tumors and most often represent extensions from ovarian, endometrial, or cervical adenocarcinomas. In one large series, 36% of ovarian and 11% of endometrial carcinomas were associated with tubal "metastases," although many of these may have represented multicentric primary cancers (Fig. 5-28).[142] Bannatyne and Russell have clearly shown in patients with ovarian carcinoma that small foci of primary carcinoma can arise in the tubal mucosa and even in the tubal serosa.[113] The same dilemma applies to bilateral tubal carcinomas.

Extragenital primary cancers with tubal metastases are much rarer and usually are mammary or gastrointestinal. The submucosal lymphatics are invaded by neoplastic cell nests that compress the mucosal plicae and replace the tubal epithelial cells (Fig. 5-29). Neoplastic cells desquamate secondarily into the tubal lumen and are subsequently carried to the peritoneal cavity, the surface of the ovary, and the uterine cavity. Direct implantation of tumor cells in the tubal mucosa or serosa is encountered, but lymphatic spread remains considerably more common. The tumor cells are disposed in cords or irregular masses, and they present the usual criteria of malignancy: nuclear hyperchromatism, anisonucleosis, and pathologic mitoses.

In situ squamous carcinoma of the endometrium and endosalpinx has been reported as an extension of invasive squamous carcinoma of the cervix.[143]

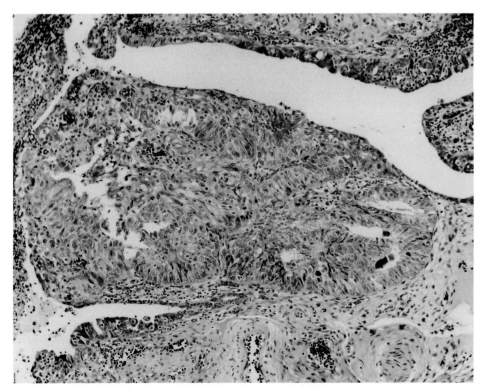

FIGURE 5-28 Endometrioid carcinoma of the fallopian tube in a patient with carcinosarcoma of the endometrium. It is uncertain whether this is a metastasis (the tumor grows predominantly beneath the mucosal surface) or an incidental separate primary tumor (note the mucosal atypical hyperplasia [*top*].)

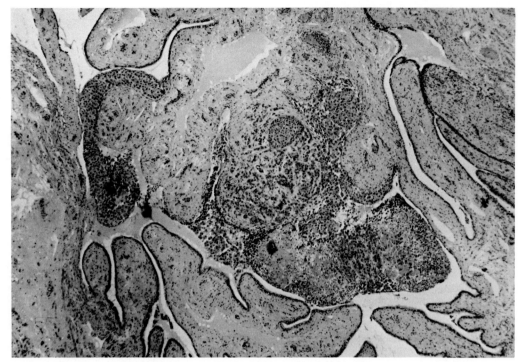

FIGURE 5-29 Tubal metastasis from adenocarcinoma of the breast. There is submucosal and lymphatic invasion and partial replacement of mucosa (*left*) by tumor cells.

References

1. Gondos B: Development of the reproductive organs. Ann Clin Lab Sci 15:363–373, 1985
2. McLean JM: Embryology and anatomy of the female genital tract and ovaries. In Fox H, ed. Haines and Taylor: Obstetrical and gynaecological pathology, 3rd ed, pp 1–50. London, Churchill Livingstone, 1987
3. Eddy CA, Pauerstein CJ: Anatomy and physiology of the fallopian tube. Clin Obstet Gynecol 26:1177–1193, 1980
4. Merchant RN, Prabhu SR, Chougale A: Uterotubal junction: Morphology and clinical aspects. Int J Fertil 28:199–205, 1983
5. Wydrzynski M: Anatomical principles of microsurgery of the tubal arteries. Anat Clin 7:233–236, 1985
6. Koritke JG, Gilley JY, Leissner P: La microvascularisation de la muqueuse tubaire et ses variations au cours du cycle ovarien chez la femme. Z Zellforsch 88:48–56, 1968
7. Helm G: Adrenergic and peptidergic neuromuscular mechanisms in the human fallopian tube, with special regard to cyclic influences. Acta Obstet Gynecol Scand (Suppl) 104:1–23, 1981
8. Donnez J, Casanas-Roux F, Caprasse J et al: Cyclic changes in ciliation, cell height, and mitotic activity in human tubal epithelium during reproductive life. Fertil Steril 43:554–559, 1985
9. Jansen RP: Endocrine response in the fallopian tube. Endocr Rev 5:525–551, 1984
10. Verhage HG, Bareither ML, Jaffe RC, Akbar M: Cyclic changes in ciliation, secretion and cell height of the oviductal epithelium in women. Am J Anat 156:505–521, 1979
11. Pollow K, Inthraphuvasak J, Grill HJ, Manz B: Estradiol and progesterone binding components in the cytosol of normal human fallopian tubes. J Steroid Biochem 16:429–435, 1982
12. Patek E, Nilsson L, Johannisson E: Scanning electron microscopic study of the human fallopian tube: I. The proliferative and secretory stages. II. Fetal life, reproductive life, and postmenopause. Fertil Steril 23:459–465, 719–733, 1972
13. Kugler P: Zur histochemie der flimmerzellen der menschlichen endosalpinx. Histochemistry 73:137–150, 1981
14. Lurie M, Tur-Kaspa I, Weill S et al: Ciliary ultrastructure of respiratory and fallopian tube epithelium in a sterile woman with Kartagener's syndrome: A quantitative estimation. Chest 95:578–581, 1989
15. Wollen AL, Flood PR, Sandvei R: Altered ciliary substructure in the endosalpinx in women using an IUCD. Acta Obstet Gynecol Scand 69:307–312, 1990
16. Andrews MC: Epithelial changes in the puerperal fallopian tubes. Am J Obstet Gynecol 62:28–37, 1951
17. Morris H, Emms M, Visser T, Timme A: Lymphoid tissue of the normal fallopian tube: A form of mucosal-associated lymphoid tissue (MALT)? Int J Gynecol Pathol 5:11–22, 1986
18. Richardson DA, Evans MI, Talerman A, Maroulis GB: Segmental absence of the mid-portion of the fallopian tube. Fertil Steril 37:577–579, 1982
19. Carosso C, Rickenbacher J: [A peculiar abnormality of the fallopian tube: induced by embryonic kidney tumor?] Schweiz Med Wochenschr 119:1548–1554, 1989
20. DeCherney AH, Cholst I, Naftolin F: Structure and function of the fallopian tubes following exposure to diethylstilbestrol (DES) during gestation. Fertil Steril 36:741–745, 1981
21. Rosenow PJ, Esterly JR: Heterotopic fallopian tube. Am J Obstet Gynecol 127:442–443, 1977
22. Silverberg SG, Frable WJ: Tubal prolapse into vaginal vault after hysterectomy. Arch Pathol 97:100–103, 1974
23. Youssef AF, Fayad MM, Shafeek MA: Torsion of the fallopian tube: A clinico-pathological study. Acta Obstet Gynecol Scand 41:292–309, 1962
24. Chambers JT, Thiagarajah S, Kitchin JD III: Torsion of the normal fallopian tube in pregnancy. Obstet Gynecol 54:487–489, 1979
25. Blickstein I, Lancet M, Rozenman D, Nissim F: Isolated ne-

crosis of the tubal fimbriae in a prepubertal girl. Z Kinderchir 44:172–173, 1989

26. Abraham JL, Spore WW, Benirschke K: Cysticercosis of the fallopian tube: Histology and microanalysis. Hum Pathol 13:665–670, 1982

27. Saffos RO, Rhatigan RM: Unilateral salpingitis due to *Enterobius vermicularis*. Am J Clin Pathol 67:296–299, 1977

28. Winkler B, Crum CP: *Chlamydia trachomatis* infection of the female genital tract: Pathogenetic and clinicopathologic correlations. Pathol Annu 22(1):193–223, 1987

29. Patton DI, Moore DE, Spadoni IR et al: A comparison of the fallopian tube's response to overt and silent salpingitis. Obstet Gynecol 73:622–630, 1989

30. Thor AD, Young RH, Clement PB: Pathology of the fallopian tube, broad ligament, peritoneum, and pelvic soft tissues. Hum Pathol 22:856–867, 1991

31. Holmes KK, Eschenbach DA, Knapp JS: Salpingitis: Overview of etiology and epidemiology. Am J Obstet Gynecol 138:893–900, 1980

32. Mårdh PA: An overview of infectious agents of salpingitis, their biology, and recent advances in methods of detection. Am J Obstet Gynecol 138:933–951, 1980

33. Sheppard BL, Bonnar J: The effect of the progesterone-releasing intrauterine device on uterine endometrium and fallopian tube epithelium. Arch Toxicol 5(Suppl):231–234, 1982

34. Beerthuizen RJ, Van Wijck JAM, Eskes TKAB et al: IUD and salpingitis: A prospective study of pathomorphological changes in the oviducts in IUD-users. Eur J Obstet Gynecol Reprod Biol 13:31–41, 1982

35. Vanlancker M, Dierick AM, Thiery M, Claeys G: Histologic and microbiologic findings in the fallopian tubes of IUD users. Adv Contracept 3:147–157, 1987

36. Scott WC: Pelvic abscess in association with intrauterine contraceptive device. Am J Obstet Gynecol 131:149–156, 1978

37. Golde SH, Israel R, Ledger WJ: Unilateral tuboovarian abscess: A distinct entity. Am J Obstet Gynecol 127:807–810, 1977

38. Burkman R, Schlesselman S, McCaffrey L et al: The relationship of genital tract actinomycetes and the development of pelvic inflammatory disease. Am J Obstet Gynecol 143:585–589, 1982

39. Hsu CT, Roan CH, Rai SY et al: Actinomycosis affecting the fallopian tube and ovary: Report of 3 cases, with special reference to 2 cases following IUD application. Asia Oceania J Obstet Gynaecol 14:275–284, 1988

40. Lukasik J: A comparative evaluation of the bacteriological flora of the uterine cervix and fallopian tubes in cases of salpingitis. Am J Obstet Gynecol 87:1028–1036, 1963

41. Kiviat NB, Wølner-Hanssen P, Eschenbach DA et al: Endometrial histopathology in patients with culture-proved upper genital tract infection and laparoscopically diagnosed acute salpingitis. Am J Surg Pathol 14:167–175, 1990

42. Phillips AJ, d'Ablaing G III: Acute salpingitis subsequent to tubal ligation. Obstet Gynecol 67:55S–58S, 1986

43. Ginsburg DS, Stern JL, Hamod KA et al: Tubo-ovarian abscess: A retrospective review. Am J Obstet Gynecol 138:1055–1058, 1980

44. Hager WD, Eschenbach DA, Spence MR, Sweet RL: Criteria for diagnosis and grading of salpingitis. Obstet Gynecol 61:113–114, 1983

45. Monif GRG: Clinical staging of acute bacterial salpingitis and its therapeutic ramifications. Am J Obstet Gynecol 143:489–495, 1982

46. David A, Garcia C-R, Czernobilsky B: Human hydrosalpinx. Histologic study and chemical composition of fluid. Am J Obstet Gynecol 105:400–411, 1969

47. Otubu JA, Winston RM, Wineman M, Ryder T: Morphology of human and experimental hydrosalpinges: A comparative study. Afr J Med Med Sci 16:79–88, 1987

48. Winston RM: Progress in tubal surgery. Clin Obstet Gynaecol 8:653–679, 1981

49. Boer-Meisel ME, te Velde ER, Habbema JD, Kardaun JW: Predicting the pregnancy outcome in patients treated for hydrosalpinx: A prospective study. Fertil Steril 45:23–29, 1986

50. Chiari H: Zur pathologischen Anatomie des Eileiter Catarrhs. Z Heilk 8:457–473, 1887

51. Punnonen R, Söderström KO: Inflammatory etiology of salpingitis isthmica nodosa: A clinical, histological and ultrastructural study. Acta Eur Fertil 17:199–203, 1986

52. Cioltei A, Tasca L, Titiriga L, Maakaron G et al: Nodular salpingitis and tubal endometriosis. I. Comparative clinical study. II. Diagnosis and differential diagnosis. Acta Eur Fertil 10:135–141, 147–160, 1979

53. Neumann HO: Salpingitis isthmica nodosa and adenomyosis. Arch Gynaekol 139:358–412, 1959

54. Nogales-Ortiz F, Tarancon I, Nogales FF Jr: The pathology of female genital tuberculosis: A 31-year study of 1436 cases. Obstet Gynecol 53:422–428, 1979

55. Franco V, Florena AM, Guarneri G, Gargano G: Xanthogranulomatous salpingitis: Case report and review of the literature. Acta Eur Fertil 21:197–199, 1990

56. Klempner LB, Giglio PG, Niebles A: Malacoplakia of the ovary. Obstet Gynecol 69:537–540, 1987

57. Clement PB, Young RH, Scully RE: Necrotic pseudoxanthomatous nodules of ovary and peritoneum in endometriosis. Am J Surg Pathol 12:390–397, 1988

58. Herrera GA, Reimann BE, Greenberg HL, Miles PA: Pigmentosis tubae, a new entity: Light and electron microscopic study. Obstet Gynecol 61:80S–83S, 1983

59. David MP, Ben-Zwi D, Langer L: Tubal intramural polyps and their relationship to infertility. Fertil Steril 35:526–531, 1981

60. Stock RJ: Postsalpingectomy endometriosis: A reassessment. Obstet Gynecol 60:560–570, 1982

61. Minh H-N, Smadja A, Orcel L: Réflexions à propos de l'histogénèse de l'endométriose tubaire. Gynecologie 42:284–288, 1991

62. McCausland A: Endosalpingosis ("endosalpingoblastosis") following laparoscopic tubal coagulation as an etiologic factor of ectopic pregnancy. Am J Obstet Gynecol 143:12–24, 1982

63. Laros RK, Zatuchni GI, Andros GJ: Puerperal tubal ligation: Morbidity, histology and bacteriology. Obstet Gynecol 41:397–403, 1973

64. Rubin A, Czernobilsky B: Tubal ligation: A bacteriologic, histologic and clinical study. Obstet Gynecol 36:199–203, 1970

65. Rewell RE: Extra-uterine decidua. J Pathol 105:219–222, 1971

66. Rock JA, Bergquist CA, Zacur HA, Parmley TH et al: Tubal anastomosis following unipolar cautery. Fertil Steril 37:613–618, 1982

67. Vasquez G, Winston RML, Boeckx W, Brosens I: Tubal lesions subsequent to sterilization and their relation to fertility after attempts at reversal. Am J Obstet Gynecol 138:86–92, 1980

68. Stock RJ: Histopathologic changes in fallopian tubes subsequent to sterilization procedures. Int J Gynecol Pathol 2:13–27, 1983

69. Donnez J, Casanas-Roux F, Férin J, Thomas K: Tubal polyps, epithelial inclusions and endometriosis after tubal sterilization. Fertil Steril 41:564–568, 1984

70. Fayez JA, Suliman SO: Infertility surgery of the oviduct: Comparison between macrosurgery and microsurgery. Fertil Steril 37:73–78, 1982

71. Tran DK, Tourame P, Oliveiro JF et al: Pathologie du segment isthmo-interstitiel de l'oviducte et microchirurgie. Gynecologie 37:192–197, 1986

72. Wiedemann R, Scheidel P, Wiesinger H, Hepp H: [Pathology of proximal tubal occlusion—morphologic evaluation. Results following microsurgical anastomosis.] Geburtshilfe Frauenheilkd 47:96–100, 1987

73. Trimbos-Kemper T, Trimbos JB, van Hall E: Etiological factors in tubal infertility. Fertil Steril 37:384–388, 1982

74. Sulak PJ, Letterie GS, Coddington CC et al: Histology of proximal tubal occlusion. Fertil Steril 48:437–440, 1987

75. Letterie GS, Sakas EL: Histology of proximal tubal obstruc-

tion in cases of unsuccessful tubal canalization. Fertil Steril 56:831–835, 1991

76. Winston RML: Microsurgery for tubal and ovarian disease. Ann Chir Gynaecol 71:97–102, 1982
77. De Brux J, Palmer R, Monteforte C, Cristofaro D: Pronostic histologique et fonctionnel des lésions tubaires dans la stérilité. Gynécol Obstét 68:11–24, 1969
78. Wu CH, Gocial B: A pelvic scoring system for infertility surgery. Int J Fertil 33:341–346, 1988
79. Hershlag A, Seifer DB, Carcangiu ML et al: Salpingoscopy: Light microscopic and electron microscopic correlations. Obstet Gynecol 77:399–405, 1991
80. Tam PP, Mao KR, Lai FM: The ultrastructural changes of the mucosa of blocked fallopian tubes. Br J Obstet Gynaecol 95:802–807, 1988
81. Siegler AM: Replacement, repair and removal of fallopian tubes. Fertil Steril 37:611–612, 1982
82. Trimbos-Kemper TCM, Trimbos JB, van Hall EV: Management of infertile patients with unilateral tubal pathology by paradoxical oophorectomy. Fertil Steril 37:623–626, 1982
83. Crissman JD, Handwerker D: Leiomyoma of uterine tube: Report of a case. Am J Obstet Gynecol 126:1046, 1976
84. Moore OA, Waxman M, Udoffia C: Leiomyoma of the fallopian tube: A cause of tubal pregnancy. Am J Obstet Gynecol 134:101–102, 1979
85. Youngs LA, Taylor HB: Adenomatoid tumors of the uterus and fallopian tube. Am J Clin Pathol 48:537–545, 1967
86. Barwick KW, Madri JA: An immunohistochemical study of adenomatoid tumors utilizing keratin and factor VIII antibodies: Evidence for a mesothelial origin. Lab Invest 47:276–280, 1982
87. Taxy JB, Battifora H, Oyasu R: Adenomatoid tumors: A light microscopic, histochemical, and ultrastructural study. Cancer 34:306–316, 1974
88. Heller DS, Rubinstein N, Dikman S et al: Adenomatous polyp of the fallopian tube: A case report. J Reprod Med 36:82–84, 1991
89. Chen KT: Bilateral papillary adenofibroma of the fallopian tube. Am J Clin Pathol 75:229–231, 1981
90. De La Fuente AA: Benign mixed Müllerian tumour-adenofibroma of the fallopian tube. Histopathology 6:661–666, 1982
91. Gisser SD: Obstructing fallopian tube papilloma. Int J Gynecol Pathol 5:179–182, 1986
92. Kaspersen P, Buhl L, Møller BR: Fallopian tube papilloma in a patient with primary sterility. Acta Obstet Gynecol Scand 67:93–94, 1988
93. Bartnik J, Powell WS, Moriber-Katz S, Amenta PS: Metaplastic papillary tumor of the fallopian tube: Case report, immunohistochemical features, and review of the literature. Arch Pathol Lab Med 113:545–547, 1989
94. Keeney GI, Thrasher TV: Metaplastic papillary tumor of the fallopian tube: A case report with ultrastructure. Int J Gynecol Pathol 7:86–92, 1988
95. Kutteh WH, Albert T: Mature cystic teratoma of the fallopian tube associated with an ectopic pregnancy. Obstet Gynecol 78:984–986, 1991
96. Baginski L, Yazigi R, Sandstad J: Immature (malignant) teratoma of the fallopian tube. Am J Obstet Gynecol 160:671–672, 1989
97. Joglekar VM: Haemangioma of the fallopian tube. Br J Obstet Gynaecol 86:823–825, 1979
98. Dede JA, Janovski NA: Lipoma of the uterine tube: A gynecologic rarity. Obstet Gynecol 22:461–467, 1963
99. Seidner HM, Thompson JR: Fibroma of the fallopian tube. Am J Obstet Gynecol 79:32–33, 1960
100. Okagaki T, Richart RM: Neurilemoma of the fallopian tube. Am J Obstet Gynecol 106:929, 1970
101. Griffith LM, Carcangiu ML: Sex cord tumor with annular tubules associated with endometriosis of the fallopian tube. Am J Clin Pathol 96:259–262, 1991
102. King A, Seraj IM, Thrasher T et al: Fallopian tube carcinoma: A clinicopathological study of 17 cases. Gynecol Oncol 33:351–355, 1989
103. Rosenblatt KA, Weiss NS, Schwartz SM: Incidence of ma-

lignant fallopian tube tumors. Gynecol Oncol 35:236–239, 1989

104. Hirai Y, Kaku S, Teshima H et al: Clinical study of primary carcinoma of the fallopian tube: Experience with 15 cases. Gynecol Oncol 34:20–26, 1989
105. Hanton EM, Malkasian GD Jr, Dahlin DC, Pratt JH: Primary carcinoma of the fallopian tube. Am J Obstet Gynecol 94:832–839, 1966
106. Anbrokh YM: Histological characteristics and questions concerning histogenesis of cancer of the fallopian tubes. Neoplasma 17:631–640, 1970
107. Jones OV: Primary carcinoma of the uterine tube. Obstet Gynecol 26:122–129, 1965
108. Dougherty CM, Cotten NM: Proliferative epithelial lesions of the uterine tube. I. Adenomatous hyperplasia. Obstet Gynecol 24:849–854, 1964
109. Dallenbach-Hellweg G, Niehoff B: Das tubenepithel in korrelation zu histologischen befunden an endometrium und ovar. Virchows Arch A Pathol Anat Histopathol 354:66–79, 1971
110. Stern J, Buscema J, Parmley T, Woodruff JD et al: Atypical epithelial proliferations in the fallopian tube. Am J Obstet Gynecol 140:309–312, 1981
111. Robey SS, Silva EG: Epithelial hyperplasia of the fallopian tube: Its association with serous borderline tumors of the ovary. Int J Gynecol Pathol 8:214–220, 1989
112. Moore SW, Enterline HH: Significance of proliferative epithelial lesions of the uterine tube. Obstet Gynecol 45:385–390, 1975
113. Bannatyne P, Russell P: Early adenocarcinoma of the fallopian tubes: A case for multifocal tumorigenesis. Diagn Gynecol Obstet 3:49–60, 1981
114. McCarthy JH, Aga R: A fallopian tube lesion of borderline malignancy associated with pseudomyxoma peritonei. Histopathology 13:223–225, 1988
115. Friedmann W, Minguillon C, Wessel J et al: [Pseudomyxoma peritonei caused by proliferating mucinous adenoma of the fimbria mucosa]. Geburtshilfe Frauenheilkd 50:579–580, 1990
116. Tokunaga T, Miyazaki K, Okamura H: Pathology of the fallopian tube. Curr Opin Obstet Gynecol 3(4):574–579, 1991
117. Hirai Y, Chen JT, Hamada T et al: Clinical and cytologic aspects of primary fallopian tube carcinoma: A report of ten cases. Acta Cytol 31:834–840, 1987
118. Kübler HC, Kühn W, Rummel HH, Schmidt W: [Diagnosis of occult fallopian tube cancers by intraoperative peritoneal cytology]. Geburtshilfe Frauenheilkd 48:116–118, 1988
119. Yoonessi M: Carcinoma of the fallopian tube. Obstet Gynecol Surv 34:257–270, 1979
120. Rorat E, Wallach RC: Endometrioid carcinoma of the fallopian tube: Pathology and clinical outcome. Int J Gynaecol Obstet 32:163–167, 1990
121. Seraj IM, Chase DR, King A: Endometrioid carcinoma of the oviduct. Gynecol Oncol 41:152–155, 1991
122. Daya D, Young RH, Scully RE: Endometrioid carcinoma of the fallopian tube resembling an adnexal tumor of probable wolffian origin: A report of six cases. Int J Gynecol Pathol 11:122–130, 1992
123. Voet RI, Lifshitz S: Primary clear cell adenocarcinoma of the fallopian tube: Light microscopic and ultrastructural findings. Int J Gynecol Pathol 1:292–298, 1982
124. Hovadhanakul P, Nuerenberger SP, Ritter PJ et al: Primary transitional cell carcinoma of the fallopian tube associated with primary carcinomas of the ovary and endometrium. Gynecol Oncol 4:138–143, 1976
125. Herbold DR, Axelrod JH, Bobowski SJ et al: Glassy cell carcinoma of the fallopian tube. Int J Gynecol Pathol 7:384–390, 1988
126. Malinak LR, Miller GV, Armstrong JT: Primary squamous cell carcinoma of the fallopian tube. Am J Obstet Gynecol 95:1167–1168, 1966
127. Jackson-York GL, Ramzy I: Synchronous papillary mucinous adenocarcinoma of the endocervix and fallopian tubes. Int J Gynecol Pathol 11:63–67, 1992
128. McMurray EH, Jacobs AJ, Perez CA et al: Carcinoma of the

fallopian tube: Management and sites of failure. Cancer 58:2070–2075, 1986

129. Muntz HG, Tarraza HM, Granai CO et al: Primary adenocarcinoma of the fallopian tube. Eur J Gynaecol Oncol 10:239–249, 1989

130. Gurney H, Murphy D, Crowther D: The management of primary fallopian tube carcinoma. Br J Obstet Gynaecol 97:822–826, 1990

131. Tamimi HK, Figge DC: Adenocarcinoma of the uterine tube: Potential for lymph node metastases. Am J Obstet Gynecol 141:132–137, 1981

132. Semrad N, Watring W, Fu YS et al: Fallopian tube adenocarcinoma: Common extraperitoneal recurrence. Gynecol Oncol 24:230–235, 1986

133. Schiller HM, Silverberg SG: Staging and prognosis in primary carcinoma of the fallopian tube. Cancer 28:389–395, 1971

134. Barakat RR, Rubin SC, Saigo PE et al: Cisplatin-based combination chemotherapy in carcinoma of the fallopian tube. Gynecol Oncol 42:156–160, 1991

135. Muntz HG, Tarraza HM, Goff BA et al: Combination chemotherapy in advanced adenocarcinoma of the fallopian tube. Gynecol Oncol 40:268–273, 1991

136. Halligan AW, McGuinness EP: Malignant fibrous histiocytoma of the fallopian tube. Br J Obstet Gynaecol 97:275–276, 1990

137. Muntz HG, Rutgers JL, Tarraza HM, Fuller AF Jr: Carcinosarcomas and mixed müllerian tumors of the fallopian tube. Gynecol Oncol 34:109–115, 1989

138. Seraj IM, King A, Chase D: Malignant mixed müllerian tumor of the oviduct. Gynecol Oncol 37:296–301, 1990

139. Van Dijk CM, Kooijman CD, van Lindert AC: Malignant mixed müllerian tumour of the fallopian tube. Histopathology 16:300–302, 1990

140. Ober WB, Maier RC: Gestational choriocarcinoma of the fallopian tube. Diagn Gynecol Obstet 3:213–231, 1981

141. Borg G, Ribon P, Hervé C: [Tubal choriocarcinoma]. Rev Fr Gynécol Obstét 82:45–59, 1987

142. Woodruff JD, Julian CG: Multiple malignancy in the upper genital canal. Am J Obstet Gynecol 103:810–822, 1969

143. Kanbour AI, Stock RJ: Squamous cell carcinoma in situ of the endometrium and fallopian tube as superficial extension of invasive cervical carcinoma. Cancer 42:570–580, 1978

Pathology in Gynecology and Obstetrics, Fourth Edition, edited by Claude Gompel and Steven G. Silverberg. J. B. Lippincott Company, Philadelphia © 1994.

6 | *The Ovary*

Charles Zaloudek

EMBRYOLOGY

The embryonic development of the ovary begins in an undifferentiated stage that is similar for the male and female genitalia. The undifferentiated gonad consists of an accumulation of mesenchymal cells covered by coelomic (germinal) epithelium. It forms an elongated bulge on the ventral surface of the mesonephros. Early in embryonic life, around the 32nd day, the primordial germ cells migrate from the yolk sac entoderm into the mesenchyme of the genital crest, passing through the root of the mesentery (Fig. 6-1). The primitive gonad begins to differentiate along ovarian lines in the seventh week. According to the most accepted embryologic theory, the migration of the primordial germ cells is accompanied by the growth of groups of cells (sex cords) from the germinal epithelium into the underlying mesenchyme (Fig. 6-2). Some of the epithelial cells invest the germ cells and differentiate into granulosa cells. The rest degenerate, except for remnants in the ovarian medulla (the rete ovarii). There may be limited downgrowth of epithelial cells from the germinal epithelium throughout embryonic life. An alternative embryologic view is that the coelomic epithelium does not contribute to the formation of the sex cords. Instead, the primordial germ cells, after migrating into the gonadal mesenchyme, play the role of organizer and induce the differentiation of the granulosa cells. This theory holds that the entire ovary, except for the germinal epithelium, is of mesenchymal origin.

Whatever their derivation, the granulosa cells become organized around the oocytes during the third trimester to form the follicles. The perifollicular stroma is derived from the gonadal mesenchyme. It is disposed around the follicles in concentric layers and constitutes the richly vascularized theca interna and the fibrous theca externa. The theca appears to represent a transformation of stromal cells that is induced by adjacent granulosa cells.

ANATOMY

The ovary has an ovoid shape and a bosselated surface. It is firm and pink or tan. During the period of gonadal activity, the ovary weighs 5 to 8 g. It increases in volume at the time of ovulation and during pregnancy. The presence of follicles of different sizes occasionally conveys a false impression that cysts are present. A diminution in size begins around age 30. The ovary atrophies after menopause and becomes small, firm, and pearly gray-white.

The ovary is situated in the retrouterine space behind and above the fallopian tube, behind the broad ligament, and in front of the rectum. It is fixed to the broad ligament at its anterior border and to the fibrous connective tissue of the mesovarium. It is attached to the uterine cornu by the utero-ovarian ligament, to the tube by the tubo-ovarian ligament, and to the lateral pelvic wall by the infundibulopelvic ligament.

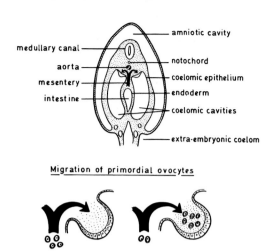

Migration of primordial ovocytes

FIGURE 6-1 Migration of primordial oocytes from the roof of the mesentery to the genital crest.

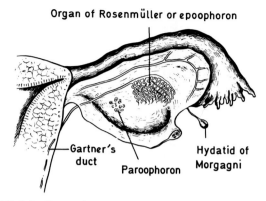

FIGURE 6-3 Parovarian organs.

The ovarian artery, a branch of the abdominal aorta, runs along the anterior border of the ovary and anastomoses with the ovarian branch of the uterine artery. About 10 arterial branches arise from this arcade and penetrate the ovary. The veins meet at the hilus, where they form a rich plexus that drains into the right and left utero-ovarian veins. The lymphatics follow the course of the veins and drain into the lumbar nodes. Nerves arise from the lumboaortic and renal plexi and enter the ovary from the ovarian plexus.

Several parovarian structures are important to the pathologist (Fig. 6-3). The *epoöphoron* is a mesonephric remnant composed of a series of parallel tubules opening into a duct that courses along the fallopian tube in the mesovarium. The epoöphoron is lined by a simple cylindrical epithelium and is surrounded by a connective tissue network containing smooth muscle fibers. The *paroöphoron,* situated in the broad ligament adjacent to the epoöphoron, is most prominent in the fetus or infant and is composed of a few tubules that are histologically similar to the epoöphoron. In contrast to the two previous structures, the *hydatid of Morgagni* is of müllerian origin. It is a small, smooth-walled cyst attached to the tubal fimbria. Its epithelium resembles that of the

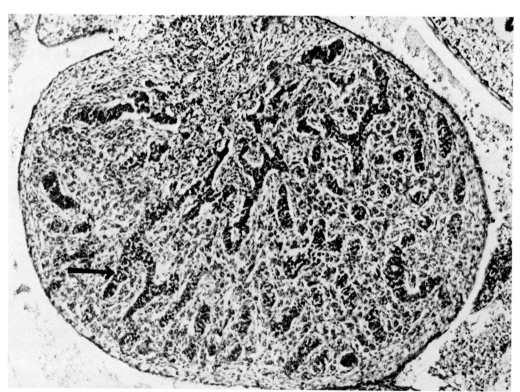

FIGURE 6-2 Fetal ovary showing sex cords.

fallopian tube and responds to hormonal stimuli in a similar manner. It may become greatly distended with clear fluid.

HISTOLOGY

The ovary consists of a stromal mass containing the follicles, vessels, and nerves. The coelomic surface epithelium is conspicuous in the infant but often is flattened and difficult to identify in the postmenopausal ovary (Fig. 6-4).

The external, or cortical, zone is composed of a stroma of fusiform connective tissue cells between which are bundles of collagen fibers. The cortex contains follicles in different stages of maturation. These follicles are numerous in infants and young adults, but their number decreases progressively with age and they disappear by menopause. The primordial follicle consists of an oocyte surrounded by a layer of cuboidal granulosa cells (Fig. 6-5). In the course of follicular maturation, the granulosa cells multiply and the granulosa cell layer becomes thickened (Fig. 6-6). It consists of round cells with regular, dark nuclei that are compressed one against the other. The oocyte becomes localized at one pole, where the granulosa proliferates to form the cumulus oophorus. When the follicle becomes mature, small spaces called *Call-Exner bodies* appear among the granulosa cells (Fig. 6-7). At the same time, a central cavity containing estrogen-rich follicular fluid develops. The stromal cells surrounding the follicle differentiate into the theca interna (Fig. 6-8). These cells sometimes assume an epithelioid appearance. They contain lipid granules when the follicle is ma-

ture, and they are surrounded by numerous capillaries that insinuate themselves between the cell cords. Mature follicles are known as *graafian follicles.*

At ovulation, the mature follicle opens at the surface of the ovary and releases its oocyte. When the oocyte leaves the follicle, the opening through which it is extruded is closed by a fibrin plug, producing the follicular stigma. The empty follicle forms a festooned vesicle, which is the beginning of the corpus luteum. After the oocyte is expelled, the granulosa becomes vascularized by capillaries from the theca interna. This vascularization may give rise to hemorrhage, which collects in the lumen of the developing corpus luteum. As the corpus luteum develops, the granulosa cells become luteinized. They have abundant pale eosinophilic cytoplasm that contains small lipid droplets (Fig. 6-9A).

Ultrastructurally, the luteinized granulosa cells have abundant smooth and rough endoplasmic reticulum arranged in whorls or in parallel arrays (Fig. 6-9B). Mitochondria are numerous and have tubular cristae. The Golgi complex is well developed and there are numerous lipid droplets. The theca cells are enlarged and luteinized, but they are smaller than luteinized granulosa cells (Fig. 6-10). The luteinized theca cells often have an epithelioid appearance and may be referred to as *theca lutein cells.*

The mature corpus luteum forms a mass of up to 1.5 cm in diameter. It appears macroscopically as a large yellow structure with a central fibrous or cystic focus (Fig. 6-11). If pregnancy does not occur, the corpus luteum involutes, with degeneration of the luteinized cells and fibrosis, ultimately resulting in a convoluted, hyalinized scar known as a *corpus albicans.*

If pregnancy occurs, a corpus luteum of preg-

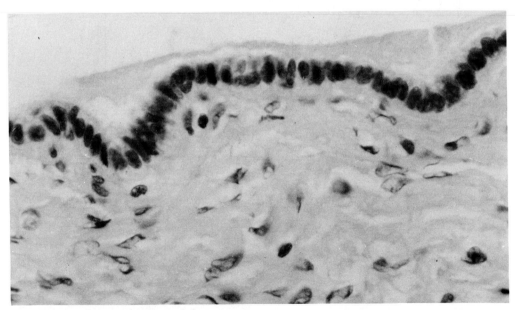

FIGURE 6-4 Surface epithelium of the ovary.

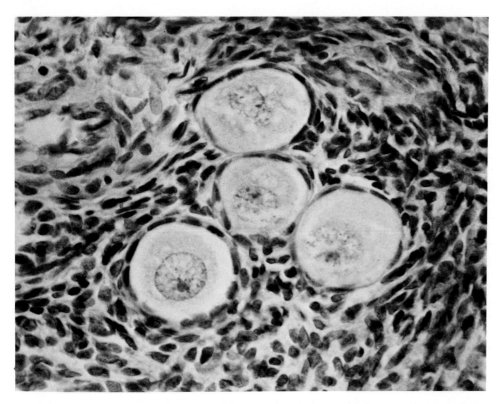

FIGURE 6-5 Primordial follicles. Oocytes are surrounded by a single layer of granulosa cells.

nancy evolves. It occupies almost half the ovary and is golden-yellow with a fibrinohemorrhagic or cystic center. The luteinized cells contain eosinophilic hyaline inclusions and lipid droplets. Regression of the corpus luteum begins after the third month of pregnancy. At the eighth month, the corpus luteum of pregnancy is only 1 or 2 cm in diameter and it subsequently undergoes total regression and fibrosis. Clusters of decidual cells are frequently present in the subcoelomic stroma in pregnant women. These

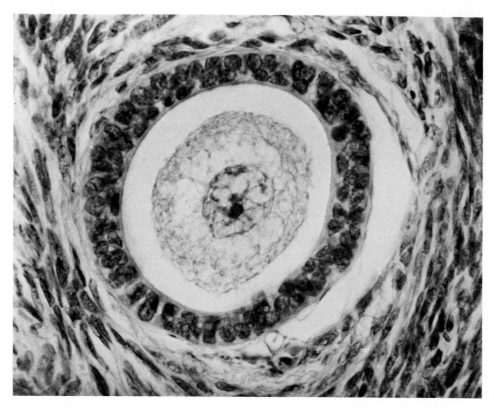

FIGURE 6-6 Oocyte surrounded by several layers of granulosa cells in primary follicle.

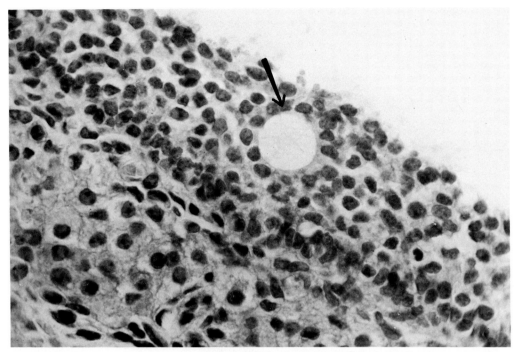

FIGURE 6-7 Graafian follicle with a Call-Exner body (*arrow*).

decidualized stromal cells have regular round nuclei and abundant eosinophilic cytoplasm.

Most of the 400,000 follicles present at birth degenerate rather than mature. Death of the ovum precedes degeneration of the follicle, which is manifested by nuclear or cytoplasmic vacuolization, condensation of the chromatin, and thickening and hyalinization of the follicular basement membrane.

The resulting structure is called an *atretic follicle*. The wall of the atretic follicle consists of granulosa cells or, when these have disappeared, of theca interna cells. As degeneration of the follicle continues, it becomes fibrotic, and the structure finally remaining is the corpus atreticum, composed of hyalinized connective tissue.

(*Text continued on page 320.*)

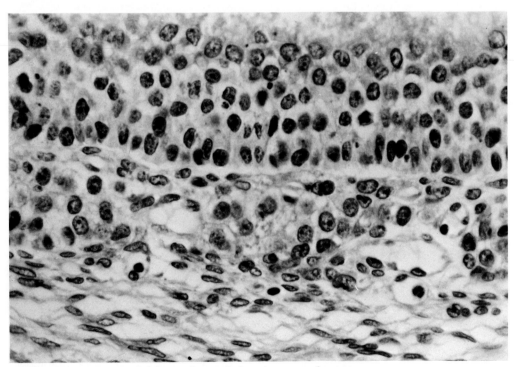

FIGURE 6-8 Graafian follicle: granulosa and theca interna and externa.

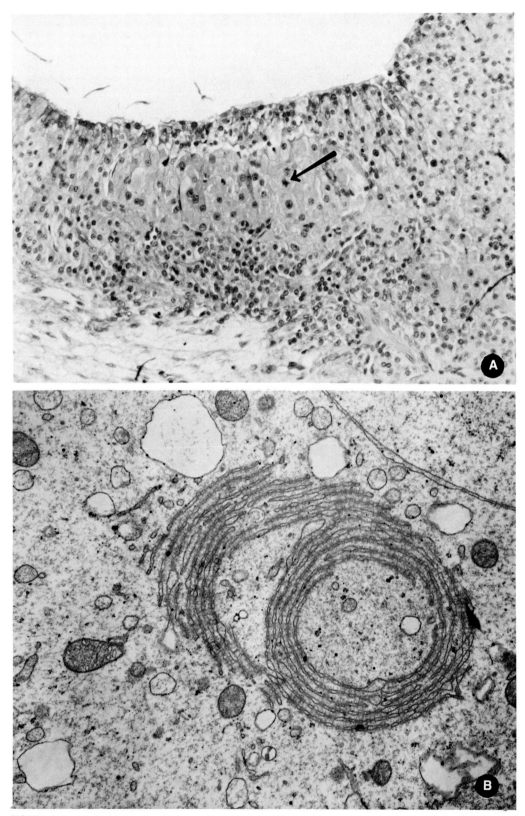

FIGURE 6-9 **(A)** Luteinized granulosa cells (*arrow*). **(B)** Whorled arrangement of annulate lamellae in luteinized granulosa cells (**B**×17,500).

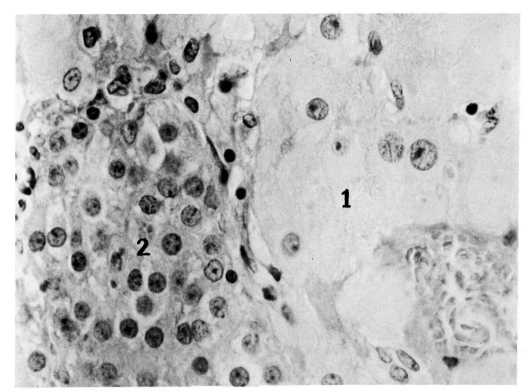

FIGURE 6-10 Wall of corpus luteum: luteinized granulosa cells (*1*) and theca cells (*2*).

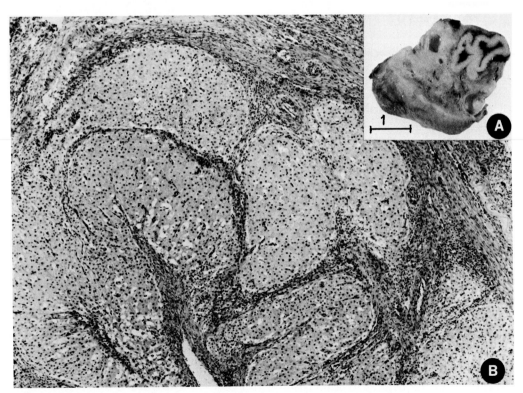

FIGURE 6-11 Mature corpus luteum. **(A)** Macroscopic appearance. **(B)** Microscopic appearance.

The medulla of the ovary is composed of stromal cells, blood vessels, lymphatics, and nerves. The hilum contains hilus cells and embryonic residua. Hilus cells are found adjacent to nonmyelinated nerves in the hilum in more than 80% of ovaries. They are round or oval cells with granular eosinophilic cytoplasm and a central round nucleus. The cytoplasm contains small brown lipochrome granules, small eosinophilic hyaline spheres, and crystals of Reinke (Fig. 6-12). The latter are eosinophilic proteinaceous rods 10 to 30 µm in length. Electron microscopy reveals that Reinke crystals have a hexagonal internal pattern.[1] Elementary tubular inclusions may be precursors of the crystals; they correspond to the eosinophilic, hyaline bodies observed by light microscopy. In addition to the crystals, the cytoplasm contains prominent smooth endoplasmic reticulum and mitochondria with tubular cristae.

The *rete ovarii*, which is the ovarian homologue of the rete testis, is an embryonic remnant with no known function. It is found in the hilum of the ovary and consists of slit-like tubules lined by cuboidal epithelial cells (Fig. 6-13). The rete tubules are surrounded by spindle-shaped stromal cells. Cysts of the rete ovarii are an occasional cause of ovarian enlargement.[2]

MALFORMATIONS AND ATROPHY

The *congenital absence* of one or both ovaries is rare. The chromosomal pattern in such cases is of female type, and the secondary sexual characteristics are typically female as well. The absence of one ovary is usually clinically inapparent because the single ovary present is capable of adequately performing the functions of both. *Ovarian agenesis* differs from the congenital absence of both ovaries in that the gonads are present but rudimentary, and there are various associated somatic malformations such as pyloric stenosis, coarctation of the aorta, cataracts, and osteoporosis.

Ovarian atrophy may be seen during the reproductive years as a morphologic manifestation of the clinical syndrome of ovarian failure. Some cases are associated with antiovarian antibodies[3-7] and may be accompanied by diabetes mellitus, hypothyroidism, adrenal cortical hypofunction, or several of these conditions, all apparently on the basis of autoimmune disease. The etiology of other cases of ovarian failure (eg, primary amenorrhea, secondary amenorrhea, or premature menopause) is unknown. The triad of endogenous hypergonadotropinemia, hyporeceptivity of the ovaries to stimulation with exogenous gonadotropins, and a histologic picture showing noncystic, unstimulated follicles has been called the *gonadotropin-resistant ovary syndrome.*[8] Hypogonadotropic ovarian failure is caused by an abnormality of the pituitary or hypothalamus that prevents normal production of gonadotropins. The ovary contains many primordial follicles, but developing follicles are not present. As many as 30% to 40% of patients with primary ovarian failure have abnormal sex chromosomes, dysgenetic gonads, or both. Finally, iatrogenic factors such as radiation therapy, chemotherapy, or surgery affecting the ovarian blood vessels can result in ovarian atrophy.

Supernumerary ovaries arise as a result of reduplication of the primitive gonadal precursors.[9-13] They are extremely rare. *Accessory ovaries* are a more frequent finding, consisting of islands of ovarian tissue attached or adjacent to the normal ovary.[14,15] So-called ectopic ovarian tissue is a characteristic of the *ovarian remnant syndrome,* in which ovarian tissue is unintentionally left in the pelvis during a technically difficult oophorectomy.[16-19] Cysts or neoplasms may develop in aberrant ovarian parenchyma, whatever its origin.

INFLAMMATORY DISEASES

Inflammatory diseases of the ovary are much rarer than salpingitis, and in most cases they are part of the clinicopathologic picture of pelvic inflammatory disease. The etiologic agents are the same as those commonly encountered in salpingitis. More rarely, ovarian infections result from the hematogenous dissemination of organisms from a distant site.

Acute Oophoritis

Acute oophoritis occasionally accompanies acute salpingitis. When the ovary is involved by an inflammatory process, it is enlarged and hyperemic, and the inflammatory exudate is accompanied by adhesions among the ovary, the tube, and the adjacent peritoneum. Occasionally, an abscess develops, although abscesses confined to the ovary are considerably rarer than tubo-ovarian abscesses.[20,21] Most ovarian abscesses develop following a surgical procedure or an abortion. An abscess consists of polymorphonuclear leukocytes, lymphocytes, plasma cells, histiocytes, and necrotic cellular debris within a richly vascularized and congested connective tissue framework. Although an abscess may rupture into the pelvis and cause peritonitis, it usually undergoes resorption and fibrosis.

Chronic Oophoritis

In chronic oophoritis, the ovary is small and fibrotic and usually adheres to adjacent tissues. Sterility is a common clinical complication. Macroscopically, the ovary is often involved in a mass of adhesions, which may form a fibrotic bloc that involves the tube. *Tuberculosis* of the ovary is characterized by the presence of epithelioid granulomas with giant cells in the ovarian parenchyma (Fig. 6-14). Tuberculous oophoritis is part of the spectrum of adnexal tuberculosis, but the ovary is less frequently involved than the tube or the endometrium. Ovarian *actinomycosis* pre-

sents as a gray abscess containing purulent granular tissue surrounded by a fibrous wall.[22] Microscopic examination reveals a granuloma, the center of which is occupied by mycelial filaments and the periphery by epithelioid cells, a few giant cells, plasma cells, and lymphocytes. The tube is often involved. The infection is generally secondary to uterine acti-

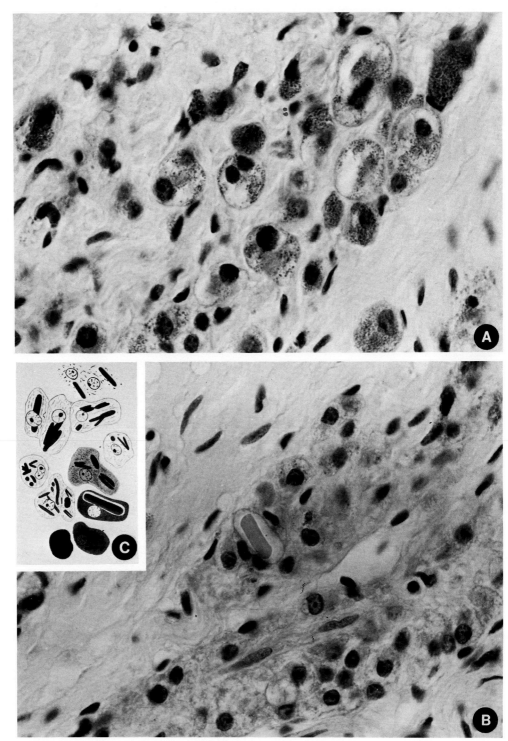

FIGURE 6-12 Ovarian hilar cells. **(A,B)** Two different views of the same cells show detail of cells and Reinke crystals. **(C)** Detail of original plate published by Reinke.

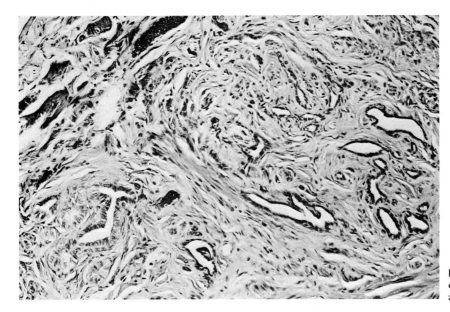

FIGURE 6-13 The rete ovarii is composed of tubules that are lined by cuboidal cells and surrounded by stromal cells.

nomycosis, which occurs after abortive procedures or in patients with an intrauterine device (IUD). *Luetic* oophoritis, or ovarian gumma, is extremely rare. Ovarian *schistosomiasis* is encountered in those parts of the world where this infection is endemic.[23,24] The schistosome ova are found within the epithelioid granulomata. Ovarian *xanthogranulomatous* reactions are rare and their etiology is unknown.[25]

NONNEOPLASTIC CYSTS AND TUMORS

Germinal Inclusion Cyst

Invaginations of the surface epithelium may be incorporated into the cortex of the ovary. Such inclusions are most numerous in conditions that cause an

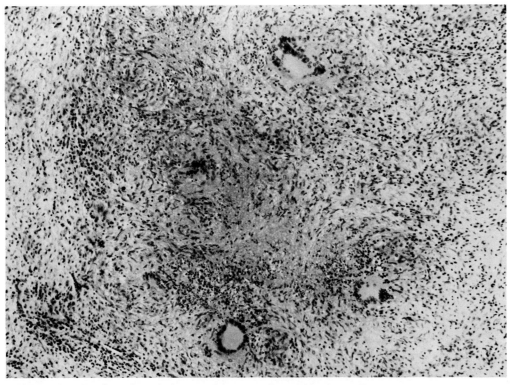

FIGURE 6-14 Ovarian tuberculosis: necrotizing granuloma with giant cells.

inflammatory or fibrotic reaction in the ovary, such as pelvic inflammatory disease or endometriosis. When epithelial inclusions lose their connection with the surface and fluid accumulates within them, a germinal inclusion cyst is formed (Fig. 6-15). Germinal inclusion cysts are common, generally small and multiple, and usually have no clinical significance. Degenerative changes, such as atrophy of the epithelial lining secondary to intracystic fluid pressure and calcification with psammoma body formation, are often seen. Tubal metaplasia of the epithelial lining is frequent. Other types of metaplasia occur, including transitional and squamous metaplasia. *Epidermoid cysts* are lined by stratified squamous epithelium. In contrast to the dermoid cyst, or benign cystic teratoma, no skin appendages are present. Some consider epidermoid cysts to be of teratomatous origin, but such cysts may arise by squamous metaplasia in germinal inclusions.[26,27]

Follicular Cyst

The most common type of ovarian cyst is the follicular cyst. These cysts develop in the ovarian cortex and may be seen beneath the surface of the ovary as translucent nodules. Clinically significant follicular cysts range from 3 to 10 cm in diameter. They have a smooth white lining and contain clear yellow or hemorrhagic fluid. Most follicular cysts develop in adults, but they also occur in neonatal and premenarchal children, in whom they account for 30% to 50% of cases of ovarian enlargement. Microscopically, the lining of a follicular cyst is composed of granulosa and theca cells separated by a basal lamina, as in a normal follicle. The granulosa cells may be proliferative and exhibit mitotic figures. Cyto-

logic evaluation of the cyst fluid may be confusing when the lining exhibits marked proliferative activity.[28,29] The cyst lining may atrophy or even disappear due to the pressure exerted by the intracystic fluid. When the lining is atrophied or reduced to a single cell layer, the follicular origin of the cyst is difficult to prove, and the lesion should be classified as a simple cyst. Follicular cysts in which the granulosa cells are luteinized are called *granulosa lutein cysts*. *Theca lutein cysts* exhibit luteinization predominantly in the theca cell layer of the follicle. Multiple theca lutein cysts are discussed below. Exceptionally large follicular cysts are occasionally discovered during pregnancy or in the puerperium.[30] Such cysts are hormonally inactive. They are distinctive because of their size and because the cells lining them are atypical and luteinized, without clear distinction between the granulosa and theca cell layers.

Hyperreactio Luteinalis (Multiple Bilateral Theca Lutein Cysts)

Massive bilateral ovarian enlargement secondary to multiple theca lutein cysts usually is observed in women with gestational trophoblastic disease; it develops in about 25% of such patients.[31] It occurs in other conditions associated with an increased level of human chorionic gonadotropin, such as fetal hydrops and multiple gestations, and it is rarely seen in singleton gestations.[32] The *ovarian hyperstimulation syndrome*, which occurs in women undergoing ovulation induction for infertility, has similar ovarian pathology.[33]

The ovarian enlargement is usually asymptomatic. Hemorrhage into the cysts may cause pain, and torsion or rupture causes acute abdominal symp-

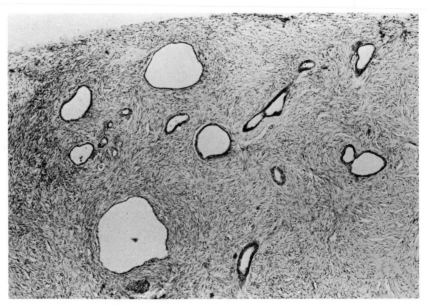

FIGURE 6-15 Multiple epithelial inclusions in cortical stroma.

toms. Signs of virilization are observed in about 25% of cases not associated with gestational trophoblastic disease. The ovaries are large, edematous, and congested (Color Figure 6-1). They contain numerous cysts measuring up to 3 to 4 cm in diameter. A corpus luteum is identified in some cases. Microscopically, the theca cell layer of the cysts is luteinized (Fig. 6-16). The granulosa cell layer shows a variable degree of luteinization, and the stroma is edematous. The ovarian cysts regress after delivery, so treatment is conservative once the diagnosis is established. Accurate diagnosis of hyperreactio luteinalis, particularly in those cases not associated with trophoblastic disease, is important if excessive surgery is to be avoided.[32]

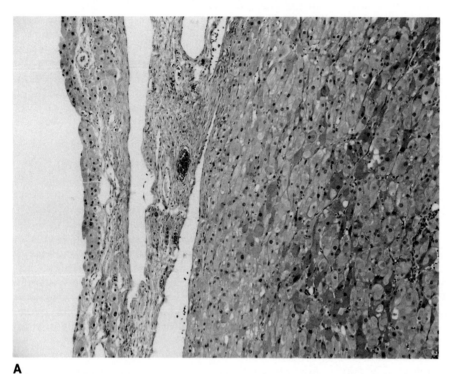

A

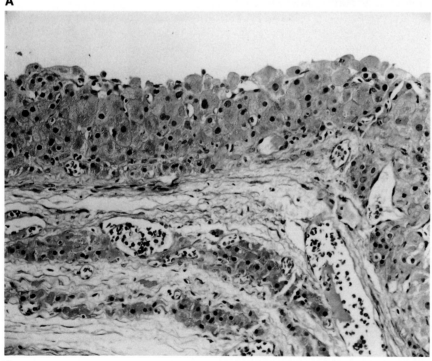

B

FIGURE 6-16 Hyperreactio luteinalis. **(A)** Low-magnification view showing thin-walled cyst and solid nodule. **(B)** Detail of cyst wall showing luteinization of lining and wall of follicle.

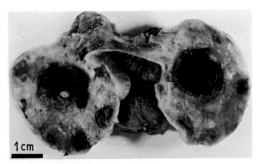

FIGURE 6-17 Hemorrhagic corpus luteum cyst.

Cysts of the Corpus Luteum

A *cystic corpus luteum* is the result of the accumulation of fluid and fibrin in the center of a corpus luteum. The central cavity may be large enough to be interpreted as a true cyst. The lining exhibits the typical microscopic features of a corpus luteum.

A *corpus luteum cyst* is formed when there is hemorrhage into the center of a corpus luteum. Early on, the cyst contains an organizing hematoma (Fig. 6-17). The lumen is surrounded by fibrin and luteinized granulosa and theca cells (Fig. 6-18). Over time, the blood is resorbed and the cyst fluid becomes clear or yellow. The cyst wall is then composed of fibrous tissue and involuting luteinized cells. If a central cavity remains after a corpus luteum cyst involutes and becomes fibrotic, it is designated as a *corpus albicans cyst*.

Cysts derived from the corpus luteum are usually asymptomatic. Occasionally, such cysts must be excised because they rupture and cause peritoneal hemorrhage.

Luteoma of Pregnancy

The luteoma of pregnancy is not a true neoplasm; it is a nodular hyperplastic reaction that becomes ap-

parent during the last trimester of pregnancy and regresses spontaneously after delivery.[31,34,35] Its development depends on human chorionic gonadotropin. The paucity of cases reported in the literature is probably not representative of the true incidence of this lesion.

Clinical Findings

Luteoma occurs in pregnant women 19 to 41 years of age. Most patients have had more than one previous pregnancy, and the average age is 27 to 28 years. Most patients are black. Maternal virilization develops in the third trimester in 30% of women with luteoma of pregnancy.[34] Androgen levels, when measured in such patients, are elevated. Sixty-five percent of the female infants born to virilized mothers are masculinized.[34] Male infants are unaffected. Most luteomas are nonpalpable and are discovered unexpectedly during the course of a cesarean section or tubal ligation.

Macroscopic Appearance

Luteoma of pregnancy produces unilateral (two thirds of cases) or bilateral nodular ovarian enlargement. On cross section, one or more soft nodules are noted within the cortex or medulla of the ovary (Fig. 6-19A). The nodules are solid and measure 1 to 20 cm in diameter; most measure 6 to 10 cm. They are gray, tan, brown, or yellow and may contain small areas of hemorrhage or necrosis.

Microscopic Appearance

The luteoma of pregnancy is composed of sheets and nests of uniform polyhedral cells with granular eosinophilic cytoplasm and central small round vesicular nuclei (see Fig. 6-19B). There is minimal nuclear atypia, but mitotic figures (1 to 2 per 10 high-power fields) are readily identified. The luteoma of preg-

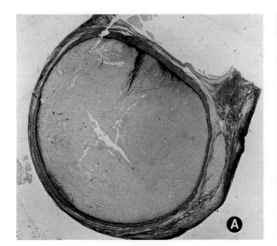
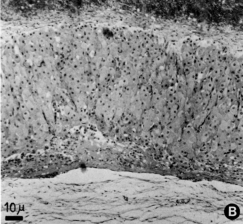

FIGURE 6-18 Corpus luteum cyst. **(A)** General appearance. **(B)** Microscopic appearance of the wall.

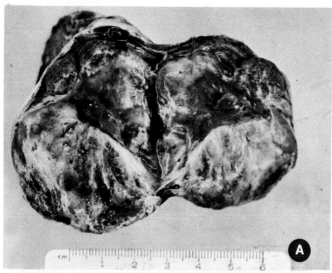

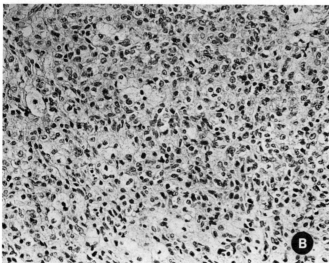

FIGURE 6-19 Luteoma of pregnancy. **(A)** Macroscopic appearance. **(B)** Microscopic appearance. **(A** courtesy of the late Dr. J. Holyoke, St. Joseph Hospital, Denver, CO).

nancy may be formed by nodular proliferation of luteinized stromal cells or by nodular hyperplastic proliferation of luteinized theca cells in cystic and atretic follicles.

Differential Diagnosis

The main differential diagnostic consideration is a Leydig cell tumor of hilar or non-hilar type.[36–38] The clinical setting and the presence of multiple and often bilateral nodules points to the correct diagnosis. Leydig cell tumors are unilateral and unifocal. Intracytoplasmic crystals of Reinke must be identified for the diagnosis of a non-hilar Leydig cell tumor. Hilar Leydig cell tumors are found in a different part of the ovary than the luteoma of pregnancy, which is located in the cortex or medulla. A luteinized thecoma has a fibromatous or thecomatous background stroma, which is not seen in association with a luteoma.[39,40] Hyperreactio luteinalis occurs in a different gestational setting from pregnancy luteoma (as discussed earlier) and is cystic and always bilateral.

Clinical Behavior and Treatment

The development and maintenance of a luteoma of pregnancy depends on the presence of human chorionic gonadotropin. The lesion involutes in the immediate postpartum period, when levels of this hormone drop. Degenerative changes occur as early as 5 days after delivery.[35] Most luteomas reported in the literature have been treated by unilateral salpingo-oophorectomy.[34,35,41] This is excessive treatment, considering the natural history of spontaneous involution. A nodule should be biopsied; if the pathologist is able to make an intraoperative diagnosis of luteoma of pregnancy, further surgery is unnecessary.

Polycystic Ovary Syndrome (Stein-Leventhal Syndrome)

In 1935, Stein and Leventhal described a syndrome consisting of bilateral polycystic ovaries and "menstrual irregularity featuring amenorrhea, a history of sterility, masculine type hirsutism, and, less consistently, retarded breast development and obesity."[42] The polycystic ovary syndrome accounts for 1% to 3% of female infertility.[43–49] The most popular theories consider the etiology to be disordered steroidogenesis and alterations in hypothalamic-pituitary-ovarian relations. Insulin resistance plays a role in some cases.[50] It is not certain whether the ovarian morphology is primary or secondary to the hormonal disturbances. It is generally agreed that the ovary is the site of increased androgen synthesis and inefficient estrogen synthesis. Hormonal studies show increased levels of androstenedione, testosterone, and other androgens. Levels of luteinizing hormone and pregnanetriol are also increased, and estrogen levels are normal or slightly increased with an increased proportion of estrone. Levels of follicle-stimulating hormone and progesterone are decreased.

Cystic ovaries may be associated with normal or abnormal ovarian function (Fig. 6-20). The Stein-Leventhal syndrome is only part of a larger spectrum of clinical conditions associated with cystic ovaries. There is no constant relation between the appearance of the ovaries and the clinical setting.

Macroscopic Appearance

Both ovaries are enlarged and may even be larger than the uterus. They are oval and have a thick, pearly white tunica. Cysts may be visible beneath the surface, but they often are not. Sectioning reveals a dense white tunica and many small cortical cysts measuring about 1 cm in diameter. Corpora lutea are absent.

Microscopic Appearance

There is marked subcapsular fibrosis. Primordial follicles are present in normal numbers, but primary and small antral follicles are absent or decreased. There is prominent hyperplasia of the cortical and medullary stroma. Cystic follicles with a luteinized theca interna are numerous (Fig. 6-21). Evidence of ovulation, such as a corpus luteum, is absent in classic cases.

Treatment

Treatment depends on whether the goal is to ameliorate hirsutism or induce ovulation.[44,45] Hirsutism is treated by ovarian suppression with oral contraceptives or by administration of corticosteroids. Weight loss may be helpful. Methods of ovulation induction include administration of corticosteroids, clomiphene citrate, bromocriptine, or gonadotropins with or without gonadotropin-releasing hormone agonists. Wedge resection of the ovaries or laparoscopic treatments may be used if medical management is ineffective.

Stromal Hyperplasia and Hyperthecosis

Ovarian stromal hyperplasia and hyperthecosis are found in some women with metabolic or endocrine disorders, such as obesity, hypertension, insulin resistance, and virilization.[51,52] The same ovarian morphology is observed as an incidental finding in women with no clinical abnormalities.[53] Ovaries that exhibit *stromal hyperplasia* are moderately enlarged and nodular. The cut surface is homogeneous and tan or brown, and the corticomedullary junction is ill-defined (Color Figure 6-2). Microscopically, there is hyperplasia of the stromal cells, which often form nodular aggregates (Fig. 6-22). *Hyperthecosis* is characterized by the presence of small clusters of luteinized stromal cells among the hyperplastic stromal cells. These cells have round or ovoid nuclei and abundant eosinophilic cytoplasm (Fig. 6-23). No crystals of Reinke are identified. There is immunoreactivity for enzymes that catalyze 17α-hydroxylation but not aromatization in the luteinized stromal cells of hyperthecosis.[51] No such immunoreactivity is observed in the nonluteinized stromal cells in hyperthecosis or stromal hyperplasia. These observations support the concept that the luteinized stromal cells produce the androstenedione that is found in increased amounts in some women with hyperthecosis. The excess androgen is converted to estrogen in the periphery, increasing the risk of hyperplasia and carcinoma of the endometrium.[51]

Massive Edema

Massive ovarian edema is a rare condition that occurs in young women.[54–57] It is characterized clinically by acute abdominal symptoms and the presence of a solid pelvic mass. The ovary is enlarged, with an average diameter of 11.5 cm, and has a smooth, glistening pink-yellow cut surface (Color Figure 6-3).[57] Microscopically, there is marked diffuse edema and the blood vessels are congested and dilated. Luteinization of the stroma is attributed to edema and can cause virilization. The most likely cause of massive ovarian edema is partial torsion of the mesovarium with vascular compression. *Ovarian fibromatosis* is a related condition in which the ovary is enlarged by a proliferation of small fibroblastic cells.[57] These cells surround normal ovarian structures and are associated with variable collagen deposition and edema.

Endometriosis

Endometriosis is a common condition, estimated to occur in 15% of the female population. The main clinical symptoms are pelvic pain, dysmenorrhea, dyspareunia, and infertility. The ovaries are involved in about 50% of women with endometriosis. Macroscopically, endometriosis of the ovary presents as small white or red plaques on the ovarian surface, as

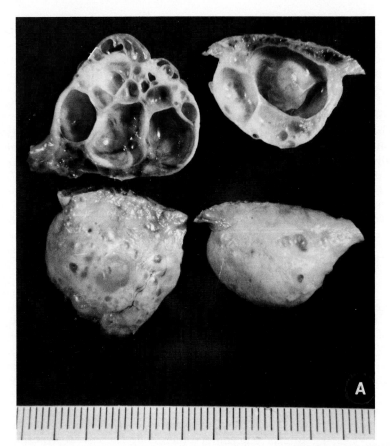

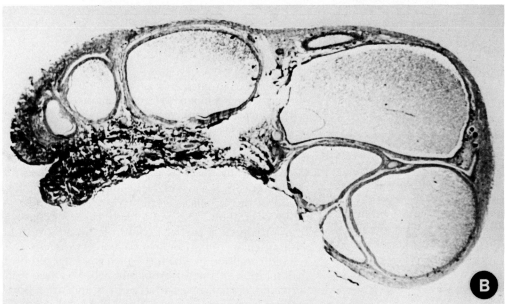

FIGURE 6-20 **(A)** Senile polycystic ovaries. **(B)** Polycystic ovary of newborn infant.

hemorrhagic foci within the ovarian parenchyma, or as cysts. The cysts have a red granular lining and are filled with a red-brown fluid that gives them the name *chocolate cysts* (Color Figure 6-4). The wall is thick, gray-white, and fibrous. Adhesions between the ovaries and adjacent structures, especially the fallopian tubes, are common. Microscopically, endome-

triosis is characterized by the presence of endometrial glands and stroma within the ovarian parenchyma or serosa. Hemorrhage and hemosiderin or hemofuscin often are present, and fibrosis, histiocytic reaction, and chronic inflammation commonly occur. The morphology may be obscured by degenerative or reparative changes. The lining of endome-

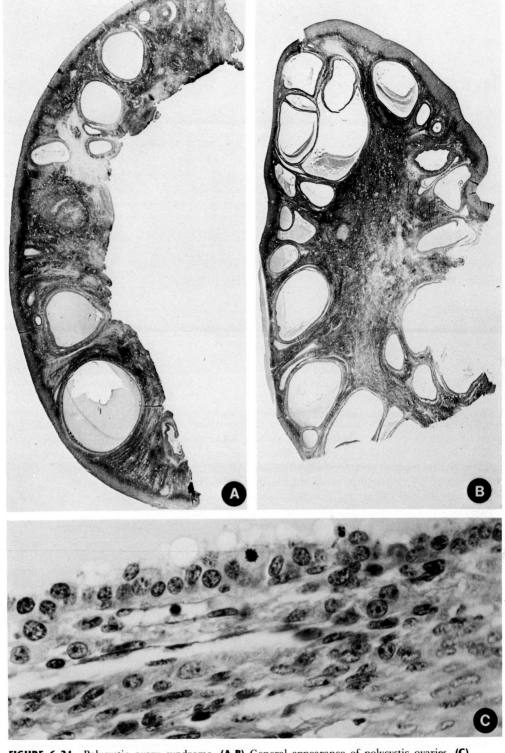

FIGURE 6-21 Polycystic ovary syndrome. **(A,B)** General appearance of polycystic ovaries. **(C)** Wall of a cyst showing mitotic figures in granulosa cells and luteinization of the theca interna.

trioid cysts is often partly or completely denuded and replaced by granulation tissue, fibroblastic proliferation, or histiocytes. Such areas can be designated as "consistent with endometriosis" even though the endometrial glands and stroma have been obliterated, provided that the clinical setting is appropri-

ate. The formation of pseudoxanthomatous nodules with central necrosis is an unusual manifestation of advanced degeneration in endometriosis.[58]

Endometriosis is a frequent finding in the ovaries or pelvis in women with clear cell or endometrioid carcinoma. Less often, a neoplasm arises di-

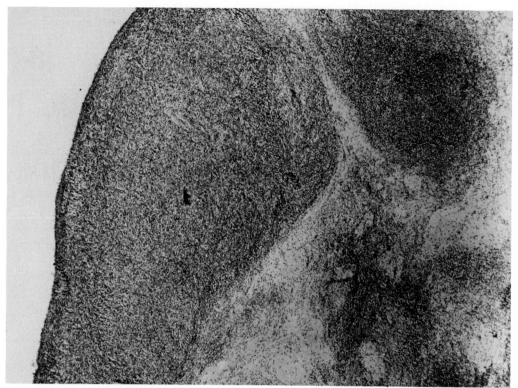

FIGURE 6-22 Ovarian cortical stromal hyperplasia.

rectly from endometriosis; this occurs in less than 1% of women with endometriosis.[59] The tumors most likely to originate in endometriosis are endometrioid carcinoma, clear cell carcinoma, and carcinosarcoma.[60] Cytoplasmic eosinophilia and nuclear enlargement and pleomorphism are common in endometriosis. These changes generally occur in areas of inflammation, degeneration, and regeneration and represent a reactive change. There is marked atypia in 3% to 4% of cases of ovarian endometriosis.[61] Most examples of markedly atypical endometriosis are due to an extreme reactive change, but some may be preneoplastic. If there is marked atypia in the absence of inflammation, the endometriosis should be excised completely and the patient followed carefully.[62] Malignant neoplasms such as clear cell carcinoma and endometrioid carcinoma may arise in atypical endometriosis.[62,63]

OVARIAN NEOPLASMS

Most primary ovarian neoplasms are derived from one of the following three sources:

1. The coelomic surface epithelium covering the ovary
2. The ovarian stroma, the sex cords, or both
3. The germ cells.[64]

A few rare ovarian tumors cannot be categorized easily. The gonadoblastoma, for example, contains germ cells and sex cord stromal elements. Many tumors that are not specific for the ovary, such as soft-tissue tumors and lymphomas, may arise there, and a significant proportion of ovarian neoplasms are metastatic from some other site.

Epithelial Tumors

Tumors of surface epithelial origin comprise 60% of all ovarian neoplasms and an even greater proportion of ovarian malignant neoplasms (Table 6-1). They occur predominantly in adults, with the malignant forms generally appearing later in life (Fig. 6-24). They are more likely to be bilateral than tumors in the other major groups. Epithelial tumors are classified according to the predominant pattern of differentiation of the neoplastic cells (Table 6-2).[64] *Serous tumors* are the most common epithelial tumors. Their epithelium resembles that of the fallopian tube, with an admixture of ciliated, muciparous, and intercalated cells. The tumor is *mucinous* if the epithelium is endocervical in type, is composed of tall columnar mucinous cells, or contains intestinal-type epithelium with goblet cells. *Endometrioid tumors* are composed of tall columnar cells similar to those seen in proliferative-phase endometrium or endometrial carcinoma. *Clear cell tumors,* formerly misclassified as of mesonephric origin, are closely related to the endometrioid group, as are the rare stromal sarcomas and mixed mesodermal tumors. Tumors whose epithelial elements are urothelial in appearance, resembling the transitional cell lining of

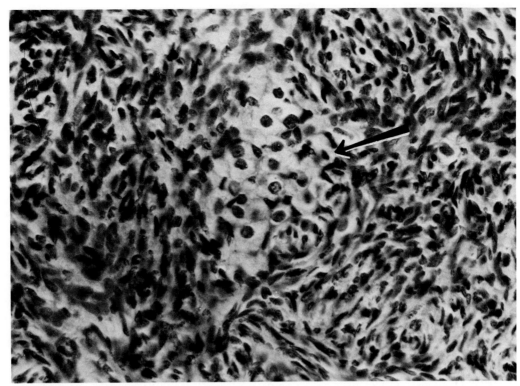

FIGURE 6-23 Hyperthecosis: ovarian cortical stromal hyperplasia with luteinized cells (*arrow*).

the urinary bladder, are known as *Brenner tumors,* or, if no benign Brenner elements are present, as *transitional cell carcinoma.* Tumors that contain two or more prominent patterns of differentiation are termed *mixed epithelial tumors.* A significant proportion of malignant epithelial tumors are so undifferentiated that they cannot, and for prognostic purposes should not, be included in the above groups. They are designated as *undifferentiated carcinoma.*

Except for undifferentiated carcinoma, each of the tumor types is subdivided into *benign, low malignant potential (LMP),* and *malignant (carcinoma)* categories (Table 6-3). In practice, serous and mucinous tumors are the only ones in which examples in all three categories are common. Most Brenner tumors

TABLE 6-1
Malignant Tumors of the Ovary: Approximate Prevalence, Bilaterality, and Survival (Literature Review)

Type of Tumor	Prevalence	Bilaterality (%)	5-Year Survival (%)
Serous LMP	10–15	60	95
Serous carcinoma	25–35	60	20
Mucinous LMP	5–10	20	95
Mucinous carcinoma	5–10	20	45
Endometrioid carcinoma	15–30	30	50
Clear cell carcinoma	4–6	10–30	40
Undifferentiated carcinoma	5–10	55	10
Dysgerminoma	1–2	10–20	90
Yolk sac tumor	<1	<5	>50
Immature teratoma	<1	<5	>50
Secondary malignant teratoma	<1	0	15
Granulosa cell tumor	2–3	5	90
Sertoli-Leydig cell tumor	<1	5	90

LMP, low malignant potential.

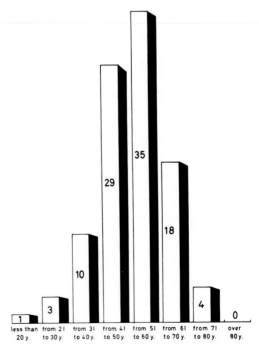

FIGURE 6-24 Primary ovarian carcinoma. The frequency (percentage) is shown as a function of age.

TABLE 6-2
Epithelial Tumors of the Ovary

Serous tumors
Mucinous tumors
   Endocervical-like
   Intestinal-type
Endometrioid tumors
   Adenofibroma
   Adenosarcoma
   Carcinoma and LMP
   Carcinosarcoma
   Endometrial stromal sarcoma
Clear cell tumors
Transitional cell tumors
   Brenner tumors
   Transitional cell carcinoma
Squamous cell tumors
Mixed epithelial tumors
Undifferentiated carcinoma
Unclassified

are benign, and most endometrioid and clear cell tumors are malignant.

Clinical Findings

Epithelial tumors of the ovary cause such protean symptoms that even the malignant variants are often not detected until late in their evolution. Menstrual abnormalities are frequent, and, as the neoplasm enlarges, compression of adjacent structures causes pelvic discomfort, pain, pressure, or urinary frequency. Torsion or rupture may precipitate acute abdominal symptoms. Neoplasms that are larger than 15 cm in diameter distend the abdomen, may be palpated by the patient, and may cause gastrointestinal symptoms. Ascites may occur in women with benign tumors but is more often observed in women whose tumors are malignant. Ascites produces progressive abdominal distention with disturbances of gastrointestinal function and nausea and vomiting. Only a minority of epithelial tumors are detected during routine examination of an asymptomatic patient. Ovarian enlargement of any degree in women older than 45 years prompts consideration of ovarian cancer and calls for further evaluation. Functional cysts (eg, follicular and luteal cysts) may enlarge the ovary in women of reproductive age. Functional cysts rarely exceed 5 to 7 cm in diameter, and they generally resolve within 4 to 6 weeks. A large mass that does not involute or that exhibits sonographic features suggestive of a neoplasm must be further evaluated. The CA-125 monoclonal antibody test is useful in the evaluation of women with epithelial tumors.[65] This test detects an antigenic determinant on a high-molecular-weight glycoprotein. Increased levels of CA-125 are typically observed in women with malignant epithelial tumors. The test is not specific, however, because elevated levels of CA-125 are also detected in pregnancy and in women with endometriosis, lupus, and other benign conditions.

Clinical Behavior and Treatment

Benign tumors are treated conservatively by cystectomy or unilateral salpingo-oophorectomy. They do not recur or metastasize.

Women with *epithelial tumors of LMP* have a favorable prognosis. Total abdominal hysterectomy and bilateral salpingo-oophorectomy is the standard surgical treatment. Extraovarian tumor is resected if possible, but aggressive cytoreduction is not indicated.[66] Women with tumors of LMP typically are in

TABLE 6-3
Histogenesis and Nomenclature of Differentiated Surface Epithelial Tumors

Pathway of Differentiation	Benign Tumor	Tumor of LMP	Malignant Tumor

Tubal	Serous
	  Cystadenoma
	  Adenofibroma
	  Surface papilloma
		Serous tumor of LMP	Serous carcinoma
			Serous surface papillary
			  carcinoma

Endocervical or intestinal	Mucinous
	  Cystadenoma
	  Adenofibroma
		Mucinous tumor of LMP
		  Intestinal-type
		  Müllerian-type
			Mucinous carcinoma

Endometrial	Endometrioid adenofibroma	Endometrioid tumor of LMP	Endometrioid carcinoma
			  Adenosarcoma
			  Carcinosarcoma
			  Stromal sarcoma

Clear cell	Clear cell adenofibroma	Clear cell tumor of LMP	Clear cell carcinoma
Transitional	Brenner tumor	Intermediate Brenner tumor Proliferating LMP	Malignant Brenner tumor Transitional cell carcinoma

LMP, low malignant potential.

their early 40s. Many women with these neoplasms are of reproductive age, and conservation of fertility often is an issue. Unilateral salpingo-oophorectomy, or, in some circumstances, cystectomy, is a valid treatment alternative in young women with localized (stage IA) disease.[67,68]

The *serous tumor of LMP* is the most common tumor of LMP in most[68-73] but not all[74-76] studies. Survival approaches 100% in women with localized tumors (stage I and IIA), and adjuvant therapy is not indicated.[77,78] Those with more extensive tumors have a significant risk of recurrence, and as many as 20% die of tumor.[77] Tumor progression is indolent, and most deaths occur more than 5 years after initial diagnosis.[79] The role of chemotherapy and radiation therapy in the treatment of tumors of LMP is controversial. There are some reports that extraovarian tumor deposits respond to chemotherapy, but neither chemotherapy nor radiation therapy has been shown to increase the likelihood of survival in women with advanced stage serous tumors of LMP.[77,80,81] Surgical resection of extraovarian tumor appears to be the most effective treatment for symptomatic women with progressive or recurrent tumor.

Mucinous tumor of LMP has a favorable prognosis. Most mucinous tumors of LMP are confined to one ovary at diagnosis (stage IA), and 5-year survival rates exceed 95%.[70,82,83] Most deaths from mucinous tumors of LMP occur in women who have pseudomyxoma peritonei.[75,84,85] There is no effective treatment for this condition, and most patients have slowly progressive disease that results in death after many years.[86]

Clinical studies of other types of epithelial tumors of LMP, such as *endometrioid*,[87,88] *clear cell*,[89] and *Brenner* types,[90-93] are limited. Most of these tumors are confined to one ovary at diagnosis, and tumor-associated deaths are rare.

Invasive carcinoma of the ovary spreads by direct invasion to adjacent organs such as the large and small intestines, the uterus and fallopian tubes, and the urinary bladder. Dissemination by way of the peritoneal fluid to (or multifocal tumor development in) the omentum (Fig. 6-25), the peritoneum, the serosal surfaces of the abdominal viscera, and the diaphragm is one of the most characteristic features of carcinoma of the ovary, and it explains why most ovarian cancers are in a high clinical stage when they are first detected. Lymph node metastases involve the abdominal (ie, hypogastric, iliac, and aortic) and thoracic chains. Distant metastases are observed most often in the lungs, pleura, and pericardium. Supraclavicular lymph node involvement may be the first sign of distant spread. The pathologic stage at operation is the single most important prognostic factor (Table 6-4).

The treatment of carcinoma of the ovary is primarily surgical. The standard operation is hysterectomy with bilateral salpingo-oophorectomy and, usually, omentectomy. If disseminated carcinoma is present, the surgeon should remove as much tumor as possible to facilitate subsequent chemotherapy or radiation therapy. Conservative surgery can be considered for young women who require conservation of fertility. Such patients can be treated by unilateral salpingo-oophorectomy if their carcinoma is stage IA and well differentiated. Systemic platinum-based combination chemotherapy is used to treat women with high-grade stage IA carcinoma and women who have advanced carcinoma.[94-96] Such therapy results in a complete clinical remission in about 50% of women with advanced cancer, but only about 30% of such patients have a pathologic complete remission documented by second-look laparotomy with multiple biopsies.[94,97-100] Women whose tumors contain a predominant (>50%) transitional cell component may be more likely to respond favorably to chemotherapy.[101] Other forms of treatment that are used in women with ovarian cancer include intraperitoneal chemotherapy,[102-104] intraperitoneal therapy with radiocolloids,[105-107] and external-beam radiation therapy.[108-111]

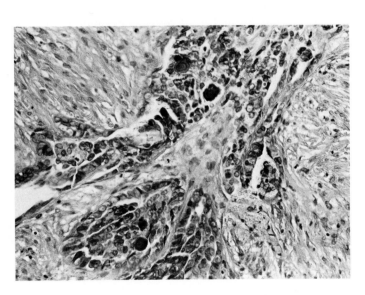

FIGURE 6-25 Omental metastasis of serous carcinoma with psammoma bodies.

TABLE 6-4
FIGO Staging of Carcinoma of the Ovary

Stage I Growth limited to the ovaries
    IA. Growth limited to one ovary; no ascites; no tumor on the external surface; capsule intact
    IB. Growth limited to both ovaries; no ascites; no tumor on the external surface; capsule intact
    IC. Growth involving one or both ovaries but with tumor on the surface, or with capsule ruptured, or with ascites containing malignant cells, or with positive peritoneal washings
Stage II Growth involving one or both ovaries with pelvic extension
    IIA. Extension and/or metastasis to the uterus and/or tubes only
    IIB. Extension to other pelvic tissues
    IIC. Stage IIA or IIB plus tumor on the surface, or ruptured capsule, or ascites with malignant cells, or positive peritoneal washings
Stage III Growth involving one or both ovaries with peritoneal implants outside the pelvis and/or positive retroperitoneal or inguinal nodes; superficial liver metastasis; limited to the true pelvis but with extension to small bowel or omentum
    IIIA. Limited to true pelvis with negative nodes, but with microscopic seeding of abdominal peritoneal surfaces
    IIIB. Implants on abdominal peritoneal surfaces not exceeding 2 cm in diameter, negative nodes
    IIIC. Abdominal implants > 2 cm in diameter and/or positive retroperitoneal or inguinal lymph nodes
Stage IV Growth involving one or both ovaries with distant metastasis outside the peritoneal cavity

Pathologic Examination

The treatment and prognosis of ovarian neoplasms is based on accurate surgical staging and a thorough pathologic evaluation. Careful gross examination is the first step in the pathologic examination. The tumor is weighed and measured, and its exterior is examined. The appearance of the tumor capsule is particularly important because capsular rupture or tumor growth on the surface of the ovary affects the stage (see Table 6-4). Next, the tumor is sectioned at 1-cm intervals, and the cut surfaces are examined and described. Tissue for microscopic examination is taken from cyst walls, solid and papillary areas, and any unusual areas (eg, zones of hemorrhage or calcification). Representative sampling is generally ensured if a block is taken for each centimeter of tumor diameter. Most immunohistochemical stains useful in the diagnosis of ovarian neoplasms are performed on fixed tissue. Tissue need not be frozen for immunohistochemistry unless a lymphoma is suspected. Tissue can be fixed in glutaraldehyde for electron microscopic study if the gross or frozen-section examination suggests a diagnostic problem that might be resolved by ultrastructural study. DNA ploidy and cell cycle measurements appear to have prognostic value in epithelial tumors, so the tissue submitted for analysis should be fresh (see Chap. 12).[112-121] Neither the measurement of estrogen and progesterone levels nor the study of oncogenes is routine in the evaluation of ovarian tumors, and tissue need not be submitted for such tests unless required by a protocol.[122] The clinical significance of histopathologic grading of invasive carcinomas is poorly understood, in part because different series use different grading systems (eg, architectural, cytologic, or combined). In general, the differences in survival between well- and poorly differentiated cancers seen in older reports disappear in series of cases treated with modern chemotherapeutic regimens.[122]

Serous Tumors

Serous neoplasms constitute about 25% of all benign and malignant ovarian neoplasms, making them the most common of the ovarian neoplasms. They represent 20% of benign and 40% of malignant primary tumors of the ovary. Of all serous tumors, 50% are benign, 15% are of LMP, and 35% are invasive carcinomas.[123,124] Benign serous tumors and serous tumors of LMP arise most often in premenopausal women. Serous carcinoma occurs predominantly in older women. Epithelial tumors in general are uncommon in children.[125-127] The incidence of bilaterality is high; it is about 20% in benign serous tumors and 40% to 60% in borderline and malignant serous tumors.

Macroscopic Appearance. *Serous cystadenoma* varies in appearance. It may be a unilocular cyst with a smooth shiny surface that is stretched by the tension of the intracystic fluid (Fig. 6-26). Other cases are multilocular and composed of pale yellow or gray-white cysts of variable size (Fig. 6-27). The cut surface reveals fascicles of homogeneous white fibrous tissue between the cysts. Small coarse papillae may be present on the interior surface of the cyst walls (Fig. 6-28). An *adenofibroma* is a predominantly solid fibrous tumor that has a convoluted, clefted surface and multiple small cysts within its fibrous stroma. A *cystadenofibroma* is similar, except that the cystic component occupies a significant proportion of the neoplasm. The *surface papilloma* is an uncommon serous neoplasm that grows predominantly on the surface of the ovary and lacks a cystic component. It is composed of finger-like papillary projections. Large, fleshy papillae, invasion through the cyst wall with proliferation of papillae on the external surface, and solid areas are signs of probable malignancy. Solid and papillary areas should always be sampled carefully for microscopic examination.

Serous tumor of LMP resembles serous carcinoma in many respects. It is frequently large and bilateral, with areas of cystic and papillary growth (Color Figure 6-5). Tumor is present on the external surface of the ovary in about 40% of cases. Unlike carcinoma, an LMP tumor rarely has solid areas or foci of hemorrhage and necrosis. Microscopic analysis is the only certain way to determine whether a serous tumor is an LMP neoplasm or a carcinoma.

Serous carcinoma is usually large and is often bi-

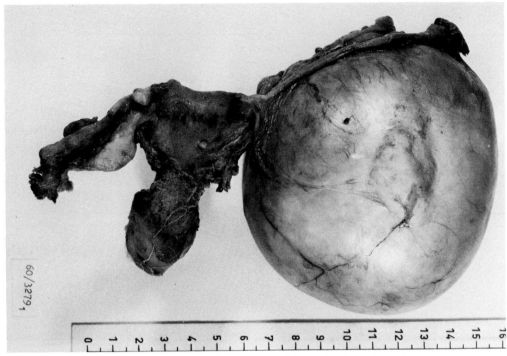

FIGURE 6-26 Serous cystadenoma (scale shown here and throughout chapter is in cm).

lateral. It exhibits a mixture of cystic, papillary, and solid growth patterns (Figs. 6-29 and 6-30). The carcinoma often invades through the ovarian capsule and grows on the surface of the ovary. The *serous surface papillary carcinoma* grows predominantly on the surface of the ovary and lacks an intracystic component.[128-131] Foci of necrosis and hemorrhage are common in serous carcinoma.

Microscopic Appearance. The epithelial lining of a *serous cystadenoma* may resemble the germinal epithelium, but it always contains at least a few foci of tubal-type epithelium, illustrating its metaplastic potential. In a typical serous cystadenoma, tubal-type

epithelium predominates; the lining is composed of tall ciliated and non-ciliated columnar cells with elongated nuclei (Fig. 6-31). The numbers of intercalated and clear cells are fewer. If the cyst is under tension, the epithelium becomes flattened, and the various cell types are no longer recognizable. The epithelium is surrounded by a variable amount of fibrous ovarian stroma. The stroma is the dominant component of the neoplasm in a *serous adenofibroma*. The epithelium lines glands and cysts within the stroma and covers the surface of the neoplasm. A *serous cystadenofibroma* is similar, except that cystic spaces comprise a dominant portion of the neoplasm (Fig. 6-32).

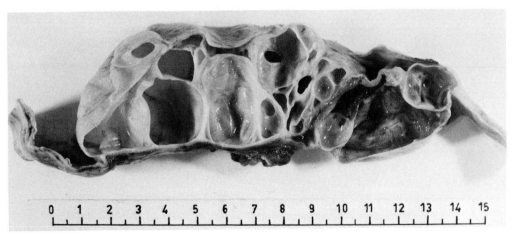

FIGURE 6-27 Serous cystadenoma. There are multiple cysts with a smooth lining.

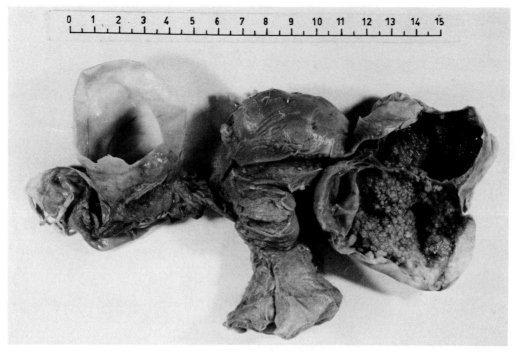

FIGURE 6-28 Cut surfaces of serous cystadenomas, showing blunt papillary structures (*right*) and a smooth-walled unilocular cyst (*left*).

Psammoma bodies are small, whorled, calcified structures. They are numerous in some serous tumors and may be found in cellular and acellular areas. They probably arise as products of cellular degeneration. Ultrastructural and x-ray diffraction studies indicate that psammoma bodies are composed of calcium apatite and that the initial site of calcium deposition is the lipid-rich vesicles in tumor cells and histiocytes.[132] The presence of psammoma bodies in a tumor strongly suggests a serous neoplasm, but it does not differentiate a benign tumor from a malignant tumor. Psammoma bodies are fre-

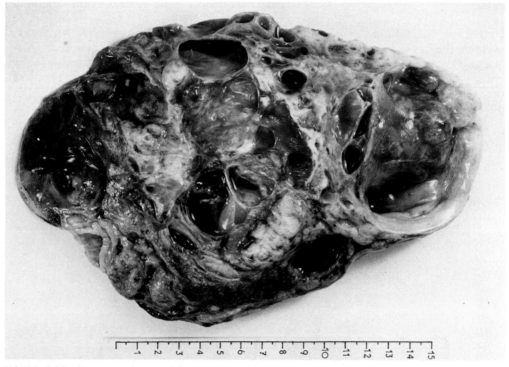

FIGURE 6-29 Serous carcinoma. Solid, fleshy areas alternate with cysts.

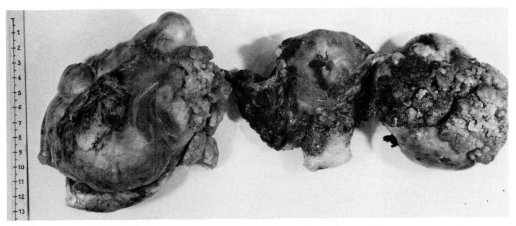

FIGURE 6-30 Serous carcinoma involving both ovaries. Note the surface papillary tumor growth.

quently encountered in nonneoplastic lesions, such as germinal inclusion cysts.

A *serous tumor of LMP* is composed of the same cell types as a benign serous tumor, but with fewer ciliated cells and some evidence of proliferative activity.[70,73,79,133] The cells are stratified into several layers, forming tufts from which clusters of cells are detached into the cystic lumina (Fig. 6-33). Complex papillary and glandular patterns of growth are typical (Fig. 6-34), and the formation of secondary cysts is a characteristic feature. The tumor cells are cytologically atypical, and mitotic figures are present, but neither of these features is as pronounced

as in serous carcinoma. Most significantly, true stromal invasion is not identified. Glands encountered within the stroma are the result of tangential cutting of complicated infoldings; they do not have an infiltrative appearance, and they are separated from each other by bands of stroma that show no evidence of reaction to the tumor. Some borderline serous tumors have sufficient stroma to be regarded as cystadenofibromas.[134]

Microscopic stromal invasion is an infrequent finding in a serous tumor of LMP.[135,136] When it occurs, nests and cords of cells with eosinophilic cytoplasm, round vesicular nuclei, and prominent nucleoli in-

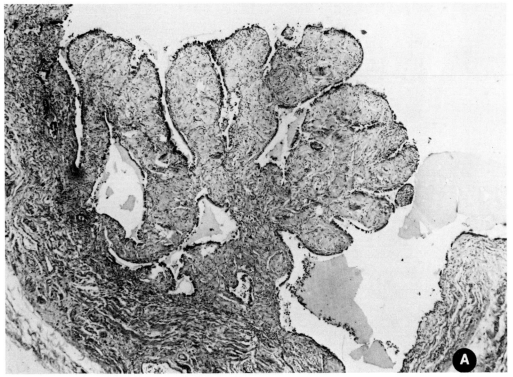

FIGURE 6-31 Serous cystadenoma. **(A)** General appearance, illustrating blunt papillae covered by a single layer of epithelial cells. **(B)** Detail of epithelium.

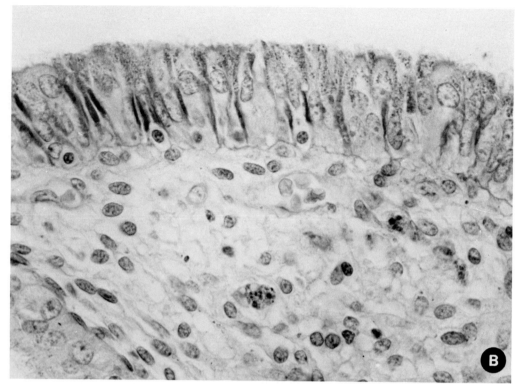

FIGURE 6-31(B) *(continued)*

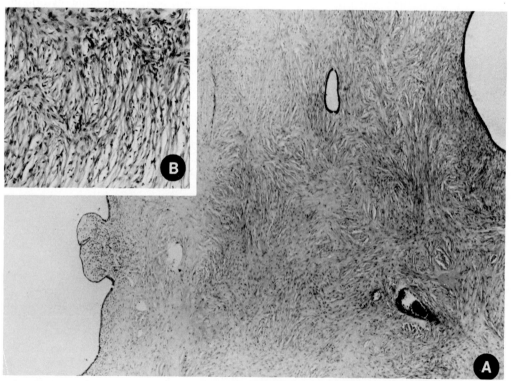

FIGURE 6-32 Serous cystadenofibroma. **(A)** Low-magnification view illustrating cystic spaces and abundant stroma. **(B)** Detail of stroma.

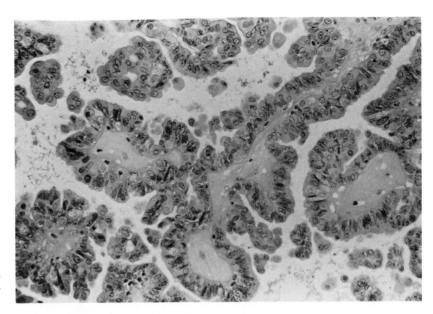

FIGURE 6-33 Serous tumor of low malignant potential, illustrating mild atypia, stratification, and detachment of cells into lumen.

vade the fibrous stroma between cysts lined by noninvasive serous LMP (Fig. 6-35). The areas of invasion are microscopic (smaller than 3 mm), and there is no stromal reaction. The clinical outcome is comparable to that observed in noninvasive serous tumors of LMP of the same clinical stage.[79,135,136]

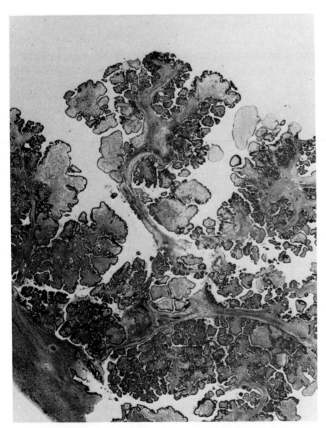

FIGURE 6-34 Serous tumor of low malignant potential with a complex papillary pattern.

Peritoneal tumor deposits are common in women with serous tumors of LMP. It is uncertain whether they represent implants from the ovarian tumor or sites of synchronous peritoneal neoplasia. Three types of deposits are described by Bell and colleagues: noninvasive epithelial, noninvasive desmoplastic, and invasive.[137]

Noninvasive epithelial implants contain a papillary epithelial proliferation of LMP on the peritoneal surface or in a circumscribed subsurface cyst. Desmoplastic implants contain papillae and glands trapped and compressed by fibrous tissue. Such implants are superficial and sharply circumscribed from the surrounding tissues. Invasive implants, which are better thought of as invasive serous carcinoma, contain irregular nests of epithelium that infiltrate underlying tissues. Marked nuclear atypia is often noted in invasive implants. Women with invasive implants also have noninvasive implants, so extensive sampling is necessary to detect them. Some researchers have observed a correlation between the histology of the peritoneal deposits and the clinical course,[137] but others have not.[138,139] The morphology of the peritoneal deposits should be evaluated carefully for invasion, although its significance is uncertain. Peritoneal deposits from a serous tumor of LMP must be differentiated from endosalpingiosis, a benign condition that is most commonly observed in the peritoneum and ovary. It is characterized by small cysts and simple papillae that are lined by cytologically bland ciliated columnar epithelial cells of tubal type. Psammoma bodies may be present, and fibrosis and chronic inflammation often surround the nests of epithelium. In contrast to a serous tumor of LMP, the cells are not stratified, there is no proliferative activity, and there is no cytologic atypia. Endosalpingiosis is discussed in more detail in Chapter 7.

Serous carcinoma is composed in part of papillae

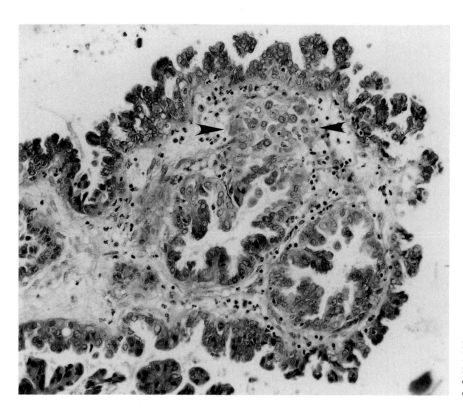

FIGURE 6-35 Serous tumor of low malignant potential with microscopic stromal invasion (*top center*). The invasive cells have large vesicular nuclei and abundant eosinophilic cytoplasm.

lined by stratified cells of serous type (Figs. 6-36 through 6-38). Ciliated cells are rare, and the degree of cytologic atypia and mitotic activity varies. In addition to papillae, the tumor may contain glands, solid cell cords, or sheets of cells, with the prominence of these patterns increasing as differentiation decreases (Figs. 6-39 and 6-40). The epithelium diffusely infiltrates a fibrotic stroma. Squamous differentiation is occasionally observed in serous carcinoma.[140] In rare cases, a serous carcinoma contains so many psammoma bodies that they dominate the histologic picture.[141]

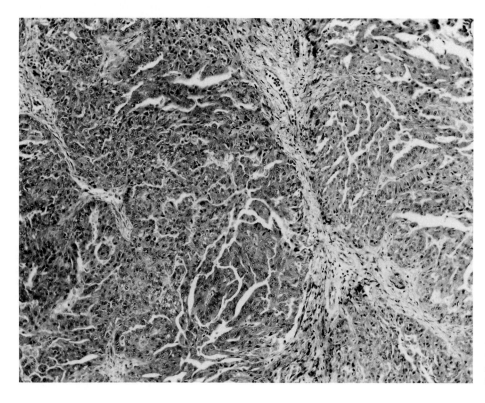

FIGURE 6-36 Serous carcinoma. Large masses of tumor cells with irregular slit-like spaces representing remnants of papillae. Compare with the more regular villoglandular architecture seen in Figure 6-50A (same magnification).

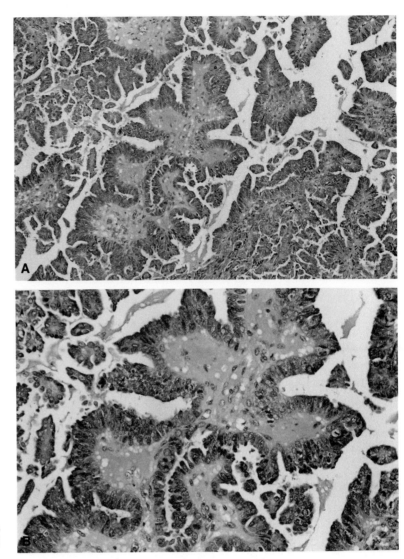

FIGURE 6-37 Moderately differentiated serous carcinoma. **(A)** Complex papillary structures. **(B)** Papillae lined by stratified, atypical cells.

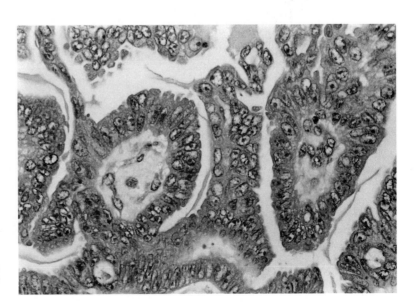

FIGURE 6-38 Moderately differentiated serous carcinoma with typical nuclear morphology. The vesicular nuclei contain prominent nucleoli.

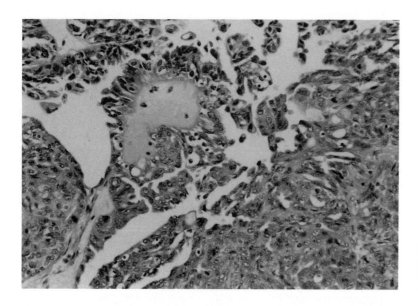

FIGURE 6-39 Serous carcinoma. Papillae are present in this poorly differentiated carcinoma (*center*), but areas of solid growth are prominent (*left* and *right*).

Ultrastructural study confirms the resemblance between a serous tumor and tubal epithelium. The papillae are lined by ciliated columnar cells, non-ciliated cells with apical microvilli, and cuboidal basal cells (Fig. 6-41).[129,142–144] As expected, cytoplasmic and nuclear anomalies become more pronounced with the progression from benign tumor to tumor of LMP to carcinoma, and specific cell structures, such as cilia, are observed with decreasing frequency.

Differential Diagnosis. The differential diagnosis of serous tumor of LMP includes müllerian mucinous tumor of LMP and Sertoli-Leydig cell tumor with prominent retiform differentiation. *Müllerian mucinous tumors of LMP* comprise 10% to 15% of all mucinous tumors of LMP.[145] Like serous tumors of LMP, they are frequently bilateral, grow in a complex papillary pattern with epithelial budding, contain indifferent cells with eosinophilic cytoplasm, and

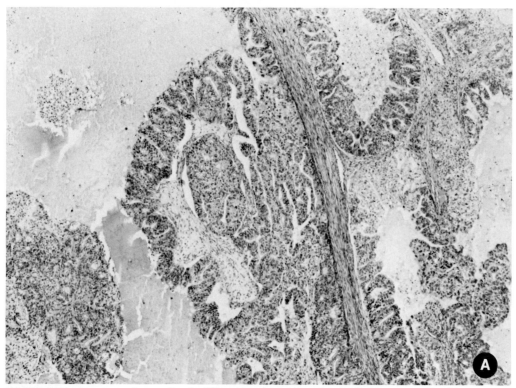

FIGURE 6-40 Serous carcinoma. Poorly differentiated carcinoma in which the cysts are lined by irregular micropapillae, glands, and solid sheets of cells.

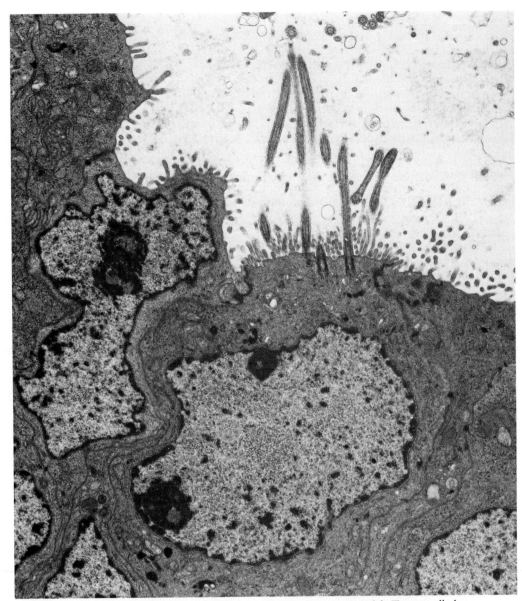

FIGURE 6-41 Ultrastructure of a serous tumor of low malignant potential. Tumor cells have cilia, microvilli, irregular nuclei with marginated chromatin, and prominent nucleoli (×10,000). (Courtesy of Dr. J. M. Orenstein, George Washington University, Washington, DC).

may be associated with peritoneal implants. Unlike serous tumor of LMP, the predominant tumor cell is a columnar mucinous cell of endocervical type. A *Sertoli-Leydig cell tumor* may be confused with a serous tumor if it exhibits exceptionally prominent retiform differentiation.[146] Patients with Sertoli-Leydig cell tumors tend to be younger than patients with serous tumors. In addition to retiform tubules, Sertoli-Leydig cell tumors contain, at least focally, typical Sertoli tubules, primitive stromal cells, and Leydig cells.

The main diagnostic problem in serous carcinoma is to differentiate it from other types of surface epithelial carcinoma. Interobserver agreement in the classification of serous carcinoma is only about 70%.[147] The classification of surface epithelial carcinomas of the ovary, particularly of poorly differentiated examples, is imprecise because their morphologic features overlap. Serous carcinoma most often is confused with endometrioid carcinoma and undifferentiated carcinoma. *Endometrioid carcinoma* is more likely to be unilateral, confined to the pelvis, and associated with a synchronous endometrial carcinoma. It is composed of columnar cells that grow in glands and trabeculae, and it frequently contains areas of squamous differentiation. Prominent nucleoli, which are characteristic of serous carcinoma, are not a usual feature of endometrioid carcinoma. Poorly differentiated carcinomas that grow as sheets of malignant cells are best classified as *undifferentiated carcinoma.*[122]

Mucinous Tumors

Mucinous cystadenoma is one of the most common ovarian neoplasms. It is about as prevalent as serous cystadenoma and comprises about 20% of all benign ovarian tumors. Malignant mucinous tumors are considerably less numerous than their serous counterparts. Mucinous carcinoma constitutes 5% to 15% of primary malignant ovarian tumors, and the mucinous tumor of LMP is equally common.

Macroscopic Appearance. *Mucinous cystadenoma* is a cystic neoplasm with a smooth, blue-white or gray external surface that is covered by numerous blood vessels. Most examples are smaller than 10 cm in diameter, but huge tumors with weights of up to 100 kg have been reported. The tumor may be firm, rubbery, or soft, depending on the amount of mucin within the cysts and the abundance of stroma. The cut surface features smooth, thin-walled cysts ranging from a few millimeters to several centimeters in diameter (Fig. 6-42). An occasional tumor is a single large unilocular cyst. The mucoid material within the cysts may be clear, yellow and turbid, or, if there has been hemorrhage into the cyst, red-brown. *Mucinous cystadenofibroma* is a solid neoplasm that contains mucin-filled cystic spaces. Benign mucinous tumors are usually unilateral; only about 5% are bilateral.

Mucinous intestinal tumors of LMP average 15 cm in diameter, and less than 10% are bilateral. They are multilocular cystic neoplasms (Color Figure 6-6), about half of which contain solid areas. The cysts contain mucoid material and generally have a smooth lining (Fig. 6-43). Intracystic papillary projections are present in only a minority of tumors. The less common mucinous LMP tumor, the *mucinous müllerian tumor of LMP*, tends to be smaller than the mucinous intestinal LMP tumor. It is more frequently bilateral and is often paucilocular, with grossly apparent intracystic papillae. *Mucinous carcinoma* is a multilocular cystic neoplasm that averages 15 to 20 cm in diameter. Firm, solid areas are slightly more common in mucinous carcinoma than in mucinous tumor of LMP, and the carcinoma is more likely to contain foci of hemorrhage and necrosis. The tumor extends to the ovarian surface in less than 10% of cases, and about 10% of cases are bilateral.

Microscopic Appearance. *Mucinous cystadenoma* typically is lined by a single layer of columnar mucinous cells of endocervical type. The cells have clear cytoplasm and a small, oval, basal nucleus (Fig. 6-44). Small papillae with a well-defined fibrovascular core are present in some neoplasms. The cytoplasmic mucin stains to a variable degree with periodic acid-Schiff stain, alcian blue stain, and mucicarmine stain. With increasing intracystic pressure, the lining cells become cuboidal or flattened and may disappear completely. Intestinal-type epithelium with goblet and endocrine cells is found in many mucinous cystadenomas.[148,149] The stroma is moderately cellular and focally edematous. The amount of stroma occasionally is sufficient to warrant designating a neoplasm as a *mucinous adenofibroma* or

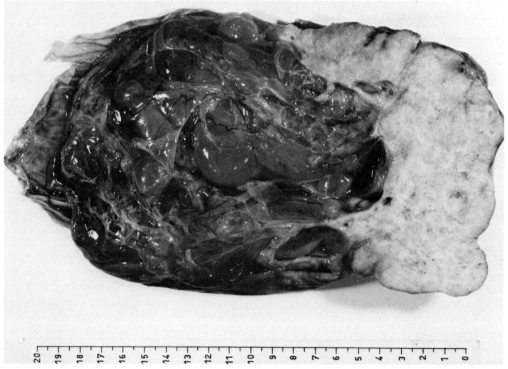

FIGURE 6-42 Mucinous cystadenoma. Thin-walled cysts contain viscous mucin.

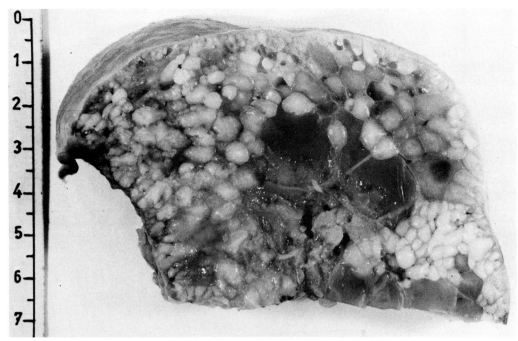

FIGURE 6-43 Mucinous tumor of low malignant potential. The cut surface shows translucent grape-like cysts filled with mucin.

cystadenofibroma.[150,151] Luteinized stromal cells are a common finding in mucinous tumors.

There are two types of *mucinous tumor of LMP* (see earlier discussion). The more common type is composed of proliferating mucinous epithelium in which *intestinal* differentiation predominates.[82,83] The epithelium lines secondary cysts and papillary infoldings supported by fine, connective tissue cores. The mucinous epithelium contains goblet cells, en-

docrine cells, and, rarely, Paneth's cells.[148,152–157] The epithelial cells are immunoreactive for carcino-embryonic antigen, exhibit slight to moderate atypia, have occasional mitotic figures, and are stratified into two or three (and occasionally more) layers (Fig. 6-45). A second type of mucinous tumor of LMP, the *müllerian mucinous tumor of LMP*, makes up 15% of mucinous tumors of LMP.[145] It exhibits a papillary growth pattern similar to that seen in the serous

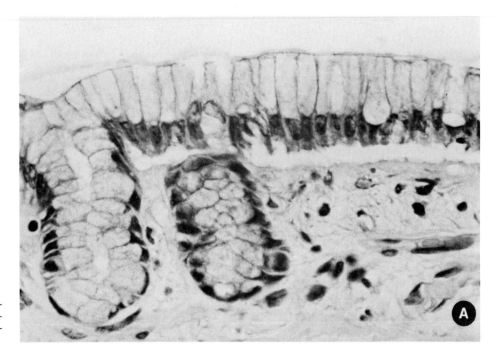

FIGURE 6-44 Mucinous cystadenoma. The epithelium is composed of endocervical-type columnar cells.

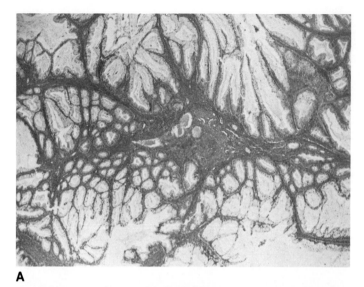

A

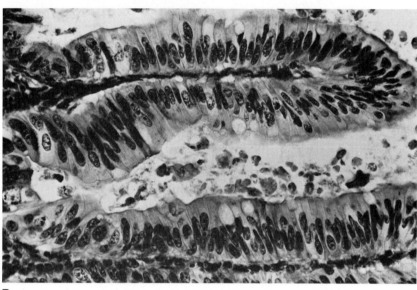

B

FIGURE 6-45 Mucinous intestinal tumor of low malignant potential. **(A)** Low-magnification view showing general architecture, with formation of complex papillae and cysts and absence of stromal invasion. **(B)** The cells have hyperchromatic, mildly atypical nuclei and are stratified into two or three layers. Note the goblet cells.

tumor of LMP (Fig. 6-46). The papillae are lined by columnar mucinous cells of endocervical type. The incidence of bilaterality is greater in this type of mucinous LMP tumor, and peritoneal implants are detected in about one third of cases. The prognosis is favorable, even for patients with extraovarian tumor deposits. Stromal invasion is not present in either type of mucinous tumor of LMP. Pseudocribriform patterns and secondary cyst formation may simulate invasion and should not be misinterpreted.

Mucinous carcinoma is composed of irregular cysts and glands lined by an atypical epithelium, which often is stratified into four or more cell layers (Fig. 6-47). The tumor cells have enlarged, hyperchromatic nuclei, prominent nucleoli, and frequent mitoses. There is less intracytoplasmic mucin than in a mucinous tumor of LMP. The main criterion of invasive carcinoma is the presence of stromal invasion by irregular epithelial cords and nests. Many authors accept the presence of marked cytologic atypia or of atypical epithelial cells stratified into four or more

cell layers, even in the absence of demonstrable stromal invasion.[82,83,158,159] The presence of a true cribriform pattern with intraglandular bridging or of areas in which glands are arranged back-to-back without intervening stroma indicates invasion.

Rare mucinous tumors contain solid *mural nodules* composed of sarcoma-like connective tissue,[160] sarcoma,[161,162] or anaplastic carcinoma.[163–166] Tumors with sarcoma-like nodules have a benign clinical evolution and are interpreted as representing a reactive process, whereas mural nodules composed of sarcoma or anaplastic carcinoma are cytologically malignant, invasive, and capable of metastasis. Immunoreactivity with antibodies against cytokeratin and other markers of epithelial differentiation is helpful in recognizing anaplastic carcinoma.

Electron microscopy reveals a variety of cell types in mucinous tumors of the ovary.[143,167] Most mucinous cystadenomas are lined by endocervical-type cells. The supranuclear cytoplasm of these cells contains numerous uniform mucin droplets and mem-

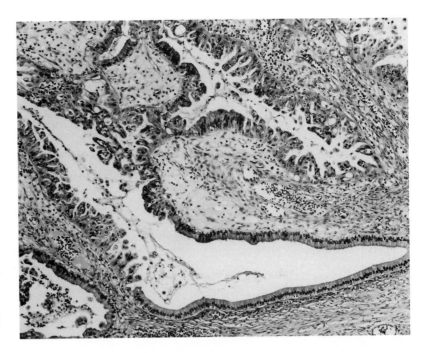

FIGURE 6-46 Mucinous müllerian tumor of low malignant potential. Endocervical-type mucinous epithelium shows focal stratification, tufting, and mild nuclear atypia. Mucin and neutrophils are present in the lumina, and neutrophils are present in the stroma.

brane-bound structures containing fibrillar material, and their apical surface is covered by microvilli. Intestinal types of epithelial cells are seen in many mucinous cystadenomas. Four types of intestinal cells are present:

Goblet cells, which contain irregular mucin droplets that sometimes coalesce into a supranuclear or apical globule

Absorptive cells, which are covered by microvilli having prominent core rootlets

Cells that are intermediate between goblet and absorptive cells

Endocrine cells.

Endocrine cells are situated adjacent to the basal lamina and contain distinctive electron-dense cytoplasmic granules. A mixture of intestinal and endocervical-type cells invariably is present in mucinous intestinal tumors of LMP (Fig. 6-48), but goblet cells and argentaffin cells are absent by light microscopy in the mucinous müllerian LMP tumor.[145] Intestinal-type cells predominate in mucinous carcinoma, with endocervical-type cells being found only focally and only in well-differentiated carcinoma. Ultrastructural studies confirm the light microscopic finding of increased anaplasia in the progression from benign to high-grade malignant mucinous tumors.

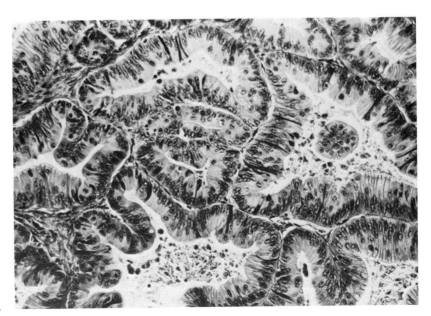

FIGURE 6-47 Mucinous carcinoma.

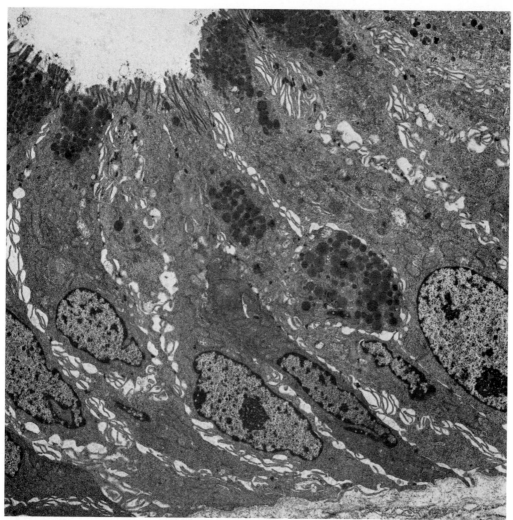

FIGURE 6-48 Ultrastructure of intestinal-type cells in a mucinous tumor of low malignant potential. The cells have microvilli with prominent core rootlets, and they contain electron-dense mucin vacuoles (×5200). (Courtesy of Dr. J. M. Orenstein, George Washington University, Washington, DC)

Pseudomyxoma Peritonei as a Complication of Mucinous Tumors. When the wall of a mucinous tumor perforates, mucin and tumor cells escape. Extracystic collections of mucin within the substance of the ovary are designated as *pseudomyxoma of the ovary*.[85] *Pseudomyxoma peritonei* is an infrequent condition characterized by accumulation of mucus and small numbers of tumor cells within the peritoneal cavity.[84,85,168,169] It is usually produced by slow leakage of mucus from a mucinous tumor of LMP or a well-differentiated mucinous carcinoma. In some cases, tumor cells escape the ovary and become implanted in the peritoneal cavity, where they grow independently. An alternative histogenetic theory is that multiple foci of mesothelial mucinous metaplasia occur in these patients, along with intraperitoneal mucin secretion.[169] Pseudomyxoma often develops early in the natural history of the ovarian tumor; in most reports, intraoperative rupture of a mucinous tumor is not followed by development of pseudo-

myxoma peritonei. Because this condition may be a complication of a ruptured mucinous tumor of the appendix, the appendicular region must be examined in patients with pseudomyxoma peritonei whether or not they have ovarian lesions. When both appendiceal and ovarian tumors are present, the appendix may be the primary site.[170] A huge volume of mucoid material may fill the peritoneal cavity in women with pseudomyxoma peritonei of ovarian or appendiceal etiology. Treatment usually fails to prevent multiple recurrences, and patients have a prolonged but uncomfortable survival.[84,86]

Differential Diagnosis. It is difficult to differentiate mucinous carcinoma from metastatic intestinal adenocarcinoma.[171,172] Bilaterality and multinodularity suggest metastatic adenocarcinoma. Unfortunately, metastatic intestinal adenocarcinoma often is unilateral and at least partly cystic, simulating primary mucinous carcinoma. The presence of mucinous cells of endocervical type in the tumor is evidence that the neoplasm is primary in the ovary. Glands and cysts lined by intestinal-type cells that resemble those in a mucinous tumor of LMP or even a benign mucinous cystadenoma are not conclusive evidence of a primary ovarian neoplasm, because such areas occur in metastatic intestinal adenocarcinoma. Special stains for mucin and carcinoembryonic antigen are not helpful in the differential diagnosis, because they are positive in both primary and metastatic mucinous tumors. It may be impossible to arrive at the correct diagnosis without knowledge of the clinical history and operative findings. Parenchymal liver metastases are uncommon in women with mucinous carcinoma of the ovary, and their discovery suggests a primary tumor of the intestine, pancreas, or biliary tract.

Endometrioid Tumors

Benign and borderline endometrioid tumors are rare. In contrast to serous and mucinous tumors, most endometrioid neoplasms are invasive carcinomas.[124] Endometrioid carcinoma, a neoplasm that histologically resembles the usual adenocarcinoma of the endometrium, is the second most frequent type of ovarian carcinoma, comprising 12% to 30% of all malignant epithelial tumors of the ovary.[173] Endometriosis, in the ovary or elsewhere in the pelvis, is common in women with endometrioid tumors.[174] Some endometrioid tumors arise in endometriosis, but most are of surface epithelial origin.

Macroscopic Appearance. *Benign and LMP endometrioid tumors* usually have a fibrous stromal component that dominates their appearance.[87,88,134,151,175] They average 8 to 10 cm in diameter and are firm, tan, solid neoplasms, many of which contain cysts of variable size. *Endometrioid carcinoma* is typically a cystic neoplasm 10 to 20 cm in diameter.[174,176–179] It contains soft or firm, tan, solid nodular regions. Some examples are predominantly solid. As many as 30% are bilateral.

Microscopic Appearance. *Benign endometrioid tumors* are virtually all adenofibromas.[151,175] They are composed of fibrous stroma within which there are glands lined by a single layer of endometrial-type cells. These are columnar cells, with basophilic or amphophilic cytoplasm and fusiform nuclei. The nuclei may be pseudostratified, as in proliferative endometrium, but mitotic figures are not seen.

The epithelial component of an *endometrioid tumor of LMP* resembles hyperplastic endometrium, with the degree of glandular crowding and cytologic atypia usually approximating that observed in atypical hyperplasia (Fig. 6-49).[87,88,134,175] Squamous metaplasia is a common finding. Most endometrioid tumors of LMP have a prominent fibrous stromal component and are appropriately classified as adenofibroma or cystadenofibroma of LMP. A significant minority are partly or exclusively papillary, with intracystic growth. Nuclear atypia and frequent mitotic figures may be noted, but there is no stromal invasion.

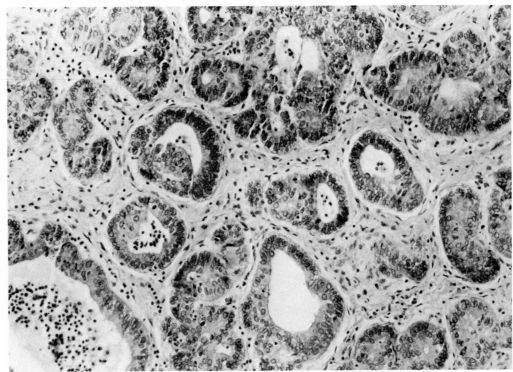

FIGURE 6-49 Endometrioid tumor of low malignant potential. The glands resemble hyperplastic endometrium and are surrounded by fibrous stroma.

Endometrioid carcinoma is a glandular neoplasm that resembles adenocarcinoma of the endometrium.[174,176–178,180] The glands generally are small and round, and they are lined by columnar cells with large atypical oval nuclei and basophilic cytoplasm (Fig. 6-50). The cells grow in single or multiple layers. Papillae, when present, are blunter and lined by less stratified cells than those observed in serous carcinoma. These cells are taller and more uniform, and they rarely exfoliate. Foci of squamous differentiation are present in 25% to 50% of endometrioid carcinomas.[176,181]

Differential Diagnosis. The differential diagnosis includes metastatic endometrial adenocarcinoma, metastatic adenocarcinoma from the large intestine, yolk sac tumor, and, particularly when luteinized stromal cells are present, a Sertoli-Leydig cell tumor. *Metastatic endometrial adenocarcinoma* must be excluded before a diagnosis of endometrioid carcinoma is made. This can pose difficulties, because simultaneous primary carcinomas in the endometrium and ovary are not infrequent.[182] If the carcinoma in the endometrium is small and superficial, both tumors generally are regarded as primary. On the other hand, if the endometrial tumor is of high grade and invades the myometrium, it is likely that the ovarian tumor is metastatic. *Metastatic colorectal carcinoma* is typically bilateral, exhibits extensive necrosis, and lacks squamous metaplasia.[171] The *endometrioid variant of yolk sac tumor* occurs in young women and children, is generally mixed with other more typical patterns of yolk sac tumor, and exhibits positive immunoreactivity for α-fetoprotein.[183] In contrast to a Sertoli-Leydig cell tumor, the sertoliform variant of endometrioid carcinoma arises in postmenopausal women and does not cause hormonal symptoms.[184–186] Characteristic areas of endometrioid carcinoma with squamous metaplasia or an adenofibromatous pattern generally are present. *Serous and mucinous carcinomas* of the ovary must be excluded, particularly if papillary foci are present; mixed patterns are common.

Clear Cell Tumors

Nearly all clear cell tumors are invasive carcinomas. Clear cell carcinomas comprise 5% to 10% of all ovarian cancers.[176,178,187–191] Benign and borderline variants occur but are rare.[89,134,151,192] Initially described as tumors of mesonephric origin, clear cell tumors are now known to be surface epithelial neoplasms closely related to the endometrioid tumors.[193] Evidence for the surface epithelial origin of clear cell tumors includes the frequent coexistence of clear cell carcinoma and other types of surface epithelial carcinoma, the frequent presence of pelvic endometriosis in women with ovarian clear cell carcinoma, and the light and electron microscopic similarity between clear cell carcinoma of the ovary and clear cell carcinoma in other sites (eg, endometrium, cervix, and vagina) where the tumor is clearly of müllerian rather than mesonephric derivation.

Macroscopic Appearance. Most *benign clear cell tumors* are unilateral. They are 3 to 15 cm in diameter and have solid white or tan cut surfaces that contain tiny cysts filled with clear fluid. *Clear cell tumors of LMP* are similar in appearance. They measure 7 to 32 cm, with an average diameter of 14 to 15 cm. The cut surface is predominantly solid, but it contains cysts of small to medium size. Most tumors are unilateral.

The macroscopic appearance of *clear cell carcinoma* is not specific. Most are cystic tumors with solid gray-tan nodules in their walls, or they are entirely solid. Bilaterality is uncommon in neoplasms that are confined to the ovaries (stage I), but it is seen in as many as 30% of cases when tumors of all stages are considered.

Microscopic Appearance. The diagnosis of a benign or LMP clear cell tumor should be made only after thorough histologic study, because clear cell carcinoma may contain bland areas. All *benign clear cell tumors* are adenofibromas. Small cysts or tubules lined by clear or hobnail cells are uniformly distributed within a fibrous stroma. Neither cytologic atypia nor mitotic activity is present.[89,151,192] The *clear cell tumor of LMP* is an adenofibromatous neoplasm.[73,89,134,192] It is composed of tubules that are distributed irregularly in a fibrous stroma. The tubules are lined by a multilayered or tufted epithelium, or there is modest mitotic activity and mild or moderate nuclear atypia. Areas of benign clear cell adenofibroma frequently are admixed.[89] There is no evidence of stromal invasion. Clear cell tumors that exhibit marked nuclear atypia or contain many mitotic figures are best classified as clear cell carcinoma, even if stromal invasion is not recognized.

Clear cell carcinoma contains clear cells and hobnail cells (Figs. 6-51 and 6-52).[176,187–189,191,193–195] One or the other may predominate, or both cell types may be prominent. The clear cells are polygonal, with abundant clear cytoplasm and central vesicular nuclei. Hobnail cells are columnar cells with granular eosinophilic or clear cytoplasm and apical nuclei that project into the lumina (see Fig. 6-51). Rare clear cell carcinomas are composed predominantly of polygonal cells with abundant eosinophilic (so-called oxyphilic) cytoplasm.[196] The growth pattern may be tubular, papillary, solid, or, frequently, mixed (see Fig. 6-52). The clear cells contain abundant glycogen, which is recognizable with special staining procedures (diastase-labile periodic acid-Schiff stain positivity).

Ultrastructurally, the cells have irregular short microvilli that contain filaments. The cells are joined by desmosomes. The dominant electron microscopic feature is the presence of abundant cytoplasmic gly-

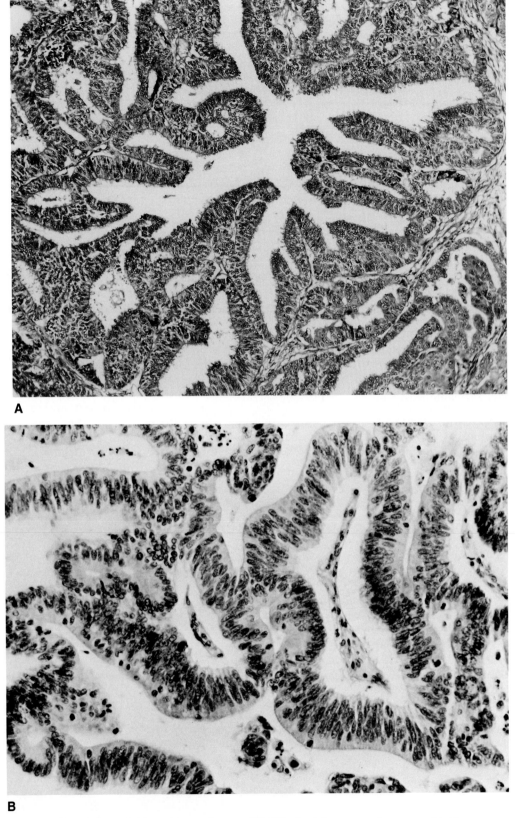

FIGURE 6-50 Endometrioid carcinoma of ovary. **(A)** Villoglandular pattern (compare with Fig. 6-36). **(B)** Detail showing orientation of cells perpendicular to basement membrane.

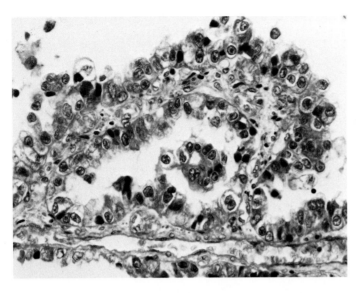

FIGURE 6-51 Clear cell carcinoma, showing clear and hobnail cells.

cogen.[197-199] The cytoplasm also contains a modest amount of rough endoplasmic reticulum, which may be stacked, and ribosomes and polyribosomes are readily identified. The Golgi is well developed, and the cytoplasm contains small mitochondria and, occasionally, bundles of microfilaments. The nuclei are irregular and round or oval. The nucleoli are prominent and homogeneous.

Differential Diagnosis. Clear cell carcinoma was confused with yolk sac tumor for many years. This differential diagnosis is crucial, however, because the treatments are different. *Yolk sac tumor* typically occurs in women younger than 30 years, whereas clear cell carcinoma occurs in women with an average age of 50 to 55 years. Serum levels of α-fetoprotein are elevated in patients with yolk sac tumor, but not in those with clear cell carcinoma. There typically is greater cytologic atypia and mitotic activity in a yolk sac tumor, which often contains areas of embryonal stroma. Immunohistochemical staining, particularly for α-fetoprotein and α$_1$-antitrypsin, is helpful.[200] *Renal cell carcinoma*, which typically has a clear cell appearance, rarely metastasizes to the ovary and is not a practical diagnostic consideration.[201]

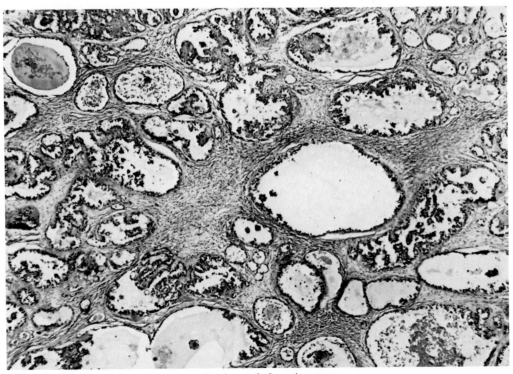

FIGURE 6-52 Clear cell carcinoma growing in a tubulocystic pattern.

Brenner Tumor and Transitional Cell Carcinoma

The Brenner tumor is a solid or partially cystic fibroepithelial tumor composed of nests of transitional epithelial cells in a connective tissue stroma.[202–208] It is an uncommon but not rare tumor, comprising about 2% of all ovarian tumors. Many Brenner tumors are found during surgery for another gynecologic problem or at autopsy. About 20% are associated with a mucinous cystadenoma or other epithelial tumor. Most Brenner tumors are benign, but intermediate (eg, proliferating or LMP) and malignant Brenner tumors can occur.[90–93,209–212] A malignant tumor composed of transitional epithelium within which no residual benign Brenner tumor can be identified is termed a *transitional cell carcinoma of the ovary.*[213]

Macroscopic Appearance. The typical *benign Brenner tumor* is a unilateral, firm, fibrous tumor that is pale yellow or light gray; it resembles a fibroma (Fig. 6-53). Occasionally, the tumor is cystic, and about 5% of Brenner tumors are bilateral.[214] Most of these tumors are 1 to 2 cm in diameter, but they can measure more than 10 cm. The Brenner tumor is usually found alone in the ovarian parenchyma but may occur in the wall of a mucinous cystadenoma or in association with a benign cystic teratoma.

Intermediate Brenner tumors are 8 to 28 cm in diameter, with an average size of 14 cm. Some are entirely solid, but most are partly or mainly cystic, with white or tan solid areas in their walls and polypoid or

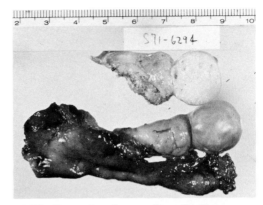

FIGURE 6-53 External and cut surface of a Brenner tumor.

papillary masses projecting into the cyst lumens. The *malignant Brenner tumor* ranges from 5 to 22 cm in diameter, with an average diameter of 15 cm. Most are partly cystic. The solid areas are gray, yellow, or tan and often contain calcifications.

Microscopic Appearance. The *benign Brenner tumor* contains nests and cords of large polyhedral epithelial cells that resemble urothelial cells (Fig. 6-54). Some cells have clear cytoplasm and elongated, grooved nuclei, whereas others have a squamoid appearance, with a suggestion of cytoplasmic keratinization. Occasionally, the transitional cell nests are cystic, and some are lined by metaplastic columnar mucinous cells (Fig. 6-55). The epithelial cells in the Brenner tumor are similar to those seen in the Walthard's cell rest, which is a coelomic inclusion

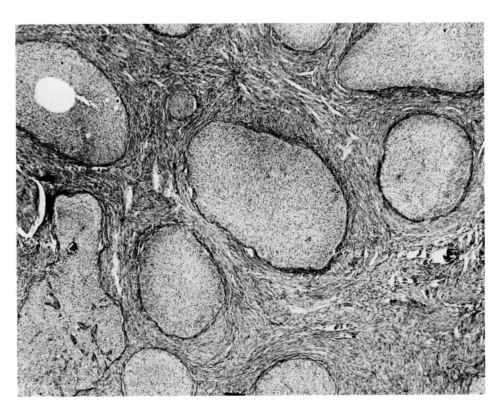

FIGURE 6-54 Brenner tumor. Nests of transitional epithelium are surrounded by fibrous stroma.

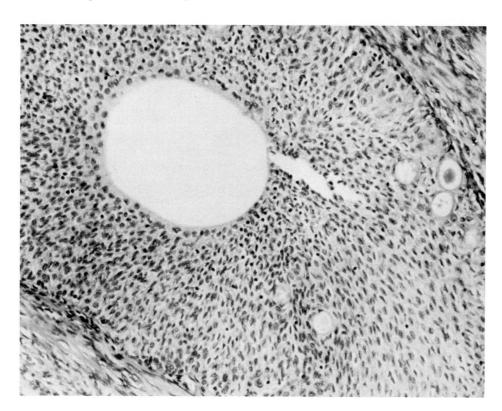

FIGURE 6-55 Brenner tumor. Nest of transitional epithelium with a central cystic space lined by columnar cells.

found uncommonly beneath the surface epithelium of the ovary and more frequently in the fallopian tube or the broad ligament (Fig. 6-56).[215,216] The nests of epithelial cells are dispersed in a fibrous stroma that contains fascicles of collagen fibers and, occasionally, luteinized stromal cells.

Intermediate Brenner tumors exhibit proliferative activity and resemble noninvasive papillary transitional cell carcinoma of the urinary bladder. The *proliferating Brenner tumor* resembles a low-grade papillary transitional cell carcinoma of the urinary bladder.[90-93] The papillary stalks are composed of delicate fibrovascular cores covered by stratified polygonal cells with uniform, slightly atypical nuclei. Mitotic figures are present but usually are not numerous. There may be marked epithelial proliferation, but it is entirely circumscribed or intracystic, and stromal invasion is not present (Fig. 6-57). Benign Brenner tumor is identified adjacent to or admixed with most proliferating Brenner tumors. Some researchers suggest that a *Brenner tumor of LMP* should be differentiated from the proliferating Brenner tumor on the basis of greater cytologic atypia in the former.[93] There are no significant clinical or macroscopic differences between these types of intermediate Brenner tumor, and the validity of the subdivision is unproved.

Malignant Brenner tumor resembles a high-grade transitional cell carcinoma of the bladder.[91,210-212,217] The tumor cells have pleomorphic, atypical nuclei, and the malignant transitional epithelium infiltrates the stroma (Fig. 6-58). Squamous and glandular differentiation is common in malignant Brenner tumor, and calcifications are noted in most. Benign or pro-

liferating Brenner tumor must be identified in or adjacent to these carcinomas for a diagnosis of malignant Brenner tumor. *Transitional cell carcinoma* of the ovary is indistinguishable in appearance from malignant Brenner tumor, except that benign or proliferating Brenner tumor is not present.[210] The distinction between malignant Brenner tumor and transitional cell carcinoma has clinical significance. Transitional cell carcinoma exhibits more aggressive biologic behavior but is more likely to respond to chemotherapy.[213] The microscopic appearance of the metastases is important in transitional cell carcinoma because the presence of nontransitional cell types of carcinoma, such as serous carcinoma, is associated with an unfavorable outcome.[213]

Undifferentiated Carcinoma

These predominantly solid tumors constitute 5% to 10% of ovarian cancers.[218] They are characterized by the growth of poorly differentiated glands, large nests or sheets of pleomorphic epithelial cells (Fig. 6-59), or small nests, cords, or single files of malignant cells disseminated in an abundant fibrous stroma. Marked cellular atypia, bizarre giant cells, and atypical mitoses are frequent. The carcinoma is too poorly differentiated to be recognized as one of the specific types described above. Undifferentiated carcinoma grows rapidly, and there is usually extraovarian spread at the time of diagnosis. These neoplasms have the poorest prognosis of any surface epithelial carcinoma of the ovary (5-year survival is 10% or less).

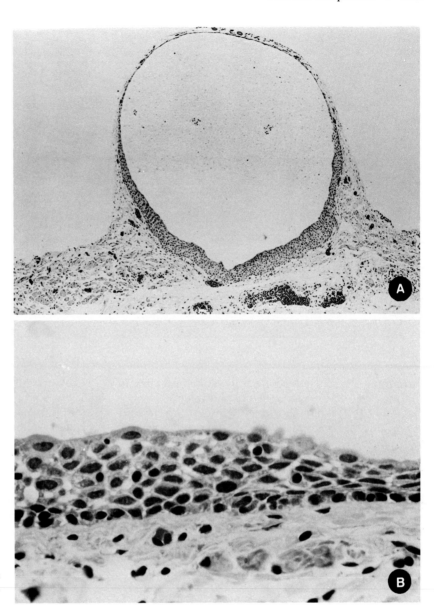

FIGURE 6-56 **(A)** Cystic Walthard cell rest in tubal serosa lined by transitional epithelium. **(B)** Detail of lining epithelium.

Carcinosarcoma, Adenosarcoma, and Endometrial Stromal Sarcoma

Carcinosarcoma (malignant mixed mesodermal tumor) and endometrial stromal sarcoma arise by neometaplasia or from endometriosis and accordingly are classified with the neoplasms of surface epithelial origin. Their clinical behavior is similar to that of their more frequent uterine counterparts, and they are discussed in more detail in Chapter 4.

Carcinosarcoma is found predominantly in postmenopausal women who present with pelvic pain, abdominal distention, or weight loss.[219–229] An adnexal mass is generally palpable, and a significant percentage of patients have ascites. At operation, more than 80% of the tumors have spread beyond the ovary, and bilateral ovarian involvement is common. The tumor is large, with an average diameter of 15 cm. The most typical appearance is that of a cyst with solid gray or tan mural nodules, but some tumors are completely solid. Hemorrhage and necrosis frequently are present. Microscopically, carcinosarcoma is a biphasic neoplasm that has epithelial and mesenchymal components (Color Figure 6-7). The epithelial component can be any type of surface epithelial carcinoma, but serous, endometrioid, and undifferentiated carcinoma are most frequent. The mesenchymal component is sarcomatous, and as a rule a mixture of several types of sarcoma is present. The types that are most common are fibrosarcoma, endometrioid stromal sarcoma, leiomyosarcoma, chondrosarcoma, and rhabdomyosarcoma. Immunohistochemical testing for cytokeratin and other epithelial markers helps identify the epithelial component in a predominantly mesenchymal neoplasm.[230,231] Immunostains for myoglobin and desmin help identify rhabdomyoblasts.[230–232] Women with carcinosarcoma of the ovary have a poor prognosis, and more than 75% of these women die within 1 year of diagnosis.

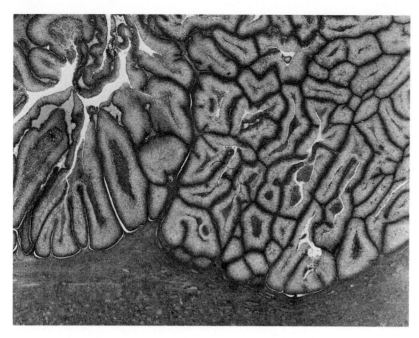

FIGURE 6-57 Proliferating Brenner tumor.

Carcinosarcoma may respond to combination chemotherapy, but the response is not durable.[233]

The *differential diagnosis* between carcinosarcoma and immature teratoma is important because the treatment and prognosis are different. Carcinosarcoma occurs in postmenopausal women, whereas immature teratoma arises in children and young women. Both tumors contain epithelium and mesenchyme, but these elements are adult and cytologically malignant in carcinosarcoma, and embryonal in teratoma.[225] Immature neuroepithelium, which is prominent in immature teratoma, is not observed in carcinosarcoma of the ovary.

Adenosarcoma of the ovary is an intermediate type of mixed mesodermal tumor. It has a sarcomatous mesenchymal component, but the epithelium is benign.[234,235] The stroma, which is fibrous or resembles endometrial stroma, is most cellular around the epithelium. Adenosarcoma is capable of local spread and metastasis, but most patients survive.[234,235]

Endometrial stromal sarcoma arises in women who average 54 years of age.[236,237] The main symptoms are abdominal swelling or pain. There is bilateral ovarian involvement in 50% of women with stromal sarcoma, extraovarian spread in nearly 80%, and pelvic endometriosis in a high proportion of cases. The tumors average 11 cm in diameter, and most are partly cystic or entirely solid. The cut surfaces are tan, yellow, or white, and hemorrhage or necrosis is often noted. Low-grade stromal sarcoma is composed of cells that resemble proliferative-phase endometrial stromal cells.[236,237] They have uniform round, oval, or spindled dark nuclei, inconspicuous nucleoli, and scanty cytoplasm with ill defined cell borders. Cytologic atypia is minimal, and mitotic figures are infrequent. Nests and cords of tumor cells infiltrate the ovarian parenchyma. Vascular invasion is prominent once the tumor invades beyond the ovary. High-grade stromal sarcoma is composed of cells that are more atypical and generally exhibit greater mitotic activity.[237] Women with low-grade stromal sarcoma have a relatively favorable prognosis, even when there is extraovarian spread.[237] The value of treatment with progesterone, radiation therapy, or chemotherapy is unclear, although beneficial results are observed in some patients. High-grade stromal sarcoma pursues a more aggressive clinical course.

The main differential diagnosis is endometrial stromal sarcoma of the uterus metastatic to the ovary and thecoma. Endometrial stromal sarcoma of the uterus frequently invades the adnexa, including the ovary. Women with stromal sarcoma of the ovary often have stromal sarcoma of the uterus, and it is difficult to determine whether the tumor in the ovary represents a metastasis or a separate primary site. Certainly, any woman with stromal sarcoma of the ovary should undergo careful evaluation of the uterus, and hysterectomy should be part of the surgical treatment.[237] Low-grade stromal sarcoma of the ovary often contains fibrous areas that raise the question of thecoma. Thorough histologic evaluation reveals more typical areas of stromal sarcoma. Thecoma, unlike stromal sarcoma, is rarely bilateral and rarely associated with endometriosis, and it almost never infiltrates into ovarian stroma or veins.

Aspiration Biopsy Cytology of Epithelial Tumors

Ovarian tumors usually are not aspirated in the United States, for several reasons. Women with these neoplasms undergo laparotomy for diagnosis and treatment regardless of the results of aspiration. In addition, there is concern that a cystic ovarian neoplasm may rupture or leak during or after aspiration. Nevertheless, ovarian masses occasionally are aspirated, and aspiration cytology can be useful in the follow-up of patients with malignant tumors.[238–241]

Aspirates from benign epithelial tumors are usually of low cellularity. They contain occasional sheets or papillary clusters of cohesive epithelial cells with uniform normochromatic nuclei and a variable amount of cytoplasm (Color Figure 6-8). Ciliated cells are observed in aspirates from women with serous tumors. The cells from mucinous tumors have a honeycomb arrangement when seen on end, and they contain mucin vacuoles (Color Figure 6-9).

Malignant tumors yield more cellular aspirates. In serous carcinoma, papillary clusters, irregular sheets and balls of cells, and loosely cohesive groups of cells are seen (Color Figure 6-10). The nuclei are large, hyperchromatic, and more variable than in benign neoplasms. Mucinous carcinoma is characterized by irregular clusters of cells with hyperchromatic, atypical nuclei and variably sized cytoplasmic mucin vacuoles. Recognizable glands are often identified in aspirates from endometrioid carcinoma, and foci of squamous differentiation may be present (Color Figure 6-11). Aspirates from clear cell carcinoma contain polygonal cells with abundant clear or granular eosinophilic cytoplasm.

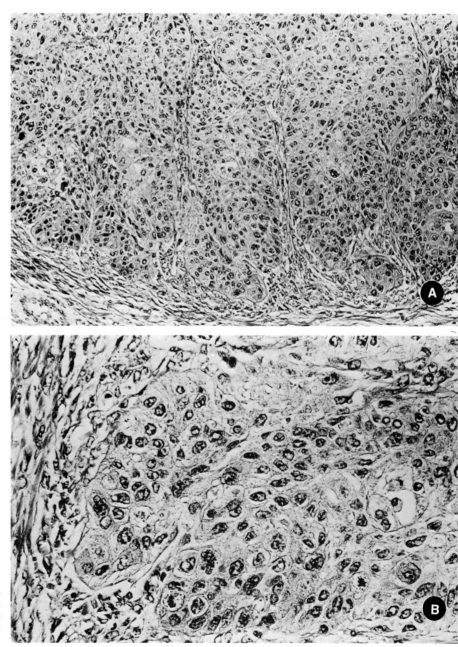

FIGURE 6-58 **(A)** Malignant Brenner tumor. Cytologically malignant transitional epithelium invades the ovarian stroma. **(B)** Detail of malignant cells.

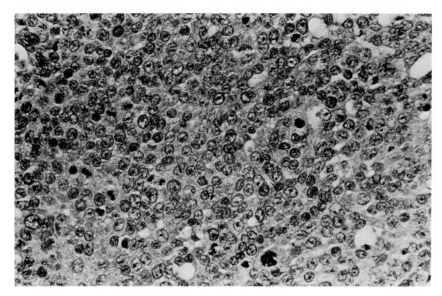

FIGURE 6-59 Undifferentiated carcinoma. This sheet of malignant epithelial cells has no specific pattern of differentiation.

Sex Cord/Stromal Tumors

The neoplasms discussed in this section are derived from the sex cords or ovarian mesenchyme (Table 6-5). They comprise 5% to 12% of all ovarian neoplasms.[242-244] The benign tumors in the fibroma-thecoma group are common. Other sex cord stromal tumors and mesenchymal tumors are uncommon or rare. The most frequent malignant ovarian sex cord stromal tumor is the granulosa cell tumor.

Adult Granulosa Cell Tumor

Granulosa cell tumor is the most common malignant sex cord stromal tumor. It constitutes 1% to 2% of all ovarian tumors.[242,244,245] There are two histologic types of granulosa cell tumor. The *adult type,* discussed in this section, is the most frequent. It develops almost exclusively in women who are 20 years of age or older. The *juvenile granulosa cell tumor,* discussed in the next section, occurs mainly in children, but occasional cases are observed in mature women.

Clinical Findings. Adult granulosa cell tumors occur in women 15 to 80 years of age. The average patient age is about 52 years, and more than half are postmenopausal.[246-250] Granulosa cell tumors occasionally are detected in pregnant women (in about 1% to 2% of cases).[246,248,251] Postmenopausal bleeding is the most frequent symptom in older women. Premenopausal women generally have disturbances of menstruation, such as menorrhagia, metrorrhagia, or amenorrhea. There is a relation between estrogen-producing tumors of the ovary and endometrial hyperplasia and carcinoma. A third or more of women with granulosa cell tumors of the ovary have endometrial hyperplasia.[246,249,250] Endometrial adenocarcinoma, which is usually well-differentiated and superficial, is detected in 2% to 13% of patients.[248-250,252] About 25% of patients have only nonspecific symptoms such as abdominal distention or abdominal pain. Acute abdominal symptoms caused by rupture or torsion of the tumor occur in 5% to 10% of cases.[250] The duration of symptoms is 6 months or less in half of the patients.[252] An adnexal mass is palpable in 60% of women with granulosa tumors. Many novel substances have been detected in the serum of patients with granulosa cell tumors, including müllerian-inhibiting substance,[253] inhibin,[254] and follicle regulatory protein.[255] One or

TABLE 6-5
Sex Cord/Stromal Tumors

Granulosa cell tumor
  Adult type
  Juvenile type
Thecoma-fibroma group
  Thecoma
    Typical
    Luteinized
  Fibroma
    Typical
    Cellular
  Fibrosarcoma
  Fibrothecoma
  Stromal tumor with minor sex cord elements
  Sclerosing stromal tumor
Sertoli cell tumor
Sertoli-Leydig cell tumor
  Well differentiated
  Intermediate differentiation
  Poorly differentiated
  Retiform
  . . . with heterologous elements.
Sex cord tumor with annular tubules (SCTAT)
Gynandroblastoma
Lipid cell (steroid cell) tumor
  Unclassified
  Stromal luteoma
  Leydig cell tumor
Soft tissue tumor not specific to ovary
Unclassified

more of these may prove to be a useful tumor marker.

Rarely, granulosa cell tumors produce androgenic hormones that cause varying degrees of virilization.[249,251,256-258] Androgenic granulosa cell tumors occur at all ages, but 70% occur in women 15 to 35 years of age.[257] The most frequent symptoms caused by androgenic granulosa tumors are hirsutism, enlargement of the clitoris, deepening of the voice, and amenorrhea.

Eighty to 90% of granulosa cell tumors are confined to the ovary (stage I) at the time of diagnosis.[248,250,252] Bilateral tumors are uncommon (<5%). Extraovarian spread, when observed, is to the peritoneum and liver.[249,259]

Macroscopic Appearance. Granulosa cell tumors vary from small, incidentally discovered nodules a few millimeters in diameter to large neoplasms 30 cm or greater in diameter. Granulosa cell tumors may be entirely solid, but most are partly or largely cystic (Color Figure 6-12). The solid areas are pink, tan, brown, or light yellow and can be firm or soft. Zones of necrosis and hemorrhagic regions are frequent. The cysts typically contain clear or yellow fluid, but intracystic hemorrhage is common. Rare granulosa cell tumors are very large and entirely cystic with a thin tan wall. An increased proportion of such tumors are androgenic.[257,258]

Microscopic Appearance. The neoplastic cells resemble normal granulosa cells. They are small, round, cuboidal, or fusiform and are uniform in size. The nuclei are round or oval and hyperchromatic, and they frequently have longitudinal grooves and a single nucleolus (Figs. 6-60 and 6-62*B*). The cytoplasm is pale, and cell borders are ill defined. Luteinized cells with abundant eosinophilic cytoplasm are present in some neoplasms, particularly in those that occur in pregnant women and in those that cause androgenic symptoms.[257,260] Mitotic figures, nuclear pleomorphism, and atypia are uncommon.

The varied histologic appearance of these neoplasms is due to the arrangement of the tumor cells. Many patterns have been described, but they frequently are mixed and have no prognostic significance. The *microfollicular* pattern is most typical (see Fig. 6-60). Cuboidal or cylindrical granulosa cells grow around small spaces (Call-Exner bodies) that contain eosinophilic material and cellular debris. The Call-Exner bodies are distributed among cords and sheets of granulosa cells. The *macrofollicular* pattern is composed of variably sized follicles lined by stratified granulosa cells. The *trabecular* pattern contains long simple or stratified cords of granulosa cells surrounded by stroma (Fig. 6-61). The *insular* pattern is distinguished by nests and islands of granulosa cells within the stroma. The cells grow in disorganized sheets in the *solid* or *diffuse* pattern (Fig. 6-62), whereas they form irregular undulating cords in the *gyriform* or *watered-silk pattern.* Granu-

losa cell tumors contain a variable amount of fibrothecomatous stroma, which has no effect on the clinical behavior of the tumor.

Immunocytochemical studies reveal that neoplastic granulosa cells react with antibodies to vimentin.[261-264] The results with antikeratin antibodies depend on the antibody that is used. A negative reaction generally is obtained with polyclonal antibodies, but monoclonal antibodies against the low-molecular-weight cytokeratins 8 and 18 (Cam 5.2, AE1/3) are positive in 30% to 60% of granulosa tumors.[261-264] Of the positive tumors, about half are diffusely positive, and the other half contain only focally reactive cells. Other antibodies that are reported to react with granulosa cell tumors are desmoplakin (in frozen sections) and S-100 protein.[261,265] Granulosa cell tumors give a negative reaction with antibodies to epithelial membrane antigen, carcinoembryonic antigen, monoclonal antibody B72.3, and neuron-specific enolase.[261,263]

Electron microscopic study discloses that the tumor cells have hyperchromatic nuclei. The cytoplasm contains numerous intermediate filaments, ribosomes, and round or elongated mitochondria. The Golgi complex is well developed, and there are many desmosomes between the tumor cells. Scattered cells contain mitochondria with tubular cristae, smooth endoplasmic reticulum, and lipid droplets.[265-267] The latter cells probably are the site of hormone production.

More than 80% of granulosa cell tumors are diploid.[248,268-270] Ploidy analysis does not appear to provide significant prognostic information.[268,270,271] Karyotype analysis of several granulosa cell tumors and other types of stromal tumors revealed trisomy 12.[272,273] Additional tumors need to be studied to verify that this finding is characteristic of granulosa cell tumor.

The cytology of granulosa cell tumor is similar in peritoneal fluid specimens and aspirates.[274-278] The nuclei are small, round or oval, and hyperchromatic. Some nuclei have longitudinal grooves, and most contain small nucleoli. The cells typically have scanty amphophilic cytoplasm. Smears prepared from aspirates are hypercellular and contain clumps of cells and individual cells (Color Figure 6-13). Microfollicular structures are a helpful diagnostic feature if present.

Differential Diagnosis. The differential diagnosis includes undifferentiated carcinoma, malignant lymphoma, primary or metastatic carcinoid, small cell carcinoma, and granulosa cell proliferations of pregnancy. *Metastatic adenocarcinoma* and *primary undifferentiated carcinoma* are the neoplasms most frequently misdiagnosed as granulosa cell tumor. Carcinoma cells have large, atypical, pleomorphic nuclei, and mitotic figures are frequent. Because most granulosa cell tumors are DNA diploid, the presence of a DNA aneuploid cell population should prompt consideration of a carcinoma.[271] Mucin often can be

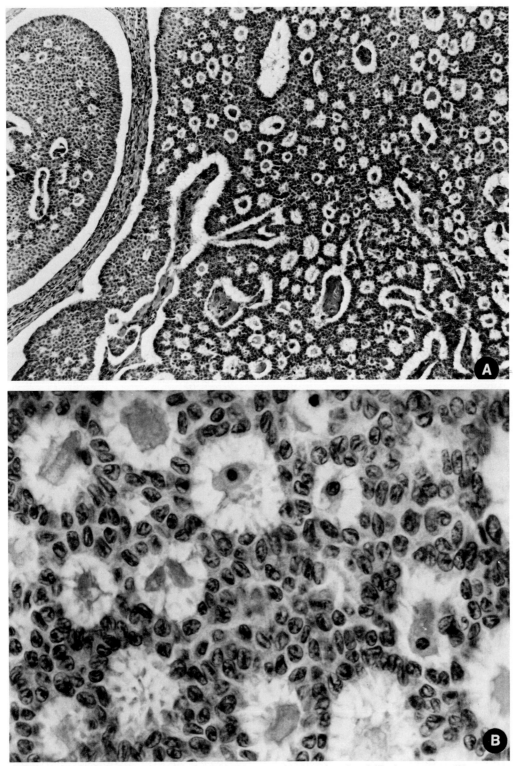

FIGURE 6-60 **(A)** Granulosa cell tumor growing in a predominantly microfollicular pattern. **(B)** High magnification view showing Call-Exner bodies and tumor cells with characteristic grooved nuclei.

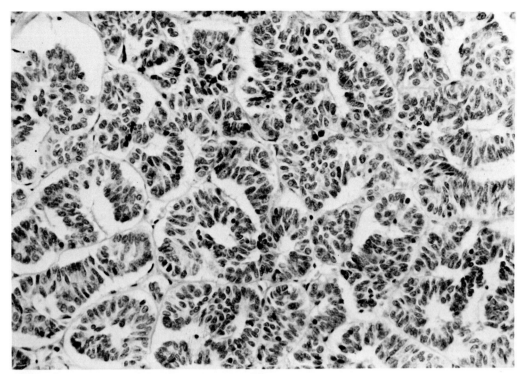

FIGURE 6-61 Granulosa cell tumor: trabecular pattern.

identified in carcinoma cells or glands with appropriate special stains. Carcinoma cells have a different immunophenotype than granulosa cells. Carcinoma cells typically give a positive reaction with cytokeratin, epithelial membrane antigen, monoclonal antibody B72.3, and carcinoembryonic antigen, and may be vimentin negative. Adult granulosa cell tumors may exhibit cytokeratin positivity and generally are vimentin positive, but they do not react with the other antibodies.

Lymphoma can mimic a granulosa cell tumor growing in a diffuse pattern. Lymphoma usually is bilateral, and typically there is extensive extraovarian disease. Lymphoma cells are noncohesive and lack nuclear grooves. They have coarser nuclear chromatin than granulosa cells. Immunostains for cytokeratin and vimentin are negative, whereas those for leukocyte common antigen and other hematopoietic antigens are positive.

Carcinoid tumors have small, round, dense nuclei, instead of the ovoid, grooved nuclei typical of granulosa cells. The neurosecretory granules in their cytoplasm can be identified by argentaffin or argyrophil stains or by electron microscopy. Immunostains for chromogranin are positive. Primary ovarian carcinoids are unilateral, homogeneous, and often associated with other teratomatous elements. Metastatic carcinoids usually are bilateral and multinodular.

Small cell carcinoma of the ovary resembles granulosa cell tumor because it grows in a diffuse pattern and may contain macrofollicles. It occurs in a younger population than does adult granulosa cell tumor (nearly all patients are younger than 40 years), and patients with small cell carcinoma often have hypercalcemia. The tumor cell nuclei are not grooved and are more variable and hyperchromatic than they are in granulosa cell tumor. Mitotic figures are more frequent. Except for the macrofollicles, none of the typical patterns of granulosa cell tumor is present. The immunohistochemical features overlap with granulosa cell tumor, but there is a greater percentage of cytokeratin positivity, and many small cell carcinomas are neuron-specific enolase or chromogranin positive.

Granulosa cell proliferation in the ovary of a pregnant woman can resemble a small adult granulosa cell tumor.[279] Such proliferations are small, multifocal, confined to the antrum of an atretic follicle, and do not exhibit the typical morphology of a granulosa cell tumor in pregnancy.[260] For the differential diagnosis with *Sertoli-Leydig cell tumor,* see the section on that tumor.

Clinical Behavior and Treatment. The standard treatment for granulosa cell tumor is total abdominal hysterectomy and bilateral salpingo-oophorectomy. Unilateral salpingo-oophorectomy is acceptable treatment for young women with stage IA neoplasms if conservation of fertility is wanted. In one series, however, several women treated by unilateral salpingo-oophorectomy had a recurrence in the female genital tract at a site that would have been removed by hysterectomy and bilateral salpingo-oophorectomy.[248] It is unclear how many of these were really

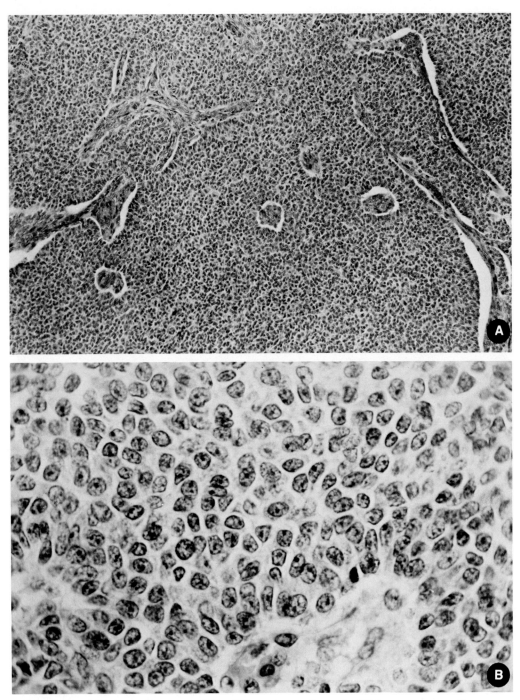

FIGURE 6-62 Granulosa cell tumor: solid or diffuse pattern of growth. **(A)** Low-power magnification. **(B)** Detail.

granulosa cell tumors. Neither adjuvant chemotherapy nor postoperative radiation therapy is administered to patients with stage IA granulosa cell tumors. Metastases are almost uniformly intra-abdominal, and, because of the slow growth rate of these neoplasms, surgical excision is the most appropriate treatment. About two thirds of patients with advanced or recurrent granulosa cell tumor respond to chemotherapy with cisplatin, doxorubicin, and cyclophosphamide or a similar regimen, but long-term complete remissions are unusual.[280] The effectiveness of radiation therapy in the treatment of advanced or recurrent disease is unclear, but it is frequently advocated.[248,250]

All granulosa cell tumors should be regarded as neoplasms of LMP, although most have a benign clinical evolution. Overall, 20% to 30% of adult granulosa cell tumors recur.[247–250] The recurrence rate is about 10% for stage IA tumors.[247] When intra-abdominal spread is present at diagnosis (stage

III), about two thirds of the patients die of tumor.[247,248] Granulosa cell tumors grow slowly, and metastases frequently are detected more than 5 years after initial treatment.[248,250] Disease-free intervals of more than 20 years followed by recurrence are not rare.

The prognosis is difficult to determine, but some pathologic features correlate with clinical outcome.[247,249,250] Large tumors (greater than 15 cm in diameter), bilateral tumors, and those that have ruptured or spread beyond the ovary have a less favorable prognosis. Granulosa cell tumors with moderate or marked atypia or with more than 2 mitotic figures per 10 high-power fields are more likely to recur. There is no correlation between the microscopic pattern and the clinical outcome. The ploidy cannot be used to predict the prognosis.[268,270]

Juvenile Granulosa Cell Tumor

Less than 5% of granulosa cell tumors occur in children and teenagers. A few of these are similar to the granulosa cell tumor seen in adults,[281] but most have distinctive clinical and pathologic features and have been termed *juvenile granulosa cell tumors.*[281-285] Infrequent examples of juvenile granulosa cell tumor are found in women older than 18 years.

Clinical Findings. Juvenile granulosa cell tumors occur over a wide spectrum of patient ages. They have been described in a stillborn infant and in a 67-year-old woman.[281,282] The average patient age is 15 years, and most juvenile granulosa cell tumors occur in children.[281-285]

More than 75% of premenarchal girls with granulosa cell tumors have isosexual precocious pseudopuberty, as manifested by development of the breasts, growth of pubic and axillary hair, endometrial proliferation with anovulatory bleeding, and increased bone age. A vaginal smear typically shows estrogen effect. Older children have menstrual abnormalities, abdominal distention, or a palpable abdominal mass. An adnexal mass is palpable in more than 70% of patients. Occasional patients develop acute abdominal symptoms due to torsion or rupture of their tumors. At operation, juvenile granulosa cell tumors are unilateral, and more than 95% are confined to the ovary (stage I). The prognosis is worse for patients with positive peritoneal cytology (stage IC), so it is important to examine peritoneal washings for the presence of tumor cells. Juvenile granulosa cell tumors occasionally are found in patients with Ollier's or Maffucci's syndromes.[282,284,286,287]

Macroscopic Appearance. The tumors measure 2.5 to 30 cm in diameter; the average diameter is 12 cm. Most are solid with cystic areas, but some are entirely solid, and a small percentage are largely cystic. The solid areas are nodular and yellow or tan. Hemorrhage is seen in about half of the tumors, and necrosis in a few of them.

Microscopic Appearance. Many juvenile granulosa cell tumors have a lobulated or nodular appearance at low magnification. Macrofollicular and solid growth patterns dominate the histologic picture (Fig. 6-63). The macrofollicles are lined by one or more layers of neoplastic granulosa cells. The follicles are uniform in some tumors and irregular in shape and size in others. The neoplastic cells are large, with round, dark nuclei, and a variable amount of cytoplasm. Nuclear grooves usually are not seen in juve-

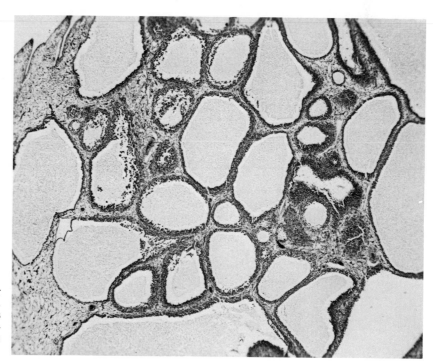

FIGURE 6-63 Juvenile granulosa cell tumor with a macrofollicular pattern of growth. (Zaloudek CJ, Norris HJ: Granulosa tumors of the ovary in children: A clinical and pathologic study of 32 cases. Am J Surg Pathol 6: 503–512, 1982)

nile granulosa cell tumors. Most neoplasms contain luteinized cells (Fig. 6-64). Cytologic atypia and mitotic activity are increased compared with adult granulosa cell tumors. There are an average of 6 mitotic figures per 10 high-power microscopic fields.

Few immunocytochemical studies have been performed on juvenile granulosa cell tumors. The tumor cells are vimentin positive and carcinoembryonic antigen negative.[261,285] Cells that react with antibodies against low-molecular-weight cytokeratins and neuron-specific enolase are found in about 50% of juvenile granulosa cell tumors.[261,285]

Ultrastructurally, the cytoplasm of nonluteinized tumor cells contains rough endoplasmic reticulum, free ribosomes, small mitochondria, and inconspicuous smooth endoplasmic reticulum. The cells are joined by immature desmosomal attachments. Other cells contain organelles associated with steroid production, including large mitochondria (some with tubular cristae), abundant smooth endoplasmic reticulum, and large lipid droplets.

Tumor cell DNA content does not appear to correlate with clinical behavior. About 40% of juvenile granulosa cell tumors contain an aneuploid cell population, but the clinical outcome is equally favorable in diploid and aneuploid tumors.[288]

Cytologic study reveals granulosa cells in aggregates, singly, or in irregular clusters.[289] The nuclei are central and have fine chromatin and small nucleoli. Nuclear grooves are absent. There is a moderate amount of granular cytoplasm.

Differential Diagnosis. The main differential diagnostic considerations are adult granulosa cell tumor and small cell carcinoma. In the first case, the age of the patient is helpful, because *adult granulosa cell tumors* occur in older patients. Juvenile tumors are composed of larger, more pleomorphic granulosa cells, and there is greater nuclear atypia and mitotic activity. Luteinized cells are more frequent in juvenile granulosa cells. At low magnification, juvenile granulosa cell tumor has a lobulated or nodular growth pattern that is not seen in adult tumors. Finally, the typical patterns observed in adult granulosa cell tumors are not seen in juvenile tumors, in which macrofollicular and diffuse patterns dominate. There are many similarities between *small cell carcinoma* and juvenile granulosa cell tumor, and it can be difficult to differentiate between them. Both neoplasms develop mainly in young patients, but small cell carcinoma is associated with hypercalcemia in 60% of cases, whereas juvenile granulosa cell tumor produces symptoms caused by abnormal estrogen production. Small cell carcinoma grows in a diffuse pattern and may contain irregular macrofollicles. It does not exhibit the nodular low-power pattern seen in juvenile granulosa cell tumor. Mitotic activity generally is more pronounced in small cell carcinoma, and atypical mitotic figures are more likely. Immunohistochemistry can be helpful in the differential diagnosis.[261] Small cell carcinoma is more likely to be cytokeratin positive. In contrast to granulosa cell tumor, about 50% of small cell carcinomas are vimentin negative. Many small cell carcinomas are chromogranin positive; granulosa cell tumor does not react with this antibody.

Clinical Behavior and Treatment. Most juvenile granulosa cell tumors are confined to one ovary (stage IA) at diagnosis and are treated successfully by

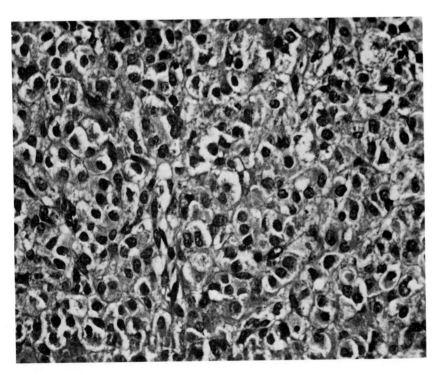

FIGURE 6-64 Juvenile granulosa cell tumor. The tumor cells are partly luteinized and have a moderate amount of granular eosinophilic cytoplasm.

unilateral salpingo-oophorectomy. Because of the young age of most patients, hysterectomy and bilateral salpingo-oophorectomy is reserved for those few patients who have advanced disease (stage II or III). The long-term survival in large series is greater than 90%.[281,282,285] Patients with positive peritoneal cytology or extraovarian tumor spread have an increased risk of recurrence.[282] Recurrence and death from tumor takes place within 3 years of diagnosis. No effective treatment for recurrent or metastatic neoplasms has been identified.

Thecoma

The thecoma is a neoplasm derived from the ovarian stroma that contains cells resembling those of the theca interna. Thecomas constitute about 7% of all sex cord stromal tumors of the ovary.[290]

Clinical Findings. Thecomas occur in women 20 to 80 years of age. Most patients are perimenopausal or postmenopausal, with an average age of slightly greater than 50 years.[245,246,252,290] Luteinized thecomas occur in somewhat younger women, and more than 30% are detected in patients younger than 30.[40] The clinical presentation depends on the patient's menopausal status. Postmenopausal patients typically present with postmenopausal bleeding, although about 25% of these patients have only nonspecific symptoms such as abdominal distention. Premenopausal women frequently have menstrual abnormalities such as irregular bleeding or amenorrhea, pelvic or abdominal pain, or abdominal distention. A few thecomas, usually of the luteinized type, are virilizing.[40,251] Endometrial hyperplasia is detected in about 15% of women with thecomas and as many as 26% to 29% have endometrial carcinoma.[252,291] At operation, 5% of patients have bilateral tumors.[245,246] Extraovarian spread does not occur except in rare malignant tumors with thecomatous features.

Macroscopic Appearance. Thecomas range from small, incidentally discovered tumors less than 1 cm in diameter to large neoplasms more than 20 cm in diameter. The average diameter is 7 cm. The consistency ranges from firm to hard. The cut surface is gray, tan, white, or yellow (Fig. 6-65 and Color Figure 6-14). Thecomas often contain cysts of various sizes containing yellow serous fluid. Calcified regions may be present.

Microscopic Appearance. Thecomas are composed of irregular, whorled, anastomosing fascicles of ovoid or fusiform cells that frequently are separated by hyalinized connective tissue plaques (see Fig. 6-65). The tumor cells have round or oval nuclei containing finely dispersed chromatin. The cytoplasm is slightly eosinophilic and can be homogeneous or vacuolated. Fat stains performed on unfixed frozen sec-

tions demonstrate cytoplasmic lipid droplets. Reticulin stains reveal a fibrillar network surrounding individual theca cells. A rich capillary network is present between the bundles of theca cells. Rare tumors in young women contain extensive areas of calcification.[292]

Variably sized clusters of polygonal luteinized stromal cells are found in some stromal tumors. Such tumors are referred to as *luteinized thecomas*, whether the background stromal pattern is that of thecoma, fibrothecoma, or fibroma.[39,40] Luteinized thecomas can produce estrogenic (50%) or androgenic (11%) effects or can be nonfunctional (39%).[40] Nearly all androgenic thecomas are luteinized thecomas.

Rare stromal tumors containing theca cells or luteinized cells invade adjacent organs, recur after adequate excision, or metastasize. Features that raise the possibility of malignancy include large size, hypercellularity, and frequent mitotic figures (4 or more mitotic figures per 10 high-power fields).[40,293]

Immunostains for vimentin are positive in thecoma, whereas those for cytokeratin are negative.[262] Immunostains for enzymes involved in steroidogenesis reveal that thecoma contains the enzymes required for cholesterol side-chain cleavage and 17α-hydroxylation but that an enzyme required for aromatization of androgen to estradiol is absent.[294] This suggests that the tumor cells, like the theca cells in the normal ovary, are capable of producing androgens, but that conversion to estrogen takes place elsewhere, within the ovary or in the periphery.

Electron microscopy discloses a spectrum of cell types, including some with features of smooth muscle cells.[267,295,296] Spindle-shaped mesenchymal cells with prominent Golgi complexes, short branching profiles of rough endoplasmic reticulum, and occasional lipid droplets predominate. Cells with abundant 10-nm intermediate filaments are found, as are cells with dilated smooth endoplasmic reticulum, lipid, and large mitochondria with tubular or straight cristae.

A cytogenetic abnormality, trisomy 12, is reported to characterize thecoma and several other sex cord stromal tumors.[272,297,298]

Differential Diagnosis. The histologic appearance of thecoma overlaps with that of fibroma. The term *fibrothecoma* is commonly used for a fibroma that contains occasional, plump, spindled theca cells. Such tumors generally are hormonally inactive.

Clinical Behavior and Treatment. Thecomas are almost invariably benign neoplasms, and surgical excision is the appropriate treatment. Rare malignant tumors with unequivocal thecomatous differentiation have been described.[40,242,251,293] However, most neoplasms reported as "malignant thecoma" are sarcomatoid granulosa cell tumors, fibrosarcomas, or other types of malignant mesenchymal tumors.

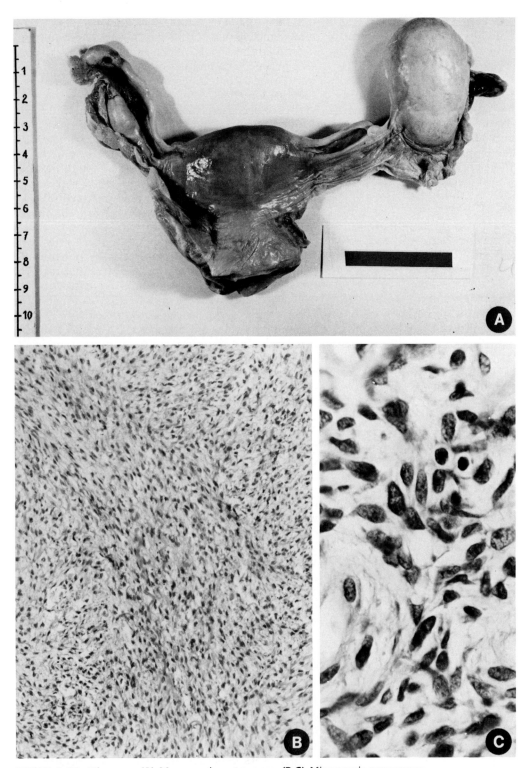

FIGURE 6-65 Thecoma. **(A)** Macroscopic appearance. **(B,C)** Microscopic appearance.

Fibroma and Related Neoplasms

The fibroma is a benign tumor that is composed of fibroblasts and collagen fibers and arises in the ovarian stroma. It represents 1% to 5% of all ovarian tumors and is by far the most common sex cord stromal tumor.[243,290] Malignant fibroblastic tumors of the ovary are rare.[299]

Clinical Findings. The clinical presentation is not specific. Fibroma occurs in patients 20 to 80 years of age, with an average age of slightly less than 50 years.[290] Many fibromas are asymptomatic and are discovered at operation for some other problem. Large tumors cause abdominal discomfort or distention and about 30% are associated with ascites.

Meigs' syndrome is a condition in which an ovarian fibroma is accompanied by ascites and hydrothorax.

Macroscopic Appearance. The fibroma is a firm, white tumor with a smooth, multinodular surface. Many fibromas are smaller than 1 cm in diameter, but tumors larger than 10 cm are not uncommon. The cut surface is solid and pearly white (Fig. 6-66A). There may be foci of necrosis and hemorrhage in large tumors. Five to 10% of fibromas are bilateral. Cellular fibroma and fibrosarcoma are larger and softer.

Microscopic Appearance. Fibromas are composed of spindle cells that grow in whorled and anastomosing bundles (see Fig. 6-66B). The nuclei are fusiform and uniform from cell to cell. A variable amount of collagenous stroma is admixed with the fibroblastic tumor cells; the stroma is occasionally so prominent that it dominates the histologic picture. Occasionally, small irregular or tubular collections of sex cord cells are present within a fibroma or fibrothecoma. Rare sex cord elements do not adversely affect the prognosis of such tumors, which are designated as *fibromas with sex cord elements.*[300]

Rare fibroblastic tumors are hypercellular neoplasms in which the spindle-shaped cells are arranged in a herringbone or storiform pattern. Hypercellular fibroblastic tumors that exhibit mild to moderate nuclear atypia and 3 or fewer mitotic figures per 10 high-power fields are designated as *cellular fibromas.* Those in which the degree of nuclear atypia is moderate or marked and in which there are 4 or more mitotic figures per 10 high-power fields are designated as *fibrosarcoma.*[299]

Ultrastructural studies suggest that fibromas and thecomas are derived from the same cell type and that they differ only in the proportion of collagen-forming and steroid-forming cells.[267,295] Cytogenetic studies reveal that trisomy 12 is a consistent abnormality in ovarian fibroma.[272,273,297]

Clinical Behavior and Treatment. The fibroma is a benign neoplasm that is treated adequately by surgical excision. Cellular fibroma is capable of locally aggressive growth if it is incompletely excised. Fibrosarcoma is a malignant mesenchymal tumor with a poor prognosis. It is treated by complete excision and chemotherapy.[299]

Sclerosing Stromal Tumor

The sclerosing stromal tumor is an uncommon benign tumor that arises predominantly in young women in the second and third decades of life.[301–304] The most typical presentation is with menstrual irregularity and pelvic pain. Sclerosing stromal tumors range from 1.5 to 17 cm in diameter. They typically are solid, firm neoplasms with nodular white or yellow cut surfaces. Rare examples are cystic.[305] At low magnification, sclerosing stromal tumor has a pseudolobular appearance produced by an admixture of densely cellular nodules and less cellular fibrous or edematous zones (Fig. 6-67). The cellular population ranges from spindle-shaped fibroblastic cells to polygonal cells with eosinophilic or vacuolated cytoplasm. Most tumor cells are vimentin positive. Scattered cells display smooth muscle differentiation, which can be demonstrated by immunohistochemistry or electron microscopy.[306] A tendency to sclerosis and to marked vascularity is typical. The sclerosing stromal tumor is benign and is treated by excision.

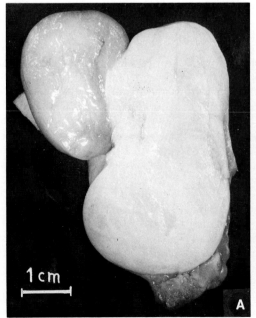
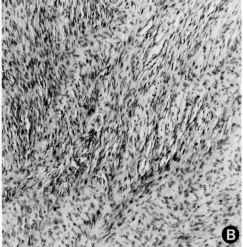

1 cm

FIGURE 6-66 Ovarian fibroma. **(A)** Macroscopic appearance. **(B)** Microscopic appearance.

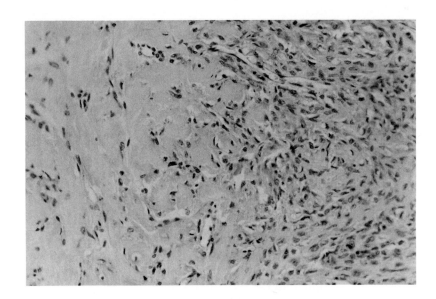

FIGURE 6-67 Sclerosing stromal tumor. The cellular region is shown on the right, and the acellular hyalinized area with prominent vessels is on the left.

The main differential diagnosis is with massive edema, which also occurs in young women. Sclerosing stromal tumor is an expansile neoplasm that displaces normal ovarian structures. In contrast, the latter are present within areas of massive edema. We have seen Krukenberg's tumors initially misdiagnosed as sclerosing stromal tumors; a stain for mucin should prevent this error.

Sertoli-Leydig Cell Tumor

Sertoli-Leydig cell tumors are rare neoplasms, comprising less than 1% of ovarian tumors. About one half are virilizing. They are classified into two main clinicopathologic groups: (1) well-differentiated Sertoli-Leydig cell tumors (10% of the total); and (2) Sertoli-Leydig cell tumors of intermediate and poor differentiation. About 25% of the latter contain areas of heterologous or retiform differentiation.

Clinical Findings. Sertoli-Leydig cell tumors typically arise in young women, but they occasionally are detected in children and in women over 60 years of age. The average age is 24 years, and 75% of patients are younger than 30.[133,307,308] Women with well-differentiated Sertoli-Leydig cell tumors average 40 years of age, 10 to 15 years older than those with the more common intermediate and poorly differentiated tumors.[133,307,308] Sertoli-Leydig cell tumors that contain areas of retiform differentiation develop in young patients; the average age is 16 years.[146,309,310]

About 50% of Sertoli-Leydig cell tumors are hormonally active.[133,307,308] These tumors cause symptoms that range from menstrual disorders to virilization. Common menstrual abnormalities include irregular bleeding, oligomenorrhea or amenorrhea, and, in older women, postmenopausal bleeding. Well-developed features of virilization are observed in about 40% of patients, who most typically have amenorrhea, deepening of the voice, and hirsutism. Other signs of virilization include temporal alopecia, hypertrophy of the clitoris, and acne. Serum levels of testosterone and urine levels of 17-ketosteroids are increased in virilized patients.

The 50% of patients whose tumors are not hormonally active present with nonspecific findings such as abdominal distention, abdominal mass, or abdominal pain. Five to 10% of patients present with acute abdominal symptoms caused by torsion or rupture of the tumor. Sertoli-Leydig cell tumors occasionally are discovered in asymptomatic women. Rare examples produce α-fetoprotein, which is useful as a tumor marker.[146,309–315]

At operation, Sertoli-Leydig cell tumors are nearly always confined to one ovary. Extraovarian spread is uncommon. Tumor rupture is an important adverse prognostic finding; it is detected in 5% to 15% of cases.[307]

Macroscopic Appearance. The well-differentiated Sertoli-Leydig cell tumor presents as an encapsulated unilateral mass 1.5 to 10 cm in diameter.[316] The average diameter is 5 cm. Well-differentiated tumors are generally solid and have a yellow or yellow-tan cut surface.

Intermediate and poorly differentiated tumors are larger. They range from small tumors less than 1 cm in diameter to large neoplasms 35 cm in diameter. The average diameter is 15 cm. Poorly differentiated tumors tend to be larger than those of intermediate differentiation, but there is considerable overlap. Most Sertoli-Leydig cell tumors are partly solid and partly cystic, but tumors that are mainly solid or mainly cystic are not uncommon. Solid areas vary from firm to soft and are gray-pink, yellow, or orange.

Microscopic Appearance. The *well-differentiated Sertoli-Leydig cell tumor* contains well-formed hollow or

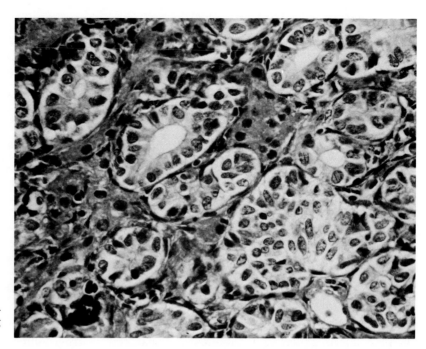

FIGURE 6-68 Well-differentiated Sertoli-Leydig cell tumor. Sertoli tubules and Leydig cells can be seen.

closed tubules lined by columnar Sertoli cells. These are admixed with large, polygonal cells with eosinophilic cytoplasm, compatible with Leydig cells (Fig. 6-68) and mature fibrous stroma. Crystals of Reinke are only rarely identified within the Leydig cells. Cytologic atypia and mitotic activity are minimal.

There are well-formed Sertoli tubules in some *intermediate and poorly differentiated Sertoli-Leydig cell tumors,* but in most tumors the Sertoli cells are organized in solid cords (Fig. 6-69). Retiform tubules are present in 10% to 25% of intermediate and poorly differentiated neoplasms and occasionally are the dominant histologic finding. Retiform tubules are long and branching and are lined by low columnar to cuboidal cells with scanty cytoplasm and hyper-

chromatic, oval nuclei (Fig. 6-70). Papillae often are present within retiform tubules. Mitotic figures generally are inconspicuous in tubular cells of all types, but there are numerous mitotic figures in occasional tumors with retiform tubules. Some tumors contain tubules lined by cytologically atypical Sertoli cells, but this does not appear to be of prognostic significance. The tubules are set in a background of immature gonadal stroma and Leydig cells. It is the presence of immature stroma that sets intermediate and poorly differentiated Sertoli-Leydig cell tumors apart from the well-differentiated neoplasms (Fig. 6-71).[133] The stroma is most prominent in poorly differentiated neoplasms, where it constitutes the bulk of the tumor. Sertoli tubules and Leydig cells are often inconspicuous in poorly differentiated neo-

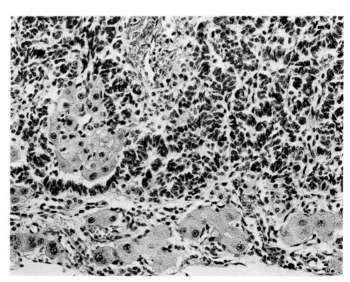

FIGURE 6-69 Intermediate Sertoli-Leydig cell tumor with clusters of Leydig cells and cord-like arrangements of Sertoli cells.

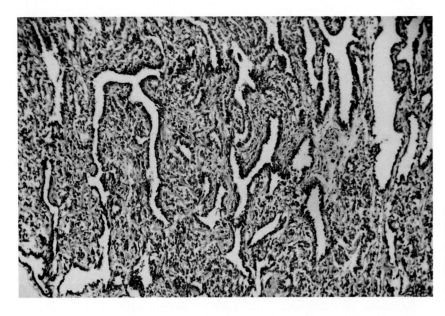

FIGURE 6-70 Retiform tubules in a Sertoli-Leydig cell tumor. The tubules are branching and are lined by cuboidal epithelial cells. (Zaloudek CJ, Norris HJ: Sertoli-Leydig tumors of the ovary: A clinicopathologic study of 64 intermediate and poorly differentiated neoplasms. Am J Surg Pathol 6:503–512, 1982)

plasms. There generally is minimal stromal cell atypia, but mitotic figures, which average 4 to 5 per 10 high-power fields, are easy to find. Heterologous elements are present in 20% to 25% of intermediate and poorly differentiated Sertoli-Leydig cell tumors. Mucinous epithelium of intestinal type is the most common of these (Fig. 6-72), but carcinoid, neuroblasts, cartilage, and striated muscle also have been described.[133,317,318]

The neoplastic Sertoli cells within the tubules react with antibodies to cytokeratin, whereas the stromal cells and Leydig cells, which are cytokeratin negative, react with antibodies to vimentin.[262,264] Rare Sertoli-Leydig cell tumors secrete α-fetoprotein. Immunostains for α-fetoprotein are positive in Leydig cells, Sertoli cells, or so-called hepatoid cells in such neoplasms.[312–315] The gastrointestinal epithelium in heterologous tumors contains cells that are argyrophilic and immunoreactive for chromogranin, serotonin, and peptides such as corticotropin, somatostatin, and calcitonin.[319] Testosterone is present in Leydig cells and in stromal cells and Sertoli cells.[320] There is immunoreactivity with antibodies against P-450 cytochromes in Leydig cells, Sertoli cells, and stromal cells, indicating that all are potential sites of steroidogenesis.[321]

Ultrastructural studies confirm that the Leydig cells are a source of hormone secretion. Leydig cells contain the prominent vesicular smooth endoplasmic reticulum and mitochondria with tubular cristae that characterize steroid hormone-producing cells.[322,323] Sertoli cells are surrounded by a basal lamina, and there are desmosomes between the cells. Their cytoplasm contains small mitochondria, rare smooth vesicles, and occasional microfilaments. Some cells contain lipid droplets.

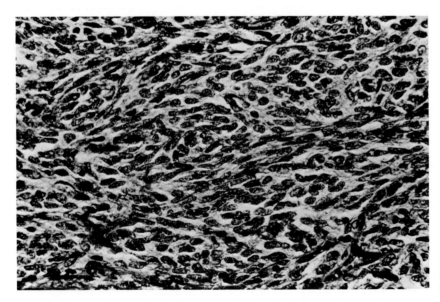

FIGURE 6-71 Immature gonadal stroma in a poorly differentiated Sertoli-Leydig cell tumor.

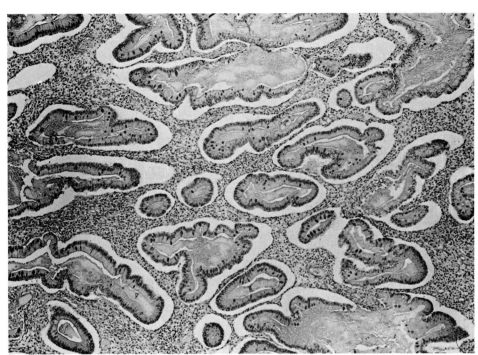

FIGURE 6-72 Sertoli-Leydig cell tumor: heterologous mucinous epithelium (mucicarmine stain).

Differential Diagnosis. The differential diagnosis of Sertoli-Leydig cell tumor includes granulosa cell tumor and unclassified sex cord/stromal tumors, endometrioid carcinoma, metastatic adenocarcinoma, and yolk sac tumor.

Granulosa cell tumor and Sertoli-Leydig cell tumor commonly contain small areas resembling the other tumor type. Well-formed tubules and Leydig cells are not seen in granulosa cell tumor, and the typical histologic patterns of granulosa cell tumor are not seen in a Sertoli-Leydig cell tumor. Heterologous differentiation is unique to the Sertoli-Leydig cell tumor. A small proportion of sex cord/stromal tumors are too poorly differentiated to designate except as unclassified sex cord/stromal tumors.

Endometrioid carcinoma can simulate a Sertoli-Leydig cell tumor, particularly when luteinized stromal cells are present within or around it.[185,186] These tumors occur in an older patient population and are hormonally inactive. They often are bilateral and associated with pelvic endometriosis. Sertoliform endometrioid carcinomas are mixed with more typical areas of endometrioid carcinoma, contain squamous metaplasia, and lack the immature stroma that characterizes a Sertoli-Leydig cell tumor.

Metastatic adenocarcinoma, particularly the tubular Krukenberg tumor, can raise the question of Sertoli-Leydig cell tumor.[324] Most cases of metastatic carcinoma are detected in older patients, and the metastatic deposits are multifocal and bilateral. The tubules are lined by cytologically malignant cells that exhibit a degree of nuclear atypia and mitotic activity not seen in the Sertoli cells lining the tubules of a Sertoli-Leydig cell tumor.

When a retiform tubular pattern is prominent, a Sertoli-Leydig cell tumor can be confused with a *yolk sac tumor,* or even with a serous epithelial tumor. The presence of virilizing clinical symptoms and of areas of more typical Sertoli-Leydig cell differentiation is helpful in arriving at the correct diagnosis. Yolk sac tumors have a primitive embryonal stroma and generally contain cells that exhibit greater cytologic atypia and mitotic activity than is seen in a Sertoli-Leydig cell tumor. Immunohistochemistry typically demonstrates α-fetoprotein in a yolk sac tumor, but rare Sertoli-Leydig cell tumors also contain this substance.

Clinical Behavior and Treatment. The treatment is mainly surgical. Unilateral salpingo-oophorectomy is sufficient in most cases.[133,307] Total abdominal hysterectomy is warranted in older patients and in those with unfavorable prognostic findings, such as rupture, extraovarian spread, a poorly differentiated neoplasm with frequent stromal cell mitoses, or heterologous mesenchymal differentiation (eg, cartilage or skeletal muscle, or foci of neuroblastoma).[133,307]

Well-differentiated Sertoli-Leydig cell tumors do not recur or metastasize after adequate excision.[133,316] Most intermediate and poorly differentiated Sertoli-Leydig cell tumors follow a benign clinical evolution, and excision of the neoplasm brings about disappearance of many of the symptoms of virilization and a return to normal hormonal activity. The 5-year survival in one report was 92%, whereas in another study 18% of the tumors were clinically malignant.[133,307] Most recurrences are detected within the first 5 years after treatment. Chemotherapy appears beneficial in about half of the patients who receive it.[280,307]

Leydig Cell Tumor

Nearly all ovarian Leydig cell tumors arise in the hilus of the ovary, presumably from hilus cells.[36,325] Leydig cell tumors in this location are sometimes referred to as *hilus cell tumors.* Occasional Leydig cell tumors originate from the ovarian stroma and are designated as *non-hilar* or *stromal Leydig cell tumors.*[37,38,40]

Clinical Findings. Most Leydig cell tumors are discovered in postmenopausal women; the average age is 58 years.[36,325] The typical clinical presentation is with hirsutism or true masculinization (ie, acne, masculine voice, and clitoral hypertrophy), which regresses after resection of the tumor. Serum levels of testosterone are elevated, but levels of urinary 17-ketosteroids generally are within normal limits.[36] Amenorrhea is common in premenopausal women, and older women frequently have postmenopausal bleeding. Study of the endometrium reveals hyperplasia in a high percentage of cases, a finding that is most likely secondary to peripheral conversion of testosterone to estrogen. In many cases, symptoms are present for several years before the diagnosis is established. Leydig cell tumors usually are too small to be palpable. They are detected because of the hormonal symptoms that they cause or are an incidental finding at operation for some other reason.

Macroscopic Appearance. These neoplasms present as small spherical brown or yellow-brown masses situated in the ovarian hilus or, rarely, in the medulla and cortex. They are poorly delimited from surrounding tissues and are of homogeneous consistency. The average diameter is 3 to 5 cm, with tumors as small as 0.7 cm and as large as 15 cm having been reported. Virtually all are unilateral.

Microscopic Appearance. Hilar Leydig cell tumors are unencapsulated and are composed of round or polygonal cells that are similar to the hilus cells present in the normal ovary.[36,325] Neoplastic cells are sometimes increased in size and are irregular in shape. Their nucleus is small, round, and hyperchromatic. The cytoplasm is granular and eosinophilic (Fig. 6-73). Some cells contain lipid droplets, and many contain yellow-brown lipochrome pigment, which is responsible for the color of the tumor. Reinke crystals are rod-like structures with round or square ends (Fig. 6-74). These can be identified in the cytoplasm of the tumor cells in about 50% of hilar Leydig cell tumors. The cytoplasm often contains round, eosinophilic, hyaline spheres.

There are two types of non-hilar Leydig cell tumors. Pure *non-hilar Leydig cell tumors* are composed exclusively of Leydig cells.[37] *Stromal Leydig cell tumors* contain Leydig cells mixed with a fibromatous or thecomatous stromal component.[38,40] By definition, crystals of Reinke must be identified within tumor cell cytoplasm for diagnosis of a non-hilar Leydig cell tumor. Because only 50% of hilar Leydig cell tumors contain crystals, some non-hilar Leydig cell tumors undoubtedly are unrecognized and are classified as stromal luteoma[326] or luteinized thecoma.[40]

Electron microscopic studies reveal abundant agranular endoplasmic reticulum and many large mitochondria. The crystals of Reinke are composed of a protein lattice, and the intracellular pigment granules appear similar to those of testicular Leydig cells.[327–329]

Differential Diagnosis. The main differential diagnostic consideration in hilar Leydig cell tumor is *hilus cell hyperplasia.* Hilus cell hyperplasia is typically bilateral and does not form a visible tumor.

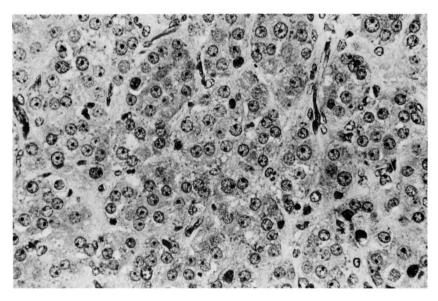

FIGURE 6-73 Hilar Leydig cell tumor composed of uniform polygonal cells.

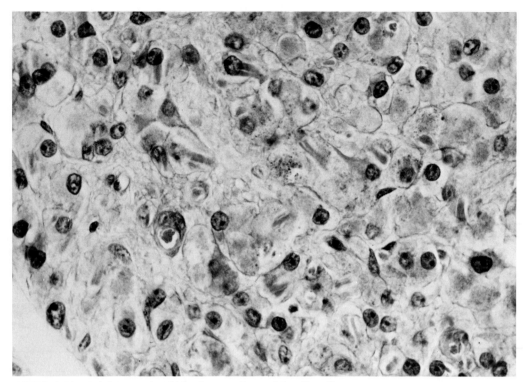

FIGURE 6-74 Reinke crystals within the cytoplasm of Leydig cells.

Microscopically, hilus cell hyperplasia is multinodular and bears a normal relation to the nerves in the ovarian hilus. Hilar Leydig cell tumors are unilateral and grossly visible, and they displace normal hilar structures. Non-hilar Leydig cell tumors must be differentiated from *stromal luteoma*[326] and stromal Leydig cell tumors from *luteinized thecoma*.[40] This distinction rests on the identification of crystals of Reinke within Leydig cells in Leydig cell tumors.

Clinical Behavior and Treatment. Malignant Leydig cell tumors are rare; only two cases have been reported.[36,325] Virtually all Leydig cell tumors are clinically benign and are cured by surgical excision.[36–38,40,325]

Stromal Luteoma

The stromal luteoma is an uncommon neoplasm that occurs predominantly in postmenopausal women.[326] Most patients have abnormal uterine bleeding, and an endometrial biopsy often reveals hyperplasia. Rare stromal luteomas are virilizing. One third of these tumors are an incidental finding at operation or autopsy. The stromal luteoma is a small unilateral neoplasm; all reported examples are less than 3 cm in diameter. The cut surface is gray, white, yellow, or brown. The tumor is located in the ovarian stroma and is composed of cells that resemble Leydig cells. They are polygonal, with granular eosinophilic cytoplasm and small, round, centrally placed nuclei. Dif-

ferentiation from a Leydig cell tumor is based on the non-hilar location of the stromal luteoma and on the absence of cytoplasmic crystals of Reinke. Other ovarian abnormalities typically are present, including stromal hyperthecosis, which is often bilateral, and hilus cell hyperplasia. The stromal luteoma is a benign neoplasm.

Sertoli Cell Tumor

Pure Sertoli cell tumors are rare. They differ from Sertoli-Leydig cell tumor by virtue of the absence of Leydig cells and of immature gonadal stroma.

Clinical Findings. Sertoli cell tumors most often arise in women of reproductive age. Most patients are in their mid-30s, but these neoplasms can occur in children and postmenopausal women.[330,331] Two thirds of the tumors are hormonally active. Of these, 70% secrete estrogen and 30% produce androgens. Patients with hormone-secreting neoplasms present with irregular bleeding, precocious pseudopuberty, or virilization, depending on their age and the type and amount of hormone that is secreted. The one third of patients with hormonally inactive neoplasms have nonspecific symptoms such as pain or abdominal swelling. Small tumors may be incidental findings.

Macroscopic Appearance. Sertoli cell tumors are unilateral, circumscribed tumors with an average diameter of 5 to 7 cm. Their cut surfaces are fleshy and tan or yellow, with cysts present in some neoplasms.

Microscopic Appearance. These neoplasms are composed of Sertoli cells and a supporting connective tissue framework. Leydig cells and immature stromal cells are absent. The Sertoli cells are columnar, with small, round to oval nuclei and granular eosinophilic or clear cytoplasm. They line elongated tubules or are arranged in solid cords that are two or three cells thick. This arrangement is referred to as a *simple tubular pattern* in contrast to the *complex tubular pattern* that is more characteristic of the closely related sex cord tumor with annular tubules. Some Sertoli cell tumors are composed of tubules that are lined by cells with abundant, clear, lipid-rich cytoplasm (Fig. 6-75). Such neoplasms are referred to as *lipid-rich Sertoli cell tumors.*

Clinical Behavior and Treatment. Most Sertoli cell tumors have a benign evolution and are treated adequately by unilateral salpingo-oophorectomy.[330,331] Rare poorly differentiated or invasive neoplasms recur or metastasize and cause the patient's death.

Sex Cord Tumor With Annular Tubules

The sex cord tumor with annular tubules (SCTAT) is designated as an unclassified sex cord/stromal tumor because the most appropriate classification is a point of controversy. Some authors view the SCTAT as a granulosa cell tumor,[332–335] whereas others consider it to be a variant of the Sertoli cell tumor.[330,336]

Clinical Findings. The SCTAT occurs in two clinical settings. First, about one third occur in women with the *Peutz-Jeghers syndrome,* a hereditary condition characterized by the presence of mucocutaneous melanin pigmentation and hamartomatous intestinal polyps.[333,337] Virtually all female patients with this syndrome have SCTATs, which are usually microscopic, multicentric, and bilateral. Most are asymptomatic and are discovered incidentally. SCTATs also occur in patients who do not have the Peutz-Jeghers syndrome.[330,333,334,337,338] In the latter setting, the neoplasms are discovered in patients 6 to 76 years of age. The average age is 36 years.[337] Premenarchal girls may have precocious pseudopuberty.[333,337] Older patients frequently have menstrual dysfunction or postmenopausal bleeding, depending on their age. An adnexal mass is palpable in about 50% of patients. A novel assay for müllerian-inhibiting substance revealed an increased serum level of that substance in one patient with a SCTAT.[253] SCTATs that are not associated with the Peutz-Jeghers syndrome generally are unilateral, solitary, and grossly apparent.

Macroscopic Appearance. In patients with the Peutz-Jeghers syndrome, the neoplasms are small and sometimes microscopic. They are multifocal, frequently bilateral, tan or yellow solid tumors (Color Figure 6-15). Foci of calcification are often present. Neoplasms that are not associated with the Peutz-Jeghers syndrome vary more in appearance, ranging from less than 1 cm to 20 cm in diameter, with fleshy, tan, or yellow cut surfaces.

Microscopic Appearance. SCTATs are composed of simple or, more frequently, complex annular tubules set in a fibrous stroma (Fig. 6-76). The tumor cells are columnar, with clear cytoplasm and hyperchromatic, round, basal nuclei (Fig. 6-77). Atypia and mitotic figures are rare. Tubular lumina are often absent. In solid areas, apposed columnar tumor cells have a paired arrangement, with their nuclei located at opposite poles of the cells. Round cores of hyaline material are present within the nests of cells, and similar material may form part of the stroma of larger neoplasms.

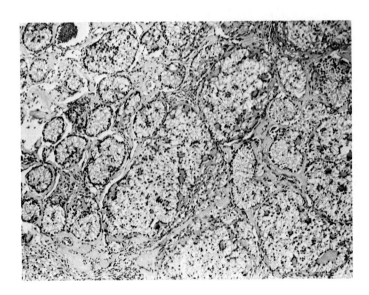

FIGURE 6-75 Sertoli cell tumor with abundant lipid-rich cytoplasm.

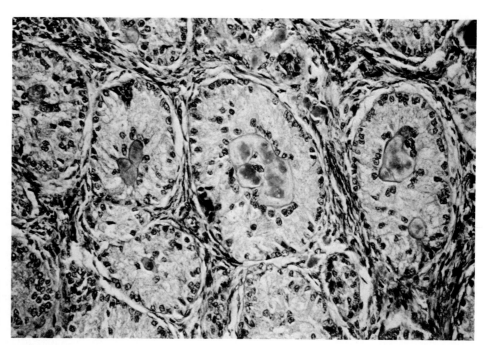

FIGURE 6-76 This sex cord tumor with annular tubules had the characteristic multifocal pattern of tumors associated with Peutz-Jeghers syndrome.

The immunocytochemical features of the SCTAT have not been characterized adequately, but many cases have been studied with the electron microscope.[330,332,334-336,339] Basement membrane material surrounds tumor cell nests and fills the central spaces within the nests, forming the hyaline cores seen by light microscopy. Most tumor cells contain cytoplasmic filaments. Some authors interpret bundles of filaments as Charcot-Böttcher filaments and conclude that SCTATs are Sertoli cell tumors.[330,336,339] Others do not identify Charcot-Böttcher filaments and interpret the ultrastructure as most compatible with that of a granulosa cell tumor.[332,334,335]

Cytologically, the SCTAT resembles a granulosa cell tumor. The tumor cells are small, with uniform nuclei and scanty pale cytoplasm. They are arranged singly, in trabeculae, in solid groups, or in rosette-like structures. The latter are reminiscent of the Call-Exner body seen in granulosa cell tumor. Hyaline cores, if present within the rosettes, may provide a clue to the correct diagnosis.[340]

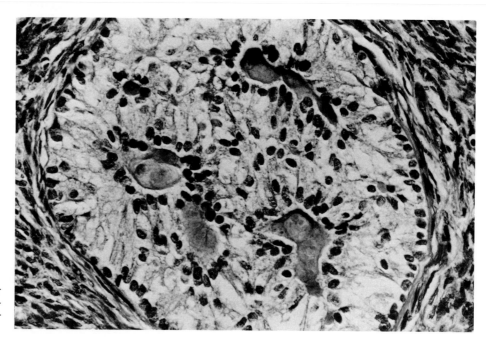

FIGURE 6-77 Sex cord tumor with annular tubules showing hyaline deposits and antipodal arrangement of cells.

Clinical Behavior and Treatment. The SCTAT is almost invariably an incidental finding in patients with the Peutz-Jeghers syndrome. The tumors are too small to palpate, and they rarely produce sufficient estrogen to cause symptoms. No treatment is necessary for asymptomatic patients.[337] Some patients with Peutz-Jeghers syndrome develop minimal deviation adenocarcinoma of the endocervix, so lifetime surveillance by a gynecologist is appropriate. A second, extremely rare sex cord/stromal tumor of the ovary occurs in children with Peutz-Jeghers syndrome and causes sexual precocity.[341]

In patients who do not have the Peutz-Jeghers syndrome, SCTAT is unilateral. Young women with localized disease (stage IA) can be treated by salpingo-oophorectomy. Older women and those with more advanced tumors are treated by hysterectomy and bilateral salpingo-oophorectomy. About 15% of SCTATs not associated with Peutz-Jeghers syndrome are clinically malignant.[337,338] It is difficult to predict which tumors will metastasize, but those in which frequent mitotic figures or stromal invasion are identified should be regarded with suspicion.

Lipid Cell Tumors (Steroid Cell Tumors)

Lipid cell or steroid cell tumors are a heterogeneous group of stromal tumors that cannot be more specifically classified. Most of the tumors in this group are composed of a mixture of cells resembling Leydig cells and cells resembling adrenal cortical cells.[342,343]

Clinical Findings. Lipid cell tumors occur in patients 3 to 80 years of age. The average age is 45 years. Most patients are virilized or hirsute. Other presentations include abdominal swelling or pain, menstrual dysfunction, or postmenopausal bleeding. Levels of urinary 17-ketosteroids and serum testosterone typically are elevated.[342,343] Most tumors are confined to the ovaries at diagnosis, and bilateral tumors are rare (6% of cases).[342] Pelvic, peritoneal, or distant metastases are present in 10% to 20% of patients.[342,343]

Macroscopic Appearance. Lipid cell tumors range from less than 1 cm to more than 20 cm in diameter. The average size is about 7 cm. Most are solid and have tan, yellow, or orange cut surfaces. Hemorrhage and necrosis are present in less than 25% of lipid cell tumors.

Microscopic Appearance. Some tumor cells resemble Leydig cells except that crystals of Reinke are not present. These cells are polygonal, with abundant eosinophilic cytoplasm and central round nuclei that contain a small nucleolus. The second major cell type resembles an adrenal cortical cell and has abundant vacuolated pale cytoplasm and a central vesicular nucleus (Fig. 6-78). A mixture of these two cell types is typical, but one or the other may predominate. Fat stains are positive in most adrenal-type cells. Mitotic figures are infrequent in lipid cell tumors, and nuclear atypia is absent or modest. Markedly atypical cells and frequent mitotic figures are observed in a minority of cases.

Immunohistochemical analysis for steroidogenic enzymes reveals intense staining of the tumor cells, which is compatible with steroid production.[321] Electron microscopic study provides evidence of steroid production within the tumor cells.[344] They contain abundant smooth endoplasmic reticulum, numerous mitochondria with tubular cristae, lipid droplets, and dense lysosomal bodies.

Clinical Behavior and Treatment. Young patients with stage IA neoplasms can be treated by salpingo-oophorectomy. Older patients and those with advanced tumors are treated by hysterectomy and bilateral salpingo-oophorectomy. Hirsutism and signs of virilization generally regress after removal of the

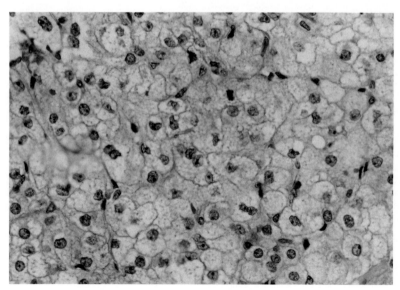

FIGURE 6-78 Lipid cell tumor: adrenal type cells with abundant foamy cytoplasm.

tumor. A significant proportion of lipid cell tumors (25% to 43%) are clinically malignant.[342,343] Recurrences generally are detected within the first several years after initial treatment, but about 20% are not detected for 5 years or more.[342] Pathologic features that help identify malignant lipid cell tumors include large size, the presence of hemorrhage or necrosis, 2 or more mitotic figures per 10 high-power fields, and moderate or marked nuclear atypia.

Gynandroblastoma

The gynandroblastoma is a rare ovarian tumor in which there are substantial areas of "testicular" (Sertoli cell or Sertoli-Leydig cell) and granulosa cell differentiation. Only about a dozen cases are well documented in the literature.[345–347] Clinically, most patients with gynandroblastoma have symptoms of masculinization. The tumor is unilateral and 1 to 18 cm in diameter.[345] The exterior is smooth, and the cut surface is cystic and multilocular, with interspersed solid white or yellow areas of variable prominence. Microscopically, tubular and cord-like structures similar to those seen in a well-differentiated Sertoli or Sertoli-Leydig cell tumor are present in intimate relation with solid nests and sheets of typical granulosa cells, within which Call-Exner bodies frequently are found. The stroma may be inconspicuous or may consist of spindle-shaped cells resembling theca cells. Occasional luteinized cells or Leydig cells are seen. All elements of the tumor are well differentiated, and cytologic atypia is minimal. All gynandroblastomas thus far reported have been clinically benign. The treatment is surgical excision.

Other Nonepithelial Tumors

Nonspecific Mesenchymal Tumors

Virtually any type of soft tissue tumor can arise in the ovary. These tumors do not differ in appearance or behavior from similar neoplasms that occur elsewhere in the body. Smooth muscle tumors are the most common mesenchymal tumors of the ovary. Most are benign leiomyomas,[348,349] but leiomyosarcoma[350–352] is sometimes observed. The lipoleiomyoma is an unusual neoplasm composed of fat and smooth muscle.[353,354] Hemangioma and myxoma are other types of benign soft tissue tumor that are seen in the ovary.[355–357] Primary sarcomas of the ovary are rare.[221,358] This group includes fibrosarcoma and endometrial stromal sarcoma, which were discussed earlier in this chapter, and rhabdomyosarcoma,[359] chondrosarcoma,[360] osteosarcoma,[361] and malignant schwannoma.[362]

Malignant Lymphoma

Less than 1% of women with lymphoma have the initial presentation of their disease in the ovary.[363] Such women present with an abdominal or pelvic mass or pelvic pain and have unilateral or bilateral ovarian tumors at laparotomy. Extraovarian lymphoma is observed at operation or shortly thereafter in most cases, indicating that ovarian lymphoma is usually part of a disseminated disease process. A few long-term survivors treated only by oophorectomy never develop extraovarian lymphoma, indicating that rare cases of primary ovarian lymphoma do occur.[363–365] Both ovaries are involved in more than 50% of cases. The tumors measure 2 cm to more than 20 cm in diameter, with an average diameter of about 15 cm. The cut surface is fleshy and pink, tan, or gray. Microscopically, all ovarian lymphomas are of the non-Hodgkin's type; Hodgkin's disease is not reported in the ovary.[363–366]

Small non-cleaved cell lymphoma of Burkitt's or non-Burkitt's type occurs with greatest frequency in children and young women and is characterized by a diffuse proliferation of small non-cleaved lymphoid cells. Mitotic figures are frequent, and phagocytic histiocytes often are present in large numbers, producing the starry-sky appearance typical of this lymphoma.

Large cell lymphoma is most common in adults. It is diffuse and composed of large cleaved or non-cleaved lymphoid cells or of immunoblasts (Fig. 6-79). The latter have vesicular nuclei with a prominent nucleolus and a moderate amount of basophilic cytoplasm. Lymphoma of the ovary rarely exhibits a follicular pattern. All immunophenotyped ovarian lymphomas have been of B-cell type.[367,368] Survival depends on the clinical stage and the histologic type of the lymphoma.[363–366] *Leukemia* can involve the ovary, and a few examples of *granulocytic sarcoma* of the ovary have been reported.

Small Cell Carcinoma

Small cell carcinoma is a biologically aggressive neoplasm of uncertain histogenesis that occurs predominantly in young women.[369–374]

Clinical Features. Small cell carcinoma occurs in women 13 to 55 years of age, but most of these tumors arise in young women who are younger than 30.[370–372] The average age is 25 years. The typical clinical presentation is with abdominal pain, nausea or vomiting, or an abdominal mass. About two thirds of patients have hypercalcemia, but this is rarely responsible for the presenting symptoms. Most tumors are confined to the ovary at diagnosis, though extraovarian spread is not unusual. Bilateral tumors are uncommon except in patients with extensive intra-abdominal tumor dissemination.

Macroscopic Appearance. Small cell carcinoma measures 8 to 27 cm, with an average diameter of 15 cm. It is a solid, nodular, gray or tan tumor that contains small cysts. Zones of hemorrhage and necrosis are common.

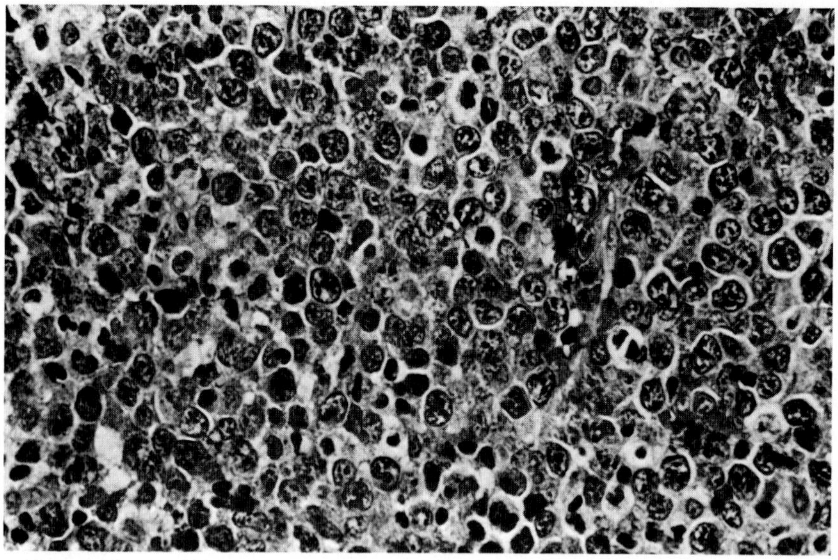

FIGURE 6-79 Large cell lymphoma involving the ovary.

Microscopic Appearance. Most tumors are composed of uniform small cells with round, oval, or fusiform nuclei and scanty cytoplasm (Color Figure 6-16). The nuclei are hyperchromatic, but the chromatin is fine. Nucleoli, if present, are small. Nuclear grooves are uncommon. There are frequent mitotic figures. Irregular follicle-like structures filled with lightly eosinophilic material are a characteristic finding in small cell carcinoma. There is focal or extensive variation from the typical morphology in one third of these neoplasms. Some tumors contain a malignant spindle cell component, and others contain large cells with abundant eosinophilic cytoplasm and vesicular nuclei with prominent nucleoli.[369,372]

Immunohistochemical testing for low-molecular-weight cytokeratins generally is positive.[261,372] One third of small cell carcinomas are immunoreactive for epithelial membrane antigen, and more than half react with antibodies against vimentin.[261,372] Neuron-specific enolase is positive in more than two thirds of small cell carcinomas, and occasional tumors are immunoreactive for parathyroid hormone.[261,371] Testing for α-fetoprotein is negative, but there is focal weak reactivity with antibodies against α1-antitrypsin in some tumors.[372]

Ultrastructurally, small cell carcinoma has features of an epithelial neoplasm.[370-373] Groups of tumor cells are delimited by a discontinuous basal lamina, and there are desmosome-like junctions between adjacent cells. Lumina are rare, and the cells lining them have microvilli. The nuclei frequently are indented, and some contain nucleoli. The most characteristic ultrastructural feature is the presence of prominent, dilated cisterns of rough endoplasmic reticulum filled with amorphous, moderately electron-dense material. Phagolysosomes, polyribosomes, and mitochondria are noted. Dense-core neurosecretory granules were observed in 3 of 4 tumors studied by one group,[371] but were not detected by others,[370,372,373] despite a careful search for them.

The morphology is variously interpreted as suggesting that small cell carcinoma is a type of sex cord stromal tumor,[373] a neuroendocrine tumor,[371] or a germ cell tumor related to yolk sac tumor.[372] The histogenesis is uncertain, and small cell carcinoma is designated as an unclassified ovarian carcinoma.

Differential Diagnosis. The main differential diagnostic considerations are malignant lymphoma and juvenile granulosa cell tumor. In contrast to small cell carcinoma, *lymphoma* is commonly bilateral and frequently involves the abdominal lymph nodes or the spleen. Immunohistochemical staining is helpful, because lymphoma reacts with leukocyte common antigen and various B-cell antibodies, whereas small cell carcinoma reacts with cytokeratin and neuron-specific enolase.

The differentiation from *juvenile granulosa cell tumor* can be difficult, particularly if macrofollicular structures are present in the tumor. Juvenile granulosa cell tumor frequently produces estrogenic symptoms, whereas small cell carcinoma causes hypercalcemia. Luteinized tumor cells are not present in small cell carcinoma. The pattern of immunoreactivity of the neoplasm can be helpful. Juvenile granulosa cell tumor is more likely to be vimentin positive, and small cell carcinoma is more likely to be cytokeratin positive or to exhibit a positive reaction for epithelial membrane antigen.[261] Both neoplasms are immunoreactive for neuron-specific enolase.[261] The demonstration by electron microscopy of dilated rough endoplasmic reticulum containing amorphous material favors a diagnosis of small cell carcinoma.

Undifferentiated carcinoma occasionally is considered in the differential diagnosis. It occurs in older women, is more pleomorphic, and usually contains some foci of differentiated epithelial carcinoma. *Metastatic small cell carcinoma* of bronchial or other origin lacks follicular structures, occurs in older women, is usually bilateral, and contains dense-core neurosecretory granules that are revealed by electron microscopy.

Clinical Behavior and Treatment. Small cell carcinoma is an aggressive neoplasm with high mortality even when disease is localized at diagnosis.[369] Although the average patient is young, the optimal surgical treatment probably is hysterectomy with bilateral salpingo-oophorectomy. There is no effective adjuvant treatment. The response to radiation therapy or chemotherapy is limited,[370,374] and overall survival is less than 20%.[370–372,374]

Germ Cell Tumors

Tumors derived directly from germ cells include dysgerminoma and embryonal carcinoma. Germ cell tumors also include those tumors derived indirectly from germ cells by embryonic (eg, teratoma) or extraembryonic (eg, choriocarcinoma and yolk sac tumor) differentiation (Table 6-6). Benign cystic teratomas are among the most common ovarian tumors.[243] Malignant germ cell tumors are rare and occur most often in children and in women younger than 30 years.

Dysgerminoma

Dysgerminoma is the most common malignant germ cell tumor of the ovary.[243,244,375,376] Nevertheless, it is a rare neoplasm, accounting for only 1% to 2% of all malignant ovarian tumors.

Clinical Features. Dysgerminoma develops mainly in children and young women.[18,377–381] Nearly all patients are between 5 and 55 years of age. The average age is 22 years, and 85% to 90% of patients are 30 years of age or younger.[382]

The clinical presentation is nonspecific. The

TABLE 6-6
Germ Cell Tumors

Dysgerminoma
Yolk sac tumor (endodermal sinus tumor)
Embryonal carcinoma
Polyembryoma
Choriocarcinoma
Teratoma
  Immature
  Mature
    Solid
    Cystic (dermoid cyst)
  Monodermal
    Struma ovarii
    Carcinoid
    Neuroectodermal tumor
Mixed germ cell tumor
Gonadoblastoma

most common symptoms are abdominal mass, increasing abdominal girth, and abdominal pain.[377,378,381,383] Twenty percent of patients have menstrual abnormalities.[379] Hormonally active tumors are rare, and patients with these tumors have secondary amenorrhea and increased levels of human chorionic gonadotropin.[384,385] Some patients with dysgerminoma have elevated levels of serum lactic dehydrogenase, which can serve as a useful tumor marker.[386,387] Levels of serum α-fetoprotein are within normal limits.[386] The average duration of symptoms before diagnosis is about 5 months.[378] Dysgerminoma is the most frequent malignant neoplasm arising in patients with gonadal dysgenesis.[380,382,388]

Most patients with dysgerminoma have localized disease. Tumor is confined to the ovaries (stage I) in 70% to 80% of cases.[377,378,381,386] Dysgerminoma is typically unilateral, but in contrast to other types of malignant germ cell tumors, bilateral growth (stage IB) occurs in 5% to 10% of cases.[377,381] Involvement of the contralateral ovary can be detected only by microscopic examination in about 50% of the bilateral cases. Biopsy of a grossly normal contralateral ovary is therefore frequently recommended if treatment is to be by unilateral salpingo-oophorectomy.[377,389] Dysgerminoma metastasizes by way of the lymphatics to the para-aortic lymph nodes.[380,386]

Macroscopic Appearance. Dysgerminoma occurs more frequently in the right ovary than in the left.[382] It is a firm, nodular tumor with smooth surfaces. It is usually large when detected, with an average diameter of 15 cm. The cut surface is fleshy and gray, tan, or white (Color Figure 6-17). Some tumors have a lobulated appearance. Hemorrhage and necrosis are common in large tumors.

Microscopic Appearance. The microscopic appearance is identical to that of seminoma of the testis. The tumor cells are medium-sized and polyhedral with round, vesicular nuclei that have reticular chromatin and prominent nucleoli. Mitotic figures are frequent. The cytoplasm, which is best preserved in tissue fixed in Bouin's or B-5 fixative, is abundant and clear or granular (Fig. 6-80). Cytoplasmic glycogen is found in some tumors. The tumor cells grow in cords or irregular nests separated by fibrous septa (Fig. 6-81). A lymphocytic infiltrate, located predominantly within the septa, is a consistent finding. Lymphoid follicles with germinal centers may be present. Epithelioid cells, multinucleated giant cells, and granulomas are seen in some tumors. Rarely, a granulomatous or fibrous reaction is extensive enough to obscure the underlying neoplastic cells. Zones of necrosis are found in some neoplasms, especially the large ones. Neoplasms in which the degree of atypia is greater than usual and in which there is a high mitotic rate (more than 30 mitotic figures per 10 high-power fields) have been termed *anaplastic dysgerminoma* by some authors; however, the prog-

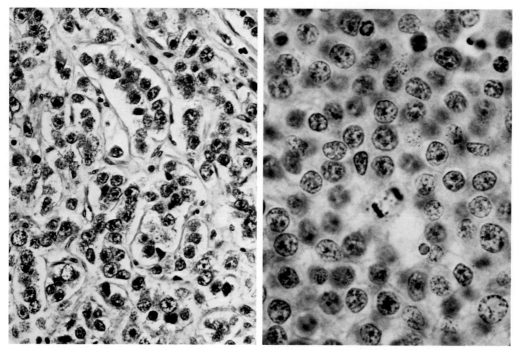

FIGURE 6-80 Dysgerminoma. Note the vesicular nuclei and clear cytoplasm.

nosis in such cases is comparable to that of typical dysgerminoma.[378] About 5% of dysgerminomas contain syncytiotrophoblastic giant cells (Fig. 6-82). No other nondysgerminomatous differentiation is found in these tumors, which are termed *dysgerminoma with syncytiotrophoblastic giant cells.*[385]

The immunohistochemistry of dysgerminoma is similar to that of testicular seminoma. Monoclonal antibodies against cytokeratin are particularly useful because germinoma cells give a negative reaction, whereas embryonal carcinoma, yolk sac tumor, and surface epithelial carcinomas exhibit positive cyto-

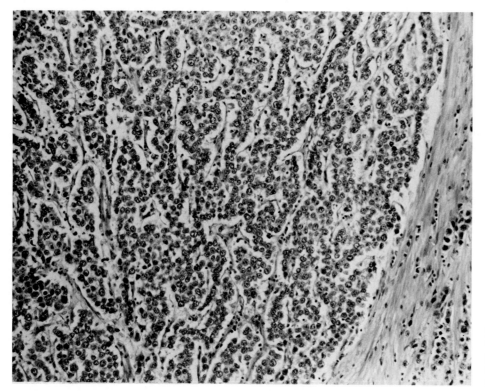

FIGURE 6-81 Dysgerminoma. This microscopic pattern shows the characteristic nests of germinoma cells separated by delicate fibrous septa.

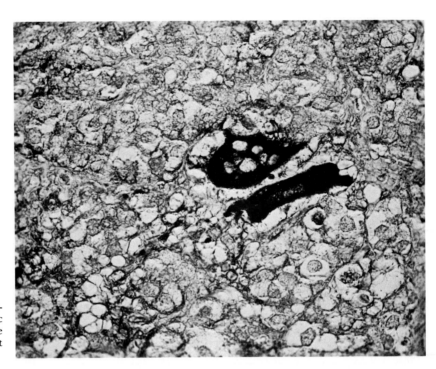

FIGURE 6-82 Dysgerminoma. An immunocytochemical reaction for human chorionic gonadotropin yields a positive reaction in the cytoplasm of the syncytiotrophoblastic giant cells.

plasmic staining.[390] Germinoma cells exhibit a positive reaction for placental alkaline phosphatase, as do other types of malignant germ cell tumors.[391,392] The syncytiotrophoblastic giant cells that rarely occur in dysgerminoma exhibit positive cytoplasmic staining for human chorionic gonadotropin.[385] Barring one exceptional case, the mononuclear germinoma cells are negative for human chorionic gonadotropin.[393] Immunostains for α-fetoprotein are negative.

Ultrastructurally, dysgerminoma cells most closely resemble oogonia.[394] They are polygonal with round central nuclei, prominent irregular nucleoli, and sparse cytoplasmic organelles. The cytoplasm contains scattered polyribosomes, annulate lamellae, scattered lysosomes, and aggregates of glycogen. There are rare desmosome-like attachments between cells.

Dysgerminoma has a characteristic cytologic appearance.[395,396] Tumor cells are found singly and in small sheets. They have large round nuclei with prominent nucleoli and a moderate amount of clear (alcohol-fixed) or basophilic (air-dried) cytoplasm (Color Figure 6-18). There is a characteristic basophilic, striated background in fine-needle aspirates that is best appreciated in air-dried smears. Lymphocytes and, in some cases, epithelioid cells are admixed with the dysgerminoma cells.

Ploidy analysis of dysgerminoma reveals that there are no diploid tumors.[397] Most dysgerminomas are aneuploid, but a sizable minority have a DNA index around 2 and may be polyploid. There is no correlation between the ploidy and the prognosis.

Differential Diagnosis. Dysgerminoma has a characteristic microscopic appearance, and most cases are easily recognized. The differential diagnosis includes embryonal carcinoma, clear cell carcinoma, malignant lymphoma, and metastatic malignant melanoma.

Patients with *embryonal carcinoma* frequently have symptoms caused by tumor secretion of human chorionic gonadotropin.[398] The tumor cells have irregular, pleomorphic nuclei. They grow in cohesive sheets and may form abortive glands. Immunostains for cytokeratin and α-fetoprotein are positive in mononuclear tumor cells. Syncytiotrophoblastic giant cells are almost always present in embryonal carcinoma, but they are rarely seen in dysgerminoma. There is no lymphocytic or granulomatous infiltrate. Ovarian embryonal carcinoma is a much rarer tumor than dysgerminoma.

Clear cell carcinoma occurs in an older age group than dysgerminoma and is more frequently bilateral. Carcinoma cells are more cohesive and frequently form glands and papillae. Immunostains for cytokeratin and other epithelial markers are positive.

Lymphoma may occur in the same age group as dysgerminoma.[363–365,399] Involvement of the ovaries is generally secondary; bilateral ovarian involvement is associated with lymphadenopathy or involvement of other extranodal sites. Malignant lymphocytes are smaller than dysgerminoma cells, and the nuclei contain coarse chromatin clumps and have less prominent nucleoli. Lymphoma cells infiltrate the ovarian stroma and surround, but often do not displace, normal ovarian structures. The fibrous septa that are characteristic of dysgerminoma are not present. Immunostains for leukocyte common antigen are positive, and the presence of other lymphocyte antigens usually can be demonstrated.

Metastatic melanoma most often is bilateral and multinodular.[400] Melanoma cells frequently have prominent eosinophilic macronucleoli and intranuclear inclusions of cytoplasm. The amphophilic or eosinophilic cytoplasm may contain melanin pigment. Positive immunostains using the HMB-45 antibody and antibodies against S-100 protein are of great assistance in correctly identifying melanoma.

Clinical Behavior and Treatment. Dysgerminoma has a favorable prognosis; the 5-year survival rate exceeds 90%.[377,379,380,383] Until recently, dysgerminoma was treated by surgical removal of the tumor followed by radiation of the pelvis and para-aortic lymph nodes. This treatment gave excellent results even in patients with extraovarian tumor spread.[378,401] Patients with unilateral encapsulated dysgerminoma (stage IA) have an excellent prognosis when treated by unilateral salpingo-oophorectomy without any adjuvant therapy.[377,381] This is the preferred treatment for such patients, who have a 5-year survival rate of greater than 95%.[386,389] Some authorities advocate biopsy of the contralateral ovary even if it appears normal because of the risk (about 5%) of occult dysgerminoma.[377] There is a slightly increased risk of local recurrence with conservative therapy, but survival is not compromised because relapses can be treated effectively.[377,379] Most recurrences are detected within 2 years, with a maximum time to recurrence of 4 years.[379,402] The standard treatment for advanced disease (stage >IA) is total abdominal hysterectomy, bilateral salpingo-oophorectomy, limited debulking, and additional treatment with chemotherapy or radiation therapy. If preservation of fertility is of paramount importance, the uterus and one ovary, if uninvolved by tumor, may be conserved.[386] Chemotherapy, especially cisplatin-based regimens, is highly effective against dysgerminoma.[403,404] The combination of bleomycin, etoposide, and cisplatin, for example, was used successfully to treat more than 90% of patients with advanced (stage III and IV) dysgerminoma.[405] Chemotherapy is more effective than radiation therapy if there is bulky tumor or if there are multiple sites of involvement. Normal menses and pregnancy are possible after radiation therapy,[378,379] but chemotherapy may pose less risk of infertility.[386,406] Chemotherapy will probably replace radiation therapy as the first-line postsurgical treatment for dysgerminoma, except when there are only small localized masses of recurrent or residual disease.[386]

Yolk Sac Tumor (Endodermal Sinus Tumor)

Yolk sac tumor is the second most common malignant germ cell tumor of the ovary. It constitutes about 1% of ovarian cancers.[375] Originally described as a tumor of mesonephric origin, it is now known to develop by differentiation of malignant germ cells into extraembryonic yolk sac structures.[407,408]

Clinical Features. Yolk sac tumors occur almost exclusively in children and young women.[409–413] Patients generally are between 5 and 45 years of age; the median age is 19 years. The tumor occurs infrequently in women older than 45.

The clinical signs are nonspecific. Most patients complain of abdominal pain.[411] Abdominal distention or a palpable abdominal mass is commonly noted.[413] About one third of patients have a fever of unexplained origin.[409] Tumor rupture or torsion produces acute abdominal symptoms in 10% of patients. Abnormal vaginal bleeding is an uncommon symptom that occurs in only about 5% of cases. The duration of symptoms is typically short, ranging from days in patients with acute abdominal symptoms to 3 months.[412] Alpha-fetoprotein is detected in the serum of most patients with yolk sac tumors.[409,412,414] Some patients have increased levels of CA-125 antigen.[414]

About 50% of patients have tumor confined to the ovary at diagnosis.[409–411] Involvement of the contralateral ovary is not seen except in advanced cases with extensive metastases.[411] It is therefore not necessary to biopsy or excise the contralateral ovary in patients with yolk sac tumor. Extraovarian spread is to the peritoneum and omentum, the para-aortic lymph nodes, and the liver. Extraovarian disease is confined to the pelvis (stage II) in about 10% of cases. More extensive metastases are present in the remaining 40%.

Macroscopic Appearance. Yolk sac tumors are large, with an average diameter of 16 cm.[409,411,412] The cut surface is predominantly solid with multiple small cysts. The tumors have a variegated appearance, with tan, white, and gray tissue admixed with areas of hemorrhage and necrosis.

Microscopic Appearance. Four major microscopic patterns have been described, and most neoplasms show a mixture of patterns.[411] The *reticular* pattern is most common. It is composed of a loose sieve-like meshwork of microcystic spaces lined by a single layer of flattened or cuboidal cells with clear or amphophilic cytoplasm and atypical, hyperchromatic nuclei (Fig. 6-83). The *festoon* or *pseudopapillary* pattern is composed of anastomosing spaces and papillae lined by columnar cells with clear or amphophilic cytoplasm and fusiform, hyperchromatic nuclei. Schiller-Duval bodies are papillary structures with a vascular, mesenchymal core covered by flattened to columnar tumor cells that project into tubules or cystic spaces (Fig. 6-84). Schiller-Duval bodies are characteristic of yolk sac tumor and are observed in two thirds of cases. In the *polyvesicular vitelline* pattern, cysts lined by cuboidal or columnar epithelial cells are surrounded by variably cellular mesenchymal stroma.[415] The *solid* pattern is characterized by sheets of small to medium-sized undifferentiated cells with a moderate amount of ampho-

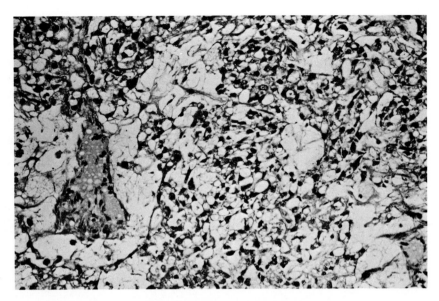

FIGURE 6-83 Yolk sac tumor, growing in a predominantly reticular pattern.

philic or clear cytoplasm. A constant finding in yolk sac tumors is eosinophilic, periodic acid-Schiff (PAS)-positive, diastase-resistant hyaline globules (see Fig. 6-84A). These globules are most numerous in the reticular and festoon patterns. Abundant extracellular hyaline PAS-positive material, usually seen in reticular or solid areas, is a characteristic finding in yolk sac tumors.[412,416] This material, which ultrastructurally resembles basement membrane and is composed of laminin and type IV collagen, has been interpreted as indicative of parietal yolk sac differentiation.[416] Small enteric glands lined by columnar cells and goblet cells are seen in 50% of yolk sac tumors. Myxoid stroma containing spindle or stellate cells is prominent in 25% of yolk sac tumors.[409] The spindle cells react with antibodies to cytokeratin and vimentin.[417] They may give rise to the differentiated mesenchymal components (eg, cartilage, striated muscle, and bone) that occasionally are seen in yolk sac tumors. The spindle cell component appears to be more resistant to chemotherapy than the epithelium. Luteinized stromal cells are present in or around 15% to 20% of yolk sac tumors. Syncytiotrophoblastic giant cells are present in rare cases.[412,418]

Several unusual growth patterns have been described. These are usually admixed with more typical patterns, facilitating their recognition as yolk sac tumors. *Hepatoid* yolk sac tumors are composed of sheets of large polygonal cells that resemble liver cells (Color Figure 6-19).[419] They have abundant eosinophilic or clear cytoplasm, well-defined cell borders, round central nuclei, and prominent nucleoli. *Glandular* yolk sac tumors are composed predominantly of glands of endometrioid[183] (Color Figure 6-20) or intestinal[420,421] type.

The immunocytochemical reaction that best characterizes yolk sac tumor is a positive reaction with antibodies against α-fetoprotein. Positive staining is observed in more than 75% of yolk sac tu-

mors and is seen in tumor cell cytoplasm, in secretions within cyst and gland lumina, and in some hyaline bodies.[200,411–413,418] Tumor cells with hepatoid, endometrioid, and intestinal patterns are positive for α-fetoprotein. Immunostains for α₁-antitrypsin,[419,422] cytokeratin,[417,418] and placental alkaline phosphatase[391,392] are positive. The extracellular hyaline material in yolk sac tumors is laminin-positive.[416] Immunostains for human chorionic gonadotropin are negative except for positive cytoplasmic staining in the syncytiotrophoblastic giant cells that are rarely seen in yolk sac tumors.[412,413]

Ultrastructurally, yolk sac tumor cells vary in size and shape. The nuclei are irregular but relatively uniform in size. Prominent nucleoli are present only in a minority of tumor cells. There are microvilli on the luminal surfaces of the cells. Adjacent cells are joined by tight junctions at their luminal borders and by desmosomes elsewhere. The cytoplasm contains uniform mitochondria, abundant glycogen that may be present in large aggregates, and rough endoplasmic reticulum that is focally dilated and filled with electron-dense material. Two ultrastructural features are characteristic of yolk sac tumor.[407,415,416,423,424] First, there is abundant extracellular, amorphous, electron-dense, basement-membrane-like material. Second, intracytoplasmic electron-dense material forms rounded aggregates that are not membrane-bound and that correspond to the hyaline bodies seen by light microscopy.

The cytologic appearance of yolk sac tumor is similar in body cavity fluids and in fine-needle aspirates.[423,425,426] Tumor cells are arranged in clusters, with few isolated single cells. They have primitive nuclei and prominent nucleoli. Two cell types have been described. One has distinct cell borders and homogeneous cytoplasm with occasional small vacuoles. The other has indistinct cell borders and many variably sized cytoplasmic vacuoles, producing a bubbly

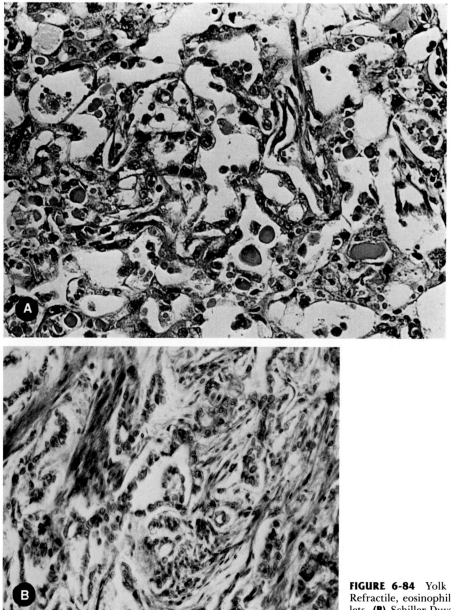

FIGURE 6-84 Yolk sac tumor. **(A)** Refractile, eosinophilic hyaline droplets. **(B)** Schiller-Duval body.

appearance. The distinctive intracytoplasmic and extracellular hyaline bodies and extracellular eosinophilic hyaline material are best visualized in air-dried smears.[423]

Nuclear DNA content has been analyzed in only a few yolk sac tumors.[427] Most are aneuploid, but the ploidy correlates poorly with the clinical outcome.

Differential Diagnosis. The differential diagnosis of yolk sac tumor includes clear cell carcinoma, other types of surface epithelial carcinoma, and embryonal carcinoma. Before Teilum showed that yolk sac tumor was of germ cell origin, pathologists thought that yolk sac tumor and clear cell (or meso-

nephroid) carcinoma were variants of the same neoplasm.[408]

Clear cell carcinoma occurs in an older patient population than yolk sac tumor and is more likely to be bilateral. Tubules and papillae are lined by cells with clear cytoplasm and by distinctive hobnail cells. Solid areas in clear cell carcinoma are composed of sheets of polygonal cells with clear cytoplasm and uniform nuclei. In yolk sac tumor, the solid areas contain sheets of small to medium-sized cells with primitive nuclei and frequent mitotic figures. The primitive spindle cell stroma seen in yolk sac tumor is absent in clear cell carcinoma, as are the characteristic growth patterns of yolk sac tumor, including Schiller-Duval bodies. Hyaline globules and extracellular hyaline material may be present in clear cell carcinoma and are a potential cause of diagnostic difficulty.[428] Immunostains may help to differentiate between clear cell carcinoma and yolk sac tumor: a positive stain for α-fetoprotein coupled with a negative reaction with the Leu-M1 antibody is reported to characterize yolk sac tumor.[200]

Rare examples of yolk sac tumor contain areas of glandular growth that resemble *endometrioid carcinoma*.[183] The youth of the patient, the aggressive nature of the tumor, the presence of other patterns of yolk sac tumor, and positive immunostains for α-fetoprotein and α₁-antitrypsin support a diagnosis of yolk sac tumor. Rare epithelial *hepatoid carcinomas* occur in the ovary.[429] These are differentiated from yolk sac tumor by their occurrence in an older patient population and by the absence of other typical patterns of yolk sac tumor.

Embryonal carcinoma is a malignant germ cell tumor that is closely related to yolk sac tumor. Embryonal carcinoma cells are larger and more pleomorphic, however, and grow mainly in a solid pattern, with only rare and poorly formed glands. Syncytiotrophoblastic cells, which secrete human chorionic gonadotropin, are frequently present. As a result, hormonally induced symptoms are common in patients with embryonal carcinoma but rare in those with yolk sac tumor.

Clinical Behavior and Treatment.

The prognosis of yolk sac tumor was poor before the widespread use of combination chemotherapy. The clinical course was characterized by rapid growth, development of metastases, and high mortality, even when the tumor appeared localized at operation. Kurman and Norris reported only a 13% 3-year survival in a large series of patients, most of whom did not receive adequate chemotherapy.[411] Yolk sac tumors are rarely bilateral, so unilateral salpingo-oophorectomy with limited debulking of extraovarian tumor is the recommended initial surgical treatment. Radiation therapy is ineffective in the treatment of yolk sac tumor.[409,430] The development of multiagent chemotherapy has radically altered the prognosis for patients with yolk sac tumor. Adjuvant vincristine, dactinomycin, and cyclophosphamide administered to patients with stage I neoplasms results in a survival rate of about 80%, and survival of patients with advanced disease approaches 50%.[409,431,432] Recent experience with chemotherapy regimens containing cisplatin document comparable results in stage I and improved survival in patients with advanced disease.[433–438] Measurement of serum α-fetoprotein levels is an effective method of monitoring the response to treatment.[414] An increase in the α-fetoprotein level may indicate the presence of recurrent tumor long before there is any clinical or radiologic evidence of recurrence. The role of second-look laparotomy is unclear.[436] Residual tumor has been identified in a few patients at second-look surgery despite a negative α-fetoprotein result.[439]

Embryonal Carcinoma

Embryonal carcinoma occurs only rarely in the ovary. The ovarian neoplasm is morphologically identical to embryonal carcinoma of the testis.

Clinical Features.

Embryonal carcinoma occurs in children and young women.[398,412,413] The age ranges from 4 to 28 years, with a median age of 15 years. The most common presentation is with a pelvic or abdominal mass. More than 50% of patients complain of abdominal pain. Hormonally mediated symptoms are noted in 60% of cases. Pregnancy tests are frequently positive, and serum levels of human chorionic gonadotropin-β (β-hCG) are elevated in most patients.[398] Half of the premenarchal patients present with precocious pseudopuberty.[398] Postpubertal patients typically have menstrual abnormalities. Most embryonal carcinomas of the ovary produce α-fetoprotein. In patients with this neoplasm, β-hCG and α-fetoprotein are useful tumor markers.

Tumor is confined to one ovary (stage IA) in 60% of cases.[398] No bilateral (stage IB) cases have been reported. Metastatic spread is to the pelvic and abdominal peritoneum.

Macroscopic Appearance.

Embryonal carcinoma is a soft, solid neoplasm. The average diameter is 17 cm. The cut surface is fleshy and tan or gray. Areas of hemorrhage and necrosis are almost always present, as are small cysts.

Microscopic Appearance.

The tumor cells grow predominantly in sheets and nests. There are occasional clefts, glands, or papillary structures. The neoplastic cells have large, vesicular nuclei with coarse chromatin and one or two prominent nucleoli. The cytoplasm is abundant and clear or amphophilic (Fig. 6-85). Syncytiotrophoblastic giant cells are present in most embryonal carcinomas. They are admixed with the mononuclear embryonal carcinoma cells or, more frequently, are seen at the periphery of the cell nests. The stroma is loose and edematous or cellular, composed of small, primitive-appearing spindle cells.

Immunocytochemical studies reveal human chorionic gonadotropin within the cytoplasm of the syncytiotrophoblastic giant cells.[398,412,413] Occasional large mononuclear cells are positive for human chorionic gonadotropin. Such cells react with antibodies to human placental lactogen and most likely are intermediate trophoblastic cells. Alpha-fetoprotein is detected within mononuclear embryonal carcinoma cells in 70% of cases.[398]

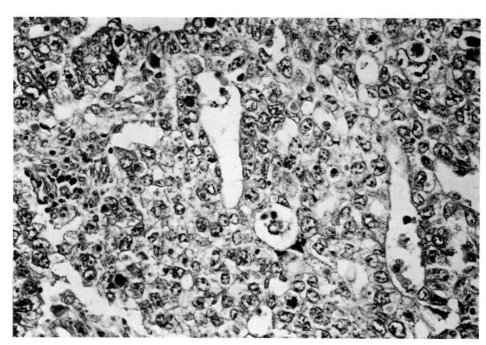

FIGURE 6-85 Embryonal carcinoma. Sheets of large atypical cells and poorly formed glandular clefts.

Differential Diagnosis. The differential diagnosis includes dysgerminoma and poorly differentiated carcinoma of surface epithelial origin. Embryonal carcinoma cells are more irregular than *dysgerminoma* cells; the nuclei are more pleomorphic, and the cytoplasm is more amphophilic. Glands and papillae are not seen in dysgerminoma. In contrast to embryonal carcinoma, dysgerminoma cells do not react with antibodies to cytokeratin or α-fetoprotein. Syncytiotrophoblastic giant cells are found much more frequently in embryonal carcinoma. *Poorly differentiated carcinoma* of surface epithelial origin occurs in an older age group than embryonal carcinoma and frequently is bilateral. No syncytiotrophoblastic giant cells are present, and immunostains for α-fetoprotein and hCG are negative.

Clinical Behavior and Treatment. Localized embryonal carcinoma is treated by unilateral salpingo-oophorectomy. Bilaterality has not been reported, and biopsy of the contralateral ovary is not recommended. Standard surgical treatment of advanced (stage >IA) disease is total abdominal hysterectomy, bilateral salpingo-oophorectomy, and limited debulking. Unilateral salpingo-oophorectomy and limited debulking surgery followed by chemotherapy can be considered for advanced tumors when conservation of fertility is important, if the contralateral ovary and uterus are uninvolved.

Before effective combination chemotherapy was available, embryonal carcinoma often progressed rapidly. Survival in stage IA was only 50%.[398] Combination chemotherapy is effective in embryonal carcinoma but response rates are difficult to determine because embryonal carcinoma of the ovary is so rare. Some patients with advanced disease can be cured with cisplatin-based chemotherapy regimens.[438]

Serum assays for human chorionic gonadotropin and α-fetoprotein are useful in the evaluation and follow-up of patients with embryonal carcinoma. If serum levels of either or both markers remain elevated after treatment, or if they become elevated during follow-up, the patient has recurrent or metastatic tumor. Serum markers are a sensitive method of monitoring patients with embryonal carcinoma because increased levels often are noted weeks or months before a recurrence is detected by clinical or radiographic examination.

Choriocarcinoma

Pure primary ovarian choriocarcinoma of germ cell origin is extremely rare.[375,440,441] Only 0.04% of ovarian tumors on file at the Armed Forces Institute of Pathology were choriocarcinomas.[375] Choriocarcinoma is seen more frequently as a component of a mixed germ cell tumor.

Clinical Features. Choriocarcinoma of the ovary occurs only in children and young women. Presenting symptoms include abdominal pain and abdominal bleeding. Premenarchal children may have precocious pseudopuberty.[440] Pregnancy tests are positive, and serum levels of β-hCG are elevated.[440,442,443]

Macroscopic Appearance. Choriocarcinoma is a large, soft, purple-red tumor between 4 and 25 cm in diameter.[440] The cut surface is hemorrhagic and necrotic.

Microscopic Appearance. A large portion of the tumor is hemorrhagic and necrotic. Viable tumor cells are best seen at the periphery, where cytotrophoblastic and syncytiotrophoblastic cells grow in a plexiform pattern. The cytotrophoblastic cells have abundant, clear cytoplasm and well-defined cell borders. They have irregular vesicular nuclei, some of which have prominent macronucleoli. The syncytiotrophoblastic cells have multiple hyperchromatic nuclei and abundant basophilic or amphophilic vacuolated cytoplasm. Immunostains for human chorionic gonadotropin disclose a positive cytoplasmic reaction in the syncytiotrophoblastic giant cells.[443]

Differential Diagnosis. *Gestational choriocarcinoma* is the most important differential diagnostic consideration. If the patient is premenarchal, the choriocarcinoma is of germ cell origin.[440,441] Metastatic or primary gestational choriocarcinoma is as common as primary choriocarcinoma of germ cell origin in young women.[441] There are no morphologic differences between gestational choriocarcinoma and choriocarcinoma of germ cell origin. The clinical history may help in the differential diagnosis. The choriocarcinoma can be proved to be of gestational origin if a paternal component can be identified in the tumor cell genome by DNA analysis.[444]

Clinical Behavior and Treatment. Choriocarcinoma of the ovary is treated by surgical excision followed by combination chemotherapy. Most patients are children or young women, so unilateral salpingo-oophorectomy is the surgery of choice. Total abdominal hysterectomy and bilateral salpingo-oophorectomy may be required if the contralateral ovary or uterus is involved. Favorable results have been described, even with suboptimal chemotherapy.[440] Recent reports indicate that patients with advanced disease can be treated successfully with platinum-containing chemotherapy protocols.[438]

Teratoma

The benign cystic teratoma (or dermoid cyst) is the most common ovarian neoplasm. It comprises between 26% and 44% of all ovarian tumors.[243,244] The other types of teratoma are all uncommon. Teratomas originate from germ cells. They have a female sex chromatin pattern (positive), and nearly all cases have a 46,XX karyotype. Experimental studies suggest that most teratomas originate by parthenogenesis from single haploid germ cells.[445] Restriction fragment length polymorphism analysis supports an origin from a single germ cell after the first meiotic division, with failure of the second meiotic division.[446] Some teratomas may originate from cells that have failed to complete the first meiotic division.[446]

Mature (Benign) Teratoma. These are cystic or, rarely, solid tumors containing tissues derived from the three embryonic germ layers: ectoderm, mesoderm, and endoderm. The common benign cystic teratoma is frequently referred to as a *dermoid cyst.*

Clinical Features. Benign teratomas occur in patients of all ages, but 85% are detected in patients between 20 and 50 years of age.[244] The peak incidence is in patients between 20 and 29 years of age. Benign teratomas grow slowly, and small neoplasms are asymptomatic. Symptoms such as pelvic pressure or pain appear when the tumor attains a large size. About 10% of benign cystic teratomas are bilateral.[376] Potentially serious complications include torsion and rupture.

Macroscopic Appearance. Benign teratomas range in size from small neoplasms several centimeters in diameter to large neoplasms weighing several kilograms. They are round, and their surfaces are smooth. Their consistency varies from firm to soft. The cut surface has a unilocular or multilocular cystic appearance (Color Figure 6-21). The cysts contain tufts of hair, yellow grumous material, or oily or serous liquid. Firm, white cartilage, gritty bone, and intact teeth may be identified (Fig. 6-86). Soft, gelatinous, gray-tan material corresponding to glial tissue, and brown, translucent zones of thyroid tissue frequently are present. Dense, solid foci within an otherwise cystic teratoma are unusual and should be sampled carefully for histologic study. A few mature (benign) teratomas are entirely solid, but these can be differentiated from immature teratoma only by microscopic study.

Microscopic Appearance. Benign teratomas contain a variable admixture of ectodermal, mesodermal, and endodermal structures. Ectodermal derivatives such as skin, hair follicles, and adnexal sebaceous and sweat glands are encountered most often (Fig. 6-87). When they are the main structures, the tumor is commonly referred to as a *dermoid cyst.* Other commonly observed tissues include neural (usually glial) tissue, choroid plexus, digestive tract mucosa (including endocrine cells), respiratory mucosa, renal tissue, adipose tissue, smooth or striated muscle, peripheral nerve, thyroid tissue, dental structures, bone or cartilage, and a loose connective tissue framework that surrounds the other elements (Figs. 6-88 and 6-89). Individual tissues occasionally dominate to the extent that the tumor can be considered a monodermal teratoma. Cystic spaces lined by flattened epithelium or granulation tissue and surrounded by multinucleated giant cells and lipophages are found in some teratomas. The foreign-body granulomatous reaction is caused by disruption of the epithelium with liberation of the cyst contents into the surrounding tissue.

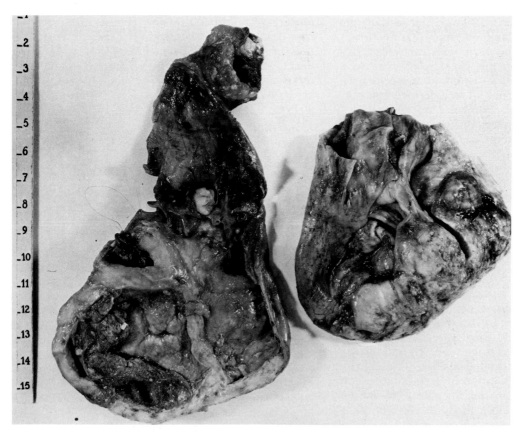

FIGURE 6-86 Macroscopic appearance of an ovarian teratoma, showing an abortive tooth.

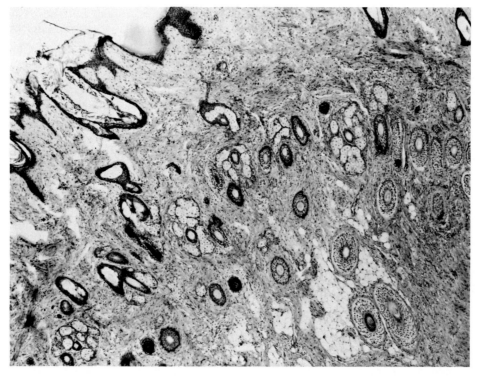

FIGURE 6-87 Squamous epithelium, sebaceous and sweat glands, and hair follicles in a benign cystic teratoma.

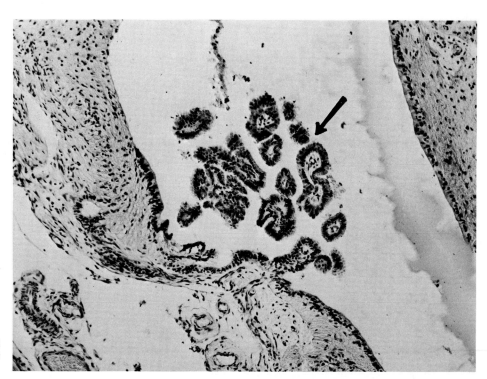

FIGURE 6-88 Glia and choroid plexus (*arrow*) in a benign cystic teratoma.

Clinical Behavior and Treatment. Mature teratomas are benign neoplasms and can be treated conservatively. Cystectomy is adequate treatment, particularly in children and young women. Peritoneal glial implants are detected in rare patients with mature solid teratoma of the ovary.[447,448] The implants are composed of mature glia (grade 0) and do not adversely affect survival.

Malignant transformation occurs in 1% to 3% of benign cystic teratomas.[449,450] This complication is typically seen in postmenopausal women, but it also occurs in premenopausal women and children. In contrast to immature teratoma, which is composed of embryonal tissues, the malignant tumors that arise in benign cystic teratoma resemble typical adult neoplasms. Squamous carcinoma is the most common malignant tumor arising in a benign cystic teratoma, accounting for about 90% of cases.[451,452] The remainder are adenocarcinoma, sarcoma, melanoma, or other rare tumor types.[453,454] The prognosis for patients with a malignant neoplasm arising in a benign cystic teratoma is unfavorable; most die within 1 year of diagnosis.

Immature Teratoma. Immature teratoma is the third most common malignant germ cell tumor of the ovary, representing 20% of such tumors at a major cancer center.[431]

Clinical Features. Immature teratoma occurs in children and young adults. The age of occurrence ranges from 6 to 40 years, with an average age of about 20 years.[431,455-459] The clinical presentation is with abdominal pain, palpable abdominal mass, or abdominal distention. Rare patients have acute abdominal symptoms due to torsion or rupture of the neoplasm.[460] The duration of symptoms ranges from 1 day to 6 months, with an average of 1 month.[460] Serum levels of α-fetoprotein are elevated in 30% to 50% of patients and may serve as a useful tumor marker.[460-462] Levels of the tumor marker CA-125 are frequently elevated in patients with immature teratoma.[461] Localized tumors (stage I) are found in 50% to 80% of patients. Bilateral (stage IB) immature teratoma is not reported. The contralateral ovary is only involved in patients with advanced disease, in whom its involvement reflects metastatic spread.[457,459,460] Metastatic spread is transcoelomic to the pelvic and abdominal peritoneum and the omentum. A benign cystic teratoma is present in the contralateral ovary in 10% to 15% of cases.[457,460,463]

Macroscopic Appearance. These are unilateral tumors of firm consistency. They range from 6 to 30 cm in diameter; the average diameter is 18 cm. The cut surface typically is partly cystic and partly solid. Cysts bearing a resemblance to a dermoid cyst are noted in 26% of cases.[463] The solid portion of the tumor is gray to brown and varies from soft and fleshy to hard and gritty. Chondroid differentiation is occasionally identified as a hard gray or white translucent area.

Microscopic Appearance. Tissues derived from all three germ cell layers are present, but ectodermal and mesodermal derivatives predominate. Typical

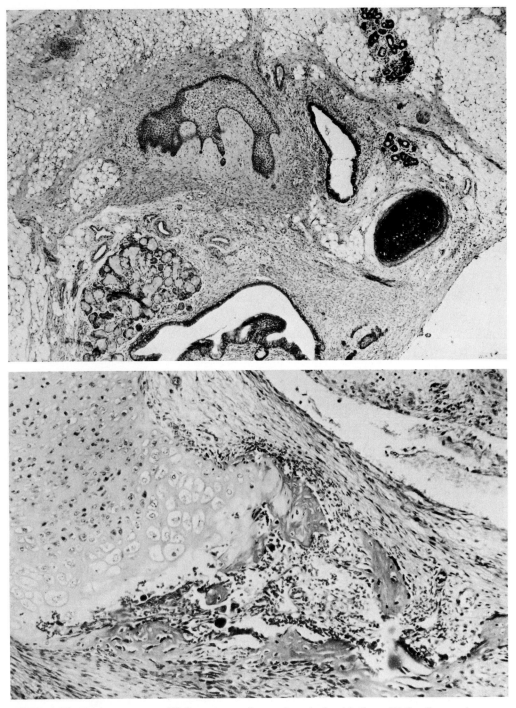

FIGURE 6-89 Benign teratoma. **(A)** Squamous and gastrointestinal epithelium. **(B)** Cartilage and bone.

ectodermal derivatives include skin, skin appendages, and neuroectoderm. Neuroectodermal elements are the most easily recognized and measured immature tissues (Fig. 6-90). They include sheets of immature neuroepithelium, neuroepithelial tubules (Fig. 6-91) and rosettes, neuroblastic elements, immature glia, and primitive retina with melanin pigmentation. The most common mesodermal tissues include cartilage, bone, and embryonal stroma. Embryonal stroma, a

readily identified indicator of immaturity, is composed of small, densely cellular fusiform cells that exhibit mitotic activity. Endodermal differentiation is mainly represented by intestinal and bronchial structures. Immature teratoma must be graded because the prognosis depends on the grade and stage. Immaturity is measured using a grading system that rates teratomas from grade 0 (a neoplasm composed entirely of mature tissues) to grade

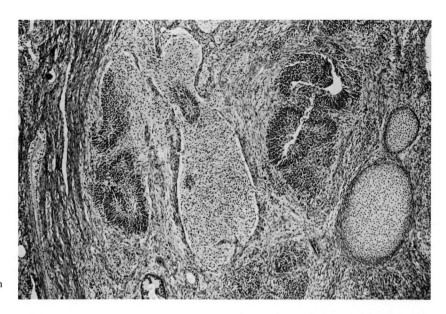

FIGURE 6-90 Immature teratoma with neuroepithelium and embryonal cartilage.

3 (a neoplasm containing abundant immature tissue; Table 6-7).[459] Metastases from an immature teratoma may be grade 0, but the primary ovarian neoplasm must, by definition, be grade 1, 2, or 3 (Fig. 6-92).

Rare examples of immature teratoma are composed predominantly or entirely of immature neuroectodermal structures including sheets of small round cells, primitive neuroepithelium, rosettes, and glia.[455,464] Such neoplasms have been termed *malignant neuroectodermal tumor*.[464]

Immunohistochemical evaluation of immature teratoma reveals positive staining of glia with antibodies to glial fibrillary acidic protein (GFAP).[225,465,466] Fibrillary and cell body staining are encountered. This reaction occasionally helps identify inconspicuous foci of glial differentiation. Primitive neuroepithelial elements do not stain with GFAP. There is a positive staining reaction with antibodies to neurofilaments in some tumors.[225,465] Neuron-specific enolase stains glial elements and, with less intensity, neuroepithelium.[465] Endodermal derivatives such as intestinal and respiratory epithelium contain argyrophilic cells, which react with a variety of antibodies against neurohormonal peptides.[225] In accord with the clinical finding of increased serum α-fetoprotein in as many as 50% of cases, there is positive staining for α-fetoprotein in such yolk sac endodermal derivatives as gland-like vesicles, intestinal epithelium, and liver.[225,462]

Electron microscopic study reveals glial elements, immature neuronal cells, occasional immature ependymal-type cells, and primitive undifferentiated cells.[465]

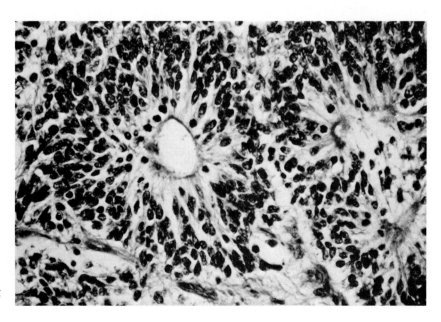

FIGURE 6-91 Neuroepithelium forming tubules in an immature teratoma.

TABLE 6-7
Histologic Grading of Immature Teratoma of the Ovary

Grade	Immature Tissue	Neuroepithelium
0	Mature tissues only	None
1	+	Rare, not more than 1 LPF per slide
2	++	Common, not more than 3 LPF per slide
3	+++	Prominent, 4 or more LPF per slide

LPF, low-power field(s).

Differential Diagnosis. Immature teratoma must be differentiated from mature cystic or solid teratoma and from carcinosarcoma. Most *mature teratomas* are predominantly cystic. They contain only mature tissues, which tend to be arranged in an organized pattern. In contrast, immature teratoma is likely to have extensive areas of solid growth. Disorganized immature tissues are admixed with mature elements. Immature neuroepithelium is the most common immature element, but it should not be confused with mature cerebellar tissue. Primitive embryonal stroma is frequently noted. *Carcinosarcoma* is a highly malignant neoplasm of surface epithelial derivation. It occurs almost exclusively in postmenopausal women and is composed of malignant adult neoplastic epithelium and mesenchyme, often including heterologous elements. Immunohistochemistry may help in the differential diagnosis, because carcinosarcoma does not display immunoreactivity to neurohormonal peptides, α-fetoprotein, neurofilaments, or GFAP. Finally, immature teratoma is a frequent constituent of

mixed germ cell tumor, so adequate sampling to exclude other tumor types is essential for accurate diagnosis.

Clinical Behavior and Treatment. Conservation of fertility is important in most patients, so surgical treatment should be conservative. Patients with localized (stage IA) tumors can be treated by unilateral salpingo-oophorectomy. Involvement of the contralateral ovary is so rare that biopsy is unnecessary. A tumor in the contralateral ovary is most likely a benign cystic teratoma, which should be managed by cystectomy.[460] More advanced tumors are treated by unilateral salpingo-oophorectomy and excision of extraovarian tumor. Effective chemotherapy is available, and if the contralateral ovary is not involved it may be conserved. If preservation of fertility is not an issue, or if the contralateral ovary is involved, hysterectomy and bilateral salpingo-oophorectomy are appropriate. A study conducted at the Armed Forces Institute of Pathology before the availability of effective chemotherapy provides a historical baseline for prognosis in immature teratoma.[459] Survival depended on stage and grade. Survival in stage IA was 100% for grade 1, 70% for grade 2, and 33% for grade 3 tumors. Survival with advanced disease was about 50%, but too few tumors were studied to relate both grade and stage to prognosis. Based on these historical results, treatment of stage IA, grade 1 immature teratoma is by surgery alone. Patients with stage IA, grade 3 immature teratoma and those with advanced disease receive chemotherapy. Treatment of patients with stage IA, grade 2 tumors is controversial, with some authors advocating chemotherapy[460,461,467] and others not.[455,456] The combination of vincristine, dactinomycin, and cyclophosphamide, as well as cisplatin-containing regimens and

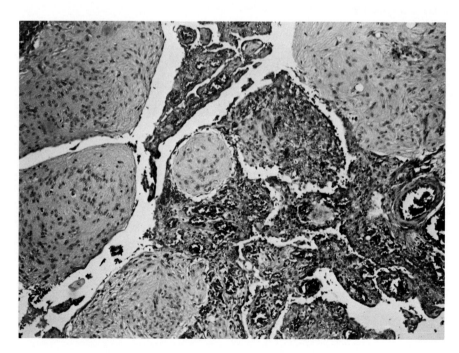

FIGURE 6-92 This peritoneal implant, which was derived from an immature teratoma, is composed entirely of benign glial tissue with reactive mesothelial and vascular hyperplasia.

doxorubicin, are effective adjuvant chemotherapies, with survival rates of 90% to 100% in patients with localized disease.[468] Patients who have residual gross tumor or recurrent tumor have a less favorable outcome. About 55% of such patients can be cured with chemotherapy regimens that include cisplatin.[438]

The prognosis in immature teratoma depends on the stage and grade of the primary tumor and on the grade of the peritoneal implants. In some instances, the peritoneal implants contain only mature tissues; such implants usually are composed exclusively or partly of mature glia (see Fig. 6-92). Grade 0 implants behave in a clinically benign manner and do not adversely affect the prognosis.[448,457,459,460,469–471]

Monodermal Teratomas

Struma Ovarii. Struma ovarii is a monodermal teratoma composed totally or in overwhelming proportion of thyroid tissue.[472] It accounts for 1% to 3% of benign teratomas of the ovary. The term *struma ovarii* is not used for dermoid cysts that contain small areas of thyroid tissue or for teratomas composed predominantly of other elements. Adequately documented cases producing hyperthyroidism are rare.

Most strumas are encapsulated neoplasms several centimeters in diameter. On cross section, they are red, with a shiny, meaty appearance (Fig. 6-93). Microscopic examination shows normal thyroid tissue (see Fig. 6-93) or thyroid tissue showing degenerative changes such as hemorrhage, cyst formation, and fibrosis. Microfollicular adenomatoid nodules may resemble granulosa cell tumor or carcinoid, creating a possible source of confusion. Immunohistochemical staining for thyroglobulin reveals a positive reaction in struma ovarii, confirming the diagnosis.

The clinical behavior is benign, and simple excision is adequate treatment. Any of the histologic types of thyroid carcinoma may arise in a struma. Most examples have been classified as carcinoma on histologic grounds alone, but cases with metastases have been reported.[472–477] Malignant struma is treated by total hysterectomy with bilateral salpingo-oophorectomy, thyroidectomy, and therapeutic doses of iodine 131.

Carcinoid Tumor. Carcinoid tumors of the ovary are rare. They are considered to be monodermal teratomas because most are associated with other teratomatous elements. Pure carcinoids occur in the ovary; most of these probably develop in and subsequently overgrow a teratoma. It is theoretically possible for a carcinoid to arise from neuroendocrine cells in mucinous tumors.

Most patients present with nonspecific symptoms. The carcinoid syndrome occurs in about one third of patients with insular carcinoid, mainly those with large neoplasms.[478] It is rarely associated with other types of primary ovarian carcinoid. The clinical presentation can be dramatic with flushing, diarrhea, and heart disease. The carcinoid syndrome can occur in the absence of metastases because venous blood from the ovaries does not pass through the liver. Metastatic intestinal or bronchial carcinoids also may be encountered in the ovary. These, too, may be associated with the carcinoid syndrome.

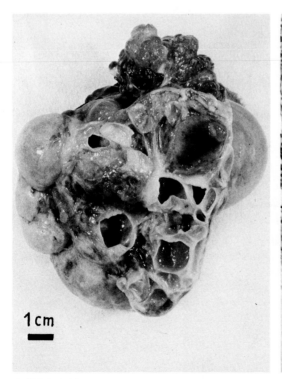
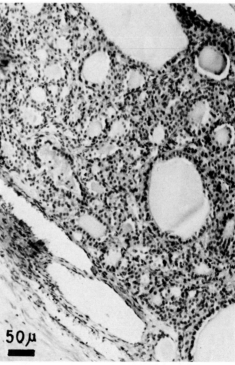

FIGURE 6-93 Struma ovarii: gross and microscopic appearance.

Carcinoids are firm, tan or yellow, solid tumors. They are unilateral and frequently arise in the wall of a benign cystic teratoma. They are composed of uniform round or cuboidal cells with round nuclei, coarse nuclear chromatin, and a moderate amount of clear or eosinophilic cytoplasm (Fig. 6-94). Fine, dark granules can be demonstrated in the cytoplasm by argentaffin or argyrophil stains. Many peptide hormones can be detected in carcinoid cells by immunohistochemistry, and neuroendocrine granules are observed in ultrastructural studies (Fig. 6-95).[479,480] Four main microscopic patterns have been described, and mixed patterns often are noted. The *insular* pattern is most common and is composed of sheets and islands of neoplastic cells surrounded by fibrous stroma.[478] The cells grow in ribbons in the *trabecular* pattern (see Fig. 6-94B).[481,482] *Strumal carcinoid* contains carcinoid and thyroid follicular epithelium that are intimately admixed, at least fo-

cally (Color Figures 6-22 and 6-23).[483–485] Finally, rare cases of primary *mucinous carcinoid* arise in the ovary.[486,487] These contain glands lined by columnar or cuboidal cells and goblet cells. Metastasis from a mucinous carcinoid tumor of the appendix must be excluded.

Teratomatous elements are often found adjacent to an ovarian carcinoid. Their identification is important evidence that the neoplasm is primary in the ovary and not metastatic. Unlike the primary ovarian carcinoid, metastatic tumors are usually bilateral, multinodular, and unassociated with other teratomatous elements. An extraovarian primary can be demonstrated by appropriate clinical studies.[480,488]

The primary ovarian carcinoid is a slowly growing neoplasm that is treated adequately by excision. Most are unilateral, and salpingo-oophorectomy is appropriate treatment for young patients. Carcinoid tumor of the ovary has a favorable prognosis. Metastases and tumor-related deaths are infre-

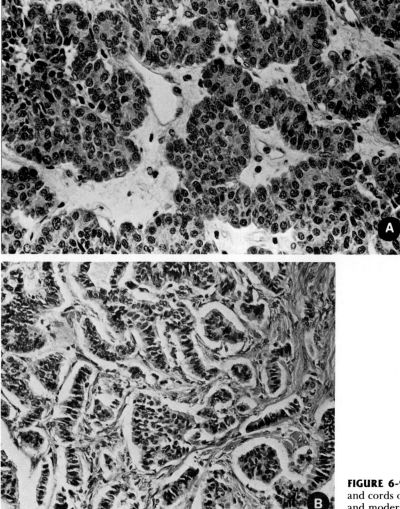

FIGURE 6-94 Carcinoid tumor. **(A)** Nests and cords of cells with regular, round nuclei and moderate amounts of eosinophilic cytoplasm. **(B)** Trabecular growth pattern.

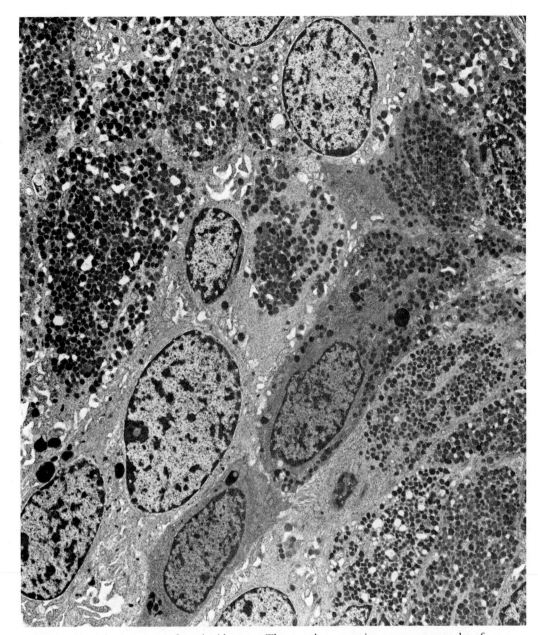

FIGURE 6-95 Ultrastructure of carcinoid tumor. The cytoplasm contains numerous granules of varying electron density and bundles of microfilaments (×5200). (Courtesy of Dr. J. M. Orenstein, George Washington University, Washington, DC).

quent. Based on the limited information in the literature, mucinous carcinoid may exhibit more aggressive behavior than other types of carcinoid. In the absence of metastases, symptoms abate rapidly after removal of the neoplasm.

Malignant Mixed Germ Cell Tumor

Malignant mixed germ cell tumors are composed of mixtures of the various pure types of germ cell tumor. Such neoplasms comprise 5% to 20% of all malignant germ cell tumors.[489,490] The presence of benign teratomatous elements does not qualify a neoplasm for inclusion in this category.

Clinical Features. Mixed germ cell tumors occur in children and in young women 5 to 33 years of age. The average patient age is 16 years. The most typical clinical presentation is with a palpable abdominal mass and abdominal pain. Acute abdominal symptoms occur in 15% to 20% of patients. Precocious pseudopuberty is detected in one third of prepubertal children with mixed germ cell tumors.[489] Older children and adults may have amenorrhea or abnormal vaginal bleeding. A positive pregnancy test or an increased level of serum human chorionic gonadotropin is discovered in 50% of patients, and the serum levels of α-fetoprotein are elevated in 50% of patients. The duration of symptoms is 1 day to 6 months, with an average of 4 weeks.[490] Most patients (57% to 66%) have stage I tumors at diagnosis.[489,490]

Macroscopic Appearance. Mixed germ cell tumors are large neoplasms. Their average diameter is 15 cm; fewer than 10% measure less than 10 cm in diameter. The appearance of the cut surface depends on the elements that are present. Areas of dysgerminoma are fleshy and gray or tan. Yolk sac tumor is variable in color and contains small cysts. Choriocarcinoma is hemorrhagic. Immature teratoma is white or tan and often contains cysts and translucent areas of cartilaginous differentiation. Most mixed germ cell tumors are unilateral. A small percentage of the tumors that contain dysgerminoma are bilateral.[490]

Microscopic Appearance. About 80% of mixed germ cell tumors contain two malignant elements. Three germ cell elements are found in 15% of these neoplasms, and the remainder contain four or more different elements. The various elements may be admixed or they may be found in separate, adjacent parts of the tumor (Fig. 6-96). Dysgerminoma is the most frequent element in mixed germ cell tumor. Yolk sac tumor and immature teratoma are each found in more than 50% of mixed germ cell tumors. Embryonal carcinoma, choriocarcinoma, and polyembryoma are observed less frequently.[489-491]

Clinical Behavior and Treatment. Early reports suggested that the prognosis depended on the size of the tumor, its stage, and the types and amounts of the various germ cell components.[489,492] More recent reports describing patients who received modern combination chemotherapy indicate that stage is the only significant determinant of prognosis.[490]

The initial treatment of malignant mixed germ cell tumor is surgical. Tumors confined to one ovary (stage IA) are treated by unilateral salpingo-oophorectomy. The standard treatment for those patients with more advanced tumors is total abdominal hysterectomy and bilateral salpingo-oophorectomy. Conservation of an uninvolved uterus and a contralateral ovary can be considered in some patients with advanced disease if conservation of fertility is desired. More than 50% of stage I tumors treated by surgery alone recur, indicating that occult metastases are present at diagnosis in most cases.[489,490,492] All patients therefore require postoperative chemotherapy, except those whose tumors are stage IA and contain only dysgerminoma and grade I immature teratoma. More than 70% of stage I patients treated with combination chemotherapy are cured.[490] Patients with more advanced tumors have a survival rate of about 50%.[438,467,490]

Gonadoblastoma

Gonadoblastoma is a rare tumor composed of germ cells and sex cord cells.[493-496] It arises almost exclusively in abnormal gonads.[496-498]

Clinical Features. Gonadoblastoma has been detected over a wide age group, ranging from 6 months to 45 years. The average age at diagnosis is 18 years, and 80% of patients are less than 20 years old.[497] The most common clinical presentation is with primary or, less often, secondary amenorrhea. Occasional tumors are detected during a physical examination, at operation for an acute abdomen, or during evaluation of adnexal calcifications detected on abdominal or pelvic radiographs. Most patients are phenotypic females, but gonadoblastoma also occurs in phenotypic males. Phenotypic females have a normal or short vagina that ends in a small cervix. The uterus is small in 75% of patients, and the fallopian tubes are small or rudimentary in 35%. Many patients are mildly virilized.[496] The most common

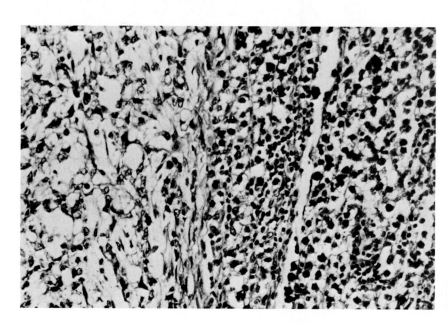

FIGURE 6-96 Malignant mixed germ cell tumor: yolk sac tumor (*left*) and dysgerminoma (*right*).

karyotypes are 46,XY and 45,X/46,XY. A Y chromosome or a Y-chromosome fragment is detected in more than 90% of patients.[497]

Macroscopic Appearance. Gonadoblastoma arises in abnormal gonads, including streak gonads, indeterminate gonads, and dysgenetic testes.[496] The neoplasms are small, ranging from microscopic to 2 to 3 cm in diameter. More than 40% are bilateral. The cut surface is tan or white and often there are visible calcified areas.

Microscopic Appearance. Gonadoblastoma is composed of nests of germ cells and sex cord cells. The germ cells are large, polygonal cells with abundant clear cytoplasm, vesicular nuclei, and prominent nucleoli (Fig. 6-97). They resemble germinoma cells. They are surrounded by smaller cells of sex cord origin, which may resemble granulosa or Sertoli cells. They surround a single germ cell, a group of germ cells, or a small space containing eosinophilic hyaline material (see Fig. 6-97). The stroma between the epithelial nests is frequently luteinized in postpubertal patients, and there are many microcalcifications.

Immunocytochemical testing reveals that the sex cord elements react with antibodies to vimentin and cytokeratin. The hyaline material reacts with anti-laminin antibodies, compatible with basement membrane material.[499] The germ cells resemble dysgerminoma cells by electron microscopy.[493,499] The sex cord cells contain cytoplasmic bundles of Charcot-Böttcher filaments, a finding compatible with differentiation toward Sertoli cells.[499]

Differential Diagnosis. Rare examples of other types of *combined germ cell-stromal tumors* have been described, including a neoplasm with an epithelial component.[500,501] The absence of cell nests and the hyaline cores within them serves to differentiate such neoplasms from gonadoblastoma. Sex cord tumor with annular tubules (SCTAT) is differentiated from gonadoblastoma and from the other types of combined tumors by the absence of germ cells. Microscopic gonadoblastoma-like lesions occur in fetal and infant ovaries in the absence of genetic abnormalities. These lesions are associated with follicular atresia, and their relation with gonadoblastoma is unclear.[502,503]

Clinical Behavior and Treatment. Gonadoblastoma is benign unless overgrown by a germinoma or some other type of malignant germ cell tumor. Bilateral gonadectomy is indicated when a gonadoblastoma is discovered.[497,498] The gonads are nonfunctional from a reproductive point of view. Gonadoblastoma is frequently bilateral, and removal of both gonads precludes virilization or evolution of a malignant germ cell tumor. The risk that a malignant germ cell tumor will arise in an abnormal gonad in a patient with a Y chromosome is estimated at 25%.[504] Most of the malignant germ cell

tumors that arise in gonadoblastoma are germinomas,[496,497,505] but other, more aggressive, types of germ cell tumor occur.[496,497,505,506] We have seen a single case of Sertoli-Leydig cell tumor arising in a gonadoblastoma.

Metastatic Tumors

Gastrointestinal, breast, and uterine carcinomas frequently metastasize to the ovaries.[171,201,507–513] Although metastatic cancer comprises 10% of all ovarian cancers seen in surgical material, the percentage of metastatic tumors that pose diagnostic problems, presenting clinically as primary ovarian neoplasms, is much smaller.

In older series compiled when the primary endocrinologic treatment for breast cancer was surgical removal of the ovaries, 30% to 50% of the metastatic cancers identified in the ovaries were from the breast (Fig. 6-98). These were usually incidental microscopic findings in grossly unremarkable or slightly enlarged ovaries. Large metastatic deposits easily mistaken for primary neoplasms were rare. Antiestrogenic drugs such as tamoxifen have largely replaced oophorectomy in the endocrinologic treatment of breast cancer, and the surgical pathologist now sees ovarian metastases from breast cancer only occasionally.[510,513] In modern surgical series, most metastatic neoplasms detected in the ovaries are from gastrointestinal primary sites.[171,201,507–509,512] These not infrequently present as primary ovarian neoplasms, with the primary gastrointestinal tumor detected only after the ovarian neoplasm has been removed and studied by the pathologist. The gastrointestinal cancers responsible for ovarian metastases are metastatic from the colon and rectum, stomach and biliary tract, in order of decreasing frequency.[514]

Ovarian metastases are most likely to affect functioning ovaries. Invasion takes place by the lymphatic or hematogenous route, by serosal implantation of neoplastic cells disseminated by the fallopian tubes into the peritoneal cavity, or by direct extension from adjacent organs such as the large intestine or appendix.

Macroscopic Appearance

Metastatic ovarian cancers vary in appearance. The entire ovary may be replaced by a solid white mass of firm or rubbery consistency. Metastatic colorectal cancer often presents as a large unilocular or multilocular cystic neoplasm with solid areas. Other metastatic carcinomas form multiple nodules in the cortex and medulla and on the serosa. Small metastases may not be readily visible because their color and consistency are similar to those of the surrounding ovarian parenchyma. Normal-appearing ovaries occasionally exhibit widespread lymphatic permeation by metastatic tumor.

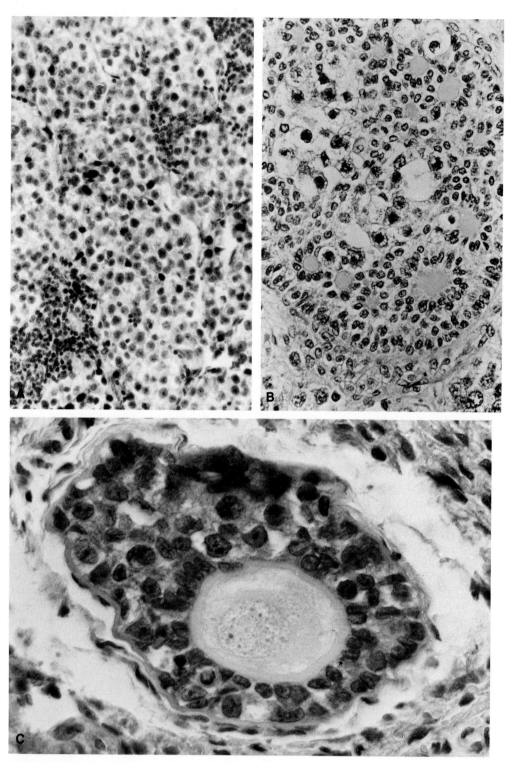

FIGURE 6-97 Gonadoblastoma. **(A)** Focus of germinoma. **(B)** Nest of sex cord elements containing scattered large germ cells. **(C)** The space surrounded by sex cord cells resembles a Call-Exner body. (Courtesy of Dr. Jean de Brux, Paris, France).

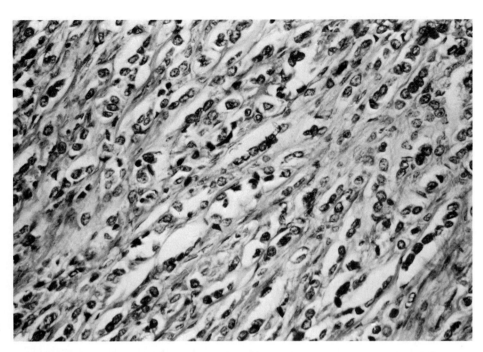

FIGURE 6-98 Metastatic breast cancer in the ovary.

When the uterus and ovaries are both involved by adenocarcinoma, it may be difficult to determine the point of origin of the tumor. Statistically, endometrial carcinoma with ovarian metastasis is more frequent than ovarian carcinoma with uterine metastasis. In most instances, however, the findings are best interpreted as simultaneous primary cancers in the endometrium and ovary. This is particularly true when the endometrial carcinoma is superficial and well differentiated, because metastases are unlikely in such a setting.

Microscopic Appearance

Metastatic carcinoma reproduces the appearance of the primary tumor to a variable degree. The most useful clue that a cancer is metastatic is that it is bilateral and multifocal. The neoplastic cells may diffusely infiltrate the parenchyma (see Fig. 6-98) or grow in discrete rounded nodules. Implants on the surface of the ovary are common. Metastatic carcinoma may be visible within lymphatic spaces in the ovary, especially the hilum, and in the mesovarium. The stromal cells in and around some metastatic cancers are luteinized. The luteinized cells occasionally secrete enough estrogen or androgen to cause clinical symptoms.

Metastatic colorectal adenocarcinoma often simulates a primary adenocarcinoma of the ovary, and the correct diagnosis can be difficult, even after microscopic examination.[171,172,507,512] This type of metastatic carcinoma typically grows in a multicystic pattern with extensive necrosis. The malignant cells lining the cystic spaces are stratified or grow in a cartwheel or cribriform pattern (Color Figure 6-24).

Metastatic colorectal cancer resembles endometrioid carcinoma if goblet cells are absent or inconspicuous. Helpful differential diagnostic features are the presence of the attributes of metastatic carcinoma listed above, segmental necrosis of glands, greater nuclear atypia than anticipated in a tumor composed of well-formed glands, and the absence of squamous metaplasia.[171] If goblet cells are present, the differential diagnosis is with mucinous carcinoma of the ovary. Many of the differential diagnostic features previously mentioned are helpful. In addition, primary mucinous carcinoma of the ovary often contains areas resembling a benign or LMP mucinous tumor, in which endocervical-type cells are present.

Metastatic carcinoid tumor is histologically identical to a primary ovarian carcinoid.[488] Bilaterality, multifocality, and the absence of other teratomatous elements suggest that a carcinoid tumor is metastatic, usually from an intestinal primary site.

Krukenberg tumor is a form of metastatic cancer in which malignant signet-ring cells invade an abundant and hypercellular stroma.[515-517] The primary carcinoma usually is located in the stomach, but signet-ring cell carcinoma of the breast, colon, and gallbladder can give rise to this type of ovarian metastasis. Krukenberg tumors are most frequent in patient populations in which there is a high incidence of gastric carcinoma, such as in women of Japanese extraction. The ovaries typically retain their shape but are symmetrically or asymmetrically enlarged. They are firm and yellow-white. The cut surface is honeycombed with small mucinous cysts, and there are foci of hemorrhage and necrosis (Fig. 6-99A). Microscopically, the signet-ring cells are found as isolated single cells, or they grow in variably sized nests, cords or tubules.

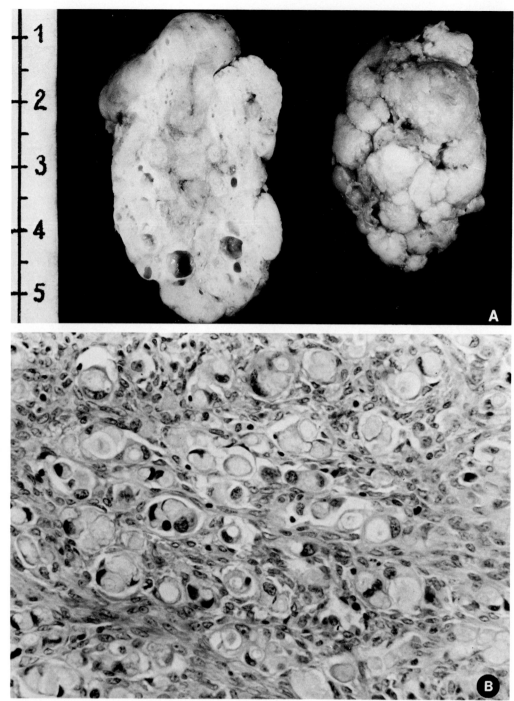

FIGURE 6-99 Ovarian metastasis from gastric carcinoma (Krukenberg tumor). **(A)** Gross appearance. **(B)** Microscopic appearance showing signet-ring cells.

A Krukenberg tumor that contains prominent tubules may be designated as a *tubular Krukenberg tumor*.[324,518] The malignant cells contain round cytoplasmic mucin globules that compress and flatten the hyperchromatic nucleus against one cell border (see Fig. 6-99*B*). The stroma is abundant and hypercellular. It is focally edematous and it may contain pools of mucin. The stroma is occasionally so prominent that it obscures the malignant cells, but they can easily be identified in sections stained with periodic ac-

id-Schiff or mucicarmine stains or with immunohistochemical stains for epithelial markers such as cytokeratin, epithelial membrane antigen, or carcinoembryonic antigen. In rare cases, an extraovarian primary tumor cannot be identified in a woman with a typical Krukenberg tumor. Such tumors have been designated as primary Krukenberg tumors. The diagnosis of primary Krukenberg tumor should be made with caution because an occult gastrointestinal primary may remain undetected even after painstaking investigation. It is best to consider all Krukenberg tumors as metastatic until proved otherwise.

Parovarian Tumors and Cysts

Almost any type of ovarian tumor can occur in the broad ligament or elsewhere in the parovarium, perhaps arising in accessory ovarian tissue. The following discussion emphasizes lesions that are encountered in these sites more frequently than in the ovary itself.

Adrenal Cortical Rests and Tumors

Accessory adrenal cortical tissue is rarely present within the ovary, but it is common in a paragonadal location. Small, circumscribed *adrenocortical rests* composed of polygonal adrenal-type cells with abundant clear, vacuolated cytoplasm and small vesicular nuclei are present in more than 20% of women (Fig. 6-100). Tumors resembling adrenal cortical adenomas may arise in this accessory adrenal tissue, and we have seen a myelolipoma develop in one case.

Hydatid of Morgagni

These common benign cysts arise from müllerian vestiges. They are situated below the fallopian tube and usually are an incidental finding. They are occasionally large enough to present clinically as an adnexal mass. They are translucent cysts, usually

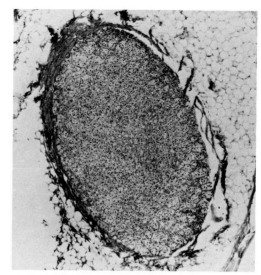

FIGURE 6-100 Parovarian adrenocortical rest.

small, that contain clear or pale yellow fluid. They may be unilocular or multilocular (Fig. 6-101). Microscopically, they are lined by cuboidal to columnar epithelium, often of tubal type, resting on a musculoconnective tissue wall.

Female Adnexal Tumor of Probable Wolffian Origin

The female adnexal tumor of probable wolffian origin is a distinctive adnexal tumor that arises within

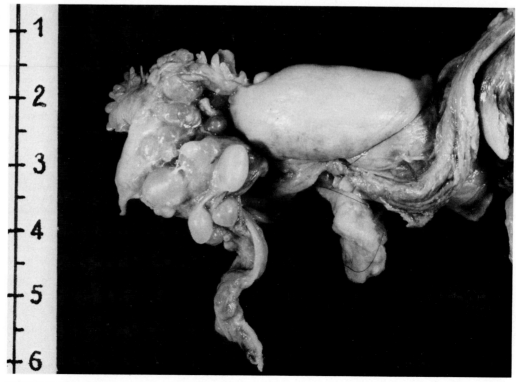

FIGURE 6-101 Parovarian cysts (hydatids of Morgagni).

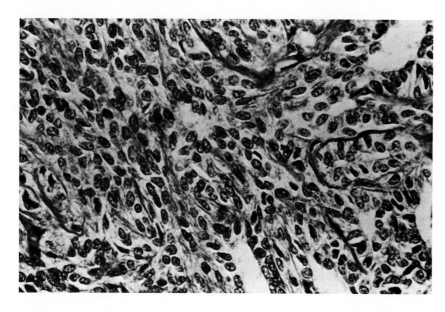

FIGURE 6-102 Adnexal tumor of probable wolffian origin (juxtaovarian tumor).

the broad ligament attached to the mesosalpinx, or within the ovary itself. It may be derived from mesonephric remnants, which are common in this area.[519-521] Most examples are found in middle-aged women, but the neoplasm occurs over a wide age range. The clinical presentation is nonspecific. The tumor is solid and ranges from 2 to 20 cm in diameter. The cut surface is solid and white or gray. The tumor is composed of uniform epithelial cells growing in diffuse, trabecular, tubular (Fig. 6-102), and microcystic patterns. Mitotic activity or cytologic atypia is uncommon. Prominent peritubular basement membranes are characteristic and are best demonstrated with the reticulin stain. Most of these neoplasms are benign, but rare malignant examples are reported. Malignant tumors of wolffian origin exhibit increased mitotic activity or cytologic atypia, overgrowth of spindle cells, or lymphatic invasion.

Adenomatoid Tumor

In the female genital tract, adenomatoid tumors are most common in the fallopian tube or the myometrium. Adenomatoid tumors rarely occur in or immediately adjacent to the ovary.[522] Most measure less than 1 to 2 cm in diameter. They are composed of tubules lined by cuboidal cells and surrounded by fibrous stroma. Adenomatoid tumors are benign neoplasms of mesothelial derivation.

Smooth Muscle Tumors of the Broad Ligament and Round Ligament

Intraligamentary leiomyomas present as firm, white, round nodules surrounded by a thin fibrous capsule. The cut surface demonstrates the typical whorled structure of a smooth muscle tumor. Microscopically, they are similar to uterine leiomyomas. Leiomyosarcoma can arise in the broad ligament.

References

1. Laffargue P, Benkoel L, Laffargue F, Casanova P, Chamlian A: Ultrastructural and enzyme histochemical study of ovarian hilar cells in women and their relationship with sympathetic nerves. Hum Pathol 9:649–659, 1978
2. Rutgers JL, Scully RE: Cysts (cystadenomas) and tumors of the rete ovarii. Int J Gynecol Pathol 7:330–342, 1988
3. Gloor E, Hurlimann J: Autoimmune oophoritis. Am J Clin Pathol 81:105–109, 1984
4. Sedmak DD, Hart WR, Tubbs RR: Autoimmune oophoritis: A histopathologic study of involved ovaries with immunologic characterization of the mononuclear cell infiltrate. Int J Gynecol Pathol 6:73–81, 1987
5. Bannatyne P, Russell P, Shearman RP: Autoimmune oophoritis: A clinicopathologic assessment of 12 cases. Int J Gynecol Pathol 9:191–207, 1990
6. Damewood MD, Zacur HA, Hoffman GJ, Rock JA: Circulating antiovarian antibodies in premature ovarian failure. Obstet Gynecol 68:850–854, 1986
7. Alper MM, Garner PR: Premature ovarian failure: Its relationship to autoimmune disease. Obstet Gynecol 66:27–30, 1985
8. Russell P, Bannatyne P, Shearman RP, Fraser IS, Corbett P: Premature hypergonadotropic ovarian failure: Clinicopathological study of 19 cases. Int J Gynecol Pathol 1:185–201, 1982
9. Cruikshank SH, Van Drie DM: Supernumerary ovaries: Update and review. Obstet Gynecol 60:126–129, 1982
10. Cruikshank S: Supernumerary ovary: Embryology. Int J Gynaecol Obstet 34:175–178, 1991
11. Alpern HD: Supernumerary ovary: A case report. J Reprod Med 32:932–934, 1987
12. Harlass F, Magelssen D, Soisson AP: Supernumerary ovary: A case report. J Reprod Med 32:459–461, 1987
13. Lee B, Gore BZ: A case of supernumerary ovary. Obstet Gynecol 64:738–740, 1984
14. Heller DS, Harpaz N, Breakstone B: Neoplasms arising in ectopic ovaries: A case of Brenner tumor in an accessory ovary. Int J Gynecol Pathol 9:185–189, 1990
15. Schultze H, Fenger C: Accessory ovary. Acta Obstet Gynecol Scand 65:503–504, 1986
16. Price FV, Edwards R, Buchsbaum HJ: Ovarian remnant syndrome: Difficulties in diagnosis and management. Obstet Gynecol Surv 45:151–156, 1990

17. Pettit PD, Lee RA: Ovarian remnant syndrome: Diagnostic dilemma and surgical challenge. Obstet Gynecol 71:580–583, 1988

18. Steege JF: Ovarian remnant syndrome. Obstet Gynecol 70:64–67, 1987

19. Symmonds RE, Pettit PDM: Ovarian remnant syndrome. Obstet Gynecol 54:174–177, 1979

20. Wetchler SJ, Dunn LJ: Ovarian abscess: Report of a case and review of the literature. Obstet Gynecol Surv 40:476–485, 1985

21. Willson JR, Black JR: Ovarian abscess. Am J Obstet Gynecol 90:34–43, 1964

22. Hoffman MS, Roberts WS, Solomon P, Gunasekarin S, Cavanagh D: Advanced pelvic actinoycotic pelvic inflammatory disease simulating gynecologic malignancy: A report of two cases. J Reprod Med 36:543–545, 1991

23. Bahary CM, Ovadia Y, Neri A: *Schistosoma mansoni* of the ovary. Am J Obstet Gynecol 98:290–292, 1967

24. Mahmood K: Granulomatous oophoritis due to *Schistosoma mansoni*. Am J Obstet Gynecol 123:919–920, 1975

25. Pace EH, Voet RL, Melancon JT: Xanthogranulomatous oophoritis: An inflammatory pseudotumor of the ovary. Int J Gynecol Pathol 3:398–402, 1984

26. Nogales FF, Silverberg SG: Epidermoid cysts of the ovary: A report of five cases with histogenetic considerations and ultrastructural findings. Am J Obstet Gynecol 124:523–528, 1976

27. Young RH, Prat J, Scully RE: Epidermoid cysts of the ovary: A report of three cases with comments on histogenesis. Am J Clin Pathol 73:272–276, 1980

28. Stanley MW, Horwitz CA, Frable WJ: Cellular follicular cyst of the ovary: Fluid cytology mimicking malignancy. Diagn Cytopathol 7:48–52, 1991

29. Selvaggi SM: Fine-needle aspiration cytology of ovarian follicle cysts with cellular atypia from reproductive-age patients. Diagn Cytopathol 7:189–192, 1991

30. Clement PB, Scully RE: Large solitary luteinized follicle cyst of pregnancy and puerperium: A clinicopathological analysis of eight cases. Am J Surg Pathol 4:431–438, 1980

31. Clement PB, Young RH, Scully RE: Nontrophoblastic pathology of the female genital tract and peritoneum associated with pregnancy. Semin Diagn Pathol 6:372–406, 1989

32. Wajda KJ, Lucas JG, Marsh WL Jr: Hyperreactio luteinalis: Benign disorder masquerading as an ovarian neoplasm. Arch Pathol Lab Med 113:921–925, 1989

33. Ovarian hyperstimulation syndrome. Lancet 338:1111–1112, 1991

34. Garcia-Bunuel R, Berek JS, Woodruff JD: Luteomas of pregnancy. Obstet Gynecol 45:407–414, 1975

35. Norris HJ, Taylor HB: Nodular theca-lutein hyperplasia of pregnancy (so-called "pregnancy luteoma"): A clinical and pathologic study of 15 cases. Am J Clin Pathol 47:557–566, 1967

36. Paraskevas M, Scully RE: Hilus cell tumor of the ovary: A clinicopathological analysis of 12 Reinke crystal-positive cases and nine crystal-negative cases. Int J Gynecol Pathol 8:299–310, 1989

37. Roth LM, Sternberg WH: Ovarian stromal tumors containing Leydig cells. II. Pure Leydig cell tumors, non-hilar type. Cancer 32:952–960, 1973

38. Sternberg WH, Roth LM: Ovarian stromal tumors containing Leydig cells. I. Stromal-Leydig tumor and non-neoplastic transformation of ovarian stroma to Leydig cells. Cancer 32:940–951, 1973

39. Roth LM, Sternberg WH: Partly luteinized theca cell tumor of the ovary. Cancer 51:1697–1704, 1983

40. Zhang J, Young RH, Arseneau J, Scully RE: Ovarian stromal tumors containing lutein or Leydig cells (luteinized thecomas and stromal Leydig tumors): A clinicopathological analysis of 50 cases. Int J Gynecol Pathol 1:270–285, 1982

41. Heller DS, Frydman CP, Klein MJ, Bleiweiss IJ, Bacall C: Luteoma of pregnancy. Mt Sinai J Med 57:40–42, 1990

42. Stein IF, Leventhal ML: Amenorrhea associated with bilateral polycystic ovaries. Am J Obstet Gynecol 29:181–191, 1935

43. Devaney K, Tavassoli FA: Immunohistochemistry as a diagnostic aid in the interpretation of unusual mesenchymal tumors of the uterus. Mod Pathol 4:225–231, 1991

44. McKenna JT: Pathogenesis and treatment of polycystic ovarian syndrome. N Engl J Med 318:558–562, 1988

45. Goldzieher JW, Young RL: Selected aspects of polycystic ovarian disease. Endocrinol Metab Clin North Am 21:141–171, 1992

46. Biggs JSG: Polycystic ovarian disease: Current concepts. Aust N Z J Obstet Gynaecol 21:26–36, 1981

47. Coney P: Polycystic ovarian disease: Current concepts of pathophysiology and therapy. Fertil Steril 42:667–682, 1984

48. Mauvais-Jarvis P, Bricaire J: Pathophysiology of polycystic ovary syndrome. J Steroid Biochem 33:791–794, 1989

49. Hutchinson-Williams KA, DeCherney AH: Pathogenesis and treatment of polycystic ovary disease. Int J Fertil 32:421–430, 1987

50. Nader S: Polycystic ovary syndrome and the androgen-insulin connection. Am J Obstet Gynecol 165:346–348, 1991

51. Sasano H, Fukunaga M, Rojas M, Silverberg SG: Hyperthecosis of the ovary: Clinicopathologic study of 19 cases with immunohistochemical analysis of steroidogenic enzymes. Int J Gynecol Pathol 8:311–320, 1989

52. Dunaif A, Hoffman AR, Scully RE et al: Clinical, biochemical and ovarian morphologic features in women with acanthosis nigricans and masculinization. Obstet Gynecol 66:545–552, 1985

53. Boss JH, Scully RE, Wegner KH, Cohen RB: Structural variations in the adult ovary: Clinical significance. Obstet Gynecol 25:747–764, 1965

54. Chervenak FA, Castadot M, Wiederman J, Sedlis A: Massive ovarian edema: A review of world's literature and report of two cases. Obstet Gynecol Surv 35:677–684, 1980

55. Kanbour AI, Salazar H, Tobon H: Massive ovarian edema: A non-neoplastic pelvic mass of young women. Arch Pathol Lab Med 103:42–45, 1979

56. Roth LM, Deaton RL, Sternberg WH: Massive ovarian edema: A clinicopathologic study of five cases including ultrastructural observations and review of the literature. Am J Surg Pathol 3:11–21, 1979

57. Young RH, Scully RE: Fibromatosis and massive edema of the ovary, possibly related entities: A report of 14 cases of fibromatosis and 11 cases of massive edema. Int J Gynecol Pathol 3:153–178, 1984

58. Clement PB, Young RH, Scully RE: Necrotic pseudoxanthomatous nodules of ovary and peritoneum in endometriosis. Am J Surg Pathol 12:390–397, 1988

59. Mostoufizadeh M, Scully RE: Malignant tumors arising in endometriosis. Clin Obstet Gynecol 23:951–963, 1980

60. Heaps JM, Nieberg RK, Berek JS: Malignant neoplasms arising in endometriosis. Obstet Gynecol 75:1023–1028, 1990

61. Czernobilsky B, Morris WJ: A histologic study of ovarian endometriosis with emphasis on hyperplastic and atypical changes. Obstet Gynecol 53:318–323, 1979

62. LaGrenade A, Silverberg SG: Ovarian tumors associated with atypical endometriosis. Hum Pathol 19:1080–1084, 1988

63. Moll UM, Chumas JC, Chalas E, Mann WJ: Ovarian carcinoma arising in atypical endometriosis. Obstet Gynecol 75:537–539, 1990

64. Scully RE: Tumors of the ovary and maldeveloped gonads (AFIP Fascicle 16, 2nd series). Washington, DC, Armed Forces Institute of Pathology, 1979

65. Jacobs I, Bast RC Jr: The CA 125 tumor-associated antigen: A review of the literature. Hum Reprod 4:1–12, 1989

66. Chien RT, Rettenmaier MA, Micha JP, DiSaia PJ: Ovarian epithelial tumors of low malignant potential. Surg Gynecol Obstet 169:143–146, 1989

67. Lim-Tan SK, Cajigas HE, Scully RE: Ovarian cystectomy for serous borderline tumors: A follow-up study of 35 cases. Obstet Gynecol 72:775–781, 1988
68. Rice LW, Berkowitz RS, Mark SD, Yavner DL, Lage JM: Epithelial ovarian tumors of borderline malignancy. Gynecol Oncol 39:195–198, 1990
69. Chambers JT, Merino MJ, Kohorn EI, Schwartz PE: Borderline ovarian tumors. Am J Obstet Gynecol 159:1088–1094, 1988
70. Bostwick DG, Tazelaar HD, Ballon SC, Hendrickson MR, Kempson RL: Ovarian epithelial tumors of borderline malignancy: A clinical and pathologic study of 109 cases. Cancer 58:2052–2065, 1986
71. Nikrui N: Survey of clinical behavior of patients with borderline epithelial tumors of the ovary. Gynecol Oncol 12:107–119, 1981
72. Barnhill D, Heller P, Brzozowski P, Advani H, Gallup D, Park R: Epithelial ovarian carcinoma of low malignant potential. Obstet Gynecol 65:53–59, 1985
73. Russell P: The pathological assessment of ovarian neoplasms. II. The proliferating "epithelial" tumors. Pathology 11:251–282, 1979
74. Tasker M, Langley FA: The outlook for women with borderline epithelial tumours of the ovary. Br J Obstet Gynaecol 92:969–973, 1985
75. Kliman L, Rome RM, Fortune DW: Low malignant potential tumors of the ovary: A study of 76 cases. Obstet Gynecol 68:338–344, 1986
76. Nakashima N, Nagasaka T, Oiwa N et al: Ovarian epithelial tumors of borderline malignancy in Japan. Gynecol Oncol 38:90–98, 1990
77. Massad LS Jr, Hunter VJ, Szpak CA, Clarke-Pearson DL, Creasman WT: Epithelial ovarian tumors of low malignant potential. Obstet Gynecol 78:1027–1032, 1991
78. Manchul LA, Simm J, Levin W et al: Borderline epithelial ovarian tumors: A review of 81 cases with an assessment of the impact of treatment. Int J Radiat Oncol Biol Phys 22:867–874, 1992
79. Katzenstein AL, Mazur MT, Morgan TE, Kao MS: Proliferative serous tumors of the ovary: Histologic features and prognosis. Am J Surg Pathol 2:339–355, 1978
80. Fort MG, Pierce VK, Saigo PE, Hoskins WJ, Lewis JL Jr: Evidence for the efficacy of adjuvant therapy in epithelial ovarian tumors of low malignant potential. Gynecol Oncol 32:269–272, 1989
81. Sutton GP, Bundy BN, Omura GA, Yordan EL, Beecham JB, Bonfiglio T: Stage III ovarian tumors of low malignant potential treated with cisplatin combination therapy (a Gynecologic Oncology Group study). Gynecol Oncol 41:230–233, 1991
82. Hart WR, Norris HJ: Borderline and malignant mucinous tumors of the ovary: Histologic criteria and clinical behavior. Cancer 31:1031–1045, 1973
83. Chaitin BA, Gershenson DM, Evans HL: Mucinous tumors of the ovary: A clinicopathologic study of 70 cases. Cancer 55:1958–1962, 1985
84. Michael H, Sutton G, Roth LM: Ovarian carcinoma with extracellular mucin production: reassessment of "pseudomyxoma ovarii et peritonei." Int J Gynecol Pathol 6:298–312, 1987
85. Kahn MA, Demopoulos RI: Mucinous ovarian tumors with pseudomyxoma peritonei: A clinicopathological study. Int J Gynecol Pathol 11:15–23, 1992
86. Mann WJ Jr, Wagner J, Chumas J, Chalas E: The management of pseudomyxoma peritonei. Cancer 66:1636–1640, 1990
87. Synder RR, Norris HJ, Tavassoli F: Endometrioid proliferative and low malignant potential tumors of the ovary: A clinicopathologic study of 46 cases. Am J Surg Pathol 12:661–671, 1988
88. Bell DA, Scully RE: Atypical and borderline endometrioid adenofibromas of the ovary: A report of 27 cases. Am J Surg Pathol 9:205–214, 1985
89. Bell DA, Scully RE: Benign and borderline clear cell adenofibromas of the ovary. Cancer 56:2911–2931, 1985
90. Hallgrimsson J, Scully RE: Borderline and malignant Brenner tumours of the ovary: A report of 15 cases. Acta Pathol Microbiol Scand [A] 80(Suppl 233):56–66, 1972
91. Woodruff JD, Dietrich D, Genadry R, Parmley TH: Proliferative and malignant Brenner tumors: Review of 47 cases. Am J Obstet Gynecol 141:118–125, 1981
92. Miles PA, Norris HJ: Proliferative and malignant Brenner tumors of the ovary. Cancer 30:174–186, 1972
93. Roth LM, Dallenbach-Hellweg G, Czernobilsky B: Ovarian Brenner tumors. I. Metaplastic, proliferating, and low malignant potential. Cancer 562:582–591, 1985
94. Ozols RF, Young RC: Chemotherapy of ovarian cancer. Semin Oncol 18:222–232, 1991
95. Gershenson DM, Wharton JT, Copeland LJ et al: Treatment of advanced epithelial ovarian cancer with cisplatin and cyclophosphamide. Gynecol Oncol 32:336–341, 1989
96. Sutton GP, Stehman FB, Einhorn LH, Roth LM, Blessing JA, Ehrlich CE: Ten-year follow-up of patients receiving cisplatin, doxorubicin, and cyclophosphamide chemotherapy for advanced epithelial ovarian carcinoma. J Clin Oncol 7:223–229, 1989
97. Podratz KC, Malkasian GD Jr, Wieand HS et al: Recurrent disease after negative second-look laparotomy in stages III and IV ovarian carcinoma. Gynecol Oncol 29:274–282, 1988
98. Podczaski ES, Stevens CW Jr, Manetta A, Whitney CW, Larson JE, Mortel R: Use of second-look laparotomy in the management of patients with ovarian epithelial malignancies. Gynecol Oncol 28:205–214, 1987
99. Rubin SC, Hoskins WJ, Saigo PE et al: Prognostic factors for recurrence following negative second-look laparotomy in ovarian cancer patients treated with platinum-based chemotherapy. Gynecol Oncol 42:137–141, 1991
100. Gershenson DM, Copeland LJ, Wharton JT et al: Prognosis of surgically determined complete responders in advanced ovarian cancer. Cancer 55:1129–1135, 1985
101. Robey SS, Silva EG, Gershenson DM, McLemore D, el-Naggar A, Ordonez NG: Transitional cell carcinoma in high-grade high-stage ovarian carcinoma: An indicator of favorable response to chemotherapy. Cancer 63:839–847, 1989
102. Hacker NF, Berek JS, Pretorius RG, Zuckerman J, Eisenkop S, Lagasse LD: Intraperitoneal cis-platinum as salvage therapy for refractory epithelial ovarian cancer. Obstet Gynecol 70:759–764, 1987
103. Howell SB, Zimm S, Markman M et al: Long-term survival of advanced refractory ovarian carcinoma patients with small-volume disease treated with intraperitoneal chemotherapy. J Clin Oncol 5:1607–1612, 1987
104. Markman M: Intraperitoneal chemotherapy. Semin Oncol 18:248–254, 1991
105. Piver MS, Lele SB, Bakshi S, Parthasarathy KL, Emrich LJ: Five and ten year estimated survival and disease-free rates after intraperitoneal chromic phosphate: Stage I ovarian adenocarcinoma. Am J Clin Oncol 11:515–519, 1988
106. Varia M, Rosenman J, Venkatraman S et al: Intraperitoneal chromic phosphate therapy after second-look laparotomy for ovarian cancer. Cancer 61:919–927, 1988
107. Soper JT, Wilkinson RH Jr, Bandy LC, Clarke-Pearson DL, Creasman WT: Intraperitoneal chromic phosphate P 32 as salvage therapy for persistent carcinoma of the ovary after surgical restaging. Am J Obstet Gynecol 156:1153–1158, 1987
108. Lanciano RM, Randall M: Update on the role of radiotherapy in ovarian cancer. Semin Oncol 18:233–247, 1991
109. Fuller DB, Sause WT, Plenk HP, Menlove RL: Analysis of postoperative radiation therapy in stage I through III epithelial ovarian carcinoma. J Clin Oncol 5:897–905, 1987
110. Dembo AJ: Epithelial ovarian cancer: The role of radiotherapy. Int J Radiat Oncol Biol Phys 22:835–845, 1992
111. Bolis G, Zanaboni F, Vanoli P, Russo A, Franchi M,

Scarfone G, Pecorelli S: The impact of whole-abdomen radiotherapy on survival in advanced ovarian cancer patients with minimal residual disease after chemotherapy. Gynecol Oncol 39:150–154, 1990

112. Iversen OE: Prognostic value of the flow cytometric DNA index in human ovarian carcinoma. Cancer 61:971–975, 1988

113. Kallioniemi OP, Punnonen R, Mattila J, Lehtinen M, Koivula T: Prognostic significance of DNA index, multiploidy, and s-phase fraction in ovarian cancer. Cancer 61:334–339, 1988

114. Blumenfeld D, Braly PS, Ben-Ezra J, Klevecz RR: Tumor DNA content as a prognostic feature in advanced epithelial ovarian carcinoma. Gynecol Oncol 27:389–402, 1987

115. Barnabei VM, Miller DS, Bauer KD, Murad TM, Rademaker AW, Lurain JR: Flow cytometric evaluation of epithelial ovarian cancer. Am J Obstet Gynecol 162:1584–90; discus, 1990

116. Volm M, Kleine W, Pfleiderer A: Flow-cytometric prognostic factors for the survival of patients with ovarian carcinoma: A 5-year follow-up study. Gynecol Oncol 35:84–89, 1989

117. Brescia RJ, Barakat RA, Beller U et al: The prognostic significance of nuclear DNA content in malignant epithelial tumors of the ovary. Cancer 65:141–147, 1990

118. Lage JM, Weinberg DS, Huettner PC, Mark SD: Flow cytometric analysis of nuclear DNA content in ovarian tumors: Association of ploidy with tumor type, histologic grade, and clinical stage. Cancer 69:2668–2675, 1992

119. Klemi PJ, Joensuu H, Maenpää J, Kiilholma P: Influence of cellular DNA content on survival in ovarian carcinoma. Obstet Gynecol 74:200–204, 1989

120. Rodenburg CJ, Cornelisse CJ, Heintz PAM, Hermans J, Fleuren GJ: Tumor ploidy as a major prognostic factor in advanced ovarian cancer. Cancer 59:317–323, 1987

121. Murray K, Hopwood L, Volk D, Wilson JF: Cytofluorometric analysis of the DNA content in ovarian carcinoma and its relationship to patient survival. Cancer 63:2456–2460, 1989

122. Silverberg SG: Prognostic significance of pathologic features of ovarian carcinoma. Curr Top Pathol 78:85–109, 1989

123. Purola E: Serous papillary ovarian tumors: A study of 233 cases with special reference to the histological type of tumor and its influence in prognosis. Acta Obstet Gynecol Scand 42(Suppl 3):1–77, 1963

124. Russell P: The pathological assessment of ovarian neoplasms. I. Introduction to the common "epithelial" tumours and analysis of benign "epithelial" tumours. Pathology 11:5–26, 1979

125. Raney RB Jr, Sinclair L, Uri A, Schnaufer L, Cooper A, Littman P: Malignant ovarian tumors in children and adolescents. Cancer 59:1214–1220, 1987

126. Jensen RD, Norris HJ: Epithelial tumors of the ovary: Occurrence in children and adolescents less than 20 years of age. Arch Pathol 94:29–34, 1972

127. Diamond MP, Baxter JW, Peerman CG Jr, Burnett LS: Occurrence of ovarian malignancy in childhood and adolescence: A community-wide evaluation. Obstet Gynecol 71:858–860, 1988

128. Mills SE, Andersen WA, Fechner RE, Austin MB: Serous surface papillary carcinoma: A clinicopathologic study of 10 cases and comparison with stage III-IV ovarian serous carcinoma. Am J Surg Pathol 12:827–834, 1988

129. White PF, Merino MJ, Barwick KW: Serous surface papillary carcinoma of the ovary: A clinical, pathologic, ultrastructural, and immunohistochemical study of 11 cases. Pathol Annu 20(Part 1):403–418, 1985

130. Rutledge ML, Silva EG, McLemore D, el-Naggar A: Serous surface carcinoma of the ovary and peritoneum: A flow cytometric study. Pathol Annu 24(Part 2):227–235, 1989

131. Gooneratne S, Sassone M, Blaustein A, Talerman A: Serous surface papillary carcinoma of the ovary: A clinicopathologic study of 16 cases. Int J Gynecol Pathol 1:258–269, 1982

132. Ferenczy A, Talens A, Zoghby M, Hussain SS: Ultrastructural studies on the morphogenesis of psammoma bodies in ovarian serous neoplasia. Cancer 39:2451–2459, 1977

133. Zaloudek C, Norris HJ: Sertoli-Leydig tumors of the ovary: A clinicopathologic study of 64 intermediate and poorly differentiated neoplasms. Am J Surg Pathol 8:405–418, 1984

134. Kao GF, Norris HJ: Cystadenofibromas of the ovary with epithelial atypia. Am J Surg Pathol 2:357–363, 1978

135. Tavassoli FA: Serous tumor of low malignant potential with early stromal invasion (serous LMP with microinvasion). Mod Pathol 1:407–414, 1988

136. Bell DA, Scully RE: Ovarian serous borderline tumors with stromal microinvasion: A report of 21 cases. Hum Pathol 21:397–403, 1990

137. Bell DA, Weinstock MA, Scully RE: Peritoneal implants of ovarian serous borderline tumors: Histologic features and prognosis. Cancer 62:2212–2222, 1988

138. Michael H, Roth LM: Invasive and noninvasive implants in ovarian serous tumors of low malignant potential. Cancer 57:1240–1247, 1986

139. Gershenson DM, Silva EG: Serous ovarian tumors of low malignant potential with peritoneal implants. Cancer 65:578–585, 1990

140. Ulbright TM, Roth LM, Sutton GP: Papillary serous carcinoma of the ovary with squamous differentiation. Int J Gynecol Pathol 9:86–94, 1990

141. Gilks CB, Bell DA, Scully RE: Serous psammocarcinoma of the ovary and peritoneum. Int J Gynecol Pathol 9:110–121, 1990

142. Blaustein A: Papillary serous tumors of the ovary: An electron microscopic study. Gynecol Oncol 4:314–323, 1976

143. Fenoglio CM: Overview article: Ultrastructural features of the common epithelial tumors of the ovary. Ultrastruct Pathol 1:419–444, 1980

144. Klemi PJ, Nevalainen TJ: Ultrastructural and histochemical observations on serous ovarian cystadenomas. Acta Pathol Microbiol Scand [A] 86:303–312, 1978

145. Rutgers JL, Scully RE: Ovarian müllerian mucinous papillary cystadenomas of borderline malignancy: A clinicopathologic analysis. Cancer 61:340–348, 1988

146. Young RH, Scully RE: Ovarian Sertoli-Leydig cell tumors with a retiform pattern--a problem in diagnosis: A report of 25 cases. Am J Surg Pathol 7:755–771, 1983

147. Stalsberg H, Abeler V, Blom GP, Bostad L, Skarland E, Westgaard G: Observer variation in histologic classification of malignant and borderline ovarian tumors. Hum Pathol 19:1030–1035, 1988

148. Ball NJ, Robertson DI, Duggan MA, Snider DD: Intestinal differentiation in ovarian mucinous tumours. Virchows Arch A Pathol Anat Histopathol 417:197–201, 1990

149. Klemi PJ: Pathology of mucinous ovarian cystadenomas. I. Argyrophil and argentaffin cells and epithelial mucosubstances. Acta Pathol Microbiol Scand [A] 86:465–470, 1978

150. Bell DA: Mucinous adenofibromas of the ovary: A report of 10 cases. Am J Surg Pathol 15:227–232, 1991

151. Kao GF, Norris HJ: Unusual cystadenofibromas: Endometrioid, mucinous, and clear cell type. Obstet Gynecol 54:729–736, 1979

152. Sasaki E, Sasano N, Kimura N, Andoh N, Yajima A: Demonstration of neuroendocrine cells in ovarian mucinous tumors. Int J Gynecol Pathol 8:189–200, 1989

153. Aguirre P, Scully RE, Dayal Y, DeLellis RA: Mucinous tumors of the ovary with argyrophil cells: An immunohistochemical study. Am J Surg Pathol 8:345–356, 1984

154. DeBoer WG, Ma J, Nayman J: Intestine-associated antigens in ovarian tumours: An immunohistochemical study. Pathology 13:547–555, 1981

155. Louwerens JK, Schaberg A, Bosman FT: Neuroendocrine cells in cystic mucinous tumours of the ovary. Histopathology 7:389–398, 1983

156. Sporrong B, Alumets J, Clase L et al: Neurohormonal peptide immunoreactive cells in mucinous cystadenomas and cystadenocarcinomas of the ovary. Virchows Arch A Pathol Anat Histopathol 392:271–280, 1981

157. Tenti P, Aguzzi A, Riva C et al: Ovarian mucinous tumors frequently express markers of gastric, intestinal, and pancreatobiliary epithelial cells. Cancer 69:2131–2142, 1992

158. Watkin W, Silva EG, Gershenson DM: Mucinous carcinoma of the ovary: Pathologic prognostic factors. Cancer 69:208–212, 1992

159. Hart WR: Ovarian epithelial tumors of borderline malignancy (carcinomas of low malignant potential). Hum Pathol 8:541–549, 1977

160. Prat J, Scully RE: Ovarian mucinous tumors with sarcoma-like mural nodules: A report of seven cases. Cancer 44:1332–1344, 1979

161. Prat J, Scully RE: Sarcomas in ovarian mucinous tumors: A report of two cases. Cancer 44:1327–1331, 1979

162. Bruijn JA, Smit VT, Que DG, Fleuren GJ: Immunohistology of a sarcomatous mural nodule in an ovarian mucinous cystadenocarcinoma. Int J Gynecol Pathol 6:287–293, 1987

163. Sondergaard G, Kaspersen P: Ovarian and extraovarian mucinous tumors with solid mural nodules. Int J Gynecol Pathol 10:145–155, 1991

164. Czernobilsky B, Dgani R, Roth LM: Ovarian mucinous cystadenocarcinoma with mural nodule of carcinomatous derivation: A light and electron microscopic study. Cancer 51:141–148, 1983

165. Prat J, Young RH, Scully RE: Ovarian mucinous tumors with foci of anaplastic carcinoma. Cancer 50:300–304, 1982

166. Nichols GE, Mills SE, Ulbright TM, Czernobilsky B, Roth LM: Spindle cell mural nodules in cystic ovarian mucinous tumors: A clinicopathologic and immunohistochemical study of five cases. Am J Surg Pathol 15:1055–1062, 1991

167. Klemi PJ, Nevalainen TJ: Pathology of mucinous ovarian cystadenomas. 2. Ultrastructural findings. Acta Pathol Microbiol Scand [A] 86:471–481, 1978

168. Limber GK, King RE, Silverberg SG: Pseudomyxoma peritonaei: A report of ten cases. Ann Surg 178:587–593, 1973

169. Sandenbergh HA, Woodruff JD: Histogenesis of pseudomyxoma peritonei: Review of 9 cases. Obstet Gynecol 49:339–345, 1977

170. Young RH, Gilks CB, Scully RE: Mucinous tumors of the appendix associated with mucinous tumors of the ovary and pseudomyxoma peritonei: A clinicopathological analysis of 22 cases supporting an origin in the appendix. Am J Surg Pathol 15:415–429, 1991

171. Lash RH, Hart WR: Intestinal adenocarcinomas metastatic to the ovaries: A clinicopathologic evaluation of 22 cases. Am J Surg Pathol 11:114–121, 1987

172. Daya D, Nazerali L, Frank GL: Metastatic ovarian carcinoma of large intestinal origin simulating primary ovarian carcinoma: A clinicopathologic study of 25 cases. Am J Clin Pathol 97:751–758, 1992

173. Aure JC, Hoeg K, Kolstad P: Clinical and histologic studies of ovarian carcinoma: Long-term follow-up of 990 cases. Obstet Gynecol 37:1–9, 1971

174. Kline RC, Wharton JT, Atkinson EN, Burke TW, Gershenson DM, Edwards CL: Endometrioid carcinoma of the ovary: Retrospective review of 145 cases. Gynecol Oncol 39:337–346, 1990

175. Roth LM, Czernobilsky B, Langley FA: Ovarian endometrioid adenofibromatous and cystadenofibromatous tumors: Benign, proliferating, and malignant. Cancer 48:1838–1845, 1981

176. Brescia RJ, Dubin N, Demopoulos RI: Endometrioid and clear cell carcinoma of the ovary: Factors affecting survival. Int J Gynecol Pathol 8:132–138, 1989

177. Klemi PJ, Gronroos M: Endometrioid carcinoma of the ovary: A clinicopathologic, histochemical, and electron microscopic study. Obstet Gynecol 53:572–579, 1979

178. Kurman RJ, Craig JM: Endometrioid and clear cell carcinoma of the ovary. Cancer 29:1653–1664, 1972

179. Russell P: The pathological assessment of ovarian neoplasms. III. The malignant "epithelial" tumors. Pathology 11:493–532, 1979

180. Czernobilsky B: Endometrioid neoplasia of the ovary: A reappraisal. Int J Gynecol Pathol 1:203–210, 1982

181. Fu YS, Stock RJ, Reagan JW, Storaasli JP, Wentz WB: Significance of squamous components in endometrioid carcinoma of the ovary. Cancer 44:614–621, 1979

182. Eifel P, Hendrickson M, Ross J, Ballon S, Martinez A, Kempson R: Simultaneous presentation of carcinoma involving the ovary and the uterine corpus. Cancer 50:163–170, 1982

183. Clement PB, Young RH, Scully RE: Endometrioid-like variant of ovarian yolk sac tumor: A clinicopathological analysis of eight cases. Am J Surg Pathol 11:767–778, 1987

184. Aguirre P, Thor AD, Scully RE: Ovarian endometrioid carcinomas resembling sex cord-stromal tumors: An immunohistochemical study. Int J Gynecol Pathol 8:364–373, 1989

185. Roth LM, Liban E, Czernobilsky B: Ovarian endometrioid tumors mimicking Sertoli and Sertoli-Leydig cell tumors: Sertoliform variant of endometrioid carcinoma. Cancer 50:1322–1331, 1982

186. Young RH, Prat J, Scully RE: Ovarian endometrioid carcinomas resembling sex cord-stromal tumors: A clinicopathologic analysis of 13 cases. Am J Surg Pathol 6:513–522, 1982

187. Montag AG, Jenison EL, Griffiths CT, Welch WR, Lavin PT, Knapp RC: Ovarian clear cell carcinoma: A clinicopathologic analysis of 44 cases. Int J Gynecol Pathol 8:85–96, 1989

188. Crozier MA, Copeland LJ, Silva EG, Gershenson DM, Stringer CA: Clear cell carcinoma of the ovary: A study of 59 cases. Gynecol Oncol 35:199–203, 1989

189. Kennedy AW, Biscotti CV, Hart WR, Webster KD: Ovarian clear cell adenocarcinoma. Gynecol Oncol 32:342–349, 1989

190. Aure JC, Hoeg K, Kolstad P: Mesonephroid tumors of the ovary: Clinical and histopathologic studies. Obstet Gynecol 37:860–867, 1971

191. Norris HJ, Rabinowitz M: Ovarian adenocarcinoma of mesonephric type. Cancer 28:1074–1081, 1971

192. Roth LM, Langley FA, Fox H, Wheeler JE, Czernobilsky B: Ovarian clear cell adenofibromatous tumors: Benign, low malignant potential, and associated with invasive clear cell carcinoma. Cancer 53:1156–1163, 1984

193. Scully RE, Barlow JF: "Mesonephroma" of ovary: Tumor of Müllerian nature related to endometrioid carcinoma. Cancer 20:1405–1417, 1967

194. Czernobilsky B, Silverman BB, Enterline HT: Clear cell carcinoma of the ovary: A clinicopathologic analysis of pure and mixed forms and comparison with endometrioid carcinoma. Cancer 25:762–772, 1970

195. Rogers LW, Julian CG, Woodruff JD: Mesonephroid carcinoma of the ovary: A study of 95 cases from the Emil Novak Ovarian Tumor Registry. Gynecol Oncol 1:76–89, 1972

196. Young RH, Scully RE: Oxyphilic clear cell carcinoma of the ovary: A report of nine cases. Am J Surg Pathol 11:661–667, 1987

197. Ohkawa K, Amasaki H, Terashima Y, Aizawa S, Ishikawa E: Clear cell carcinoma of the ovary: Light and electron microscopic studies. Cancer 40:3019–3029, 1977

198. Salazar H, Merkow LP, Walter WS, Pardo M: Human ovarian neoplasms: Light and electron microscopic considerations. II. The clear cell tumor. Obstet Gynecol 44:551–563, 1974

199. Silverberg SG: Ultrastructure and histogenesis of clear cell carcinoma of the ovary. Am J Obstet Gynecol 115:394–400, 1973

200. Zirker TA, Silva EG, Morris M, Ordonez NG: Immunohistochemical differentiation of clear-cell carcinoma of the fe-

male genital tract and endodermal sinus tumor with the use of alpha-fetoprotein and Leu-M1. Am J Clin Pathol 91:511–514, 1989

201. Young RH, Scully RE: Metastatic tumors in the ovary: A problem-oriented approach and review of the recent literature. Semin Diagn Pathol 8:250–276, 1991

202. Yoonessi M, Abell MR: Brenner tumors of the ovary. Obstet Gynecol 54:90–96, 1979

203. Balasa RW, Adcock LL, Prem KA, Dehner LP: The Brenner tumor: A clinicopathologic review. Obstet Gynecol 50:120–128, 1977

204. Fox H, Agrawal K, Langley FA: The Brenner tumour of the ovary: A clinicopathological study of 54 cases. J Obstet Gynecol Br Commonw 79:661–665, 1972

205. Silverberg SG: Brenner tumor of the ovary: A clinicopathologic study of 60 tumors in 54 women. Cancer 28:588–596, 1971

206. Jorgensen EO, Dockerty MB, Wilson RB, Welch JS: Clinicopathologic study of 53 cases of Brenner's tumors of the ovary. Am J Obstet Gynecol 108:122–127, 1970

207. Carpen E: Brenner tumours of the ovary: A clinicopathological study. Acta Obstet Gynecol Scand Suppl 50:1–41, 1976

208. Ehrlich CE, Roth LM: The Brenner tumor: A clinicopathologic study of 57 cases. Cancer 27:332–342, 1971

209. Chen KT, Hoffmann KD: Malignant Brenner tumor of the ovary. J Surg Oncol 39:260–263, 1988

210. Austin RM, Norris HJ: Malignant Brenner tumor and transitional cell carcinoma of the ovary: A comparison. Int J Gynecol Pathol 6:29–39, 1987

211. Seldenrijk CA, Willig AP, Baak JP et al: Malignant Brenner tumor: A histologic, morphometrical, immunohistochemical, and ultrastructural study. Cancer 58:754–760, 1986

212. Roth LM, Czernobilsky B: Ovarian Brenner tumors. II. Malignant. Cancer 56:592–601, 1985

213. Silva EG, Robey-Cafferty SS, Smith TL, Gershenson DM: Ovarian carcinomas with transitional cell carcinoma pattern. Am J Clin Pathol 93:457–465, 1990

214. Lamping JD, Blythe JG: Bilateral Brenner tumors: A case report and review of the literature. Hum Pathol 8:583–585, 1977

215. Roth LM: The Brenner tumor and the Walthard cell nest: An electron microscopic study. Lab Invest 31:15–23, 1974

216. Bransilver BR, Ferenczy A, Richart RM: Brenner tumors and Walthard cell nests. Arch Pathol 98:76–86, 1974

217. Trebeck CE, Friedlander ML, Russell P, Baird PJ: Brenner tumours of the ovary: A study of the histology, immunohistochemistry and cellular DNA content in benign, borderline and malignant ovarian tumors. Pathology 19:241–246, 1987

218. Silva EG, Tornos C, Bailey MA, Morris M: Undifferentiated carcinoma of the ovary. Arch Pathol Lab Med 115:377–381, 1991

219. Dinh TV, Slavin RE, Bhagavan BS, Hannigan EV, Tiamson EM, Yandell RB: Mixed mesodermal tumors of the ovary: A clinicopathologic study of 14 cases. Obstet Gynecol 72:409–412, 1988

220. Suggs CL, Lee JL, Jr., Choi H, Lewis GC: Malignant mixed mesodermal tumors of the ovary: A report of 13 cases. Am J Clin Oncol 11:12–15, 1988

221. Shakfeh SM, Woodruff JD: Primary ovarian sarcomas: Report of 46 cases and review of the literature. Obstet Gynecol Surv 42:331–349, 1987

222. Terada KY, Johnson TL, Hopkins M, Roberts JA: Clinicopathologic features of ovarian mixed mesodermal tumors and carcinosarcomas. Gynecol Oncol 32:228–232, 1989

223. Barwick KW, Livolsi VA: Malignant mixed mesodermal tumors of the ovary: A clinicopathologic assessment of 12 cases. Am J Surg Pathol 4:37–42, 1980

224. Dehner LP, Norris HJ, Taylor HB: Carcinosarcomas and mixed mesodermal tumors of the ovary. Cancer 27:207–216, 1971

225. Calame JJ, Schaberg A: Solid teratomas and mixed Müllerian tumors of the ovary: A clinical, histological, and immunocytochemical comparative study. Gynecol Oncol 33:212–221, 1989

226. Pfeiffer P, Hardt-Madsen M, Rex S, Holund B, Bertelsen K: Malignant mixed Müllerian tumors of the ovary: Report of 13 cases. Acta Obstet Gynecol Scand 70:79–84, 1991

227. Ortega I, Nogales FF, Amerigo J, Fernandez-Sanz J: Carcinosarcomas and mixed mesodermal tumors of the ovary: A clinicopathologic study of six cases. Int J Gynaecol Obstet 15:561–565, 1978

228. Dictor M: Malignant mixed mesodermal tumor of the ovary: A report of 22 cases. Obstet Gynecol 65:720–724, 1985

229. Morrow CP, d'Ablaing G, Brady LW, Blessing JA, Hreschyshyn MM: A clinical and pathologic study of 30 cases of malignant mixed müllerian epithelial and mesenchymal ovarian tumors: A Gynecologic Oncology Group study. Gynecol Oncol 18:278–292, 1984

230. Deligdisch L, Plaxe S, Cohen CJ: Extrauterine pelvic malignant mixed mesodermal tumors: A study of 10 cases with immunohistochemistry. Int J Gynecol Pathol 7:361–372, 1988

231. Costa MJ, Khan R, Judd R: Carcinosarcoma (malignant mixed müllerian [mesodermal] tumor) of the uterus and ovary: Correlation of clinical, pathologic, and immunohistochemical features in 29 cases. Arch Pathol Lab Med 115:583–590, 1991

232. Mukai K, Varela-Duran J, Nochomovitz LE: The rhabdomyoblast in mixed Müllerian tumors of the uterus and ovary: An immunohistochemical study of myoglobin in 25 cases. Am J Clin Pathol 74:101–104, 1980

233. Andersen WA, Young DE, Peters WA, Smith EB, Bagley CM, Taylor PT Jr: Platinum-based combination chemotherapy for malignant mixed mesodermal tumors of the ovary. Gynecol Oncol 32:319–322, 1989

234. Clement PB, Scully RE: Extrauterine mesodermal (Müllerian) adenosarcoma: A clinicopathologic analysis of five cases. Am J Clin Pathol 69:276–283, 1978

235. Kao GF, Norris HJ: Benign and low grade variants of mixed mesodermal tumor (adenosarcoma) of the ovary and adnexal region. Cancer 42:1314–1324, 1978

236. Silverberg SG, Nogales FF: Endolymphatic stromal myosis of the ovary: A report of three cases and literature review. Gynecol Oncol 12:129–138, 1981

237. Young RH, Prat J, Scully RE: Endometrioid stromal sarcomas of the ovary: A clinicopathologic analysis of 23 cases. Cancer 53:1143–1155, 1984

238. Tao L-C: Transabdominal fine-needle aspiration biopsy, pp 321–367. New York: Igako-Shoin, 1990

239. Nunez C: Cytopathology and fine-needle aspiration in ovarian tumours: Its utility in diagnosis and management. Curr Top Pathol 78:69–83, 1989

240. Nadji M, Sevin B-V: Pelvic fine needle aspiration cytology in gynecology. In Linsk JA, Franzen S, eds. Clinical aspiration cytology, 2nd ed, pp 261–282. Philadelphia, JB Lippincott, 1989

241. Ganjei P, Nadji M: Aspiration cytology of ovarian neoplasms: A review. Acta Cytol 28:329–332, 1984

242. Dudzinski M, Cohen M, Ducatman B: Ovarian malignant luteinized thecoma: An unusual tumor in an adolescent. Gynecol Oncol 35:104–109, 1989

243. Katsube Y, Berg JW, Silverberg SG: Epidemiologic pathology of ovarian tumors: A histopathologic review of primary ovarian neoplasms diagnosed in the Denver Standard Metropolitan Statistical Area, 1 July–31 December 1969 and 1 July–31 December 1979. Int J Gynecol Pathol 1:3–16, 1982

244. Koonings PP, Campbell K, Mishell DR Jr, Grimes DA: Relative frequency of primary ovarian neoplasms: A 10-year review. Obstet Gynecol 74:921–926, 1989

245. Stage AH, Grafton WD: Thecomas and granulosa-theca cell tumors of the ovary: An analysis of 51 tumors. Obstet Gynecol 50:21–27, 1977

246. Anikwue C, Dawood MY, Kramer E: Granulosa and theca cell tumors. Obstet Gynecol 51:214–220, 1978

247. Bjorkholm E, Silfversward C: Prognostic factors in granulosa-cell tumors. Gynecol Oncol 11:261–274, 1981

248. Evans AT III, Gaffey TA, Malkasian GD Jr, Annegers JF: Clinicopathologic review of 118 granulosa and 82 theca cell tumors. Obstet Gynecol 55:231–238, 1980

249. Fox H, Agrawal K, Langley FA: A clinicopathologic study of 92 cases of granulosa cell tumor of the ovary with special reference to the factors influencing prognosis. Cancer 35:231–241, 1975

250. Stenwig JT, Hazekamp JT, Beecham JB: Granulosa cell tumors of the ovary: A clinicopathological study of 118 cases with long-term follow-up. Gynecol Oncol 7:136–152, 1979

251. Norris HJ, Taylor HB: Prognosis of granulosa-theca tumors of the ovary. Cancer 21:255–263, 1968

252. Bjorkholm E, Pettersson F: Granulosa cell and theca cell tumors: The clinical picture and long term outcome for the Radiumhemmet series. Acta Obstet Gynecol Scand 59:361–365, 1980

253. Gustafson ML, Lee MM, Scully RE et al: Müllerian inhibiting substance as a marker for ovarian sex-cord tumor. N Engl J Med 326:466–471, 1992

254. Lappohn RE, Burger HG, Bonma J, Bangah M, Krans M, de Bruijn HWA: Inhibin as a marker for granulosa cell tumors. N Engl J Med 321:790–793, 1989

255. Rodgers KE, Marks JF, Ellefson DD et al: Follicle regulatory protein: A novel marker for granulosa cell cancer patients. Gynecol Oncol 37:381–387, 1990

256. Jarabak J, Talerman A: Virilization due to a metastasizing granulosa cell tumor. Int J Gynecol Pathol 2:316–324, 1983

257. Nakashima N, Young RH, Scully RE: Androgenic granulosa cell tumors of the ovary: A clinicopathologic analysis of 17 cases and review of the literature. Arch Pathol Lab Med 108:786–791, 1984

258. Norris HJ, Taylor HB: Virilization associated with cystic granulosa tumors. Obstet Gynecol 34:629–635, 1969

259. Margolin KA, Pak HY, Esensten ML, Doroshow JH: Hepatic metastasis in granulosa cell tumor of the ovary. Cancer 56:691–695, 1985

260. Young RH, Dudley AG, Scully RE: Granulosa cell, Sertoli-Leydig cell, and unclassified sex cord-stromal tumors associated with pregnancy: A clinicopathological analysis of thirty-six cases. Gynecol Oncol 18:181–205, 1984

261. Aguirre P, Thor AD, Scully RE: Ovarian small cell carcinoma: Histogenetic considerations based on immunohistochemical and other findings. Am J Clin Pathol 92:140–149, 1989

262. Benjamin E, Law S, Bobrow LG: Intermediate filaments cytokeratin and vimentin in ovarian sex cord-stromal tumours with correlative studies in adult and fetal ovaries. J Pathol 152:253–263, 1987

263. Chada S, van der Kwast TH: Immunohistochemistry of ovarian granulosa cell tumours: The value of tissue specific proteins and tumour markers. Virchows Arch A Pathol Anat Histopathol 414:439–445, 1989

264. Miettinen M, Wahlstrom T, Virtanen I, Talerman A, Astengo-Osuna C: Cellular differentiation in ovarian sex-cord-stromal and germ-cell tumors studied with antibodies to intermediate-filament proteins. Am J Surg Pathol 9:640–651, 1985

265. Czernobilsky B, Moll R, Leppien G, Schweikhart G, Franke WW: Desmosomal plaque-associated vimentin filaments in human ovarian granulosa cell tumors of various histologic patterns. Am J Pathol 126:476–486, 1987

266. Gaffney EF, Majmudar B, Hertzler GL, Zane R, Furlong B, Breding E: Ovarian granulosa cell tumors—immunohistochemical localization of estradiol and ultrastructure, with functional correlations. Obstet Gynecol 61:311–319, 1983

267. Klemi PJ, Gronroos M: An ultrastructural and clinical study of theca and granulosa cell tumors. Int J Gynaecol Obstet 17:219–225, 1979

268. Hitchcock CL, Norris HJ, Khalifa MA, Wargotz ES: Flow cytometric analysis of granulosa tumors. Cancer 64:2127–2132, 1989

269. Klemi PJ, Joensuu H, Salmi T: Prognostic value of flow cytometric DNA content analysis in granulosa cell tumor of the ovary. Cancer 65:1189–1193, 1990

270. Suh KS, Silverberg SG, Rhame JG, Wilkinson DS: Granulosa cell tumor of the ovary: Histopathologic and flow cytometric analysis with clinical correlation. Arch Pathol Lab Med 114:496–501, 1990

271. Chada S, Cornelisse CJ, Schaberg A: Flow cytometric DNA ploidy analysis of ovarian granulosa cell tumors. Gynecol Oncol 36:240–245, 1990

272. Fletcher JA, Gibas Z, Donovan K et al: Ovarian granulosa-stromal cell tumors are characterized by trisomy 12. Am J Pathol 138:515–520, 1991

273. Leung WY, Schwartz PE, Ng HT, Yang-Feng TL: Trisomy 12 in benign fibroma and granulosa cell tumor of the ovary. Gynecol Oncol 38:28–31, 1990

274. Benda JA, Zaleski S: Fine needle aspiration cytologic features of hepatic metastasis of granulosa cell tumor of the ovary: Differential diagnosis. Acta Cytol 32:527–532, 1988

275. Ehya H, Lang WR: Cytology of granulosa cell tumor of the ovary. Am J Clin Pathol 85:402–405, 1986

276. Bjersing L, Frankendal B, Angstrom T: Studies on a feminizing ovarian mesenchymoma (granulosa cell tumor). I. Aspiration biopsy cytology, histology, and ultrastructure. Cancer 32:1360–1369, 1973

277. Fidler WJ: Recurrent granulosa cell tumor: Aspiration cytology findings. Acta Cytol 26:688–690, 1982

278. Ramzy I, Delaney M, Rose P: Fine needle aspiration of ovarian masses. II. Correlative cytologic and histologic study of non-neoplastic cysts and noncoelomic epithelial neoplasms. Acta Cytol 23:185–193, 1979

279. Clement PB, Young RH, Scully RE: Ovarian granulosa cell proliferations of pregnancy: A report of nine cases. Hum Pathol 19:657–662, 1988

280. Gershenson DM, Copeland LJ, Kavanagh JJ, Stringer CA, Saul PB, Wharton JT: Treatment of metastatic stromal tumors of the ovary with cisplatin, doxorubicin, and cyclophosphamide. Obstet Gynecol 70:765–769, 1987

281. Zaloudek CJ, Norris HJ: Granulosa tumors of the ovary in children: A clinical and pathologic study of 32 cases. Am J Surg Pathol 6:503–512, 1982

282. Young RH, Dickersin GR, Scully RE: Juvenile granulosa cell tumor of the ovary: A clinicopathological analysis of 125 cases. Am J Surg Pathol 8:575–596, 1984

283. Lack EE, Perez-Atayde AR, Murthy ASK, Goldstein DP, Crigler JF Jr, Vawter GF: Granulosa-theca cell tumors in premenarchal girls: A clinical and pathologic study of ten cases. Cancer 48:1846–1854, 1981

284. Vassal G, Flamant F, Caillaud JM, Demeocq F, Nihoul-Fekete C, Lemerle J: Juvenile granulosa cell tumor of the ovary in children: A clinical study of 15 cases. J Clin Oncol 6:990–995, 1988

285. Biscotti CV, Hart WR: Juvenile granulosa cell tumors of the ovary. Arch Pathol Lab Med 113:40–46, 1989

286. Velasco-Oses A, Alouso-Alvaro A, Blanco-Pozo A, Nogales FF: Ollier's disease associated with ovarian juvenile granulosa cell tumor. Cancer 62:222–225, 1988

287. Tamimi HK, Bolen JW: Enchondromatosis (Ollier's disease) and ovarian juvenile granulosa cell tumor: A case report and review of the literature. Cancer 53:1605–1608, 1984

288. Swanson SA, Norris HJ, Kelsten ML, Wheeler JE: DNA content of juvenile granulosa tumors determined by flow cytometry. Int J Gynecol Pathol 9:101–109, 1990

289. Stamp GW, Krausz T: Fine needle aspiration cytology of a recurrent juvenile granulosa cell tumor. Acta Cytol 32:533–539, 1988

290. Gee DC, Russell P: The pathological assessment of ovarian neoplasms. IV: The sex cord-stromal tumours. Pathology 13:235–255, 1981

291. Evans AT III, Gaffey TA, Malkasian GD Jr, Annegers JF: Clinicopathologic review of 118 granulosa and 82 theca cell tumors. Obstet Gynecol 55:231–238, 1980

292. Young RH, Clement PB, Scully RE: Calcified thecomas in young women: A report of four cases. Int J Gynecol Pathol 7:343–350, 1988

293. Waxman M, Vuletin JC, Ureuyo R, Belling CG: Ovarian low-grade stromal sarcoma with thecomatous features: A critical reappraisal of the so-called "malignant thecoma." Cancer 44:2206–2217, 1979

294. Sasano H, Sasano N: What's new in the localization of sex steroids in the human ovary and its tumors? Pathol Res Pract 185:942–948, 1989

295. Amin HK, Okagaki T, Richart RM: Classification of fibroma and thecoma of the ovary: An ultrastructural study. Cancer 27:438–446, 1971

296. Gaffney EF, Majmudar B, Hewan-Lowe K: Ultrastructure and immunohistochemical localization of estradiol in three thecomas. Hum Pathol 15:153–160, 1984

297. Pejovic T, Heim S, Mandahl N et al: Trisomy 12 is a consistent chromosomal aberration in benign ovarian tumors. Genes Chromosom Cancer 2:48–52, 1990

298. Mrözek K, Nedoszytko B, Babinska M et al: Trisomy of chromosome 12 in a case of thecoma of the ovary. Gynecol Oncol 36:413–416, 1990

299. Prat J, Scully RE: Cellular fibromas and fibrosarcomas of the ovary: A comparative clinicopathologic analysis of seventeen cases. Cancer 47:2663–2670, 1981

300. Young RH, Scully RE: Ovarian stromal tumors with minor sex cord elements: A report of seven cases. Int J Gynecol Pathol 2:227–234, 1983

301. Chalvardjian A, Scully RE: Sclerosing stromal tumors of the ovary. Cancer 31:664–670, 1973

302. Tiltman AJ: Sclerosing stromal tumor of the ovary. Int J Gynecol Pathol 4:362–369, 1985

303. Gee DC, Russell P: Sclerosing stromal tumours of the ovary. Histopathology 3:367–376, 1979

304. Yuen BH, Robertson DI, Clement PB, Mincey EK: Sclerosing stromal tumor of the ovary. Obstet Gynecol 60:252–256, 1982

305. Hsu C, Ma L, Mak L: Sclerosing stromal tumor of the ovary. Int J Gynecol Pathol 2:192–200, 1983

306. Saitoh A, Tsutsumi Y, Osamura RY, Watanabe K: Sclerosing stromal tumor of the ovary: Immunohistochemical and electron microscopic demonstration of smooth-muscle differentiation. Arch Pathol Lab Med 113:372–376, 1989

307. Young RH, Scully RE: Ovarian Sertoli-Leydig cell tumors: A clinicopathological analysis of 207 cases. Am J Surg Pathol 9:543–569, 1985

308. Roth LM, Anderson MC, Govan ADT, Langley FA, Gowing NFC, Woodcock AS: Sertoli-Leydig cell tumors: A clinicopathologic study of 34 cases. Cancer 48:187–197, 1981

309. Talerman A: Ovarian Sertoli-Leydig cell tumor (androblastoma) with retiform pattern: A clinicopathologic study. Cancer 60:3056–3064, 1987

310. Roth LM, Slayton RE, Brady LW, Blessing JA, Johnson G: Retiform differentiation in ovarian Sertoli-Leydig cell tumors: A clinicopathologic study of six cases from a Gynecologic Oncology Group study. Cancer 55:1093–1098, 1985

311. Tiltman A, Dehaeck K, Soeters R, Goldberg G, Levin W: Ovarian Sertoli-Leydig cell tumour with raised serum alpha fetoprotein: A case report. Virchows Arch A Pathol Anat Histopathol 410:107–112, 1986

312. Tetu B, Ordonez NG, Silva EG: Sertoli-Leydig cell tumor of the ovary with alpha-fetoprotein production. Arch Pathol Lab Med 110:65–68, 1986

313. Mann WJ, Chumas J, Rosenwaks Z, Merrill JA, Davenport D: Elevated serum alpha-fetoprotein associated with Sertoli-Leydig cell tumors of the ovary. Obstet Gynecol 67:141–144, 1986

314. Young RH, Perez-Atayde AR, Scully RE: Ovarian Sertoli-Leydig cell tumor with retiform and heterologous components: Report of a case with hepatocytic differentiation and elevated serum alpha-fetoprotein. Am J Surg Pathol 8:709–718, 1984

315. Gagnon S, Tëtu B, Silva EG, McCaughey WT: Frequency of alpha-fetoprotein production by Sertoli-Leydig cell tumors of the ovary: An immunohistochemical study of eight cases. Mod Pathol 2:63–67, 1989

316. Young RH, Scully RE: Well-differentiated ovarian Sertoli-Leydig cell tumors: A clinicopathological analysis of 23 tumors. Int J Gynecol Pathol 3:277–290, 1984

317. Young RH, Prat J, Scully RE: Ovarian Sertoli-Leydig cell tumors with heterologous elements. I. Gastrointestinal epithelium and carcinoid: A clinicopathologic analysis of 36 cases. Cancer 50:2448–2456, 1982

318. Prat J, Young RH, Scully RE: Ovarian Sertoli-Leydig cell tumors with heterologous elements. II. Cartilage and skeletal muscle: A clinicopathologic analysis of twelve cases. Cancer 50:2465–2475, 1982

319. Aguirre P, Scully RE, DeLellis RA: Ovarian heterologous Sertoli-Leydig cell tumors with gastrointestinal-type epithelium: An immunohistochemical analysis. Arch Pathol Lab Med 110:528–533, 1986

320. Kurman RJ, Andrade D, Goebelsmann U, Taylor CR: An immunohistological study of steroid localization in Sertoli-Leydig tumors of the ovary and testis. Cancer 42:1772–1783, 1978

321. Sasano H, Okamoto M, Mason JI et al: Immunohistochemical studies of steroidogenic enzymes (aromatase, 17α-hydroxylase and cholesterol side-chain cleavage cytochromes P-450) in sex cord-stromal tumors of the ovary. Hum Pathol 20:452–457, 1989

322. Roth LM, Cleary RE, Rosenfield RL: Sertoli-Leydig cell tumor of the ovary, with an associated mucinous cystadenoma: An ultrastructural and endocrine study. Lab Invest 31:648–657, 1974

323. Stegner H-E, Lisboa BP: Steroid metabolism in an androblastoma (Sertoli-Leydig cell tumor): A histopathological and biochemical study. Int J Gynecol Pathol 2:410–425, 1984

324. Bullon A, Arseneau J, Prat J, Young RH, Scully RE: Tubular Krukenberg tumor: A problem in histopathologic diagnosis. Am J Surg Pathol 5:225–232, 1981

325. Dunnihoo DR, Grieme DL, Woolf RB: Hilar-cell tumors of the ovary: Report of 2 new cases and a review of the world literature. Obstet Gynecol 27:703–713, 1966

326. Hayes MC, Scully RE: Stromal luteoma of the ovary: A clinicopathological analysis of 25 cases. Int J Gynecol Pathol 6:313–321, 1987

327. Schnoy N: Ultrastructure of a virilizing ovarian Leydig-cell tumor: Hilar cell tumor. Virchows Arch A Pathol Anat Histopathol 397:17–27, 1982

328. Sohval AR, Churg J, Cobin RH, Katz N, Gabrilove JL: Histopathology and ultrastructure of ovarian hilus cell tumor: Report of two cases. Gynecol Oncol 7:79–101, 1979

329. Paoletti M, Pridjian G, Okagaki T, Talerman A: A stromal Leydig cell tumor of the ovary occurring in a pregnant 15-year-old girl: Ultrastructural findings. Cancer 60:2806–2810, 1987

330. Tavassoli FA, Norris HJ: Sertoli tumors of the ovary: A clinicopathologic study of 28 cases with ultrastructural observations. Cancer 46:2281–2297, 1980

331. Young RH, Scully RE: Ovarian Sertoli cell tumors: A report of 10 cases. Int J Gynecol Pathol 2:349–363, 1984

332. Crissman JD, Hart WR: Ovarian sex cord tumor with annular tubules: An ultrastructural study of three cases. Am J Clin Pathol 75:11–17, 1981

333. Anderson MC, Govan ADT, Langley FA, Woodcock AS, Tyagi SP: Ovarian sex cord tumours with annular tubules. Histopathology 4:137–145, 1980

334. Hart WR, Kumar N, Crissman JD: Ovarian neoplasms resembling sex cord tumors with annular tubules. Cancer 45:2352–2363, 1980

335. Kalifat R, de Brux J: Ovarian sex cord tumor with annular tubules: An ultrastructural study. Int J Gynecol Pathol 6:380–388, 1987

336. Ahn GH, Chi JG, Lee SK: Ovarian sex cord tumor with annular tubules. Cancer 57:1066–1073, 1986

337. Young RH, Welch WR, Dickersin GR, Scully RE: Ovarian sex cord tumor with annular tubules: Review of 74 cases including 27 with Peutz-Jeghers syndrome and four with adenoma malignum of the cervix. Cancer 50:1384–1402, 1982

338. Gloor E: Ovarian sex cord tumor with annular tubules: Clinicopathologic report of two benign and one malignant cases with long follow-ups. Virchows Arch A Pathol Anat Histopathol 384:185–193, 1979

339. Astengo-Osuna C: Ovarian sex cord-stromal tumor with annular tubules: Case report with ultrastructural findings. Cancer 54:1070–1075, 1984

340. Yazdi HM: Fine needle aspiration cytology of ovarian sex cord tumor with annular tubules. Acta Cytol 31:340–344, 1987

341. Young RH, Dickersin GR, Scully RE: A distinctive ovarian sex cord-stromal tumor causing sexual precocity in the Peutz-Jeghers syndrome. Am J Surg Pathol 7:233–243, 1983

342. Hayes MC, Scully RE: Ovarian steroid cell tumors (not otherwise specified): A clinicopathological analysis of 63 cases. Am J Surg Pathol 11:835–845, 1987

343. Taylor HB, Norris HJ: Lipid cell tumors of the ovary. Cancer 20:1953–1962, 1967

344. Ishida T, Okagaki T, Tagatz GE, Jacobson ME, Doe RP: Lipid cell tumor of the ovary: An ultrastructural study. Cancer 40:234–243, 1977

345. Jaworski RC, Fryatt JJ, Turner TB, Osborn RA: Gynandroblastoma of the ovary. Pathology 18:348–351, 1986

346. Anderson MC, Rees DA: Gynandroblastoma of the ovary. Br J Obstet Gynaecol 82:68–73, 1975

347. Chalvardjian A, Derzko C: Gynandroblastoma: Its ultrastructure. Cancer 31:664–670, 1982

348. Matamala MF, Nogales FF, Aneiros J, Herraiz MA, Caracuel MD: Leiomyomas of the ovary. Int J Gynecol Pathol 7:190–196, 1988

349. Fallahzadeh H, Dockerty MB, Lee RA: Leiomyoma of the ovary: Report of five cases and review of the literature. Am J Obstet Gynecol 113:394–398, 1972

350. Friedman HD, Mazur MT: Primary ovarian leiomyosarcoma: An immunohistochemical and ultrastructural study. Arch Pathol Lab Med 115:941–945, 1991

351. Balaton A, Vaury P, Imbert MC, Mussy MA: Primary leiomyosarcoma of the ovary: A histological and immunocytochemical study. Gynecol Oncol 28:116–120, 1987

352. Nogales FF, Ayala A, Ruiz-Avila I, Sirvent JJ: Myxoid leiomyosarcoma of the ovary: Analysis of three cases. Hum Pathol 22:1268–1273, 1991

353. Mira JL: Lipoleiomyoma of the ovary: Report of a case and review of the English literature. Int J Gynecol Pathol 10:198–202, 1991

354. Dodd GD, Lancaster KT, Moulton JS: Ovarian lipoleiomyoma: A fat-containing mass in the female pelvis. AJR Am J Roentgenol 153:1007–1008, 1989

355. Alvarez M, Cerezo L: Ovarian cavernous hemangioma. Arch Pathol Lab Med 110:77–78, 1986

356. Tëtu B, Bonenfant JL: Ovarian myxoma: A study of two cases with long-term follow-up. Am J Clin Pathol 95:340–346, 1991

357. Eichhorn JH, Scully RE: Ovarian myxoma: Clinicopathologic and immunocytologic analysis of five cases and review of the literature. Int J Gynecol Pathol 10:156–169, 1991

358. Anderson B, Turner DA, Benda J: Ovarian sarcoma. Gynecol Oncol 26:183–192, 1987

359. Guerard MJ, Arguelles MA, Ferenczy A: Rhabdomyosarcoma of the ovary: Ultrastructural study of a case and review of literature. Gynecol Oncol 15:325–339, 1983

360. Talerman A, Auerback WM, Van Meurs AJ: Primary chondrosarcoma of the ovary. Histopathology 5:319–324, 1981

361. Hines JF, Compton DM, Stacy CC, Potter ME: Pure primary osteosarcoma of the ovary presenting as an extensively calcified adnexal mass: A case report and review of the literature. Gynecol Oncol 39:259–263, 1990

362. Stone GC, Bell DA, Fuller A, Dickersin GR, Scully RE: Malignant schwannoma of the ovary: Report of a case. Cancer 58:1575–1582, 1986

363. Osborne BM, Robboy SJ: Lymphomas or leukemia presenting as ovarian tumors: An analysis of 42 cases. Cancer 52:1933–1943, 1983

364. Fox H, Langley FA, Govan AD, Hill AS, Bennett MH: Malignant lymphoma presenting as an ovarian tumour: A clinicopathological analysis of 34 cases. Br J Obstet Gynaecol 95:386–390, 1988

365. Paladugu RR, Bearman RM, Rappaport H: Malignant lymphoma with primary manifestation in the gonad: A clinicopathologic study of 38 patients. Cancer 45:561–571, 1980

366. Chorlton I, Norris HJ, King FM: Malignant reticuloendothelial disease involving the ovary as a primary manifestation: A series of 19 lymphomas and 1 granulocytic sarcoma. Cancer 34:397–407, 1974

367. Linden MD, Tubbs RR, Fishleder AJ, Hart WR: Immunotypic and genotypic characterization of non-Hodgkin's lymphomas of the ovary. Am J Clin Pathol 90:156–162, 1988

368. Liang R, Chiu E, Loke SL: Non-Hodgkin's lymphomas involving the female genital tract. Hematol Oncol 8:295–299, 1990

369. Clement PB, Young RH, Scully RE: Clinical syndromes associated with tumors of the female genital tract. Semin Diagn Pathol 8:204–233, 1991

370. Dickersin GR, Kline IW, Scully RE: Small cell carcinoma of the ovary with hypercalcemia: A report of eleven cases. Cancer 49:188–197, 1982

371. Abeler V, Kjrstad KE, Nesland JM: Small cell carcinoma of the ovary: A report of six cases. Int J Gynecol Pathol 7:315–329, 1988

372. Ulbright TM, Roth LM, Stehman FB, Talerman A, Senekjian EK: Poorly differentiated (small cell) carcinoma of the ovary in young women: Evidence supporting a germ cell origin. Hum Pathol 18:175–184, 1987

373. McMahon JT, Hart WR: Ultrastructural analysis of small cell carcinomas of the ovary. Am J Clin Pathol 90:523–529, 1988

374. Senekjian EK, Weiser PA, Talerman A, Herbst AL: Vinblastine, cisplatin, cyclophosphamide, bleomycin, doxorubicin, and etoposide in the treatment of small cell carcinoma of the ovary. Cancer 64:1183–1187, 1989

375. Kurman RJ, Norris HJ: Malignant germ cell tumors of the ovary. Hum Pathol 8:551–564, 1977

376. Russell P, Painter DM: The pathological assessment of ovarian neoplasms. V. The germ cell tumours. Pathology 14:47–72, 1982

377. Asadourian LA, Taylor HB: Dysgerminoma: An analysis of 105 cases. Obstet Gynecol 33:370–379, 1969

378. Bjorkholm E, Lundell M, Gyftodimos A, Silfversward C: Dysgerminoma: The Radiumhemmet Series 1927–1984. Cancer 65:38–44, 1990

379. Buskirk SJ, Schray MF, Podratz KC et al: Ovarian dysgerminoma: A retrospective analysis of results of treatment, sites of treatment failure, and radiosensitivity. Mayo Clin Proc 62:1149–1157, 1987

380. Gallion HH, van Nagell JR Jr, Donaldson ES, Powell DE: Ovarian dysgerminoma: Report of seven cases and review of the literature. Am J Obstet Gynecol 158:591–595, 1988

381. Gordon A, Lipton D, Woodruff JD: Dysgerminoma: A review of 158 cases from the Emil Novak Ovarian Tumor Registry. Obstet Gynecol 58:497–504, 1981

382. Talerman A, Huyzinga WT, Kuipers T: Dysgerminoma: Clinicopathologic study of 22 cases. Obstet Gynecol 41:137–147, 1973

383. Krepart G, Smith JP, Rutledge F, Delclos L: The treatment of dysgerminoma of the ovary. Cancer 41:986–990, 1978

384. Kapp DS, Kohorn EI, Merino MJ, Livolsi VA: Pure dysgerminoma of the ovary with elevated serum human chorionic gonadotropin: Diagnostic and therapeutic considerations. Gynecol Oncol 20:234–244, 1985

385. Zaloudek CJ, Tavassoli FA, Norris HJ: Dysgerminoma with syncytiotrophoblastic giant cells: A histologically and clinically distinctive subtype of dysgerminoma. Am J Surg Pathol 5:361–367, 1981

386. Thomas GM, Dembo AJ, Hacker NF, DePetrillo AD: Current therapy for dysgerminoma of the ovary. Obstet Gynecol 70:268–275, 1987

387. Schwartz PE, Morris JM: Serum lactic dehydrogenase: A

tumor marker for dysgerminoma. Obstet Gynecol 72:511–515, 1988

388. Burkons DM, Hart WR: Ovarian germinomas (dysgerminomas). Obstet Gynecol 51:221–224, 1978

389. LaPolla JP, Benda J, Vigliotti AP, Anderson B: Dysgerminoma of the ovary. Obstet Gynecol 69:859–864, 1987

390. Battifora H, Sheibani K, Tubbs RR, Kopinski MI, Sun T: Antikeratin antibodies in tumor diagnosis: Distinction between seminoma and embryonal carcinoma. Cancer 54:843–848, 1984

391. Bailey D, Marks A, Stratis M, Baumal R: Immunohistochemical staining of germ cell tumors and intratubular malignant germ cells of the testis using antibody to placental alkaline phosphatase and a monoclonal anti-seminoma antibody. Mod Pathol 4:167–171, 1991

392. Manivel JC, Jessurun J, Wick MR, Dehner LP: Placental alkaline phosphatase immunoreactivity in testicular germ cell neoplasms. Am J Surg Pathol 11:21–29, 1987

393. Mullin TJ, Lankerani MR: Ovarian dysgerminoma: Immunocytochemical localization of human chorionic gonadotropin in the germinoma cell cytoplasm. Obstet Gynecol 68:80S–83S, 1986

394. Gondos B: Comparative studies of normal and neoplastic ovarian germ cells: 2. Ultrastructure and pathogenesis of dysgerminoma. Int J Gynecol Pathol 6:124–131, 1987

395. Hees K, de Jonge JP, von Kortzfleisch DH: Dysgerminoma of the ovary: Cytologic, histologic and electron microscopic study of a case. Acta Cytol 35:341–344, 1991

396. Akhtar M, Ali MA, Huq M, Bakry M: Fine-needle aspiration biopsy of seminoma and dysgerminoma: Cytologic, histologic, and electron microscopic correlations. Diagn Cytopathol 6:99–105, 1990

397. Oud PS, Soeters RP, Pahlplatz MM et al: DNA cytometry of pure dysgerminomas of the ovary. Int J Gynecol Pathol 7:258–267, 1988

398. Kurman RJ, Norris HJ: Embryonal carcinoma of the ovary: A clinicopathologic entity distinct from endodermal sinus tumor resembling embryonal carcinoma of the adult testis. Cancer 38:2420–2433, 1976

399. Rotmensch J, Woodruff JD: Lymphoma of the ovary: Report of twenty cases and update of previous series. Am J Obstet Gynecol 143:870–875, 1982

400. Young RH, Scully RE: Malignant melanoma metastatic to the ovary: A clinicopathologic analysis of 20 cases. Am J Surg Pathol 15:849–860, 1991

401. Boyes DA, Pankratz E, Galliford BW, White GW, Fairey RN: Experience with dysgerminomas at the Cancer Control Agency of British Columbia. Gynecol Oncol 6:123–129, 1978

402. Freel JH, Cassir JF, Pierve VK, Woodruff J, Lewis JL Jr: Dysgerminoma of the ovary. Cancer 43:798–805, 1979

403. Gershenson DM, Wharton JT, Kiline RC, Larson DM, Kavanagh J, Rutledge FN: Chemotherapeutic complete remission in patients with metastatic ovarian dysgerminoma. Cancer 58:2594–2599, 1986

404. Weinblatt ME, Ortega JA: Treatment of children with dysgerminoma of the ovary. Cancer 49:2608–2611, 1982

405. Williams SD, Blessing JA, Hatch KD, Homesley HD: Chemotherapy of advanced dysgerminoma: Trials of the Gynecologic Oncology Group. J Clin Oncol 9:1950–1955, 1991

406. Mitchell MF, Gershenson DM, Soeters RP, Eifel PJ, Delclos L, Wharton JT: The long-term effects of radiation therapy on patients with ovarian dysgerminoma. Cancer 67:1084–1090, 1991

407. Gonzalez-Crussi F: The human yolk sac and yolk sac (endodermal sinus) tumors. A review. Perspect Pediatr Pathol 5:179–215, 1979

408. Teilum G: Endodermal sinus tumors of the ovary and testis: Comparative morphogenesis of the so-called mesonephroma ovarii (Schiller) and extraembryonic (yolk sac-allantoic) structures of the rat's placenta. Cancer 12:1092–1105, 1959

409. Gershenson DM, del Junco G, Herson J, Rutledge FN: En-dodermal sinus tumor of the ovary: The M. D. Anderson experience. Obstet Gynecol 61:194–202, 1983

410. Kawai M, Kano T, Furuhashi Y et al: Prognostic factors in yolk sac tumors of the ovary: A clinicopathologic analysis of 29 cases. Cancer 67:184–192, 1991

411. Kurman RJ, Norris HJ: Endodermal sinus tumor of the ovary: A clinical and pathologic analysis of 71 cases. Cancer 38:2404–2419, 1976

412. Langley FA, Govan ADT, Anderson MC et al: Yolk sac and allied tumours of the ovary. Histopathology 5:389–401, 1981

413. Morris HH, La Vecchia C, Draper GJ: Endodermal sinus tumor and embryonal carcinoma of the ovary in children. Gynecol Oncol 21:7–17, 1985

414. Kawai M, Furuhashi Y, Kano T et al: Alpha-fetoprotein in malignant germ cell tumors of the ovary. Gynecol Oncol 39:160–166, 1990

415. Nogales FF, Matilla A, Nogales-Ortiz F, Galera-Davidson H: Yolk sac tumors with pure and mixed polyvesicular vitelline patterns. Hum Pathol 9:553–566, 1978

416. Ulbright TM, Roth LM, Brodhecker CA: Yolk sac differentiation in germ cell tumors: A morphologic study of 50 cases with emphasis on hepatic, enteric, and parietal yolk sac features. Am J Surg Pathol 10:151–164, 1986

417. Michael H, Ulbright TM, Brodhecker CA: The pluripotential nature of the mesenchyme-like component of yolk sac tumor. Arch Pathol Lab Med 113:1115–1119, 1989

418. Harms D, Janig U: Germ cell tumours of childhood: Report of 170 cases including 59 pure and partial yolk-sac tumours. Virchows Arch A Pathol Anat Histopathol 409:223–239, 1986

419. Prat J, Bhan AK, Dickersin GR, Robboy SJ, Scully RE: Hepatoid yolk sac tumor of the ovary (endodermal sinus tumor with hepatoid differentiation): A light microscopic, ultrastructural and immunohistochemical study of seven cases. Cancer 50:2355–2368, 1982

420. Cohen MB, Mulchahey KM, Molnar JJ: Ovarian endodermal sinus tumor with intestinal differentiation. Cancer 57:1580–1583, 1986

421. Kim CR, Hsiu JG, Given FT: Intestinal variant of ovarian endodermal sinus tumor. Gynecol Oncol 33:379–381, 1989

422. Beilby JOW, Horne CHW, Milne GD, Parkinson C: Alpha-fetoprotein, alpha-1-antitrypsin and transferrin in gonadal yolk sac tumours. J Clin Pathol 32:455–461, 1979

423. Akhtar M, Ali MA, Sackey K, Jackson D, Bakry M: Fine-needle aspiration biopsy diagnosis of endodermal sinus tumor: Histologic and ultrastructural correlations. Diagn Cytopathol 6:184–192, 1990

424. Nogales FF, Silverberg SG, Bloustein PA, Martinez-Hernandez A, Pierce GB: Yolk sac carcinoma (endodermal sinus tumor): Ultrastructure and histogenesis of gonadal and extragonadal tumors in comparison with normal human yolk sac. Cancer 39:1462–1474, 1977

425. Morimoto N, Ozawa M, Amano S: Diagnostic value of hyaline globules in endodermal sinus tumor: Report of two cases. Acta Cytol 25:417–420, 1981

426. Roncalli M, Gribaudi G, Simoncelli D, Servida E: Cytology of yolk-sac tumor of the ovary in ascitic fluid: Report of a case. Acta Cytol 32:113–116, 1988

427. Kelley JL III, Naus GJ, Christopherson WA: Endodermal sinus tumor of the ovary: A case series with flow cytometric DNA content analysis. Gynecol Oncol 42:34–38, 1991

428. Klemi PJ, Meurman L, Gronroos M, Talerman A: Clear cell (mesonephroid) tumors of the ovary with characteristics resembling endodermal sinus tumor. Int J Gynecol Pathol 1:95–100, 1982

429. Ishikura H, Scully RE: Hepatoid carcinoma of the ovary: A newly described tumor. Cancer 60:2775–2784, 1987

430. Ungerleider RS, Donaldson SS, Warnke RA, Wilbur JR: Endodermal sinus tumor: The Stanford experience and the first reported case arising in the vulva. Cancer 41:1627–1634, 1978

431. Gershenson DM, Copeland LJ, Kavanagh JJ et al: Treatment of malignant nondysgerminomatous germ cell tumors

of the ovary with vincristine, dactinomycin, and cyclophosphamide. Cancer 56:2756–2761, 1985

432. Slayton RE, Hreschyshyn MM, Silverberg SG et al: Treatment of malignant ovarian germ cell tumors: Response to vincristine, dactinomycin, and cyclophosphamide (preliminary report). Cancer 42:390–398, 1978

433. Gershenson DM, Kavanagh JJ, Copeland LJ et al: Treatment of malignant nondysgerminomatous germ cell tumors of the ovary by vinblastine, bleomycin, and cisplatin. Cancer 57:1731–1737, 1986

434. Gershenson DM, Morris M, Cangir A et al: Treatment of malignant germ cell tumors of the ovary with bleomycin, etoposide, and cisplatin. J Clin Oncol 8:715–720, 1990

435. Pippitt CH Jr, Cain JM, Hakes TB, Pierce VK, Lewis JL Jr: Primary chemotherapy and the role of second-look laparotomy in non-dysgerminomatous germ cell malignancies of the ovary. Gynecol Oncol 31:268–275, 1988

436. Sessa C, Bonazzi C, Landoni F, Pecorelli S, Sartori E, Mangioni C: Cisplatin, vinblastine, and bleomycin combination chemotherapy in endodermal sinus tumor of the ovary. Obstet Gynecol 70:220–224, 1987

437. Smales E, Peckham MJ: Chemotherapy of germ-cell ovarian tumours: First-line treatment with etoposide, bleomycin, and cisplatin or carboplatin. Eur J Clin Oncol 23:469–474, 1987

438. Williams SD, Blessing JA, Moore DH, Homesley HD, Adcock L: Cisplatin, vinblastine, and bleomycin in advanced and recurrent ovarian germ-cell tumors: A trial of the Gynecologic Oncology Group. Ann Int Med 111:22–27, 1989

439. Curtin JP, Rubin SC, Hoskins WJ, Hakes TB, Lewis JL Jr: Second-look laparotomy in endodermal sinus tumor: A report of two patients with normal levels of alpha-fetoprotein and residual tumor at reexploration. Obstet Gynecol 74:683–685, 1989

440. Axe SR, Klein VR, Woodruff JD: Choriocarcinoma of the ovary. Obstet Gynecol 66:111–114, 1985

441. Jacobs AJ, Newland JR, Green RK: Pure choriocarcinoma of the ovary. Obstet Gynecol Surv 37:603–609, 1982

442. Wheeler CA, Davis S, Degefu S, Thorneycroft IH, O'Quinn AG: Ovarian choriocarcinoma: A difficult diagnosis of an unusual tumor and a review of the hook effect. Obstet Gynecol 75:547–549, 1990

443. Vance RP, Geisinger KR: Pure nongestational choriocarcinoma of the ovary: Report of a case. Cancer 56:2321–2325, 1985

444. Fisher RA, Newlands ES, Jeffreys AJ, Boxer GM, Begent RHJ, Rustin GJS, Bagshawe KD: Gestational and nongestational trophoblastic tumors distinguished by DNA analysis. Cancer 69:839–845, 1992

445. Linder D, McCaw BK, Hecht F: Parthenogenetic origin of benign ovarian teratoma. N Engl J Med 292:63–66, 1975

446. Dahl N, Gustavson KH, Rune C, Gustavsson I, Pettersson U: Benign ovarian teratomas: An analysis of their cellular origin. Cancer Genet Cytogenet 46:115–123, 1990

447. Fanning J, Bates J: Mature solid teratoma associated with gliomatosis peritonei. Am J Obstet Gynecol 155:661–662, 1986

448. Robboy SJ, Scully RE: Ovarian teratoma with glial implants on the peritoneum: An analysis of 12 cases. Hum Pathol 1:643–653, 1970

449. Genadry R, Parmley T, Woodruff JD: Secondary malignancies in benign cystic teratomas. Gynecol Oncol 8:246–251, 1979

450. Stamp GWH, McConnell EM: Malignancy arising in cystic ovarian teratomas: A report of 24 cases. Br J Obstet Gynaecol 90:671–675, 1983

451. Amerigo J, Nogales FF, Fernandez-Sanz J, Oliva H, Velasco A: Squamous cell neoplasms arising from ovarian benign cystic teratoma. Gynecol Oncol 8:277–283, 1979

452. Krumerman MS, Chung A: Squamous carcinoma arising in benign cystic teratoma of the ovary: A report of four cases and review of the literature. Cancer 39:1237–1242, 1977

453. Cronje HS, Woodruff JD: Primary ovarian malignant melanoma arising in cystic teratoma. Gynecol Oncol 12:379–383, 1981

454. Tsukamoto N, Matsukuma K, Matsumura M, Kamura T, Matsuyama T, Kinjo M: Primary malignant melanoma arising in a cystic teratoma of the ovary. Gynecol Oncol 23:395–400, 1986

455. Nielsen SN, Gaffey TA, Malkasian GD Jr: Immature ovarian teratoma: A review of 14 cases. Mayo Clin Proc 61:110–115, 1986

456. Koulos JP, Hoffman JS, Steinhoff MM: Immature teratoma of the ovary. Gynecol Oncol 34:46–49, 1989

457. Nogales FF, Favara BE, Major FJ, Silverberg SG: Immature teratoma of the ovary with a neural component ("solid" teratoma): A clinicopathologic study of 20 cases. Hum Pathol 7:625–642, 1976

458. Nogales FF, Ortega I, Rivera F, Armas JR: Metanephrogenic tissue in immature ovarian teratoma. Am J Surg Pathol 4:297–299, 1980

459. Norris HJ, Zirkin HJ, Benson WL: Immature (malignant) teratoma of the ovary: A clinical and pathologic study of 58 cases. Cancer 37:2359–2372, 1976

460. Gershenson DM, del Junco G, Silva EG, Copeland LJ, Wharton JT, Rutledge FN: Immature teratoma of the ovary. Obstet Gynecol 68:624–629, 1986

461. Kawai M, Kano T, Furuhashi Y et al: Immature teratoma of the ovary. Gynecol Oncol 40:133–137, 1991

462. Perrone T, Steeper TA, Dehner LP: Alpha-fetoprotein localization in pure ovarian teratoma: An immunohistochemical study of 12 cases. Am J Clin Pathol 88:713–717, 1987

463. Yanai-Inbar I, Scully RE: Relation of ovarian dermoid cysts and immature teratomas: An analysis of 350 cases of immature teratoma and 10 cases of dermoid cyst with microscopic foci of immature tissue. Int J Gynecol Pathol 6:203–212, 1987

464. Aguirre P, Scully RE: Malignant neuroectodermal tumor of the ovary, a distinctive form of monodermal teratoma: report of five cases. Am J Surg Pathol 6:283–292, 1982

465. Vance RP, Geisinger KR, Randall MB, Marshall RB: Immature neural elements in immature teratomas: An immunohistochemical and ultrastructural study. Am J Clin Pathol 90:397–411, 1988

466. Steeper TA, Mukai K: Solid ovarian teratomas: an immunocytochemical study of thirteen cases with clinicopathologic correlation. Pathol Annu 19:81–92, 1984

467. Micha JP, Kucera PR, Berman ML, Romansky S, Flamm M, Reynolds J, DiSaia PJ: Malignant ovarian germ cell tumors: A review of thirty-six cases. Am J Obstet Gynecol 152:842–846, 1985

468. Vergote IB, Abeler VM, Kjrstad KE, Tropë C: Management of malignant ovarian immature teratoma: Role of adriamycin. Cancer 66:882–886, 1990

469. Harms D, Janig U, Göbel U: Gliomatosis peritonei in childhood and adolescence: Clinicopathological study of 13 cases including immunohistochemical findings. Pathol Res Pract 184:422–430, 1989

470. Nielsen SNJ, Scheithauer BW, Gaffey TA: Gliomatosis peritonei. Cancer 56:2499–2503, 1985

471. Truong LD, Jurco S, McGavran MH: Gliomatosis peritonei: Report of two cases and review of literature. Am J Surg Pathol 6:443–449, 1982

472. Hasleton PS, Kelehan P, Whittaker JS, Burslem RW, Turner L: Benign and malignant struma ovarii. Arch Pathol Lab Med 102:180–184, 1978

473. Brunskill PJ, Rollason TP, Nicholson HO: Malignant follicular variant of papillary struma ovarii. Histopathology 17:574–576, 1990

474. O'Connell ME, Fisher C, Harmer CL: Malignant struma ovarii: Presentation and management. Br J Radiol 63:360–363, 1990

475. Rosenblum NG, Livolsi VA, Edmonds PR, Mikuta JJ: Malignant struma ovarii. Gynecol Oncol 32:224–227, 1989

476. Pardo-Mindan FJ, Vazquez JJ: Malignant struma ovarii: Light and electron microscopic study. Cancer 51:337–343, 1983

477. Yannopoulos D, Yannopoulos K, Ossowski R: Malignant struma ovarii. Pathol Annu 11:403–413, 1976

478. Robboy SJ, Norris HJ, Scully RE: Insular carcinoid primary in the ovary: A clinicopathologic analysis of 48 cases. Cancer 36:404–418, 1975

479. Sporrong B, Falkmer S, Robboy SJ et al: Neurohormonal peptides in ovarian carcinoids: An immunohistochemical study of 81 primary carcinoids and of intraovarian metastases from six mid-gut carcinoids. Cancer 49:68–74, 1982

480. Serratoni FT, Robboy SJ: Ultrastructure of primary and metastatic ovarian carcinoids: Analysis of 11 cases. Cancer 36:157–160, 1975

481. Robboy SJ, Scully RE, Norris HJ: Primary trabecular carcinoid of the ovary. Obstet Gynecol 49:202–207, 1977

482. Talerman A, Evans MI: Primary trabecular carcinoid tumor of the ovary. Cancer 50:1403–1407, 1982

483. Robboy SJ, Scully RE: Strumal carcinoid of the ovary: An analysis of 50 cases of a distinctive tumor composed of thyroid tissue and carcinoid. Cancer 46:2019–2034, 1980

484. Snyder RR, Tavassoli FA: Ovarian strumal carcinoid: Immunohistochemical, ultrastructural, and clinicopathologic analysis. Int J Gynecol Pathol 5:187–201, 1986

485. Ulbright TM, Roth LM, Ehrlich CE: Ovarian strumal carcinoid: An immunocytochemical and ultrastructural study of two cases. Am J Clin Pathol 77:622–631, 1982

486. Alenghat E, Okagaki T, Talerman A: Primary mucinous carcinoid tumor of the ovary. Cancer 58:777–783, 1986

487. Wolpert HR, Fuller AF, Bell DA: Primary mucinous carcinoid tumor of the ovary: A case report. Int J Gynecol Pathol 8:156–162, 1989

488. Robboy SJ, Scully RE, Norris HJ: Carcinoid metastatic to the ovary: A clinicopathologic analysis of 35 cases. Cancer 33:798–811, 1974

489. Kurman RJ, Norris HJ: Malignant mixed germ cell tumors of the ovary: A clinical and pathologic analysis of 30 cases. Obstet Gynecol 48:579–589, 1976

490. Gershenson DM, del Junco G, Copeland LJ, Rutledge FN: Mixed germ cell tumors of the ovary. Obstet Gynecol 64:200–207, 1984

491. King ME, Hubbell MJ, Talerman A: Mixed germ cell tumor of the ovary with a prominent polyembryoma component. Int J Gynecol Pathol 10:88–95, 1991

492. Jimmerson GK, Woodruff JD: Ovarian extraembryonal teratoma. II. Endodermal sinus tumor mixed with other germ cell tumors. Am J Obstet Gynecol 127:302–305, 1977

493. Garvin AJ, Pratt-Thomas HR, Spector M, Spicer MM, Williamson HO: Gonadoblastoma: Histologic, ultrastructural, and histochemical observations in five cases. Am J Obstet Gynecol 125:459–471, 1976

494. Govan AD, Woodcock AS, Gowing NF, Langley FA, Neville AM, Anderson MC: A clinico-pathological study of gonadoblastoma. Br J Obstet Gynaecol 84:222–228, 1977

495. Woodcock AS, Govan AD, Gowing NF, Langley FA, Anderson MC: A report of the histological features in 12 cases of gonadoblastoma. Tumori 65:181–189, 1979

496. Scully RE: Gonadoblastoma: A review of 74 cases. Cancer 25:1340–1356, 1970

497. Troche V, Hernandez E: Neoplasia arising in dysgenetic gonads. Obstet Gynecol Surv 41:74–79, 1986

498. Deligdisch L, Richards CJ, Reyniak VJ: Pure gonadal dysgenesis and gonadal tumors: Report of three cases and review of literature. Mt Sinai J Med 55:313–317, 1988

499. Roth LM, Eglen DE: Gonadoblastoma: Immunohistochemical and ultrastructural observations. Int J Gynecol Pathol 8:72–81, 1989

500. Talerman A: A distinctive gonadal neoplasm related to gonadoblastoma. Cancer 30:1219–1224, 1972

501. Tavassoli FA: A combined germ cell-gonadal stromal-epithelial tumor of the ovary. Am J Surg Pathol 7:73–84, 1983

502. Kedzia H: Gonadoblastoma: Structures and background of development. Am J Obstet Gynecol 147:81–85, 1983

503. Safneck JR, deSa DJ: Structures mimicking sex cord-stromal tumours and gonadoblastomas in the ovaries of normal infants and children. Histopathology 10:909–920, 1986

504. Schellhas HF: Malignant potential of the dysgenetic gonad. Part I. Obstet Gynecol 44:298–309, 1974

505. Hart WR, Burkons DM: Germ cell neoplasms arising in gonadoblastomas. Cancer 43:669–678, 1979

506. Talerman A: Gonadoblastoma associated with embryonal carcinoma. Obstet Gynecol 43:138–142, 1974

507. Birnkrant A, Sampson J, Sugarbaker PH: Ovarian metastasis from colorectal cancer. Dis Colon Rectum 29:767–771, 1986

508. Demopoulos RI, Touger L, Dubin N: Secondary ovarian carcinoma: A clinical and pathological evaluation. Int J Gynecol Pathol 6:166–175, 1987

509. Resta L, De Benedictis G, Colucci GA et al: Secondary tumors of the ovary. III. Tumors of the gastrointestinal tract and other sites. Eur J Gynaecol Oncol 11:289–298, 1990

510. Gagnon Y, Têtu B: Ovarian metastases of breast carcinoma: A clinicopathologic study of 59 cases. Cancer 64:892–898, 1989

511. Mazur MT, Hsueh S, Gersell DJ: Metastases to the female genital tract: Analysis of 325 cases. Cancer 53:1978–1984, 1984

512. Ulbright TM, Roth LM, Stehman FB: Secondary ovarian neoplasia: A clinicopathologic study of 35 cases. Cancer 53:1164–1174, 1984

513. Young RH, Carey RW, Robboy SJ: Breast carcinoma masquerading as primary ovarian neoplasm. Cancer 48:210–212, 1981

514. Young RH, Scully RE: Ovarian metastases from carcinoma of the gallbladder and extrahepatic bile ducts simulating primary tumors of the ovary: A report of six cases. Int J Gynecol Pathol 9:60–72, 1990

515. Yakushiji M, Tazaki T, Nishimura H, Kato T: Krukenberg tumors of the ovary: A clinicopathologic analysis of 112 cases. Nippon Sanka Fujinka Gakkai Zasshi 39:479–485, 1987

516. Wong PC, Ferenczy A, Fan LD, McCaughey E: Krukenberg tumors of the ovary: Ultrastructural, histochemical and immunohistochemical studies of 15 cases. Cancer 57:751–760, 1986

517. Holtz F, Hart WR: Krukenberg tumors of the ovary: A clinicopathologic analysis of 27 cases. Cancer 50:2438–2447, 1982

518. Fung MF, Vadas G, Lotocki R, Heywood M, Krepart G: Tubular Krukenberg tumor in pregnancy with virilization. Gynecol Oncol 41:81–84, 1991

519. Kariminejad MH, Scully RE: Female adnexal tumor of probable Wollfian origin: A distinctive pathologic entity. Cancer 31:671–677, 1973

520. Young RH, Scully RE: Ovarian tumors of probable Wolffian origin: A report of 11 cases. Am J Surg Pathol 7:125–136, 1983

521. Prasad CJ, Ray JA, Kessler S: Female adnexal tumor of wolffian origin. Arch Pathol Lab Med 116:189–191, 1992

522. Young RH, Silva EG, Scully RE: Ovarian and juxtaovarian adenomatoid tumors: A report of six cases. Int J Gynecol Pathol 10:364–372, 1991

Pathology in Gynecology and Obstetrics, Fourth Edition, edited by Claude Gompel and Steven G. Silverberg. J. B. Lippincott Company, Philadelphia © 1994.

7

The Female Peritoneum

In the 1980s, several new clinicopathologic entities primarily involving the female peritoneum were described, and several other previously known conditions were characterized more fully. These findings probably were the result of the increased use of exploratory laparotomy with extensive peritoneal sampling in women with tumors of the genitalia, but they may also be partly due to an increased incidence of some of these conditions.

Because of the gynecologic emphasis of this text, conditions that affect the male and female peritoneum similarly are mentioned only briefly, whereas those that are significantly more prevalent in or limited to women are given more extensive coverage. Endometriosis, although not exclusively a peritoneal condition, is included here because most of its manifestations are related to peritoneal localizations of the disease.

EMBRYOLOGY

The peritoneum is formed from the lateral mesoderm, which splits into a somatic and a splanchnic layer. These layers are associated with the ectoderm and entoderm, respectively, and enclose the intraembryonic coelom, a cavity that later forms the pleural and peritoneal cavities. The peritoneal cavity is formed from the portion of the intraembryonic coelom that is caudal to the septum transversum. The peritoneal cavity subsequently divides into the lesser and greater sacs, which communicate through the epiploic foramen.

ANATOMY

The peritoneum is a continuous serous membrane that lines the abdominal wall (parietal peritoneum) and is reflected over the abdominal and pelvic viscera (visceral peritoneum). The space between these two layers is the peritoneal cavity. Because the two layers are normally in contact, however, this cavity is largely a potential one.

The lesser sac of the peritoneum is known as the omental bursa and is related only to the dorsal surface of the stomach and the closely surrounding structures. The remainder of the peritoneal cavity (the portion to which we refer throughout this chapter) is known as the greater sac. The abdominal viscera are either attached to the abdominal wall and partly covered by the peritoneum (the *retroperitoneal viscera*) or completely surrounded by the peritoneum and suspended from the abdominal wall by *mesenteries,* sheets of connective tissue containing blood and lymph vessels and covered by the peritoneum.

Further consideration of the complex anatomy of the peritoneum is beyond the scope of this chapter, but three points should be emphasized with particular reference to the female peritoneum. First, although in the male the peritoneum is a completely closed sac, in the female the free ends of the fallopian tubes open directly into the peritoneal cavity, providing a conduit to the external environment. Second, the pelvic peritoneum in women is considerably more irregular than that in men because of its numerous folds, fossae, recesses, and cul-de-sacs.[1] These include the vesicouterine and rectouterine cul-de-sacs; the paravesical, parauterine, pararectal, and ovarian fossae; and the tubo-ovarian recess. These complex nooks and crannies often are sites for the development of infection, adhesions, and foci of endometriosis and metastatic carcinoma. Finally, the relation of the peritoneum to the female genitalia should be considered. The germinal epithelium of the ovaries is derived from and directly continuous with the pelvic peritoneum. The serous coats of the fallopian tubes, uterine corpus, and cervix are peritoneal, and the so-called ligaments from which these various organs are suspended are covered by peritoneum. The cervix is not covered anteriorly by peritoneum, because the vesicouterine cul-de-sac extends caudad only as far as the junction between the uterine corpus and cervix.

HISTOLOGY

In its resting state, the peritoneum is lined by a single layer of low cuboidal cells, which are underlaid by a thin layer of nonspecific fibrous mesenchymal tissue. This subserous mesenchymal layer contains a small network of capillaries, lymphatics, and nerve fibers. Ultrastructurally, the mesothelial cells contain microvilli on their apical surfaces and numerous pinocytotic vesicles. The nucleus occupies a large portion of the cell, and intracytoplasmic organelles are not prominent.

CYTOLOGY

Because peritoneal mesothelial cells usually are examined cytologically in effusions, which by definition are pathologic, opportunities to observe normal cells are limited. In addition, free-floating cells in an effusion take on different characteristics from the same cells attached to a serous membrane. Therefore, the following discussion of "normal" peritoneal cytology must assume at least slight variation from the true physiologic norm.[2–4]

The mesothelial cells appear as solitary elements, gathered in small clusters, and in sheets. The individual cells generally are round to polygonal and measure from 10 to 20 μm in diameter. The nucleus is centrally located and occupies about one-half the cell diameter. The nuclear membrane is prominent, and there is a finely dispersed chromatin network with occasionally one or two prominent nucleoli. The cytoplasm is homogeneous and is basophilic to faintly eosinophilic.

The cells adhere well to one another in clusters and sheets and appear uniform in size, shape, and nuclear morphology. Papillary clusters are frequently seen in cases of "irritation" but should not be observed in the absence of pathology. In addition to mesothelial cells, macrophages and various leukocytes are frequently encountered in peritoneal fluid specimens.

INFLAMMATORY LESIONS

Although inflammatory lesions of the peritoneum are common, they are discussed here only briefly for two reasons. First, they are as likely to occur in males as in females. Second, they are usually diagnosed bacteriologically rather than histologically and only infrequently generate material for the surgical pathologist.

Peritonitis is most commonly due to infectious and chemical causes. *Infectious peritonitis* is usually bacterial and may be primary or secondary. The primary form is rare and usually is caused by pneumococci or streptococci. Secondary bacterial peritonitis usually is due to perforation of a viscus, usually within the gastrointestinal tract (eg, peptic ulcer, diverticulum, or tumor), and the resulting peritonitis is both bacterial and chemical. Bohnen and colleagues found a mortality rate of 38% in generalized peritonitis but noted a much lower mortality rate (about 10%) if the initiating condition was acute appendicitis or a perforated duodenal ulcer.[5] In women, a common cause of peritonitis is acute bacterial salpingitis. In the staging system of Monif, salpingitis with peritonitis is considered stage II salpingitis, whereas the ruptured tubo-ovarian abscess is considered stage IV and a potentially life-threatening situation (see Table 5-1).[6]

Other types of infectious peritonitis result from *tuberculosis* and *actinomycosis*. These infections may be difficult to diagnose because of the absence of an obvious primary lesion elsewhere. Singh and associates found percutaneous peritoneal biopsy helpful in making the diagnosis in 64% of patients with tuberculous peritonitis (Fig. 7-1).[7] Although acid-fast bacilli are seldom found on smears of peritoneal fluid, a culture often is more rewarding.

Chemical peritonitis may be caused by an almost endless list of agents. The most common source of chemical peritonitis is rupture of a portion of the gastrointestinal tract, but iatrogenic causes are also common. In particular, material from surgical gloves (previously talc and now more commonly starch) has been demonstrated to produce a foreign-body granulomatous response, which generally becomes evident 1 to 4 weeks after a surgical procedure. The offending agent should be demonstrable within histiocytes and foreign-body giant cells, thereby avoiding the mistaken diagnosis of an infectious granulomatous peritonitis. Sources of foreign-body granulomata in the female peritoneum include contrast media used for hysterosalpingography, contents of a ruptured ovarian dermoid cyst, and meconium disseminated at cesarean section.[8]

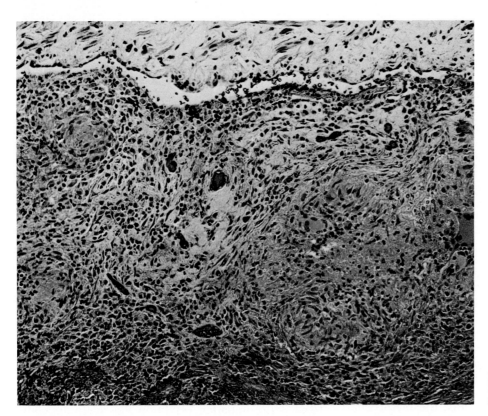

FIGURE 7-1 Peritoneal tuberculosis: granulomas on serosal surface of tube.

The peritoneum can be the site of an inflammatory response in autoimmune diseases such as *systemic lupus erythematosus* and *familial Mediterranean fever*. The latter condition, which is also known as familial recurrent polyserositis or periodic fever, is an inherited disease of unknown cause, characterized by acute self-limited attacks of fever and signs of peritonitis, pleuritis, and arthritis. Familial Mediterranean fever is clinically important because it can mimic surgical causes of peritonitis and because generalized amyloidosis tends to develop in these patients.[9]

ADHESIONS

Peritoneal adhesions unfortunately are a common problem in both men and women and are encountered frequently in the practice of surgical pathology. Although adhesions may develop as a consequence of inflammatory lesions, they most often pose a significant clinical problem after abdominopelvic operations. An extensive study of the mechanisms of development of postoperative peritoneal adhesions suggested that intraoperative bleeding is the most important etiologic factor.[10] In this study, intraoperative drying of the serosa appeared to be an important potentiating factor, and the presence of talc, infection, and tissue necrosis was important in some instances.

Although peritoneal adhesions initially are composed predominantly of proliferating fibroblasts and mesothelial cells, blood, and fibrin, they eventually become densely collagenous and can cause intestinal obstruction. The usual treatment is surgical lysis of the adhesions, and the pathologist must search the submitted material carefully for evidence of a specific cause. This is particularly true if the initial surgical operation was for cancer, because a few recurrent cancer cells may be masked by massive fibroplasia. The pathologist must be equally careful when adhesions develop in a postradiotherapeutic rather than postoperative setting. In this situation, the opposite danger exists: misdiagnosis as recurrent cancer of bizarre cellular atypias that have developed in fibroblasts or endothelial cells as a result of radiation therapy.

Other iatrogenic causes of extensive peritoneal fibrous adhesions include drugs, notably β-adrenergic blocking agents such as practolol. The generalized condition produced by these drugs has been designated *sclerosing peritonitis*.[11]

CYSTS

True peritoneal cysts are rare. Walker and Putnam analyzed 33 cases of omental, mesenteric, and retroperitoneal cysts and suggested classification of these cysts into four major groups:

1. Embryonic and developmental
2. Traumatic or acquired
3. Neoplastic
4. Infectious and degenerative.[12]

Although 27 of the 33 cases occurred in females, many cysts were of enteric, genitourinary, or lymphatic origin and thus would not qualify as being derived from the peritoneum. Most traumatic and infectious cysts are actually pseudocysts because they are not lined by epithelium or mesothelium.

The most common true cystic lesion of the peritoneum that we have encountered in women has been designated *cystic mesothelioma* or *multilocular peritoneal inclusion cysts* (see the following section on benign tumors).

HYPERPLASIAS, METAPLASIAS, AND BENIGN TUMORS

Reactive Hyperplasia

Whenever the peritoneum is irritated, the mesothelium can proliferate to an alarming degree, forming papillary, glandular, and solid structures that may be confused with malignant mesothelioma or metastatic adenocarcinoma. Rosai and Dehner noted this situation within hernia sacs,[13] but we have encountered it frequently in many other peritoneal locations. In women, reactive hyperplasia is particularly likely to be encountered in pelvic inflammatory disease. In this situation, if there are extensive adhesions between the ovary and fallopian tube, the proliferating mesothelial cells may be found at the center of the inflammatory mass and not near any obvious serosal surface, making their correct identification even more difficult. Considerable anisonucleosis and nuclear pleomorphism may be present in these hyperplastic foci, but the overall appearance is still that of mesothelial cells: polygonal cell outlines, low nuclear–cytoplasmic ratios, glassy cytoplasmic appearance, and absence of stainable mucin (Fig. 7-2). Mitoses may be present but generally are few in number.

Cytologically, the cells may appear atypical, but their mesothelial origin is usually recognizable.[2-4] They can probably best be recognized by identifying intermediate forms between the atypical, often gigantic reactive cells and other classic benign mesothelial cells (Color Figure 7-1). In addition, the large, atypical mesothelial cells, although hyperchromatic, usually lack the internal structural aberrations suggestive of malignancy, such as coarsely clumped chromatin and condensation of chromatin along the nuclear membrane. If the atypia is of inflammatory origin, large numbers of inflammatory cells are usually present in the peritoneal effusion or washing specimen, and their prominence is helpful (although not infallible) in the differential diagnosis from a malignant peritoneal process.

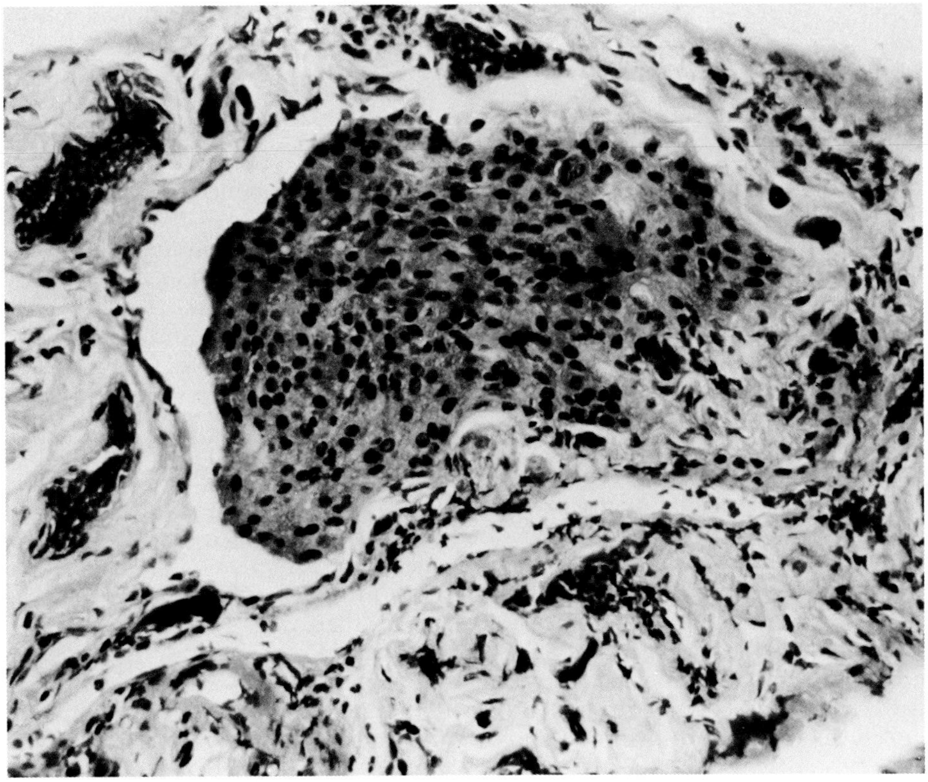

FIGURE 7-2 Mesothelial cell proliferation in hernia sac.

Flow cytometric analysis of peritoneal fluid specimens has been suggested as a useful adjunct to classic cytologic examination. Comparative studies in women with benign and malignant gynecologic diseases, however, have noted unacceptably high false-positive and false-negative results with flow cytometry.[14,15]

Endosalpingiosis

The term *endosalpingiosis* was coined by Sampson in 1930 to delineate persistent or recurrent nests of tubal epithelium in salpingectomy scars.[16] Sampson thought that these cells had an aggressive potential, and he noted similar cells in various peritoneal locations, including the ovarian surfaces. The term has subsequently come to be identified with any proliferation of müllerian-type epithelium on a peritoneal surface, although, as the name suggests, these proliferations most often are of the tubal epithelial type. Although these lesions were little more than a rarely seen histologic curiosity as recently as 20 years ago, they are being found with increasing frequency as gynecologic oncologists have become more aggressive in performing exploratory laparotomy in gynecologic cancer. Because they are encountered frequently in biopsy specimens from cases of ovarian or endometrial adenocarcinoma, often of relatively low grade, their differential diagnosis from metastatic adenocarcinoma poses an increasingly vexing problem to the pathologist.

Etiology

The causes suggested for this condition are the same as those suggested for endometriosis, and it is not unusual to find endometriosis and endosalpingiosis coexisting in a patient.[17] Because direct transitions from normal to slightly hyperplastic mesothelium to foci of endosalpingiosis can often be demonstrated, we favor the concept of a müllerian metaplastic histogenesis in most cases. We believe that endosalpingiosis frequently coexists with müllerian neoplasms of the upper female genital tract because we have encountered it in about 10% to 15% of cases of stage I serous carcinomas and borderline tumors of the ovary. This coexistence has been noted with equal or greater frequency in several published series.[18,19]

On the other hand, Zinsser and Wheeler noted the presence of tubal inflammatory disease in all cases of omental endosalpingiosis and concluded that tubal epithelial regurgitation with subsequent peritoneal implantation is the most common histogenetic pathway.[16] As in endometriosis, this question remains unresolved, and more than one etiologic mechanism may exist.

Clinical Findings

Unlike endometriosis, endosalpingiosis seems almost invariably to be a totally asymptomatic condition. Only rarely are symptomatic cases reported.[20] The lesions are discovered during the course of surgery for another condition, usually an ovarian or endometrial tumor or tubal inflammatory disease. It is surprising that this condition was not found in omental specimens at autopsy by Zinsser and Wheeler, because similar müllerian glandular inclusions have been reported in abdominal and pelvic lymph nodes in 5% to 41% of women at autopsy.[16,21]

Macroscopic Appearance

The lesions of endosalpingiosis may be grossly cystic or papillary. More often they present as small gray-white, firm, and occasionally calcified nodules measuring 1 to 2 mm in diameter (Color Figure 7-2) or as incidental findings on histologic examination of grossly unremarkable structures. They may be found on any peritoneal mesothelial surface but seem to have a predilection for the omentum, posterior uterine serosa, ovarian surface, and rectouterine cul-de-sac. The serosal surfaces of the fallopian tubes, bowel, bladder, and diaphragm are also common sites.

Microscopic Appearance

The lesions are composed of glands, papillae, cysts, and small solid cell nests. The cells are often organized as a single layer of cuboidal cells of mesothelial type but also show transitions to various types of müllerian epithelium, which by definition must include tubal epithelium (Figs. 7-3 and 7-4). When tubal metaplasia is clear-cut, one should be able to identify ciliated, secretory, and intercalated cells (Fig. 7-5). The glandular epithelium may also resemble endometrium, endocervix, or urothelium (Fig. 7-6). The latter metaplastic pathway is rare unless one includes the *Walthard's cell rests* commonly seen on the serosal surface of the fallopian tube under the rubric of endosalpingiosis.

Considerable chronic inflammation and fibrosis may accompany, entrap, and eventually obliterate the cellular elements in these proliferations. Calcification is common and usually takes the form of small concentric psammoma bodies. Sometimes it is difficult to find residual viable cells within a large mass of psammoma bodies and fibrous tissue (Fig. 7-7).

Cytologic Appearance

Because endosalpingiosis has been discussed in detail only in recent years, its cytologic appearance is still being defined.[22,23] In a peritoneal lavage spec-

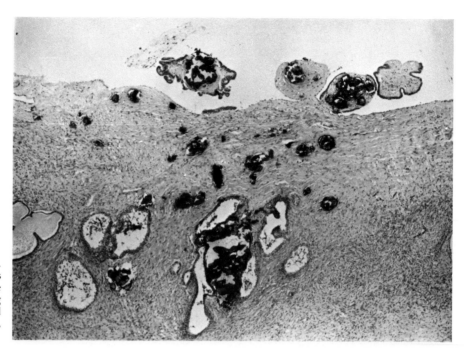

FIGURE 7-3 Endosalpingiosis of ovary. Note the numerous microcalcifications and growth both at and below the serosal surface. (Farhi DC, Silverberg SG: Pseudometastases in female genital cancer. Pathol Annu 17 [Part I]:47–76, 1982)

imen (which is the usual source of cytologic material in endosalpingiosis), the most useful diagnostic criterion is the presence of transitions from cells of epithelial, often atypical, appearance to those of classic benign mesothelial cells. Although the cells may be large and atypical, they lack the classic cytologic criteria of malignancy. Psammoma bodies may be numerous within the peritoneal cavity (Color Figures 7-3 and 7-4) and are not diagnostic of malignancy or even of neoplasia.[24] Papillary formations with

psammoma bodies may be seen in the vaginal smears of women with endosalpingiosis, and this should always be considered as an alternative to the diagnosis of carcinoma.

Differential Diagnosis

The most important differential diagnosis of endosalpingiosis is with a malignant tumor of the peritoneum, usually metastatic adenocarcinoma but occa-

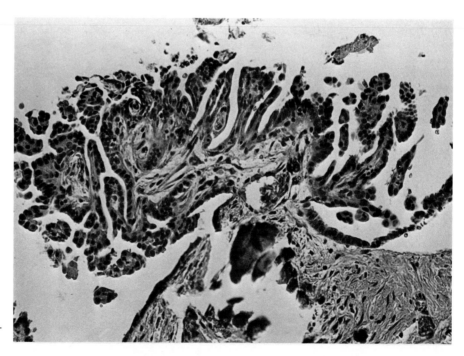

FIGURE 7-4 Endosalpingiosis of ovarian surface: detail.

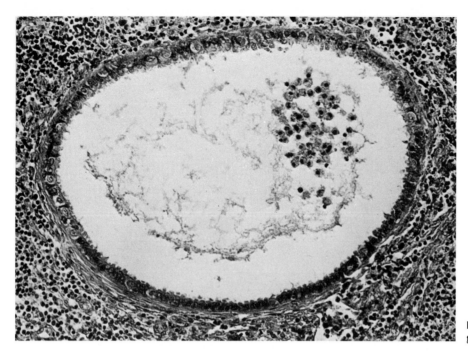

FIGURE 7-5 Detail of endosalpingiosis gland showing tubal-type epithelium.

sionally malignant mesothelioma. The finding of transitions to obvious mesothelial cells should rule out the diagnosis of metastatic carcinoma, even when a carcinoma is present in the ovary or endometrium. The absence of tumor elsewhere and the presence of tubal inflammatory disease strongly support the diagnosis of endosalpingiosis. Of equal or greater importance, in most cases, are the cytologic features of the epithelium itself. The presence of a tubal pattern, particularly if ciliated cells are numerous, is virtually diagnostic of endosalpingiosis. Even if such a pattern is not easily identified, the overall appearance should be bland, with atypia that is no more than slight to moderate and with only rare mitotic figures. There should be no destructive stromal invasion, although this may be difficult to differentiate from the inflammatory and sclerosing response by which the spontaneous regression of many foci of endosalpingiosis apparently takes place. Psammoma bodies may be seen in both endosalpingiosis and metastatic adenocarcinoma, but if the primary tumor elsewhere lacks psammoma bodies or a papillary ar-

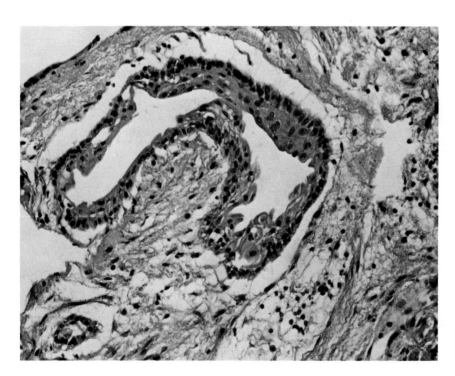

FIGURE 7-6 Endosalpingiosis of intestinal serosa showing urothelial metaplasia.

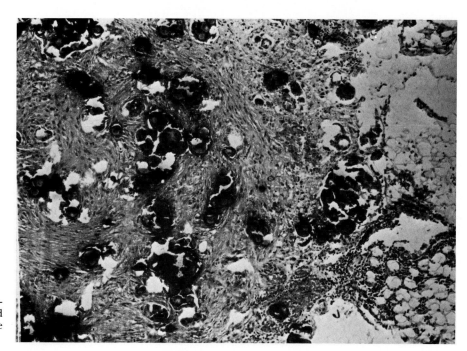

FIGURE 7-7 "Healed" endosalpingiosis of omentum, with fibrosis and microcalcifications. No residual viable cells are present.

chitecture, their presence in a mesothelial nodule otherwise consistent with endosalpingiosis would suggest benignity. The absence of a back-to-back or cribriform pattern is helpful. The differential diagnosis with malignant mesothelioma includes all these factors but is made simpler by the observation that classic mesothelioma of the peritoneum rarely occurs in women. When it does, it is almost invariably a macroscopically visible, diffuse, infiltrating tumor rather than the small, often microscopic proliferations of endosalpingiosis.

More difficult than the differentiation from metastatic adenocarcinoma is that from *serous tumor of low malignant potential (borderline tumor*[25,26] or *micropapillomatosis of low malignant potential*[27]) of the peritoneum, which may occur in the presence or absence of serous borderline tumor of the ovary. Bell and Scully have considered peritoneal proliferative lesions to be serous borderline tumors if they are composed of tubal-type epithelium exhibiting papillary projections, tufting, or detachment of cell clusters, even when they arise on the background of endosalpingiosis.[25,26] We believe that some lesions that we would consider to be atypical or even typical endosalpingiosis are overdiagnosed by these criteria (Fig. 7-8). We prefer to diagnose peritoneal borderline tumors by the same criteria used for ovarian borderline tumors (ie, cytologic criteria of malignancy without stromal invasion; see Chap. 6).

If the same criteria that are used for ovarian lesions are applied to peritoneal serous lesions, terms such as *noninvasive epithelial implants, noninvasive desmoplastic implants,* and *invasive implants* are no longer necessary.[28] These terms appear to be applied differently by different authors in describing the spectrum of neoplastic proliferations seen in various peritoneal sites in women with ovarian serous borderline tumors. We use only two diagnostic categories for these lesions—serous borderline tumor or invasive serous carcinoma (Figs. 7-9 through 7-11). Lesions with a tubal-type epithelium and a reactive stroma but without the usual architectural and cytologic features of serous carcinoma are usually regressing endosalpingiosis. Those with a reactive stroma and malignant cellular features are serous carcinomas, and serous tumors without evidence of stromal invasion but with tufting, cellular stratification and exfoliation, nuclear atypia, and mitotic activity are borderline tumors.

These distinctions are important because of differences in *prognosis*. The evolution of endosalpingiosis appears to be benign, and cases of carcinoma or borderline tumors should not be staged higher because of the finding of endosalpingiosis at exploratory laparotomy. In rare cases, the apparent development of a malignant or borderline tumor in a benign glandular inclusion has been reported (Fig. 7-12), usually when a similar tumor is present in the endometrium or ovary, and more often in a lymph node inclusion than in one of the more common sites of endosalpingiosis.[21,29] Nevertheless, the possibility of such a transformation must be kept in mind. Some or all multifocal serous carcinomas and serous borderline tumors arising from peritoneal surfaces may have developed in foci of endosalpingiosis, but this phenomenon has not been demonstrated conclusively and must remain speculative. Endosalpingiosis appears to require no treatment. Because the condition usually is diagnosed after its removal, it is difficult to be certain of its natural history if untreated. However, cases of spontaneous regression have been reported.

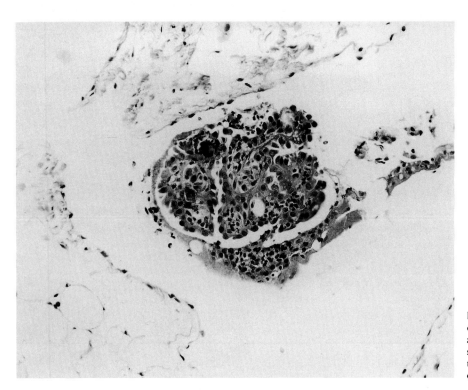

FIGURE 7-8 Atypical endosalpingiosis of omentum. There is papillary tufting and moderate nuclear atypia but no stratification or exfoliation of cell clusters. The patient had an ovarian serous tumor of low malignant potential.

The prognostic significance of peritoneal serous borderline tumors, on the other hand, is somewhat controversial. When they occur in the absence of an ovarian tumor, these tumors usually have a totally benign follow-up. Some patients may experience episodes of small bowel obstruction as a result of persistent or recurrent borderline tumors. Progression to invasive cancer and tumor-related death is rare.[25–27]

There is considerably less unanimity concerning the clinical significance of peritoneal serous borderline tumors and invasive carcinomas accompanying serous borderline tumors of the ovary. As summarized by Gershenson and Silva, some authors believe that only "invasive implants" worsen the prognosis, whereas an equal number report no significant difference in the outcome of patients with "invasive" or

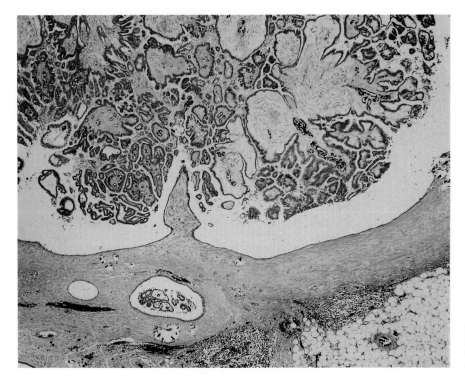

FIGURE 7-9 Serous tumor of low malignant potential in omentum. The patient had histologically identical tumors of both ovaries.

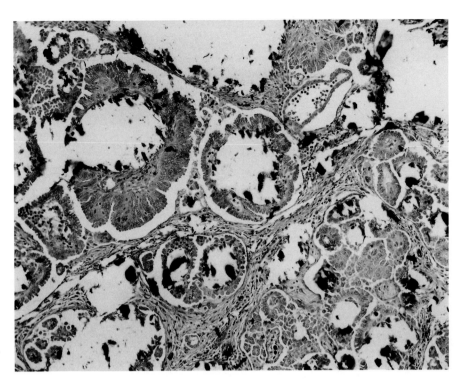

FIGURE 7-10 Serous tumor of low malignant potential in omentum. The tumor is heavily calcified, but papillary tufting, stratification, nuclear atypia, and exfoliation of cell clusters are easily seen. There is no stromal invasion. The patient had an ovarian serous tumor of low malignant potential.

"noninvasive" implants.[30] These differences may be based on differing diagnostic criteria or merely on the small numbers of cases in most reported series. In a review of my (SGS) recent, equally small, and unreported material, we found that patients with either of these lesions fared equally well.

Another controversial aspect of these "implants" is their *pathogenesis*. Many authors (including ourselves) have believed that they represent multifocal primary peritoneal neoplasia (the so-called field effect), but Segal and Hart have presented strong evidence in favor of their being true implants from the primary ovarian borderline tumor.[31] In their series, peritoneal implants were found in 29 of 47 patients (62%) whose ovarian tumors were found to have exophytic growth on the serosal surface, compared with 2 of 51 patients (4%) without exophytic tumor. Until this question is resolved completely, we

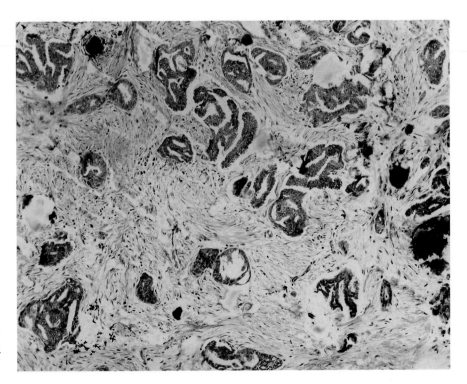

FIGURE 7-11 Invasive serous carcinoma of omentum. The patient had a synchronous ovarian serous tumor of low malignant potential.

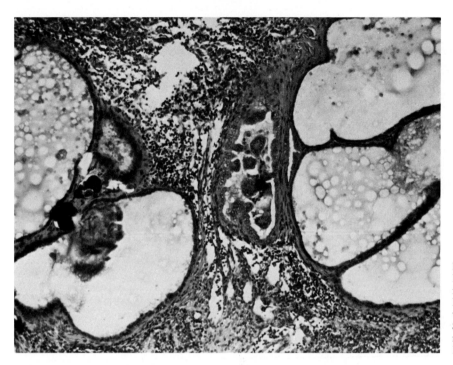

FIGURE 7-12 Development of a border-line serous tumor in an otherwise typical focus of endosalpingiosis (*right*) in a pelvic lymph node. A borderline serous tumor was also present in the ovary. (Farhi DC, Silverberg SG: Pseudometastases in female genital cancer. Pathol Annu 17 [Part I]:47–76, 1982)

recommend the designation of these lesions as peritoneal serous borderline tumors or as invasive serous carcinoma—which are strictly morphologic diagnoses—rather than as noninvasive or invasive implants, which implies a specific pathogenesis. Primary serous carcinoma of the peritoneum is a different lesion from a clinical point of view and is discussed later in this chapter.

Benign glandular inclusions of müllerian type occur frequently in pelvic and paraortic lymph nodes of women (Fig. 7-13).[21,32,33] The same diagnostic criteria for differentiation of endosalpingiosis from

metastatic adenocarcinoma should be applied in this situation (Fig. 7-14). An additional helpful observation is the involvement of the subcapsular sinusoid in metastatic cancer versus its lack of involvement by the benign glandular inclusions.

Another differential diagnosis of endosalpingiosis is endometriosis. The two conditions coexist and probably have identical pathogenetic mechanisms, and the distinction may be more apparent than real. However, it should be attempted because endometriosis is related clinically to infertility, pain, and other symptoms, and endosalpingiosis is not. In endometri-

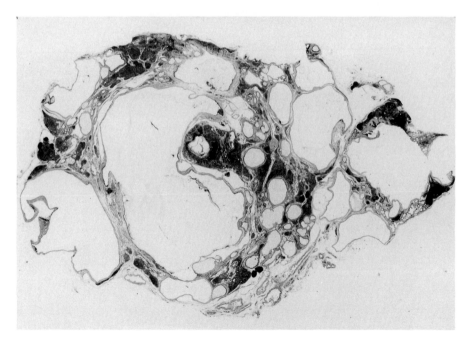

FIGURE 7-13 Pelvic lymph node largely replaced by benign glandular inclusions, lined by flattened and tubal-type epithelium.

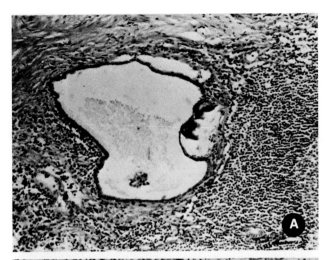

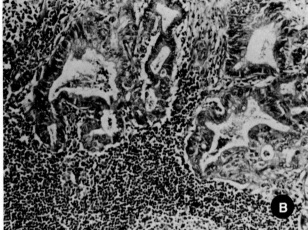

FIGURE 7-14 Comparison of benign glandular inclusion **(A)** and metastatic adenocarcinoma **(B)** in a pelvic lymph node. Both illustrations are from the same node. (Farhi DC, Silverberg SG: Pseudometastases in female genital cancer. Pathol Annu 17 [Part I]:47–76, 1982)

osis, the classic triad of endometrial epithelium, endometrial stroma, and old or recent hemorrhage should be present, whereas in endosalpingiosis the epithelium is more commonly of tubal type and, even when endometrial, should not be surrounded by stroma and hemorrhage.

Endometriosis

Endometriosis is one of the most common—and most important clinically—of those peritoneal conditions limited to or markedly more common in women. Endometriosis is not found only in peritoneal sites, however, and although we have included it among the metaplasias, its pathogenesis is uncertain.

Endometriosis is defined most simply as the presence of benign endometrial epithelium and stroma in an ectopic site. The condition has been divided into *endometriosis interna* (or *adenomyosis*), which involves the myometrium, and *endometriosis externa*, which generally is found in extrauterine localizations but is also found in the uterine serosa in the absence of myometrial involvement. Adenomyosis is discussed in Chapter 4; our discussion here is confined to the external variant of endometriosis. Sites other than the uterine serosa are, in descending order of frequency, the ovary, pelvic peritoneum, rectovaginal septum, fallopian tube, rectum and sigmoid, cervix, uterine ligament, vagina, other pelvic and abdominal locations, and rare scattered sites entirely outside the pelvis and abdomen.[34-38]

Pathogenesis

The pathogenesis of endometriosis has been debated for more than half a century, and the issue is by no means settled. There is ample clinical and experimental evidence favoring each of the main theories of pathogenesis. These theories are:

1. Retrograde menstruation and implantation
2. Coelomic metaplasia
3. Lymphatic or hematogenous dissemination.

Theory of Implantation. Sampson was the first major figure to champion the theory of implantation.[39] He hypothesized that retrograde menstruation with expulsion of endometrial fragments through the tubal lumina into the peritoneal cavity would lead to implantation and development of these fragments in most of the common sites of endometriosis.[40] This theory corresponds well with the usual distribution of clinical endometriosis and with experimental studies that induce endometriosis by implantation in animals and humans.[41,42] The implantation theory is also supported by reports of so-called scar endometriosis, in which the lesion develops in a surgical scar related to an episiotomy, a recently cauterized cervix, or an excised Bartholin's gland.[43]

Opponents of this theory point to the rarity of documented retrograde menstruation, the apparent lack of viability in most fragments of menstrual endometrium, and the occasional foci of endometriosis in sites where retrograde menstruation would not be likely to play a role (eg, pleuropulmonary endometriosis).[38]

Theory of Coelomic Metaplasia. Meyer adapted the theory of coelomic metaplasia from the ideas of von Recklinghausen.[44] The theory proposes that the peritoneal mesothelium undergoes müllerian metaplasia into endometrial-type tissues. It is supported by the knowledge that the müllerian ducts and the peritoneal serosa have a common coelomic origin. Other supportive data (which usually are anecdotal) include the development of endometriosis in patients without intrauterine endometrium[45] and the association of endometriosis with other types of epithelial and mesenchymal proliferations presumably derived by mesothelial metaplasia.[17,46] This theory might explain intrathoracic endometriosis, because all but two of the reported cases have been pleural or subpleural.[38] However, even rarer localizations that are not abdominal, pelvic, or thoracic would be difficult to explain using this theory.

Theory of Lymphatic or Hematogenous Dissemination. A theory of lymphatic or hematogenous dissemination would appear to explain those rare cases that are dissonant with the other two theories. Endometrial fragments can be found in myometrial vascular spaces during menstruation and in other phases of the menstrual cycle,[47,48] and endometriosis in pelvic lymph nodes has been attributed to lymphatic spread.[49] Most of the common pelvic and abdominal sites of endometriosis, however, are better explained by one or both of the previously cited theories.

Other Theories. Other phenomena have been invoked to explain why endometriosis develops in some women but not in others. The theory of metaplasia, in particular, cannot explain the absence of endometriosis in normal males and premenarchal females without an additional hormonal explanation. The few cases reported in males and in phenotypic females with gonadal dysgenesis generally have been associated with the use of exogenous hormones.[50,51] Studies in monkeys have indicated that although implantation endometriosis can be initiated without ovarian steroid hormones, maintenance depends on estrogen, progesterone, or both.[52] However, almost all studies of hormone receptors in human endometriosis have found that these receptors are present in lower concentrations in ectopic endometrium than in normal intrauterine endometrium in the same patients and may be absent entirely from the endometriotic foci.[53–56]

A heritable tendency toward the development of endometriosis has been suggested,[57,58] and immunologic abnormalities have been noted in patients with endometriosis.[59–61] These factors may be causative or secondary.

Symptoms

Endometriosis appears during the period of gonadal activity and stabilizes or regresses after a natural or artificial menopause. Some cases are asymptomatic and represent incidental surgical findings, whereas others cause painful pelvic manifestations connected with the menstrual cycle and show signs of compression of adjacent organs. The most frequent clinical manifestations are dysmenorrhea, menometrorrhagia, dyspareunia, infertility, and lumbar or rectal pain.[34,35,62,63]

The pain associated with endometriosis is usually aggravated during menstruation and appears to be due to bleeding into and around the foci of disease. Some studies suggest that dysmenorrhea is a consequence of the prostaglandins produced by the endometriotic implants, but other studies indicate that women with and without endometriosis have no significant differences in prostaglandin levels.[64] The pathogenesis of the other symptoms, particularly infertility, is equally difficult to explain. Although infertility in anatomically advanced cases of endometriosis is probably best attributed to replacement or obstruction of normal reproductive structures, the infertility frequently encountered in the presence of minimal endometriosis remains to be explained.[65] Various types of ovulatory dysfunction, including luteinization of an unruptured follicle (the so-called LUF syndrome), have been suggested as the cause of infertility in these cases, as have increased prostaglandin production and autoimmunity to endometrial or ovarian tissue.[34,59,60]

Other clinical manifestations of endometriosis are based on specific locations. For example, endometriosis has been reported to cause ureteral obstruction and to mimic acute appendicitis and rectosigmoid carcinoma.[36]

Clinical Staging

Classification of the severity of endometriosis is important in determining prognosis and treatment and in comparing different methods of treatment. The system of classification of pelvic endometriosis most frequently used is the revised classification of the American Fertility Society (Table 7-1).[66] Extrapelvic endometriosis has been classified by Markham and colleagues (Table 7-2).[67]

Macroscopic Appearance

Endometriosis presents diffusely or as isolated nodules that vary in size but generally do not surpass a few millimeters in diameter. Appearance and size vary with the phase of the menstrual cycle; the nodules become congested and painful during the menstrual phase. In the ovary, endometriosis presents as firm red-brown or blue cysts of several millimeters in diameter on the surface of the organ.[68] A section made through these foci reveals white or yellow tissue surrounding a more hemorrhagic central zone. When these tissues are voluminous, they may occupy a large part of the ovary and deeply invade the cortex. These cysts contain altered blood and their contents often are brown, prompting the common term, *chocolate cysts of the ovary* (see Color Figure 6-4). They are distended during menstrual periods and may rupture or develop fistulas into the ovarian stroma or the pelvic peritoneal cavity.

In the uterosacral ligaments, the rectovaginal septum, the round ligaments, and the umbilicus, foci of endometriosis are single or multiple small, blue nodules. The nodules vary in size, and the largest may be palpable. When they appear under the peritoneal or tubal serosa, these nodules have a stellate aspect with blue centers. More rarely, tubal endome-

TABLE 7-1
American Fertility Society Classification of Endometriosis: 1985

Disorder		Extent	
Endometriosis	<1 cm	1–3 cm	>3 cm
Peritoneum			
Superficial	1	2	4
Deep	2	4	6
Ovary			
R Superficial	1	2	4
Deep	4	16	20
L Superficial	1	2	4
Deep	4	16	20

	Partial		Complete
Posterior Cul-de-sac Obliteration	4		40

Adhesions	<1/3 Enclosure	1/3–2/3 Enclosure	>2/3 Enclosure
Ovary			
R Filmy	1	2	4
Dense	4	8	16
L Filmy	1	2	4
Dense	4	8	16
Tube			
R Filmy	1	2	4
Dense	4*	8*	16
L Filmy	1	2	4
Dense	4*	8*	16

*If the fimbriated end of the fallopian tube is completely enclosed, change the point assignment to 16.

Total of Above: 1–5 = stage I (minimal); 6–15 = stage II (mild); 16–40 = stage III (Moderate); > 40 = stage IV (severe).

American Fertility Society: Classification of endometriosis: 1985. Fertil Steril 43:351–352, 1985

TABLE 7-2
Classification and Staging of Extrapelvic Endometriosis

Classification of Extrapelvic Endometriosis
  Class I: Endometriosis involving the intestinal tract
  Class U: Endometriosis involving the urinary tract
  Class L: Endometriosis involving the lung and thoracic cage
  Class O: Endometriosis involving other sites outside the abdominal cavity

Staging of Extrapelvic Endometriosis
  Stage I No organ defect
    1. Extrinsic: surface of organ (serosa, pleura)
       a. <1 cm lesion
       b. 1 to 4 cm lesion
       c. >4 cm lesion
    2. Intrinsic: mucosal, muscle, parenchyma
       a. <1 cm lesion
       b. 1 to 4 cm lesion
       c. >4 cm lesion
  Stage II Organ defect*
    1. Extrinsic: surface of organ (serosa, pleura)
       a. <1 cm lesion
       b. 1 to 4 cm lesion
       c. >4 cm lesion
    2. Intrinsic: mucosal, muscle, parenchyma
       a. <1 cm lesion
       b. 1 to 4 cm lesion
       c. >4 cm lesion

*Organ defect would depend on the organ of involvement and would include but not be limited to obstruction and partial obstruction of the urinary tract and the intestinal tract and hemothorax, hemoptysis, and pneumothorax resulting from pulmonary involvement.

Markham SM, Carpenter SE, Rock JA. Extrapelvic endometriosis. Obstet Gynecol Clin North Am 1989;16(1):193.

triosis simulates a hematosalpinx. This deeply pigmented appearance, although characteristic of mature lesions, may not be seen in early lesions such as those often encountered in laparoscopic staging procedures.[69–71] These initial lesions may be white, yellow, or red and may progress to the brown or blue appearance with time. The pain associated with the menstrual period is caused by the vascular tension that results from the periodic growth of these masses. The vulvar localization, of which relatively few cases have been reported, occurs mainly in women who have sustained obstetric vulvar trauma or an episiotomy. It often is not associated with involvement of the usual pelvic sites.[36]

Similarly, superficial cervical endometriosis is common after endometrial curettage combined with cervical conization, whereas deep cervical involvement usually is an extension from the cul-de-sac.[36] Intestinal, ureteral, pleural, pulmonary, and cutaneous localizations have been described (Color Figure 7-5).

Microscopic Appearance

Endometriosis is composed of glands, cellular stroma, and, in some cases, smooth muscle fibers (Fig. 7-15). The glands are lined by columnar, cuboidal, or flattened epithelial cells. The ciliated cells found in normal endometrium are also found in endometriosis. The stroma may be difficult to find or may be considerably more abundant than the glandular component. Unlike adenomyosis, the endometrium in external endometriosis generally responds to ovarian hormones and may show secretory changes in the second half of the cycle and decidual transformation during pregnancy.

Endometriosis is difficult to recognize when repeated hemorrhages have modified the tissue, leaving only glands lined by flattened epithelium or cysts completely devoid of epithelium. If hemorrhage is pronounced, macrophages laden with hemosiderin or, more commonly, lipofuscin or hemofuscin are found in the stroma. These cells are characteristic and may be the only clue to the diagnosis. However, if extensive sectioning fails to reveal glands or stroma of endometrial type, the diagnosis of endometriosis can only be suggested rather than confirmed.

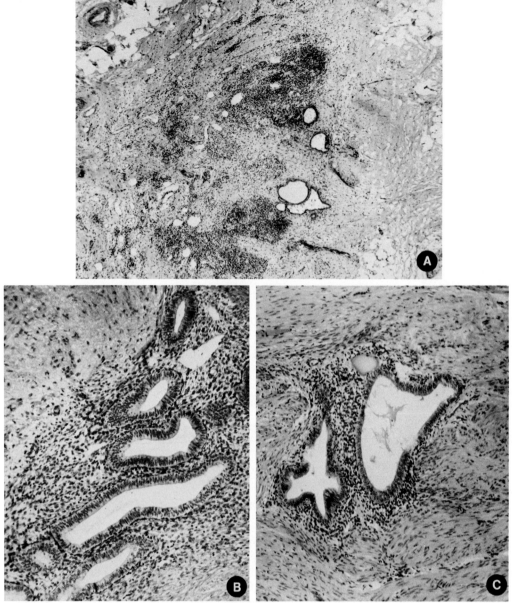

FIGURE 7-15 Endometriosis. **(A)** Lymph node; **(B)** rectal wall; and **(C)** sigmoid.

Several variations in appearance have been characterized recently. *Stromal endometriosis,* in which glands cannot be identified, is most common in the ovary and the cervix.[72] The absence of glands leads to a differential diagnosis with low-grade endometrial stromal sarcoma and other stromal neoplasms, including sex cord-stromal tumors in the ovary and Kaposi's sarcoma in the cervix.[36,72] *Necrotic pseudo-xanthomatous nodules* are apparently a manifestation of end-stage endometriosis and are seen particularly in perimenopausal and postmenopausal women.[73] These nodules involve the ovaries and peritoneum and consist of central necrosis surrounded by palisaded pseudoxanthoma cells, hyalinized fibrous tissue, or both. Typical endometriosis is found elsewhere. *Endomyometriosis* is a variant in which exten-

sive proliferation of smooth muscle results in the formation of uterus-like masses in the ovary, broad ligament, omentum, and other locations.[74] An alternative explanation for these masses is that they are congenital malformations. Other variations seen in endometriosis include stromal calcification, ossification, myxoid change, and inflammatory infiltrates, the latter possibly following superimposed infection.

Hormonal lesions may be reflected in the ectopic endometrium. For example, varying degrees of endometrial hyperplasia may be seen, particularly in ovarian endometriosis, and may coexist with similar images of hyperplasia in the intrauterine endometrium. Rare cases of endometriosis—again particularly in the ovarian localization—show marked cytologic atypia of the glandular epithelium without architectural evidence of hyperplasia or carcinoma (Fig. 7-16). This *atypical endometriosis*, which should be diagnosed only when the atypia is not a reaction to underlying inflammation, has been reported as coexisting with and progressing to carcinoma, usually of the clear cell or endometrioid type (Fig. 7-17) .[75,76] Chalas and colleagues have suggested that a high AgNOR (silver-staining nucleolar organizing region) count in atypical endometriosis may predict the development of carcinoma.[76]

Finally, peripheral reactive fibrosis is often seen and contributes to the increase in volume of the mass. Extensive fibrous adhesions may form, even to the point of causing a "frozen pelvis." Neither the formation of these adhesions nor the perineural or vascular invasion occasionally encountered in otherwise typical endometriosis should by itself be accepted as evidence of malignancy.[36]

Cytologic Examination

Cytologic examination is rarely performed in endometriosis. The overall appearance is benign, and epithelial and stromal cells may be seen.[38] Ceroid or iron pigment in histiocytes may falsely suggest the diagnosis of malignant melanoma.[77] Increased numbers of macrophages may be seen in peritoneal fluids from infertile endometriosis patients.[78]

Malignant Transformation

Ectopic endometrium shares with intrauterine endometrium the ability to undergo malignant change, although this transformation occurs in less than 1% of patients with endometriosis. Mostoufizadeh and Scully, for example, found 11 cases of carcinoma in more than 1800 reported cases of ovarian endometriosis.[79] Brooks and Wheeler pointed out that almost one fourth of the cases of malignant tumors arising in endometriosis were in extraovarian sites.[80]

Endometrioid carcinoma of the ovary may be of endometriotic origin, but this can be proved in only a small proportion of cases (up to 24% of cases reported in the literature). Clear cell carcinoma and mucinous müllerian borderline tumor are the only other ovarian epithelial tumors frequently associated with endometriosis (see Chap. 6). Proof of malignant transformation in endometriosis should consist of the two strict criteria formulated by Sampson: the presence of a focus of benign endometriosis at the origin of the tumor, and the demonstration of transition between the benign and malignant zones (Fig. 7-18). A malignant tumor may arise from any of the constituents of endometriosis: glandular epithelium, endometrial stroma, or smooth muscle fibers. Carcinomatous transformation of the glandular epithelium is most common. The appearance of stromal sarcoma, leiomyosarcoma, carcinosarcoma, or adenosarcoma is more unusual.

Treatment

There are strong proponents of both medical and surgical treatment for endometriosis. Medical treatment includes oral contraceptives, other progestational agents, and danazol, a synthetic steroid derivative of ethisterone with antigonadotropic properties.[62,81] Other agents are Gn-RH-a, a long-acting

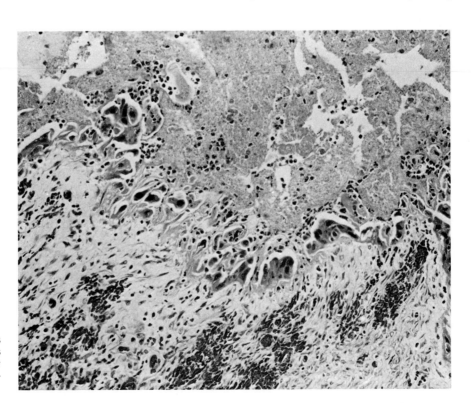

FIGURE 7-16 Atypical endometriosis of ovary. Bizarre proliferated cells project into a blood-filled cavity. They are underlaid by hemorrhagic endometrial stroma.

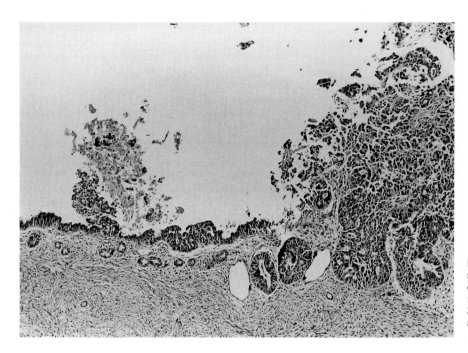

FIGURE 7-17 Ovarian cyst lining shows atypical endometriosis (*left*) in continuity with endometrioid carcinoma (*right*). (LaGrenade A, Silverberg SG: Ovarian tumors associated with atypical endometriosis. Hum Pathol 19:1080–1084, 1988)

gonadotropin-releasing hormone agonist, and gestrinone, an antiprogesterone steroid.[81–83] The results of different therapeutic measures are just beginning to be compared by the standardized approach permitted by the new clinical staging system (see Table 7-1).

The histologic changes brought about by the long-term administration of progestational agents are the same in clinical endometriosis and in the experimental disease in monkeys: decidual reaction followed by necrosis and fibrosis of the endometriotic foci. With danazol therapy, a pseudomenopause is created; small lesions regress completely, whereas large and thick-walled lesions decrease in size and may develop new adhesions.[62] The uterus, tubes, and ovaries atrophy with this form of treatment. Similar changes are seen in gestrinone-treated patients. Some lesions, however, show no change after therapy. The effectiveness of medical therapy can be monitored in some cases by serial determinations of plasma CA-125 levels.[84]

Surgical treatment is often necessary for diag-

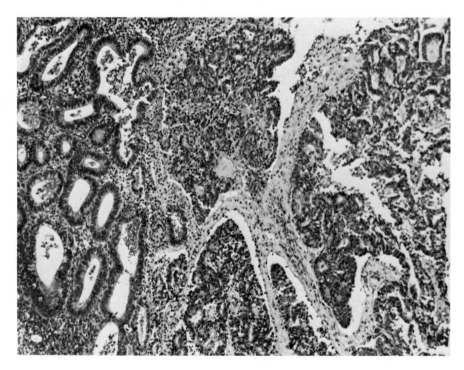

FIGURE 7-18 Adenocarcinoma (*right*) arising in endometriosis (*left*) of the vaginal wall. This patient had a synchronous carcinoma of the intrauterine endometrium without myometrial invasion.

nostic purposes and is indicated in the event of failure of hormonal therapy.[65,85] Surgery sometimes becomes necessary in the event of a serious complication such as obstruction or massive hemorrhage. The surgery may be local if the focus is easily resectable, or radical if the lesion is extensive or diffuse. Both medical and surgical therapies are more effective in cases of mild endometriosis. Clinical recurrence is frequent. In a review of the literature, Wheeler and Malinak found recurrence rates of 2% to 47% after conservative surgery, 17% to 29% after the establishment of pseudopregnancy with progestational agents, and 39% after danazol therapy.[86]

Endocervicosis

Far rarer than endosalpingiosis and endometriosis is a lesion known as endocervicosis, in which benign müllerian metaplasia results in the formation of mucinous epithelium resembling that of the endocervix. This lesion is usually an incidental finding in pelvic lymph nodes or the pelvic peritoneum but has been reported as a symptomatic mass in the posterior wall of the urinary bladder.[87,88] The differential diagnosis is with metastatic (or, in the bladder, primary) mucinous adenocarcinoma.

Leiomyomatosis Peritonealis Disseminata

A rare condition, leiomyomatosis peritonealis disseminata is found in women of reproductive age and is characterized by the presence of widespread peritoneal nodules. Although the first case was reported in 1952, subsequent case reports have accumulated so slowly that the 1982 report by Tavassoli and Norris[89] of 20 cases comprised about half of the reported cases in the literature at that time,[90] and only about 20 additional cases have been reported since then.[91] The condition has stimulated discussion, however, because of the discrepancy between the gross appearance of the lesions, which resemble a disseminated malignant tumor, and their uniformly benign evolution.

The condition occurs in women of reproductive age, many of whom are pregnant or postpartum (43% of cases) or taking contraceptive steroids or other hormones (27%) at the time of diagnosis.[91] The lesions are usually discovered incidentally, often at the time of cesarean section, laparoscopic tubal ligation, or other exploratory procedures associated with pregnancy. Because this lesion is often associated with unusual hormonal situations, it is widely assumed that its pathogenesis is related to hormonal imbalances. Fujii and colleagues were able to induce peritoneal nodules containing smooth muscle cells in guinea pigs by administering estrogen and progesterone.[92] The origin of the lesions appears to be in the subcoelomic mesenchyme, as discussed in detail by Ober and Black.[93]

Clinical Findings

Clinically, these are generally asymptomatic lesions that are discovered at the time of an exploratory procedure, usually a cesarean section or postpartum tubal ligation. Women with abdominal or pelvic symptoms almost always have coexistent disease such as endometriosis or uterine leiomyomata.[22,91]

Macroscopic Appearance

Macroscopically, there is a frightening picture of dozens to hundreds of small, well-demarcated, firm, gray to white nodules diffusely involving the peritoneal surfaces. These nodules usually measure 2 to 3 mm in diameter but may grow as large as 2 to 3 cm or even larger.

Microscopic Appearance

Microscopically, the nodules are composed of well-circumscribed whorled masses of uniform and benign-appearing smooth muscle cells (Fig. 7-19). Decidual cells may be admixed in those cases occurring in pregnant or postpartum women. Pleomorphism, nuclear atypia, and mitotic figures are absent or minimal. Collagenous sclerosis and inflammation may be present, but necrosis is absent. Foci of endometriosis or endosalpingiosis are present in continuity with the nodules in 10% of the cases.[94]

Ultrastructurally, the typical appearance is that of smooth muscle cells, with myofibrils, dense bodies, pinocytotic vesicles, and basal lamina. Some researchers have commented on the presence of cells resembling myofibroblasts and decidual cells, and of endometriosis.[46,89]

The evolution of these lesions has been generally benign, although two reported cases have been interpreted as progressing to leiomyosarcoma.[95,96] In several cases, the lesions have been shown to regress after the cessation of the abnormal hormonal stimulus (termination of pregnancy or of oral contraception). In a few cases, the lesions have recurred (or persisted) with a subsequent pregnancy. This association with hormonal stimuli is consistent with the presence of estrogen and progesterone receptors in the smooth muscle cells of the lesion.[97] It would appear from the reported cases that treatment should be conservative.

Deciduosis

Just as the subcoelomic mesenchyme apparently can proliferate and result in the development of smooth muscle nodules, a somewhat different pathway of development may produce solitary or multiple nodules of decidua in pregnant women.[94,98–100] As in leiomyomatosis peritonealis disseminata, these nodules are almost always asymptomatic findings discovered during the course of laparotomy for other indications,

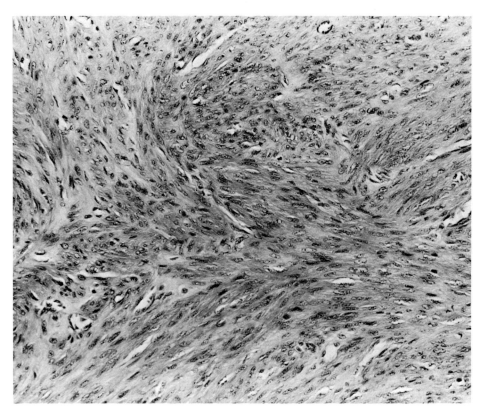

FIGURE 7-19 Benign smooth muscle proliferation in leiomyomatosis peritonealis disseminata.

although rare cases have been associated with massive intraperitoneal hemorrhage.[98,99] Similar foci of ectopic decidua may be seen in the cervix, the fallopian tubes, and pelvic and paraortic lymph nodes (Fig. 7-20). In one series, they were found in the tubal serosa in 5.5% of postpartum tubal ligation specimens.[98] In these situations, their major significance is the possibility of being misinterpreted as carcinoma, usually of squamous type.[100] Because decidual cells may show some cytologic atypia, the differential diagnosis depends on their low nuclear–cytoplasmic ratio, voluminous glassy eosinophilic cytoplasm, sharply demarcated cell borders, lack of intercellular bridges, and absence of destructive or proliferative stromal invasion. If doubt remains, the lack of immunoreactivity of decidual cells for cytokeratins should be helpful.

Splenosis

Splenosis is a rare condition in which traumatic splenic rupture results in the implantation of splenic fragments throughout the peritoneal cavity.[101] It is no more common in women than in men but is notable in women because of its tendency to mimic endometriosis in its gross appearance. The nodules usually are an incidental finding at laparotomy and involve, in descending frequency, the small bowel, omentum, parietal peritoneum and large intestinal serosa, and diaphragm. Their dark purple color may suggest hemorrhagic foci of endometriosis. Histologic examination quickly resolves this problem.

Benign Mesotheliomas

For many years, when the term *mesothelioma* was used to refer to a peritoneal lesion, the assumption was made that this represented a diffuse malignant process. In the past few decades, it has become apparent that a large variety of benign peritoneal mesotheliomas may be encountered and that they are far more common in women than the classic malignant mesothelioma.

Four benign or putatively benign patterns of peritoneal mesothelioma have been delineated: localized fibrous tumors, papillary mesotheliomas, cystic mesotheliomas, and adenomatoid tumors. The *localized fibrous tumor* is a common tumor of the pleura and a rarity in the peritoneum.[102,103] It is not limited to or overwhelmingly more common in women. Its other names, localized fibrous mesothelioma and submesothelioma, reflect the debate between advocates of a mesothelial origin and a fibroblastic derivation. The most recent ultrastructural and immunohistochemical (keratin-negative, vimentin-positive) studies support the latter theory.[103] As the name used here suggests, the lesion is localized, solitary, and composed of a uniform spindle cell proliferation with varying amounts of collagen. A focally or diffusely prominent hemangiopericytic pattern is often present. Atypia and mitotic activity are minimal, and lesions studied by flow cytometry have been diploid.[103] The evolution is benign.

The *adenomatoid tumor* has been convincingly demonstrated to be of peritoneal mesothelial origin, but it is almost always found in women in the fallo-

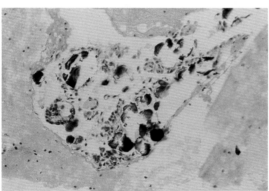

Color Figure 7-1

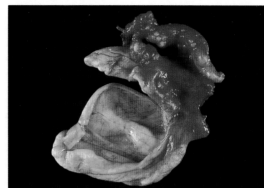

Color Figure 7-2

Color Figure 7-3

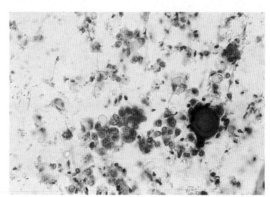

Color Figure 7-4

Color Figure 7-1   Reactive mesothelial cell atypia.

Color Figure 7-2   Endosalpingiosis of the tubal serosa accompanying a benign ovarian cyst.

Color Figure 7-3   Endosalpingiosis. Psammoma bodies and a few benign cells in peritoneal fluid cell block.

Color Figure 7-4   Endosalpingiosis in peritoneal washing: benign cells and psammoma body.

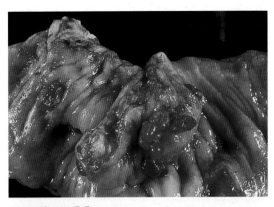

Color Figure 7-5

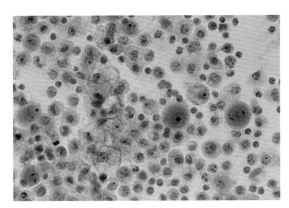

Color Figure 7-6

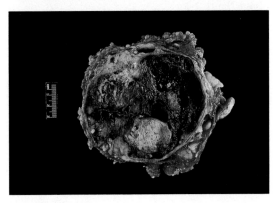

Color Figure 7-7

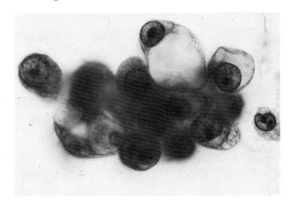

Color Figure 7-8

Color Figure 7-5 Intestinal endometriosis. Nodular red serosal lesions extend through the bowel wall and ulcerate the mucosa.

Color Figure 7-6 Malignant mesothelioma. Mesothelial cells range from small to large and bizarre.

Color Figure 7-7 Serous carcinoma of mesentery. Patient had undergone a hysterectomy with bilateral salpingo-oophorectomy for benign disease 14 years earlier (see Fig. 7-27 for microscopic appearance).

Color Figure 7-8 Metastatic adenocarcinoma in peritoneal fluid: mucin-secreting malignant cells. (Courtesy of Dr. Poonam Chandra, George Washington University, Washington, DC)

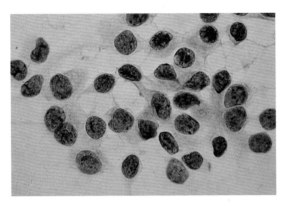

Color Figure 10-1

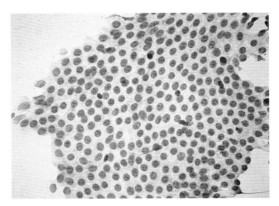

Color Figure 10-2

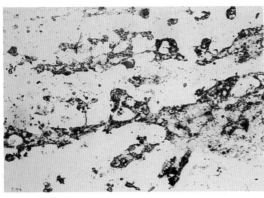

Color Figure 10-3

Color Figure 10-4

Color Figure 10-1 Fine-needle aspirate from infiltrating duct carcinoma. Poorly cohesive cells with increased nuclear–cytoplasmic ratios and nuclear hyperchromatism are shown. This tumor was moderately well differentiated.

Color Figure 10-2 Fine-needle aspirate from poorly differentiated infiltrating duct carcinoma. There is increased pleomorphism compared with that shown in Color Figure 10-1.

Color Figure 10-3 Fat necrosis: smear shows necroinflammatory background with no ductal cells.

Color Figure 10-4 Fine-needle aspirate from fibroadenoma. A large sheet of uniform ductal epithelial cells is shown in a honeycomb array, with peripheral blunt branches.

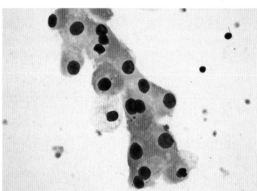

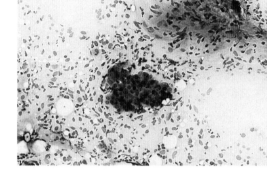

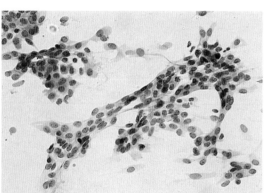

Color Figure 10-5

Color Figure 10-6

Color Figure 10-7

Color Figure 10-8

Color Figure 10-5 Lactational hyperplasia. An air-dried Diff-Quick-stained smear shows poorly cohesive ductal cells with mildly atypical nuclei and intracytoplasmic lipid vacuoles.

Color Figure 10-6 Low-grade phyllodes tumor. Cytologic picture of benign ductal cells and hypercellular stroma.

Color Figure 10-7 Intraductal papilloma: benign ductal cells showing apocrine metaplasia in smear from nipple discharge.

Color Figure 10-8 Nipple adenoma (subareolar papillomatosis). Intraoperative smear of biopsy specimen emphasizes cytologic benignity.

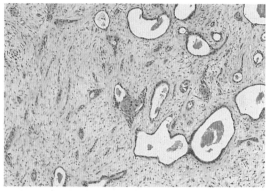

Color Figure 10-9

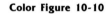

Color Figure 10-10

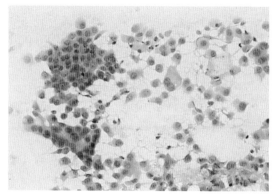

Color Figure 10-11

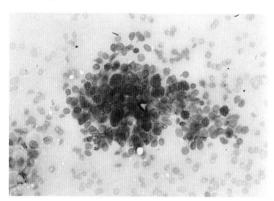

Color Figure 10-12

Color Figure 10-9 Syringomatous adenoma of nipple. Infiltrating dilated and comma-shaped glandular structures, some with squamous metaplasia, in a nonreactive stroma. (Courtesy of Dr. Mirka Jones, Armed Forces Institute of Pathology, Washington, D.C.)

Color Figure 10-10 Collagenous spherulosis. This was an incidental microscopic finding in a breast biopsy performed for another indication.

Color Figure 10-11 Intraductal carcinoma. Smear shows cohesive and dyshesive malignant ductal cells.

Color Figure 10-12 Adenoid cystic carcinoma. Smear from fine-needle aspirate shows small, uniform tumor cells in hyaline background. (Courtesy of Dr. Sana Tabbara, The George Washington University Medical Center, Washington DC)

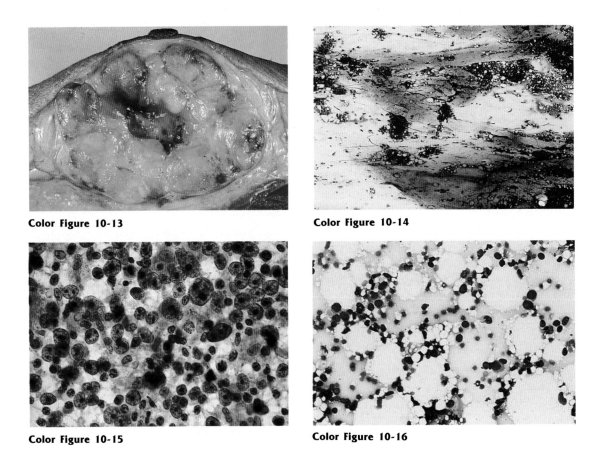

Color Figure 10-13

Color Figure 10-14

Color Figure 10-15

Color Figure 10-16

Color Figure 10-13 Mucinous carcinoma. A large, well-circumscribed, gelatinous gross appearance is typical.

Color Figure 10-14 Mucinous carcinoma. Smear shows clusters of small tumor cells in voluminous extracellular mucinous background (Diff-Quick stain).

Color Figure 10-15 Medullary carcinoma. Cytologic appearance of large, bizarre, dyshesive carcinoma cells and small lymphocytes.

Color Figure 10-16 Infiltrating lobular carcinoma. The most cellular region of a paucicellular smear shows small tumor cells in small clusters and as single cells.

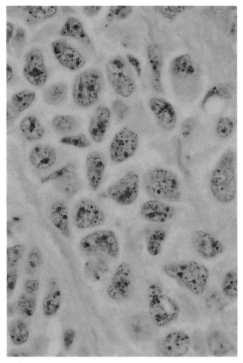

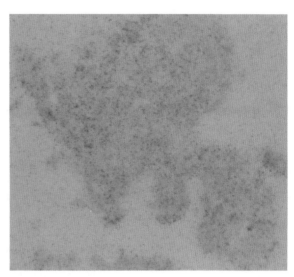

Color Figure 12-1

Color Figure 12-2

Color Figure 12-1 AgNORs in serous papillary adenocarcinoma of the ovary. The specimen was fixed in 10% formalin for 18 hours and then embedded in wax. AgNORs are seen as black dots. They sometimes appear in aggregates within the nucleus.

Color Figure 12-2 Simultaneous immunohistochemistry and in situ hybridization of c-*myc* in serous papillary adenocarcinoma of the human ovary. The brown colorimetric diaminobenzidine reaction represents immunoreactivity of c-*myc,* and the black dots represent hybridization signals on autoradiography. This technique allows the expression of c-*myc* at mRNA and protein levels in the same tumor cells.

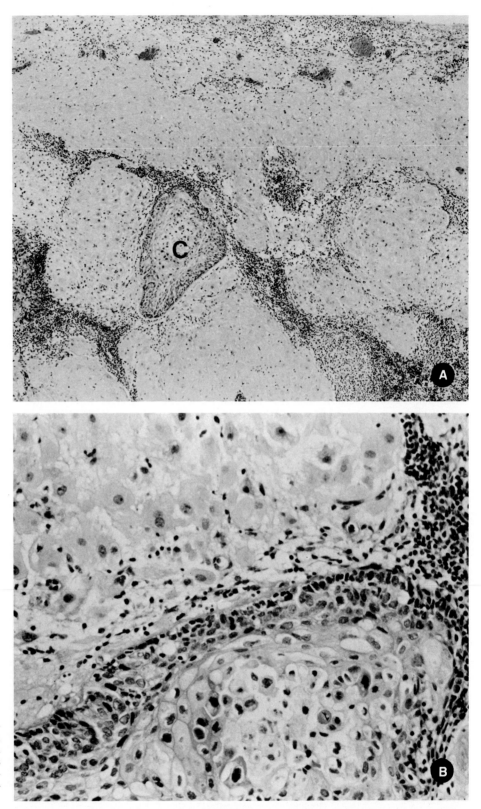

FIGURE 7-20 Decidua and metastatic cervical squamous carcinoma in pelvic lymph node of pregnant patient. **(A)** Low-power (single focus of carcinoma is marked *C*); **(B)** detail with decidua (*top*) and carcinoma (*below*).

pian tube or the uterine corpus. However, structures resembling those seen in adenomatoid tumors have been induced experimentally in animals in subperitoneal nodules produced by sex steroids, and rare examples of adenomatoid tumor arising in peritoneal sites outside the uterus and fallopian tube have been reported.[104,105] For further discussion of this tumor, see Chapters 4 and 5.

Since the initial case report in 1952, more than 120 cases of *cystic mesothelioma* have been reported, most in young or middle-aged women.[91,106–110] These tumors present as multiloculated cystic masses in the abdomen and pelvis, with the usual clinical complaint of pain or a palpable mass. They vary in size, ranging from smaller than 1 cm in diameter to 20 cm or greater, whereas the individual cysts comprising the tumor vary in diameter from millimeters to centimeters (Fig. 7-21). The cysts contain thin watery secretions and are lined predominantly by a single layer of flattened to cuboidal mesothelial-like cells (Fig. 7-22). Occasional papillary tufts may be encountered (Fig. 7-23), as may foci of squamous metaplasia and mild to moderate cytologic atypia with occasional mitotic figures. The stroma between the cysts is generally thin and collagenous to myxoid. It may contain focal mild inflammatory cell infiltration.

Ultrastructurally, the lining cells of the cysts are confirmed to be of mesothelial origin by the presence of microvilli, desmosomes, and intracytoplasmic microfilaments.[106,107] About 40% of patients with adequate follow-up data have experienced recurrences, often after several years, but there are no reports of distant metastasis or death due to the tumor. The main differential diagnosis is with *cystic lymphangioma,* which is grossly and microscopically similar but occurs predominantly in males and children, and often in the mesentery.[110] Histologic and ultrastructural distinctions are based on the fact that the cystic lymphangioma is lined by endothelial rather than mesothelial cells and contains smooth muscle within the intercystic stroma. Unlike cystic mesothelioma, the lymphangiomas rarely recur.[110]

The main controversy surrounding this lesion concerns its fundamental nature. The term *cystic* or *multicystic mesothelioma* is used by those investigators who consider it a neoplasm,[108] whereas the term *multilocular peritoneal inclusion cysts* is preferred by those who conclude that these cases are reactive.[91,109] The latter view is encouraged by the finding that a history of previous abdominal surgery, pelvic inflammatory disease, or endometriosis was present in 84% of cases in one large series.[109] Those who take the former view are happier to quote the lower figure of 27% in another series.[108] The recurrence rate of 40% supports the neoplastic adherents, whereas their opponents state that these recurrences are merely examples of reactions to new adhesions formed at surgery. To make matters more confusing, some supporters of the reactive origin hypothesis claim that rare cases of true multicystic mesotheliomas do exist and can be recognized by the presence of markedly atypical mesothelial cells and the absence of a prominent inflammatory component.[91] We have not been able to appreciate this difference. We use the term *cystic mesothelioma,* and, whatever its origin, we emphasize the frequently recurrent but benign evolution of this lesion.

The most difficult benign mesotheliomas to characterize are those with a papillary architecture. Foyle and colleagues have divided papillary tumors of the peritoneum occurring in women into four groups.[102] *Diffuse papillary mesothelioma* is the least common type and is identical to the diffuse malignant mesothelioma known for decades and occurring far more frequently in men. *Papillary carcinoma* refers to a malignant tumor identical to serous carcinoma of the ovary but occurring in patients without

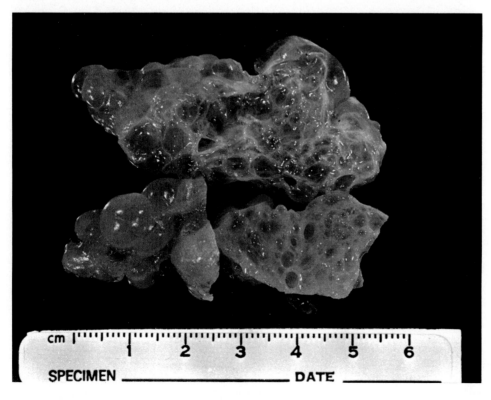

FIGURE 7-21 Macroscopic appearance of cystic mesothelioma.

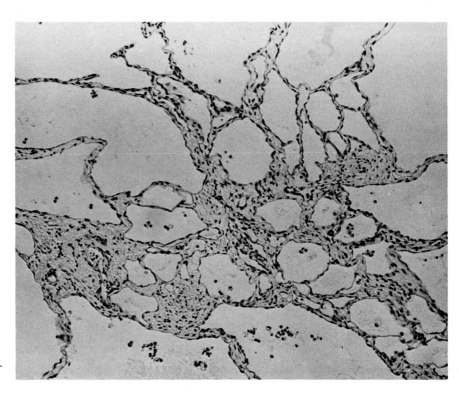

FIGURE 7-22 Low-power photomicrograph of cystic mesothelioma.

an ovarian primary tumor. *Atypical diffuse mesothelioma* was the term used to describe lesions intermediate in appearance between the first two. Because these are all malignant tumors, they are discussed in a later section of this chapter. More pertinent to the present section is the fourth group, *well-differentiated diffuse papillary mesothelioma.* As the name indicates, these are diffuse papillary proliferations that are confined to the omentum or are widespread on peritoneal surfaces. The experience of Foyle's group was subsequently updated to 22 cases,[111] and a total of about 35 cases have been published.[106,112–114] Although some of these mesotheliomas occurred in men and in postmenopausal women, the usual presentation was as an incidental finding in women of reproductive age. The lesions usually are multiple and small, although solitary lesions with an identical histologic appearance were described by Goepel.[112]

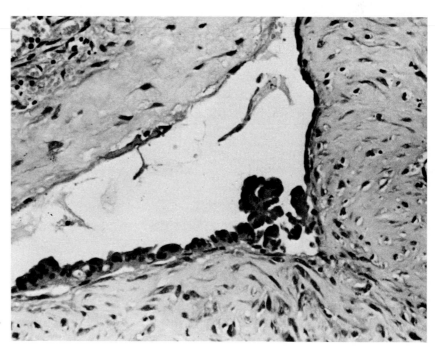

FIGURE 7-23 Cystic mesothelioma. Detail shows focal slightly atypical proliferation of mesothelial cells.

The most commonly involved sites are the omentum and pelvic peritoneum.

Histologically, these tumors are tubulopapillary or purely papillary. The papillary areas show coarse branching fronds with prominent fibrovascular cores. The lining cells are low cuboidal and uniform, with generally inconspicuous nucleoli and few mitotic figures (Fig. 7-24). In the tubular areas, there may be slightly more pleomorphism, but always less than in malignant diffuse mesothelioma. The absence of cell stratification, necrosis, and stromal invasion is helpful in the differential diagnosis. So few of these benign mesotheliomas have been reported that their cytologic appearance is poorly characterized.[113] We would, however, expect it to appear somewhat similar to reactive mesothelial hyperplasia and endosalpingiosis.

When all the lesions found in a patient are typical of well-differentiated diffuse papillary mesothelioma, the evolution appears to be benign, although persistence or recurrence has been noted for as long as 29 years.[102] However, these lesions have coexisted with or evolved into diffuse malignant mesothelioma in some patients.[91,114] Other patients have died, usually after a protracted course, although it is unclear whether the tumor or its therapy was most responsible.[111] All lesions should be removed and examined histologically, and the prognosis should be determined by the histologically most aggressive pattern.

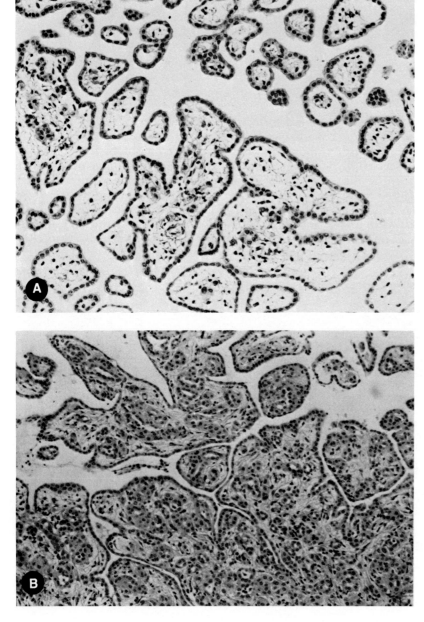

FIGURE 7-24 Well-differentiated papillary mesothelioma. **(A)** Papillary pattern; **(B)** tubulopapillary pattern. (**A:** Foyle A, Al-Jabi M, McCaughey WTE: Papillary peritoneal tumors in women. Am J Surg Pathol 5:241–249, 1981. **A** and **B** courtesy of Dr. W.T.E. McCaughey.)

MALIGNANT TUMORS

Malignant Mesothelioma

Malignant mesothelioma is a tumor that has been studied for many years, but a somewhat recent observation has been its rarity in women. Kannerstein and Churg, for example, encountered only 6 women among 83 patients with pathologically confirmed malignant peritoneal mesotheliomas.[115] Similarly, only 3 of 25 papillary peritoneal tumors in women reported by Foyle and associates were classic malignant mesotheliomas.[102] Because of the relative paucity of these tumors among women, they are not covered in detail in this chapter. They must be considered briefly, however, because of their importance in the differential diagnosis of benign mesothelial hyperplasias, metaplasias, and tumors, on the one hand, and metastatic and primary peritoneal carcinomas on the other.

Unlike these lesions in the differential diagnosis, classic malignant mesothelioma in women is associated with asbestos exposure, as it is in its more common manifestation in men.[107] The tumor is virtually always symptomatic because of its diffuse and invasive nature.

Macroscopic Appearance

Macroscopically, the diffuse tumor involvement of peritoneal surfaces presents with small nodules and large plaque-like masses. Intraperitoneal viscera are matted together by masses of tumor and are frequently invaded. Nodal and distant metastases generally present as a late event.

Microscopic Appearance

As in the more common pleural tumors, the microscopic picture varies from a purely epithelial to a mixed epithelial-sarcomatoid pattern (Fig. 7-25). The pure sarcomatoid pattern is rare.[116,117] In the epithelial pattern, papillae, tubules, and solid nests are seen. Psammoma bodies may be encountered, but these are more common in papillary adenocarcinomas. The cells show the usual cytologic criteria of malignancy.

Differential Diagnosis

The differential diagnosis is with benign mesothelial proliferations and carcinomas. The gross appearance, the presence of stromal invasion, and the finding of extensive necrosis, cell stratification, nuclear enlargement, hyperchromatism, and frequent mitotic figures generally are sufficient to establish the malignant nature of the process. At the cytologic level, this distinction may be much more difficult, but the presence of large clusters of cells, multinucleated cells, and malignant-appearing nuclei in some cells should suggest the diagnosis.

The differential diagnosis from adenocarcinoma is even more difficult, and it is not uncommon for

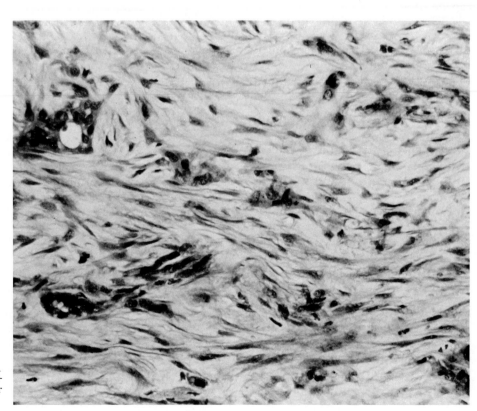

FIGURE 7-25 Malignant mesothelioma, showing malignant tubular and stromal elements.

the final diagnosis not to be established until postmortem examination. At the light microscopic level, the presence of malignant stromal cells is virtually diagnostic (save for the rare possibility of a metastatic carcinosarcoma), but more commonly the tumors are of pure epithelial type. Histochemical, immunohistochemical, and ultrastructural criteria have been suggested by various researchers, but we have found none of them to be infallible. At the histochemical level, Kannerstein and Churg emphasized the presence of intracytoplasmic colloidal iron-positive secretion, which was removed by hyaluronidase in many of their mesotheliomas.[115] In metastatic epithelial neoplasms, the mucosubstances present were not dissolved by hyaluronidase. Immunohistochemically, the most useful antigens have been carcinoembryonic antigen (CEA), Leu-M1 (CD15), TAG-72 (recognized by monoclonal antibody B72.3), and the antigen recognized by monoclonal antibody BER-EP4, all of which are demonstrable in most adenocarcinomas and in few or no mesotheliomas.[118,119]

Ultrastructurally, the emphasis has been on the presence in mesotheliomas of long and slender microvilli without a glycocalyx (Fig. 7-26), the quantitative increase in the numbers of intermediate filaments in mesotheliomas compared with adenocarcinomas, and the absence of specific findings seen in some adenocarcinomas, such as abundant mucin, numerous cilia, glycocalyx, rootlets of microvilli, and neurosecretory-type dense core granules.[118,120,121] When ultrastructural examination is available, it is probably the most reliable study that can be used.

The cytologic differential diagnosis is difficult.[2,3,122] In most instances, the pathologist is able to suggest but not make the unequivocal diagnosis of malignant mesothelioma on examination of an ascitic fluid specimen (Color Figure 7-6). Numerous papillary clusters of cells showing the usual cytologic criteria of malignancy should be present. The clusters are often large and demonstrate a three-dimensional morphology compared with the generally flat clusters of benign mesothelial cells. The individual cells are considerably larger than benign mesothelial cells, but unlike the cells of a metastatic adenocarcinoma, they show apparent transitions to cells with obvious mesothelial morphology (ie, abundant cytoplasm, a distinct, clear cell border, and a small nucleus). The cytoplasm is occasionally vacuolated, but usually much less so than in adenocarcinoma. However, a secretory type of peritoneal mesothelioma has been reported, in which many vacuoles of mucolipid are present.[123] Occasionally, prominent microvilli can be observed at the light microscopic level in cytologic material. If a cell block is prepared, some of the histochemical and immunohistochemical techniques mentioned previously may be used, and ultrastructural and flow cytometric study of cells from an effusion may be helpful.

Prognosis and Treatment

The prognosis of malignant mesothelioma is dismal. Although distant metastases may develop as a late event or not at all, the extensive local progression of the tumor almost invariably leads to death within a few years of diagnosis. Treatment is largely supportive.

Adenocarcinoma of Presumed Mesothelial Origin

Although it has been accepted for some time that many, if not all, of the malignant "epithelial" tumors of the ovary are ultimately of mesothelial origin, it is only within the past few years that evidence has accumulated to suggest that similar tumors may arise outside the ovaries.

Their pathogenesis is probably analogous to that of endosalpingiosis and some cases of endometriosis and involves a simultaneous or sequential process of metaplasia and neoplasia. Although any of the histologic patterns of "epithelial" ovarian cancer (serous, mucinous, endometrioid, clear cell, transitional cell, and mixed mesodermal) may be encountered as a primary extraovarian mesothelial-derived tumor, the vast majority are serous. Ovarian serous carcinomas usually are widely disseminated in the peritoneal cavity at the time of diagnosis, and it is possible that this phenomenon represents a multifocal origin rather than an ovarian primary with metastases.[124,125] Similarly, we believe it is likely that the "intra-abdominal carcinomatosis after prophylactic oophorectomy in ovarian-cancer-prone families" reported by Tobacman and colleagues[126] and the "serous surface papillary carcinomas of the ovary" reported by Gooneratne and associates[127] represent the same entity, as do the "papillary carcinomas of the peritoneum" of Foyle and colleagues.[102]

The clinical presentation and gross appearance of these lesions are identical to those of metastatic serous carcinoma of ovarian origin, with the following exceptions: the ovaries are absent, having been removed previously, usually for benign disease (Color Figure 7-7); the ovaries are present but uninvolved with tumor; or the ovaries are present and only minimally involved. In the latter situation, a case can be made that ovarian surface involvement, even if limited to microscopic foci, represents the source of the peritoneal dissemination.[127] The proportion of disseminated serous carcinomas diagnosed as extraovarian in origin varies from 7% to 18% in recently published series from different countries, with the difference more likely due to varying diagnostic criteria than to true geographic variation.[128-131] The criteria for the diagnosis of primary extraovarian carcinoma used by the Gynecologic Oncology Group are reproduced here:

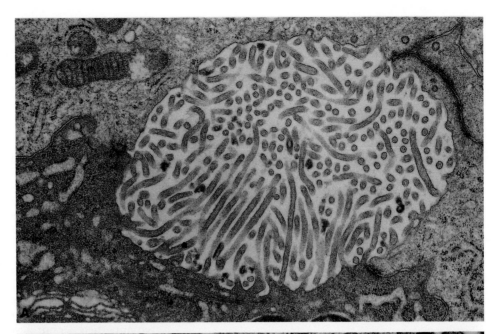

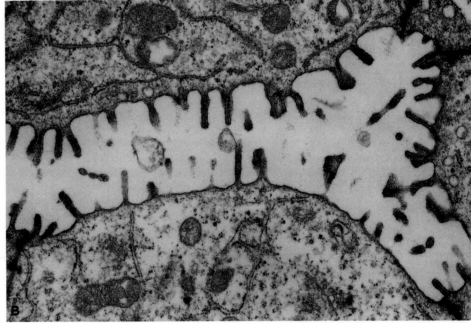

FIGURE 7-26 Electron micrographs of the lumina of malignant mesothelioma **(A)** and serous carcinoma of ovary **(B).** The height to width ratio of microvilli in **A** exceeds 10:1, compared with about 4:1 for microvilli of the serous carcinoma. Note the glycocalyx coating the microvilli in the lower figure only. (×25,000; courtesy of Jan M. Orenstein, MD, PhD, George Washington University, Washington, DC)

Both ovaries are either physiologically normal in size or enlarged by a benign process. In the judgment of the surgeon and the pathologist, the bulky tumor is in the peritoneum and the degree of tumor involvement at one or more extraovarian sites is greater than on the surface of either ovary.

Microscopically, the ovarian component is one of the following: (1) nonexistent; (2) confined to ovarian surface epithelium with no evidence of cortical invasion; (3) involves ovarian surface and underlying cortical stroma but with any given tumor size less than 5 × 5 mm; (4) tumor less than 5 × 5 mm within ovarian substance associated with or without surface disease.

The histological and cytological characteristics of the tumor are predominantly serous type—that is, similar or identical to ovarian serous papillary adenocarcinoma, any grade.

Patients who had an oophorectomy performed prior to the diagnosis of extraovarian peritoneal serous papillary carcinoma (EPSPC) must fit one of the following two categories: (1) the pathology report is required to document benign ovaries, and all slides of normal ovaries must be submitted for review if the oophorectomy was performed within five years of the diagnosis of EPSPC; (2) if the oophorectomy occurred more than five years prior to the diagnosis of EPSPC, the pathology report of the benign ovaries is required, and an attempt to obtain the slides must be made.

Microscopic Appearance

Microscopically, these tumors are identical to serous carcinomas of ovarian origin (Fig. 7-27). They are usually poorly differentiated, lack the malignant stromal elements that may be seen in malignant mesothelioma, and are much more likely to contain numerous psammoma bodies than are classic malignant mesotheliomas.

Ultrastructural Findings

Ultrastructural study of a few cases has shown the presence of the type of secretory granules commonly encountered in ovarian serous carcinomas, as well as shorter and blunter microvilli than those of classic mesotheliomas.

Immunohistochemical Findings

Immunohistochemical results are similar to those for ovarian serous carcinoma and aid in the distinction from malignant mesothelioma (see Malignant Meso-

thelioma earlier in this chapter). A panel of immunohistochemical markers including CEA and Leu-M1 can be used to differentiate small tumor nodules (positive for both) from benign epithelial and mesothelial proliferations.[132]

Prognosis

The prognosis in these cases was originally thought to be worse than that for correspondingly disseminated ovarian serous carcinoma, but most recent studies have indicated that the response rates to platinum-based chemotherapeutic regimens and the ultimate survival are comparable.[128–131]

Foyle and colleagues, in their report of 25 papillary peritoneal tumors in women, grouped 4 cases under the classification of "atypical diffuse mesothelioma."[102] These tumors were said to occupy an intermediate position histologically between typical diffuse malignant mesothelioma and the papillary carcinomas that we have just described. One of the patients died within a year, but the other 3 patients demonstrated a more prolonged course. Although such an intermediate group probably exists, we advise caution in making this diagnosis because we recently encountered an identical tumor that eventually proved to be a metastatic pancreatic carcinoma.

Finally, primary peritoneal malignant tumors of ovarian type occasionally are of histologic types other than serous, such as mucinous and clear cell adenocarcinomas (Fig. 7-28).[133,134] Unlike extraovarian serous carcinomas, these tumors usually form a solitary mass and are found most frequently in the retroperitoneum or mesentery. Their natural

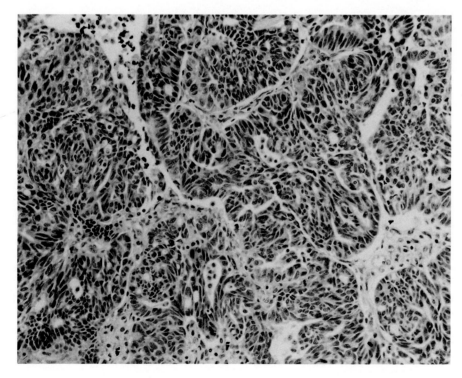

FIGURE 7-27 Serous carcinoma of the peritoneum. This patient had undergone bilateral oophorectomy 14 years earlier for a benign condition (see Color Figure 7-7).

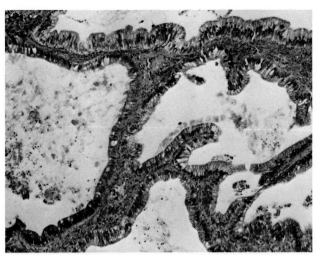

FIGURE 7-28 Retroperitoneal borderline mucinous tumor. The ovaries were grossly normal. (Farhi DC, Silverberg SG: Pesudometastases in female genital cancer. Pathol Annu 17 [Part I]:47–76, 1982)

history remains poorly defined because of the small number of cases reported. Benign epithelial tumors of ovarian type are reported in peritoneal and retroperitoneal locations.[135]

Metastatic Tumors

Although we have devoted a large portion of this chapter to the discussion of primary malignant peritoneal tumors, the pathologist encounters metastases to the peritoneum far more frequently. The differential diagnosis of metastatic carcinoma includes many of the reactive, metaplastic, and neoplastic conditions described in this chapter, and it is always important to consider the possibility of these conditions before rendering a diagnosis of metastatic carcinomatosis, with its attendant dramatic therapeutic and prognostic implications.

Any malignant tumor may metastasize to the peritoneum. In women, the cancers most likely to be discovered on biopsy are those of the ovary, endometrium, and large intestine. The metastatic breast cancers formerly encountered during oophorectomy or adrenalectomy have declined in number with the decreased popularity of these operations, and metastatic breast cancer is encountered in the peritoneum by the surgical pathologist today primarily in cases in which it results in intestinal obstruction. Cervical carcinomas seldom metastasize to the peritoneum, although peritoneal wash cytologies may be positive. Positive findings are more common with cervical adenocarcinoma than with squamous cell carcinoma.[136]

Clinically, metastatic peritoneal cancer is often manifested by increased abdominal girth secondary to ascites. About as often, the metastatic disease is asymptomatic and is detected by biopsy at the time of exploratory laparotomy or by cytologic examination of peritoneal fluid.

Macroscopic Appearance

Macroscopically, metastatic cancer may vary from grossly undetectable to multiple pearly white nodules of a few millimeters each to massive peritoneal plaques with extensive adhesions leading to a "frozen pelvis." This latter appearance is encountered more frequently with ovarian tumors than with other primaries.

Microscopic Appearance

The microscopic appearance of the metastatic tumor should be similar to that of the primary tumor from which it arose. This is important in the differential diagnosis, because foci of endosalpingiosis are often identified by their different appearance from the primary endometrial or cervical tumor with which they may be associated. In the differential diagnosis of metastatic serous ovarian carcinoma, the presence of a papillary architecture and psammoma bodies in endosalpingiosis may be confusing. Any peritoneal nodules associated with borderline ovarian tumors (see Chap. 6) should be carefully classified as benign, borderline, or invasive malignant, although, as discussed earlier, it is unclear whether invasive "implants" augur a worse prognosis than borderline ones.[30]

Cytologic Diagnosis

Cytologic diagnosis of metastatic carcinoma in peritoneal fluids is one of the most difficult problems in the field of diagnostic cytology. There are many benign conditions that can result in the observation of atypical mesothelial cells in a peritoneal fluid, and some of these conditions (such as endosalpingiosis) seem to occur with greater frequency in women who have female genital cancer. It behooves the pathologist not to overdiagnose such a specimen as malignant, even if he or she is tempted to do so by knowledge of the presence of a primary carcinoma. A cytologic diagnosis of metastatic carcinoma should depend on the presence of several groups of cells with clearly malignant features, such as cellular enlargement, increased nuclear—cytoplasmic ratio, an abnormal, coarsely clumped chromatin pattern, and abnormal mitotic figures (Fig. 7-29 and Color Figure 7-8). Other useful findings include the production of mucin and the presence of many cell aggregates with a three-dimensional configuration and of two or more sex chromatin bodies in a single cell.[2–4] Although these characteristics identify most metastatic cancers in women, other findings may point to specific tumor types: melanin pigment in malignant melanoma, bizarre spindle cells in metastatic sarcomas, and so-called Indian-filing in some cases of metastatic mammary carcinoma.

Among primary carcinomas of the female genital tract, peritoneal cytologic findings are positive in at least one half of the cases of ovarian carcinoma,[137,138] less frequently in endometrial carcinoma,[139,140] and

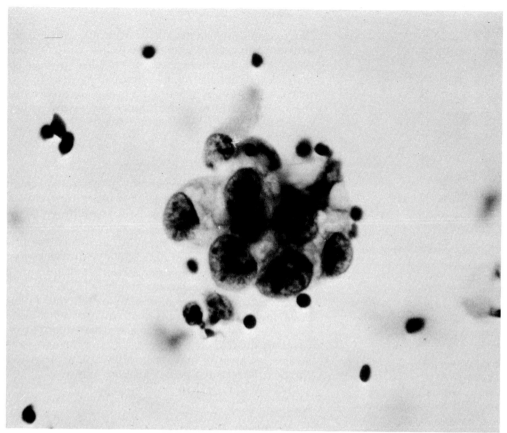

FIGURE 7-29 Cluster of malignant cells in peritoneal fluid from a woman with primary adenocarcinoma of the endometrium.

least frequently (less than 10% of cases) in carcinoma of the cervix.[136] The prognostic significance of a positive peritoneal cytology in these tumors has been debated, but in general it seems to correlate best with high-stage and high-grade tumors and may add fairly little to an already poor prognosis. In ovarian cancer, however, the FIGO (International Federation of Gynecology and Obstetrics) staging system recommends that a stage I or II cancer be assigned to subgroup Ic or IIc on the basis of a positive peritoneal cytology or the presence of ascitic fluid.

Special Variants

Two rare but interesting conditions that should be considered under the heading of metastatic tumors to the peritoneum are *pseudomyxoma peritonei* and *gliomatosis peritonei*. The former term refers to a clinical syndrome of mucinous ascites of any origin, but most often the syndrome is associated with a mucinous tumor of the ovary or appendix (and often both). The pathogenesis of the peritoneal lesion is controversial. Some investigators consider these associated ovarian and appendiceal tumors to be borderline or low-grade malignant,[141] whereas others are equally convinced of their benignity.[142] The peritoneal lesions may represent metastases but may also represent a metaplastic phenomenon such as has been suggested in cases of endosalpingiosis and en-

dometriosis. Young and colleagues have recently postulated that when pseudomyxoma peritonei occurs in association with mucinous tumors of both the ovary and appendix, the appendiceal tumor represents the origin of the peritoneal lesion.[143] In any event, pseudomyxoma peritonei presents grossly as loculated, yellow-brown, glairy mucus on peritoneal surfaces, often leading to dense adhesions and an "omental cake." Microscopically, mucinous cells that generally show minimal atypia are found (sometimes with difficulty) floating in large pools of extracellular mucin. The condition is generally considered to be incurable, but patients may survive with persistent disease for many years. Repeated paracenteses with intraperitoneal installation of chemotherapeutic agents or hyaluronidase may be helpful.

The term *gliomatosis peritonei* refers to the presence of benign glial implants on peritoneal surfaces in association with an immature teratoma of the ovary (see Chap. 6). This tumor seems to have a peculiar tendency to mature into benign tissues. In one large series, extraovarian tumor foci usually were better differentiated than the associated primary ovarian tumors.[144] Mature components other than glia may be seen, and the phenomenon has been seen in lymph nodes and other metastatic sites (Fig. 7-30), but the usual presentation is that of multiple, small peritoneal nodules composed of histologically benign neuroglia (Fig. 7-31). If the glial implants are

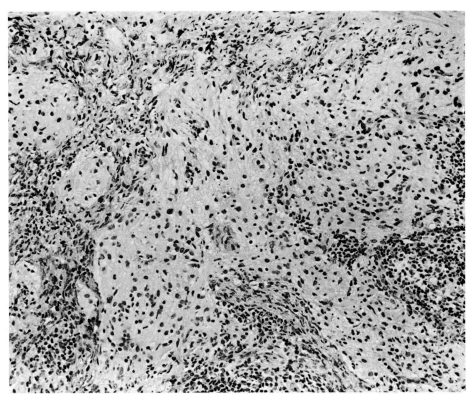

FIGURE 7-30 Mature glial tissue in the sinusoids of a pelvic lymph node. The patient had immature teratoma of the ovary.

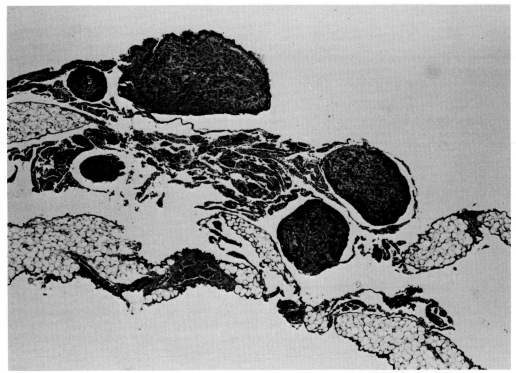

FIGURE 7-31 Multiple peritoneal nodules of benign glial tissue (gliomatosis peritonei) associated with ovarian immature teratoma.

all mature (grade 0), they do not unfavorably influence the prognosis, which then depends largely on the grade of the primary ovarian tumor.[144–146] Multiagent chemotherapy is instituted if the primary tumor is of high grade or if immature implants are found, but in a grade I immature teratoma of the ovary with only grade 0 implants, the prognosis is excellent without any adjuvant therapy. Second-look laparotomies in these latter patients generally have shown either persistence or regression (but not growth) of the implants.[147]

References

1. Kamina P, Dufrenot A, de Tourris H: Fosses, récessus et culs-de-sac du peritoine pelvien chez la femme. J Gynécol Obstét Biol Réprod 8:393–398, 1979
2. Koss LG: Diagnostic cytology and its histopathologic bases, 4th ed. Philadelphia, JB Lippincott, 1992:629–642.
3. Naylor B: Pleural, peritoneal and pericardial fluids. In Bibbo M, ed. Comprehensive cytopathology, pp 541–614. Philadelphia, WB Saunders, 1991
4. Zuna RE, Mitchell ML: Cytologic findings in peritoneal washings associated with benign gynecologic disease. Acta Cytol 32:139–147, 1988
5. Bohnen J, Boulanger M, Meakins JL, McLean PH: Prognosis in generalized peritonitis: Relation to cause and risk factors. Arch Surg 118:285–290, 1983
6. Monif GRG: Clinical staging of acute bacterial salpingitis and its therapeutic ramifications. Am J Obstet Gynecol 143:489–495, 1982
7. Singh MM, Bhargava AN, Jain KP: Tuberculous peritonitis. An evaluation of pathogenetic mechanisms, diagnostic procedures and therapeutic measures. N Engl J Med 281:1091–1094, 1969
8. Freedman SI, Ang EP, Herz MG et al: Meconium granulomas in post-cesarean section patients. Obstet Gynecol 59:383–385, 1982
9. Meyerhoff J: Familial Mediterranean fever: Report of a large family, review of the literature, and discussion of the frequency of amyloidosis. Medicine 59:66–77, 1980
10. Ryan GB, Grobéty J, Majno G: Postoperative peritoneal adhesions: A study of the mechanisms. Am J Pathol 65:117–148, 1971
11. Eltringham WK, Espiner HJ, Windsor CWO et al: Sclerosing peritonitis due to practolol: A report on 9 cases and their surgical management. Br J Surg 64:229–235, 1977
12. Walker AR, Putnam TC: Omental, mesenteric and retroperitoneal cysts: A clinical study of 33 new cases. Ann Surg 178:13–19, 1973
13. Rosai J, Dehner LP: Nodular mesothelial hyperplasia in hernia sacs: A benign reactive condition simulating a neoplastic process. Cancer 35:165–175, 1975
14. Finn CB, Ward K, Luesley DM et al: Qualitative and quantitative analysis of peritoneal fluids from women with gynecologic disease: Comparison of cytology and flow cytometry for the detection of malignancy in lavage and ascitic fluids. Anal Quant Cytol Histol 13:182–186, 1991
15. Jones MA, Hitchcox S, D'Ascanio P et al: Flow cytometric DNA analysis versus cytology in the evaluation of peritoneal fluids. Gynecol Oncol 43:226–232, 1991
16. Zinsser KR, Wheeler JE: Endosalpingiosis in the omentum: A study of autopsy and surgical material. Am J Surg Pathol 6:109–117, 1982
17. Kerner H, Gaton E, Czernobilsky B: Unusual ovarian, tubal and pelvic mesothelial inclusions in patients with endometriosis. Histopathology 5:277–283, 1981
18. McCaughey WTE, Kirk ME, Lester W et al: Peritoneal epithelial lesions associated with proliferative serous tumours of the ovary. Histopathology 8:195–208, 1984
19. Copeland LJ, Silva EG, Gershenson DM et al: The significance of müllerian inclusions found at second-look laparotomy in patients with epithelial ovarian neoplasms. Obstet Gynecol 71:763–770, 1988
20. Onybeke W, Brescia R, Eng K, Quagliarello J: Symptomatic endosalpingiosis in a postmenopausal woman. Am J Obstet Gynecol 156:924–926, 1987
21. Farhi DC, Silverberg SG: Pseudometastases in female genital cancer. Pathol Annu 17 (I):47–76, 1982
22. Sidawy MK, Silverberg SG: Endosalpingiosis in female peritoneal washings: A diagnostic pitfall. Int J Gynecol Pathol 6:340–346, 1987
23. Sneige N, Fernandez T, Copeland LJ, Katz RL: Müllerian inclusions in peritoneal washings: Potential source of error in cytologic diagnosis. Acta Cytol 30:271–276, 1986
24. Holmes MD, Levin HS: Endosalpingiosis. Cleve Clin J Med 48:345–352, 1981
25. Bell DA, Scully RE: Benign and borderline serous lesions of the peritoneum in women. Pathol Annu 24(2):1–21, 1989
26. Bell DA, Scully RE: Serous borderline tumors of the peritoneum. Am J Surg Pathol 14:230–239, 1990
27. Biscotti CV, Hart WR: Peritoneal serous micropapillomatosis of low malignant potential (serous borderline tumors of the peritoneum): A clinicopathologic study of 17 cases. Am J Surg Pathol 16:467–475, 1992
28. Bell DA, Weinstock MA, Scully RE: Peritoneal implants of ovarian serous borderline tumors: Histologic features and prognosis. Cancer 62:2212–2222, 1988
29. Shiraki M, Otis CN, Donovan JT, Powell JL: Ovarian serous borderline epithelial tumors with multiple retroperitoneal nodal involvement: Metastasis or malignant transformation of epithelial glandular inclusions? Gynecol Oncol 46:255–258, 1992
30. Gershenson DM, Silva EG: Serous ovarian tumors of low malignant potential with peritoneal implants. Cancer 65:578–585, 1990
31. Segal GH, Hart WR: Ovarian serous tumors of low malignant potential (serous borderline tumors). The relationship of exophytic surface tumor to peritoneal "implants." Am J Surg Pathol 16:577–583, 1992
32. Shen SC, Bansal M, Purrazzella R et al: Benign glandular inclusions in lymph nodes, endosalpingiosis, and salpingitis isthmica nodosa in a young girl with clear cell adenocarcinoma of the cervix. Am J Surg Pathol 7:293–300, 1983
33. Ehrmann RI, Federschneider JM, Knapp RC: Distinguishing lymph node metastases from benign glandular inclusions in low-grade ovarian carcinoma. Am J Obstet Gynecol 136:737–746, 1980
34. Brosens I, Koninckx P, Boeckx W: Endometriosis. Clin Obstet Gynaecol 8(3):639–651, 1981
35. Ranney B: Endometriosis: Pathogenesis, symptoms, and findings. Clin Obstet Gynecol 23:865–874, 1980
36. Clement PB: Pathology of endometriosis. Pathol Annu 25(1):245–295, 1990
37. Lawrence HC III: Pulmonary endometriosis in pregnancy. Am J Obstet Gynecol 159:733–734, 1988
38. Zaatari GS, Gupta PK, Bhagavan BS, Jarboe BR: Cytopathology of pleural endometriosis. Acta Cytol 26:227–232, 1982
39. Sampson JA: Development of the implantation theory for the origin of peritoneal endometriosis. Am J Obstet Gynecol 40:549–557, 1940
40. Halme J, Hammond MG, Hulka JF et al: Retrograde menstruation in healthy women and in endometriosis. Obstet Gynecol 64:151–154, 1980
41. Ridley JH, Edwards IK: Experimental endometriosis in the human. Am J Obstet Gynecol 76:738–790, 1958
42. Scott RB, Wharton LR Jr: Effects of progesterone and norethindrone on experimental endometriosis in monkeys. Am J Obstet Gynecol 84:867–875, 1962
43. Chatterjee SK: Scar endometriosis: A clinicopathologic study of 17 cases. Obstet Gynecol 56:81–84, 1980

44. Meyer R: In Lubarsch H, ed. Handbuch d. spez. Path Anat u. Histol, vol 7, part 1. Berlin, Springer, 1930

45. El-Mahgoub S, Yaseen S: A positive proof for the theory of coelomic metaplasia. Am J Obstet Gynecol 137:137–140, 1980

46. Kuo T, London SN, Dinh TV: Endometriosis occurring in leiomyomatosis peritonealis disseminata: Ultrastructural study and histogenetic consideration. Am J Surg Pathol 4:197–204, 1980

47. Sahin AA, Silva EG, Landon G et al: Endometrial tissue in myometrial vessels not associated with menstruation. Int J Gynecol Pathol 8:139–146, 1989

48. Banks ER, Mills SE, Frierson HF Jr: Uterine intravascular menstrual endometrium simulating malignancy. Am J Surg Pathol 15:407–412, 1991

49. Javert CT: Pathogenesis of endometriosis based on endometrial homeoplasia, direct extension, exfoliation and implantation, lymphatic and hematogenous metastasis. Cancer 2:399–410, 1949

50. Beckman EN, Leonard GL, Pintado SO, Sternberg WH: Endometriosis of the prostate. Am J Surg Pathol 9:374–379, 1985

51. Binns BA, Banerjee R: Endometriosis with Turner's syndrome treated with cyclical oestrogen/progesterone: Case report. Br J Obstet Gynaecol 90:581–582, 1983

52. Dizerega GS, Barber DL, Hodgen GD: Endometriosis: Role of ovarian steroids in initiation, maintenance, and suppression. Fertil Steril 33:649–653, 1980

53. Bergqvist A, Rannevik G, Thorell J: Estrogen and progesterone cytosol receptor concentration in endometriotic tissue and intrauterine endometrium. Acta Obstet Gynecol Scand Suppl 101:53–58, 1981

54. Jänne O, Kauppila A, Kokko E et al: Estrogen and progestin receptors in endometriosis lesions: Comparison with endometrial tissue. Am J Obstet Gynecol 141:562–566, 1981

55. Bur ME, Greene GL, Press MF: Estrogen receptor localization in formalin-fixed, paraffin-embedded endometrium and endometriotic tissues. Int J Gynecol Pathol 6:140–151, 1987

56. Lyndrup J, Thorpe S, Glenthøj A et al: Altered progesterone/estrogen receptor ratios in endometriosis: A comparative study of steroid receptors and morphology in endometriosis and endometrium. Acta Obstet Gynecol Scand 66:625–629, 1987

57. Malinak LR, Buttram VC JR, Elias S, Simpson JL: Heritable aspects of endometriosis. II. Clinical characteristics of familial endometriosis. Am J Obstet Gynecol 137:332–337, 1980

58. Simpson JL, Elias S, Malinak LR, Buttram VC Jr: Heritable aspects of endometriosis. I. Genetic studies. Am J Obstet Gynecol 137:327–331, 1980

59. Dmowski WP, Gebel HM, Rawlins RG: Immunologic aspects of endometriosis. Obstet Gynecol Clin North Am 16(1):93–104, 1989

60. Saifuddin A, Buckley CH, Fox H: Immunoglobulin content of the endometrium in women with endometriosis. Int J Gynecol Pathol 2:255–263, 1983

61. Steele RW, Dmowski WP, Marmer DJ: Immunologic aspects of human endometriosis. Am J Reprod Immunol 6:33–36, 1984

62. Dmowski WP: Current concepts in the management of endometriosis. Obstetrics and Gynecology Annual 10:279–311, 1981

63. Wilson EA, ed: Endometriosis. New York, Alan R. Liss, 1987

64. Halme J: Basic research in endometriosis. Obstetrics and Gynecology Annual 14:288–309, 1985

65. Candiani GB, Vercellini P, Fedele L et al: Mild endometriosis and infertility: A critical review of epidemiologic data, diagnostic pitfalls, and classification limits. Obstet Gynecol Surv 46:374–382, 1991

66. American Fertility Society: Classification of endometriosis: 1985. Fertil Steril 43:351–352, 1985

67. Markham SM, Carpenter SE, Rock JA: Extrapelvic endometriosis. Obstet Gynecol Clin North Am 16(1):193–220, 1989

68. Egger H, Weigmann P: Clinical and surgical aspects of ovarian endometriotic cysts. Arch Gynecol 233:37–45, 1982

69. Audebert AJM: Endométriose externe: Pathogénie, diagnostic et classification. Gynecologie 42:278–283, 1991

70. Jansen RPS, Russell P: Nonpigmented endometriosis: Clinical, laparoscopic, and pathologic definition. Am J Obstet Gynecol 155:1154–1159, 1986

71. Redwine DB: Age-related evolution in color appearance of endometriosis. Fertil Steril 48:1062–1063, 1987

72. Clement PB, Young RH, Scully RE: Stromal endometriosis of the uterine cervix: A variant of endometriosis that may simulate a sarcoma. Am J Surg Pathol 14:449–455, 1990

73. Clement PB, Young RH, Scully RE: Necrotic pseudoxanthomatous nodules of ovary and peritoneum in endometriosis. Am J Surg Pathol 12:390–397, 1988

74. Pueblitz-Peredo S, Luévano-Flores E, Rincón-Taracena R, Ochoa-Carillo FJ: Uteruslike mass of the ovary: Endomyometriosis or congenital malformation? A case with a discussion of histogenesis. Arch Pathol Lab Med 109:361–364, 1985

75. LaGrenade A, Silverberg SG: Ovarian tumors associated with atypical endometriosis. Hum Pathol 19:1080–1084, 1988

76. Chalas E, Chumas J, Barbieri R, Mann WJ: Nucleolar organizer regions in endometriosis, atypical endometriosis, and clear cell and endometrioid carcinomas. Gynecol Oncol 40:260–263, 1991

77. Gaulier A, Jouret-Mourin A, Marsan C: Peritoneal endometriosis: Report of a case with cytologic, cytochemical and histopathologic study. Acta Cytol 27:446–449, 1983

78. Haney AF, Muscato JF, Weinberg JB: Peritoneal fluid cell populations in infertility patients. Fertil Steril 35:696–698, 1981

79. Mostoufizadeh M, Scully RE: Malignant tumors arising in endometriosis. Clin Obstet Gynecol 23:951–963, 1980

80. Brooks JJ, Wheeler JE: Malignancy arising in extragonadal endometriosis. Cancer 40:3065–3073, 1977

81. Brosens IA, Verleyen A, Cornillie F: The morphologic effect of short-term medical therapy of endometriosis. Am J Obstet Gynecol 157:1215–1221, 1987

82. Cornillie FJ, Brosens A, Vasquez G, Riphagen I: Histologic and ultrastructural changes in human endometriotic implants treated with the antiprogesterone steroid ethylnorgestrinone (gestrinone) during 2 months. Int J Gynecol Pathol 5:95–109, 1986

83. Metzger DA, Luciano AA: Hormonal therapy of endometriosis. Obstet Gynecol Clin North Am 16(1):105–122, 1989

84. Dawood MY, Khan-Dawood FS, Ramos J: Plasma and peritoneal fluid levels of CA 125 in women with endometriosis. Am J Obstet Gynecol 159:1526–1531, 1988

85. Candiani GB, Vercellini P, Fedele L et al: Conservative surgical treatment for severe endometriosis in infertile women: Are we making progress? Obstet Gynecol Surv 46:490–498, 1992

86. Wheeler JM, Malinak R: Recurrent endometriosis: Incidence, management, and prognosis. Am J Obstet Gynecol 146:247–252, 1983

87. Baird D, Reddick RL: Extraovarian mucinous metaplasia in a patient with bilateral mucinous borderline tumors: A case report. Int J Gynecol Pathol 10:96–103, 1991

88. Clement PB, Young RH: Endocervicosis of the urinary bladder: A report of six cases of a benign müllerian lesion that may mimic adenocarcinoma. Am J Surg Pathol 16:533–542, 1992

89. Tavassoli FA, Norris HJ: Peritoneal leiomyomatosis (leiomyomatosis peritonealis disseminata): A clinicopathologic study of 20 cases with ultrastructural observations. Int J Gynecol Pathol 1:59–74, 1982

90. Williams LJ Jr, Pavlick FJ: Leiomyomatosis peritonealis dis-

seminata: Two case reports and a review of the medical literature. Cancer 45:1726–1733, 1980

91. Thor AD, Young RH, Clement PB: Pathology of the fallopian tube, broad ligament, peritoneum, and pelvic soft tissues. Hum Pathol 22:856–867, 1991

92. Fujii S, Nakashima N, Okamura H et al: Progesterone-induced smooth muscle-like cells in the subperitoneal nodules produced by estrogen. Am J Obstet Gynecol 139:164–172, 1981

93. Ober WB, Black MB: Neoplasms of the subcoelomic mesenchyme. Arch Pathol 59:698–705, 1955

94. Clement PB, Young RH, Scully RE: Nontrophoblastic pathology of the female genital tract and peritoneum associated with pregnancy. Semin Diagn Pathol 6:372–406, 1989

95. Rubin SC, Wheeler JE, Mikuta JJ: Malignant leiomyomatosis peritonealis disseminata. Obstet Gynecol 68:126–129, 1986

96. Akkersdijk GJM, Flu PK, Giard RWM et al: Malignant leiomyomatosis peritonealis disseminata. Am J Obstet Gynecol 163:591–593, 1990

97. Due W, Pickartz H: Immunohistologic detection of estrogen and progesterone receptors in disseminated peritoneal leiomyomatosis. Int J Gynecol Pathol 8:46–53, 1989

98. Zaytsev P, Taxy JB: Pregnancy-associated ectopic decidua. Am J Surg Pathol 11:526–530, 1987

99. Young RH: Pregnancy-associated lesions of the female genital tract. Irish J Med Sci 157(Suppl 7):24–29, 1988

100. Cobb CJ: Ectopic decidua and metastatic squamous carcinoma: Presentation in a single pelvic lymph node. J Surg Oncol 38:126–129, 1988

101. Watson WJ, Sundwall DA, Bensen WL: Splenosis mimicking endometriosis. Obstet Gynecol 59(Suppl):51S–53S, 1982

102. Foyle A, Al-Jabi M, McCaughey WTE: Papillary peritoneal tumors in women. Am J Surg Pathol 5:241–249, 1981

103. El-Naggar AK, Ro JY, Ayala AG et al: Localized fibrous tumor of the serosal cavities: Immunohistochemical, electron microscopic, and flow-cytometric DNA study. Am J Clin Pathol 92:561–565, 1989

104. Fujii S, Konishi I, Ban C, Okamura H: Adenomatoid tumor-like structures in the subperitoneal nodules produced by sex steroids. Am J Obstet Gynecol 145:850–856, 1983

105. Bergholz M, Altmannsberger M, Schaver A: Benign mesothelioma of the cul-de-sac: A tumor with misleading histologic pattern in an unusual localization. Gynecol Oncol 11:393–395, 1981

106. Dumke K, Schnoy N, Specht G, Buse H: Comparative light and electron microscopic studies of cystic and papillary tumors of the peritoneum. Virchows Arch A Pathol Anat Histopathol 399:25–39, 1983

107. Katsube Y, Mukai K, Silverberg SG: Cystic mesothelioma of the peritoneum: A report of five cases and review of the literature. Cancer 50:1615–1622, 1982

108. Weiss SW, Tavassoli FA: Multicystic mesothelioma: An analysis of pathologic findings and biologic behavior in 37 cases. Am J Surg Pathol 12:737–746, 1988

109. Ross MJ, Welch WR, Scully RE: Multilocular peritoneal inclusion cysts (so-called cystic mesotheliomas). Cancer 64:1336–1346, 1989

110. Carpenter HA, Lancaster JR, Lee RA: Multilocular cysts of the peritoneum. Mayo Clin Proc 57:634–638, 1982

111. Daya D, McCaughey WTE: Well-differentiated papillary mesothelioma of the peritoneum: A clinicopathologic study of 22 cases. Cancer 65:292–296, 1990

112. Goepel JR: Benign papillary mesothelioma of peritoneum: A histological, histochemical and ultrastructural study of six cases. Histopathology 5:21–30, 1981

113. Shapiro SP, Nunez C: Psammoma bodies in the cervicovaginal smear in association with a papillary tumor of the peritoneum. Obstet Gynecol 61:130–134, 1983

114. Burrig K, Pfitzer P, Hort W: Well-differentiated papillary mesothelioma of the peritoneum: A borderline mesothelioma. Virchows Arch A Pathol Anat Histopathol 417:443–447, 1990

115. Kannerstein M, Churg J: Peritoneal mesothelioma. Hum Pathol 8:83–94, 1977

116. Bolen JW, Thorning D: Mesothelioma: A light and electron microscopical study concerning histogenetic relationships between the epithelial and the mesenchymal variants. Am J Surg Pathol 4:451–464, 1980

117. Suzuki Y: Pathology of human malignant mesothelioma. Semin Oncol 8:268–282, 1981

118. Wick MR, Loy T, Mills SE et al: Malignant epithelioid pleural mesothelioma versus peripheral pulmonary adenocarcinoma: A histochemical, ultrastructural, and immunohistologic study of 103 cases. Hum Pathol 21:759–766, 1990

119. Gaffey MJ, Mills SE, Swanson PE et al: Immunoreactivity for BER-EP4 in adenocarcinomas, adenomatoid tumors, and malignant mesotheliomas. Am J Surg Pathol 16:593–599, 1992

120. Warhol MJ, Hunter NJ, Corson JM: An ultrastructural comparison of mesotheliomas and adenocarcinomas of the ovary and endometrium. Int J Gynecol Pathol 1:125–134, 1982

121. Burns TR, Greenberg SD, Mace ML, Johnson EH: Ultrastructural diagnosis of epithelial malignant mesothelioma. Cancer 56:2036–2040, 1985

122. Kwee WS, Veldhuizen RW, Alons CA et al: Quantitative and qualitative differences between benign and malignant mesothelial cells in pleural fluid. Acta Cytol 26:401–416, 1982

123. Boon ME, Posthuma HS, Ruiter DJ, von Andel JG: Secreting peritoneal mesothelioma: Report of a case with cytological, ultrastructural, morphometric and histological studies. Virchows Arch A Pathol Anat Histopathol 392:33–44, 1981

124. Genadry R, Poliakoff S, Rotmensch J et al: Primary papillary peritoneal neoplasia. Obstet Gynecol 58:730–734, 1981

125. Katsube Y, Berg JW, Silverberg SG: Epidemiologic pathology of ovarian tumors: A histopathologic review of primary ovarian neoplasms diagnosed in the Denver Standard Metropolitan Statistical Area, 1 July–31 December 1969 and 1 July–31 December 1979. Int J Gynecol Pathol 1:3–16, 1982

126. Tobacman JK, Tucker MA, Kase R et al: Intra-abdominal carcinomatosis after prophylactic oophorectomy in ovarian-cancer-prone families. Lancet II:795, 1982

127. Gooneratne S, Sassone S, Blaustein A, Talerman A: Serous surface papillary carcinoma of the ovary: A clinicopathologic study of 16 cases. Int J Gynecol Pathol 1:258–269, 1982

128. Lele SB, Piver MS, Matharu J, Tsukada Y: Peritoneal papillary carcinoma. Gynecol Oncol 31:315–320, 1988

129. Dalrymple JC, Bannatyne P, Russell P et al: Extraovarian peritoneal serous papillary carcinoma: A clinicopathologic study of 31 cases. Cancer 64:110–115, 1989

130. Altaras MM, Aviram R, Cohen I et al: Primary peritoneal papillary serous adenocarcinoma: Clinical and management aspects. Gynecol Oncol 40:230–236, 1991

131. Fromm GL, Gershenson DM, Silva EG: Papillary serous carcinoma of the peritoneum. Obstet Gynecol 75:89–95, 1990

132. Manivel JC, Wick MR, Coffin CM, Dehner LP: Immunohistochemistry in the differential diagnosis in the second-look operation for ovarian carcinomas. Int J Gynecol Pathol 8:103–113, 1989

133. Nelson H, Benjamin B, Alberty R: Primary retroperitoneal mucinous cystadenocarcinoma. Cancer 61:2117–2121, 1988

134. Evans H, Yates WA, Palmer WE et al: Clear cell carcinoma of the sigmoid mesocolon: A tumor of the secondary müllerian system. Am J Obstet Gynecol 162:161–163, 1990

135. Pennell TC, Gusdon JP Jr: Retroperitoneal mucinous cystadenoma. Am J Obstet Gynecol 160:1229–1231, 1989

136. Abu-Ghazaleh S, Johnston W, Creasman WT: The significance of peritoneal cytology in patients with carcinoma of the cervix. Gynecol Oncol 17:139–148, 1984

137. Mangioni C, Bolis G, Incalci MD, Molteni P et al: Laparoscopy and peritoneal cytology as markers in the follow-up of ovarian epithelial tumors. Recent Results Cancer Res 68:146–151, 1979

138. Yoshimura S, Scully RE, Taft PD, Herrington JB: Peritoneal fluid cytology in patients with ovarian cancer. Gynecol Oncol 17:161–167, 1984

139. Kadar N, Homesley HD, Malfetano JH: Positive peritoneal cytology is an adverse factor in endometrial carcinoma only if there is other evidence of extrauterine disease. Gynecol Oncol 46:145–149, 1992

140. Lurain JR: The significance of positive peritoneal cytology in endometrial cancer (Editorial). Gynecol Oncol 46:143–144, 1992

141. Limber GK, King RE, Silverberg SG: Pseudomyxoma peritonaei: A report of ten cases. Ann Surg 178:587–593, 1973

142. Sandenberg HA, Woodruff JD: Histogenesis of pseudomyxoma peritonei: Review of 9 cases. Obstet Gynecol 49:339–345, 1977

143. Young RH, Gilks CB, Scully RE: Mucinous tumors of the appendix associated with mucinous tumors of the ovary and pseudomyxoma peritonei: A clinicopathologic analysis of 22 cases supporting an origin in the appendix. Am J Surg Pathol 15:415–429, 1991

144. Nogales FF Jr, Favara BE, Major FJ, Silverberg SG: Immature teratoma of the ovary with a neural component ("solid" teratoma): A clinicopathologic study of 20 cases. Hum Pathol 7:625–642, 1976

145. Robboy SJ, Scully RE: Ovarian teratoma with glial implants on the peritoneum. Hum Pathol 1:643–653, 1970

146. Harms D, Janig U, Göbel U: Gliomatosis peritonei in childhood and adolescence: Clinicopathological study of 13 cases including immunohistochemical findings. Pathol Res Pract 184:422–430, 1989

147. Heydenrych JJ, Villet WT, du Toit DF: Gliomatosis peritonei: The value of a "second look" operation. J Surg Oncol 12:119–125, 1979

Pathology in Gynecology and Obstetrics, Fourth Edition,
edited by Claude Gompel and Steven G. Silverberg.
J. B. Lippincott Company, Philadelphia © 1994.

8

The Placenta

Janice M. Lage

The placenta is the most vital fetal organ: a fetus cannot survive without its placenta. The placenta serves the most basic metabolic needs of the fetus, including respiration, nourishment, and excretion. A diseased placenta will continue to function to some extent until it is destroyed completely. The fetal sequelae resulting from placental compromise depend on the severity of the insult, the adequacy of residual placental function, and the time remaining in utero. In many cases, the delivered placenta contains a morphologic record of the antecedent intrauterine events.

Because the placenta is the most accessible of all fetal organs and contains a record of intrauterine events, it should not be routinely discarded at delivery. All placentas should be examined by the attendant at delivery, usually the obstetrician-gynecologist. In most cases, the newborn is healthy, and the placenta, being normal on examination, may be discarded after neonatal well-being has been ensured. Unfortunately, untoward outcomes do occur, and the placentas from these deliveries should be examined by a pathologist. Table 8-1 lists the indications for placental examination by a pathologist.

Because medicolegal concerns focus attention on placental examination as a morphologic record of antenatal conditions and intrapartum events, it is essential that the practicing general pathologist perform an adequate gross examination and take appropriate samples for microscopic examination. In addition, photographs of any gross placental lesions, particularly those associated with fetal or neonatal death, may be pivotal in the outcome of a legal action.

This chapter provides a basic description of placental pathology, focusing on the salient gross and microscopic placental lesions encountered in daily practice. The intricacies of placental embryology are well-covered elsewhere and are not included in this book. Many excellent texts are available to aid the examiner in evaluating particularly difficult or unusual specimens.[12,13,17,48]

EARLY DEVELOPMENT

By accessing the maternal circulatory system, the placenta obtains essential biological support for the fetus. This is first achieved by implantation of the blastocyst into the uterine endometrium, which begins around postovulatory day 6 or 7 and is completed near day 10 (menstrual cycle day 24).[1-2] The blastocyst burrows into the decidualized endometrium, and its trophoblastic shell initially proliferates radially, forming the scaffolding for the definitive villi that begin to develop during the second week after implantation. By the third week, blood lakes created between invading villi coalesce, forming the intervillous space (Fig. 8-1). Invagination of the extraembryonic mesenchyme into the villi initiates the development of villous capillaries. Developing fetal blood cells appear in primitive villous capillaries about 28 days after conception (Fig. 8-2).[3]

The definitive placenta forms from the basally oriented villi of the chorion frondosum (Fig. 8-3). Peripheral divisions of the main stem villi form secondary and tertiary villi. This villous branching expands the interface between the fetal trophoblast and the maternal blood, enhancing transfer of oxygen and nutrients. Those villi directed toward the endometrial cavity, the chorion laeve, atrophy due to inadequate nutrition.

The implantation site contains cytotrophoblast, syncytiotrophoblast, and intermediate trophoblast, with the latter predominating (Fig. 8-4). Mononuclear trophoblast invades the maternal spiral arteries. This trophoblastic invasion of the maternal spiral arteries peaks at the 12th week and continues, progressing to the level of the junction between the spiral arteries and the myometrial radial arteries.[2] Intravascular trophoblast invades outwardly through the vessel walls, splaying apart and destroying muscular and elastic fibers. Concomitantly, endometrial stromal trophoblast invades the spiral arterial walls from the endometrial stroma. The destructive vascular invasion by trophoblast eventuates in markedly dilated, fibrotic vessel walls, which increase uteroplacental blood flow while precluding vasoconstriction. Between the 14th and 20th weeks, a second wave of trophoblast invades deeper into myometrial segments of the spiral arteries, further enhancing blood flow.

TYPES OF TROPHOBLAST

By microscopy, three types of trophoblast are identified: cytotrophoblast, syncytiotrophoblast (syncytium), and intermediate trophoblast (Fig. 8-5). The cytotrophoblast forms single, polygonal to oval cells with vesicular nuclei, prominent nucleoli, moderate amount of clear to granular cytoplasm, and distinct cell borders. Cytotrophoblastic mitotic activity is brisk during the first trimester and virtually inapparent by term. The syncytiotrophoblast represents an amalgamation of cytotrophoblastic cells forming a large, multinucleated "cell" with abundant, dense, amphophilic to violaceous cytoplasm with multiple vacuoles. The nuclei shrink, resulting in more condensed, pyknotic chromatin. The syncytiotrophoblast is incapable of cell division but remains metabolically active. The third type of trophoblast, previously termed *X cells*, is now known as *intermediate trophoblast*.[4] This trophoblast is characterized by discrete cells, which may be uninucleate, binucleate, or multinucleate. Their cell shape ranges from round and polygonal with abundant eosinophilic to amphophilic cytoplasm to spindle-shaped with attenuated cytoplasm. Nuclei of the intermediate trophoblast are hyperchromatic and may be lobulated. Nucleoli are inconspicuous.

Trophoblast may be divided into two groups: villous or extravillous. Villous trophoblast encompasses that trophoblast overlying the villi: cytotrophoblast, syncytiotrophoblast, and scant intermediate trophoblast (see Fig. 8-5). Most extravillous trophoblast is

TABLE 8-1
Indications for Placental Examination

Fetal Indications
  Untoward obstetric outcome
  Stillbirth
  Small or large neonate for gestational age
  Known or suspected intrauterine infection, maternal toxoplasmosis
  Malformations or deformations, oligohydramnios, chromosomal anomalies
  Multiple gestation

Maternal Indications
  Abnormal pregnancy: poor fetal growth, hyperemesis, α-fetoprotein abnormalities
  Preterm labor
  Premature rupture of membranes
  Abruption or unexplained vaginal bleeding
  Maternal fever, septicemia, chorioamnionitis
  Maternal disorders affecting pregnancy: preeclampsia/eclampsia, hypertension, diabetes, blood dyscrasias, malignancy

Placental Indications
  Cloudy, foul-smelling membranes
  Excessively large or small placenta for gestational age
  Abnormalities of shape
  Placental hematoma(s) and thrombi
  Abnormalities of umbilical cord: cysts, knots, single umbilical artery, webs, bands
  Abnormalities of chorionic membranes: white spots on fetal surface, yellow streaking, extrachorial gestation, cysts

intermediate trophoblast with some syncytiotrophoblast and cytotrophoblast (see Fig. 8-4). Extravillous trophoblast may be found in the uterine implantation site, both intravascularly and within endometrial stroma and myometrium, placental septa, and placental membranes.

ANATOMY

Viewed from the maternal surface, the placental disc is formed of 15 to 20 so-called maternal cotyledons, nodules of villous tissue created and demarcated by the *placental septa* (see Fig. 8-4). The placental septa are infoldings of decidua and implantation-site trophoblast that are pulled up into the placental parenchyma by their attachment to more slowly growing anchoring villi. The maternal cotyledons have no functional significance (see Fig. 8-3).

In contrast, a *fetal cotyledon* describes all villous tissues derived from a main stem villus (see Fig. 8-3) and consists of an anatomic unit with a single stem artery from one of the umbilical arteries. A placental *lobule* is the villous tissues derived from a secondary stem villus. The functional unit of the placenta is the *tertiary villus*, also called the *terminal villus*. Fetal metabolic needs are satisfied by active and passive transport of nutrients, gases, and hormones across the vasculosyncytial membranes of terminal villi.

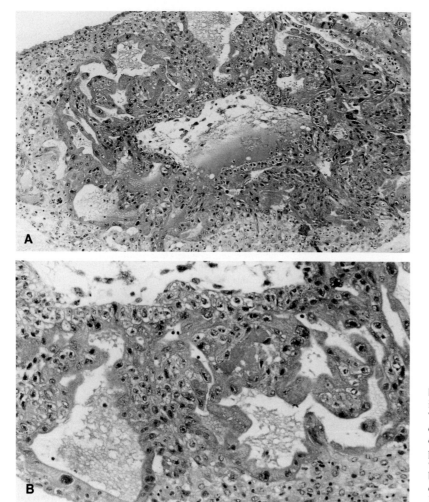

FIGURE 8-1 **(A)** Day 10 to 11. The blastocyst is embedded in the superficial endometrium. The embryo is not present in the exocoelomic cavity in this section. The trophoblastic shell is composed of syncytiotrophoblast and cytotrophoblast. **(B)** Blood lacunae are formed by invading cytotrophoblast and syncytiotrophoblast. (Lage JM. Diagnostic dilemmas in gynecologic and obstetric pathology. Semin Diagn Pathol 7(2):146–155, 1990)

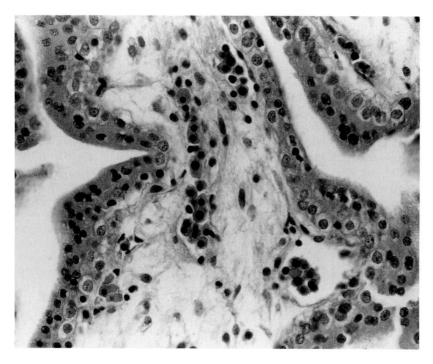

FIGURE 8-2 An immature villus with villous capillaries containing nucleated red blood cells. The villus surface is composed of two layers: inner cytotrophoblast and outer syncytiotrophoblast. The stroma contains fibroblastic stromal cells and macrophages (Hofbauer cells).

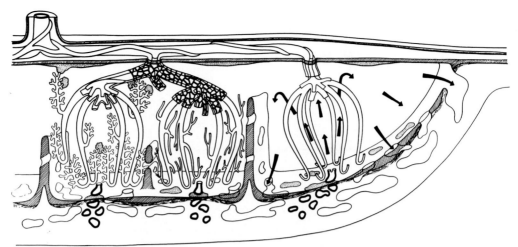

FIGURE 8-3 Placental structure. *Top*: The umbilical cord inserts into the chorionic plate (amnion, chorionic vessels [*light lines*] from umbilical cord arteries and vein, and chorion). Umbilical arteries branch onto the surface of the chorionic plate and penetrate the placental villous parenchyma. They divide with the villous branches to the tertiary villus, where the vessels closely approximate the maternal intervillous space, then pass back to the chorionic plate, ultimately fusing to form the umbilical vein. The basal plate is the interface between the placental villous tissue and maternal endometrium. Maternal uteroplacental arteries or spiral arteries (*heavy lines*) perfuse the intervillous spaces, and uteroplacental veins (superficial endometrial sinusoids, *light lines*) drain blood from the intervillous spaces. Fetal cotyledons may be single (*right*) or multiple (*left*). The maternal cotyledon is outlined by slanted lines. Arrows indicate direction of maternal blood flow.

The size of tertiary villi decreases throughout gestation. In the first trimester, the tertiary villi measure 170 μm in diameter; by second trimester, 70 μm; and by term, 40 μm. The presence and number of syncytiotrophoblastic knots reflects villous maturation: the closer to term, the more syncytial knots. A placenta may be described as immature or mature based on villous size and amount of syncytial knots. Mature placentas, usually after 34 weeks' gestation, contain small tertiary villi, and there is close approximation of capillary vascular endothelium to attenuated syncytium facing the maternal intervillous space. There is scant villous mesoderm, little if any

cytotrophoblast, and syncytial knots on roughly 30% to 40% of villi. Placentas lacking these features are termed *immature*. Placental maturity does not connote gestational maturity. A term placenta associated with fetal α-thalassemia will remain histologically immature even when delivery occurs at 40 weeks' gestation.

The umbilical cord contains two arteries carrying deoxygenated blood from the fetus to the placenta, and one vein carrying oxygenated blood from the placenta back to the fetus. The extraplacental fetal membranes are composed of amnion, chorion, and decidua. The umbilical cord and extraplacental membranes may be described as placental adnexa.

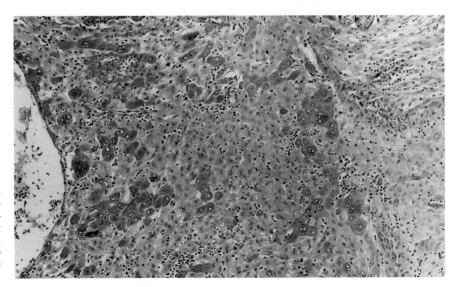

FIGURE 8-4 Decidualized endometrium with implantation-site trophoblast composed of mononucleated and multinucleated trophoblast. This histologic finding confirms intrauterine pregnancy. (Lage JM. Diagnostic dilemmas in gynecologic and obstetric pathology. Semin Diagn Pathol 7(2):146–155, 1990)

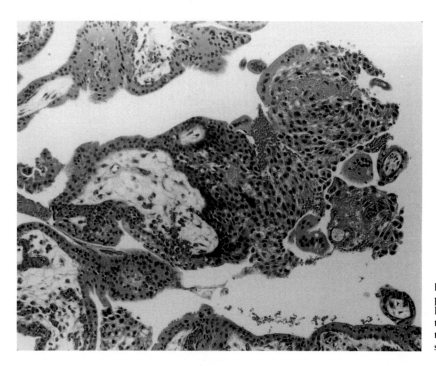

FIGURE 8-5 First-trimester villus with basal proliferation of cytotrophoblast (nearest villus), intermediate trophoblast (central core of trophoblast), and multinucleated syncytiotrophoblast (facing the maternal intervillous space).

EVALUATION OF EARLY CONCEPTUSES: SPONTANEOUS ABORTUSES, ELECTIVE TERMINATIONS, AND ECTOPIC PREGNANCIES

The pathologist's role in the evaluation of uterine curettings from an early conceptus is to document the presence and normality of fetal tissues: embryo, villi, or trophoblast (see Fig. 8-4). The gross specimen should be examined by someone with knowledge of normal fetal and placental morphology. Fetal tissues recognized grossly or found microscopically confirm intrauterine pregnancy. Identifying placental villous tissue verifies intrauterine pregnancy; however, any gross diagnosis requires microscopic confirmation because decidua may simulate villi. Implantation-site trophoblast or syncytiotrophoblast alone also confirms intrauterine pregnancy.

The extent of microscopic examination is determined by the nature of the specimen. In most institutions, identification of grossly normal fetal and villous tissues appears adequate in elective terminations of pregnancy with no abnormal maternal or fetal history. Microscopic examination is reserved for specimens with abnormal clinical history, gross fetoplacental abnormalities, or scant tissue. Although uterine curettings after a spontaneous abortion or complete abortion may contain only scant villous tissue, this is not the case for curettings from an elective termination (therapeutic abortion). In this case, identification of only a small amount of placental tissue is abnormal, and the following possibilities should be considered: clinically unknown or unsus-

pected spontaneous or missed abortion, ectopic pregnancy, or incomplete uterine evacuation. When confirmation of intrauterine pregnancy is lacking (ie, no fetal or villous tissue and no trophoblast), the pathologist is obligated to notify the clinician that an ectopic pregnancy cannot be excluded regardless of the clinical circumstances. An immediate verbal report regarding the possibility of ectopic pregnancy must be given. The clinician also should be notified when the pathologist suspects that the uterine curettings contain a paucity of villous tissue for the gestational age in an elective termination.

Microscopic examination of all spontaneous abortuses is required to document the presence of villous tissues and to exclude hydatidiform mole. Cytogenetic analysis of fetal or placental tissues should always be performed after the third spontaneous abortion or when gross fetal anomalies are present. Excellent recent texts describe normal fetal histology and development.[5,6]

The villi of a missed or spontaneous abortus may be small and sclerotic or large and edematous. In the *hydropic abortus,* the villi are diffusely enlarged and balloon-shaped, but the villous trophoblast is attenuated (see Fig. 8-6). Villous cavitation, both real and as a result of tangential sectioning of the chorion plate, may be apparent. Diagnosis of hydatidiform mole is excluded as there is no trophoblast hyperplasia. More than 50% of missed abortions have chromosomal anomalies.[7] Excluding triploidy and partial hydatidiform moles, chromosomal anomalies such as autosomal trisomies, 45,X, tetraploidy, and mosaicisms are not associated with specific villous morphologic alterations.[7]

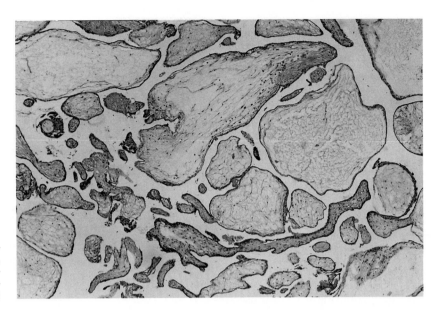

FIGURE 8-6 Hydropic abortus with a spectrum of villus sizes, attenuated trophoblast, and focal cavitation. (Lage JM. Diagnostic dilemmas in gynecologic and obstetric pathology. Semin Diagn Pathol 7(2):146–155, 1990)

GROSS EXAMINATION

There are many protocols for gross placental examination. An example is provided in Appendix 8-1. The placenta can be kept refrigerated for several days without significant destruction of morphology. The two most important physical requirements for gross examination are appropriate gear designed to protect the prosector from blood splashes (eg, goggles, mask, hat, gloves, gown, and shoe covers) and a large sink with running water and an adjacent cleared surface.

Placental dimensions are measured and the disc shape recorded. Fetal surface, membranes, and cord are examined. The umbilical cord is measured and the number of vessels recorded. One or two sections of umbilical cord are taken, preferably not from the placental insertion site. A membrane roll (or jellyroll) is prepared and fixed. The adnexa are then trimmed and the placental disc weighed. The placenta is turned over and the maternal surface examined. Any blood clots are measured and noted. The completeness of the maternal surface is assessed. Slicing the entire disc from decidua to chorionic plate allows inspection and palpation of parenchyma. The color of the villous parenchyma is recorded. All lesions, particularly infarcts, thrombi, hematomas, or undefined nodularity, are measured and described. If no lesions are identified, three routine cassettes containing the following should be submitted:

1. Umbilical cord and membrane roll
2. Random section of peripheral parenchyma (avoid atrophic areas)
3. Random section of central parenchyma.

Any gross lesion should be sampled for microscopic examination. Transverse parenchymal sections should include the full thickness from chorionic plate to the basal plate, with chorionic plate vessels cut in cross section if possible. Representative tissue blocks (or the entire placenta) should be fixed overnight and trimmed the next day. Placental parenchyma is excessively bloody and requires prolonged fixation. Fresh tissues submitted for routine processing and sectioning the following day usually result in inadequate fixation and, although interpretable, are suboptimal.

Placental Weight

The weight of a normal placenta increases with gestational age. Published charts compare normal placental weights by gestational age for whites and blacks.[9] These weights are based on trimmed, unfixed placentas. Roughly, by 20 weeks' gestational age, the placental weight should not exceed 150 g, or, at 30 weeks' gestational age, 375 g.[8] A term placenta weighs 400 to 600 g. A heavy placenta, or *placentomegaly*, is associated with maternal and fetal disorders, some of which are listed in Table 8-2. Most common is fetal macrosomia, which results from maternal diabetes or, less frequently, from Beckwith-Wiedemann syndrome.[10] A metabolic storage disorder may be diagnosed by unusual vacuolation of villous and extravillous trophoblast and villous stromal cells (see Fig. 8-7).[11] A small placenta is often associated with a small baby, suggesting intrauterine growth retardation. Others have dismissed the value of placental weights, suggesting that differences from the norm may be accounted for by variation in the amount of fetal blood retained in the placenta, a function of the time of cord clamping.[12]

TABLE 8-2
Conditions Associated With Placentomegaly

Diabetes mellitus, maternal
Blood dyscrasia, fetal-maternal
Neoplasm, fetal or maternal
Storage disorder, fetal
Chronic fetal infection
Fetal macrosomia
Multiple gestations
Anemia, maternal or fetal
Hydrops fetalis, not otherwise specified

Placental Shape

Placental shapes vary greatly. Some shapes are variants of normal with no clinical significance, whereas others are associated with potential fetal morbidity and mortality. Figure 8-8 illustrates the spectrum of singleton placental forms. Placentas usually are discoid and can be as large as 15 to 20 cm at term.

Succenturiate or Accessory Placenta (Placenta Succenturiata)

Extra lobules of placental parenchyma separated from the main disc are termed *accessory* or *succenturiate lobes* and constitute the most common variation of placental shape in singletons (Fig. 8-9). Succenturiate placentation occurs in roughly 3% of placentas.[13] It refers to a single (and rarely multiple), detached, smaller placental lobule, whose connection to the main disc is by way of chorionic vessels in the fetal membranes with minimal or no underlying parenchyma (see Fig. 8-9). The umbilical cord tends to insert centrally into the main mass. In most, the membranous chorionic vessels are completely unprotected by underlying villous parenchyma, placing them at risk for rupture, particularly when crossing the cervical os. Antepartum traumatic (iatrogenic) rupture of such vessels has resulted in rapid fetal exsanguination and death. In addition to fetal risks in succenturiate placentation, severance and retention of the accessory lobe may result in postpartum maternal hemorrhage.

Bilobate or Bipartite Placenta (Placenta Bilobata)

The bilobed or bipartite placenta consists of two separate placental masses of equal size joined by an isthmus composed of thinned parenchyma or membranes (Fig. 8-10). The umbilical cord tends to insert near the center of the isthmus or on the membranes near the isthmus. This type of placentation generally is not associated with poor fetal outcome. Depending on the architecture of the umbilical and chorionic vessels, there is some potential for antepartum disruption similar to that caused by the succenturiate placenta (Fig. 8-11). Bilobate placentation has been associated with older women of high gravidity, with infertility, and with increased manual placental extraction.[14] *Trilobate* and *multilobate* placentas are similar to bilobate placentas except that three or more lobes of similar sizes are present. The multiplex placentations (*placenta duplex, triplex,* and *multiplex*) are similar to the multilobed placentas except that in multiplex placentas each lobule is perfused directly from the umbilical cord rather than through chorionic vessels derived from the single dominant lobe as in multipartite placentations.

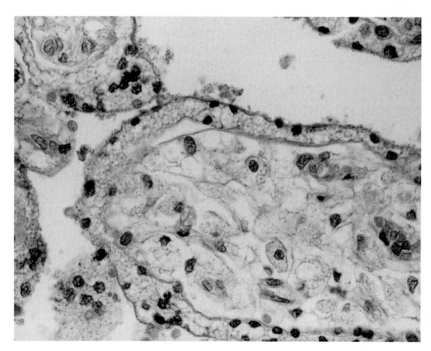

FIGURE 8-7 Fetal storage disorder, a GM$_1$ gangliosidase deficiency, is reflected in vacuolation of villous syncytiotrophoblast and stromal cells. Both cytotrophoblast and intermediate trophoblast of basal plate (not shown here) were vacuolated.

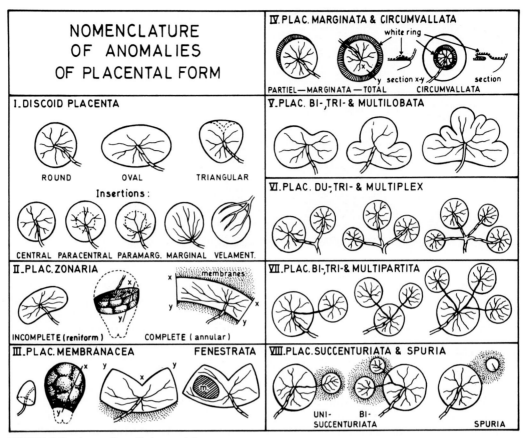

FIGURE 8-8 Anomalies of placental form.

Other Abnormal Placental Shapes

The most extreme form of multilobation is the *placenta membranacea (diffusa)*. This type of placentation is common in animals and is the norm for sheep. In our experience, placenta membranacea has an incidence of roughly 1 in 20,000 to 30,000 births. The placenta consists of numerous (15 to 30), 2- to 3-cm masses of chorionic villi dispersed throughout the entire gestational sac. It is as if the chorion laeve failed to atrophy and a single dominant placental disc never formed. Each lobule of villi tends to have a single chorionic artery and vein connecting directly to the umbilical cord or to another lobule. Placenta membranacea usually is placenta previa and may well be placenta accreta. It is associated with increased vaginal bleeding during pregnancy and, more commonly, with postpartum bleeding, often due to retained placental tissues.

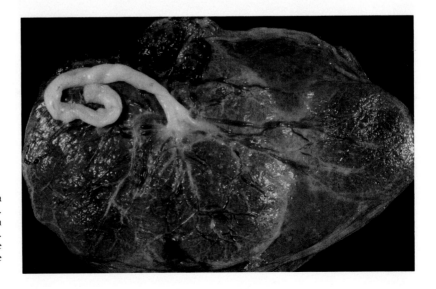

FIGURE 8-9 Succenturiate placenta (placenta succenturiata), a variant of placenta bipartita. Chorionic vessels travel unsupported through the placental membranes to the accessory lobe. Vessels of the accessory lobe unite with those of the main disc on the chorionic plate before entering the umbilical cord.

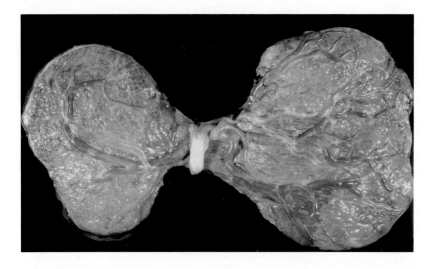

FIGURE 8-10 Bilobed placenta (placenta bipartita). The umbilical cord inserts centrally into membranes between the two placental discs.

In the *ring-shaped* placenta (*complete placenta zonaria*), the villous tissue is annular, forming a doughnut-like ring. When fixed, it can stand up on its own. This type of placentation is uncommon and in our experience occurs in about 1 in 50,000 births. The umbilical cord may insert onto the membranes.

A *fenestrate* placenta (*placenta fenestrata*) has a localized, approximately 2-cm, round to oval absence of villous tissue, generally within a central or paracentral portion of the chorionic plate. This curious villous defect has not been ascribed to any known predisposing factors.

Abnormal Membrane Insertions

In normal *marginal insertion*, the placental membranes insert at the edge of the chorionic plate. *Placenta extrachorialis* describes the general category of abnormal membrane insertion, of which there are two main types: *circummarginate (placenta marginata)* and *circumvallate (placenta vallata*; see Fig. 8-8). In the circummarginate placenta, the membrane insertion appears normal except that there is a 1- to 2-cm white plaque along a portion or the entire circumference of the chorionic plate (Fig. 8-12). On microscopy, this subchorionic white plaque consists of maternal decidua and some implantation-site trophoblast with the placental villi tucked under the intervening endometrium. There seem to be minimal sequelae associated with circummarginate membrane insertion.

In contrast, in circumvallate membrane insertion the extraplacental membranes are folded back onto themselves resulting in a deep "V" on the fetal surface, distal to which a layer of endometrium is sandwiched between the extraplacental membranes and the marginal chorionic villi (Fig. 8-13). Circumvallate placentation may be associated with prior marginal placental separation. Pregnancy outcome generally is normal. A full spectrum of intermediate forms of membrane insertions ranging from circummarginate to circumvallate have been observed.

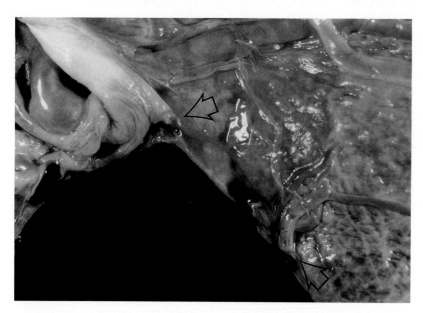

FIGURE 8-11 This umbilical artery is lacerated at the umbilical cord insertion site (same placenta as in Fig. 8-10).

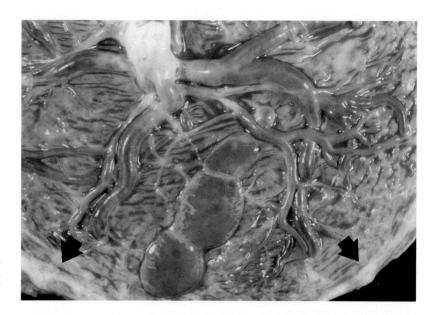

FIGURE 8-12 Circummarginate membrane insertion is indicated by the rim of white tissue at the placental margin (*arrows*). Innocuous subchorionic cysts are seen on the fetal surface.

PLACENTA CRETA

Placenta accreta refers to an abnormal adherence of the placenta to the uterus after delivery of the fetus. It is a clinical diagnosis. Pathologists have proffered a variety of histologic criteria to support its diagnosis. The most common, a lack of decidua intervening between villi and myometrium, may be a subjective call. Any placental tissue remaining in the uterus after the third stage of delivery implies abnormal adherence. By this definition, villous tissue in a postpartum hysterectomy specimen connotes placenta accreta. Villi may be implanted directly onto myometrium, with little to no intervening fibrin, implantation-site trophoblast, or decidua. Most commonly, the retained villi are associated with scant implantation-site trophoblast and fibrin, with minimal, if any,

decidua. Placenta accreta may be focal or extensive, involving the entire placenta. Most often, placenta accreta is focal, and the scant amount of residual villous tissues in a postpartum hysterectomy belies the gravity of this potentially life-threatening process.

Placenta increta refers to villi within the myometrium, usually involving previous cesarean section or myomectomy scars. In some, there is no history of previous uterine instrumentation. The placentation of all ectopic pregnancy sites including fallopian tubes, cornua, and cervix is increta or percreta.

The most severe and life-threatening abnormal placentation is *placenta percreta,* in which villi penetrate through the uterine wall to the serosa. Placenta percreta may cause bleeding at any point in gestation, with severe postpartum hemorrhage occurring if manual or surgical placental extraction is attempted. All forms of placenta creta are associated

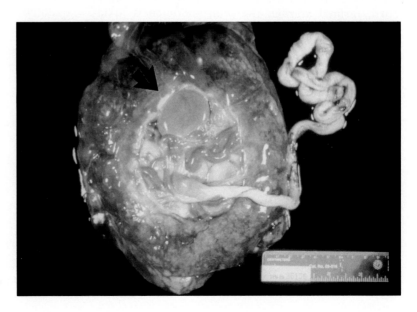

FIGURE 8-13 Circumvallate membrane insertion. Placental membranes are doubled back onto the fetal surface (*arrow*).

with increased postpartum bleeding, which may necessitate hysterectomy for control. Uterine inversion, although uncommon, is a serious and potentially lethal complication resulting from failure to diagnose placenta creta.

UMBILICAL CORD

The normal umbilical cord measures 40 to 70 cm in length at term, is 1 to 2 cm in diameter, and contains three vessels. The umbilical vessels are cushioned within Wharton's jelly, a myxomatous substance providing structural support. The amnion forming the surface of the cord is contiguous with the amnion of the placental membranes.

Gross structural abnormalities of the cord involve its insertion into the placental disc, the number and structure of vessels and vestigial remnants, its shape, and intrinsic tumors. The most common abnormality of the cord, inflammation of cord vessels relating to chorioamnionitis, is presented in the section dealing with placental infections.

Umbilical cords measuring less than 40 cm in length are arbitrarily designated *short*, whereas those more than 70 cm in length are called *long*. An umbilical cord that appears short at placental examination may simply be incomplete, with a section of cord having been submitted for blood gas analysis or an unusually long portion left attached (temporarily) to the infant. Truly short cords have been associated with congenital anomalies such as gastroschisis, amnionic band syndrome, abnormal fetal brain development, and low intelligence quotients in childhood.[15] They generally are associated with a lack of fetal movement, whereas long cords have been associated with excessive fetal movement. Entrapment of fetal parts (nuchal cord), formation of true knots, and cord prolapse are the main risks associated with a long cord. In the rare total absence of the umbilical cord, termed *acordia*, the fetal abdomen is juxtaposed to the placenta (Fig. 8-14). These fetuses generally do not survive.

Normally, the umbilical cord inserts centrally or slightly eccentrically into the chorionic plate (see Fig. 8-9). Insertion at the edge of the placental disc is termed *marginal* (battledore), and occurs in around 6% of cases. Studies analyzing the association between marginal cord insertion and fetal sequelae have yielded conflicting results. Recently, Davies found marginal cord insertion associated with fetal growth retardation.[16]

In 1% of placentas, the cord inserts directly into the fetal membranes. This is called *membranous* (velamentous) insertion. The fetal vessels may be traumatized or compressed due to a lack of underlying placental parenchyma (Fig. 8-15).[17] Membranous insertion of the cord in twins is seven times more common than in singletons. Membranous vessels crossing over the cervical os, *vasa previa*, may be ruptured during labor or delivery, leading to fatal fetal exsanguination. Robinson found fetal structural deformities, including hip dislocation and skull malformations, associated with membranous cord insertion.[18]

The normal cord contains two arteries and one vein. Absence of one umbilical artery, termed *single umbilical artery*, occurs in 1% of placentas and is more frequent in twins and in whites.[19,20] It is associated with congenital anomalies, most often involving the genitourinary and cardiovascular systems, chromosomal anomalies, stillbirth, and neonatal death. Leung found renal anomalies in 19% of fetuses with single umbilical artery who were studied by obstetric ultrasonography.[19] Others have suggested that there is no predilection for specific types of anomalies associated with single umbilical artery.[17] Because the umbilical arteries may fuse near the chorionic insertion site, sections of cord documenting vascular content should be taken proximal to the insertion site. In some states in the United States, the delivering physician is required by law to document the number of umbilical cord vessels at birth.

A *true knot* in the umbilical cord is found in about 1% of deliveries and most often is inconsequential. Normally, a true knot slides up and down

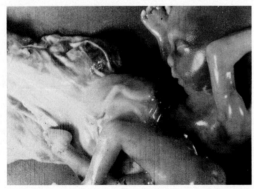

FIGURE 8-14 In the total absence of the umbilical cord (acordia), the fetal abdomen is juxtaposed to chorionic vessels.

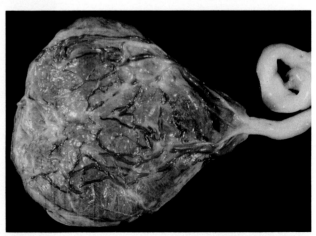

FIGURE 8-15 Membranous insertion of umbilical cord.

the cord and does not restrict blood flow. Umbilical cords with two or three knots, or a knot "tied twice" have been observed. True knots are an uncommon cause of intrauterine fetal death (Fig. 8-16). A true knot is described as occlusive when associated with a marked narrowing of the cord on one side of the knot and dilatation on the other. The *false knot* is not a knot at all (Fig. 8-17). It consists of a varicosity or tortuosity of an umbilical vessel and, unless associated with a thrombus, leads to no sequelae.

Vascular structural abnormalities of cord vessels include thrombosis, stenosis, and aneurysms. Complete thrombosis of the umbilical vein is lethal. Partial thrombosis may result in placental hydrops (Fig. 8-18). Thrombosis of one umbilical artery is not life-threatening. Occasionally, an umbilical artery is stenotic. Arterial stenosis has been suggested as a cause of single umbilical artery. Aneurysms of the umbilical vein have been associated with fetal systemic vascular malformations (Fig. 8-18).

In its early form, the primitive umbilical cord contains the omphalomesenteric duct, the allantoic duct, and the vitelline artery and vein. The *omphalomesenteric duct* connects the fetal yolk sac with the small intestine at the site of a Meckel's diverticulum. It atrophies during the 7th to 16th week. Vestigial remnants of the omphalomesenteric duct may be found in the periphery of the cord in Wharton's jelly near the amnionic surface. The duct is lined by cuboidal to columnar, intestinal-type epithelium, often

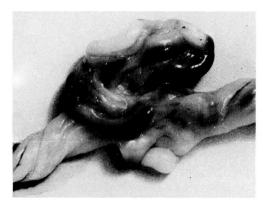

FIGURE 8-17 False knot of umbilical cord.

mucin-containing, which may be hyperplastic or metaplastic. Adenomas of small or large intestinal-type epithelium and a variety of mesodermally derived composite lesions, parallelling those of a Meckel's diverticulum, may develop within omphalomesenteric duct remnants (Fig. 8-19). In rare cases, such a lesion prolapses out the omphalomesenteric duct, through Wharton's jelly, and onto the cord surface, forming a pedunculated, beefy-red polyp.

Remnants of the *allantoic duct* are more common but less interesting. In early fetal life, the allantoic duct serves as a conduit for the fetal bladder. True to its association with the urinary tract, it is lined by a transitional-type epithelium that remains flat to cuboidal, with scant clear cytoplasm. The duct is often encountered in routine sections of the umbilical cord, lying between the umbilical arteries. Remnants of the vitelline vessels may be found in the term cord. They have no known clinical significance in the mature placenta.

There are rare umbilical cord cysts containing Wharton's jelly (Fig. 8-20). The more exotic, benign vascular tumors of the umbilical cord include *hemangiomas* (angiomyxomas) and *teratomas*. Although most cord hemangiomas are benign, the larger ones

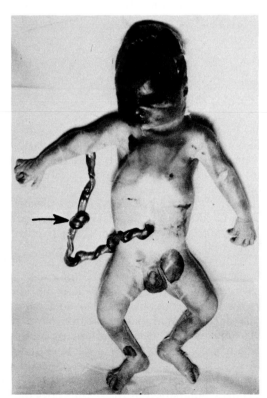

FIGURE 8-16 True knot in umbilical cord resulting in fetal death in utero.

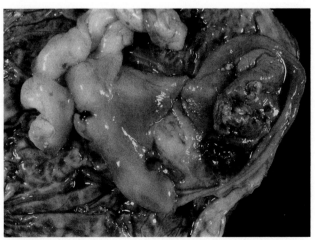

FIGURE 8-18 Aneurysm of umbilical vein associated with a large thrombus.

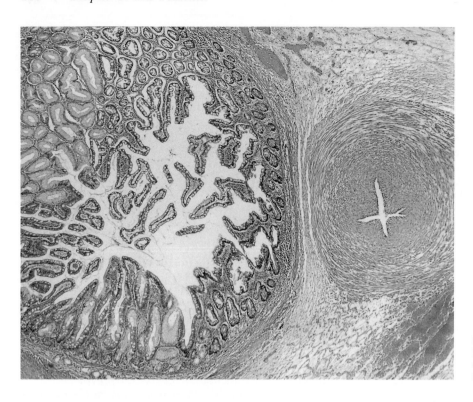

FIGURE 8-19 Intestinal-type epithelium within an omphalomesenteric duct remnant of an umbilical cord in a term infant.

may shunt blood or compress umbilical cord blood flow (Fig. 8-21). Some have obstructed delivery or have been associated with stillbirth.[21,22] Rare umbilical cord teratomas have been reported.[23] Some of these may represent included twins.

Bacteria can infect the cord, giving it an overall cloudy appearance. In contrast, *fungal colonization* by *Candida* species produces multiple, creamy yellow nodules, typically 3 to 4 mm in diameter and located just under the amnion. By microscopy, spores and hyphal forms are seen on hematoxylin and eosin-stained sections (Fig. 8-22) and are highlighted by periodic acid-Schiff or silver stains. The newborn may have disseminated skin nodules or may be totally normal. Candidal septicemia and pneumonia are rare.

The amnion of the cord may undergo metaplastic changes, including squamous metaplasia and columnar metaplasia (see discussion later in this chapter). Deposits of amnion nodosum are usually located at the base of the cord, although the amnion overlying the chorionic plate tends to be involved more extensively. Amnionic bands may entwine, constrict, or occlude the cord.

PLACENTAL MEMBRANES

The fetus floats in amnionic fluid enclosed within the amnionic cavity. The amnionic sac enlarges and obliterates the chorionic cavity and fuses with the chorion. The uterine cavity itself is obliterated near the end of the third month by the fusion of the chorion laeve and its attached decidua capsularis to the decidua vera (decidua parietalis). The amnion, chorion laeve, and decidua form the extraplacental membranes.

The amnion is composed of a single layer of flattened to cuboidal epithelial cells (amniocytes) atop a mesoblastic connective tissue layer. The chorion contains extravillous trophoblast and is adjacent to the maternal decidua. Within the chorion laeve of the extraplacental membranes are remnants of atrophic villi. The decidua is composed of decidualized endometrial stroma, endometrial glands, and spiral arteries. Macrophages are present in all three layers. Microscopic examination of the membranes provides valuable information about acute and chronic placental infection, meconium or blood exposure, ma-

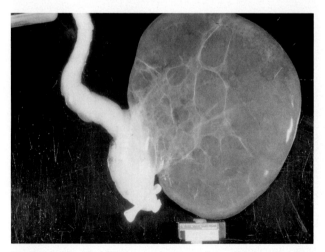

FIGURE 8-20 Umbilical cord cyst containing Wharton's jelly.

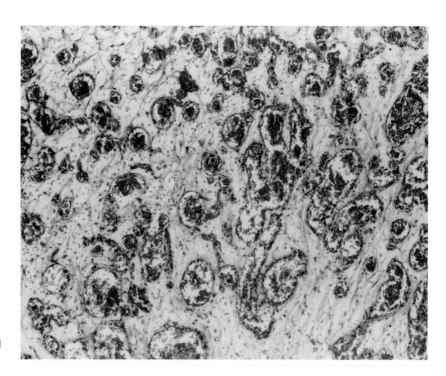

FIGURE 8-21 Hemangioma of umbilical cord.

ternal disorders affecting uteroplacental perfusion, and the amount of amnionic fluid.

Chorioamnionits

Chorioamnionitis is diagnosed pathologically by maternal leukocytes infiltrating into the chorioamnionic membranes. Chorioamnionitis is rare in the first trimester. In the second trimester, it is a common cause of premature labor, premature rupture of membranes, and stillbirth. At term, it is often observed histologically but is rarely associated with poor neonatal outcome if delivery is achieved within the first 24 hours.[24] Chorioamnionitis is discussed in more detail in the section on placental infections.

Meconium

Fresh meconium is dark green and viscous. It is water-soluble and easily cleared in tissue processing. In

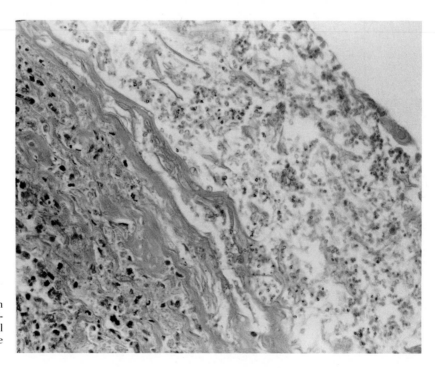

FIGURE 8-22 Umbilical cord with collection of spores and hyphal forms of *Candida* species on surface of cord. There is superficial invasion of the umbilical cord and acute inflammation.

histologic sections, it is light yellow, finely granular, dusty, and far less bright yellow than hematoidin. Hemosiderin is coarsely granular and yellow-brown to brown and, unlike meconium, is refractile.

The timing and response to meconium exposure in vivo is not well characterized. Apparently, meconium initially causes focal epithelial necrosis, followed by amnionic columnar metaplasia with ballooning and cytoplasmic vacuolization.[17] Associated subamnionic macrophages engulf meconium pigment (Fig. 8-23). Imbued meconium can be found in macrophages of the chorion, umbilical cord, or decidua. The high degree of water solubility accounts for the marked disparity between the intense green to brown discoloration of the fetal surface in meconium-stained placentas and for the subtlety of histologic findings.

In vitro studies suggest that meconium appears within chorionic macrophages about 3 hours after fetal release (see Fig. 8-23).[25] There is some evidence to suggest that meconium induces necrosis of umbilical cord vascular smooth muscle, thereby causing vasospasm and decreasing fetal blood flow.[26] Meconium staining of the placenta is not invariably associated with fetal meconium aspiration.[27]

All green-stained placentas are not the result of meconium passage. Green discoloration may reflect hemosiderin deposits from metabolized blood of placental thrombi, hematomas, abruptions, fetal hemolysis, and marginal hemorrhages. Sometimes it is difficult to differentiate meconium from hemosiderin; in such cases, an iron stain is helpful.

Amnion Nodosum

Amnion nodosum consists of nodular deposits of fetal vernix caseosum and debris atop ulcerated amnion (Fig. 8-24). It is always associated with oligohydramnios. The deposits may be numerous (more than 100), elevated, yellow to cream-colored. They measure 2 to 5 mm in diameter. In contrast to squamous metaplasia, they are easily removed by firm scraping. Although they center around the umbilical cord insertion and extend centrifugally from the juxtaumbilical chorionic plate, some deposits may be found on the extraplacental membranes.

Microscopic examination often reveals an ulcerated amnion, which may be attenuated but intact. The nodule consists of an eosinophilic hump of debris: parakeratotic fetal squames, hair, and amorphous granular material (Fig. 8-25). At the edges, regenerating amnion may partially cover the nodule. Amnion nodosum, apart from its association with oligohydramnios, is related to structural anomalies of the fetal urinary tract and may result from bilateral renal agenesis, cystic dysplastic kidneys, ureteral atresia or agenesis (bilateral), absence of the urinary bladder, posterior urethral valves with marked obstruction, urethral stenosis, or atresia. Oligohydramnios from preterm rupture of membranes usually results in fewer deposits of amnion nodosum than does bilateral renal agenesis. Amnion nodosum should prompt careful monitoring and evaluation of the newborn's urinary tract.

Squamous Metaplasia

Squamous metaplasia may involve the amnion of the umbilical cord and the placental membranes. It is grossly similar to amnion nodosum except that the nodules are smaller and whiter. Firm scraping will not remove a nodule of squamous metaplasia because it is an inherent part of the amnion. By microscopy, it consists of multilayered squamous epithelium

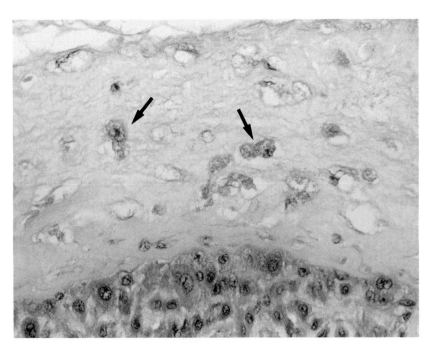

FIGURE 8-23 Placental membranes with subamnionic macrophages imbued with finely particulate, granular meconium (*arrows*). Meconium is also present in superficial macrophages in the chorion. Amnionic epithelium is avulsed.

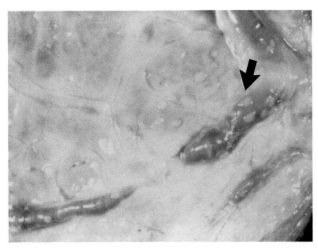

FIGURE 8-24 Fetal surface of placenta showing nodular deposits of amnion nodosum on amnion overlying chorionic vessels (*arrow*). Fetus had bilateral renal agenesis.

complete with keratohyalin granules and occasionally with dense ortho- or parakeratosis (Fig. 8-26). It has no known clinical significance and its importance derives from differentiating it from amnion nodosum. Microscopy should be performed in all cases of nodular deposits on the fetal surface.

Amnionic Vacuolization

Fetal gastroschisis is associated with a distinctive vacuolization of the amnion. The eosinophilic cytoplasm of the amnion contains a single vacuole or a few small to medium-sized clear vacuoles. In contrast to the columnar metaplasia associated with meconium exposure, the nuclei of amnionic vacuolization in gastroschisis are normal and not pyknotic. This type of vacuolization generally is not found with fetal omphalocele.

Amnionic Band Syndrome

Amnionic band syndrome (amnion rupture sequence) results from a premature rupture of the amnion. The fetus is no longer housed in the amnionic cavity, but within a cavity lined by subamnionic connective tissues or chorion.[28] The strings or bands of the ruptured amnion and its connective tissue may entrap, disrupt, or amputate developing fetal structures. The resultant malformations depend on the timing of the rupture and the site of entrapment. Rupture in early gestation leads to major malformations, such as craniofacial defects, some types of encephaloceles and meningoceles, and possibly gastroschisis. Usually severe oligohydramnios ensues, with resultant pulmonary hypoplasia, positional deformations of extremities, and Potter facies. Amputation of an arm, leg, or even the head may occur. The fetus, even with good Apgar scores at birth, often dies shortly after birth of pulmonary insufficiency.

Rupture later in pregnancy is less destructive, although bands may entrap fingers, toes, or feet, resulting in amputation, constriction, or deformation (Fig. 8-27). Examination of the placenta shows avulsion of the amnion with erosion of the subamnionic connective tissue. Remnants of amnionic bands encircle the base of the umbilical cord or entrap fetal parts. Amputated fetal parts may become attached to the placenta or may be free-floating, delivered with the placenta and adnexa.[29] Rarely, the infant adheres to the placenta. Defects associated with amnionic

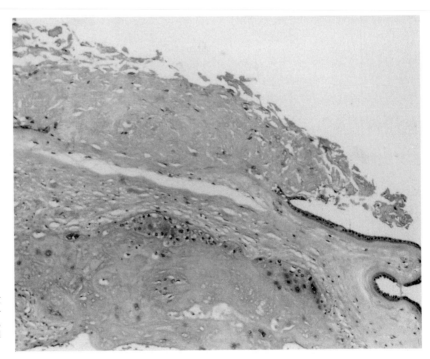

FIGURE 8-25 Amnion nodosum involving the placental chorionic plate. Ulcerated amnion is replaced by a mound of fetal squames, debris, and lanugo. Fetus had bilateral renal agenesis.

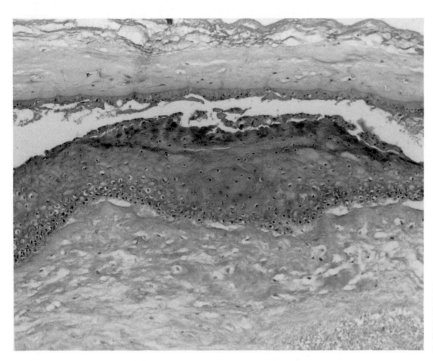

FIGURE 8-26 Membrane roll showing squamous metaplasia of amnion (*center*). Amnion is converted into squamous epithelium complete with keratohyalin granules and parakeratosis. The normal amnion is opposite the nodule of squamous metaplasia.

band formation are sporadic and, in most cases, are not associated with chromosomal anomalies or recurrences. Although it was initially feared that second-trimester amniocentesis would result in an increase in amnionic band formation, no such association has been observed.[30]

Decidual Vasculopathy

Pathology in the decidual vessels of the extraplacental membranes (decidua parietalis) provides data

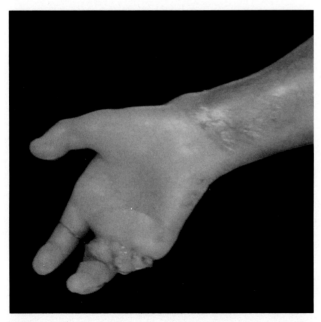

FIGURE 8-27 Fetal hand with amnionic band constricting the fingers, deforming and amputating the digits.

regarding the status of maternal circulation during gestation. *Decidual vasculopathy* (or *early atheromatous change, acute atherosis*) is a pathologic finding in abnormal placentas that affects maternal vessels that do not undergo the physiologic vascular changes of pregnancy. It is not found in normal, uncomplicated pregnancies.[31] Decidual vasculopathy is most commonly associated with preeclampsia, eclampsia, small-for-gestational-age infants,[31–33] and hypertension.[34–35] It is found less frequently with diabetes mellitus,[34,36] collagen vascular diseases such as lupus erythematosus,[37] and renal disorders. Even among women with preeclampsia, only 25% have decidual vasculopathy in random sections of the membranes. Submitting an extra sample of the membrane roll increases the diagnostic yield; two samples of the membrane roll should be submitted for microscopic examination in high-risk placentas.

Microscopically, decidual vasculopathy takes three distinct forms:

1. Thickening or hyalinization of arteriolar vessel walls with mild perivascular mononuclear cell infiltrate
2. Marked arteriolar wall thickening with onion-skinning (Fig. 8-28)
3. Moderate arteriolar wall thickening with fibrinoid necrosis, focal or complete occlusion of vascular lumen, infiltrate of mononuclear cells (lymphocytes and plasma cells), and lipid-rich macrophages (lipophages; Figs. 8-29 and 8-30). In rare cases, the macrophages contain cholesterol clefts.

Finding vasculopathy in the maternal decidual vessels of the extraplacental membranes is important because it reflects the status of the vessels in the pla-

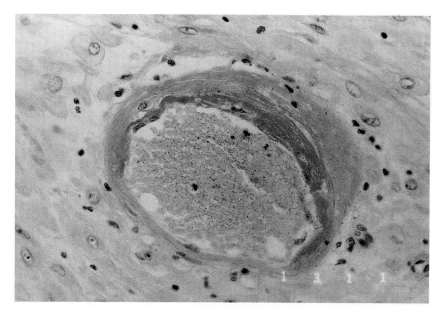

FIGURE 8-28 Decidual vasculopathy with marked dilation of decidual arteriole, hyalinization of vessel wall, dense crescentic fibrin deposit, and sparse mononuclear cell infiltrate. Section taken from extraplacental membranes.

cental bed of the implantation site. The vascular lesions of preeclampsia affect the spiral arteries of the decidua parietalis (away from the implantation site), the basal arteries, and the deep myometrial portions of the spiral arteries serving the implantation site.[38] Khong found that acute atherosis also involved the decidual segments of the spiral arteries of the placental bed in pregnancies complicated by preeclampsia or small-for-gestational-age infants (Fig. 8-30).[39] Destruction of vascular walls by fibrinoid necrosis with focal or complete luminal occlusion or thrombosis decreases placental perfusion and results in parenchymal infarcts. It has been suggested that decidual vasculopathy represents the localized results of an inappropriate fetal-maternal immunologic re-

action because it is histologically similar to the vascular lesions of allograft transplant rejection.[40]

MULTIPLE GESTATION AND ITS COMPLICATIONS

Twin gestations provide an opportunity to study the interactions of nature and nurture in forming human life. Because the uterus was designed to support one gestation at a time, twins constitute a reproductive error. Prematurity is the rule in twin births, with perinatal mortality rates three times higher than in singletons.[41–43] Congenital malformations,

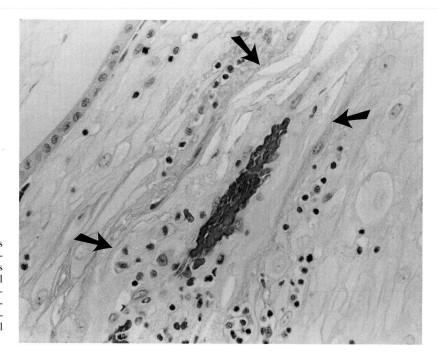

FIGURE 8-29 Extraplacental membranes showing decidual vasculopathy with expansion of maternal vessel (*arrows*) by numerous macrophages, some containing cholesterol clefts, embedded in loose eosinophilic fibrinoid material. There is moderate mononuclear cell infiltrate of vessel and surrounding decidua. Amnion (*upper left*) and minimal chorion can be seen.

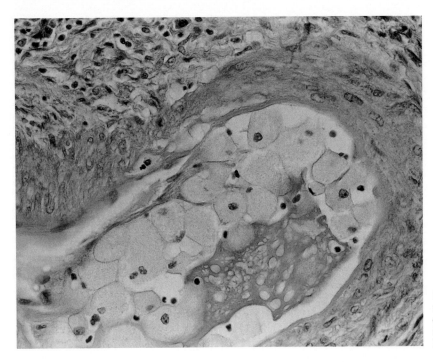

FIGURE 8-30 Decidual vasculopathy with numerous lipophages, scattered mononuclear cells, and central fibrin. Section of decidua from the basal plate of placenta subtending a large placental infarct.

particularly congenital heart disease and central nervous system anomalies, occur more frequently in identical twins.[44]

Twin gestations are the most common type of multiple gestation. In Western countries, there is 1 twin birth for every 80 births.[45] Naturally occurring births of higher order are significantly less common, with the frequency of triplets at $1:80^2$, quadruplets, $1:80^3$, and quintuplets, $1:80^4$.

There are two types of twins: monozygous and dizygous. *Monozygous twins* (identical twins) are derived from the fertilization of one oocyte by one spermatozoon and are genetically identical. *Dizygous twins* (fraternal twins) are derived from two separate fertilization events: two different oocytes are fertilized by two different spermatozoa. Dizygous twins are no more alike than any other full sibling pair. There are rare cases of half-identical twins derived from fertilization of an ova and its polar body. Even more rare are cases of twin ova fertilized by spermatozoa from different fathers.

The rate of monozygous twinning is relatively constant throughout the world at 3.5 per 1000 births and is not associated with any known predisposing factors.[43,44,46] Depending on the population, monozygotes account for as many as one-third of all twin births. In contrast, the incidence of dizygous twinning depends on multiple factors. Dizygous twinning increases with family history of twins, advanced maternal age (highest between ages 35 and 40), increased parity, and exposure to exogenous gonadotropins. Among whites, dizygotic twinning occurs in about 8 per 1000 births. Asian women have a rate one half as frequent, and black women twice as great.[46] In Nigeria, where the rate of dizygous twinning is at its highest, twin births in the Yoruba tribe account for 1 per 22 to 25 births.[46,47]

The most common question posed on the birth of twins is whether the twins are identical or fraternal. Twins derived from a single zygote are genetically identical and monozygous.[45] Those from two different zygotes (dizygous) are fraternal. Examination of the placenta in conjunction with knowledge of the sex of each twin allows ascertainment of zygosity in about 55% of twin births.[49] In a series of 250 consecutive twin placentas past 20 weeks' gestational age, 1.5% were monoamnionic-monochorionic; 29.6% were diamnionic-monochorionic; 34% were diamnionic-dichorionic, fused; and 35.2% were diamnionic-dichorionic, separate.[50] Further evaluation of the twins in this series from the eastern United States revealed that 41% were monozygous and 59% dizygous. Of the monozygous twins, 70% were monochorionic and 30% dichorionic, with fused or separate placentas. All dizygous twins had dichorionic placentation.

The physical characteristics of the twin placenta or placentas depend on the zygosity, the proximity of the two implantation sites, and the time of fission of the zygote in monozygous twins (Table 8-3). A twin or multiple gestation may have one or more amnion, chorion, and placental mass. Placentation is the term used to describe the anatomic relations among these various elements. In some instances, zygosity may be inferred from knowledge of placentation.

The timing of zygote fission determines the type of placentation. Four potential types of placentation may form in monozygous twins (see Table 8-3).[45,50] If the blastocyst divides before the 3rd day, the placentas are indistinct from those of dizgyous twins: each twin has its own amnion, chorion, and placental disc, and the placenta is termed *diamnionic-dichorionic*. Proximity of uterine implantation sites determines whether each disc remains separate or fuses

TABLE 8-3
Relationship Between Number of Placental Discs, Composition of Dividing Septum, and Inferred Zygosity

Type of Twin Placenta(s)	Number of Placental Masses	Dividing Septum	Amnions in Dividing Septum	Chorions in Dividing Septum	Zygosity
Monoamnionic-monochorionic	1	No	—	—	Monozygous
Diamnionic-monochorionic	1	Yes	2	0	Monozygous
Diamnionic-dichorionic, fused	Apparently 1*	Yes	2	2	Monozygous or dizygous
Diamnionic-dichorionic, separate	2	No†	—	—	Monozygous or dizygous

*The two fused placentas often resemble one large placental disc.
†Although separate diamnionic-dichorionic placentas will ultimately contain areas of placental fusion either of the extraplacental membranes or of the discs themselves, there is no dividing septum.

(Figs. 8-31 through 8-33). When the twinning event occurs after the chorion has already formed, between the 3rd to 8th day, both fetuses will share the same chorion, but each will have its own amnion. This type of placenta is called *diamnionic-monochorionic* (Fig. 8-34). Division of the blastocyst after formation of amnion and chorion, between the 8th and 13th days, yields two fetuses housed within the same chorioamnion, termed *monoamnionic-monochorionic* (Fig. 8-35). Although there are four types of placentation associated with monozygous twinning, only in monochorionic placentation is monozygosity ensured. Zygosity cannot be determined from placental examination in dichorionic placentation, because monozygous and dizygous gestations may result in dichorionic placentation.

Only two types of placentas may form in dizygous gestations (see Table 8-3 and Figs. 8-31 through 8-33). Because the conceptuses are derived from separate fertilizations, each forms a separate placenta with a separate amnion, chorion, and placental disc. Due to space constraints, the two placentas eventually come in contact with each other. In some cases, this involves only the extraplacental

membranes, and both discs remain separate (see Fig. 8-31). In others, large portions of the placental discs fuse, giving the impression of one placenta (see Fig. 8-32). Except in rare cases, two separate placentas imply diamnionic-dichorionic placentation. A recently reported bipartite diamnionic-monochorionic placenta was an exception to this rule.[51]

For placentas with dividing septa, a membrane roll (jelly-roll) should be prepared from the intact septum. Although a T section of the septum with underlying chorion has been recommended, we find that it disrupts the vasculature of the chorionic plate and, depending on how tightly it is rolled, may be somewhat difficult to interpret. After taking tissue for a membrane roll, the septum should then be examined grossly to ascertain its composition. The septum from dichorionic placentas is relatively opaque and contains two amnions and two chorions (Fig. 8-36), with a few scattered villi from either side (Fig. 8-37). The latter finding is particularly helpful when the septum has been severely disrupted during delivery. The septum of a monochorionic placenta, however, is translucent, composed of only two layers of amnion, and devoid of chorion or chorionic villi

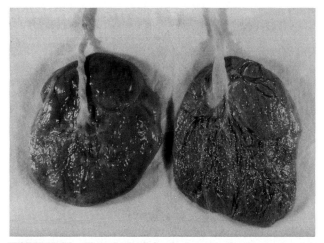

FIGURE 8-31 Diamnionic-dichorionic twin placentas, separate. Placenta on left had chorioamnionitis and meconium within amnionic macrophages. Placenta on right was normal.

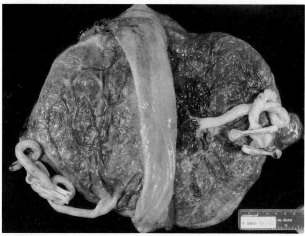

FIGURE 8-32 Diamnionic-dichorionic twin placentas, fused. Dividing septum is composed of two layers of amnion and two layers of chorion.

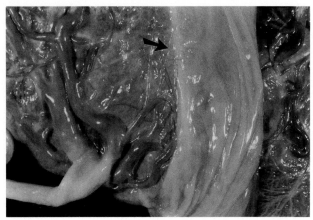

FIGURE 8-33 Closer view of Figure 8-32. The dividing septum is opaque, and the junction between the two placentas forms a ridge at the base of the septum (*right of arrow*) that is characteristic of fused dichorionic placentas. Tiny chorionic vessels course along the chorionic surface and onto the dividing septum for a short distance (*arrow*).

(Fig. 8-38). Microscopic confirmation offers histologic documentation.

Examination of placentas from multiple gestations such as triplet (Fig. 8-39) and quadruplet (Fig. 8-40) gestations is performed similarly to that of twin gestations. The pathologist must note the exact source of sections, particularly with respect to the dividing septa, on gross sketch and on tissue cassettes and slides.

Conjoined Twins

Conjoined twins are formed by incomplete fission of an embryo late in development, on or after the 13th day of gestation.[45] They are uncommon, occurring once in every 100,000 births. More than 70% are fe-

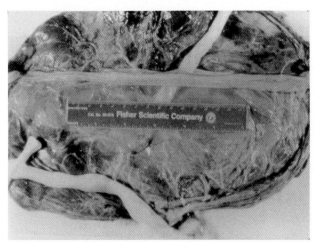

FIGURE 8-34 Diamnionic-monochorionic twin placenta with translucent dividing septum composed of two layers of amnion. (Lavery PJ, ed: The human placenta. Rockville, MD, Aspen, 1987)

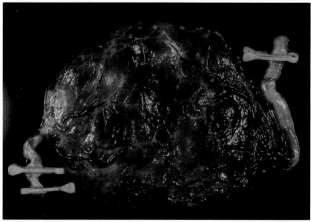

FIGURE 8-35 Monoamnionic-monochorionic twin placenta. There is no dividing septum in this type of placentation. (Lavery PJ, ed: The human placenta. Rockville, MD, Aspen, 1987)

male, for unknown reasons.[45] Their placentation is always monochorionic. Although there is great variety in the joining sites, most show partial to complete fusion of the chest, termed *thoracopagii*. In some, only part of the body was duplicated, with the remainder remaining singleton (Fig. 8-41). Associated umbilical cord anomalies include partial or complete fusion or forking (Fig. 8-42).

Vascular Anastomoses in Twin Placentas

Virtually all monochorionic placentas contain vascular anastomoses linking the fetal circulations,[52] but they are less frequent in monoamnionic-monochorionic placentas.[53] Most fused dichorionic placentas have no vascular anastomoses between the two fetal circulations, although exceptions have been reported.[54,55]

Vascular anastomoses across the chorionic plate are visible on gross inspection. Most frequently these take the form of arterial-to-arterial or venous-to-venous connections. Less common are arterial-to-venous or venous-to-arterial anastomoses. The easiest way to check for suspected anastomoses is by visual inspection of the fetal surface, and then by injecting air (20 to 40 mL) into a large chorionic vessel while constricting the umbilical cord. Vascular anastomoses are demonstrated when air tracks from vessels on one twin to those of the co-twin. Reinjection confirms initial impressions. If needed, radiographs of barium-injected anastomoses can serve as a permanent record.

The consequences of these vascular links depend largely on their nature, number, and net circulatory result. Those that connect vessels of similar pressures (eg, artery-artery or vein-vein) are of little consequence. If unbalanced, potentially life-threatening sequelae may result from shunting of blood from one twin to the other by artery-vein or vein-artery anastomoses.

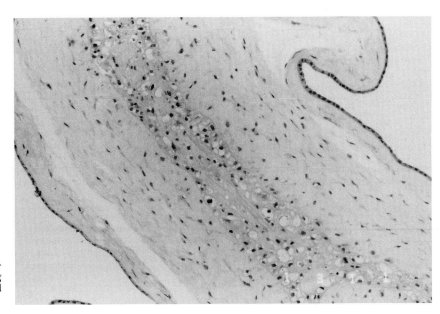

FIGURE 8-36 Dividing septum in diamnionic-dichorionic twin placentas showing two amnions (*lower left* and *upper right*) and partial fusion of the two chorions (*center*).

Dizygous twins usually have completely separate placental circulatory systems. Joining of the fetal circulations in dizygous twins may result in blood group chimerism, identified by two red blood cell groups in one twin. Precursor blood cells are passed between fetuses at a stage when the tolerance of the immature immune system allows these cells to engraft and proliferate. More than 30 pairs of such dizygous twins with blood group chimerism have been described.[45,48,56] Vascular anastomoses have been documented in fused placentas from dichorionic twins.[54,55]

Twin Transfusion Syndrome

The twin transfusion syndrome, a consequence of unidirectional blood shunting between the twins by unbalanced chorionic anastomoses, is one of the most serious hazards of monochorionic twining. The risk is greatest in diamnionic-monochorionic twins, in whom the incidence is 5% to 16%.[56,57] In its extreme form, both twins die.[58] The donor twin transfuses the recipient twin with every beat of its heart. The donor becomes malnourished, small, pale, and growth-retarded (Fig. 8-43), eventuating in a severely anemic fetus with high output heart failure. There is massive extramedullary hematopoiesis in virtually all organs, including the placenta. The recipient becomes plethoric and macrosomic, developing congestive heart failure with hepatomegaly due to volume overload (see Fig. 8-43). The pathology of the monochorionic placenta in twin transfusion syndrome reflects the circulatory status, the donor's portion being pale, hydropic, and immature, with

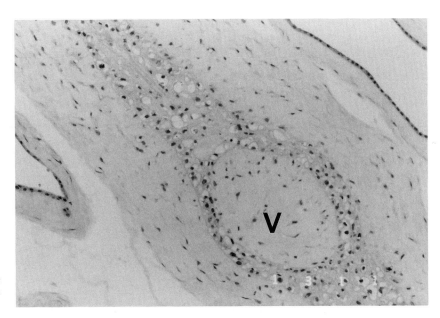

FIGURE 8-37 A residual villus (*V*) from the chorion laeve within the dividing septum confirms dichorionic placentation.

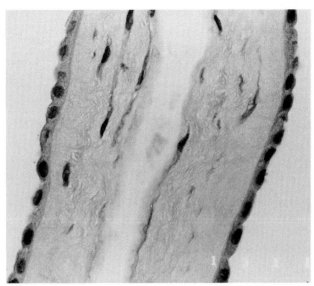

FIGURE 8-38 Dividing septum of the diamnionic-monochorionic placenta. The septum is composed of two layers of amnion and is totally devoid of chorion.

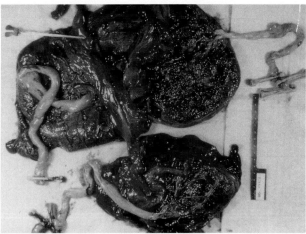

FIGURE 8-40 Quadruplet placenta. Three infants were live-born, and one died in utero. The placenta of the stillborn fetus is indicated by the probe.

villous vessels packed with extramedullary hematopoiesis (Figs. 8-44 through 8-46). The recipient's portion is congested and more mature (see Figs. 8-44 and 8-45). On the death of one twin, usually the recipient, the shunting temporarily reverses and finally stops. The pathology observed depends on when the sequence is interrupted, either by delivery or fetal death, and, if death occurs, on the interval between fetal death and delivery.

Acardiac Twin

The formation of an acardiac twin, formerly called an *acardiac monster,* is another disastrous consequence of vascular anastomoses in monochorionic twins. As the name implies, this twin has no heart or has a rudimentary heart; often, the twin has no head (Fig. 8-47). The incidence of this abnormality is 1 in 100 monozygous twin gestations or 1 in 30,000 deliveries.[48] Recent Doppler studies have proved the long-believed but previously unsubstantiated theory regarding the etiology of the acardiac twin: it is caused by a reversal of vascular perfusion.[59] The acardiac twin is perfused by vascular anastomoses from its partner's placenta rather than from its own placenta (see Fig. 8-47). This results in two problems: (1) the acardiac twin receives blood by the umbilical arteries rather than by the umbilical vein, and (2) the blood it receives is low in oxygen, having already passed through the co-twin's body. The lower extremities get the first pass of blood and are the most normal morphologically. Those structures perfused later are less normal, and the last on the line are overtly malformed, atretic, or absent (agenesis). Thus, the heart and head are usually substantially malformed or absent. Some acardiac twins are remarkably dysmorphic, composed of a ball with skin enclosing a mass of disorganized visceral, cartilaginous, and bony structures, prompting some to

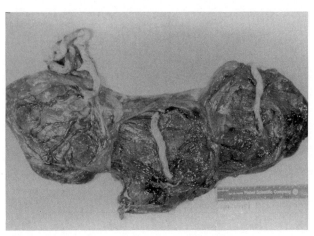

FIGURE 8-39 Triplet placenta, triamnionic-trichorionic.

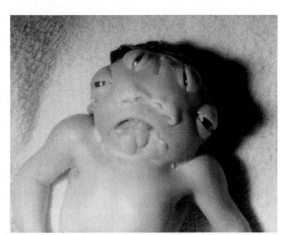

FIGURE 8-41 Anencephalic partially conjoined twins with duplication of head and upper spine. Remainder of fetal corpus was singleton. (Courtesy of Dr. Kristina Amyot, Albany, New York)

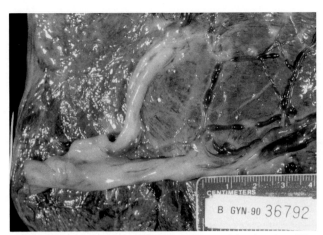

FIGURE 8-42 Forked umbilical cord in conjoined twins. The smaller cord contained a single umbilical artery.

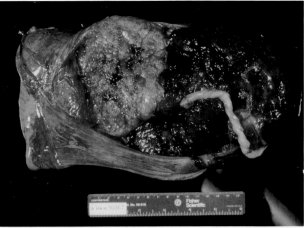

FIGURE 8-44 Maternal surface of monochorionic twin placenta in twin transfusion syndrome. The donor portion (*left*) is small, pale, and spongy. The recipient portion (*right*) is enlarged, congested, and hemorrhagic. The umbilical cord is reflected over the maternal surface.

question whether a birth certificate should be issued for the acardiac co-twin.

Fetus in Fetu

Fetus in fetu refers to a monozygous twin that grew within the body of its co-twin. It generally is found within the abdomen of its co-twin;[60] Dr. Shirley G. Driscoll saw such a fetus in the neck of a stillbirth (personal communication). Cytogenetic analysis of a pair of such twins demonstrated that the liveborn twin and included *fetus in fetu* had identical karyotypes.[60] Although both are monozygous twins, the acardiac is differentiated from the *fetus in fetu* by physical separation from its partner. Yet some *feti in fetu* contain morphologic anomalies that closely resemble those of acardiac twins.[59,60] It appears that these commonalities may result from a reversal of

blood perfusion patterns similar to that described in acardiac twins.

Congenital Malformations

Although twinning itself, particularly monozygous twinning, constitutes a reproductive error, additional congenital malformations are two to three times more frequent in twins than singleton.[61] Among twins, malformation rates are highest in monozygous twins. These malformations include anencephaly (see Fig. 8-41), holoprosencephaly, cloacal exstrophy, Vater association, sirenomelia, and sacrococcygeal teratoma. Velamentous insertion of the umbilical cord and single umbilical artery are seven times more frequent in twins.[48] It is possible that the single umbilical artery in twins results from perturbations

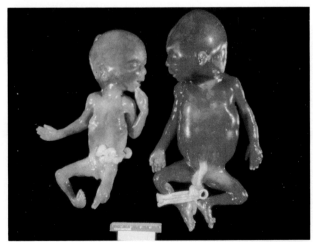

FIGURE 8-43 Monozygous twins with twin transfusion syndrome. There is a marked discrepancy between fetal sizes. The donor twin (*left*) is small and undernourished. Oligohydramnios is reflected by positional deformation of right foot (talipes equinovarus deformity). The left foot was amputated during delivery. The recipient twin (*right*) is hydropic with visceromegaly.

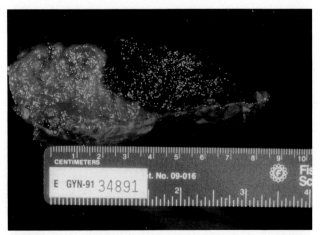

FIGURE 8-45 Cross section of placenta showing marked contrast of donor placental parenchyma (*right*) and recipient placental parenchyma (*left*). The same specimen is shown in Figure 8-44.

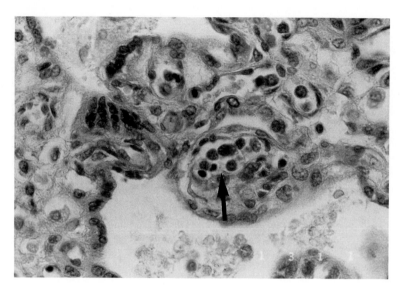

FIGURE 8-46 Donor placenta of twin transfusion syndrome with erythroblasts in fetal capillaries (*arrows*),

of placental growth and may not be associated with the same incidence and severity of congenital anomalies as in singletons.

Fetal Death in Utero

Perinatal mortality in recognized twin gestations is about 10%.[17] Early fetal loss is far greater. In a seminal ultrasonographic study, 71% of twin gestations diagnosed before 10 weeks' gestation were delivered as singletons.[62] One twin "vanished" before delivery. However, all twin gestations diagnosed after 15 weeks' gestation were delivered as twins. Overall perinatal mortality rates are roughly twice as high in monochorionic twins compared with dichorionic twins, with monoamnionic twins having the highest perinatal mortality rate.[63] Monoamnionic twins are prone to premature delivery, fetal death in utero

(presumably related to cord accident), and lower birth weights.[64] In a recent study, monoamnionic monochorionic twins of more than 20 weeks' gestational age showed 65% double survival rate and 70% overall survival.[64] Similar fetal death rates of 10% to 40% have been reported for monoamnionic twins.[65,66]

Fetus Compressus and Fetus Papyraceous

When death occurs in one twin during the first 3 months, all fetoplacental remnants may be resorbed. Death later in gestation results in a compressed but intact fetus, encased within the membranes, termed *fetus compressus* (Figs. 8-48 and 8-49). Further desiccation of fetal tissues results in a paper-thin, macerated, mummy-like appearance, termed *fetus papyraceous* (Fig. 8-50). There is significant overlap between these two categories. At delivery of a term

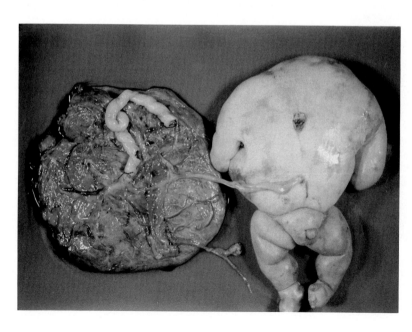

FIGURE 8-47 Acardiac twin showing umbilical vasculature derived from placental chorionic vascular anastomoses. The lower body is more completely formed than the upper body. (Courtesy of Dr. David Genest, Boston, Massachusetts)

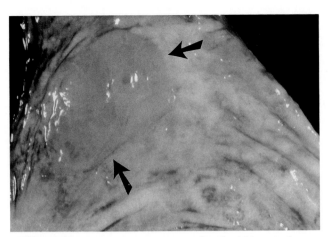

FIGURE 8-48 A fetus compressus enclosed within membranes (*arrows*). The extraplacental membranes of the surviving co-twin encircle the fetus compressus and its atrophic placenta.

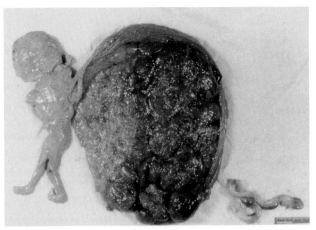

FIGURE 8-50 Maternal surface of monochorionic twin placenta with one twin a fetus papyraceus. The portion of the placenta supplying the fetus papyraceus was thin, fibrotic, and avascular. The surviving co-twin was healthy at birth.

gestation in which there was early intrauterine death of a co-twin, it is often hard to find any evidence of the antecedent twin, sometimes called a "vanishing twin" (see Fig. 8-48). Radiographs of the placenta and membranes may be helpful in disclosing fetal bones. Microscopic examination of a thickening or focal opacity of the fetal membranes may reveal cartilage and bony remnants.[67]

Placental villi of the dead twin may be recognized, particularly if the fetus survived well into the later half of gestation. If fetal death occurs within 1 month of delivery, the villi most commonly are smaller than expected for gestational age, with large syncytiotrophoblastic knots and recanalized blood vessels. Villous vascular recanalization, termed *hemorrhagic endovasculitis*, initially was thought to be associated with and causal of, rather than incidental to, fetal death in utero.[68] By microscopy, recanalization of the chorionic stem vessels by proliferating endothelium results in the formation of small blood-filled channels (Fig. 8-51). The muscular coat remains rel-

atively unperturbed. Apparent extravasation of entrapped and fragmented red blood cells creates a buckshot appearance. Subsequent studies demonstrated identical pathology in normal placentas that were maintained by artificial perfusion for a few days after delivery, implying that the initiating event is cessation of fetal circulation.[69]

PLACENTAL INFECTIONS

General Concepts

The two main types of fetoplacental infection are *acute infection* and *chronic infection*. Infections may involve both placenta and fetus, or one alone. There are two main routes of placental infection: ascending and hematogenous. *Ascending infections* are transmitted by the vagina and cervix directly into chorioamnion or by intermediary endometrial decidua. *Hematogenous infections* are caused by maternal blood-borne pathogens entering the intervillous space and crossing into placental villi, or by infection of decidua, which leads to involvement of placental structures. Ascending infections tend to be acute, whereas hematogenous infections more commonly are chronic.

Acute Chorioamnionitis

Acute chorioamnionitis is the most common cause of preterm birth throughout the world. Although pathologists and clinicians both diagnose chorioamnionitis, they do not use the same criteria.[70] Clinically, chorioamnionitis is diagnosed based on signs and symptoms of maternal infection, such as fever and tachycardia without an extrauterine source, bacteria on cultures or Gram stain of amnionic fluid, or foul-

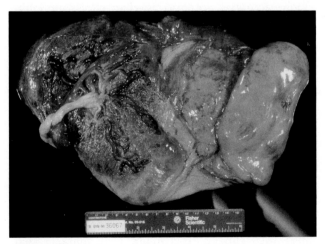

FIGURE 8-49 A fetus compressus that is slightly more mature than fetus in Figure 8-48 is enclosed within fetal membranes (*right*).

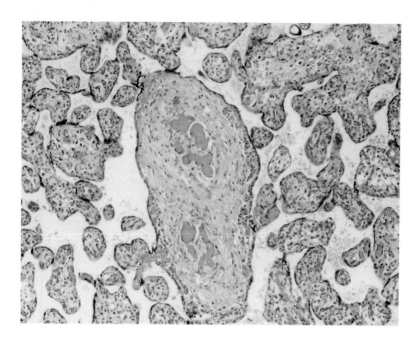

FIGURE 8-51 Vascular recanalization of chorionic stem vessel following fetal death in utero. Endothelial proliferation following cessation of fetal circulation results in repartitioning of vessel lumen.

smelling placenta at delivery. Clinically apparent chorioamnionitis has an incidence of 123 per 1000 births.

Pathologic diagnosis of chorioamnionitis, based on inflammatory cells in the placental membranes, occurs in 18% of term deliveries and in 32% of preterm deliveries.[71] Chorioamnionitis was found in 7.5% of placentas from elective cesarean deliveries performed before labor began.[71] In recent studies, 44%[72] to 72%[73] of placentas with histologically confirmed chorioamnionitis contained pathogenic organisms. This rate increased to 82% when there was a clinical diagnosis of chorioamnionitis.[73] In the latter study, more than 50% of pathogens were anaerobes.[73] The pathogens catalogued in individual studies vary depending on the patient populations, on whether anaerobic cultures were performed, and in some instances on the specific interests of the investigators. Organisms commonly isolated include *Staphylococcus epidermidis,* Gram-positive anaerobic cocci, group B β-hemolytic streptococcus, *Escherichia coli, Staphylococcus aureus, Listeria monocytogenes, Bacteroides* species, *Gardnerella vaginalis, Neisseria gonorrhoeae, Ureaplasma urealyticum,* and *Mycoplasma hominis.*

Chorioamnionitis is the most frequent pathologic diagnosis of placentas examined and is associated with increased neonatal morbidity in some studies.[72] However, chorioamnionitis is rarely associated with infants who develop signs of birth asphyxia (metabolic acidemia, seizures in the immediate newborn period, or Apgar scores of 3 or less)[24] in *term* gestations.[74] Recent studies suggest that no untoward fetal outcome is associated with chorioamnionitis if delivery is achieved within 24 hours.[75] Antepartum or neonatal death from intrauterine infection is uncommon. When it does occur, antemortem or postmortem blood cultures (in neonatal sepsis) and lung cultures (in congenital aspiration pneumonia) often reveal the same pathogens as those cultured from placenta or cervix. These results support the clinical view that chorioamnionitis is strongly associated with placental and, less commonly, fetal infections. One caveat must be added: as with other organ systems, all inflammatory lesions are not infectious in etiology. The possibility of membranitis resulting from noninfectious causes such as trauma or autoimmune processes cannot be excluded.

The controversy regarding rupture of membranes and chorioamnionitis is like the story of the chicken and the egg: Which came first? It seems logical that rupture of the membranes allows vaginal flora access to the amnionic cavity. It is just as plausible that infection may spread through contiguous structures to the amnionic cavity when the membranes are intact. Chorioamnionitis has been found with and without membrane rupture. The most widely accepted scenario is that chorioamnionitis weakens the membranes, inciting subsequent rupture.

Pathology of the Placenta in Chorioamnionitis

Grossly, chorioamnionitis is characterized by a heavy placenta with thickened, yellow-white to tan, cloudy membranes that may be foul-smelling (Fig. 8-52). A variety of pathologic terms have been used to describe its associated microscopic findings. *Acute chorioamnionitis* is defined by *maternal* leukocytic infiltrate of chorioamnion (Figs. 8-53 through 8-55). The term *chorionitis* may be applied to neutrophilic infiltrates confined to the chorion that have not crossed into the subamnionic connective tissue. The incidence and relevance of chorioamnionitis compared with chorionitis are not well characterized. Applicable factors may include the extent of membrane sampling, the proximity to the site of mem-

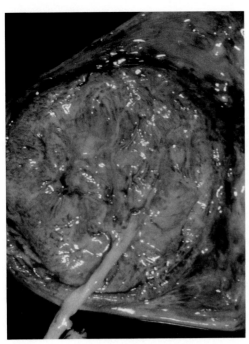

FIGURE 8-52 Fetal surface of placenta with chorioamnionitis. Membranes are thickened, opaque, and yellow-white.

brane rupture, and the duration of infection. Membrane rolls prepared from the site of rupture enhance the diagnostic yield.[76] Sometimes chorioamnionitis is not evident in the membrane roll, although it can be inferred by chorionic plate inflammation or umbilical vasculitis. Deciduitis, composed of neutrophils migrating from decidual vessels, invariably accompanies chorioamnionitis and chorionitis (see Fig. 8-53).

Umbilical Cord Inflammation (Funisitis)

Migration of *fetal leukocytes* through the muscular walls of the umbilical vessels, usually through the umbilical vein first and then through the arteries, is termed *umbilical cord vasculitis* or *funisitis* (Figs. 8-56 and 8-57). *Umbilical phlebitis* refers to inflammation involving the umbilical vein. A cord with extensive inflammation in which all the vessels and Wharton's jelly contain migrating fetal neutrophils may be described as umbilical panvasculitis and perivasculitis.

In long-standing umbilical inflammation, rings of degenerating inflammatory cells encircle the umbilical vessels in a pattern similar to an Ouchterlony immunodiffusion plate. Calcification may develop. Although most umbilical cord inflammation involves fetal leukocytes, in syphilis and toxoplasmosis the infiltrate may be lymphoplasmocytic. Although it is commonly believed that acute chorioamnionitis precedes funisitis, the temporal relations between these lesions are not well characterized. It is probably safe to assume that in most cases umbilical inflammation implies some sort of fetoplacental infection.

Chorionic Plate Vasculitis

In a fashion analogous to that of the umbilical cord, migration of *fetal leukocytes* from the chorionic vessels through the muscular walls toward the amnion constitutes *chorionic vasculitis*. It has been suggested that the hallmarks of ascending infection follow an ordered sequence: deciduitis, chorioamnionitis, and umbilical cord vasculitis, with chorionic plate vasculitis last in the sequence. This may be true, but there is no evidence documenting this sequence.

Villous Edema

Villous edema results from accumulation of excess stromal fluid and is characterized by a punched-out, Swiss-cheese appearance of the villous stroma (Fig. 8-58). It may be found in many pathologic states including those causing hydrops fetalis: blood dyscrasias, fetoplacental infection, and congenital anoma-

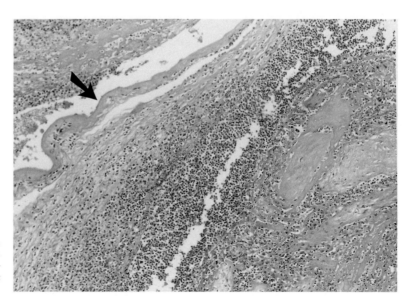

FIGURE 8-53 Extraplacental membrane roll showing chorioamnionitis with necrotic amnion (*arrow*) and dense neutrophilic infiltrate of amnion, chorion, and maternal decidua. Sclerotic villi of chorion laeve are visible (*right*).

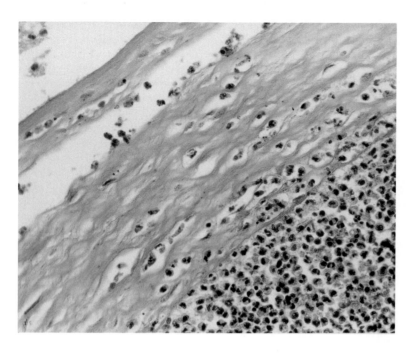

FIGURE 8-54 A high-power magnification of Figure 8-53 showing inflammation of the amnion. There is a large collection of neutrophils (*lower right*) between the amnion and underlying chorion (not pictured).

lies, particularly those impeding venous return to the heart. Naeye found villous edema in 87% of placentas with chorioamnionitis.[77] Its severity and extent were associated positively with the cord arterial blood pH values, low Apgar scores, vigorous resuscitation at birth, need for assisted ventilation later, frequency of hyaline membrane disease, and neonatal mortality.[77]

Acute Fetal Infection

Transplacental passage of particularly virulent organisms results in acute fetal infection (early onset neonatal sepsis) in 3 to 5 births per 1000. The fetus is infected by swallowing or aspirating infected amnionic fluid or hematogenously through infection of placental villi, umbilical cord vessels, or chorionic plate vessels. Fetal infection generally is manifested by congenital fetal aspiration pneumonia resulting from inhalation of infected amnionic fluid containing viable bacterial organisms (Fig. 8-59). Swallowing of infected fluid results in bacterial colonization of the gastrointestinal tract with subsequent parenchymal invasion producing enteritis, pancreatitis, or rarely gastritis. Bacteria can be identified by lung, blood, or spleen cultures.

Beta-hemolytic streptococcus is the prototypic organism for this condition. Despite early and appro-

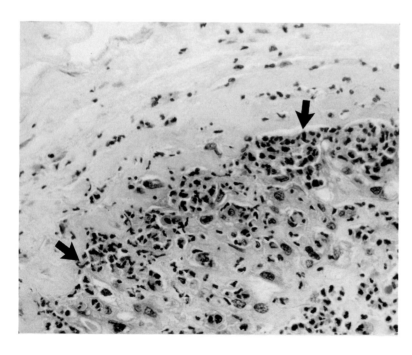

FIGURE 8-55 Chorioamnionitis showing maternal neutrophils invading from the decidua through the chorion (*arrow*) and into the amnion (*upper left*).

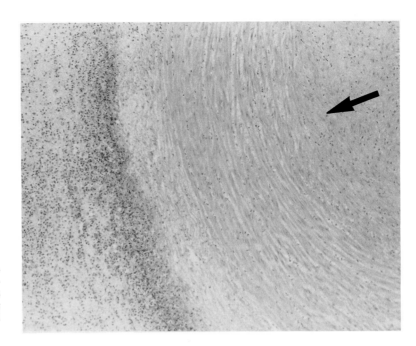

FIGURE 8-56 Umbilical cord with funisitis showing marked, concentric, neutrophilic inflammation of the umbilical artery with fetal neutrophils migrating from the vessel lumen to the amnionic cavity. The arrow indicates the direction of fetal neutrophilic migration.

priate pharmacotherapy, there is a high perinatal mortality rate associated with acute fetal infection, particularly in preterm neonates. Other commonly identified organisms include *Staphylococcus epidermidis, Escherichia coli* and *Ureaplasma urealyticum.*[78]

Chronic Fetal Infection

Chronic fetal infections may involve the fetoplacental unit or the fetus or placenta alone. In chronic fetoplacental infection, clinically apparent disease occurs in 1 to 2 births per 1000. The placental villi become colonized, and the infection may remain localized within the villi or may spread systemically by accessing fetal villous vasculature. With some infectious agents (eg, herpes simplex), the fetus may succumb to systemic disease in utero even though the delivered placenta shows minimal stigmata of infection.

Chronic Villitis

The hallmark of chronic placental infection is *chronic villitis.* Chronic villitis is defined by a mononuclear inflammatory cell infiltrate involving villi (Fig. 8-60). It may be focal or diffuse and is often basal. The infiltrate consists mostly of lymphocytes and mononuclear histiocytic cells, with occasional plasma cells.

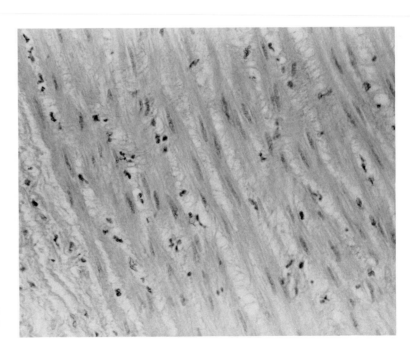

FIGURE 8-57 High-power magnification of same specimen as Figure 8-56 showing fetal neutrophils between the muscle fibers of the umbilical artery.

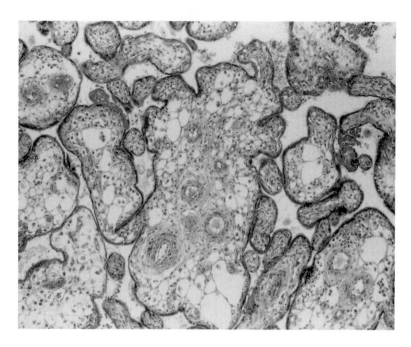

FIGURE 8-58 Villous edema involving a second-trimester placenta. Villous stromal edema forms collections of clear spaces, giving a "Swiss cheese" appearance to the stroma.

Immunohistochemical studies of these lesions demonstrate predominantly helper T lymphocytes and activated macrophages that react with monoclonal antibodies to D-related human leukocyte antigen.[79]

The incidence of chronic villitis depends on the population studied and the number of sections examined per placenta. In general, about 10% of placentas contain chronic villitis. Prevalances of 13.6%[80] and 7.6%[81] have been reported. In a recent study examining an average of 13.4 blocks per placenta, chronic villitis was identified by histology or immunohistochemistry in 76% of normal term placentas.[82]

Although chronic villitis is a common and distinct pathologic lesion, pathogens are rarely found. Characteristic infiltrates are associated with some agents, but inferences of a specific organism based on villous histopathology in the absence of diagnostic pathogens remains speculative. Assays of umbilical cord immunoglobulin M (IgM) values as an index of fetal infection document increased IgM values in less than 10% of cases with chronic villitis.[83] This has led some to proffer that chronic villitis, although definitely associated with infection in some placentas, is most commonly the result of an immunologic reaction.[79] Others counter this notion by suggesting that the immunologic reaction results from, or is associated with, the placental infection.

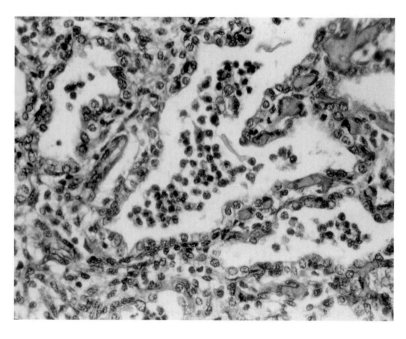

FIGURE 8-59 Fetal lung with congenital aspiration pneumonia. Numerous maternal neutrophils and fetal squames are aspirated into fetal alveoli. Interstitial fetal neutrophils were present elsewhere.

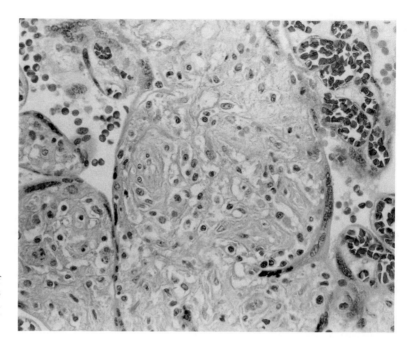

FIGURE 8-60 Term placenta with focus of chronic villitis characterized by expanded villous stroma with mononuclear cell infiltrate composed of lymphocytes and histiocytes. Plasma cells may be seen in some cases.

Chronic Chorioamnionitis

Chronic chorioamnionitis, a condition of uncertain etiology, is defined by chronic inflammatory cells within the chorioamnion (Fig. 8-61). In a recent study of chronic chorioamnionitis, no specific pathogen was identified.[84] Chronic chorioamnionitis with chronic umbilical panvasculitis and perivasculitis is commonly associated with spirochetal infections, such as by *Treponema pallidum*.

Chronic Fetal Infection

The most common signs of fetal infection in utero include growth retardation and preterm birth. An enlarged placenta (placentomegaly), particularly with hydrops or chronic villitis, suggests fetal infection. Autopsy findings in fetal or neonatal death due to infection include hydrops, jaundice, purpura, skin rashes, eye lesions, hepatosplenomegaly, central nervous system anomalies, and parenchymal plasma cells.

Specific Pathogens

Bacterial Organisms

Beta-Hemolytic Streptococcus. More than 50% of serious neonatal infections are caused by group B

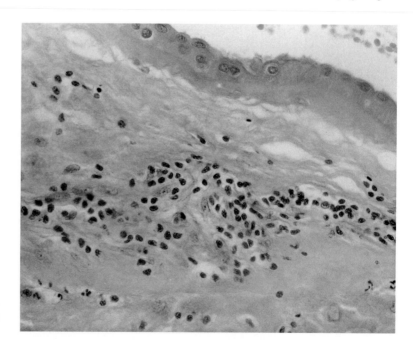

FIGURE 8-61 Chronic chorioamnionitis characterized by lymphocytic infiltrate of the chorion and amnion.

β-hemolytic streptococcus. Maternal colonization ranges from 5% to 50% with perinatal transmission rates of 0.5%.[85] In the United States, 3 of every 1000 infants develops a streptococcal congenital aspiration pneumonia, sepsis, or meningitis.[86] Despite appropriate treatment, the combined neonatal morbidity and mortality rate associated with group B β-hemolytic streptococcal infection exceeds 50%. Although β-hemolytic streptococcus is the most common offender, *Staphylococcus aureus* is moving to the top of the list at some centers. Novak and Platt found chorioamnionitis in 64% of placentas associated with early onset group B streptococcal neonatal sepsis, funisitis in 27%, and organisms on the fetal membranes in 41%.[87] Villous edema was present and was focal in 23% and diffuse in 18%.[87]

Grossly, placentas with streptococcal infection have cloudy membranes and may be heavy for gestational age. Occasionally, the membranes are yellow-white, opaque, and foul-smelling. Early infection, particularly in immature placentas, may be inapparent on gross examination.

Microscopy shows chorioamnionitis ranging from mild or moderate chorionitis to severe, necrotizing chorioamnionitis with numerous bacterial colonies (Fig. 8-62; see also Figs. 8-53 and 8-54). The umbilical cord shows panvasculitis and perivasculitis, often with concentric rings of inflammatory cells and many necrotic surrounding cord vessels (see Figs. 8-56 and 8-57). The most intense inflammation is directed toward the amnionic surface. In some instances, cocciform bacterial colonies sit atop the amnion with little underlying inflammation (see Fig. 8-62). We have seen rare cases of fetal death from congenital aspiration pneumonia with culture-proved β-hemolytic streptococcus infection of lung and spleen without any significant placental inflamma-

tion. The villi in streptococcal infections are often edematous and have a Swiss-cheese appearance (see Fig. 8-58). Septic intervillositis and fetal chorionic vasculitis with thrombus formation occur in advanced cases.

Listeria Monocytogenes.

Listeria monocytogenes is a diphtheroid bacillus responsible for outbreaks of listeriosis. It has been associated with abortions and fetal death in cattle and other animals, including humans. It is a facultative intracellular bacterium whose eradication requires macrophage- and T-cell-mediated immunity. Growth of *L. monocytogenes* is enhanced by cold temperatures. Maternal infection usually occurs after consumption of milk, milk products such as cheese, and meat products contaminated by infected manure. Maternal infection results in decidual seeding that spreads to involve the placenta. Intrauterine fetal infection carries a high perinatal mortality rate. In an infected fetus or a stillborn or liveborn delivered with disseminated disease, the condition is termed *granulomatosis infantiseptica.*[88]

Placental pathology is virtually pathognomonic in fully developed listeriosis. Macroscopically, multiple, small, yellow-white foci dot the cut surfaces of the placental villi. By microscopy, these consist of multifocal, villous micro- to macroabscesses with villous necrosis; smaller lesions show acute villitis (Fig. 8-63). Neutrophils and fibrin surround affected villi, and a characteristic acute villitis develops. Numerous neutrophils accumulate in an artificially created subtrophoblastic space and then invade the villous stroma. Occasionally, multinucleated giant cells are formed in villous abscesses (see Fig. 8-63). Sometimes there is chorioamnionitis, but it is far less extensive than in the average β-hemolytic streptococcal chorioamnionitis. The diphtheroid organisms of lis-

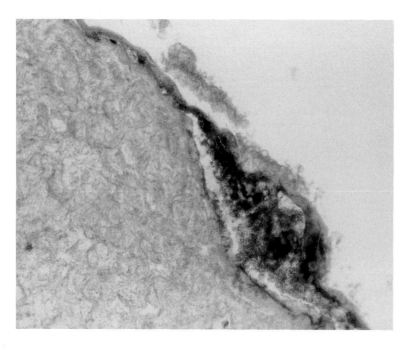

FIGURE 8-62 Amnion of extraplacental membranes showing a large subepithelial collection of cocciform bacterial colonies.

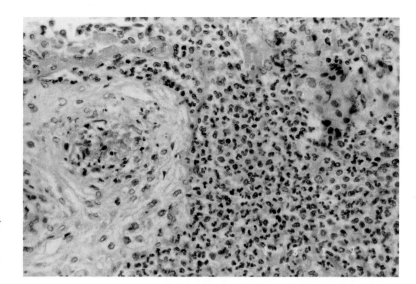

FIGURE 8-63 Acute intervillositis with slight acute villitis in a placenta infected with *Listeria monocytogenes.* There is a massive accumulation of maternal leukocytes in the intervillous space, with focal acute inflammation involving the villus (*left*). A poorly formed multinucleated giant cell can be seen (*upper right*).

teriosis seem to accumulate and proliferate preferentially in the amnion overlying the chorionic plate or in the villous abscesses, and, although difficult to identify in some cases, they are best highlighted by Brown-Brenn or Gram stains. Cold-enrichment of the placenta (ie, storage in the refrigerator overnight or on a long weekend) favors demonstration of organisms.

Syphilis. Syphilis, a disease thought to be relegated to historical texts, has made a dramatic resurgence within our communities. The smallest of us have taken the lion's share of the burden, since unrecognized congenital syphilis may be lethal in utero.

Treponema pallidum, the spirochete that causes syphilis, is hematogenously transmitted to the placenta during maternal spirochetemia. Although it was suggested that infection could not occur in early gestation, this is not the case. Grossly, placentas infected with syphilis are pale, bulky, edematous, and heavy. Focal lesions are not recognized.

Early infection with *T. pallidum,* as with *Toxoplasma* species, may invoke no inflammatory response. Abundant spirochetes, best seen on Warthin-Starry stains, are found in Wharton's jelly and are totally devoid of surrounding host reaction. As infection continues, a chronic necrotizing funisitis develops,[89] often containing lymphocytes, plasma cells, and much karyorrhectic debris. Necrotizing funisitis is not specific for syphilis because it may develop in viral and bacterial infections. The placenta reflects the spirochetal infection and the associated fetal anemia by showing a characteristic chronic villous vasculitis (Fig. 8-64). Villous capillaries contain circulating nucleated red blood cells and erythroblasts.

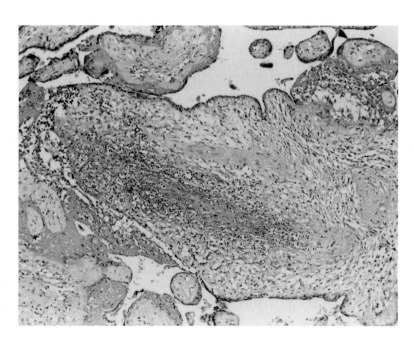

FIGURE 8-64 Necrotizing villous vasculitis in a near-term placenta infected with syphilis. Villi are expanded by a mononuclear cell infiltrate that is centered on and destroying vessel walls. The hydropic fetus was stillborn.

Other Bacteria, Genital Mycoplasma, Ureaplasma, and Chlamydia. Placental infections caused by virtually all known fetal and neonatal pathogens have been described. The literature is replete with case reports demonstrating the pathology associated with specific agents. In *Ureaplasma urealyticum, Mycoplasma hominis,* and *Chlamydia* placental infections, the placental pathology is nonspecific, usually consisting of chorioamnionitis and funisitis. Further data regarding these agents can be found elsewhere.[78]

Viral Infections

Cytomegalovirus. Cytomegalovirus (CMV), one of the *Herpesviridiae,* is the most common cause of perinatal infections, with an incidence ranging from 8 to 22.2 per 1000 births. In the United States, 3000 to 4000 infants are born each year with symptomatic disease.[90] In many, congenital CMV infection is unrecognized. Late sequelae include unilateral or bilateral deafness, blindness, and mental retardation. Virus reaches the placenta by hematogenous dissemination during the viremic phase of primary or recurrent maternal infection. A maternal-fetal transmission rate of 20% to 50% has been reported.[91] Although fetal infection may occur at any time during gestation, the greatest sequelae are associated with infection in early and mid-gestation, particularly when the mother is unsensitized. Neonatal CMV infection is common and is associated with minimal or no sequelae.

Grossly, the placenta infected with CMV may be small, normal, or large for gestational age. In recent and severe infection, it is commonly edematous, pale, and heavy, particularly when fetal anemia is present. In early infections, the placental weight may be normal.

CMV is a major cause of chronic villitis. Microscopically, CMV is characterized by a necrotizing villitis, described by some as "acute" and by others as "chronic" (Figs. 8-65 and 8-66). It is "acute" in the sense that the infection is active and ongoing, and "chronic" because lymphocytes and plasma cells constitute the inflammatory infiltrate. The villi are edematous and show foci of ongoing, active villous destruction with thrombosis of villous capillaries, necrosis of stroma and overlying trophoblast, lymphocytic and plasmacytic infiltration, hemosiderin deposition, calcification, and stromal hyalinization. Over time, there is villous stromal scarring (see Figs. 8-65 and 8-66). The severe, destructive lesions may be focal, with remaining villi relatively normal or slightly hypercellular. CMV is diagnosed by finding the pathognomonic violaceous, intranuclear and cytoplasmic inclusions in endothelial cells, stromal cells, Hofbauer cells or, much less commonly, trophoblast. The stromal Hofbauer cells may be prominent, showing unusual configurations.[92,93] Villous endothelial destruction results in an acute vasculitis that progresses to an obliterative vasculitis. Viral inclusions may be found in decidua, amnionic macrophages, and amnion.[94] The stromal inflammatory cells have been characterized as T cells and fetal plasma cells, the latter secreting IgG and IgM.[92] If no inclusions are identified in initial sections of necrotizing villitis, additional villous tissue should be examined microscopically. Newer approaches to the diagnosis of viral placentitis include immunoperoxidase staining, in situ hybridization, and polymerase chain reaction.

In long-standing lesions, viral inclusions may be inconspicuous or absent. The necrotizing deciduitis associated with CMV placentitis supports the notion that fetal CMV infection may result from reactivation of latent virus in the endometrium.[95] There has been

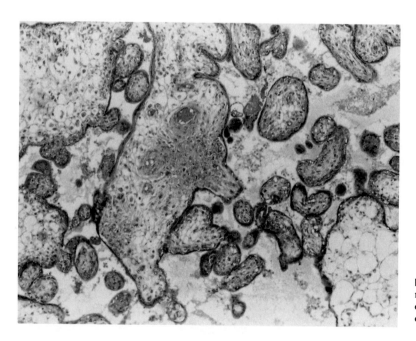

FIGURE 8-65 Acute necrotizing villitis in cytomegalovirus infection of placenta. Note the villous edema of the surrounding villi. The central villus depicts two foci of villous necrosis.

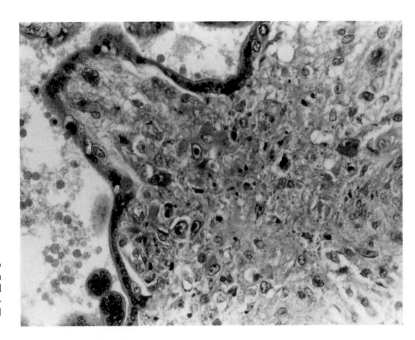

FIGURE 8-66 A magnification of Figure 8-65 demonstrating effects of cytomegalovirus infection of placenta. Villous stroma is necrotic and eosinophilic, and stromal cells contain both "owl-eye" intranuclear and granular cytoplasmic viral inclusions.

some correlation between the extent and severity of placental involvement and the clinical outcome.[96] In lethal congenital CMV infections, the fetus is jaundiced and anemic and has hepatosplenomegaly. Viral inclusions are found in the epithelia and mesenchyme of many fetal organs, including the lung, thymus, thyroid follicles, pancreatic and bile ducts, glomeruli, and renal tubules. Central nervous system involvement may result in hydrocephalus, microcephaly, and microcalcifications. Surviving children may have cataracts, chorioretinitis, and deafness.

Herpes Simplex Virus Types 1 and 2. The incidence of neonatal herpes simplex virus (HSV) infections is estimated to range from 1 in 2500 to 1 in 10,000 deliveries.[97-99] Eighty percent of HSV infection in the neonate is of type 2, and 20% is type 1. In the United States, 16.4% of adults are seropositive for HSV type 2.[100] Asymptomatic shedding of virus occurs in 0.35% to 2.3% of pregnant women.[101,102] Fetal transmission of HSV in a primary maternal infection is associated with an increased frequency of spontaneous abortions, congenital malformations, and stillbirth.[97,98] Maternal seropositivity for HSV type 2, but not for HSV type 1, reduces the neonatal transmission of HSV type 2 infection.[102] Recurrent infection is the most common form of infection during pregnancy.[100,102] Perinatal transmission occurs in 33% of women with a primary infection, compared with 3% with reactivated infection.[101] HSV is most commonly acquired intrapartum, although rare cases of hematogenous dissemination have been documented. Neonatal HSV infection is associated with a 50% mortality rate despite treatment with vidarabine or acyclovir.[103]

The hallmarks of antenatal HSV infection of the placenta are not well characterized. Even when the fetus is stillborn and when autopsy discloses multifocal destructive hepatic and pulmonic parenchymal lesions, placental findings may be minimal and nonspecific (Fig. 8-67). Typical ground-glass nuclear inclusions of HSV in the placenta are rare.[104,105] Inclusions have been demonstrated in chorion.[105] Garcia described a placenta infected with HSV that showed intranuclear inclusions in decidual cells, chronic chorioamnionitis, chronic lymphoplasmacytic villitis with Langhans'-type giant cells containing necrotic foci centered on villous vessels, and villous trophoblast necrosis with fibrin deposition.[106] A recent study of neonatal HSV infections depicted villous stromal cells containing viral antigens by immunohistochemistry and virions by electron microscopy.[107] Others have reported acute or subacute necrotizing membranitis with amnionic necrosis,[96,104,108] mononuclear or plasmacytic chronic chorioamnionitis,[108] agglutination of villi, fibrinoid necrosis or thrombosis of villous vessels, bland placental necrosis,[96,109] and necrotizing deciduitis. Benirschke illustrates a remarkable plasmacytic infiltrate of membranes with a subamnionic blister.[17] Herpetic placentas can be identified by polymerase chain reaction,[110] and infected cells may be mapped by directly labeled oligonucleotide probes.[111]

The infant may develop vesicular skin lesions, hepatoadrenal necrosis, and meningoencephalitis. In lethal cases, the fetal lung and liver show extensive geographic necrosis with residual ground-glass nuclear inclusions at the periphery of necrotic zones (see Fig. 8-67).

Varicella. Chickenpox is caused by infection by varicella-zoster virus, another member of the *Herpesviridae*. Congenital fetal infection results from intrauterine transmission of maternal infection by viremia

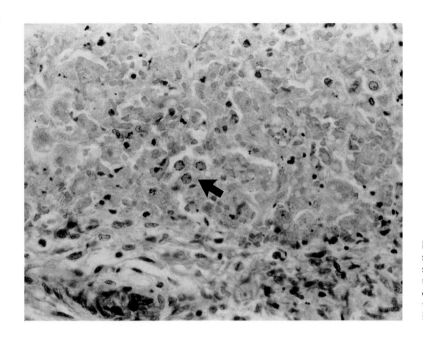

FIGURE 8-67 Neonatal liver in congenital herpes simplex virus 2 infection. There were large, sharply demarcated areas of hepatic necrosis containing ground-glass nuclear inclusions (*arrow* indicates three involved cells). The infant died 3 weeks after birth from a systemic herpetic infection.

in an unsensitized gravida. Primary infection occurs at an incidence of 1 to 5 per 10,000 pregnancies,[112,113] with perinatal transmission in 26%.[114] Infection in the first trimester may be associated with chorioretinitis, cataracts, cutaneous scars, and limb hypoplasia.[115,116] Neonates infected antepartum may be born with the chickenpox rash or may develop it within a week or so after birth.

Placental findings depend on the duration of infection and, as in all viral infections, the extent to which the placenta is sampled for microscopic examination. In one case, villous involvement produced grossly recognized "rice seeds."[117] Varicella may be characterized by acute necrotizing villitis or granulomatous villitis. Early lesions are composed of focal, acute, necrotizing villitis that is similar to but not associated with the degree of destructive necrosis found in CMV infection. Even in these early lesions, multinucleated histiocytic giant cells may be striking (Fig. 8-68). Along with eosinophilic intranuclear viral inclusions, these cells help to differentiate varicella from CMV placentitis. As the disease progresses, an extensive granulomatous villitis develops.

Parvovirus B-19. Parvovirus B-19 was discovered serendipitously in 1975 during screening of blood for hepatitis B.[118] It is the cause of the childhood exanthem erythema infectiosum, also known as *fifth disease*. It also causes aplastic crisis in chronic hemolytic anemia, a chronic rheumatoid arthritis, and

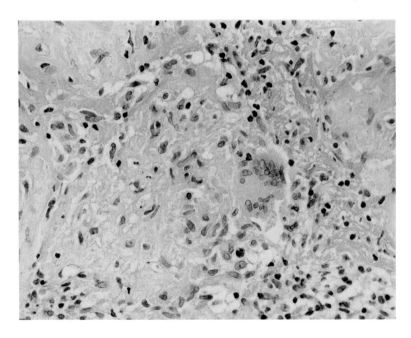

FIGURE 8-68 Placenta in congenital varicella-zoster infection. Villous outlines are obscured by a dense, fibrinous exudate containing mononuclear cells and a multinucleated giant cell. Villous parenchyma showed slight liquefaction. Apart from this focus, the other villi showed only chronic villitis. The baby was hospitalized for chickenpox 6 days after delivery.

chronic bone marrow suppression. Its association with spontaneous abortion is well-described in the veterinary literature. In humans, it has been reported to cause spontaneous abortions and nonimmune hydrops fetalis due to aplastic anemia or myocarditis. Congenital parvovirus infection has been diagnosed and treated successfully in utero.[119] In children, apart from fever, catarrhal symptoms, and a rash, it is a benign disease with anemia occurring only rarely.

Placental infection is most likely to occur by a hematogenous route in a nonsensitized woman. In a study of 10 women with clinically proved disease, fetal transmission was documented in 3 cases, and anomalies were described in 1 fetus.[120] The placental pathology mirrors the degree of fetal anemia. The placenta may be heavy, bulky, and pale. Fetal villous capillaries contain numerous nucleated red blood cells with erythroblasts. Erythropoiesis may be found in the villi. Parvovirus infection involves red blood cell precursors and nucleated red blood cells. Infected nuclei are enlarged and distended by a homogeneous, glassy-red to violaceous, intranuclear inclusion. These inclusions are like those of HSV infection except that they are more violaceous. It is uncommon to see these affected cells in the placenta, even when there is extensive fetal involvement. We have seen similar inclusions in developing fetal organs such as the lung, thyroid, kidney, and skeletal muscle. It appears that the inclusions may involve a variety of immature fetal mesenchymal and epithelial cells, not only the red blood cells within these structures.

Depending on the fixative used, similar-appearing cells are found in early first-trimester placentas in which the nucleated red blood cells are derived from the yolk sac. It is not clear whether all such placentas contain parvovirus infection, or whether this unusual nuclear appearance is the result of erythroblastosis of yolk sac or villous stromal origin. Similarly, certain decalcifying solutions used in our institution for bone marrow decalcification create intranuclear inclusions in erythroid precursors that are indistinguishable from parvovirus. After excluding other causes of hemolytic and nonhemolytic hydrops, parvovirus infection should be considered if a hydropic placenta contains numerous nucleated red blood cells. In formalin-fixed tissues, pathognomonic viral inclusions are sufficient for a diagnosis of parvovirus infection. If parvovirus is suspected, serologic analysis of maternal or fetal IgM and IgG for parvovirus-specific antibodies or a polymerase chain reaction for parvoviral DNA in placenta or fetal tissues should be performed.

Hepatitis B.

Hepatitis B infection may be transmitted hematogenously to the placenta and fetus. Asymptomatic hepatitis B infection was found in 0.66% of women in a low-risk group.[121] Although the infection usually develops postnatally, presumably by enteric infection, rare transplacental infec-

tion has been documented, suggesting that the placenta serves as an intermediary.[122]

Placental findings in congenital hepatitis B infection are primarily related to elevated maternal bilirubin levels. Khudr and Benirschke described bilirubin in chorionic macrophages and villous Hofbauer cells.[123] In a severe case, villous tissue curetted from an icteric woman was deep yellow-green, and the villi had bile pigments by microscopy.[17] Apart from placental cells stained by bile and villous edema,[124] specific placental parenchymal changes do not seem to occur in most cases of hepatitis B infection.

Human Immunodeficiency Virus (HIV).

The World Health Organization estimates that more than 3 million women of reproductive age are infected with human immunodeficiency virus.[125] Maternal to fetal transmission of the human immunodeficiency virus type 1 (HIV-1), which causes the acquired immune deficiency syndrome (AIDS), occurs in about 24% to 30% of cases.[126,127] Perinatal transmission increases as maternal CD4 lymphocyte counts decrease.[128] It is estimated that 0.05% of all neonates born in the United States are infected with the HIV virus.[128] Within a group of high-risk women, 7.1% were found to be antibody-positive.[129] Neonatal seroconversion in congenital infection may not occur until after infancy. In a recent study, measurement of neonatal HIV-IgA levels showed a high overall sensitivity and specificity for determining neonatal infection.[130] Life expectancy is severely reduced both for the mother and infected neonate. Treatment is supportive at best, and no cure or preventive vaccine has been developed.

Although many investigators have examined carefully the placentas of women with known HIV positivity or AIDS, few morphologic findings have been described. This may reflect an inability to determine which placentas are infected, or it may be that infection results in minimal placental pathology. Jauniaux and colleagues studied placentas from 49 HIV-infected mothers and found no distinct lesions.[131] This agrees with our experience. Lewis and associates found HIV in trophoblast, Hofbauer cells, and embryonic blood cell precursors using immunocytochemistry and in situ hybridization.[127] Villous destruction does not seem to occur in HIV infection. As with all human tissues, full protective precautions must be taken; in placental examination, this includes gown, gloves, mask, and eye protection.

Rubella.

The highest incidence and greatest severity of sequelae result from congenital rubella infection during the first trimester. As with all viral placentitides, the pathology depends on the severity and stage of maternal or placental infection. In acute maternal infection, the placenta tends to be smaller than normal. Gross lesions are not observed. Microscopy shows focal necrotizing villitis with acute villous endovasculitis; the latter is characteristic of congenital rubella infection.[132] Severe endothelial necrosis of villous vessels may fragment red blood cells but is not associated with villous stromal hemorrhage. Additional vascular pathology includes endothelial cushions and old calcified thrombi.[93] Obliteration of villous blood flow results in shrunken, avascular villi, and villous agglutination may result from trophoblast injury with subsequent fibrin deposition. Eosinophilic cytoplasmic viral inclusions may be found in endothelial cells, stromal cells, macrophages, and trophoblast.[133,134] In contrast to CMV placentitis, the villitis of rubella is not associated with stromal hemosiderin deposition or villous edema.

The fetal sequelae of congenital rubella infection depend on the gestational age of the fetus. Fetal death in utero may occur when infection occurs in the first trimester. Just as in the placenta, the virus is vasculotropic, destroying fetal blood vessel walls and resulting in ischemia and parenchymal organ abnormalities. Nonlethal sequelae of early infection include the following:

> Congenital malformations, particularly involving the cardiovascular system
> Intrauterine growth retardation
> Interstitial pneumonitis
> Hepatomegaly with parenchymal necrosis
> Focal extramedullary hematopoiesis
> Periportal round cell infiltrates
> Bile stasis and jaundice
> Splenomegaly with anemia, purpura, and thrombocytopenia
> Small, fibrotic spleen
> Cataracts
> Deafness
> Microcephaly and mental retardation.

Plasma cells in fetal lymph nodes connote premature B cell maturation. Widespread immunization of children for rubella has decreased the incidence of overt congenital rubella infections. The long-term effects of live vaccines remain unknown. Reinfection of previously immunized women has been reported.[135,136]

Other Viral Infections. In general, viral infection of the placenta results in villous destruction with mononuclear and plasma cell infiltrates, in viral inclusions with or without giant cells, and in villous agglutination. In *mumps* infection, presence of the paramyxovirus can be inferred by eosinophilic cytoplasmic inclusions in villous fibroblasts and decidual cells.[137] Maternal-fetal transmission of *measles* infection was associated with fetal stillbirth in one reported case. Measles viral antigens were found in the syncytiotrophoblast and decidua by immunoperoxidase and immunofluorescence studies.[138] There were agglutination of villi with trophoblast necrosis, diffuse intervillous fibrin, and mononuclear cells.[138] Placental infection by the *Epstein-Barr virus* in maternal infectious mononucleosis resulted in perivasculitis

and necrotizing deciduitis, acute chorionitis, villous edema, necrotic trophoblast, and obliterative villous vasculitis with mononuclear and plasmacytic inflammation.[139,140]

No specific placental lesions are described for the picornavirus infections of *poliomyelitis, ECHO virus,* and *Coxsackie B virus.* Garcia and colleagues reported villitis and intervillositis in placentas with ECHO 33 and ECHO 27 infection.[141] Placental hydrops resulting from severe fetal myocarditis may develop in Coxsackie B infection.

Parasitic and Protozoan Infections

Toxoplasma gondii. In developed nations, the most common parasitic infection that the placental pathologist is likely to encounter is the coccidian *Toxoplasma gondii.* Cats serve as the primary hosts. Cultures in contact with cats, particularly cat litter boxes and outdoor sandboxes, are at risk for toxoplasma from fecal contamination by oocysts. Humans, sheep, and pigs become hosts for the secondary cycle. Congenital toxoplasmosis is more common in France due to the consumption of infected raw meat (ie, steak tartare or undercooked meat) containing cysts and tachyzoites. Transplacental transmission in seronegative women results in primary fetal infection in about 50% of women. Fetal infection in early pregnancy may result in severe abnormalities, including hydrocephalus, seizures, central nervous system calcifications, hydrops fetalis, and chorioretinitis leading to blindness. Transmission is more common later in pregnancy, with the consequences being less severe. In infected infants, new lesions may appear late into childhood.[142]

Placental *Toxoplasma* infection may be overlooked by the most experienced obstetric pathologist. Congenital *Toxoplasma* infections often are missed because of the total lack of inflammation surrounding the cysts and because high-power examination ($\times$200 to 400) is required to identify the organisms.

Grossly, the placenta in toxoplasmosis is similar to that of villitis in general: heavy, edematous, and pale. Some have a normal weight. Microscopic examination discloses villitis, with a spectrum of lesions ranging from subtle lymphocytic chronic villitis with minimal villous fibrosis to a proliferative villitis with lymphoplasmocytic infiltrates eventually terminating in fibrosis. Villous endarteritis and focal necrosis may occur.[143] The encysted organisms are 200 μm in diameter and can be found in the amnion, the subamnionic macrophages of the chorioamnionic membranes, the umbilical cord, and even within the trophoblast (Fig. 8-69).[144] Most often, the cysts and sometimes even the newly released organisms remain totally unperturbed within the subamnionic connective tissue. Occasionally slight calcification and single cell necrosis trumpet their presence. Over time, rupture of cysts with extrusion of free organisms sparks a chronic lymphoplasmocytic infiltrate. A chronic funisitis may develop in the cord. The released sin-

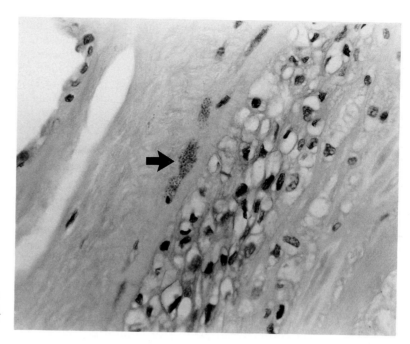

FIGURE 8-69 Congenital toxoplasmosis infection disclosing encysted organisms within macrophages (*arrow*) of subamnionic connective tissues of extraplacental membranes.

gle, small, crescent-shaped organisms are 2 to 4 μm by 4 to 8 μm. Periodic acid-Schiff stains are positive. The decidua shows chronic lymphoplasmacytic inflammation and rarely contains parasites.

Chagas' Disease. Maternal–fetal transmission of Chagas' disease, caused by infection with *Trypanosoma cruzi,* occurs by hematogenous dissemination to the placenta. The trypanosome infects trophoblast and Hofbauer cells, and then enters the fetal circulation. Infected placentas are heavy and pale, showing a chronic destructive villitis with fibrin deposition and intervillositis, ending in villous destruction with scarring.[145,146]

Villitis of Unknown Etiology

Unfortunately, all discussions of chronic villitis must end with villitis of unknown etiology. In placentas with genuine chronic villitis, failure to identify the offending agent by morphologic recognition of the organism, by history, or by serologic studies occurs in 6% to 33.8% of cases.[147] In 1973, Altshuler coined the term *villitis of unknown etiology* to describe such cases.[148] Russell found focal chronic villitis of unknown etiology in 7.6% of placentas.[81] It has been associated with fetal growth retardation and perinatal mortality and may recur in subsequent gestations.[80,81,149] It is not clear whether the villitis is due to an unknown infection or is the result of an immune-mediated phenomenon.[147] Some suggest that an unrecognized infection invokes an immune response, whereas others opine that the entire process is immunologic and devoid of an infectious component.[147,150] Clearly, further investigation is warranted.

Fungal Infections

Organisms of *Candida* species are the most common fungi to involve the placenta and its adnexa. This infection is described and illustrated earlier in this chapter in the section on the umbilical cord.

PARENCHYMAL PLACENTAL LESIONS

Infarcts

In the placenta, as in other tissues, infarcts occur when perfusion stops. Inciting events in the placenta include alterations in maternal blood flow through the maternal uterine arteries and premature separation of the placenta from its implantation site. Most infarcts result from disturbances in uteroplacental perfusion and are associated most frequently with maternal disorders such as preeclampsia. In preeclampsia and other diseases, decidual vasculopathy (atheromatous change) of the uterine vessels diminishes the luminal diameter, obstructing and ultimately preventing adequate placental perfusion. At this point, infarction occurs. Much less commonly, infarcts are associated with a retroplacental hematoma. Infarcts may occur anywhere within the villous parenchyma, but they are more frequently basal and peripheral.

Placental infarcts are uncommon in immature placentas. At term, small infarcts occupying less than 5% of the total parenchyma may be found in 25% of placentas and are inconsequential.[151] The significance of a placental infarct depends on many factors: most important are the number and extent of the in-

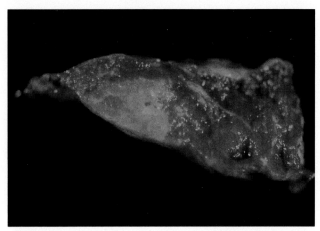

FIGURE 8-70 Placenta with wedge-shaped marginal infarct.

farcts. When more than 10% of the placenta is infarcted, fetal well-being is jeopardized. There is a rough correlation between the quantity of infarcted villous tissue and the degree of fetal compromise.

Placental infarcts take on a variety of gross and microscopic appearances. On gross examination, a recent, fresh infarct is well-demarcated, beefy red, and more firm than the surrounding parenchyma (Fig. 8-70). In fresh infarcts, demarcation from normal parenchyma is more easily palpated than visualized. As the infarct ages, it becomes brown and then turns yellow to white. The oldest infarcts look like white scars.

On microscopic examination, the villi in a recent infarct are crowded together, diminishing the normal intervillous space (Fig. 8-71). The villous vessels are congested and dilated, and blood may extravasate into the stroma. Trophoblast nuclei become hyperchromatic, and karyorrhexis ensues (Fig. 8-72). Scant fibrin is deposited at the periphery of

the infarct and in the intervillous space. Usually there is a minimal to slight maternal neutrophilic infiltrate surrounding the infarct, although it may be totally absent.

Less commonly, infarcts result from decreased maternal villous perfusion due to the interposition of an underlying retroplacental hematoma. Blanc has suggested that a villous infarct associated with a retroplacental hematoma evinces similar but slightly different histology: The intervillous space between infarcted villi is enlarged and congested when the infarct is due to retroplacental hematoma and is collapsed when it is a result of maternal vasculopathy.[152]

As the infarct ages, there is a loss of nuclei in the trophoblast and villous stromal and vascular cells, and the dead villi eventually become pale pink on hematoxylin-eosin staining (Figs. 8-73 and 8-74A). The fetal stem artery of the infarcted villi thromboses. Later, the infarct consists of pale white scaffolds of "ghost villi" outlined by fibrin. Viable villi adjacent to an infarct are small, containing more multinucleated syncytial giant cells than those distant from the infarct.

Infarcts are more frequent when there is a maternal history of preeclampsia or hypertension.[151] Large areas of infarcted villi encircling small foci of preserved villi are most commonly associated with severe obstruction of maternal blood flow to the placenta, which may result in intrauterine death, fetal hypoxia, or growth retardation.[151] Most commonly, the pathology of the affected maternal vessels is not evident in the decidua underlying the infarct, although occasionally the superficial decidual vessels show characteristic vasculopathic changes. The identification of decidual vasculopathy is enhanced by examination of the decidua parietalis (in the extraplacental membranes). If present, decidual vasculopathy suggests a similar affliction in some retroplacental implantation-site vessels.

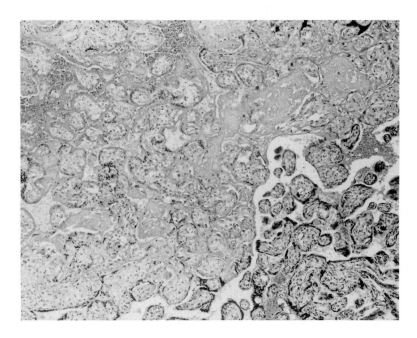

FIGURE 8-71 Recent villous infarct, low-power magnification, characterized by villous crowding with interspersed fibrin and early trophoblast necrosis.

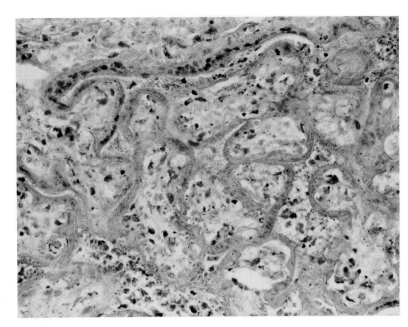

FIGURE 8-72 Recent villous infarct (higher power magnification of specimen in Fig. 8-71), showing focal pallor of trophoblast nuclei, trophoblast necrosis, villous stromal necrosis with nuclear debris, and fragmentation of nuclei in intervillous space.

Fibrin Deposition

Intervillous fibrin deposition occurs in 22% of term placentas and, less commonly, in preterm placentas or in those pregnancies complicated by preeclampsia, essential hypertension, or diabetes mellitus.[12,13,153] Most term placentas contain some subchorionic fibrin grossly recognizable as tiny, white to yellow subchorionic streaks on the fetal surface. Many have a 1- to 2-cm plaque of subchorionic fibrin that is inconsequential. Naeye has correlated an absence of subchorionic fibrin with fetal hypoactivity, cerebral palsy, low childhood intelligence quotient, fetal hypotonia, trisomy 21, and short umbilical cord.[154]

Microscopically, fibrin is often found in the subchorionic space. Not uncommonly, tiny foci of fibrin deposition surround scattered villi within the placental parenchyma. It is believed that eddy currents are greatest under the chorionic plate, resulting in some destruction of the trophoblast surface with adherence of fibrin and platelets. Occasionally, villi underlying a subchorionic plaque become entrapped within the fibrin. Although fibrin is acellular, it may entrap maternal red blood cells. Fibrin deposits on villous trophoblast and intermediate trophoblast (from the placental septa and cell islands) invoke trophoblastic proliferation to some extent, possibly as a reaction to the fibrin stranglehold (see Fig.

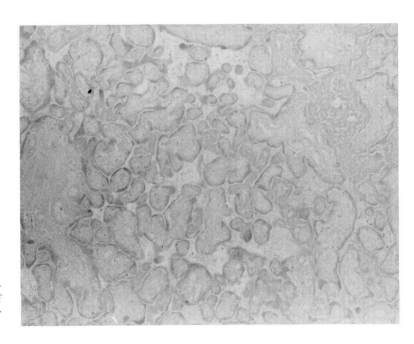

FIGURE 8-73 Remote villous infarct, low-power magnification, with bland homogenization of villous stroma and few trophoblastic nuclear outlines remaining.

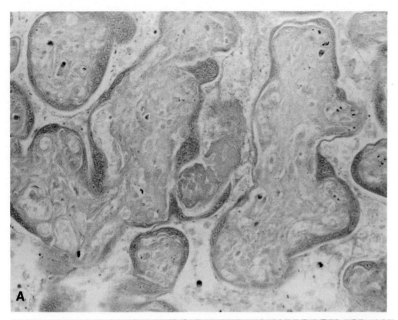

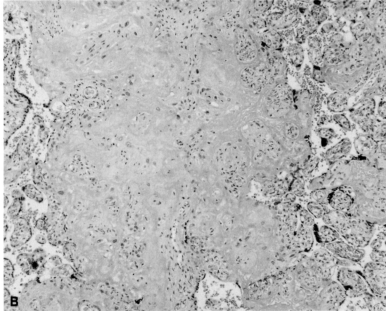

FIGURE 8-74 **(A)** Remote villous infarct (higher magnification of specimen in Fig. 8-73) showing crowded villi, amorphous stroma with few cellular outlines, and ghost nuclei of syncytiotrophoblast. **(B)** Intervillous fibrin deposition: fibrin encircles normal villi, invoking a proliferation of intermediate trophoblast.

8-74*B*). The proliferating trophoblast, usually intermediate trophoblast, may mimic primary and metastatic malignancy by its cytologic atypia and mitotic activity.

There are unusual states of extensive fibrin deposition in which virtually all the villi are surrounded by a fibrin blanket, described by some as "massive intervillous fibrin deposition" (the so-called glitter infarct).[155] It is often associated with excessive decidual fibrin deposition with chronic inflammation and infarction of basal villi, termed *maternal floor infarction*.[17] There appears to be a relation between the two, because they often coexist in the same pla-

centa. Both are associated with fetal growth retardation and poor perinatal outcome, and they may recur in subsequent pregnancies. In many, the fetus is stillborn. It is unclear whether the stillbirth is the result of, or etiology for, both maternal floor infarction and massive intervillous fibrin deposition.

Placental Hematomas and Abruption

Placental hematomas occur at many sites. Grossly, a hematoma may be *retroplacental, marginal, retromembranous,* or *subamnionic* (Fig. 8-75). All are derived

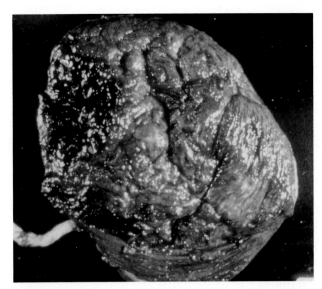

FIGURE 8-75 Retroplacental hematoma (*upper left*) and marginal hematoma (*lower left*) viewed from maternal surface of placenta.

from maternal blood except for the subamnionic hematoma, which is fetal in origin and often results from undue traction on the umbilical cord to hasten placental delivery. Microscopic examination of placental hematomas shows layering of fibrin and red blood cells (Fig. 8-76).

The most dangerous of the placental hematomas, *massive retroplacental hematoma*, usually results from a tear in a decidual spiral artery. The leaking blood forms a large retroplacental blood clot. The hematoma may be large enough to dissect the placenta entirely off the decidua, resulting in a complete abruption and total loss of placental perfusion, which, without immediate delivery, leads to fetal death in utero. If the placenta remains partially attached (partial abruption), the villous tissue overlying the abruption usually becomes infarcted.

Retroplacental hematomas occur in 4.5% of placentas.[13] The incidence increases threefold in pregnancies complicated by preeclampsia.[13] Retroplacental hematomas, particularly when large, are associated with increased perinatal mortality. A diagnosis of retroplacental hematoma may be obvious in a placenta with attached hematoma, or it may be inferred based on the amount of clotted blood received with a placenta in the specimen container, or based on the presence of a large, fixed, smooth depression on the maternal surface indicating its former location. All retroplacental hematomas should be described, measured, and recorded. Although there is often an association between a retroplacental hematoma and a clinical diagnosis of abruption, the two do not go hand in hand. A clinical diagnosis of abruption may be associated with a placenta showing no pathologic evidence of hematoma, and the corollary is true: a retroplacental hematoma may not be associated with a clinical diagnosis of, or sequelae from, abruption.

The so-called marginal sinus bleed or tear is a small hematoma that sometimes develops along the placental margin (see Fig. 8-75). The blood spreads centrifugally, extending retromembranously and retroplacentally. A large marginal hematoma may result in antepartum maternal hemorrhage with "port wine" amnionic fluid. If the hematoma is long-standing, there may be hemosiderin deposition in macrophages of membranes and decidua. This hematoma is of no clinical significance to the fetus.

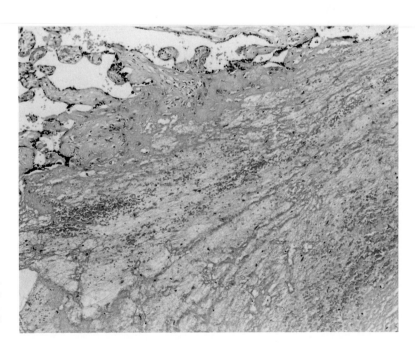

FIGURE 8-76 Microscopy of retroplacental hematoma showing layers of fibrin and red blood cells separating basal plate from maternal decidua. This case was associated with a clinical diagnosis of abruption.

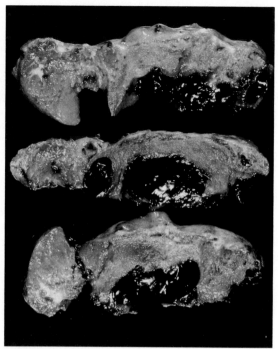

FIGURE 8-77 Placenta with multiple large, recent intervillous thrombi associated with infarction of surrounding villi.

Intervillous and Subchorionic Thrombi

An *intervillous thrombus* is a space-occupying, intraplacental blood clot that displaces surrounding villi. Intervillous thrombi may be single or multiple and usually are situated midway between the chorionic plate and the basal plate (Fig. 8-77). They commonly measure 1 to 2 cm in diameter but may exceed 3 to 4 cm. Intervillous thrombi are found in up to 40% of all placentas.[13] When fresh, an intervillous thrombus is mahogany-red, soft, and gelatinous (see Fig. 8-77). Over time, the thrombus firms as the blood components layer out, and a laminated appearance ensues. The initial mahogany-red color fades to white. Sometimes an intervillous thrombus may be difficult to differentiate grossly from an infarct.

Microscopically, it is composed of red blood cells and fibrin (Fig. 8-78). An aged thrombus is laminated, with alternating layers of red blood cells and fibrin (Fig. 8-79). Intervillous thrombi never organize. The blood of an intervillous thrombus is a mixture of maternal and fetal blood. Fetal blood loss into an intervillous thrombus is purported to cause fetal-maternal hemorrhage[156] and may prompt maternal sensitization to fetal red blood cell antigens.[157] Surrounding villi are displaced but usually are not infarcted. Occasionally, stromal villous hemorrhages are found.

Massive subchorial thrombosis, which is greater than 1 cm in thickness, has been called *Breus' mole.* It represents a recent subchorionic thrombus that protrudes into the amnionic cavity or down to the basal plate, or both. As it matures, it becomes laminated and may enlarge, displacing and disrupting a large amount of normal parenchyma. These thrombi are associated with fetal death in utero and are maternal in origin.[13,48,158]

Fetal Artery Thrombosis

Thrombosis of a fetal artery results in loss of fetal villous perfusion. The involved villi are grossly similar to infarcted villi. The lesion is pyramidal, appearing triangular on full-thickness cross sections, with its apex pointing to the chorionic plate. As the lesion ages, the villi become white and shrink.

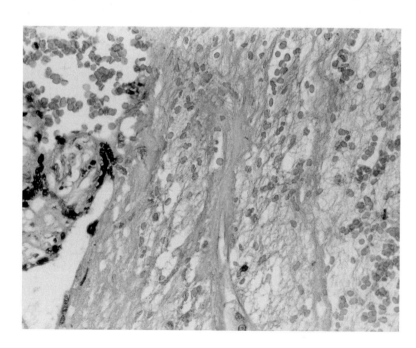

FIGURE 8-78 Recent intervillous thrombus with fibrin entrapping red blood cells. Adjacent villus is viable.

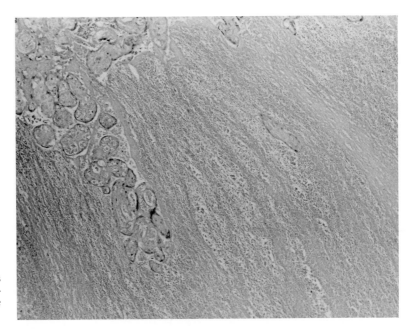

FIGURE 8-79 An older, laminated intervillous thrombus showing thick layers of fibrin and entrapped red blood cells. Adjacent villi are infarcted.

Microscopically, the thrombosis may involve a fetal chorionic artery or, just distal to that, a mainstem villous artery (Fig. 8-80). The villi most distal to the thrombosis are completely avascular, with those more proximal showing fibromuscular sclerosis of stem villous vessels, most likely a reactive change (Fig. 8-81). In distal villi, fibrous obliteration of the villous vessels is accompanied by stromal hyalinization. In some foci, maternal perfusion of the intervillous space continues, and the syncytiotrophoblast remains viable and may form large knots. A localized fetal artery thrombosis is more common in diabetics[13,36] and occurs in 4.5% of full-term placentas.[13] In some placentas, thrombosis of 20% to 30% of the villi apparently has been inconsequential to the fetus.[12] Greater degrees of villous avascularity, approaching 50%, have resulted in fetal death.[12]

PLACENTAL PATHOLOGY ASSOCIATED WITH MATERNAL AND FETAL DISORDERS

Maternal Disorders

The scope of this chapter allows only an introduction to the placental findings associated with maternal disorders. The most common maternal conditions affecting the placenta—preeclampsia, essential hypertension, diabetes mellitus, and maternal malig-

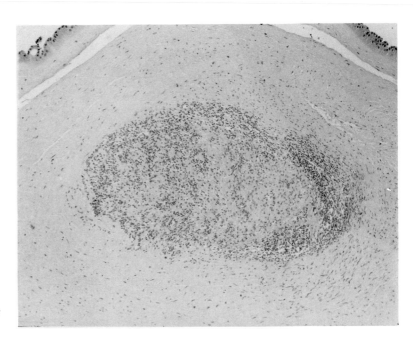

FIGURE 8-80 Thrombosis of a fetal artery of the chorionic plate.

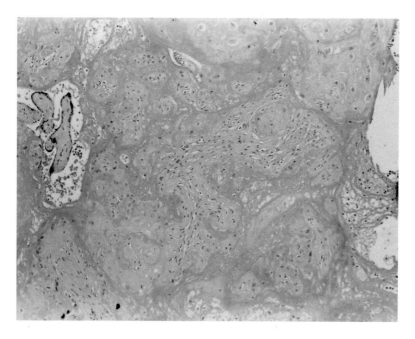

FIGURE 8-81 Villi distal to the thrombus depicted in Figure 8-80. There is dense intervillous fibrin deposition and fibromuscular sclerosis. Note the lack of villous blood vessels and a few uninvolved villi (*left*).

nancy—are discussed in this section. For a review of other less common maternal diseases such as intrahepatic cholestasis of pregnancy,[12] sickle cell disease and trait (Fig. 8-82),[159–163] maternofetal rhesus incompatibility,[17,164] systemic lupus erythematosus,[12,13] and maternal exposure to toxins,[12,13] the reader should consult the literature cited.

Preeclampsia (Toxemia of Pregnancy) and Eclampsia

Preeclampsia is one of the most serious maternal disorders whose onset is occasioned solely by pregnancy. Preeclampsia is defined by hypertension and protein-uria or generalized edema developing after 20 weeks' gestation. It becomes eclampsia when accompanied by a maternal seizure. Despite extensive research, the etiology of preeclampsia remains unknown.

Although the literature reviewing placental pathology associated with preeclampsia is voluminous, much of it remains conflicting. Most investigators agree that in preeclampsia the placenta tends to be smaller than normal, and that infarcts, particularly recent ones, and retroplacental hematomas are more common.[12,165,166] The amount and extent of infarction seem proportional to the severity of preeclampsia: 33% of placentas in mild preeclamptics have infarcts, compared with 60% for those with severe disease.[12] Apart from these lesions, the noninfarcted

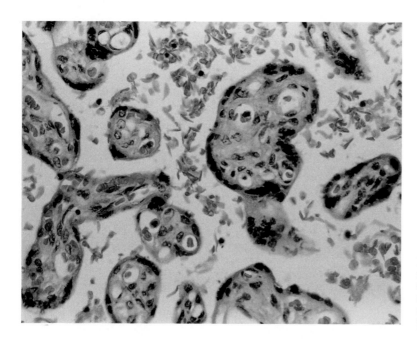

FIGURE 8-82 Maternal sickle cell disease. The maternal red blood cells in the intervillous space are sickled. Fetal hemoglobin F protects fetal cells against sickling, and the fetal status with regard to sickle cell trait or disease cannot be ascertained by placental examination.

villi tend to have a more prominent cytotrophoblastic layer and a thickened basement membrane.[12] In some, there are excessive syncytiotrophoblastic knots (so-called Tenney-Parker knots; Fig. 8-83), decreased number of and smaller villous vessels, and narrowing of fetal stem arteries.[167–169] Maternal vascular changes, known as decidual vasculopathy (eg, acute atherosis, acute atheromatous changes), are presented in the preceding section on the fetal membranes. It has been suggested that many of the placental changes in preeclamptics result from the lack of a second wave of trophoblastic invasion of maternal myometrial arteries: The vascular muscle and elastic lamina remain intact. This precludes further vascular dilatation and increased placental perfusion, which are essential for normal fetal growth in later pregnancy.

Essential Hypertension

Clinically, the term *essential hypertension* refers to hypertension preceding 20 weeks' gestation. Pregnancy-induced hypertension is defined as hypertension occurring later in pregnancy and unaccompanied by proteinuria and edema. The placental findings in essential hypertension are similar to those of preeclampsia: infarcts, retroplacental hematomas, increased cytotrophoblast, and thickening of the trophoblastic basement membrane. In addition, and differentiating it from preeclampsia, an unusual form of decidual vasculopathy (hyperplastic arteriosclerosis) has been described in essential hypertension. It consists of vessels with increased overall diameter, markedly thickened glassy-eosinophilic walls, and proliferations of the intima that result in luminal narrowing and uteroplacental ischemia.[170–172] Hyperplastic arteriosclerosis is best observed in the uterine radial arteries and is seen less frequently in the intra-myometrial implantation-site vessels. There appear to be minimal fetal sequelae in pregnancies with uncomplicated essential hypertension.[12,173,174]

Diabetes Mellitus

Maternal diabetes mellitus is associated with fetal macrosomia and increased neonatal morbidity. In general, the placental hallmark of maternal diabetes mellitus, whether gestational or not, is placentomegaly. Some of the largest and heaviest placentas, excluding those from erythroblastosis fetalis, are from diabetic mothers. The placenta is bulky and thickened by edematous villi. In some, the placenta is normal or small for gestational age. Single umbilical artery is 3 to 5 times more common in diabetics, as are some congenital malformations, particularly those involving the cardiovascular system.[36,175] The cord itself, like the macrosomic placenta and fetus, is larger than expected.

Microscopically, the increased villous bulk is translated into villous immaturity and villous edema. The cytotrophoblastic layer is prominent and shows persistent mitotic activity. The trophoblastic basement membrane is thickened. Fibrinoid necrosis of villi is more common in diabetics.[176] In addition to acute atherosis, Driscoll has described an additional type of decidual vasculopathy in 50% of diabetics consisting of arteriolar medial hypertrophy, hyalinization, and onion-skinning.[36]

Hydrops Placentalis: Immune and Nonimmune

Within this broad category are a large number of lethal or severely debilitating fetal diseases, the pathol-

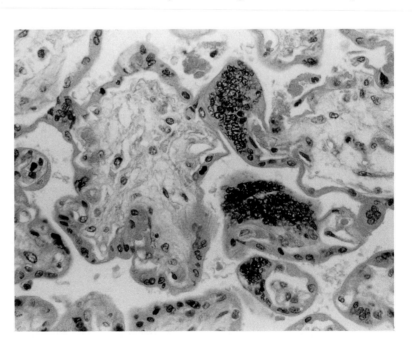

FIGURE 8-83 Tenney-Parker syncytiotrophoblastic knots in placenta from a woman with preeclampsia.

ogy of which directly involves, or is reflected in, the placenta. Extreme villous edema has been termed *villous hydrops* or *hydatid change* and refers to an excessive accumulation of clear watery fluid resulting in the formation of grossly visible, swollen, grape-like placental villi. Villous hydrops may be diagnosed early in gestation by obstetric ultrasonography and is often associated with hydrops fetalis, a condition consisting of an abnormal accumulation of watery, serous fluid in the fetal tissues.

Hydropic placentas tend to be large, heavy, bulky, pale, and spongy. Microscopically, the villi are immature and edematous. The cytotrophoblast is conspicuous, and cell proliferation is evidenced by increased mitotic activity. Fetal capillaries contain nucleated fetal red blood cells and erythroblasts (see Fig. 8-46). In many instances, the placental changes reflect fetal anemia, heart failure, or increased venous pressures. For a concise and clear review of the pathophysiology of fetal hydrops, the reader is referred to the recent comprehensive article by Machim.[177]

Formerly, the most common cause of hydrops placentalis was Rhesus blood group incompatibility. With the advent of the immune globulin preparation (RhoGAM) in the 1960s, the incidence of maternal sensitization has decreased markedly. Because of improved diagnosis and treatment of affected fetuses, marked placental hydrops due to Rh disease is uncommon. Leading the list of causes of placental hydrops are congenital malformations with and without associated genetic disorders, infections, α-thalassemia, blood group incompatibilities due to ABO and Kell antigens, red cell dyscrasias, congenital nephrotic syndrome (Finnish nephrosis), fetal-maternal hemorrhage, and storage disorders.

OTHER VASCULAR LESIONS OF THE PLACENTA

Chorangiosis is a term describing a distinct increase in the number of villous vessels, which has been correlated with poor neonatal outcome (Fig. 8-84).[178] The validity of this lesion has been challenged by some who claim that it represents filling and distension of previously collapsed vessels. Chorangiosis defined by Altshuler's criteria of "ten villi, each with ten or more vascular channels in ten or more noninfarcted and nonischemic zones of at least three different placental areas" (using a 10× objective) is uncommon in routine placental material. The rarity of this lesion in our experience and its association with high-risk pregnancies lends support to the contention that increased villous vascularity relates to poor neonatal outcome. Clearly, further investigation is warranted.

PLACENTAL CALCIFICATION

Calcification of the placenta increases throughout gestation. First-trimester placentas are rarely calcified. Scattered calcific deposits occur in the second trimester, and by term most placentas have scattered calcifications. Ultrasonographic determination of placental calcification is expressed as grades ranging from 1 to 3. Neither histologic nor ultrasonographic assessments of placental calcifications can be used to determine pulmonary maturity. Although the amount of placental calcification is variable, there are no studies demonstrating a relation between calcification and neonatal outcome.

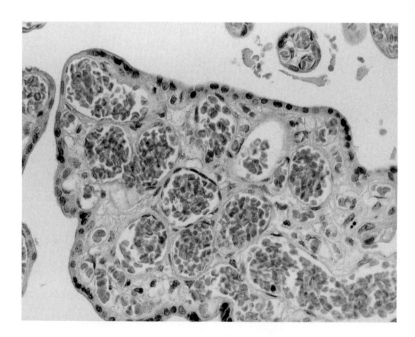

FIGURE 8-84 Chorangiosis of placenta depicting a villus with more than 10 vessels. Diagnosis requires multiple fields containing similar such villi.

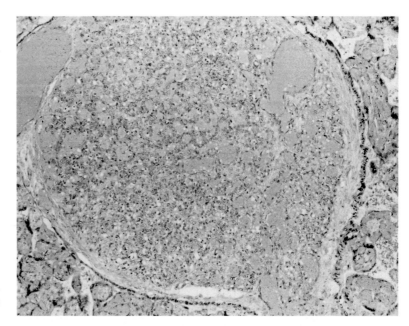

FIGURE 8-85 Microscopic chorangioma illustrating vascular proliferation within the confines of a single villus.

TUMORS OF THE PLACENTA

Benign Tumors

The most common benign tumor to involve the placenta is a *chorangioma*. It is composed of a localized proliferation of fetal blood vessels and villous stroma, generally occurring within the confines of one or a few villi. Most are small and recognized by microscopy alone (Fig. 8-85). Large tumors may form a rounded mass, bulging into the amniotic cavity (Fig. 8-86). Such large tumors are often associated with polyhydramnios and hydrops fetalis from vascular shunting; thrombocytopenia, hemolysis, or disseminated intravascular coagulation; and, in some, intrauterine death. Although mitotic activity may be brisk in some chorangiomas, no metastases have been reported.

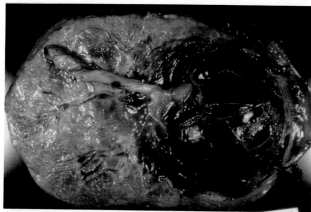

FIGURE 8-86 Large chorangioma of the placenta forming a hemorrhagic mass that bulges from the fetal surface toward the amnionic cavity.

Uncommonly, *placental teratomas* have been found embedded between the amnion and the chorion in the placenta or in subamnionic location in the umbilical cord. Their histopathology is akin to that of the mature (cystic) teratoma of the ovary: skin and fat are virtually always present. No malignant placental teratoma has been reported. The origin of placental teratomas is controversial. Faulty migration of germ cells from the yolk sac represents the most likely theory, with unrecognized twin gestations (similar to acardiac fetuses) remaining an alternative mechanism.[179]

Malignant Tumors

Melanoma is reported to be the most common malignant tumor to metastasize to the placenta,[180] although in our practice metastatic breast carcinoma is more common by far. Any hematogenously disseminated tumor may metastasize to the placenta, and a gynecologic malignant tumor may involve the placenta by direct extension. Circulating malignant cells from fetal tumors such as neuroblastoma and lymphoma can escape the confines of the villous capillaries and invade the stroma. Choriocarcinoma is discussed below.

GESTATIONAL TROPHOBLASTIC DISEASES

Hydatidiform mole, the most common gestational trophoblastic tumor, results from an abnormal fertilization event. In hydatidiform moles, as in the other trophoblastic tumors, neoplasia is due to uncontrolled trophoblastic proliferation. Trophoblastic tumors may be subclassified dichotomously as tumors with villi–hydatidiform mole, partial and complete; and tumors without villi–choriocarcinoma and placental site trophoblastic tumor. The World Health Organization classification of gestational trophoblastic tumors is presented in Table 8-4.

Based on genetic and morphologic criteria, hydatidiform moles are divided into two types: partial hydatidiform mole and complete hydatidiform mole.[181,182] A pathologic distinction between these hydatidiform moles is necessary as they are associated with differing clinical outcomes. A 10% to 30% incidence of gestational trophoblastic disease follows complete mole, compared with 5% for partial mole.[183] Although its overall incidence may be falling, choriocarcinoma may develop after complete mole;[184] however, it rarely occurs after partial mole.[185]

The *incidence* of molar pregnancies varies throughout the world, ranging from 1 in 4500 deliveries in the United States[186] to 1 in 1300 deliveries in Israel[187] and 1 in 85 to 373 deliveries in Indonesia.[188] The mean age of women with partial and complete moles is similar, near 28 years.[183] Women with complete or partial mole are more likely to have a personal or family history of previous gestational trophoblastic disease, and personal history of two or more previous spontaneous miscarriages, infertility and smoking.[189] Having had one complete mole increases a patient's risk of a subsequent mole by 100-fold. Both groups tend to present with abnormal vaginal bleeding, with complete mole more commonly associated with increased uterine size for dates, toxemia, thyrotoxicosis, theca lutein cysts and hyperemesis.[190]

The standard *treatment* for both types of hydatidiform mole is uterine evacuation, generally by dilatation and curettage. Follow-up consists of monitoring serum or urine β human chorionic gonadotropin (hCG) levels. Although spontaneous remission follows most molar evacuations, any consistent plateau or rise in hCG values should prompt treatment with chemotherapy.

There are marked *genetic* differences in hydatidiform moles. The complete mole is diploid by cytogenetic studies[191] and generally is diploid or tetraploid by flow cytometric studies (Fig. 8-87). In

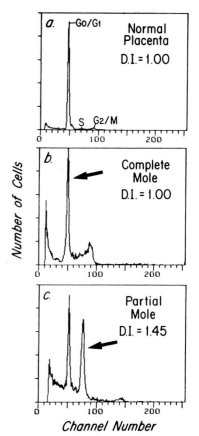

FIGURE 8-87 DNA histograms. **(A)** Diploid hydropic abortus. **(B)** Diploid complete hydatidiform mole. **(C)** Triploid partial hydatidiform mole. Channel number reflects nuclear DNA content. The DNA index (D.I.) is the ratio of the test sample modal G0/G1 DNA content to control (diploid) modal G0/G1 DNA content. G0/G1 peaks of complete mole **(B)** and partial mole **(C)** are indicated by arrows. The G0/G1 peak of the complete mole contains the same DNA content as the added control lymphocytes; therefore, the D.I. = 1.0. (Lage JM, Driscoll SG, Yauner DL, Olivier AP, Mark SD, Weinberg DS. Hydatiform moles: application of flow cytometry in diagnosis. Am J Clin Pathol 89: 596–600, 1988)

contrast to the genotype of normal diploid placenta, the 46 chromosomes of a complete mole are totally paternal in origin, termed androgenetic.[191] About 90% of complete moles are derived from the fertilization of an empty ovum by a haploid spermatozoon which then duplicates its DNA (homozygous complete mole). The remaining 10% are produced from fertilization of an empty ovum by two different spermatozoa resulting in a mixture of homozygous and heterozygous alleles (heterozygous complete mole). There is no difference in the natural history of homozygous versus heterozygous complete moles. Maternal mitochondrial DNA is preserved in complete mole, supporting the postulated "empty-ovum" theory.[192]

In contrast, the partial mole is triploid, having 69 chromosomes: the maternal pronucleus with its haploid DNA is conserved and, instead of fertilization by one haploid set of paternal DNA, *two* haploid sets of paternal DNA are added.[181] Thus, there is a

TABLE 8-4
World Health Organization Classification of Gestational Trophoblastic Diseases

Hydatidiform mole
  Complete
  Partial
Invasive hydatidiform mole
Choriocarcinoma
Placental site trophoblastic tumor
Trophoblastic lesions, miscellaneous
  Exaggerated placental site
  Placental site nodule or plaque
Unclassified trophoblastic lesion

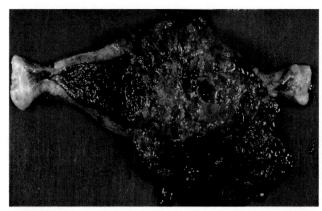

FIGURE 8-88 Complete hydatidiform mole in a gravid hysterectomy specimen.

predominance of paternal DNA in partial and complete mole. In the partial mole, the retained maternal haploid component serves to mollify the histologic expression and natural history of the disease.

Complete Hydatidiform Mole

Pathology

The complete mole has such a characteristic *macroscopic appearance* that it may be diagnosed by the ultrasonographer, attendant at delivery, or pathologist (Fig. 8-88). The placenta is voluminous, far exceeding that expected for gestational age. The villi swell, forming numerous grossly recognizable vesicles (Fig. 8-89). The size of the vesicles depends on the age of the mole and the manner of evacuation, and the largest villous vesicle averages 1.6 cm in maximum diameter.[183] No fetal parts are found.

Microscopic examination discloses diffuse, marked villous enlargement due to massive stromal edema.

The edema displaces the mesenchymal stroma centrally, creating an acellular clear space called a central cistern (villous cavitation). There is marked proliferation of cyto- and syncytiotrophoblast (Fig. 8-90). Some villi have remnants of villous vessels with degenerating nucleated red blood cells. Well-formed villous vessels with abundant nucleated red blood cells are not characteristic of complete hydatidiform mole. The endomyometrial implantation site contains large, hyperchromatic trophoblast.

Evolution

Most women with complete mole undergo spontaneous gonadotropin remission after molar evacuation. In 10% to 30%, chemotherapy is required to eradicate residual molar villi or trophoblast.[183,190] The incidence of pathologically confirmed choriocarcinoma after complete mole seems to be decreasing in the United States, developing in less than 1% to 2%. In a recent study of 150 women with complete mole followed at a trophoblastic disease center, 33 received chemotherapy for persistence, and none developed choriocarcinoma.[184]

Most commonly, there is no attempt to obtain tissue for pathologic evaluation of metastases because the risks of operation outweigh the information gained. Accordingly, the clinical term "persistent gestational trophoblastic disease (or tumor)" was coined to encompass all types of molar residua. The chemotherapeutic regimens used to treat persistent disease are based on a variety of clinical parameters, focusing on the clinical extent of disease, hCG values, and type of antecedent gestation.

Endometrial curettings in patients with persistent gestational trophoblastic disease after complete hydatidiform mole usually contain residual molar villi and avillous, or implantation-site, trophoblast. Frank choriocarcinoma is rare. A diagnosis of choriocarcinoma should be contemplated only after the

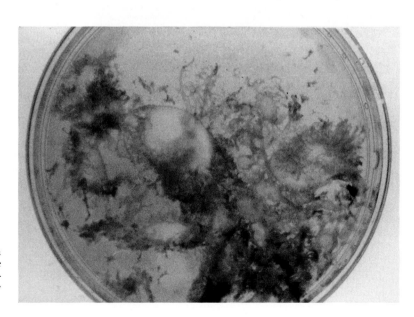

FIGURE 8-89 Molar villi floated in saline in a petri dish (same specimen as in Fig. 8-88). Villi are swollen, filled with fluid, and covered by hyperplastic trophoblast that may be recognized grossly as fibrillary projections from villous surfaces.

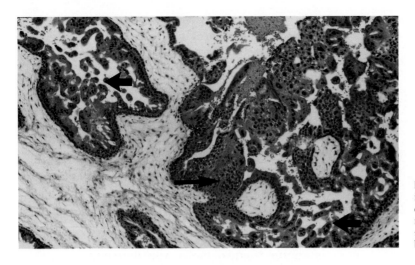

FIGURE 8-90 Complete hydatidiform mole showing collapsed villus with prominent uninucleate cytotrophoblast hyperplasia (*long arrow*) and multinucleated syncytiotrophoblast hyperplasia (*short arrows*). Villous stroma lacks blood vessels and red blood cells.

entire specimen has been carefully examined microscopically and the possibility of residual villous tissue is excluded (see section on choriocarcinoma). A pathologic diagnosis of choriocarcinoma significantly alters clinical treatment.

Complete Hydatidiform Mole in a Twin Gestation

Because twinning occurs with a frequency of 1 in 80 gestations, it is not too uncommon for a complete mole to be accompanied by a normal twin. About 1% to 2% of hydatidiform moles are from twin gestations.[183,193] Interpretation of pathology in such cases is facilitated by previous ultrasonographic recognition of a twin gestation, by receipt of a hysterectomy specimen (Fig. 8-91), or by knowledge of a liveborn normal co-twin.

If the mole is evacuated by curettage and the abnormal, molar villi are admixed with normal villi,

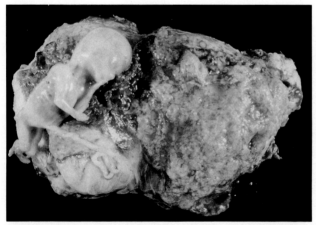

FIGURE 8-91 Gravid hysterectomy showing twin pregnancy: complete hydatidiform mole and and normal twin with umbilical cord and placenta intact. (Lage JM, Mark SD, Roberts DJ, Goldstein DP, Bernstein MR, Berkowitz RS: A flow cytometric study of 137 fresh hydropic placentas: correlation between types of hydatidiform moles and nuclear DNA ploidy. Obstet Gynecol 79:403–410, 1992)

the initial gross examination may point to partial mole. Microscopically, the complete mole is differentiated from partial mole by much more exuberant trophoblastic hyperplasia involving cytotrophoblast and syncytiotrophoblast, and more extensive and pronounced villous cavitation. The complete mole lacks villous scalloping and the two populations of villi characteristic of partial mole (vide infra). In contrast to partial mole, a twin fetus accompanying complete mole is generally without congenital anomalies.

Partial Hydatidiform Mole

A partial hydatidiform mole is derived from an abnormal conceptus that contains an extra haploid set of DNA, is termed triploid (see Fig. 8-87), and has a total of 69 chromosomes. Both the fetus and its placenta are triploid and abnormal. By *gross examination,* the amount of villous tissue in most partial moles is greater than expected for gestational age. In one study, the average maximum villous diameter was 0.51 cm.[183] Fetal tissues are virtually always present and often anomalous.

Though a partial mole may be suspected on gross examination, the diagnosis rests with *microscopy* (Table 8-5). In contrast to the diffuse villous enlargement of the complete mole, there are two populations of villi in partial moles, with some enlarged and some normal to small and sclerotic[181,182] (Fig. 8-92). The villous outline is scalloped (Fig. 8-93) resulting in stromal trophoblastic inclusions (Fig. 8-94). The sine qua non of partial mole is focal trophoblastic hyperplasia (Fig. 8-95; see also Fig. 8-92). The trophoblast hyperplasia ranges from minimal to moderate and chiefly involves the syncytiotrophoblast (see Fig. 8-95). Frank villous cavitation occurs, but to a much lesser degree. Villous blood vessels contain nucleated red blood cells. In older, late second trimester partial moles, villous vessels may form bizarre, gaping, anastomotic channels[182] reminiscent of vascular malformations (Fig. 8-96). Although fragmented and occa-

TABLE 8-5
Gross and Microscopic Differences Between Hydropic Abortus, Partial Hydatidiform Mole, and Complete Hydatidiform Mole

	Hydropic Abortus	*Partial Hydatidiform Mole*	*Complete Hydatidiform Mole*
Amount of Tissue	Scant	Increased for gestational age	Markedly increased
Villous Swelling	Diffuse swelling, involves chorion laeve	Two populations with focal villous swelling	Diffuse swelling
Villous Cavitation	Focal	Focal	Common to extensive
Trophoblast Hyperplasia	None	Focal, involving syncytiotrophoblast	Extensive
Villous Scalloping and Villous Stromal Inclusions	Usually balloon-shaped villi, no scalloping	Focal	Absent
Fetal Tissue	Usually absent, trisomy 18 a notable exception	Usually intact or fragmented fetal parts	Absent
DNA Content	Diploid, often with abnormal karyotype	Triploid: 69 XXX, 69 XXY, rarely 69 XYY	Diploid, paternal

sionally autolyzed, fetal tissues usually are found in partial moles. In older fetuses, anomalies may involve any organ system, but fusion of the fingers or toes, termed syndactyly, is a tipoff to triploidy.[194,195] The implantation site usually contains enlarged, somewhat hyperchromatic, nuclei.

The *natural history* of partial mole is well-documented.[183,196–200] Most women with partial mole undergo spontaneous gonadotropin remission after molar evacuation. About 5%, and in some series, 1% or so, require reevacuation or chemotherapy.[193,198] Although infrequent, choriocarcinoma has followed partial mole.[185,200]

Distinction of Partial Mole from Hydropic Abortus

In many instances the most difficult diagnostic distinction for the obstetric pathologist is between the partial mole and the hydropic abortus (see Table 8-5). The villi of both are focally enlarged, edematous, and even cavitated. Microscopic examination demonstrates a total lack of trophoblastic hyperplasia in the hydropic abortus. Its villi are balloon-shaped, regular, and covered by thin, attenuated trophoblast. Most hydropic abortuses lack fetal tissues and are diploid or near-diploid by karyotype or flow cyto-

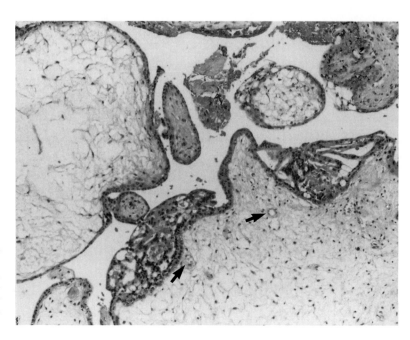

FIGURE 8-92 Partial hydatidiform mole showing two populations of villi: large, edematous villi with focal syncytiotrophoblastic hyperplasia and smaller, focally sclerotic villi. Fetal capillaries are indicated by arrows. Villous edema of villus (*upper left*) is beginning to coalesce, forming the precursor to a small, central cistern.

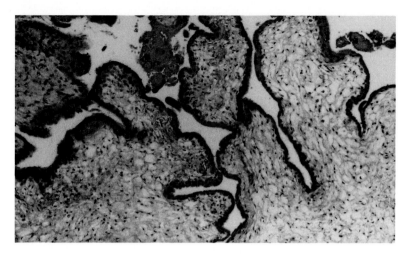

FIGURE 8-93 Partial hydatidiform mole showing enlarged villi with scalloped villous outlines.

metric analysis, although trisomy of a single or a few chromosomes is common.

In contrast, most partial moles are triploid (see Fig. 8-87). The total volume of villous tissue in partial moles far exceeds that in hydropic abortuses. Furthermore, in partial moles the villous outlines are scalloped, forming trophoblastic inclusions, and trophoblast hyperplasia is focally evident. Fetal tissues are more readily found in partial moles.

Third Type of Hydatidiform Mole

Some diploid hydatidiform moles have more phenotypic similarities to partial mole than to complete mole.[181,183,201] Some have maternal and paternal DNA.[201] This has prompted some to opine that a third category of molar gestation might exist: that of diploid partial mole. A conceptus could have a relative "predominance" of a specific paternal DNA

locus if there were a deletion of the comparable maternal locus. This uniparental disomy could result in a molar phenotype, albeit slightly different from the triploid partial mole. Because our knowledge regarding molar gestations is simplistic, any placenta with trophoblast hyperplasia that cannot be further subtyped should be diagnosed as "hydatidiform mole," and appropriate hCG monitoring should follow regardless of DNA content or parental origin.

Invasive Hydatidiform Mole

Hydatidiform moles, partial and complete, can invade the uterine wall, resulting in a tumor that is beyond the reach of the curette. Invasive mole is the most common form of persistent gestational trophoblastic disease after complete mole. Molar villi invade the myometrium in a manner identical to that of placenta increta and may even perforate the

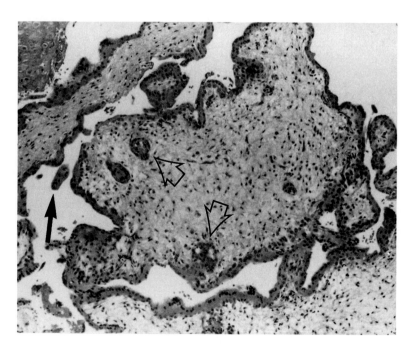

FIGURE 8-94 Partial hydatidiform mole with enlarged villus containing stromal trophoblastic inclusions (*open arrows*). Syncytiotrophoblastic notch (*closed arrow*) in intervillous space appears detached from adjacent villi.

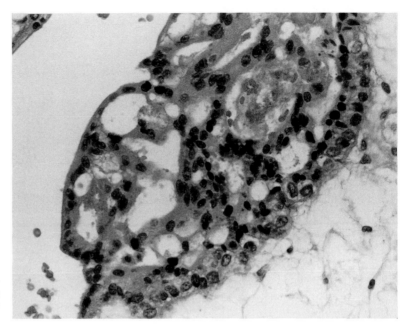

FIGURE 8-95 Partial hydatidiform mole depicting trophoblastic hyperplasia composed of mounds of lacy syncytiotrophoblast. A single layer of cytotrophoblast is present.

uterine serosa. In most cases, invasive mole is effectively treated by chemotherapy, although some require hysterectomy.

Placental Site Lesions

Placental Implantation Site and Placental Site Nodule and Plaque

The implantation site is composed predominantly of intermediate trophoblast (see Fig. 8-5). This type of trophoblast is generally uninucleate, with a single moderate-size nucleus and clear to eosinophilic cytoplasm. After fetal death, degenerative changes in the intermediate trophoblast result in marked nuclear pyknosis and hyperchromasia. Usually all implanta-

tion-site trophoblast has disappeared from the postgravid uterus by 4 to 6 weeks postpartum or postevacuation. Abnormally retained implantation-site trophoblast may form single cells or masses of cells within the endomyometrium. In the past, this was called "retained implantation-site trophoblast."

Recent studies have described another form of retained implantation-site trophoblast composed of discrete, round to oval, eosinophilic nodules with radially oriented intermediate trophoblast in a hyalinized stroma.[202,203] These nodules of intermediate trophoblast have been termed *placental site nodules (or plaques)*. A placental site nodule is depicted in Figures 8-97 and 8-98. In most cases, placental site nodules are derived from residua of placental septal trophoblast (Fig. 8-99) or from cell islands that become embedded in the endomyometrium. Signifi-

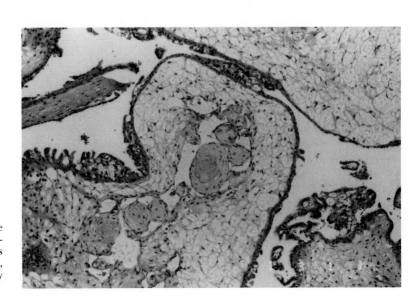

FIGURE 8-96 Partial hydatidiform mole, late second-trimester specimen, with enlarged, edematous villi containing aberrant, maze-like villous vessels, piles of hyperplastic syncytiotrophoblast, and syncytiotrophoblastic notches. Flow cytometry confirmed triploid DNA content.

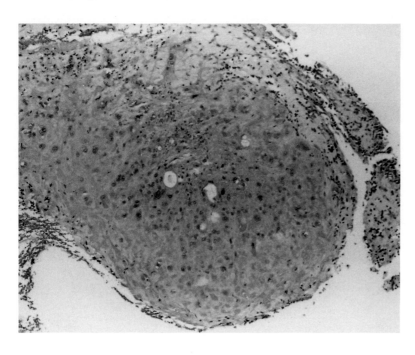

FIGURE 8-97 Placental-site nodule in endometrial curettings. Nodule is predominantly acellular, composed of eosinophilic hyalinized material with preservation of residual central intermediate trophoblast. This lesion showed positive immunostaining for keratin and human placental lactogen.

cant mitotic activity such as >1/10 to 20 high-power (×400) fields should raise the possibility of placental site trophoblastic tumor. Uterine curettage appears to be effective treatment in most cases. Careful follow-up is warranted as there is no basis for assuming that persisting placental site nodules might not serve as a precursor of, or be associated with, a placental site trophoblastic tumor in some instances.

Placental Site Trophoblastic Tumor

The placental site trophoblastic tumor (PSTT) is a rare malignant tumor developing in women who have been pregnant previously.[204–209] It is composed of intermediate trophoblast that secretes small amounts of β-hCG. Grossly, tumor nodules are hemorrhagic and fleshy and may occur at any site in the uterus. Microscopically, it consists of invasive sheets and nodules of monotonous, malignant-appearing, intermediate trophoblast that splay apart, but do not destroy, myometrial fibers (Fig. 8-100). The tumor is strongly hPL positive, with focal hCG positivity. Surgery remains the mainstay of treatment, because the tumor—unlike choriocarcinoma—responds poorly to chemotherapy. Most recurrences tend to be local, although systemic metastases may be fatal.[206,208] Only 10% to 15% of PSTTs behave malignantly, and behavior cannot always be predicted by histopathologic

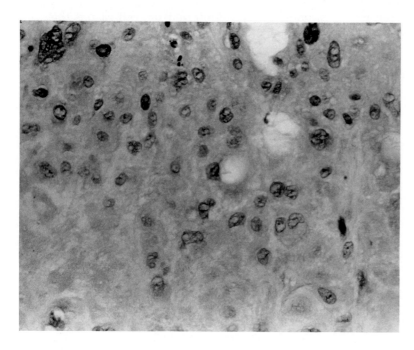

FIGURE 8-98 Placental-site nodule, higher magnification of Figure 8-97, showing loosely formed columns of uninucleate and multinucleate intermediate trophoblast without mitotic activity.

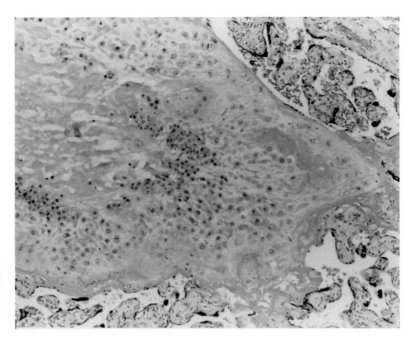

FIGURE 8-99 Placental septum from a normal term placenta showing intermediate trophoblast surrounded by acellular fibrinoid. Anchoring villi are attached to surface of placental septum. Placental-site nodules most likely represent residua of normal placental septa or cell islands.

analysis.[204–209] It has been suggested that numerous mitotic figures (over 5 per 10 high-power fields), extensive necrosis, and strong and diffuse hCG immunoreactivity are more frequently associated with malignant behavior.[207,209]

Placental site trophoblastic tumor must be differentiated from choriocarcinoma as the clinical management differs significantly. Choriocarcinoma is characterized by a proliferation of intermediate trophoblast and cytotrophoblast with foci of diagnostic syncytiotrophoblast (Fig. 8-101). Tumor necrosis and hemorrhage are pronounced. Choriocarcinoma is strongly hCG-positive by immunohistochemistry, and elevated serum β-hCG values suggest

choriocarcinoma. Placental site tumor is devoid of syncytiotrophoblast and is far less necrotic. Its tumor cells are immunoreactive for hPL with minimal hCG staining. Serum β-hCG is virtually always low in women with placental site trophoblastic tumors. Both tumors are keratin-positive.

Gestational Choriocarcinoma

Reported incidences of choriocarcinoma range from 1 in 20,000 livebirths[210] and 1 in 40,000 deliveries[186] in the United States to 1 in 570 to 1 in 1650 deliveries in Indonesia.[188] The risk of gestational chorio-

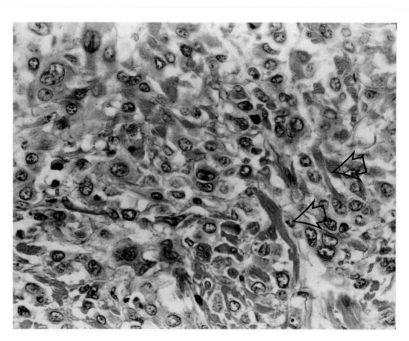

FIGURE 8-100 Placental-site trophoblastic tumor composed of sheets of intermediate trophoblast invading the myometrium. Tumor splays apart the individual myometrial myocytes (*arrows*) without inducing significant necrosis or hemorrhage.

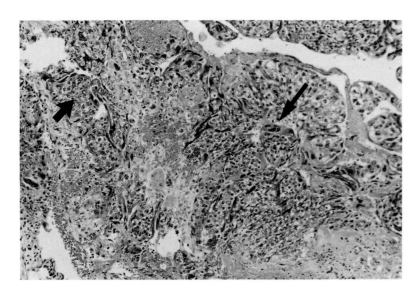

FIGURE 8-101 Choriocarcinoma showing extensive tumor necrosis and hemorrhage. Viable tumor consists of nests of cytotrophoblast (*short arrow*) capped by syncytiotrophoblast (*long arrow*).

carcinoma depends on the nature of the antecedent pregnancy: 50% of gestational choriocarcinomas follow complete hydatidiform mole, 25% follow spontaneous abortion, 22.5% follow normal pregnancy, and 2.5% follow ectopic pregnancy.[211]

Choriocarcinoma most commonly affects the uterus and is manifested by vaginal bleeding. Numerous bizarre presentations have been reported, reflecting the extent of widespread, systemic metastases present at the time of initial diagnosis. The tumor is characterized by hCG production, and hCG level relates to tumor burden.

Although postmolar gestational choriocarcinoma may be virtually uniformly cured by chemotherapy, the same is not true for choriocarcinoma developing after normal delivery. This may reflect the increased time interval between onset of tumor and diagnosis as well as differences in DNA content and parental

source. The DNA of postmolar choriocarcinoma is usually totally androgenetic, being derived from the complete mole,[212] whereas postgestational choriocarcinoma contains the normal, biparental DNA of the delivered infant or fetus.[212–214]

Grossly, choriocarcinoma is recognized by its strikingly dark red, hemorrhagic appearance. Uterine choriocarcinomas may be polypoid, projecting into the endometrial cavity, or solely intramyometrial, or diffusely replacing the entire corpus and cervix. Large areas may be necrotic. When metastatic, tumor nodules tend to be well-circumscribed, hemorrhagic and necrotic.

Microscopically, the degree of tumor necrosis, hemorrhage and infarction is unsurpassed by most malignant tumors. Diligent searching for viable tumor reveals islands of uninucleate intermediate trophoblast and cytotrophoblast alternating with

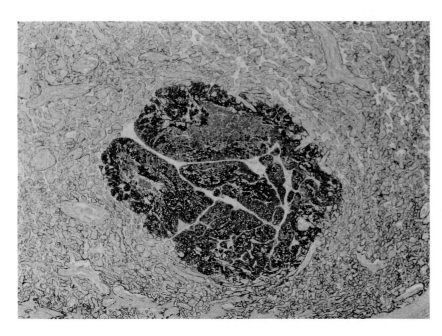

FIGURE 8-102 Choriocarcinoma in a term placenta. Keratin immunostaining (AE1/AE3 Boehringer-Mannheim, Indianapolis, IN) highlights malignant cytotrophoblast and syncytiotrophoblast surrounded by normal term villi. Tumor islands contain much central necrosis. (Lage JM, Roberts DJ. Choriocarcinoma in a term placenta: Pathologic diagnosis of tumor in an asymptomatic patient with metastatic disease. Int J Gynecol Pathol 12:80–85, 1993.)

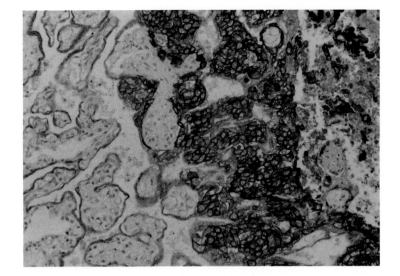

FIGURE 8-103 Choriocarcinoma in a term placenta, higher magnification of Figure 8-102, keratin immunostain (AE1/AE3, Boehringer-Mannheim, Indianapolis, IN). Tumor develops from trophoblast of normal-appearing villi and proliferates, forming avillous nodules of choriocarcinoma. Note the central necrosis of one tumor nodule at right. (Lage JM, Roberts DJ. Choriocarcinoma in a term placenta: Pathologic diagnosis of tumor in an asymptomatic patient with metastatic disease. Int J Gynecol Pathol 12:80–85, 1993.)

syncytiotrophoblast (see Fig. 8-101). The syncytiotrophoblast tends to remain peripherally located, encircling nodules of uninucleate trophoblast. Small clusters of syncytiotrophoblast demarcate the somewhat larger foci of uninucleate trophoblast giving the tumor an overall biphasic appearance. Although the cells of many undifferentiated tumors may simulate the appearance of uninucleate trophoblast, the presence of syncytiotrophoblast, characterized by multinucleation and abundant violaceous to blue cytoplasm, is required to diagnose choriocarcinoma. Syncytiotrophoblastic nuclei tend to be small and inconspicuous, with occasional eosinophilic nucleoli, although larger nuclei are sometimes seen. In contrast, the uninucleate trophoblast (cytotrophoblast and intermediate trophoblast) has greater cytologic atypia, with cells containing large, lobulated and even bizarre nuclei, coarse chromatin, and prominent nucleoli. The cytoplasm tends to be clear to granular and slightly eosinophilic in cytotrophoblast, and dense, amphophilic to eosinophilic in intermediate trophoblast.

Choriocarcinoma has a predilection for early and extensive vascular space invasion, leading to systemic metastases even when tumor volume is small. Destructive endometrial and myometrial invasion are identified in hysterectomy specimens (now rarely seen) and may be seen in uterine curettings. Large sheets of tumor cells differentiating into syncytiotrophoblast and cytotrophoblast or intermediate trophoblast, absence of villous tissue, and destructive endomyometrial invasion have been offered as criteria required for the diagnosis of choriocarcinoma in uterine curettings.[215] Choriocarcinoma is strongly immunopositive for keratin and hCG, with weak immunopositivity for hPL.

Choriocarcinoma, like the placental site tumor, is devoid of villi, the only exception being those tumors arising in association with a placenta.[216,217] In such cases, the villous origin of the malignant trophoblast is easily discerned (Figs. 8-102 and 8-103).

The presence of molar villi from a partial or complete hydatidiform mole obviates a diagnosis of choriocarcinoma, even if sheets of obviously malignant trophoblast are identified. Chemotherapy with surgery as an adjunctive modality offers cure in 81% of all women and in 71% of those with metastatic tumor.[218] Although choriocarcinoma may arise from a placenta at any point in gestation, fetal metastases are uncommon, but uniformly lethal. Presentation in an infant or fetus in the absence of any evidence of maternal tumor has been reported.[219]

References

1. Boyd JD, Hamilton WJ. The human placenta. Cambridge, W Heffer and Sons, 1970.
2. Ramsey EM. Development and anatomy of the placenta, Chapter 36, in: Haines and Taylor Obstetrical and Gynaecological Pathology, 3rd Ed. Fox, H, ed., Churchill Livingstone, Edinburgh, 1987.
3. Demir R, Kaufmann P, Castellucci M, Erbengi T, Kotowski A. Fetal vasculogenesis and angiogenesis in human placental villi. Acta Anat (Basel) 1989;136:190–203.
4. Kurman RJ, Main CWS, Chen HC. Intermediate trophoblast: A distinctive form of trophoblast with specific morphological, biochemical and functional features. Placenta 5:349, 1984.
5. Kalousek DK, Fitch N, Paradice BA. Pathology of the Human Embryo and Previable Fetus. An Atlas. Springer-Verlag, New York. 1990.
6. Moragas A, Ballabriga A, Vidal MT. Atlas of Neonatal Histopathology. W.B. Saunders Co, Philadelphia. 1977.
7. Rehder H, Coerdt W, Eggers R, Klink F, Schwinger E. Is there a correlation between morphological and cytogenetic findings in placental tissue from early missed abortions? Hum Genet 82:377–385, 1989.
8. Altshuler G. Placenta within the medicolegal imperative. Arch Pathol Lab Med 1991;115:688–95.
9. Naeye RL. Do placental weights have clinical significance? Hum Pathol 18:387–91, 1987.
10. Lage JM. Placentomegaly with massive hydrops of placental stem villi, diploid DNA content, and fetal omphaloceles: Possible association with Beckwith-Wiedemann syndrome. Hum Pathol 1991;22:591–7.

11. Roberts DR, Ampola MG, Lage JM. Diagnosis of unsuspected fetal metabolic storage disease by routine placental examination. Pediatr Path 1991;11:647–656.

12. Fox H. General Pathology of the placenta. Chapter 37. In: Obstetrical and Gynaecological Pathology. H. Fox, Ed. Vol 2. pp. 972–1000.

13. Fox H. Pathology of the placenta. Major problems in pathology series. Philadelphia, Saunders, Vol 7. 1978.

14. Fujikura T, Benson RC, Driscoll SG. The bipartite placenta and its clinical features. Am J Obstet Gynecol 107:1013–7, 1970.

15. Naeye RL. Umbilical cord length: clinical significance. J Pediatr 1985;107:278–281.

16. Davies BR, Casanueva E, Arroyo P. Placentas of small-for-dates infants: a small controlled series from Mexico City, Mexico. Am J Obstet Gynecol 1984;149:731–6.

17. Benirschke K, Kaufmann P. Pathology of the Human Placenta. 2nd Edition. Springer-Verlag, New York. 1990.

18. Robinson LK, Jones KL, Benirschke K. The nature of structural defects associated with velamentous and marginal insertion of the umbilical cord. Am J Obstet Gynecol 1983;146:191–3.

19. Leung AKC, Robson WLM. Single umbilical artery: a report of 159 cases. Am J Dis Child 1989;143:108–11.

20. Byrne J, Blanc WA. Malformations and chromosomal anomalies in spontaneously aborted fetuses with single umbilical artery. Am J Obstet Gynecol 1985;151:340–2.

21. Yavner DL, Redline RW. Angiomyxoma of the umbilical cord with massive cystic degeneration of Wharton's jelly. Arch Pathol Lab Med 1989;113:935–7.

22. Mishriki YY, Vanyshelbaum Y, Epstein H, Blanc W. Hemangioma of the umbilical cord. Pediatr Pathol 1987;7:43–9.

23. Smith D, Majmudar B. Teratoma of the umbilical cord. Hum Pathol 1985;16:190–3.

24. Maberry MC, Ramin SM, Gilstrap LC, Leveno KJ, Dax JS. Intrapartum asphyxia in pregnancies complicated by intra-amniotic infection. Obstet Gynecol 1990;76:351–4.

25. Miller PW, Coen RW, Benirschke K. Dating the time interval from meconium passage to birth. Obstet Gynecol 66:459–62, 1985.

26. Altshuler G, Hyde S. Meconium induced vasoconstriction: a potential cause of cerebral and other fetal hypoperfusion and of poor pregnancy outcome. Child Neurol 4:137–42, 1989.

27. Altshuler G, Herman A. The medicolegal imperative: placental pathology and epidemiology. In, Fetal and Neonatal Brain Injury: Mechanisms, Management and the Risk of Malpractice. DK Stevenson, and P Sunshine, eds., pp. 250–63. B.C. Decker, 1989.

28. Torpin R. Amniochorionic mesoblastic fibrous strings and amnionic bands: Associated constricting fetal malformation of fetal death. Am J Obstet Gynecol 1965;91:65–75.

29. Lage JM, vanMarter LJ, Bieber FR. Questionable role of amniocentesis in the formation of amniotic bands. J Reprod Med 1988;33:71–3.

30. Porreco RP, Young PE, Resnik R, Cousins L, Jones OW, Richards T, Kernahan C, Matson M. Reproductive outcome following amniocentesis for genetic indications. Am J Obstet Gynecol 1982;143:653–60.

31. Khong TY. Acute atherosis in pregnancies complicated by hypertension, small-for-gestational age infants, and diabetes mellitus. Arch Pathol Lab Med 115:722–5, 1991.

32. Brosens I, Dixon HG, Robertson WB. Fetal growth retardation and the arteries of the placental bed. Br J Obstet Gynaecol 84:656–63, 1977.

33. Hustin J, Foidart JM, Lambotte R. Maternal vascular lesions in preeclampsia and intrauterine growth retardation: light microscopy and immunofluorescence. Placenta 4:489–98, 1983.

34. Kitzmiller JL, Watt N, Driscoll SG. Decidual arteriopathy in hypertension and diabetes in pregnancy: immunofluorescent studies. Am J Obstet Gynecol 141:773–9, 1981.

35. Brosens I. A study of the spiral arteries of the decidua basalis in normotensive and hypertensive pregnancies. J Obstet Gynaecol Br Commonw 71:222–30, 1964.

36. Driscoll S. The pathology of pregnancy complicated by diabetes mellitus. Med Clin North Am 1965, 49:1053–67.

37. Abramowsky CR, Vegas ME, Swinehart IG, Gyves MT. Decidual vasculopathy of the placenta in lupus erythematosus. N Engl J Med 303:668–72, 1980.

38. Robertson WB. Uteroplacental vasculature. J Clin Pathol [Suppl] 10:9–17, 1976.

39. Khong TY, De Wolf F, Robertson WB, Brosens I. Inadequate maternal vascular response to placentation in pregnancies complicated by preeclampsia and by small-for-gestational age infants. Br J Obstet Gynecol 93:1049–59, 1986.

40. Labarre CA. Acute atherosis. A histopathological hallmark of immune aggression? Placenta 1988;9:95–108.

41. Hendricks CH. Twinning in relation to birth weight, mortality and congenital anomalies. Obstet Gynecol 27:47–53, 1966.

42. Leroy F. Major fetal hazards in multiple pregnancy. Acta Genet Med Gemellol Rome 25:299–306, 1976.

43. Potter EL. Twin zygosity and placental form in relation to the outcome of pregnancy. Am J Obstet Gynecol 87:566–77, 1963.

44. Hay S, Wehrung DA. Congenital malformations in twins. Am J Human Genet 1970;22:662–78.

45. Benirschke K, Kim CK. Multiple pregnancy. N Engl J Med 1974;288:1276–84, 1329–36.

46. Blumer MD. The Biology of Twinning in Man. Oxford, England, Claredon Press, 1970.

47. Nylander PPS. The value of the placenta in the determination of zygosity—a study of 1052 Nigerian twin maternities. J Obstet Gynaecol Br. Commonw 1969;76:699–04.

48. Benirschke K, Driscoll SG. The Pathology of the Human Placenta. New York, Springer-Verlag, 1967.

49. Benirschke K. Accurate recording of twin placentation. A plea to the obstetrician. Obstet Gynecol 1961A, 18:334.

50. Benirschke K. Major pathologic features of the placenta, cord and membranes. Birth Defects Original Article Series, Vol 1, No 1; April 1965, pp 52–63.

51. Kim K, Lage JM. Bipartite diamnionic monochorionic twin placenta with superficial vascular anastomoses. Hum Pathol 1991;22:501–3.

52. Aherne W, Strong SJ, Corney G. The structure of the placenta in the twin transfusion syndrome. Biol Neonate 1968;12:121–35.

53. Sekiya S, Hafez ESE. Physiomorphology of twin transfusion syndrome. Obstet Gynecol 1977;50:288–92.

54. Lage JM, vanMarter LJ, Mikhail E. Vascular anastomoses in fused, dichorionic twin placentas resulting in twin transfusion syndrome. Placenta 1989;10:55–9.

55. Robertson EG, Neer KJ. Placental injection studies in twin gestation. Am J Obstet Gynecol 1983;147:170–74.

56. Tippett P. Human chimeras. In, Chimeras in Developmental Biology. N.L. Douarin and A McLaren, eds., pp. 165–78. Academic Press, Orlando, 1984.

57. Rausen AR, Seki M. Strauss L. Twin transfusion syndrome. J Pediatr 1965;66:613–28.

58. Naeye RL. Organ abnormalities in a human parabiotic syndrome. Am J Pathol 1965;46:829–42.

59. Benson CB, Bieber RF, Genest DR, Doubilet PM. Doppler demonstration of reversed umbilical blood flow in an acardiac twin. J Clin Ultrasound 1989;17:291–5.

60. Alpers CE, Harrison MR. Fetus in fetu associated with an undescended testis. Pediatr Path 1985;4:37–46.

61. Hendricks CH. Twinning in relation to birth weight, mortality, and congenital anomalies. Obstet Gynecol 1966;27:47–53.

62. Levi S. Ultrasonic assessment of the high rate of human multiple pregnancy in the 1st trimester. J Clin Ultrasound 1976;4:3–5.

63. Benirschke K. Twin placenta in perinatal mortality. N Y State J Med 1961;61:1499–1508.

64. Tessen JA, Zlatnik FJ. Monoamnionic twins: A retrospective controlled study. Obstet Gynecol 1991;77:832–4.

65. Wensinger JA, Daly RF. Monoamniotic twins. Am J Obstet Gynecol 1962;83:1254–6.

66. Carr SR, Aronson MP, Coustan DR. Survival rates of mon-

oamniotic twins do not decrease after 30 weeks' gestation. Am J Obstet Gynecol 1990;163:719–22.

67. Jauniaux E, Elkazen N, Leroy F, Wilkin P, Rodesch F, Hustin J. Clinical and morphologic aspects of the vanishing twin phenomenon. Obstet Gynecol 1988;72:577–81.

68. Sander CH. Hemorrhagic endovasculitis and hemorrhagic villitis of the placenta. Arch Pathol Lab Med 1980;104:371–3.

69. Silver MM, Yeger H, Lines LD. Hemorrhagic endovasculitis-like lesion induced in placental organ culture. Hum Pathol 1988;19:251–6.

70. Driscoll SG. Chorioamnionitis: perinatal morbidity and mortality. Pediatr Infect Dis 1986;5:S273–5.

71. Mueller-Heuback E, Rubinstein DN, Schwarz SS. Histologic chorioamnionitis and preterm delivery in different patient populations. Obstet Gynecol 75:622–26, 1990.

72. Zhang J, Kraus FT, Aquino TI. Chorioamnionitis: A comparative histologic, bacteriologic, and clinical study. Int J Gynecol Pathol 4:1–10, 1985.

73. Pankuch GA, Appelbaum PC, Lorenz RP, Botti JJ, Schachter J, Naeye RL. Placental microbiology and histology and the pathogenesis of chorioamnionitis. Obstet Gynecol 64:802–6, 1984.

74. Utility of Umbilical Cord Blood Acid-Base Assessment. ACOG Committee Opinion: Committee on Obstetrics: Maternal and Fetal Medicine. Number 91—February 1991.

75. Hauth JC, Gilstrap LC, Hankins GDV, Connor KD. Term maternal and neonatal complications of acute chorioamnionitis. Obstet Gynecol 1985;66:59–62.

76. Salafia CM, Weigl C, Silberman L. The prevalence and distribution of acute placental inflammation in uncomplicated term pregnancies. Obstet Gynecol 1989;73:383–9.

77. Naeye RL, Maisels J, Lorenz RP, Botti JJ. The clinical significance of placental villous edema. Pediatrics 1983;71:588–94.

78. Madan E, Meyer MP, Amortequi A. Chorioamnionitis: A study of organisms isolated in perinatal autopsies. Ann Clin and Lab Sci 1988;18:39–45.

79. Labarre CA, McIntyre JA, Faulk WP. Immunohistologic evidence that villitides in human normal term placentas is an immunologic lesion. Am J Obstet Gynecol 1990;162:515–22.

80. Knox WF, Fox H. Villitis of unknown aetiology: its incidence and significance in placentae from a British population. Placenta 1984;5:395–402.

81. Russell P. Inflammatory lesions of the human placenta. III. The histopathology of villitis of unknown aetiology. Placenta 1980;1:227–44.

82. Labarrere CA, Faulk WP, McIntyre JA. Villitis in normal term human placentae: Frequency of the lesion determined by monoclonal antibody to HLA-DR antigen. J Reprod Immunol 1989;16:127–35.

83. Mortimer G, MacDonald DJ, Smeeth A. A pilot study of the frequency and significance of placental villitis. Br J of Obstet Gynaecol 1985;92:629–33.

84. Gersell DJ, Phillips NJ, Beckerman K. Chronic chorioamnionitis: A clinicopathologic study of 17 cases. Int J Gynecol Path 1991;10:217–29.

85. Singer DB, Campognone P. Perinatal group B streptococcal infection in midgestation. Pediatr Pathol 1986;5:271–6.

86. Haft RF, Kasper DL. Group B streptococcus infection in mother and child. Hospital Practice Dec 15, 1991, p. 111–34.

87. Novak RW, Platt MS. Significance of placental findings in early-onset group B streptococcal neonatal sepsis. Clin Pediatr 1985;24:256–8.

88. Barresi JA. Listeria monocytogenes: A cause of premature labor and neonatal sepsis. Am J Obstet Gynecol 1980;136:410–1.

89. Fojaco RM, Hensley GT, Moskowitz L. Congenital syphilis and necrotizing funisitis. JAMA 1989;261:1788–90.

90. Yow MD. Congenital cytomegalovirus disease: A NOW problem. J Infect Dis 1989;159:163–7.

91. Anonymous. Screening for congenital CMV. Lancet 1989;2:599–600.

92. Schwartz DA, Khan R, Stoll B. Characterization of the fetal inflammatory response to cytomegalovirus placentitis. Arch Pathol Lab Med 1992;116:21–7.

93. Blanc WA. Pathology of the placenta, membranes and umbilical cord in bacterial, fungal and viral infections in man. In Naeye RL, Kissane JM, eds. Perinatal diseases, pp 67–132. IAP Monograph Series, No. 22. Baltimore, Williams & Wilkins, 1981

94. Garcia AGP, Fonseca EF, Marques RGdS, Lobato YY. Placental morphology in cytomegalovirus infection. Placenta 1989;10:1–18.

95. Alford CA, Stagno S, Pass RF. Natural history of perinatal cytomegaloviral infection. In: Ciba Foundation Symposium 77, Excerpta Medica, Amsterdam. 1980. p 125–47.

96. Blanc WA. Pathology of the placenta and cord in some viral infections. In: Viral diseases of the fetus and newborn. Major problems in clinical pediatrics, Hanshan JB, Dregeon JA (eds). Philadelphia, W.B. Saunders, Vol 17.

97. Nahmias AJ, Keyserling HH, Kerrick G. Herpes Simples. In: Remington JS, Klein JO, eds. Infectious diseases of the fetus and newborn infant. Philadelphia, W.B. Saunders, 1983:156–90.

98. Florman AL, Gershon AA, Blackett PR, Nahmias AJ. Intrauterine infection with herpes simplex virus: resultant congenital malformations. JAMA 1973;225:129–32.

99. Stagno S, Whitley RJ. Herpesvirus infections of pregnancy. Part II: Herpes simplex virus and varicella-zoster virus infections. N Engl J Med 1985;313:1327–30.

100. Johnson RE, Nahmias AJ, Magder LS, Lee FK, Brooks, CA, Snowden Cb. A seroepidemiologic survey of the prevalence of herpes simplex virus type 2 infection in the United States. N Engl J Med 1989;321:7–12.

101. Wittek AE, Yeager AS, Au DS, Hensleigh PA. Asymptomatic shedding of herpes simplex virus from the cervix and lesion site during pregnancy: correlation of antepartum shedding with shedding at delivery. Am J Dis Child 1984;138:439–42.

102. Brown ZA, Benedetti J, Ashely R, Burchett S, Selke S, Berry S, Vontver LA, Corey L. Neonatal herpes simplex virus infection in relation to asymptomatic maternal infection at the time of labor. N Engl J Med 1991;324:1247–52.

103. Whitley R, Arvin A, Prober C, Burchett S, Corey L, Powell D, Plotkin S, Starr S, Alford C, Connor J, Jacobs R, Nahmias A, Soong SJ and the National Institute of Allergy and Infectious Diseases Collaborative Antiviral Study Group. A controlled trial comparing vidarabine with acyclovir in neonatal herpes simplex virus infection. N Engl J Med 1991;324:444–9.

104. Hain J, Doshi N, Harger JH. Ascending transcervical herpes simplex infection with intact fetal membranes. Obstet Gynecol 1980;56:106–9.

105. Herzen JL, Benirschke K. Unexpected disseminated herpes simplex infection in a newborn. Obstet Gynecol 1977;50:728–30.

106. Garcia AGP. Maternal herpes-simplex infection causing abortion. Histopathologic study of the placenta. "O Hospital" 1970;78:1267–1274.

107. Nakamura Y, Yamamoto S, Tanaka S, Yano H, Nishimura G, Saito Y, Tanaka T, Tanimura A, Hirose F, Fukuda S, Shingu M, Hashimoto T. Herpes simplex viral infection in human neonates. Hum Pathol 1985;16:1091–7.

108. Altshuler G. Pathogenesis of congenital herpesvirus infection. Am J Dis Child 1974;127:427–9.

109. Witzleben CL, Driscoll SG. Possible transplacental transmission of herpes simplex infection. Pediatr 1965;36:192–9.

110. Rogers BB, Josephson SL, Mak SK. Detection of herpes simplex virus using the polymerase chain reaction followed by endonuclease cleavage. Am J Pathol 1991;139:1–6.

111. Bruner JM. Oligonucleotide probe for herpes virus: use in paraffin sections. Mod Pathol 1990;3:635–8.

112. Sever J, White LR. Intrauterine viral infections. Annu Rev Med 1968;19:471–86.

113. Siegel M, Fuerst HT. Low birth weight and maternal virus diseases: a prospective study of rubella, measles, mumps, chickenpox, and hepatitis. JAMA 1966;197:680–4.

114. Paryani SG, Arvin AM. Consequences of varicella or herpes

zoster in pregnancy for mother and infant. Programs and Abstracts of the Twenty-Fourth Interscience Conference on Antimicrobial Agents and Chemotherapy. Washington, D.C. October 8–10, 1984.

115. Williamson A. The varicella zoster virus in the etiology of severe congenital defects. Clin Pediatr 1975;14:553–9.

116. Alkalay AL, Pomerance JJ, Rimoin DL. Fetal varicella syndrome. J Pediatr 1987;111:320–3.

117. Garcia AGP. Fetal infection in chickenpox and alastrim with histopathologic study of the placenta. Pediatr 1963;32:895–901.

118. Cossart YE, Field AM, Cant B, Widdows D. Parvovirus-like particles in human sera. Lancet 1975;1:72–3.

119. Sahakian V, Weiner CP, Naides SJ, Williamson RA, Scharosch LL. Intrauterine transfusion treatment of non-immune hydrops fetalis secondary to human parvovirus B19 infection. Am J Obstet Gynecol 1991;164:1090–1.

120. van Elsacker-Niele, AMW, Salimans MMM, Weiland HT, Vermey-Keers CHR, Anderson MJ, Versteeg. Fetal pathology in human parvovirus B19 infection. Br J Obstet Gynaecol. 1989;96:768–75.

121. Christian SS, Duff P. Is universal screening for hepatitis B infection warranted in all prenatal populations? Obstet Gynecol 1989;74:259–61.

122. Li L, Sheng M-H, Tong S-P, Chen H-Z, Wen Y-M. Transplacental transmission of hepatitis B virus. Lancet 1986;2:872.

123. Khudr G, Benirschke K. Placental lesion in viral hepatitis. Am J Obstet Gynecol 1972;40:381–4.

124. Altschuler G, Russell P. The human placental villitides: a review of chronic intrauterine infection. Current Topics in Pathology 1975;60:63–112.

125. Chin J. Current and future dimensions of the HIV/AIDS pandemic in women and children. Lancet 1990;336:221–4.

126. European Collaborative Study: Mother-to-child transmission of HIV infection. Lancet 1988;2:1039–45.

127. Lewis SH, Reynolds-Kohler C, Fox HE, Nelson JA. HIV-1 in trophoblastic and villous Hofbauer cells, and haematological precursors in eight-week fetuses. Lancet 1990;335:565–8.

128. Holmes KK. AIDS: Problems and prospects IX: The changing epidemiology of HIV transmission. Hospital Practice Nov 15, 1991;153–78.

129. Barton JJ, O'Connor TM, Cannon MJ, Weldon-Linne CM. Prevalence of human immunodeficiency virus in a general prenatal population. Am J Obstet Gynecol 1989;160:1316–24.

130. Quinn TC, Kline RL, Halsey N, Hutton N, Ruff A, Butz A, Boulos R, Modlin JF. Early diagnosis of perinatal HIV infection by detection of viral-specific IgA antibodies. JAMA 1991;266:3439–3442.

131. Jauniaux E, Nessmann C, Imbert MC, Meuris S, Puissant F, Hustin J. Morphological aspects of the placenta in HIV pregnancies. Placenta 1988;9:633–42.

132. Driscoll SG. Histopathology of gestational rubella. Am J Dis Child 1969;118:49–53.

133. Garcia AGP, Marques RLS, Lobato YY, Fonseca MEF, Wigg MD. Placental pathology in congenital rubella. Placenta 1985;6:281–5.

134. Ornoy A, Segal S, Nishmi M, Simcha A, Polishuk WZ. Fetal and placental pathology in gestational rubella. Am J Obstet Gynecol 1973;116:949–56.

135. Northrup RL, Gardner WM, Geittmann WF. Rubella reinfection during early pregnancy. Obstet Gynecol 1972;39:524–6.

136. Eilard T, Strannegard O. Rubella reinfection in pregnancy followed by transmission to the fetus. J Infect Dis 1974;129:594–6.

137. Garcia AGP, Pereira JMS, Vidigal N, Lobato YY, Pegado CS, Branco JPC. Intrauterine infection with mumps virus. Obstet Gynecol 1980;56:756–9.

138. Moroi K, Saito S, Kurata T, Sata T, Yanagida M. Fetal death associated with measles virus infection of the placenta. Am Obstet Gynecol 1991;164:1107–8.

139. Ornoy A, Dudai M, Sadovsky E. Placental and fetal pathol-

ogy in infectious mononucleosis. A possible indicator for Epstein-Barr virus teratogenicity. Diagn Gynecol Obstet 1982;4:11–6.

140. Joncas JH, Alfieri C, Leyritz-Wills M, Brochu P, Jasmin G, Boldogh I, Huang ES. Simultaneous congenital infection with Epstein-Barr virus and cytomegalovirus. N Engl J Med 1981;304:1399–1403.

141. Garcia AGP, Basso NGdaS, Fonseca MEF, Outani HN. Congenital ECHO virus infection—morphological and virological study of fetal and placental tissue. J Pathol 1990;160:123–7.

142. Koppe JG, Loewer-Sieger DH, de Roever-Bonnet H. Results of 20-year follow-up of congenital toxoplasmosis. Lancet 1986;1:254–6.

143. Elliott WG. Placental toxoplasmosis: Report of a case. Am J Clin Pathol 1970;53:413–7.

144. Werner H, Schmidtke L, Thomascheck G. Toxoplasmose-Infektion und Schwangerschaft: der histologische Nachweis des intrauterinen Infektion-sweges. Klin Wochenschr 1963;41:96–101.

145. Bittencourt AL, de Freitas LAR, Galvao MO, Jacomo K. Pneumonitis in congenital Chagas' disease: a study of ten cases. Am J Trop Med Hyg 1981;30:38–42.

146. Bittencourt AL. Congenital Chagas disease. Am J Dis Child 1976;130:97–103.

147. Labarrere CA, McIntyre JA, Faulk WP. Immunohistologic evidence that villitis in human normal term placentas in an immunologic lesion. Am J Obstet Gynecol 1990;162:515–22.

148. Altshuler G. Placental villitis of unknown etiology: harbinger of serious disease? A four months' experience of nine cases. J Reprod Med 1973;11:215–222.

149. Redline RW, Abramowsky CR. Clinical and pathological aspects of recurrent villitis. Hum Pathol 1985;16:727–31.

150. Labarrere C, Althabe O, Telenta M. Chronic villitis of unknown aetiology in placentae of idiopathic small for gestational age infants. Placenta 1982;3:309–18.

151. Fox H. The significance of placental infarction in perinatal morbidity and mortality. Biol Neonate 1967;11:87–105.

152. Blanc WA. Circulatory lesions of the human placenta in abruptio. Berh Deutsch Ges Pathol 1976;60:386–92.

153. Moe N. Depositions of fibrin and plasma proteins in the normal placenta: an immunofluorescence study. Acta Pathol Microbiol Scand 1969;76:74–88.

154. Naeye RL. The clinical significance of absent subchorionic fibrin in the placenta. Am J Clin Pathol 1990;94:196–8.

155. Labarrere C, Mullen E. Fibrinoid and trophoblastic necrosis with massive chronic intervillositis: An extreme variant of villitis of unknown etiology. Am J Reprod Immunol Microbiol 1987;15:85.

156. Kaplan C, Blanc WA, Elias J. Identification of erythrocytes in intervillous thrombi: A study using immunoperoxidase identification of hemoglobins. Hum Pathol 1982;13:554–7.

157. Batcup G, Tovey LAD, Longster G. Fetomaternal blood group incompatibility studies in placental intervillous thrombosis. Placenta 1983;4:449–54.

158. Shanklin DR, Scott JS. Massive subchorial thrombohaematoma. (Breus' mole). Br J Obstet Gynaecol 1975;82:476–87.

159. Blattner P, Dar H, Nitowsky HM. Pregnancy outcome in women with sickle cell trait. JAMA 1977;238:1392–4.

160. Bloomfield RD, Suarez JR, Malangit AC. The placenta: A diagnostic tool in sickle cell disorders. J Natl Med Assoc 1978;70:87–88.

161. Fujikura T, Froehlich L. Diagnosis of sickling by placental examination. Geographic differences in incidence. Am J Obstet Gynecol 1968;100:1122–4.

162. Platt HS. Effect of maternal sickle cell trait on perinatal mortality. Br Med J 1971;4:334–6.

163. Rimer BA. Sickle-cell trait and pregnancy: A review of a community hospital experience. Am J Obstet Gynecol 1975;123:6–11.

164. Wentworth P. The placenta in cases of hemolytic disease of the newborn. Am J Obstet Gynecol 1967;98:283–9.

165. Bartholomew RA, Colvin ED, Grimes WH Jr, Fish JS,

Lester WM, Galloway WH. Criteria by which toxemia of pregnancy may be diagnosed from unlabelled formalin-fixed placentas. Am J Obstet Gynecol 1961;82:277–90.

166. Wentworth P. Placental infarction and toxemia of pregnancy. Am J Obstet Gynecol 1967;99:318–26.

167. Risteli J, Foidart JM, Risterli L, Boniver J, Goffinet G. The basement membrane proteins laminin and type IV collagen in isolated villi in pre-eclampsia. Placenta 1984;5:541–50.

168. Las Heras J, Baskerville JC, Harding PGR, Haust MD. Morphometric studies of fetal placental stem arteries in hypertensive disorders ("toxaemia") of pregnancy. Placenta 1985;6:217–28.

169. van der Veen F, Walker S, Fox H. Endarteritis obliterans of the fetal stem arteries of the human placenta: An electron microscopic study. Placenta 1982;3:181–90.

170. Robertson WB. Uteroplacental vasculature. J Clin Pathol [Suppl] 1976;10:9–17.

171. Robertson WB, Brosens I, Dixon G. Uteroplacental vascular pathology. Eur J Obstet Gynecol Reprod Biol 1975;5:47–65.

172. Sheppard BL, Bonnar J. Uteroplacental arteries and hypertensive pregnancy. In: Pregnancy Hypertension, Bonnar J, McGilliray I, Symonds E (eds). MTP Press, Lancaster, pp 213–9.

173. Chamberlain G, Philipp E, Howlett B, Masters K. British births 1970, Volume 2, Obstetric care. Heinemann, London. 1978.

174. MacGillivray I, Campbell DM. The effect of hypertension and oedema on birth weight. In: Bonner J, MacGillivray I, Symonds EM (eds) Pregnancy Hypertension, MTP Press, Lancaster P 307–311.

175. Haust MD. Maternal diabetes mellitus—Effects on the fetus and placenta. In: Perinatal diseases. International Academy of Pathology monograph No. 22: Baltimore, Williams & Wilkins, pp 201–85.

176. Jones CJP, Fox H. Placental changes in gestational diabetes. An ultrastructural study. Obstet Gynecol 1976;48:274–80.

177. Machim GA. Hydrops revisited: Literature review of 1,414 cases published in the 1980's. Am J Med Genet 1989;34:366–90.

178. Altshuler G. Chorangiosis: an important placental sign of neonatal morbidity and mortality. Arch Pathol Lab Med 1984;108:71–74.

179. Unger JL. Placental teratoma. Am J Clin Pathol 1989;92:371–3.

180. Potter JF, Schoeneman M. Metastasis of maternal cancer to the placenta and fetus. Cancer 1970;25:380–8.

181. Szulman AE, Surti U. The syndromes of hydatidiform mole. I. Cytogenetic and morphologic correlations. Am J Obstet Gynecol 1978;131:665–71.

182. Szulman AE, Surti U. The syndromes of hydatidiform mole. II. Morphologic evolution of the complete and partial mole. Am J Obstet and Gynecol 1978;132:20–7.

183. Lage JM, Mark SD, Roberts DJ, Goldstein DP, Bernstein MR, Berkowitz RS. A flow cytometric study of 137 fresh hydropic placentas: Correlation between types of hydatidiform moles and nuclear DNA ploidy. Obstet Gynecol 1992;79:403–10.

184. Genest DR, Laborde O, Berkowitz RS, Goldstein DP, Bernstein MR, Lage JM. A clinical-pathologic study of 153 cases of complete hydatidiform mole (1980–1990): Histologic grade lacks prognostic significance. Obstet Gynecol 1991;78:402–9.

185. Gardner HAR, Lage JM. Choriocarcinoma following partial hydatidiform mole: A case report. Hum Pathol 1992;23:468–471.

186. Yen S, MacMahon B. Epidemiologic features of trophoblastic disease. Am J Obstet Gynecol 1968;101:126–32.

187. Matalon M, Modan B. Epidemiologic aspects of hydatidiform mole in Israel. Am J Obstet Gynecol 1972;112:107–12.

188. Poen HT, Kjojopranoto M. The possible etiologic factors of hydatidiform mole and choriocarcinoma. Am J Obstet Gynecol 1965;92:510–3.

189. Parazzini F, Mangili G, La Vecchia C, Negri E, Bocciolone L, Fasoli M. Risk factors for gestational trophoblastic disease: A separate analysis of complete and partial hydatidiform moles. Obstet Gynecol 1991;78:1039–45.

190. Berkowitz RS, Goldstein DP, DuBeshter B, Bernstein MR. Management of complete molar pregnancy. J Reprod Med 1987;32:634–9.

191. Kajii T, Ohama K. Androgenetic origin of hydatidiform mole. Nature 1977;268:633–4.

192. Azuma C, Saji F, Tokugawa Y, et al. Application of gene amplification by polymerase chain reaction to genetic analysis of molar mitochondrial DNA: The detection of anuclear empty ovum as the cause of complete mole. Gynecol Oncol 1991;40:29–33.

193. Lawler SD, Fisher RA, Dent J. A prospective genetic study of complete and partial hydatidiform moles. Am J Obstet Gynecol 1991;164:1270–7.

194. Wertelecki W, Graham JM, Sergovich FR. The clinical syndrome of triploidy. Obstet Gynecol 1976;47:69–76.

195. Doshi N, Surti U, Szulman AE. Morphologic anomalies in triploid liveborn fetuses. Hum Pathol 1983;14:716–23.

196. Berkowitz RS, Goldstein DP, Bernstein MR. Natural history of partial molar pregnancy. Obstet Gynecol 1983;66:667–81.

197. Szulman AE, Surti U. The clinicopathologic profile of the partial hydatidiform mole. Obstet Gynecol 1982;59:597–602.

198. Rice LW, Berkowitz RS, Lage JM, et al. Persistent gestational trophoblastic tumor after partial hydatidiform mole. Gynecol Oncol 1990;36:358–62.

199. Lage JM, Berkowitz RS, Rice LW, Goldstein DP, Bernstein MR, Weinberg DS. Flow cytometric analysis of DNA content in partial hydatidiform moles with persistent gestational trophoblastic tumor. Obstet Gynecol 1991;77:111–5.

200. Bagshawe KD, Lawler SD, Paradinas FJ, Dent J, Brown P, Boxer GM. Gestational trophoblastic tumours following initial diagnosis of partial hydatidiform mole. Lancet 1990;335:1074–6.

201. Vejerslev LO, Sunde L, Hansen BF, Larsen JK, Christensen IBJ, Larsen G. Hydatidiform mole and fetus with normal karyotype: Support of a separate entity. Obstet Gynecol 1991;77:868–74.

202. Lee KC, Chan JKC. Placental site nodule. Histopathology 1990;16:193.

203. Young RH, Kurman RJ, Scully RE. Placental site nodules and plaques: A clinicopathologic analysis of 20 cases. Am J Surg Pathol 1990;14:1001–9.

204. Heintz APM, Schaberg A, Engelsman E, van Hall EV. Placental-site trophoblastic tumor: Diagnosis, treatment, and biological behavior. Int J Gynecol Pathol 1985;4:75–82.

205. Lathrop JC, Lauchlan S, Nayak R, Ambler M. Clinical characteristics of placental site trophoblastic tumor (PSTT). Gynecol Oncol 1988;31:32–42.

206. Eckstein RP, Russell P, Friedlander ML, Tattersall MHN, Bradfield A. Metastasizing placental site trophoblastic tumor: A case study. Hum Pathol 1985;16:632–6.

207. Collins RJ, Ngan HYS, Wong LC. Placental site trophoblastic tumor: With features between an exaggerated placental site reaction and a placental site trophoblastic tumor. Int J Gynecol Pathol 1990;9:170–7.

208. Finkler NJ, Berkowitz RS, Driscoll SG, et al. Clinical experience with placental site trophoblastic tumor at the New England Trophoblastic Disease Center. Obstet Gynecol 1988;71:854–7.

209. Young RH, Kurman RJ, Scully RE. Proliferations and tumors of intermediate trophoblast of the placental site. Semin Diagn Pathol 5:223–227, 1988.

210. Brinton LA, Bracken MB, Connelly RR. Choriocarcinoma incidence in the United States. Am J Epidemiol 1986;123:1094–100.

211. Hertig AT, Mansell H. Tumors of the female sex organs. Part I. Hydatidiform mole and choriocarcinoma. In, Atlas of Tumor Pathology. Sect. IX, Fasc 33. Armed Forces of Pathology, 1956.

212. Fisher RA, Lawler SD, Povey S, Bagshawe KD. Genetically homozygous choriocarcinoma following pregnancy with hydatidiform mole. Br J Cancer 1988;58:788–92.

213. Chaganti RS, Koduru PR, Chakraborty R, Jones WB. Genetic origin of a trophoblastic choriocarcinoma. Cancer Res 1990;50:6330–3.

214. Osada H, Kawata M, Yamada M, Okumura K, Takamizawa H. Genetic identification of pregnancies responsible for choriocarcinomas after multiple pregnancies by restriction fragment length polymorphism analysis. Am J Obstet Gynecol 1991;165:682–8.

215. Elston CW, Bagshawe KD. The diagnosis of trophoblastic tumours from uterine curettings. J Clin Path 1972;25:111–8.

216. Lage JM, Roberts DJ. Choriocarcinoma in a term placenta. Pathologic diagnosis of tumor in an asymptomatic patient with metastatic disease. Int J Gynecol Pathol 1993;12:80–85.

217. Christopherson WA, Kanbour A, Szulman AE. Case Report: Choriocarcinoma in a term placenta with maternal metastases. Gynecol Oncol 1992;46:239–245.

218. Parazzini F, LaVecchia C, Pampallona S, et al. Reproductive patterns and the risk of gestational trophoblastic disease. Am J Obstet Gynecol 1985;152:866–70.

219. Avril MR, Mathieu A, Kalifa C, Caillou C. Infantile choriocarcinoma with cutaneous tumors. J Am Acad Dermatol 1986;14:918–27.

APPENDIX 8-1
Protocol for Gross Placental Examination

WOMEN'S & PERINATAL PATHOLOGY   PLACENTAL EXAMINATION

NAME   **AGE:**   Path.*

UH*   **EDC**   Date   Dr.:

HISTORY: Prenatal and labor

    INFANT: _____ lb. _____ oz.   Term   Premature   Alive

Stillborn   Macerated   Sex

Other

(Twins Sex: 1:   2:   Weight: 1:   2:   )

GROSS EXAMINATION (In case of multiple gestation, use one form for placenta of each infant):

    WEIGHT: _____ gm.   **DIMENSIONS:** _____ × _____ × _____ cm.

    CORD: _____ cm.   Insertion: _____ cm. from margin. Membranous_____

    Color: _____ No. of vessels: _____ Other: _____

    FETAL SURFACE: Color: _____ Dull: _____ Opaque Membranes: _____

Subchorionic fibrin: None: _____ Slight: _____ Moderate: _____ Extensive: _____

Other:

MEMBRANES OF SAC: Complete: _____ Uncertain: _____ Incomplete:_____

Insertion: Marginal _____% Circummarginate _____% Circumvallate _____%

Edema _____ Nearest pt. of rupture _____ cm.

Decidual Necrosis (Extent and Location):

Other:

(Twin Dividing Membranes: Amnions _____ Chorions _____)

    MATERNAL SURFACE: Complete: _____ Uncertain: _____ Incomplete: _____

Depressions: Location & Dimensions (apparent cause?):

*Designate as #1 and #2, if so labeled when received. Designate as A and B, if arbitrarily labeled.

PLACENTAL EXAMINATION (continued)

Path. #

MATERNAL SURFACE (continued):

Old Hemorrhage: _____ Dimensions _____ × _____ × _____ cm.

Retroplacental _____ Retromembranous _____ Distant from margin: _____ cm.

Recent Hemorrhage: _____ Dimensions _____ × _____ × _____ cm.

Retroplacental _____ Retromembranous _____ Distant from margin: _____ cm.

Calcification: Slight _____ Moderate _____ Extensive _____

Other:

CUT SURFACE: Color (Normal, Pale, Congested, Mottled) _____

Consistency (Spongy, Firm, Gritty) _____

Intervillous Thrombi: Laminated: Number, Dimensions _____

Not Laminated: Number, Dimensions _____

Marginal Sinus Thrombi (Describe) _____

Infarcts: Color, Dimensions & Location: _____

Other:

GROSS SUMMARY:

FINAL DIAGNOSIS:

REMARKS:

Examined by: _____

Pathology in Gynecology and Obstetrics, Fourth Edition, edited by Claude Gompel and Steven G. Silverberg. J. B. Lippincott Company, Philadelphia © 1994.

9 | *Ectopic Pregnancy*

Ectopic pregnancy is significant because of its clinical consequences and the frequency with which it occurs. About 0.3% of all pregnancies are ectopic, and the frequency is increasing worldwide.[1-4] In the United States, ectopic pregnancy accounts for up to 10% of maternal deaths, and mortality is even higher than that in black women.[1,5]

Ectopic pregnancy is the consequence of an anomaly of implantation of the ovum. For various reasons, which are not always understood, the migration of the fertilized egg is sometimes disturbed. Implantation, instead of taking place in the endometrial cavity, is brought about in a uterine cornu, the fallopian tube, or, more rarely, in the ovary, cervix, or peritoneal cavity.

Most ectopic pregnancies evolve for a period of a few weeks and are terminated by the death of the fetus, which is caused by hemorrhage or by rupture of the walls containing the ectopic conceptus (due to distention or corrosive action of the villi). However, a significant percentage of cases continue into the second or even the third trimester, and deliveries of live infants occasionally take place.

In addition to decidual transformation of the endometrium, other endometrial histologic changes may suggest the existence of an ectopic pregnancy (Arias-Stella phenomenon; see Chap. 4). The abnormal localization of the implantation site causes hemorrhage in the placenta. The decidual mucosa may separate from the endometrial wall as a single cast or as multiple fragments. This expulsion follows the death of the fetus after an interval varying from a few hours to a few days. The decidual fragments are infiltrated by leukocytes, and the glands show a regressive appearance of postmenstrual type. The absence of chorionic villi, trophoblastic cells, and fetal parts in a uterine evacuation specimen for induced abortion should always be noted and investigated thoroughly. The failure to recognize ectopic pregnancies in this situation has led to maternal death.[6]

ETIOLOGY

The etiology of ectopic pregnancy is not entirely understood, and diverse mechanisms are invoked to explain ectopic implantation of the conceptus. The migration of the ovum may be disturbed by mechanical factors, including tubal chronic inflammation, compression of the pathway of migration by intrinsic or extrinsic tumors, diverticula, or endometriosis.[7,8] The most important factor in tubal ectopic pregnancy is previous tubal inflammatory disease. This is true whether salpingitis is implicated by clinical history,[4] antibody studies for *Chlamydia trachomatis* or other organisms,[3] or direct histopathologic examination of the uninvolved tube.[8-11] A few studies have identified salpingitis in as low a proportion as 29% of the tubes involved by ectopic pregnancies.[2] However, most studies found the prevalence of salpingitis to be in the range of 90%, which was significantly greater than the percentages found for control tubes[9,11] and included even tubes that were laparoscopically normal.[10] In recurrent ectopic pregnancies in tubes previously treated conservatively, the underlying tubal disease (including salpingitis isthmica nodosa) seems to be the major causal factor.[12] In women who were exposed in utero to diethylstilbestrol (DES), tubal

515

malformations rather than inflammatory lesions appear to be responsible for the increased frequency of tubal ectopic pregnancy.[7,13]

Another suggested cause of ectopic pregnancy is the presence of ectopic endometrial tissue (endometriosis) in the tube, which favors implantation at that site, although this is an uncommon association.[4,9] In some cases, there may be increased receptivity of the tubal mucosa to ovular implantation. In other cases, delayed ovulation and inadequate development of luteal endometrium may lead to failure of normal implantation, with subsequent menstrual bleeding impeding the progress of the ovum in the tube; this mechanism is considered uncertain.[14] It is possible that still unknown anomalies of the ovum may be responsible for nidation.

Induced abortion is claimed to increase the incidence of subsequent ectopic pregnancy.[15,16] More recent studies have denied this association unless there is postabortal infection, in which case the effects are mediated through the pathway of salpingitis.[17,18]

In women with intact intrauterine contraceptive devices (IUDs), almost 5% of all pregnancies are ectopic, apparently because the IUD is far more effective in reducing intrauterine than extrauterine pregnancies.[4] However, the rate of ectopic pregnancies per thousand woman-years of IUD use is not increased.[19,20]

Other iatrogenic causes of ectopic pregnancy have been postulated. These include ovulation induction with clomiphene citrate, human pituitary gonadotropin, or human chorionic gonadotropin, suggesting that the pathogenesis involves an endocrine disturbance, such as unusually high estrogen levels;[21] in vitro fertilization with insertion of the embryo directly into the fundus, which supports the theory of retrograde menstrual flow after delayed ovulation;[22] and failed tubal sterilization procedures, particularly laparoscopic and especially electrocoagulation, emphasizing the role of mechanical tubal factors.[23]

Previous ectopic pregnancy greatly increases the risk for another ectopic gestation and for infertility.[4,8,12,24] The risk factors probably include the therapeutic tubal surgery itself and the underlying tubal inflammation that may have been responsible for the first tubal pregnancy.

TUBAL PREGNANCY

Tubal pregnancy is by far the most frequent type of ectopic pregnancy. More than 97% of 1559 ectopic pregnancies in two large series were tubal localizations.[25,26] Implantation takes place most often in the ampullary portion, less frequently in the isthmic portion, and rarely in the interstitial portion of the tube.[9,27] Bilateral tubal pregnancy has been reported in more than 150 cases.[28] Simultaneous intra- and extrauterine pregnancy has been reported in more than 500 cases.[29]

Tubal pregnancy is characterized by the following symptoms, in descending order of frequency: lower abdominal pains, bloody vaginal discharge, and periods of amenorrhea, nausea, and vomiting. The most common objective findings are cervical tenderness, uterine contractions and other signs of early pregnancy, abdominal tenderness, fluid in the abdominal cavity, and a tender adnexal mass. Rupture is accompanied by violent pains, abdominal rigidity and rebound tenderness, and signs of incipient or actual shock secondary to internal hemorrhage. Common positive findings in the clinical history include a history of infertility for several years before the current incident, a history of previous salpingitis, and, more rarely, a history of a previous ectopic pregnancy. The incidence of repeated contralateral ectopic pregnancy ranges from 7% to 27%.[25,30] Repeated ipsilateral tubal pregnancy is becoming more common after conservative operative therapy.[2,12,24]

Macroscopically, the tube is enlarged and takes an ovoid shape. The serosa is stretched and congested (Fig. 9-1). Placental villi progressively erode into the wall until they provoke rupture of the tube. In some cases, hemorrhage is so pronounced that it leads to fetal death before rupture takes place. This hemorrhage is due to destruction of an arterial or arteriolar wall and leads to weakening of the implantation of the ovum with rupture of the capsule surrounding it (Fig. 9-2).

Microscopically, in some cases, there is a well-developed decidual reaction in the submucosal stroma. This reaction is usually minimal compared with that in the endometrium, and it presents in the form of small cell nests.[31] That portion of the tubal mucosa that is not directly involved by the placental tissues shows abundant leukocytic infiltrates. The gestational tissue itself is often completely or largely intraluminal, although invasion of the tubal wall may occur earlier in isthmic than in ampullary cases.[2,8,32] Villi are sometimes found only after a protracted search or not at all, with the final histopathologic diagnosis being hematosalpinx. In conservatively treated cases (less than salpingectomy), the embryo frequently is not identified.

In other cases, fetal death is not accompanied by hemorrhage or rupture, and the fetoplacental tissues undergo fibrotic regression. The pathologist may discover hyalinized and sclerotic debris of placental villi on examination of a tube resected at a later date for other clinical indications.[33] Secondary calcification and fetal mummification are rarer sequelae.

If the trophoblastic tissues have undergone such a degree of degeneration that their hormonal activity has ceased, biological tests for pregnancy may be negative. Other diagnostic maneuvers that may be of value include endometrial curettage, examination under anesthesia, culdoscopy, and culdocentesis (aspiration of nonclotting blood is suggestive but not di-

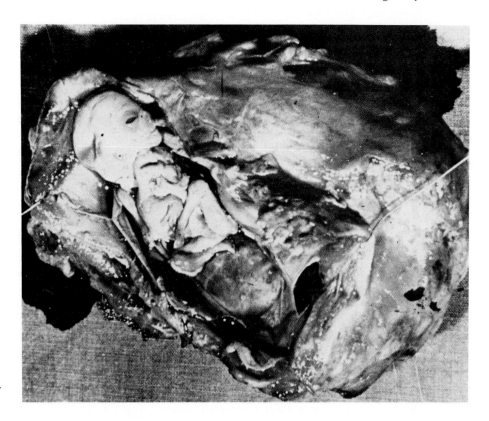

FIGURE 9-1 Ruptured tubal pregnancy.

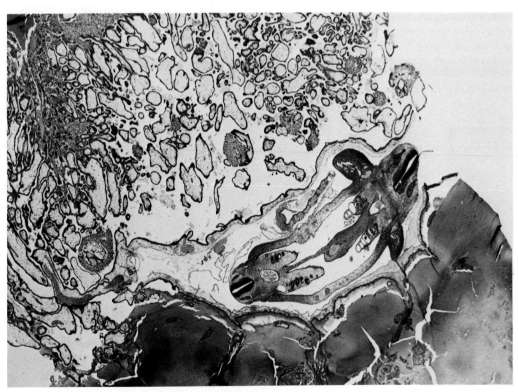

FIGURE 9-2 Tubal pregnancy: microscopic appearance.

agnostic of ectopic pregnancy). A newer modality that has been of great value is ultrasonography.[27]

The maternal mortality in tubal pregnancy is around 0.1%, and fetal mortality is nearly 100%.[5] Less than 50% of women treated for tubal pregnancy are able to conceive thereafter, and a contralateral tubal pregnancy develops in many of these women.[24,30] As a general rule, the severity of chronic inflammation in the excised tube is inversely related to the chance for a subsequent normal pregnancy.[8,30]

ANGULAR PREGNANCY

Angular or cornual pregnancy is characterized by the implantation of the ovum in a uterine cornu. This rare event generally terminates in abortion before the fourth month. Examination of the uterus reveals a soft hemorrhagic zone in one of the cornua, from which fetoplacental debris can be recovered.

INTRAMURAL PREGNANCY

Intramural pregnancy refers to a conceptus completely surrounded by myometrium and showing no connection with the endometrium or the tube. This is a rare presentation.[34] The fertilized ovum may enter the myometrium from the endometrial or serosal surface. Postulated mechanisms include adenomyosis, previous uterine trauma, abnormal endometrial glands, increased trophoblastic activity, and perforation of uterine blood vessels.

ISTHMIC PREGNANCY

Ovular implantation in the cervical canal at the isthmus is frequently complicated by hemorrhage and rupture of the uterine wall. If the pregnancy evolves, dystocic accidents such as placenta previa must be considered.

CERVICAL PREGNANCY

Development of the ovum in the cervical tissues leads to serious hemorrhages at the time of placental separation. This type of pregnancy almost always results in abortion. The maternal mortality rate is 30%.[35]

Macroscopic examination shows a voluminous, soft, hemorrhagic, and necrotic cervix contrasting with a small corpus uteri. Histologic examination confirms the diagnosis of ectopic pregnancy by demonstration of fetoplacental debris in the cervix, without corporeal attachment.

OVARIAN PREGNANCY

More than 400 cases of primary ovarian pregnancy are reported in the literature; they are estimated to account for 0.17% to 4.7% of all ectopic pregnancies.[36,37] The true value is probably closer to the lower figure. The criteria that must be satisfied before this diagnosis is made are as follows:

1. The tube must be intact and separate from the ovary, with no microscopic evidence of tubal pregnancy.
2. The gestational sac must be in the normal position of the ovary and connected to the uterus by the utero-ovarian ligament.
3. Ovarian tissue must be demonstrated in the wall of the gestational sac.

The localization of the products of conception may be intrafollicular or extrafollicular. The former is thought to be the result of a disturbance of ovulation, whereas the latter may be due to inhibition of discharge of the ovum secondary to mechanical factors (eg, inflammation, hypoplastic tube, uneven ovarian surface, or endometriosis).

Although most of these cases terminate in abortion in the first trimester, full-term live births have been reported in about 1 in 25 cases. A significant percentage of these infants are malformed.

ABDOMINAL PREGNANCY

Several hundred cases of abdominal pregnancy have been described. This presentation is said to occur once for each 15,000 live births,[38] and once for each 70 ectopic gestations.[39] It may be primary or, more often, secondary to an expelled ovarian or tubal pregnancy.

The placenta can develop among the intestinal loops or on an appendix epiploica, although it most often develops on the peritoneal surface. The pregnancy may result in a viable infant as a result of secondary vascularization from the peritoneum. About half of these infants are born alive, but most subsequently do not survive. A dead fetus, if not recognized and removed immediately, may undergo skeletonization, saponification (replacement of the soft parts by fats and soaps), suppuration or abscess formation, or lithopedion formation (sterile calcification). The maternal mortality rate is approximately 10%.[39]

References

1. Barnes AB, Wennberg CN, Barnes BA: Ectopic pregnancy: Incidence and review of determinant factors. Obstet Gynecol Surv 38:345–356, 1983

2. Pauerstein CJ, Croxatto HB, Eddy CA et al: Anatomy and pathology of tubal pregnancy. Obstet Gynecol 67:301–308, 1986

3. Walters MD, Eddy CA, Gibbs RS et al: Antibodies to *Chlamydia trachomatis* and risk for tubal pregnancy. Am J Obstet Gynecol 159:942–946, 1988

4. Mäkinen JI, Erkkola RU, Laippala PJ: Causes of the increase in the incidence of ectopic pregnancy: A study of 1017 patients from 1966 to 1985 in Turku, Finland. Am J Obstet Gynecol 160:642–646, 1989

5. Dorfman SF: Deaths from ectopic pregnancy, United States, 1979 to 1980. Obstet Gynecol 62:334–338, 1983

6. Rubin GL, Cates W Jr, Gold J et al: Fatal ectopic pregnancy after attempted legally induced abortion. JAMA 244:1705–1708, 1980

7. Russell JB: The etiology of ectopic pregnancy. Clin Obstet Gynecol 30:181–190, 1987

8. Stock RJ: Tubal pregnancy: Associated histopathology. Obstet Gynecol Clin North Am 18:73–94, 1991

9. Dubuisson JB, Aubriot FX, Vacher-Lavenu MC et al: Chronic salpingitis and extra-uterine pregnancy: Results of the histologic study of 215 tubal pregnancies. J Gynecol Obstet Biol Reprod (Paris): 16:27–31, 1987

10. Cumming DC, Honoré LH, Scott JZ, Williams KE: Microscopic evidence of silent inflammation in grossly normal fallopian tubes with ectopic pregnancy. Int J Fertil 33:324–328, 1988

11. Green LK, Kott ML: Histopathologic findings in ectopic tubal pregnancy. Int J Gynecol Pathol 8:255–262, 1989

12. Stock RJ: Histopathology of fallopian tubes with recurrent tubal pregnancy. Obstet Gynecol 75:9–14, 1990

13. DeCherney AH, Cholst I, Naftolin F: Structure and function of the fallopian tubes following exposure to diethylstilbestrol (DES) during gestation. Fertil Steril 36:741–745, 1981

14. Iffy L: Embryologic studies of time of conception in ectopic pregnancy and first-trimester abortion. Obstet Gynecol 26:490–498, 1965

15. Panayotou PP, Kaskarelis DB, Miettinen OS et al: Induced abortion and ectopic pregnancy. Am J Obstet Gynecol 114:507–510, 1972

16. Shinagawa S, Nagayama M: Cervical pregnancy as a possible sequela of induced abortion: Report of 19 cases. Am J Obstet Gynecol 105:282–284, 1969

17. Beral V: An epidemiologic study of recent trends in ectopic pregnancy. Br J Obstet Gynaecol 82:775–782, 1975

18. Chung CS, Smith RG, Steinhoff PG, Mi M-P: Induced abortion and ectopic pregnancy in subsequent pregnancies. Am J Epidemiol 115:879–887, 1982

19. Ory HW (Women's Health Study): Ectopic pregnancy and intrauterine contraceptive devices: New perspectives. Obstet Gynecol 57:137–144, 1981

20. Vessey MP, Yeates D, Flavel R: Risk of ectopic pregnancy and duration of use of an intrauterine device. Lancet 2:501–502, 1979

21. McBain JC, Evans JH, Pepperell RJ et al: An unexpectedly high rate of ectopic pregnancy following the induction of ovulation with human pituitary and chorionic gonadotropin. Br J Obstet Gynaecol 87:5–9, 1980

22. Tucker M, Smith DH, Pike I et al: Ectopic pregnancy following in-vitro fertilisation and embryo transfer (Letter). Lancet 2:1278, 1981

23. Chi IC, Laufe LE, Gardner SD et al: An epidemiologic study of risk factors associated with pregnancy following female sterilization. Am J Obstet Gynecol 136:768–773, 1980

24. Langer R, Bukovsky I, Herman A et al: Conservative surgery for tubal pregnancy. Fertil Steril 38:427–430, 1982

25. Bobrow ML, Bell HG: Ectopic pregnancy: A 16-year survey of 905 cases. Obstet Gynecol 20:500–506, 1962

26. Breen JL: A 21 year survey of 654 ectopic pregnancies. Am J Obstet Gynecol 106:1004–1019, 1970

27. Smith HJ, Hanken H, Brundelet PJ: Ultrasound diagnosis of interstitial pregnancy. Acta Obstet Gynecol Scand 60:413–416, 1981

28. Foster HM, Lakshin AS, Taylor WF: Bilateral tubal pregnancy with vaginal delivery. Obstet Gynecol 60:664–666, 1982

29. Honoré LH, Nickerson KG: Combined intrauterine and tubal ectopic pregnancy: A possible case of superfetation. Am J Obstet Gynecol 127:885–887, 1977

30. Franklin EW III, Zeiderman AM: Tubal ectopic pregnancy: Etiology and obstetric and gynecologic sequelae. Am J Obstet Gynecol 117:220–225, 1973

31. Randall S, Buckley CH, Fox H: Placentation in the fallopian tube. Int J Gynecol Pathol 6:132–139, 1987

32. Senterman M, Jibodh R, Tulandi T: Histopathologic study of ampullary and isthmic tubal ectopic pregnancy. Am J Obstet Gynecol 159:939–941, 1988

33. Burrows S, Moore W, Peckala B: Missed tubal abortion. Am J Obstet Gynecol 136:691–692, 1980

34. McGowan L: Intramural pregnancy. JAMA 192:637–639, 1965

35. Kouyoundjian AJ: Cervical pregnancy: Case report and literature review. J Natl Med Assoc 76:791–796, 1984

36. Grimes HG, Nosal RA, Gallagher JC: Ovarian pregnancy: A series of 24 cases. Obstet Gynecol 61:174–180, 1983

37. Hallatt JG: Primary ovarian pregnancy: A report of twenty-five cases. Am J Obstet Gynecol 143:55–60, 1982

38. Dehner LP: Advanced extrauterine pregnancy and the fetal death syndrome: Report of a case with clinicopathologic considerations. Obstet Gynecol 40:525–534, 1972

39. Delke I, Perez Viridiano N, Tancer ML: Abdominal pregnancy: Review of current management and addition of 10 cases. Obstet Gynecol 60:200–204, 1982

Pathology in Gynecology and Obstetrics, Fourth Edition, edited by Claude Gompel and Steven G. Silverberg. J. B. Lippincott Company, Philadelphia © 1994.

10 | *The Breast*

EMBRYOLOGY

Phylogenetically, the breast originates in sweat gland tissue and arises as a cutaneous appendage. It appears in the 8-mm embryo as a longitudinal cutaneous thickening situated on each side of the midline and extending from the axillary to the inguinal region.[1,2] These mammary crests regress rapidly except in the thoracic region, and in the 20-mm embryo the only one persisting is the precursor of the future mammary gland (Fig. 10-1). When regression is incomplete, aberrant (supernumerary) mammary glands develop.

In the fifth month of fetal life, 15 to 20 epithelial buds arise on the deep surface of the mammary crest and ramify to form the outlines of the lactiferous ducts. In the eighth month, the epithelial cords develop lumina. Proliferation of the connective tissue stroma of the central region forms the nipple. Apocrine glands develop around the nipple to form Montgomery's glands.[3] Once at this stage, the breast is not modified further until birth. At this time, under the influence of maternal hormones, the primordial lactiferous ducts ramify and briefly secrete a milky substance (colostrum or "witch's milk") containing fat globules, protein granules, and corpuscles of Donné.

At puberty, the evolution of the gland begins again and is completed. The main lactiferous ducts develop numerous prolongations (secondary lactiferous ducts) and terminate in small saccular structures lined by cuboidal epithelium (alveoli). Each main duct and its ramifications constitute a mammary lobe, of which there are 15 to 20 in each breast. The proliferation of these epithelial structures is accompanied by development of the vasculo-connective tissue framework and adipose tissue.

ANATOMY

The breast is composed of a glandular apparatus and fibroadipose tissue; it rests on a musculo-connective tissue bed.[1,2] In the center of its convex surface is an epidermis-covered, circular, pigmented region measuring about 2 cm in diameter, known as the *areola*. The nipple is situated at the center and forms a cylindrical excrescence of about 1 cm in diameter. Surrounding the nipple are the tubercles of Montgomery.[3] The arteries of the breast are branches of the internal mammary, external mammary, and intercostal arteries.

The lymphatics merit a more detailed description because they play an important role in the dissemination of malignant tumors of the breast.[4,5] Some of the perilobular, perialveolar, and ductal, and all the cutaneous lymphatics drain into the areolar plexus, from which three lymphatic groups arise: external, internal, and inferior. Many of the deep lymphatics of the breast bypass the areolar plexus and drain directly into these groups. The external mammary lymphatics form several large trunks, which flow peripherally around the external border of the pectoralis major muscle and terminate in the nodes surrounding the external mammary vessels. These nodes are in direct continuity with the other nodes of the axilla.

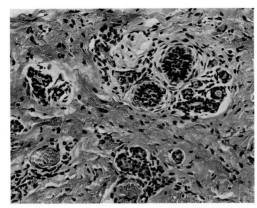

FIGURE 10-1 Fetal mammary gland.

The axillary nodes, from 10 to 30 in number, constitute five groups: (1) the group of the axillary vein; (2) the external mammary group; (3) the scapular group; (4) the central group; and (5) the subclavicular group.

The interpectoral nodes of Rotter provide a potential direct pathway to the subclavicular group, bypassing the lower axillary nodes, but they are usually of little significance. The internal mammary lymphatics arise in the internal part of the areolar plexus, traverse the intercostal spaces, and flow into the nodes of the internal mammary vessels; they measure from 1 to 3 mm each and number 6 to 8. From there, the lymphatic chains proceed into the supraclavicular lymphatic system and the mediastinal nodes.

The inferior or inframammary lymphatics originate in the deep surface of the breast and flow into the anterior pectoral nodes and then into the axillary or subclavicular nodes. There are also lymphatic trunks coursing to the supraclavicular nodes and to the lymphatics of the contralateral breast. Finally, lymphatic pathways lead to the paravertebral chains. Injection studies using colloidal gold have shown that 97% of the lymph flows to the axillary nodes and 3% to the internal mammary chain.[6] Intramammary nodes have been reported in 28% of carcinomatous breasts and were involved by metastatic cancer in one third of all cases in which they were present.[5] Intramammary nodes are also frequently encountered as mammographically detected masses in benign breasts.[7]

The nerves of the breast come from the second through sixth intercostals and from the cervical and brachial plexus.

HISTOLOGY

The main lactiferous ducts consist of a stratified lining of superficial columnar cells and deep cuboidal cells underlain by a layer of myoepithelial cells. A fibroelastic lamina surrounds this glandular structure (Fig. 10-2). The secondary lactiferous ducts are of smaller caliber but have the same structure.

The acini are composed of cuboidal cells partially surrounded by discontinuous myoepithelial cells. During the nursing period, the cuboidal cells become columnar, and their apical poles are charged with fatty secretory droplets (apocrine secretion).

The ductules or terminal ducts connect ducts with their lobules and acini. They represent the cut-off point for the elastic fibers in the periductal stroma, have the greatest proliferative activity of all mammary epithelial units, and may represent the site of origin of most breast cancers.[8,9]

Electron microscopy has permitted us to understand better the fine structure of myoepithelial and epithelial cells (Figs. 10-3 and 10-4).[10,11] The myoepithelial cells have clear cytoplasm that is poor in cellular organelles and rich in fibrillar bundles of smooth muscle type. The epithelial cells have dense to clear cytoplasm corresponding to an uneven distribution of organelles. Cytokeratin and actin filaments are visible in the cytoplasm. The morphology of the epithelial cells varies with the phase of the menstrual cycle. Estrogen stimulates epithelial proliferation corresponding to a greater RNA synthesis, with increased nuclear density and a high mitotic count. Ultrastructural studies reveal an increase in number and size of the Golgi apparatus, ribosomes, and mitochondria. Progesterone induces the dilation of ducts and secretion by the alveolar epithelial cells. Only in the third month of pregnancy and thereafter does secretory activity develop fully. Growth factors are also important in mammary development and function.[12] Argyrophilic cells are rare in normal breast tissue; some of them are hormonally active.

Premenstrual fullness is attributable to increasing interlobular edema and ductular and acinar proliferation. Steroid receptors and membrane-bound peptide receptors are involved in these mechanisms.[12]

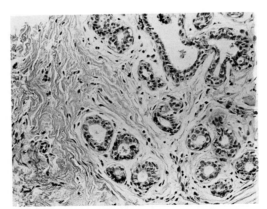

FIGURE 10-2 Normal mammary terminal ductule (*upper right*) and lobule. Note the epithelial and surrounding myoepithelial cells and the loose intralobular and dense inter- or perilobular stroma.

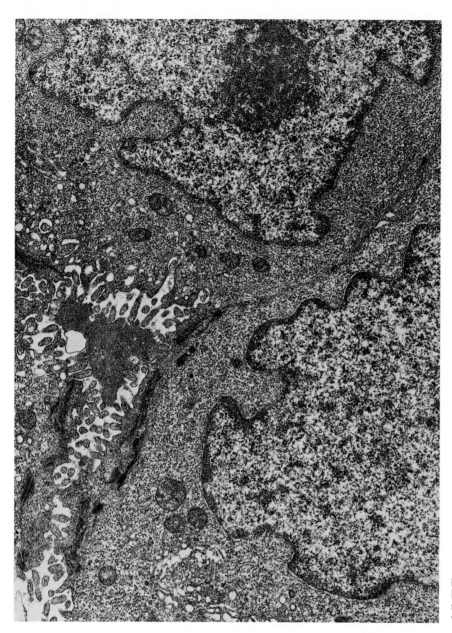

FIGURE 10-3 Electron micrograph of luminal aspect of normal mammary terminal duct. Note the numerous microvilli, tight junctions, and desmosomes.

During pregnancy, the breast undergoes a period of proliferation and remarkable hyperplasia (Fig. 10-5). These changes are a result of the activity of sex steroid hormones, prolactin, placental lactogen, and chorionic gonadotropin. The ducts form new digitations that terminate in numerous acini. During the nursing period, the epithelial cells develop marked secretory activity, with the production first of colostrum and later of milk. The secretory cells produce fat, lactose, and proteins through apocrine and merocrine mechanisms. Thus, the breast passes through three phases of development: at birth, at puberty, and during pregnancy.[12] It undergoes atrophy after the menopause (Fig. 10-6).

The intralobular connective tissue stroma is poor in collagen fibers and adipose tissue. It participates in the histophysiologic modifications of the mammary gland.[12,13] On the contrary, the perilobular connective tissue is thick and does not undergo histologic transformation during the various stages of development of the breast.

The nipple is covered by pigmented epidermis showing numerous papillae penetrating into the dermis. The stroma contains smooth muscle fibers, which constitute the areolar muscle, and accessory mammary glands derived from apocrine glands (glands of Montgomery).[3] At the periphery of the areola are found sebaceous and sweat glands and a few hair follicles.

MALFORMATIONS

Absence of the nipple (athelia) or of the breast (amastia) is rare. The latter may be unilateral or bilateral and is often associated with other congenital

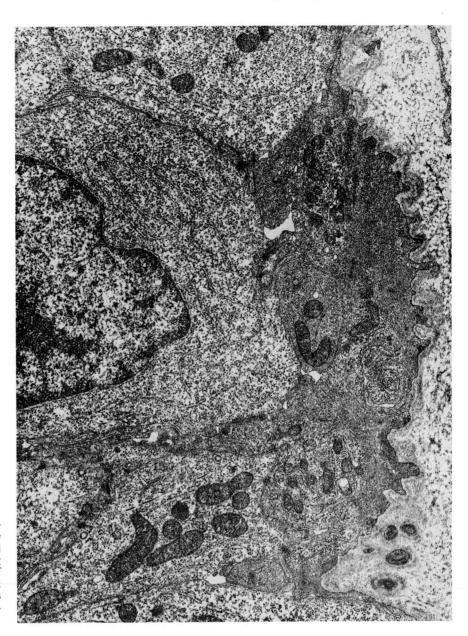

FIGURE 10-4 Basal aspect of the terminal duct shown in Figure 10-3. The dark cell at right is a myoepithelial cell, with hemidesmosomes bordering a basement membrane, to the right of which are collagen fibers. The light cells at left are the epithelial cells whose apical portions are seen in Figure 10-3.

anomalies. More common is the presence of supernumerary nipples (polythelia) or of supernumerary glands (polymastia). The aberrant formations are most often found in the path of the primitive mammary crest. They may be single or multiple, rudimentary or voluminous, and may show signs of secretory activity. They may be sites of benign or malignant tumors; axillary polymastia is a problem in this regard.

MAMMARY HYPERTROPHY

Mammary hypertrophy is found in the young girl of 8 to 10 years of age or at puberty. It is also seen in association with constitutional precocious puberty. It consists of unilateral or bilateral abnormal development of the mammary parenchyma. Before puberty,

it may be provoked by a functional ovarian tumor, a luteal cyst, an adrenal cortical tumor, or a cyst of the third ventricle. In a certain number of cases, thorough investigation fails to reveal an underlying cause. Puberty usually brings about spontaneous amelioration. Mammary hypertrophy developing after puberty advances progressively and sometimes attains monstrous proportions, necessitating surgical treatment.[14] The hypertrophy may be unilateral. Histologically, the hyperplasia involves the ducts as well as connective tissue stroma and adipose tissue.

DIAGNOSIS OF BREAST LESIONS

Tumors constitute the major category in breast pathology, and the major reason for breast diagnosis is ultimately to diagnose and treat malignant tumors.

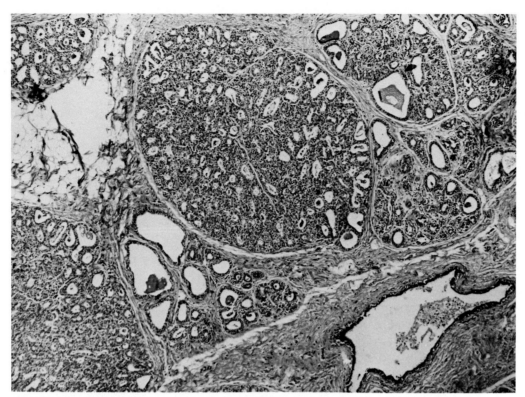

FIGURE 10-5 Lactating breast. Microscopic appearance.

The situation has changed markedly from 100 or even 20 years ago, when the patient generally presented to her physician with a self-detected mass, a biopsy was performed to determine whether the mass was cancer, and immediate operative treatment—usually without any adjuvant nonoperative therapy—was undertaken on the basis of that diagnosis.

In current practice, on the other hand, there are many variations from this classic scenario. First, most biopsies are performed in women who participate in screening programs in which abnormalities are detected radiographically, and many of these abnormalities are not palpable by the patient or the examining physician. Second, fewer and fewer operations for breast cancer are performed as one-stage procedures based on an intraoperative diagnosis. In most cases, the diagnostic procedure is separated from a subsequent therapeutic procedure by a period of days or even weeks. Third, it is now recognized that, rather than a simple diagnosis of benign versus malignant, numerous lesions exist which, although themselves benign, are premalignant or serve as markers of breasts at increased risk of developing cancer in the future. Finally, the therapeutic options for invasive cancers—as well as for preneoplastic conditions—now include various types of mastectomy and more limited operative procedures, as well as a vast array of adjuvant radiotherapeutic, hormonal, and chemotherapeutic options. The final choice or choices from this extensive menu depend on the specific diagnosis made by the pathologist and on additional features specific to each patient.

Clinical Diagnostic Techniques

As mentioned above, the classic—and for many years the only—diagnostic technique available to the clinician was inspection and palpation of the breast. At the beginning of the era of microscopic diagnosis, noted clinicians such as Velpeau could state that obvious cancers should be removed, and that there was no chance that "active and reasoned experience can ever be replaced by microscopic anatomy."[15]

In subsequent years, an extensive literature arose to prove that clinical impressions of the benignity or malignancy of palpable breast masses were often incorrect, and therefore must always be confirmed by biopsy. Even this literature is now largely of historic interest because of the decreasing proportion of mammary lesions presenting as palpable masses. Thus, a number of noninvasive techniques have arisen to assist the clinician in formulating an impression of a breast lesion.

Thermography and *infrared photography* depend on the difference between the skin temperature over a lesion and that over adjacent uninvolved breast tissue.[16] *Ultrasonography,* which uses high-frequency sound waves, is a totally noninvasive technique, like thermography, but both of these lack diagnostic precision and therefore should not be used as a

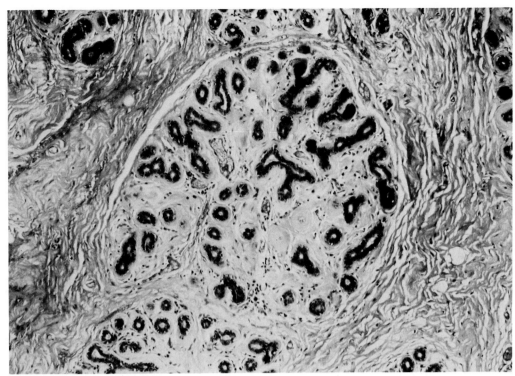

FIGURE 10-6 Perilobular fibrosis in an atrophic breast.

screening method in asymptomatic women.[16,17] *Galactography* (radiography after injection of the ducts with radiopaque dye) and *fiberoptic ductoscopy*[18] may identify lesions in cases of nipple discharge but cannot diagnose them accurately. With the latter technique, biopsy material can be obtained from the lesion. The most valuable technique is *mammography* (and its variant *xeroradiography*), a type of soft-tissue radiography of the breast. Mammography is of particular value in the detection of small, clinically impalpable malignant tumors, including those that have not yet invaded the stroma.[19–21] Although initially limited by its high percentage of error, mammography has shown a substantial change in the quality of its results because of improved image receptors and examination hardware and the increased experience of radiologists. This has been accompanied by a decrease in the dose of radiation to the patient, minimizing the potential danger of the technique. When used in conjunction with ultrasonography, which has a good ability to differentiate between solid and cystic masses, it provides complementary information. Unlike thermography, mammography has proved to be a useful technique for screening of asymptomatic women. About 25% of biopsies performed in this circumstance contain cancer, of which almost half are noninvasive.[22]

A certain diagnosis can be provided only by histologic examination. In instances of biopsy for mammographically suspicious or positive lesions, contralateral breast biopsy in patients with mammary cancer, specimens with noninfiltrating cancer, or any large biopsy with no grossly evident lesion, radiographic examination of the specimen can be an invaluable aid to the pathologist.[19,23,24]

Pathologic Diagnostic Methods

In addition to the purely clinical and noninvasive techniques discussed above—all of which essentially function to identify specific lesions for which a pathologic diagnosis must be obtained—there are numerous techniques available for transferring diagnostic tissues or cells from the patient to the pathology laboratory. These are discussed in general terms in this section, and the cytopathologic and histopathologic appearances of specific lesions are discussed under the headings of those lesions.

Fine-Needle Aspiration Biopsy

Fine-needle aspiration (FNA) cytology is easily performed, cost-effective, accurate, safe, and well accepted by patients. The technique is now well recognized after an eclipse of more than 40 years,[25] and many reports in the world literature reveal a high diagnostic efficiency.[26–29] This procedure is performed with an 18- to 22-gauge needle attached to a 20-mL syringe. Suction (which has been shown to be optional[30]) permits withdrawal of minuscule tissue fragments, which are smeared on a slide and fixed, preferably in 95% alcohol or with a commercial spray fixative. An air-drying technique can also be used with staining by the Romanovsky or Diff-Quik technique. Rapid staining and examination are useful to verify that adequate material has been obtained and, in some instances, to reassure an anxious patient. Malignant cells are recognized by their manner of desquamation in plaques and by their cytologic alterations (Fig. 10-7; Color Figures 10-1 and 10-2).

The general diagnostic criteria applied in clinical cytology are used here: variations of the nuclear shape and size, modifications of the chromatin structure, enlargement of nucleoli, staining affinities of cytoplasm, and modifications of the cellular size and form.[26,28,29] In addition to diagnosing malignancy, aspiration cytology is able to recognize some particular forms of cancer such as colloid and signet-ring cell, medullary, and papillary cancers; squamous carcinomas and comedocarcinomas; and various sarcomas (see discussions of these tumors). Immunohistochemical methods for demonstrating hormonal receptors in aspiration smears are available.[31]

FNA cytology of palpable lesions provides a simple means of differentiating between cystic and solid breast masses. Clear fluid from cystic lesions can be discarded, because experience has shown the absence of suspicious cellular elements. If a solid area remains after the aspiration, or if the mass recurs, the procedure should be repeated.[32] The technique has given excellent diagnostic results (about 10% false-negative and less than 0.1% false-positive reports) in the hands of pathologists expert in the interpretation of this material.[27] Unsatisfactory specimens are less often obtained when pathologists perform the aspiration and immediately check the material for adequacy.[28,29]

The value of FNA in the evaluation of nonpalpable lesions is less well documented. It is only by chance that the needle will penetrate a microscopic lesion in the absence of a stereotactic procedure. Hook-wire systems have improved the location of minute pathologic foci and provide a relatively stable guide for the surgeon.[33] Nevertheless, we think that FNA has not replaced open biopsy for the diagnosis of suspicious nonpalpable lesions. Negative aspirations should be evaluated in concert with the mammographic findings, because nonpalpable lesions may have been sampled inadequately.

Core-Needle Biopsy

The core-needle biopsy method, which produces best results when using a rotating trocar coupled with a motor turning at great speed, has the advantage of permitting true tissue biopsies to be obtained.[34] The disadvantage (as with other incisional techniques, including FNA) is that the specimen available may be from the tissue surrounding a lesion rather than from the lesion itself when the latter is small. FNA tends to produce more accurate results than core-needle biopsy.[27]

Cytologic Examination of Nipple Secretions

Nipple secretions may be spread on a slide, fixed in alcohol-ether or air-dried, stained, and examined.

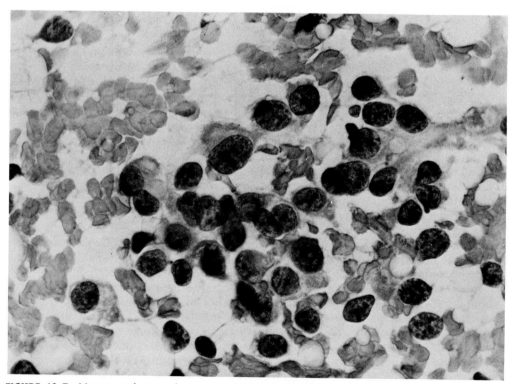

FIGURE 10-7 Mammary duct carcinoma: neoplastic cells in needle aspiration smear.

Spontaneous nipple discharge is usually produced by benign lesions involving large ducts, but cancer (usually intraductal) is occasionally the culprit.[35] When secretion is discrete, massage may be necessary. Even when this latter manipulation is used, most benign and malignant breast lesions do not produce nipple discharge. An additional disadvantage of this technique is the frequent necessity of extensive manipulation of the lesion, which may facilitate metastatic dissemination in cases of malignancy.

Open Surgical Biopsy

Open surgical biopsy remains the method of choice in many institutions. The fragment removed by the surgeon is immediately examined by the pathologist, and the most suspicious zones may be submitted for intraoperative histologic (frozen section) or cytologic examination. This technique permits rapid histologic interpretation, on the basis of which further excision, whether conservative or radical, may be planned. Immediate interpretation, however, may be difficult or even impossible; this is particularly the case for in situ carcinomas and atypical but benign intraductal lesions, some examples of sclerosing or microglandular adenosis, and paucicellular or well-differentiated infiltrating carcinomas. In these doubtful cases—and in many institutions in all cases—the surgeon must wait for the examination of permanent sections before proceeding.

In many institutions, intraoperative cytology is used as an adjunct to, or even a replacement for, the traditional frozen section examination in intraoperative pathologic consultation. The technique is more rapid than frozen section, and it enables the pathologist to study several regions of a suspicious tissue fragment. As with FNA cytology, alcohol-fixed or air-dried techniques may be used. The criteria used for diagnosis are similar to those used in FNA cytology.

Intraoperative cytology has three advantages over frozen section that are particularly important in breast pathology. First, intraoperative cytology preserves tissue from small tumors for use in adjunctive studies, such as receptor analysis and flow cytometry. Second, it eliminates diagnostic problems caused by architecturally atypical but cytologically benign lesions, such as sclerosing papillomas, radial scars, and sclerosing adenosis. Third, it avoids artifactual distortion of tissues by freezing, particularly in intraductal and intralobular lesions, in which permanent sections become difficult to interpret after such artifacts are introduced.

Accuracy rates for intraoperative cytology have been found to be comparable to those for frozen sections in the hands of experienced pathologists.[36,37] The field is perilous for the novice, however. A pathologist who is familiar with the frozen section technique should perform frozen sections and cytologic preparations in parallel for an extended period of time before electing to substitute cytology for frozen section examination.

How reliable is intraoperative diagnosis of breast lesions? Because frozen sections are performed more frequently for lesions of the breast than for any other site, this is a question that is frequently asked by the surgeon and the novice pathologist. Obviously, the adequacy of frozen section diagnosis depends largely on the pathologist's familiarity with the procedure; the institution that performs 10 procedures each year will have poorer results than the institution that performs 1000 each year. With this reservation in mind, we can summarize the classic literature as follows: false-positive diagnoses are extremely rare, false-negative diagnoses account for 0.5% to 1.5% of diagnoses reviewed, and another 1% to 3% of diagnoses are deferred to the examination of permanent sections.[36]

These published figures reflect the era in which the usual breast cancer was a large, palpable mass discovered by the patient herself or her physician. At the present time, when many tumors are "minimal" lesions discovered during the course of a screening mammographic examination, and when the practice of immediate mastectomy after frozen section has fallen into disfavor, we find that many more (up to 10% or 15%) intraoperative diagnoses are deferred, and that the false-negative rate may rise because of sampling error in macroscopically benign biopsy specimens. The main points of intraoperative pathologic consultation in many of these cases may be to confirm by immediate specimen radiography that the proper area has been removed by the surgeon, and to rule out the presence of a gross tumor that requires tissue processing for special studies. In most of these cases, gross examination alone may suffice.[38] In gross tumors, even if immediate mastectomy is not scheduled, an imprint or frozen section diagnosis is useful to confirm that the tissue sample frozen immediately for hormone receptor analysis is carcinoma and does represent viable tumor tissue.

Processing and reporting of mammographically directed biopsies represent a new and in many ways different chapter in breast biopsy pathology, and they require close cooperation among the surgeon, the radiologist, and the pathologist. Recommendations for the collaborative management of such cases have been published and are summarized in Table 10-1.[23,24,39–41] For small biopsies, all tissue received by the pathologist should be submitted for microscopic examination. With larger specimens, the submission of all areas of radiographic calcification and fibrous parenchyma in mammographically directed biopsy specimens,[40] and of 10 blocks of fibrous parenchyma in grossly lesion-free biopsy specimens resulting from the presence of a palpable mass,[41] has been demonstrated to be cost-effective and diagnostically adequate.

TABLE 10-1.
Steps in the Evaluation of Patients with Mammographically Detected Nonpalpable Lesions with Microcalcifications

1. Careful mammographic evaluation before biopsy to establish the extent of the microcalcifications
2. Biopsy with needle localization
3. Specimen radiography to confirm excision
4. Examination of the specimen radiograph by the pathologist and comparison with the gross specimen
5. Inking of the specimen margins by the pathologist followed by careful gross dissection, examination, and description
6. Submission of a portion of a grossly apparent invasive carcinoma measuring greater than 1.0 cm for ancillary studies (eg, receptors, flow cytometry)*
7. Postbiopsy mammography to confirm that all suspicious microcalcifications have been removed
8. Careful microscopic examination of permanent sections to confirm the presence of microcalcifications, diagnose any lesions present, and determine the relation of tumor (if present) to the inked resection margins.

*We [C.G., S.S.] recommend that frozen sections not be performed on specimens showing no gross tumor, an apparent intraductal lesion, or an apparent invasive carcinoma of 1.0 cm or less in greatest diameter, and that such specimens be submitted for careful microscopic examination of permanent sections, with or without intraoperative scrape or imprint cytology.

Adapted from Schnitt SJ, Silen W, Sadowsky NL et al: Ductal carcinoma in situ (intraductal carcinoma) of the breast. N Engl J Med 318:898–903, 1988

INFLAMMATORY DISEASES OF THE BREAST

Acute Mastitis

The risk of infection is greatest in the lactating gland. Obstruction of the major breast ducts may provoke milk stasis, which progresses to noninfectious mastitis and eventually to infectious mastitis. The leukocyte count is less than 10 per millimeter of milk in noninfectious mastitis but may be greater in infectious mastitis.[42] Bacterial contamination occurs through the fissured nipple and is propagated by means of the lymphatics toward the lactiferous ducts. The bacteria present are common skin inhabitants such as streptococci, *Haemophilus* species, and *Micrococcus pyogenes*. The breast is red and edematous; a purulent nipple discharge is seen. The ductal epithelium is infiltrated by leukocytes and subsequently undergoes necrosis. At this stage, the lesions may regress under the influence of antibiotics or, more rarely, progress to abscess formation. At the periphery of the suppurative zone are seen intense vascular congestion and edema and an abundant stromal histioleukocytic infiltrate. In addition to these abscesses related to the lactiferous ducts, we must mention subcutaneous abscesses (supramastitis) and deep abscesses (inframastitis).

Mondor's disease or thrombophlebitis of the superficial chest wall (thoracoepigastric) veins is a rare, usually self-limited condition.[43] The diagnosis is usually evident to the clinician, so that the pathologist rarely encounters the lesions as an excised specimen.

Histologically, it consists of an obliterative endophlebitis with thrombosis and severe alteration of the adventitia and intima. It may accompany carcinoma of the breast.[43]

Chronic Mastitis

Chronic abscess of the breast is of the same etiology as acute abscess. It consists of a purulent pocket surrounded by a thick fibrous wall. Histologic examination reveals leukocytic and histiocytic infiltration of the wall, which is dense, thick, and sclerotic.

Galactocele should be classified among the chronic abscesses.[44] It is a cystic lesion of variable dimensions containing altered liquid and viscous milk. The cyst wall consists of fibrous tissue containing leukocytes and macrophages. A prominent foreign-body giant cell reaction may be present (Fig. 10-8). Galactocele has been described in patients receiving oral contraceptives and suffering from galactorrhea. Diagnostic aspiration can cure the lesion.

Granulomatous mastitis, described by Kessler and Wolloch, is a lobular lesion characterized by noncaseous granulomas in which no organisms are identified.[45] An immunologic mechanism identical to the one observed in granulomatous thyroiditis has been suggested to explain this lesion.

Another probable autoimmune mastitis is the condition that has been called *lymphocytic mastopathy*[46] and, because of its frequent association with insulin-dependent diabetes mellitus, *diabetic mastopathy*.[47] The histologic features include lymphocytic ductitis and lobulitis with lobular atrophy and sclerosis, lymphocytic vasculitis, and dense keloid-like fibrosis (Fig. 10-9). The infiltrating lymphocytes have been described as predominantly B cells. The focal distribution of the infiltrate and the rarity of small lymphocytic lymphomas in the breast help in the differential diagnosis from malignant lymphoma.

Chronic subareolar abscess may occur in women during the reproductive years. It probably results from the obstruction of major lactiferous ducts due to foci of hyperkeratotic squamous metaplasia, a mechanism similar to the development of epidermal inclusion cysts. This obstruction creates an obstructive mastopathy with parenchymal alterations due to the granulomatous process.

Mammary tuberculosis is no longer common in Western countries. It is encountered in young women and often is secondary to pulmonary, lymph nodal, or costal tuberculosis; more rarely, it represents a solitary primary focus. It is accompanied by voluminous caseous axillary lymphadenopathy. Macroscopically, the lesion consists of soft, yellow, granular lesions disseminated in the breast. When abscesses form, they may fistulize to the skin. A sclerosing and nonabscess-forming type may simulate cancer. Histologic examination reveals Langhans' giant cell granulomata. Culture of

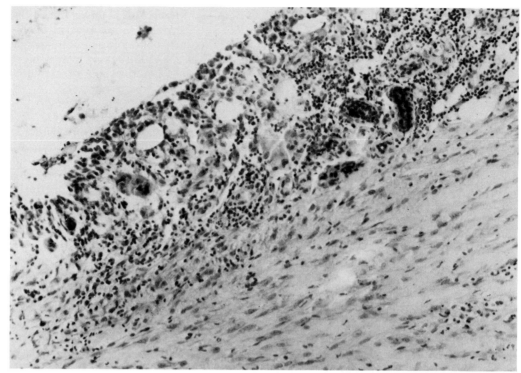

FIGURE 10-8 Galactocele wall: leukocytes, histiocytes (some multinucleated), and underlying fibrosis.

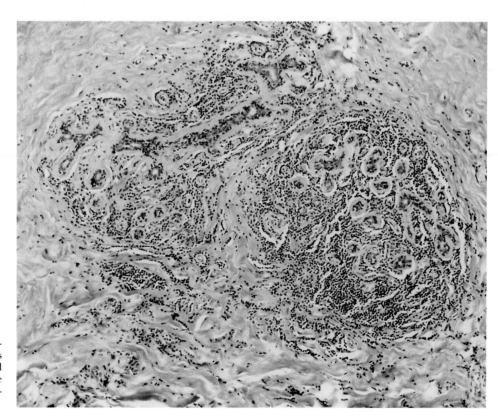

FIGURE 10-9 Lymphocytic mastopathy. Atrophic terminal ducts and lobules are surrounded and infiltrated by a dense infiltrate of small lymphocytes. This patient was not diabetic.

the tubercle bacillus or guinea pig inoculation confirms the diagnosis.

Mammary syphilis is a rare lesion. Primary chancre has been described in the older literature among wet nurses contaminated by infants with congenital syphilis. The lesion appears at the base of the nipple. Rare examples of secondary syphilis (cutaneous syphilids) and tertiary gummas have been reported.[48]

Mammary actinomycosis is rare and is secondary to a pulmonary focus. It presents as a fistulizing nodular induration. *Actinomyces bovis* may be identified in the purulent fistulous drainage.

Other inflammatory lesions that we merely mention because of their great rarity are the mammary localizations of *sarcoidosis*,[49] *blastomycosis, hydatid cyst, filariasis,* and *scleroderma. Mammary necrosis* as a complication of anticoagulant therapy with sodium warfarin (Coumadin) should be mentioned; vasculitis, thrombi, hemorrhage, and necrosis are found in these rare cases, which may represent a manifestation of a Schwartzman phenomenon.[50] *Wegener's granulomatosis* may occur in the breast,[51] as may localized vasculitis of no clinical significance.

Duct Ectasia

Mammary duct ectasia is manifested by the presence in the mature woman of dilated principal lactiferous ducts accompanied by adjacent granulomatous and chronic inflammatory lesions.[52] Synonyms are *periductal mastitis, chronic mastitis, comedomastitis, plasma cell mastitis, mastomalacia,* and *varicocele tumor.* It may be confused grossly with intraductal carcinoma. Clinically, it presents as subareolar induration accompanied by serous or sanguineous nipple discharge and retraction or deformation of the nipple. The rather slow development of these lesions and the secondary inflammatory complications clinically suggest an abscess. The complications regress after anti-inflammatory therapy but reappear periodically, the cause not having been suppressed. The nipple discharge and nipple inversion produced by duct ectasia and periductal fibrosis are not encountered in cases of fibrocystic change.

If the clinical and pathologic features of the disease are well defined, the precise mechanism of development of the lesion is not known. Is periductal inflammation the initial pathologic manifestation or is it the stasis of ductal contents? Pregnancy and lactation have been implicated in the development of the lesions, but this relation has been denied; moreover, this condition has been described in men.[53] Dixon and colleagues suggest that the primary change is periductal inflammation followed by ductal fibrosis and later ductal dilatation.[52] They have observed that the periductal inflammation is more frequent in young patients, whereas duct dilatation and secondary nipple retraction are more commonly seen in older patients.

Macroscopic Appearance. The subareolar zone is firm and shows several blue or brown voluminous ducts containing creamy or necrotic fluid. The ducts are surrounded by gray or necrotic inflammatory tissue. Compression of the dilated ducts expels the creamy discharge.

Microscopic Appearance. Two lesions are prominent: the presence of dilated ducts with thick fibrotic walls and giant cell inflammatory granulomata. The lesion appears to begin as duct dilatation, followed by rupture of the duct wall (Fig. 10-10). The cell debris, lipid contents of the duct, and lipophages spread into the adjacent stroma and induce the formation of a granulomatous inflammatory reaction, which sometimes simulates a tuberculous lesion. The granuloma organizes around lipid deposits and contains epithelioid cells and plasma cells. The abundance of plasma cells explains the term *plasma cell mastitis* that previously designated the lesion. Hemosiderin deposits are found in the macrophages. Distortion and destruction of the elastic tissue are always present. Foam cells are abundant. Retraction of the nipple is caused by secondary fibrosis. Histologic examination of the lesion erases the clinical suspicion of malignancy and avoids needless mutilative surgery.

Fat Necrosis

Fat necrosis of the breast is a lesion that frequently is mistaken for carcinoma.[54–56] This benign condition presents as a pseudotumorous mass with cutaneous retraction, ecchymoses, pain, and redness of the overlying skin. It is most commonly encountered in women with voluminous fatty breasts. In half the cases, the lesion is post-traumatic; more rarely, it may consist of necrosis secondary to an inflammatory focus. It is encountered in mastectomy specimens at a previous biopsy or FNA site and as a sequel to radiation therapy for breast cancer.[56]

Macroscopic Appearance. The biopsy specimen shows a poorly circumscribed indurated zone with yellow or gray foci of necrosis. Small cysts, fatty deposits, and hemorrhagic foci are sometimes visible. In advanced lesions, marked fibrosis, occasionally accompanied by calcification, is seen. Even on gross examination, the dense, granular, firm tissue may suggest a malignant lesion.

Microscopic Appearance. Histologic examination reveals necrosis of adipose cells with an inflammatory infiltrate rich in plasma cells, lymphocytes, and histiocytes. The macrophages are filled with lipids and appear as large cells with clear and microvacuolar cytoplasm (Fig. 10-11). Subsequently, a foreign-body granuloma rich in epithelioid cells and giant cells is formed around the fatty deposits and choles-

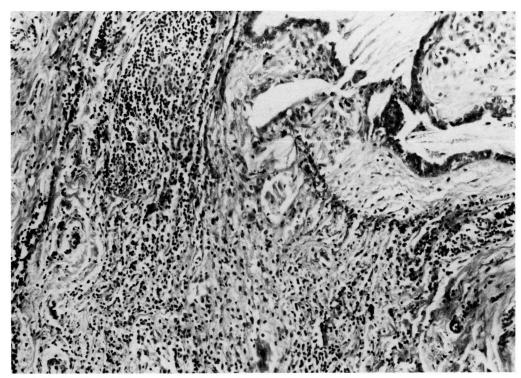

FIGURE 10-10 Plasma cell mastitis (duct ectasia).

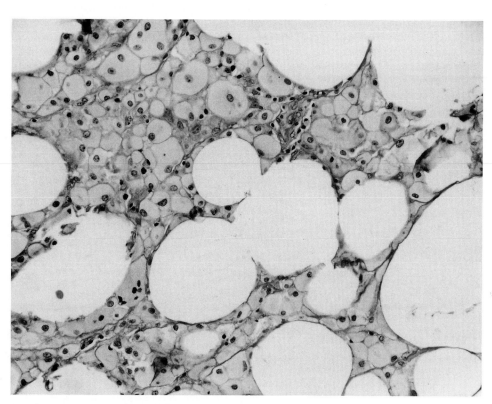

FIGURE 10-11 Fat necrosis. Adipose tissue is infiltrated by foamy macrophages.

terol crystals (Fig. 10-12). The lesion evolves toward fibrosis, which is responsible for the nipple retraction. Histologic examination is essential to arrive at the correct diagnosis and avoid overtreatment.

Duct ectasia with severe periductal mastitis is sometimes misinterpreted as fat necrosis. A clinical history of breast injury and the presence of necrosis may help to clarify the diagnosis. *Fine-needle aspiration* may provide diagnostic material, consisting of foam cells with vesicular nuclei, giant histiocytes, and leukocytes (Color Figure 10-3). Unlike carcinoma, ductal cells are absent or few in number. The evolution is benign, and local excision is curative.

Paraffinoma

For cosmetic reasons, women may receive intramammary injections or implants of paraffin or silicone. These substances may provoke the formation of chronic abscesses, foreign body granulomata, and cutaneous fistulas.[57,58] The clinical history, combined with the finding on physical examination of one or several tender, firm, well-circumscribed nodules, is usually diagnostic, but it is not rare to see carcinoma develop within a silicone granuloma.[57] The excised lesion is recognizable by the presence of a white, glistening, glairy substance, which histologically shows the foreign body surrounded by a prominent inflammatory reaction, usually with many foreign-body giant cells (Fig. 10-13). Penetration of the injected material into the thoracic wall and pleural cavity has been reported. This lesion is, fortunately, rare.

Because of recent publicity concerning leakage of silicone implants, many women are choosing to have their implants removed. The pathologist receiving specimens from such procedures should carefully examine the implants for evidence of rupture or leakage, and submit any surrounding mammary tissue received for microscopic examination.

INFARCTION

Although infarction is uncommon, it is important for two clinical reasons. The first of these is that infarcts presenting as localized masses may mimic carcinoma; they appear in young women during pregnancy or lactation[59] and usually involve fibroadenomas, adenomas, intraductal papillomas,[60] or lactating mammary tissue. Fixation of the lesion to the surrounding tissues, hardness, and sometimes enlarged axillary lymph nodes create a clinical impression of malignancy. The underlying lesion may be difficult to demonstrate if the infarct is extensive and chronic. It is sometimes difficult to determine if infarction appears in preexisting fibroadenoma or occurs in hyperplastic lobules; in the absence of pregnancy, infarction of fibroadenoma is rare. Mammary infarcts are significant in that, particularly in the older woman, they may be associated with other, potentially lethal, thromboembolic complications in other regions of the body. This is especially true in those cases that occur in women taking anticoagulant medication and in women who have Wegener's gran-

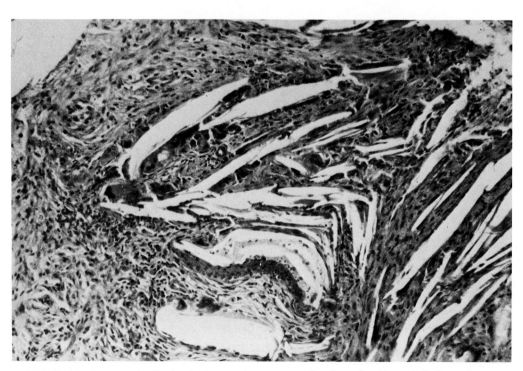

FIGURE 10-12 Fat necrosis: foreign body granuloma surrounding fatty deposits and cholesterol crystals.

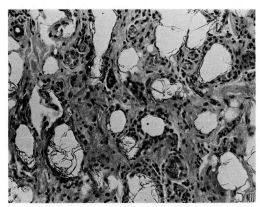

FIGURE 10-13 Paraffinoma: foreign material surrounded by histiocytes and giant cells.

ulomatosis,[51,61] thrombophlebitis migrans disseminata, and mitral stenosis with heart failure. In these situations, vascular lesions (arterial or venous) are usually prominent, whereas these are rarely found in pregnant or lactating women with a mammary infarct. Thus, the pathogenesis in the latter situation is assumed to be increased hemodynamic demand of lactating tissue. Occasionally, vascular occlusions are found in the infarcted tissues.

Macroscopic Appearance. The lesion is usually small, solitary, and well demarcated in the young woman but may involve the entire breast and the overlying skin in the older woman on oral anticoagulants. Infarction of multiple fibroadenomas has been reported.

Histologic Appearance. Ischemic necrosis, with or without extensive hemorrhage, is the main finding. "Ghost" outlines of previously viable tissue may be present if the infarct is recent. The distorted and compressed ductal formations at the periphery of the lesion should not be interpreted as infiltrating carcinoma. Squamous metaplasia of ductal epithelium may be so prominent as to provoke confusion with squamous carcinoma. Although carcinomas may, on occasion, become focally or even extensively infarcted, some evidence of the underlying tumor is always present. The persistence of a two-cell–layered epithelium argues against the malignant nature of the infarcted tissue.

MAMMARY INVOLVEMENT IN INHERITED SYSTEMIC DISEASES

The breast may be involved in several systemic diseases of inherited type. Among these manifestations are mammary subcutaneous neurofibromas in generalized neurofibromatosis, mammary fibromatosis in Gardner's syndrome,[62] and lobular agenesis in cystic fibrosis.[63] Women with the complex of cardiac and cutaneous myxomas, spotty pigmentation, endocrine overactivity, and schwannomas may have mammary manifestations including myxoid fibroadenoma, myxomatosis, and ductal adenoma with tubular features.[64,65] The skin overlying the breast may demonstrate the same lesions as extramammary skin in inherited and noninherited systemic diseases.

More importantly, benign and malignant breast lesions have been reported in women with Peutz-Jeghers and Cowden's syndromes,[64] and breast carcinoma itself is commonly familial (see the section on carcinoma).

BENIGN TUMORS

Fibroadenoma (Adenofibroma)

The fibroadenoma is a slowly growing benign lesion composed of epithelial and connective tissue elements distributed in variable proportions. It may represent a nodular hyperplasia of epithelial and stromal tissues and is not a tumor in the usual sense of the word. It is the third most commonly seen breast disease, after fibrocystic change and carcinoma. It develops in young women, particularly between 20 and 40 years of age, and rarely appears after this age. It is extremely rare in the male breast.

Etiology. Genital hormones appear to play a promotional role: the tumor develops during the period of gonadal activity, enlarges during pregnancy, and undergoes variations in volume and sensitivity in relation to the menstrual cycle. Fibroadenomas of huge dimensions may be encountered during adolescence. Estrogen administration may lead to vascular congestion, edema, and leukocytic infiltration within the tumor. Infarction may occur during pregnancy,[59] as may florid epithelial proliferation.[66] The latter has been reported with oral contraceptive agents, but a controlled study failed to confirm this as a significant finding.[67]

Clinical Appearance. Fibroadenoma is a well-circumscribed and freely movable, round, lobular tumor of a firm and elastic consistency. It does not adhere to adjacent tissues, skin, or chest wall, and it is not painful.

Macroscopic Appearance. The appearance of the tumor is characteristic. It is a well-limited, spherical, pink or white, lobular mass. When the epithelial elements are abundant, the color tends toward deep pink to light tan. Section reveals smooth, shiny fibrous tissue of lobulated structure (Fig. 10-14*A*). A leaf-like structure with deep clefts may be present. The surface of the tumor bulges above the plane of section as a consequence of the elasticity of the connective tissue framework.

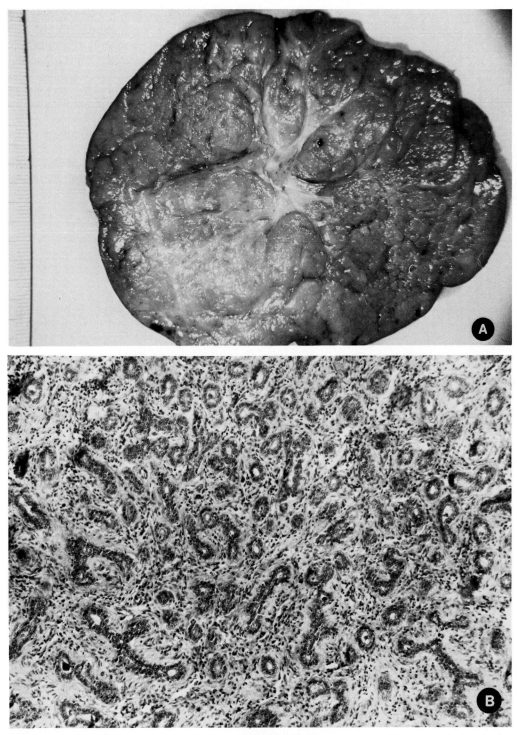

FIGURE 10-14 Pericanalicular fibroadenoma. **(A)** Macroscopic appearance. **(B)** Microscopic appearance.

Microscopic Appearance. Fibroadenomas may be subclassified according to the abundance and disposition of the epithelial formations. When these are numerous, the tumor is called a *tubular* or *pericanalicular fibroadenoma* (Fig. 10-14*B*). The tubular epithelial structures are ramified, of variable diameter, lined by columnar or cuboidal cells analogous to those of the lactiferous ducts, and surrounded by cuffs of connective tissue. Apocrine epithelium occasionally is present. The tubular lumina may be easily seen or reduced to small slits. The tubules may show varied appearances, depending on the planes in which they are sectioned.

The connective tissue framework is dense and richly cellular; the elements composing it are elongated and disposed in whorling fascicles that have a concentric disposition in the immediate vicinity of the epithelial formations. Numerous collagen fibers are present. Capillary vascularization is discrete. Foci of edema and myxoid or, more rarely, cystic degeneration may be present. Giant multinucleated cells of reactive nature have been described. In about 2% of cases, the epithelial formations are so overwhelmingly predominant and the connective tissue stroma so sparse that the tumor is known as an *adenoma*.[66,68]

In the *intracanalicular fibroadenoma*, connective tissue proliferation dominates the picture, and the epithelial tubules are compressed and deformed by the stroma (Fig. 10-15). The tubules and ducts become compressed, flattened, and curved in on themselves so that they no longer show true central lumina. Epithelial proliferation forms thin ramifying cell cords, which enclose round masses. The subclassification into pericanalicular and intracanalicular patterns, although consecrated by usage, does not imply differences in behavior and is of little practical significance.

Not too infrequently, epithelial proliferation may be seen within the fibroadenoma to a degree that appears alarming, especially when combined with moderate cytologic atypia. However, the development of carcinoma within a fibroadenoma is an extremely rare event, and these proliferative changes are of no clinical significance. True carcinomas arising in fibroadenomas are usually noninfiltrating (in situ lobular or, less frequently, intraductal carcinomas).[69,70] Rarely, pictures of squamous, cartilaginous, osseous, or adipose metaplasia are seen within the tumor.

In adolescents, fibroadenomas may grow rapidly and attain a large size, arousing clinical concern.[71] These juvenile lesions reveal marked epithelial proliferation without ductal compression and high stromal cellularity. Cellular atypia is not present. Differential diagnosis with phyllodes tumor may be considered, but the latter lesion almost always occurs in older patients and is characterized by at least focal stromal overgrowth and mild to marked stromal atypia.

A rare variant of fibroadenoma with the presence of argyrophilic cells has been reported by Azzopardi and colleagues.[72] The ductal outer layer shows a marked proliferation, which overshadows the inner layer; these large cells with a vesicular nucleus are argyrophilic with the Bodian silver impregnation technique. Azzopardi suggests a probable endocrine nature of the lesion.

Differential Diagnosis. Fibroadenoma is common and characteristic, but may on occasion pose a diagnostic problem in its distinction from phyllodes tumor, hamartoma, tubular or ductal adenoma, or adenosis tumor. The only clinically significant problem is with phyllodes tumor (see below), because the others all behave clinically like fibroadenomas.

Cytologic Appearance. In FNA biopsies or intraoperative lesional smears, cellularity is high. Broad sheets of uniform epithelial cells are present, often in a honeycomb pattern (Color Figure 10-4), and they characteristically contain numerous clefts and

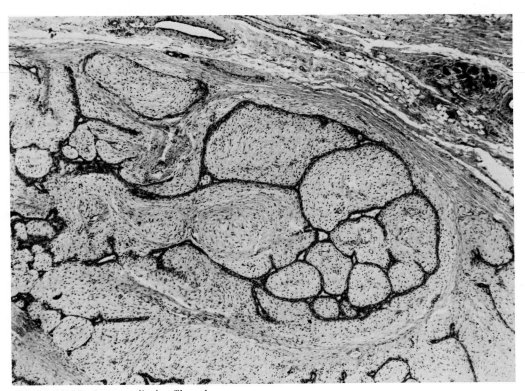

FIGURE 10-15 Intracanalicular fibroadenoma.

branches. These cell clusters are tightly cohesive, but single cells with ovoid nuclei lacking surrounding cytoplasm are also numerous, as are fragments of fibrous stroma. The apocrine cells and foam cells seen frequently in fibrocystic changes tend to be absent in fibroadenomas, but overlap occurs between the two lesions. Focal epithelial atypia is common in fibroadenomas, and may rarely lead to a misdiagnosis of carcinoma.[73] True carcinoma (almost always in situ lobular or ductal) may also be seen within a fibroadenoma, and has an excellent prognosis when treated conservatively.[69,70]

Lactational changes (Color Figure 10-5) may also mimic carcinoma, particularly in air-dried smears, because the cohesive nature of the epithelial cells is not well demonstrated. The presence of numerous intracytoplasmic lipid globules suggests the correct diagnosis.

Evolution and Prognosis. Growth is slow but may continue over a period of years to produce a voluminous tumor. These tumors stabilize or regress at the menopause, and they occasionally become calcified. The treatment of choice (mainly for diagnostic purposes) is surgical excision. These are radioresistant tumors. Although hormonal factors are thought to play a significant role in their genesis, endocrine therapy has been ineffective.

Phyllodes Tumor (Cystosarcoma Phyllodes)

Phyllodes tumor is essentially a fibroepithelial tumor characterized by marked proliferation of the connective tissue stroma and often by great size as well. It appears in middle-aged women with greatest frequency, but it has been reported in teenagers and in elderly women. Many of the cases reported in teenagers, however, are probably really examples of juvenile or giant fibroadenoma.[74] Phyllodes tumor generally contains progesterone receptors but not estrogen receptors.[75]

Phyllodes tumor characteristically grows slowly at first, and then rapidly, often attaining considerable dimensions. This tumor represents about 1% of all mammary fibroadenomas. The name of cystosarcoma phyllodes was given to this tumor by Müller, who first described it in 1838.[76] He used this term to indicate a cystic and fleshy tumor, but confusion has been caused subsequently by the implication of malignancy. In actuality, only about 10% to 25% of these tumors are malignant.[77–80] The term *phyllodes tumor* is therefore more appropriate for this lesion.

Clinical Appearance. This is a spherical, firm, usually well-circumscribed tumor, which may easily attain a diameter of 10 to 20 cm within a few months. Cutaneous ulceration, however, is a late manifestation even in these huge tumors and is of trophic rather than neoplastic character.

Macroscopic Appearance. The lesion consists of a well-circumscribed multinodular mass. Although the classic description is that of a voluminous tumor, typical lesions have been reported that measured as little as 2 cm in diameter, emphasizing the fact that it is the histologic appearance that is diagnostic. Section of the tumor reveals firm, white nodules separated by fibrous septa. In large tumors, foci of necrosis, hemorrhage, and cystic degeneration are numerous (Fig. 10-16).

Microscopic Appearance. Proliferation of stromal cells is intense, with the epithelial formations being rare and almost lost in the hyperplastic stroma. In many cases a tumor that at first appears to be purely mesenchymal reveals its true nature only after examination of many sections, when finally a few epithelial structures are found. However, it must be clear that these are an integral part of the tumors, and not merely normal ducts that have been overgrown by the tumor, before the diagnosis of phyllodes tumor is made. The connective tissue cells are large, with voluminous, elongated, and sometimes hyperchromatic nuclei and clear cytoplasm. They are disposed in anastomosing and whorled bundles that form multiple round nodules. Immunohistochemical and ultrastructural studies reveal a proliferation of myofibroblasts.[81–83] Heterologous stromal elements other than fibromyxoid tissue can be present, including bone, cartilage, and striated muscle. In some cases, the epithelial components may be abundant and form cysts and florid proliferations. Carcinoma can occur within a phyllodes tumor in rare cases.

The distinction between the benign and malignant forms is important but sometimes difficult to make. Because stromal cellular atypia immediately adjacent to the epithelial formations is common to both varieties, the regions that should be examined to make the distinction are those that are far removed from these formations, particularly at the periphery of the tumor (Fig. 10-17).

In the malignant form, cellular anarchy is more accentuated, nuclear and cytoplasmic atypia and mitotic figures are numerous, and the tumor borders tend to be infiltrating rather than well circumscribed (see Fig. 10-17). Stromal overgrowth (large regions of pure stromal proliferation) is commonly seen. Because of the frequent difficulty in dividing these tumors into benign and malignant forms, some authors prefer to include a "borderline" group for the intermediate cases. Our recommendation is to use only two categories, expressed as low-grade and high-grade tumor. In any event, the report of the pathologist to the surgeon should always state in some form the degree of histologic atypia of the tumor. However, the pathologist and surgeon must realize that cytologically benign lesions occasionally behave in a malignant fashion or recur locally as the malignant variant and, conversely, that a high percentage of malignant lesions are cured by conservative surgery.

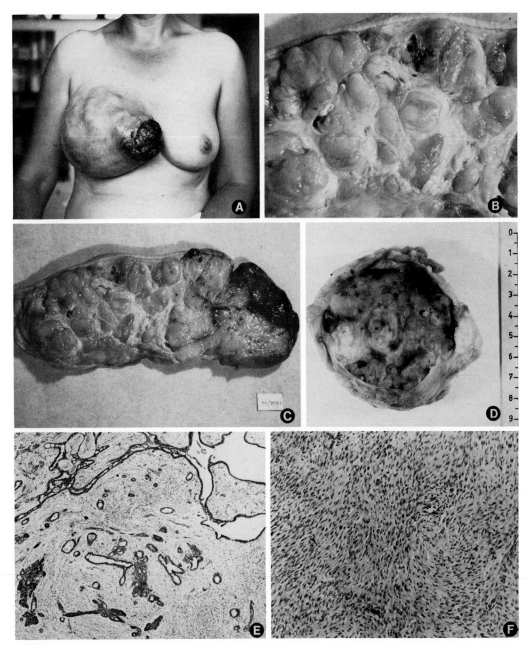

FIGURE 10-16 Cystosarcoma phyllodes: benign form.

Different prognostic factors have been tested, including tumor margins, mitotic activity, stromal overgrowth, stromal cellular atypism, and necrosis, but conflicting results have been obtained.[78–80,84,85] Ploidy studies have been found to be useful in some series[84] but not in others.[80,85]

Cytologic Appearance. A few cases have been reported in which the diagnosis was suggested by FNA cytology.[86,87] Phyllodes tumor is characterized by a high cellularity of stromal fragments with bipolar naked nuclei, clusters of ductal cells with overlapping nuclei, giant cells of foreign-body type, and foam cells (Color Figure 10-6). The appearance is similar to that described above for fibroadenoma but with more stromal cellularity and atypia.

Evolution and Prognosis. The evolution of the benign tumors is rapid; the volume and the threat of cutaneous ulceration demand rapid surgical intervention. Local recurrence after an inadequately wide excision is not uncommon but does not indicate conversion to malignancy, which rarely occurs. The malignant forms grow rapidly locally and have the potential for hematogenous metastases; the most frequent sites are lung, pleura, and bone. Lymph node metastases have been reported but are so rare that they do not constitute a significant hazard. The me-

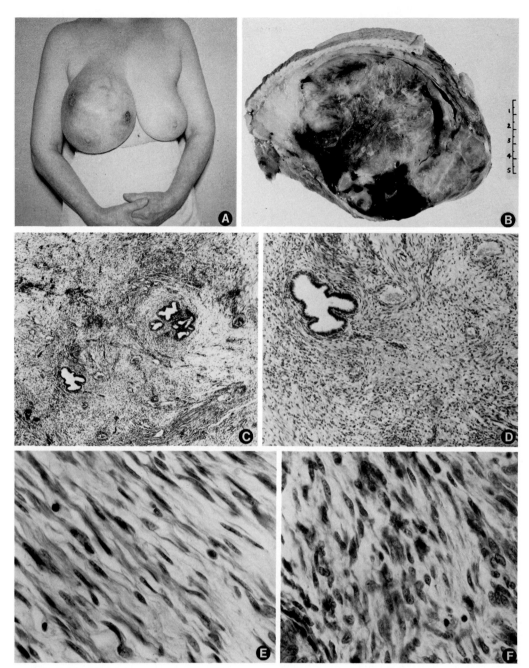

FIGURE 10-17 Cystosarcoma phyllodes: malignant form.

tastases consist histologically of the stromal elements of the tumor only, with the exception of a single reported case in which stromal and epithelial elements metastasized.[88]

Surgical treatment may consist of local excision if the tumor is benign and not too large. Voluminous or malignant phyllodes tumors are best treated by simple mastectomy. Adjuvant radiation therapy does not seem to change the prognosis.

Differential Diagnosis. Although the differential diagnosis between the benign and malignant forms (see above) is discussed extensively in the litera-

ture—albeit with no uniform conclusion—an equally vexing problem involves the distinction between a fibroadenoma with an unusual degree of stromal proliferation and the lowest grade lesion acceptable as a phyllodes tumor. In our opinion, the age of the patient (adolescent and very young women rarely have phyllodes tumors) and the size of the tumor (with 2 cm as a useful but not perfect dividing line) often are helpful adjuncts to purely histologic features. For the diagnosis of phyllodes tumor, the stromal proliferation should be diffuse rather than focal and should be accompanied by at least some cytologic atypia. Ultrastructural studies have demonstrated basement membrane reduplication at the epithelial-stromal junction in fibroadenoma and focal ruptures of basement membrane in phyllodes tumor,[83] but it remains to be seen if this can be demonstrated at the light microscopic level by immunohistochemical stains for basement membrane components. In any event, borderline tumors should be excised adequately rather than shelled out.

At the other end of the spectrum, high-grade phyllodes tumors with a sparse ductal component should be differentiated from pure fibrosarcoma, liposarcoma, and malignant fibrous histiocytoma of the breast, which generally have a poorer prognosis. Many sections may be required to demonstrate the ductal elements, which must be well within the tumor rather than entrapped at the periphery.

Intraductal Papilloma

Also known as *papillary adenoma, papillary cystadenoma,* and *dendritic adenoma,* intraductal papillomas are found within the principal lactiferous ducts and are composed of epithelial vegetations with central connective tissue axes.[89-91] These lesions are relatively uncommon. They appear at any age, but preferentially between 30 and 50 years. They frequently pose the diagnostic problem of differentiation from intraductal carcinoma. They should be differentiated from the far more common intraductal "papillomatosis," better known as *intraductal hyperplasia* or *epitheliosis,* a multicentric involvement of secondary ducts usually seen as part of the spectrum of fibrocystic changes (see below).

Clinical Appearance. This lesion manifests itself by (1) spontaneous or induced serous or bloody nipple discharge, (2) the presence of a small subareolar tumor of a few millimeters in diameter, and (3) rarely, nipple retraction. Galactography or ductoscopy often permits localization of the tumor.[18] Cytologic examination of the discharge reveals numerous epithelial cells of benign appearance.

Macroscopic Examination. Within a dilated or cystic duct is found a soft, friable, red or yellow, papillomatous formation attached by a short, thin stalk to the duct wall. These tumors usually approximate 5 mm in diameter and show superficial hemorrhagic ulceration.

Microscopic Examination. The tumor is composed of multiple papillae, each of which consists of a connective tissue axis on which are disposed the cuboidal or columnar epithelial cells (Fig. 10-18). These structures frequently ramify and are coupled together to form pseudoglandular cavities of diverse sizes and shapes; proliferation of solid cell nests is commonly seen. Apocrine metaplasia may be present, but it is much more common in the multifocal intraductal "papillomatosis" of fibrocystic change.

The cells show moderate secretory activity and are disposed in two or three layers, which include a variable number of myoepithelial cells. Bizarre and atypical nuclear and cytoplasmic anomalies are absent, and mitoses are rare. Small foci of sclerosis and hyalinization are frequently seen; these are sequelae of hemorrhage, ulceration, or arterial thrombosis in the stalks.

Cytologic Appearance. Cytologic examination of the serous or bloody nipple discharge shows uniform cells with vesicular nuclei, fine granular chromatin, and homogeneous cytoplasm (Color Figure 10-7). Nucleoli are inconspicuous. These cells are isolated or display very typical cohesive papillary structures. Distinction from carcinoma is based on the absence of nuclear and cytoplasmic atypia and the lesser degree of cellularity. Myoepithelial cells may be represented by dark, elongated, naked nuclei.

Differential Diagnosis. The distinction between a benign but moderately atypical intraductal papilloma and a low-grade intraductal papillary carcinoma may be difficult to make.[89,92-95] Benign lesions are more frequently misdiagnosed as malignant than vice versa. The presence of notable cytologic atypia (unless limited to cells showing apocrine metaplasia) should characterize an intraductal papillary lesion as malignant, as should abnormal mitotic figures, the absence of vasculo-connective tissue axes in the stalks of the papillae, and the presence of cell strands bridging the duct lumen and forming a pattern like the spokes of a cartwheel (cribriform pattern). The holes between the spokes, however, should be round and uniform, because slit-like and non-uniform spaces are frequently seen in benign papillomas and papillomatoses. Central necrosis also suggests malignancy but may be seen rarely in benign lesions. Myoepithelial cells are numerous in intraductal papillomas and absent to sparse in carcinomas, and they can be demonstrated immunohistochemically using antibodies to muscle-specific actin and, less reproducibly, to high-molecular-weight keratins and S-100 protein.[93] If myoepithelial cells are easily seen without special stains, benignity is strongly favored. Apocrine metaplasia, as mentioned previously, is far more common in benign than in malignant lesions, particularly when it is focal; the rare apocrine carcinoma shows this change diffusely. The presence of true stromal invasion, of course, characterizes a tumor as indisputably malignant. However, marked sclerosis within and around a benign intraductal papilloma occasionally produces an appearance of "pseudoinvasion," with which the pathologist must be familiar.[92] This sclerosis is usually densely hyalinized, as opposed to the more myxoid and inflamed fibroelastotic stroma of infiltrating carcinoma (Fig. 10-19).

Infarction of a papilloma, associated with marked distortion of the ductal structures, is important to recognize because it may simulate invasive

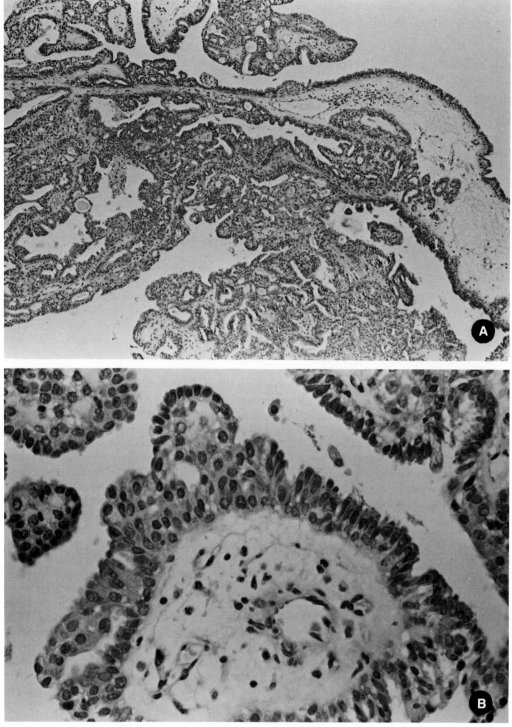

FIGURE 10-18 Intraductal papilloma. **(A)** Low-power photomicrograph—note the fibrovascular connective tissue stalks. **(B)** Detail of benign-appearing ductal epithelial cells and underlying myoepithelial cells.

carcinoma.[60] Squamous metaplasia sometimes present in papillomas should not be overdiagnosed as differentiated squamous carcinoma.[60] In metaplasia, the squamous elements are devoid of nuclear atypia and atypical mitoses.

Under the term *juvenile papillomatosis,* localized masses with grossly visible cysts (so-called "Swiss cheese" disease) and prominent intracystic and intraductal proliferations have been described in adolescents and young women (Fig. 10-20).[96] This proliferation can range from banal to florid to atypical hyperplasia. Coexistent adenosis, fibrosis, and radial

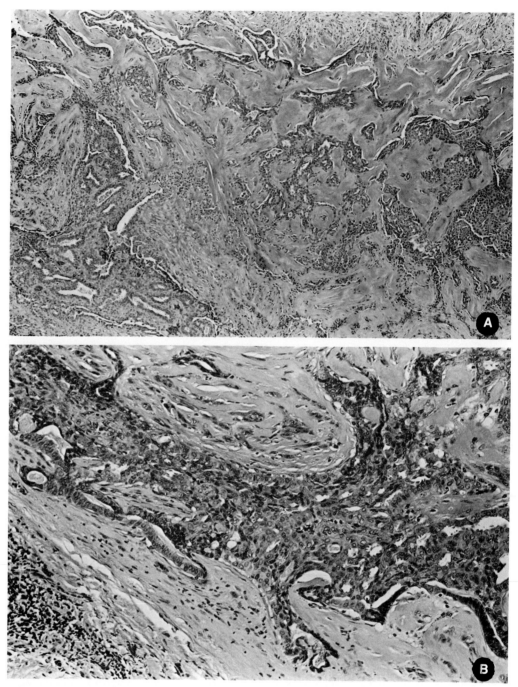

FIGURE 10-19 Sclerosing papilloma. Hyalinized stroma **(A)** within and **(B)** around the ductal proliferation creates a pseudoinfiltrative pattern. The benign cytologic appearance of the lesion is demonstrated in **B**.

scars are frequently encountered. FNA cytology confirms the benign polymorphous picture and includes many foam cells as well as normal and atypical ductal cells. This lesion should be differentiated from the diffuse "papillomatosis" accompanying fibrocystic changes in older women, in which no mass is macroscopically evident, and from solitary or multiple papillomas. Juvenile papillomatosis also occurs in adult women—up to 35 years of age in the series of Rosen and Kimmel,[96] so the name is somewhat misleading.

Long-term follow-up of these lesions is necessary because our knowledge of their malignant potential is scanty. Rosen and Kimmel suggest that carcinoma is more likely to develop in women with a positive family history and recurrent bilateral lesions.[96]

Another recently characterized lesion that probably is a variant of intraductal papilloma is *ductal adenoma of the breast*.[97] This is a lesion of medium-sized to large ducts, usually single but occasionally multiple, that is solid and may show worrisome cytologic

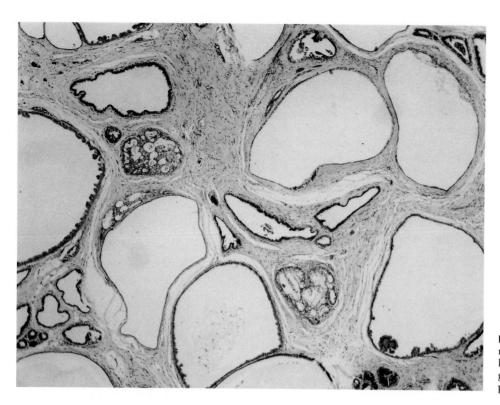

FIGURE 10-20 Juvenile papillomatosis. Multiple cystically dilated ducts show varying degrees of intracystic epithelial proliferation.

atypia and pseudoinfiltration. Myoepithelial cells and intact basement membrane can be demonstrated immunohistochemically, and the lesion does not recur after local excision.

Evolution. Although numerous studies have suggested that the multiple intraductal hyperplastic lesions of fibrocystic change probably form a continuous spectrum from benign to malignant, with the dividing line poorly defined, solitary intraductal papillomas are totally benign lesions in almost all cases.[98-100] Although some authors have noted an increased risk of subsequent carcinoma in patients treated for intraductal papilloma, others have felt that in most of these cases the original lesion was probably underdiagnosed. In any event, excision should be complete to avoid local recurrence. Actual focal or complete malignant transformation within an intraductal papilloma is rare; such a lesion should be treated as intraductal carcinoma (Fig. 10-21). In the uncommon case of multiple intraductal papillomas, the risk of subsequent carcinoma is higher than that of the usual solitary lesion.[99]

Adenoma of the Nipple

Adenoma of the nipple presents as a nodule immediately beneath the nipple, often with crusting or ulceration of the nipple, and is often misdiagnosed clinically as Paget disease or an intraductal papilloma or carcinoma. The lesion may be accompanied by a bloody discharge and soreness of the nipple and appears more frequently during the fourth and fifth decades. Synonyms are *subareolar papillomatosis, florid papillomatosis, papillary adenoma,* and *erosive adenomatosis.*

Macroscopically, the lesion is a solitary, well-circumscribed, usually solid mass with a density ranging from soft to firm. It infiltrates indistinctly the nipple and the subareolar region.

The *histologic appearance* is identical to that of hidradenoma papilliferum, a type of sweat gland adenoma, but no sweat glands are seen, and the lesion appears to arise in mammary ducts (Figs. 10-22 and 10-23). The characteristic features are ducts filled by branched papillary projections with central connective tissue axes, lined by a double layer of cells (epithelial and myoepithelial). The cells are always uniform, and mitotic activity is usually low. Necrosis is rare. Apocrine snouts, squamous cysts, solid nests of cells, and peripheral fibrosis with pseudoinvasion are frequently seen.[101-103] Fibrosis with subsequent epithelial distortion may be considerable, and it should be noted that this is not a purely intraductal lesion.

The *cytologic appearance* in FNA or intraoperative smears (Color Figure 10-8) is characterized by high cellularity, with uniform ductal epithelial cells in clusters and occasionally singly, as well as myoepithelial cells, variable numbers of inflammatory cells and macrophages, and some necrotic debris.[104] Nuclear atypia is absent or minimal.

The *evolution* of this lesion is benign, and it is cured by local excision. Because intraductal papil-

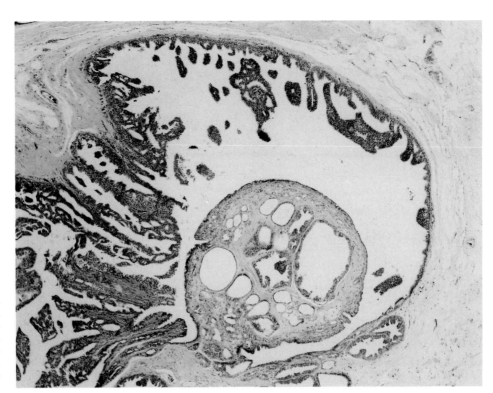

FIGURE 10-21 Intraductal papilloma (the round polypoid lesion on a stalk) coexisting in the same duct with extensive micropapillary proliferation diagnosable as intraductal carcinoma when it involves two or more complete duct profiles.

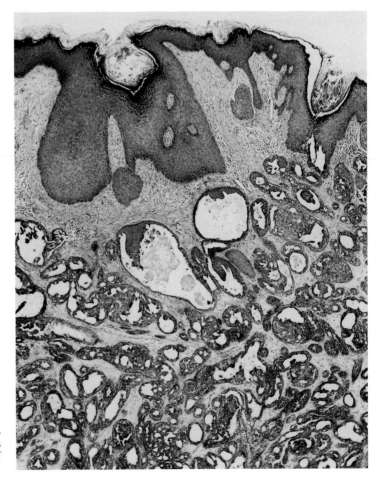

FIGURE 10-22 Adenoma of the nipple. Note the extension to the nipple epidermis. Squamous epithelium is present within some of the dilated ducts in the center of the figure. Lack of circumscription is apparent.

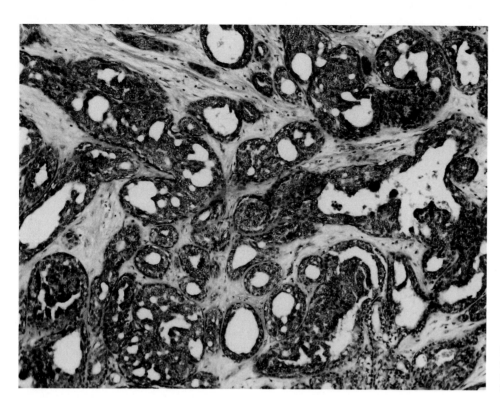

FIGURE 10-23 Adenoma of the nipple. Ducts are surrounded by prominent myoepithelial cell layer.

loma and intraductal or invasive carcinoma have been seen elsewhere in the same breast on a number of occasions, their presence should always be excluded.[101,103]

Sweat and Salivary Gland-Type Tumors

In addition to adenoma of the nipple, rarer lesions showing the histologic picture of benign sweat gland or salivary gland tumors have been reported. These include *clear cell hidradenoma* (clear cell myoepithelioma),[105] *eccrine spiradenoma*,[105] *pleomorphic adenoma* (benign mixed tumor)[106] and *syringomatous adenoma of the nipple*.[107] Follow-up of these lesions has been uniformly benign. Syringomatous adenoma of the nipple (Color Figure 10-9) is particularly important to recognize, because it may mimic certain patterns of mammary carcinoma. Diagnostic features include the typical location as well as the usual slit-like lumina, cell stratification, squamous metaplasia, absence of cytologic atypia, and lack of a stromal response.

In addition, there is a group of mammary tumors of low or incompletely characterized malignant potential that deserve mention in this section. *Adenoid cystic carcinoma* is traditionally included in the classification of ductal carcinomas and is discussed in that section. However, in many ways it should be thought of as belonging here because it is of salivary gland type.

A more recently described group of lesions that are best described here are the *myoepithelial lesions* of the breast. Tavassoli has classified these as myoepitheliosis, adenomyoepithelioma, and myoepithelial carcinoma.[108] By far the most common—although still a rare mammary lesion—is *adenomyoepithelioma*, a solitary gross tumor with well- or poorly circumscribed margins. The characteristic feature is a bimorphic cellular proliferation, with both ductal and myoepithelial cells, often arranged as ductal cell-lined tubules surrounded by concentric bands of clear myoepithelial cells (Figs. 10-24 and 10-25). The latter may be predominantly spindled and are best identified by positive immunostaining for muscle-specific actin or S-100 protein. The lesion appears to be benign, although it can recur locally if inadequately excised, and 2 of 27 adenomyoepitheliomas in Tavassoli's series had carcinoma arising within them. Three cases in this series were multifocal microscopic lesions with a similar cellular population, designated as myoepitheliosis, whereas a single case of myoepithelial carcinoma was an infiltrating malignant tumor composed purely of myoepithelial cells.

Collagenous spherulosis is another recently described lesion that has been shown to be of combined epithelial and myoepithelial cell origin.[109] It is usually an incidental microscopic finding but may rarely form a palpable mass. The characteristic microscopic feature is the presence of whorls of dense hyalinized collagen interspersed with the two cell types (Color Figure 10-10). The lesion is benign.

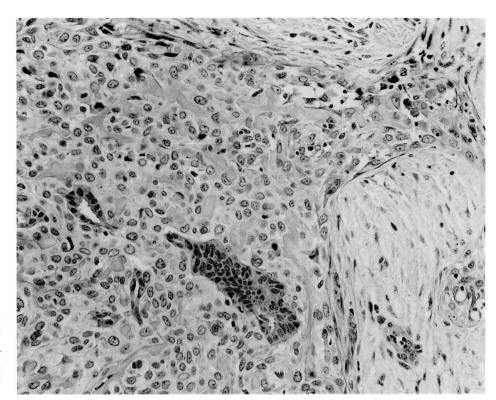

FIGURE 10-24 Adenomyoepithelioma. Bland-appearing ductal structures are surrounded by a circumscribed proliferation of ovoid myoepithelial cells, and the entire complex is bordered by fibrotic stroma.

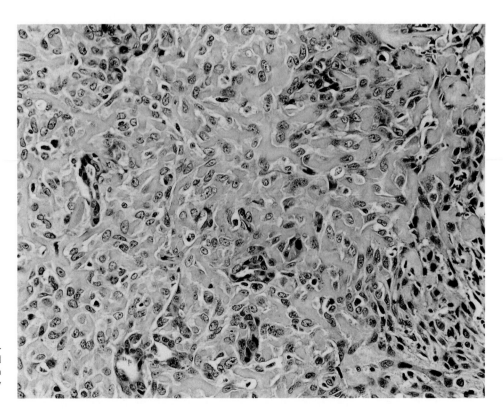

FIGURE 10-25 Adenomyoepithelioma. These myoepithelial cells are more spindled than those in Figure 10-24 and show some atypia and mitotic activity.

Lipoma

Lipoma of the breast is seen in women between 40 and 60 years of age, in the form of a well-demarcated, soft, round mass, the diameter of which is generally in the range of 1 to 5 cm. It is surrounded by a thin fibrous capsule.

The *macroscopic appearance* is clearly that of a benign lesion, and can easily be confused with normal adipose tissue except for its encapsulation. The *histologic picture* is that of banal adipose tissue. The form known as *adenolipoma* consists of a lipoma in which a few mammary lobules are found included in the tumorous fatty proliferation; this is probably better included under the heading of hamartoma.[110,111] This is also true for chondrolipoma.[112]

Hamartoma

The term *hamartoma* recently has been used to describe benign, encapsulated growths with the gross appearance of fibroadenomas but histologically resembling normal breast tissues (Fig. 10-26). This lesion differs from fibroadenoma in that the stroma does not take an active part in the tumorigenesis, fat is usually present, and apocrine metaplasia is often seen.[110,111]

Lactoma (Lactating Adenoma)

Although not a true tumor, this lesion is discussed here because it presents to the clinician as a well-defined tumorous mass during late pregnancy and lactation and is often excised for diagnostic purposes. It consists of a well-demarcated but unencapsulated, small, spherical mass composed of histologically normal-appearing lactating mammary tissue.[66,68] This is a proliferative rather than a neoplastic lesion and, as such, regresses spontaneously after the nursing period if it is untreated.

A somewhat similar lesion may be encountered in the breasts of women taking oral contraceptives or other medications, particularly antipsychotic and antihypertensive drugs.[113] The proliferation in these cases may be localized (Fig. 10-27) or diffuse and is frequently an incidental microscopic finding. Malignant transformation has not been reported.

Granular Cell Tumor

Granular cell tumor is also known as *Abrikosov's tumor* and *granular cell myoblastoma*. Almost 100 cases of granular cell tumor of the breast have been reported.[114]

The macroscopic appearance of these lesions may lead to confusion with carcinoma, because they present as firm, rounded masses that usually adhere to surrounding tissues. They appear to arise most often in the upper and medial segments of the breast. Their histologic and cytologic appearances are characteristic and allay fears about malignancy. A histologic description is given in Chapter 1.

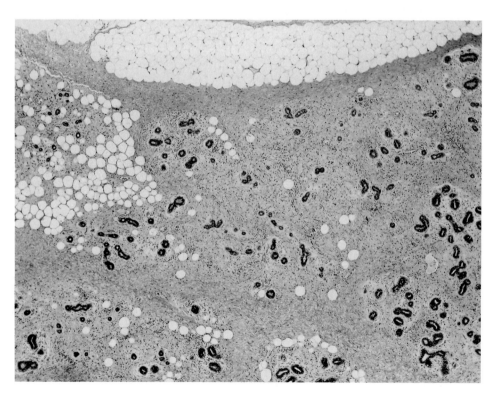

FIGURE 10-26 Hamartoma. This lesion was removed as a probable fibroadenoma. It consists of randomly scattered ductules, fibrous stroma, and fat, and it is well demarcated from adjacent adipose tissue.

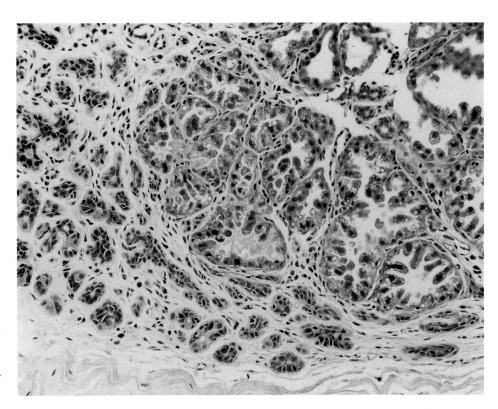

FIGURE 10-27 Secretory (lactational) hyperplasia seen focally as an incidental microscopic finding. Note the enlarged hyperchromatic nuclei, which should not raise the suspicion of carcinoma in this setting.

Leiomyoma

Rare cases of mammary leiomyoma have been described.[115] Leiomyoma develops from the chest wall musculature, smooth muscle of the skin, and vascular or areolar muscle.

Hemangioma and Related Vascular Lesions

Pathologists who were trained more than 20 years ago will remember having been taught that any vascular lesion occurring in mammary parenchyma (as opposed to the skin overlying or muscle underlying the breast proper) was by definition an angiosarcoma, regardless of how benign it might appear. This concept is of historical interest only, because a number of benign vascular lesions of the breast have now been documented. The most common of these is the *perilobular hemangioma,* a sharply circumscribed and usually perilobular lesion (Fig. 10-28) that generally measures less than 1.5 mm and is an incidental microscopic finding (angiosarcomas are large, grossly visible tumors).[116,117] Lesueur found an 11% prevalence of these lesions in a forensic autopsy series.[117] Histologically, they are identical to benign hemangiomas seen elsewhere.

Other less common vascular lesions in the breast include *venous hemangiomas,*[118] *angiomatosis*[119] (a rare lesion in which variably-sized but benign-appearing vessels are distributed uniformly through the tumor), *hemangioma with atypical histologic features*[120] (which has been shown to be benign), and *hemangiopericytoma.*[121]

A related but nonvascular lesion is *pseudoangiomatous hyperplasia of mammary stroma,* a benign keloid-like fibrosis containing slit-like spaces that are not lined by endothelial cells, as demonstrated by negative immunostaining for factor VIII-related antigen and *Ulex europaeus* lectin. This lesion was found as an incidental microscopic finding in 23% of breast biopsy specimens in one series.[122] It occasionally forms a palpable mass.

The main clinical significance of all these lesions is that they may be diagnosed by the unwary pathologist as angiosarcoma. Basically, angiosarcoma is always grossly infiltrative and is usually a large tumorous mass containing (at least focally) atypical and mitotically active endothelial cells. This tumor is discussed in greater detail later in this chapter.

Other Benign Masses

A number of other benign lesions may present as palpable or mammographically detected intramammary masses. These include normal or pathologic *intramammary lymph nodes,*[7,123] *plasma cell granuloma* (inflammatory pseudotumor),[124] *fibromatosis*[125], and *mucocele-like tumor.*[126,127] All of these resemble their counterparts seen in other parts of the body. The mucocele-like tumor is important in the differential diagnosis of mucinous carcinoma and is discussed with that tumor.

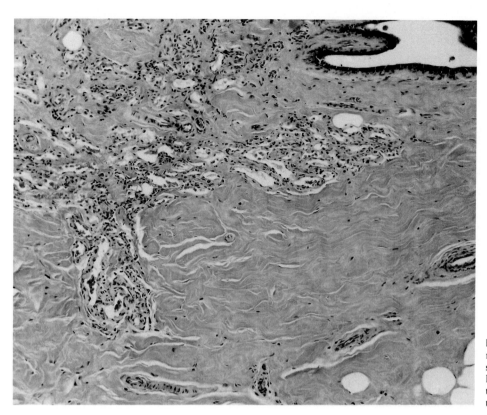

FIGURE 10-28 Perilobular hemangioma. This microscopic lesion (seen almost in its entirety here) is adjacent to a lobule, the terminal duct of which is seen in the photomicrograph.

FIBROCYSTIC CHANGES

Fibrocystic changes represent a condition formerly known under a great variety of names, including *fibrocystic disease, chronic cystic mastitis, fibrocystic mastopathy, fibrocystic dysplasia, fibroadenomatosis, mazoplasia, mastodynia, cystic dysembryoplasia, chronic mammitis, Reclus' disease,*[128] and *Schimmelbusch's disease.*[129] This multitude of names reflects the confusion in the definition of the fibrocystic complex of clinical, gross, and histopathologic changes. Because at least some of the histopathologic changes are encountered in most women in their reproductive years, the tendency—which we applaud—is not to characterize these changes as a "disease."[130,131] We do, however, continue to use the term *fibrocystic changes* diagnostically, as a means of notifying the surgeon that a submitted sample cannot be characterized as normal resting breast tissue.[132]

The main significance of the lesions discussed under this heading lies in what they do not represent—a cancerous or highly precancerous condition. However, numerous studies have demonstrated a slightly increased risk (in the range of twofold or less) of cancer development in the breasts of women bearing these lesions.[100,133,134] Whether this indicates a real premalignant potential, or merely indicates a different level of concern and follow-up of women who have had benign breast biopsies, remains to be determined. In any event, we have chosen to separate the discussion of atypical lobular and ductal hyperplasias—which are most commonly seen in association with the fibrocystic complex—because these latter lesions are (1) associated with considerably higher (on the order of fourfold) risk of subsequent cancer, and (2) more difficult to differentiate at the histopathologic level from lesions that are considered to be noninvasive cancers.

Etiology

The etiology of a non-disease is difficult to define. Nevertheless, it is clear that women with clinically significant fibrocystic changes (in other words, those who come to biopsy) are probably different in some ways from women who never develop such changes. Women in whom these same changes can be demonstrated at autopsy are also different from women in whom they cannot. It is generally agreed that the prevalence of fibrocystic lesions is probably related to hormonal disequilibria to which the breast is subject during the course of reproductive life, which in turn are related to genetic background, age, parity, lactational history, and administration of exogenous hormones.[132] In one autopsy study in which women of different racial groups were compared, those groups at greater risk for the development of breast cancer showed more fibrocystic changes.[135]

Clinical Features

The first clinical manifestation is usually the discovery by the patient of an intramammary nodule. Intracystic tension may produce discomfort and tenderness to palpation. The cysts may appear rapidly and disappear just as rapidly by rupture or resorption. Symptoms are characteristically aggravated in the premenstrual period and usually involve both breasts. The manifestations of the condition decrease after menopause.

Clinical examination reveals one or several firm, moderately movable nodules, which may give the impression of "beads on a string." Skin retraction is absent, and nipple discharge is rarely seen. The consistency of these nodules depends on the tension of the fluid within the cysts and the prominence of associated fibrosis.

Sclerosing adenosis is usually an incidental microscopic finding, but it may rarely present as a clinically detectable mass (*adenosis tumor*).[136,137] The other components of the fibrocystic process are generally incidental findings, with the exception of radial scars, which may be appreciated as individual lesions by palpation or mammography.

Many biopsies showing fibrocystic changes are obtained as the result of mammographically detected abnormalities in asymptomatic women with no palpable masses. In many instances, the primary feature that provokes the biopsy is the presence of microcalcifications.

Macroscopic Appearance

The biopsy specimen is usually characterized by the presence of small cysts in a white fibrous parenchyma. The classic color of the cysts is blue (so-called blue-dome cysts), but yellow, green, and brown cysts also are encountered. They may reach a few centimeters in diameter or may be so small that they are identified only at histologic examination. The cyst walls are small and shiny unless intraductal or intracystic proliferative lesions are present, in which case a velvety, tan to white inner surface may be seen. The intracystic fluid may be clear and straw-colored, viscous and green, or even creamy yellow or brown.

In occasional cases, multiple gross cysts with intracystic papillary proliferations are seen forming a localized mass in the breast of a young woman. This "Swiss cheese" pattern has been characterized as *juvenile papillomatosis*.[96]

Noninvasive and invasive cancers may be found within a breast biopsy in which the dominant features are fibrocystic. The pathologist should search carefully for regions of increased firmness with a granular, chalky appearance, often with yellow streaks radiating into the surrounding benign tissues. Such lesions generally prove to be infiltrating carcinomas, but radial scars may have a similar gross appearance. Intraductal carcinomas may be recognized as foci of soft papillomatous proliferation or of comedo-type necrosis within dilated ducts. Again, benign intraductal lesions can show these gross appearances, and other intraductal carcinomas may not be detect-

able grossly. Lobular carcinoma in situ is almost always an incidental microscopic finding.

Microscopic Appearance

Fibrocystic changes are characterized by the presence of several basic microscopic lesions, excluding the atypical lesions to be discussed later:

- Lactiferous cysts
- Stromal fibrosis
- Apocrine metaplasia
- Sclerosing adenosis
- Radial scars
- Secondary inflammation
- Intraductal epithelial hyperplasia.

Lactiferous Cysts

Lactiferous cysts usually are surrounded by a dense fibrous stroma (Fig. 10-29*A*). The lining epithelium may be cuboidal, flattened, or even missing entirely and replaced by a fibrous wall (Fig. 10-29*B*). Sometimes the cells become charged with lipids, are desquamated into the cyst lumina, and form plaques of large cells with finely vacuolated cytoplasm. The cysts may be isolated, compressed against each other, or ramified. They are formed from the principal or secondary lactiferous ducts and are surrounded by discrete lymphoplasmacytic infiltrates. In some cases, lipid-laden cells become agglomerated, and cholesterol crystals appear in the necrotic debris. Secondary calcification may take place in benign lesions (Fig. 10-30) but should always arouse a suspicion of malignancy.

Stromal Fibrosis

Stromal fibrosis is a constant finding, but its degree varies from one case to another and from one area to another in the same case. Fibrosis encircles the lobules and the ducts, and in a more advanced stage atrophic epithelial structures are compressed by an abundant stroma containing collagen and acid mucopolysaccharides. Hyalinization, calcification, and ossification may be observed in longstanding lesions. The reactive desmoplastic stroma associated with infiltrating carcinoma and characterized by large spindled cells in a fibroelastotic background with myxoid and inflammatory changes is by definition absent.

Apocrine Metaplasia

Apocrine metaplasia is often found in cystic epithelia. It affects primary and secondary ducts equally. The lining cells are large, with abundant pale eosinophilic cytoplasm and small round nuclei; the apical pole swells and herniates into the cyst lumen (Fig. 10-31). They may involve an entire duct or only part of a duct, and may be seen in both flat and prolifer-

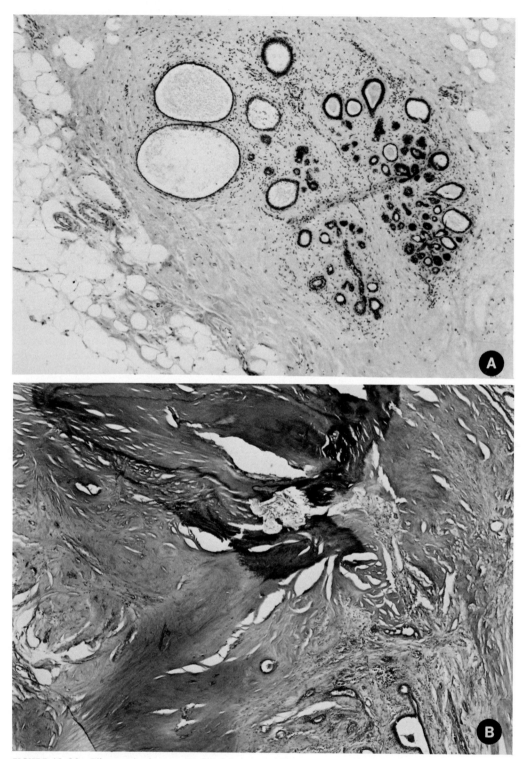

FIGURE 10-29 Fibrocystic change. **(A)** Focal duct cysts. **(B)** Secondary fibrosis and calcification.

ated epithelia. Whether these cells are truly analogous to those of apocrine sweat glands has been the subject of several investigations. Although some authors stress the similarities, most feel that the mammary cells are not truly apocrine.[138] They are actively proliferating and secreting cells, and might better be referred to as *oncocytes* because of their nu-

merous mitochondria. The apocrine cells may, on occasion, show moderate cellular atypia.

Sclerosing Adenosis

Sclerosing adenosis represents a particular clinico-pathologic picture, recognized since the 1940s, in

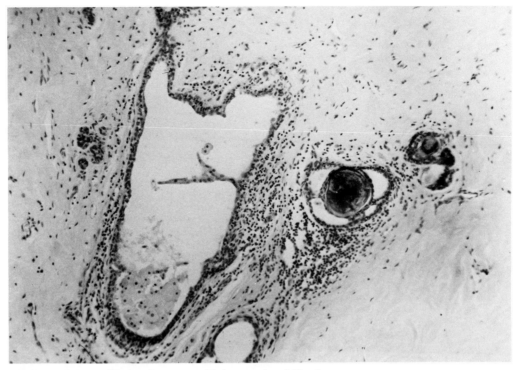

FIGURE 10-30 Lactiferous duct cysts with intracystic calcification.

which the proliferation of the myoepithelium constitutes the dominant lesion (Fig. 10-32).

In the initial phase, some ductules proliferate intensely in the form of ducts or cell cords compressed against each other. The lobular structure persists, and bizarre cell atypias are not seen. This hyperplasia involves primarily the myoepithelial cells, which are seen as elongated elements with acidophilic cytoplasm in which myofibrils are occasionally visible without special stains. This is followed by hyperplasia of the epithelial cells and proliferation originating in ductal budding. Ultrastructural studies confirm the involvement of the myoepithelial cells in the development of sclerosing adenosis.[139] Myoepithelial cells are characterized by the presence of filaments and dense bodies in the cytoplasm and are underlain by basal lamina. Their presence in these lesions can be confirmed by immunohistochemical positivity for muscle-specific actin and (less reliably) S-100 protein.

In the subsequent phase, marked interstitial fibrosis takes place, breaking up the glandular formations into such small pieces that a false appearance of neoplastic infiltration is created. On rare occasions, even perineural infiltration may be present.[140] The epithelial cords are finally completely submerged in a fibrotic and hyalinized connective tissue framework, but they always retain a vague lobular disposition.

This lesion is too frequently misdiagnosed as carcinoma, particularly on frozen section, and it is important to be aware of its existence and appearance (Table 10-2). Intraoperative or FNA cytology (smears or imprints) always appears benign.[36,137] Malignant transformation occurs extremely rarely and is usually lobular or ductal carcinoma in situ.[141,142] Atypical apocrine metaplasia is a benign but histologically worrisome focal lesion that may also be encountered within sclerosing adenosis.[143] Different opinions have been expressed concerning the existence of an elevated risk of carcinoma associated with sclerosing adenosis. Two studies provide arguments for the reassignment of sclerosing adenosis to a category of slightly elevated cancer risk.[144,145] The pathologist should perform a careful search for atypical lobular or ductal hyperplasia, which represent more grave risk factors, when sclerosing adenosis is observed.

Radial Scar

The radial scar lesion also is known as *infiltrating epitheliosis, nonencapsulated sclerosing lesion,* and *indurative mastopathy.* It is sometimes detected by mammography or may present as an incidental finding in tissues excised in cases of fibrocystic change. It is single or multiple. Its mean size is around 1 cm in diameter. Macroscopically, it consists of a firm, regular, gray-white lesion with a central depressed retraction.

Microscopically, it is characterized as a radial stellate lesion consisting of a dense, central, fibroelastotic core with entrapped ductal structures (Fig. 10-33). These structures exhibit varying degrees of adenosis, hyperplasia, and ductal cystic dilatation. The cells lining these epithelial structures generally lack cytologic atypia. Mitoses are very rare.

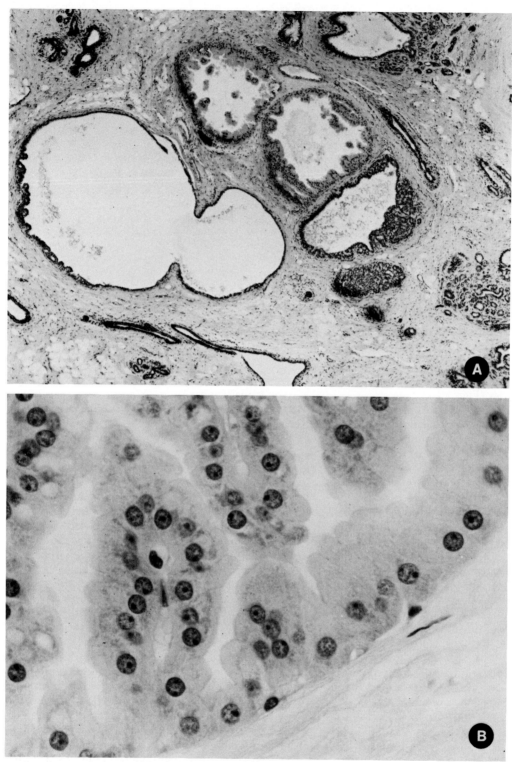

FIGURE 10-31 Apocrine metaplasia. **(A)** Low magnification. **(B)** Detail.

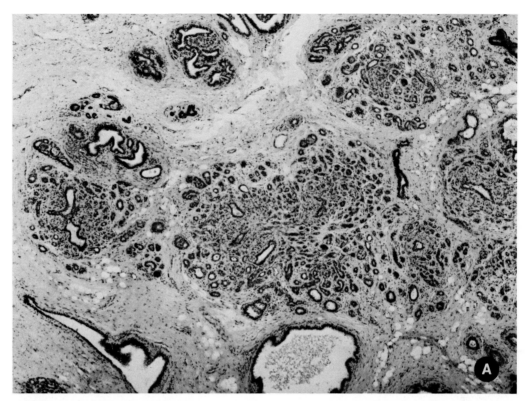

FIGURE 10-32 Sclerosing adenosis.

The lesion worries the pathologist for two reasons. First, it has some histologic similarities with tubular carcinoma, and second, for some authors it may represent a precursor of tubular or other types of carcinoma.[146,147] The absence of infiltration of the adjacent stroma and the presence of myoepithelial cells characterize a radial scar.

In any case, the lesion should be considered as part of the fibrocystic complex and shares with it the potential risks of cancer development.

Secondary Chronic Inflammation

Secondary chronic inflammation is characterized by the presence of plasma cells and polymorphonuclear leukocytes in the vicinity of ruptured cysts. It is a local complication; an inflammatory process is not an essential constituent of fibrocystic change. These reactive changes should not be confused with a primary mastitis or the inflammatory stroma accompanying a carcinoma.

Intraductal Epithelial Hyperplasia (Epitheliosis; Papillomatosis)

Intraductal epithelial hyperplasia is defined as an increase in epithelial cell numbers above the normal bilayered structure (epithelial and myoepithelial cells). It may involve the lobule, the terminal duct, or any part of the ductal system. However, the lesion by convention is considered to be a ductal rather than a lobular proliferation. The term *epithelial hyperplasia* is preferred to *epitheliosis* and *papillomatosis* because it suggests the hyperplastic character of the lesions and reflects the probable continuous progression from typical hyperplasia to atypical hyperplasia, carcinoma in situ, and eventually invasive carcinoma.

Two proposed classifications of the entire spectrum of proliferative mastopathy are summarized in Tables 10-3 and 10-4.[100,148] The distinction among these lesions involves many subjective features, and reproducibility among different observers may be difficult to obtain.[94,95] These statements are similar to those that have been made for many years with reference to intraepithelial lesions of the uterine cervix, and the same degree of caution must be exercised in the interpretation of these mammary alterations. Despite this more or less continuous spectrum, we believe that it is useful to separate the typical hyperplasias to be considered here from the atypical forms, both because the latter are defined by their distinction from in situ carcinoma and because they carry a higher risk of progression to carcinoma. Thus, a lack of resemblance to in situ carcinoma is implied in the definition of typical hyperplasia.

Typical intraductal hyperplasia is characterized by a proliferation in which there is an increase in cell numbers to more than the normal two layers (Figs. 10-34 through 10-36). There is formation of bridges, tufts, arcades, and fenestrated sheets preserving the presence of lumina in the new proliferations, as well as cell nests that appear solid in at least

(*Text continued on page 556*)

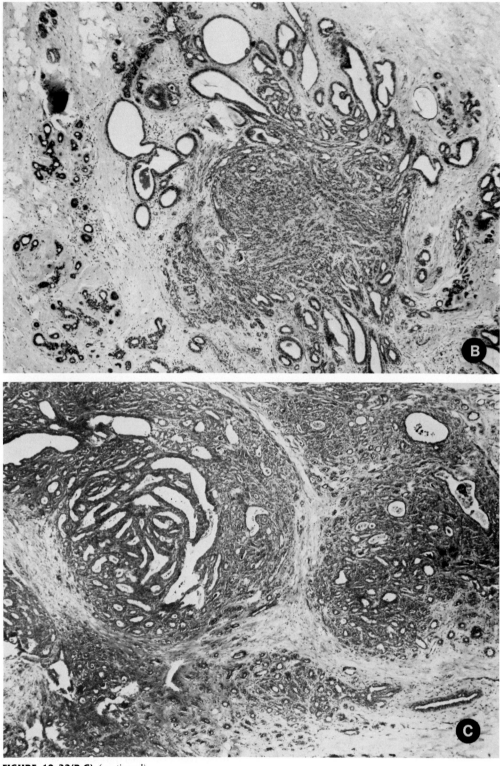

FIGURE 10-32(B,C) *(continued)*

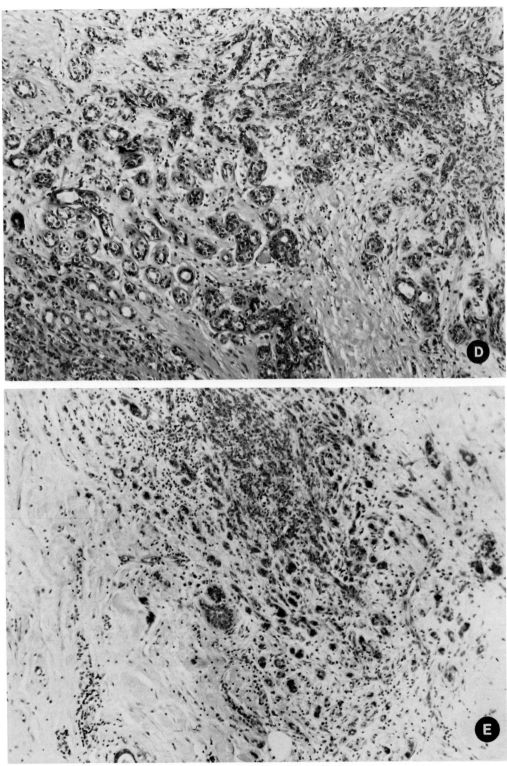

FIGURE 10-32(D,E) *(continued)*

TABLE 10-2.
Differential Diagnosis of Sclerosing Adenosis Versus Infiltrating Carcinoma

	Sclerosing Adenosis	*Carcinoma*
Distribution	Multifocal	Usually one dominant mass
Architecture	Lobular pattern preserved	Irregular
Borders	Circumscribed	Infiltrating (usually)
Lumina	Sclerosed centrally, often preserved peripherally	Uniform throughout
Swirling	Prominent	Rare
Stroma	Fibrotic, hyalinized	Fibroelastotic, myxoid, inflamed, sometimes normal; almost never hyalinized
Cell Type	Epithelial and myoepithelial	Epithelial
Nuclear Atypia	Absent to minimal	Slight to marked
Focal Apocrine Change	Frequently present	Rare

some histologic sections. The lumina generally are irregular in size and shape, with numerous compressed slit-like spaces. The cells are small, irregularly shaped, and arranged at least focally in a swirling or streaming pattern. There is a lack of cellular uniformity, so that it is usually easy to demonstrate the presence of more than one cell type, and ovoid to spindled cells are admixed with rounder ones. Nuclear hyperchromasia, prominent nucleoli, and mitotic figures are absent or present only very focally.

This discussion of ductal hyperplasia raises the question of whether similar proliferative but not atypical lesions occur in lobules. According to Page and colleagues, such lesions do not exist (or at least are not included in their classification of epithelial hyperplasia of the breast).[149] Fechner and Mills recognize *lobular hyperplasia* without atypia, but they indicate that its premalignant potential is unknown.[150] Carter also illustrates lobular hyperplasia and defines it as intralobular proliferation of cells that are not appreciably enlarged or atypical, do not distend the lobules, and are accompanied by at least some myoepithelial cells.[151] We accept this definition, along with the caveat of Fechner and Mills that we do not know the clinical significance of this lesion. It does not seem to have any association with fibrocystic changes, and it may or may not represent the lower end of the spectrum in which lobular carcinoma in situ is the other end.

Another lesion involving lobules, the clinical significance of which is also unknown, is the picture

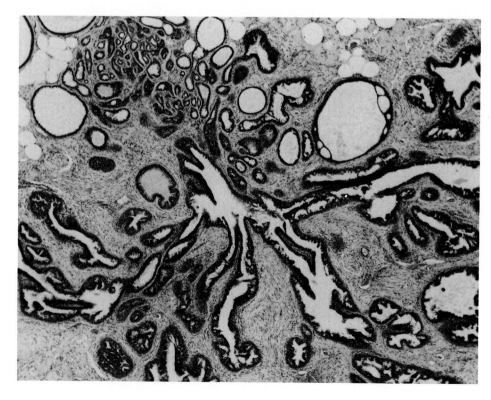

FIGURE 10-33 Radial scar. Central sclerosis and radial ductal proliferation are surrounded by foci of sclerosing adenosis and intraductal hyperplasia.

TABLE 10-3.
Mammary Epithelial Proliferative Disease Characterized by Cancer Risk

Cancer Risk	Morphologic Features
No increased risk	No proliferative disease: Adenosis (including florid) Apocrine change Duct ectasia Mild epithelial hyperplasia of usual type
Slightly (1.5–2×) increased risk	Usual hyperplasia, moderate or florid Sclerosing adenosis Papilloma
Moderately (4–5×) increased risk	Atypical ductal hyperplasia Atypical lobular hyperplasia
High (8–10×) risk	Lobular carcinoma in situ Noncomedo ductal carcinoma in situ

Adapted from Page DL, Dupont WD: Anatomic markers of human premalignancy and risk of breast carcinoma. Cancer 66:1326–1335, 1990

that has been known classically as *blunt duct adenosis* and is now more generally referred to as *unfolded lobules*.[152] These basically are cystically dilated lobules that resemble ducts but are too close to one another to represent true preexisting ducts (Fig. 10-37). Tangential sectioning of the epithelium within unfolded lobules can produce images falsely resembling hyperplasia, but true hyperplasias, including atypical hyperplasias, can develop in these structures.

ATYPICAL HYPERPLASIAS AND IN SITU CARCINOMAS

The lesions discussed in this section are intimately related to one another in three senses. First, the histologic pictures within the spectra of atypical hyperplasias and in situ carcinomas—whether for lobular or ductal lesions—are similar and pose difficult differential diagnostic problems. Second, all these lesions are associated with a markedly increased risk for the subsequent development of invasive cancer, although, as we shall see, the details of the magnitude of risk depend on the specific diagnosis and on other clinical factors, such as a family history of breast cancer. Finally, these lesions all share the property of being diagnosed most frequently by mammography or as incidental findings in breast tissues removed for other indications, rather than presenting as palpable masses.

Intraductal and intralobular carcinomas are defined as malignant transformation of the epithelium without infiltration of the underlying stroma. Although previously these lesions accounted for no more than 10% of all mammary carcinomas, they are now seen more and more frequently as the result of the widespread application of screening mammography.[98] When radiographically suspicious microcalcifications are present and biopsy is performed, more than 50% of the malignant tumors identified are noninvasive, with most of these being ductal rather than lobular.[22,98] The processing of these mammographically directed biopsies represents an important new chapter in breast pathology for the

TABLE 10-4.
Diagnostic Criteria and Cancer Risk for Nonapocrine Intraductal Hyperplasias and Carcinomas

Category	Criteria	Risk of Invasive Carcinoma
Ordinary or regular intraductal hyperplasia (IDH)	Multiple cell types, variable cellular and nuclear appearance, irregular/peripheral fenestrations, stretched or twisted epithelial bridges, focal cell streaming or spindling, unevenly distributed nuclei	2.6%
Atypical intraductal hyperplasia (AIDH)	Cell population monotonous and uniformly distributed, subtly increased nuclear–cytoplasmic ratio, round nuclei; architectural pattern of IDH or cribriform, micropapillary or stratified spindle cell papillary pattern not exceeding 2 mm in aggregate cross-sectional ductal diameters	9.8%*
Intraductal carcinoma (IDC)	Criteria for AIDH exceeding 2 mm in aggregate diameter or a cytologically obviously malignant lesion	Not stated

*Increased in the presence of sclerosing adenosis or a positive family history of breast carcinoma.

Adapted from Tavassoli FA, Norris HJ: A comparison of the results of long-term follow-up for atypical intraductal hyperplasia and intraductal hyperplasia of the breast. Cancer 65:518–529, 1990

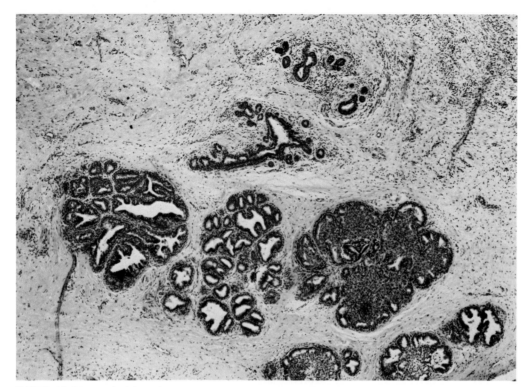

FIGURE 10-34 Typical intraductal hyperplasia of predominantly solid type.

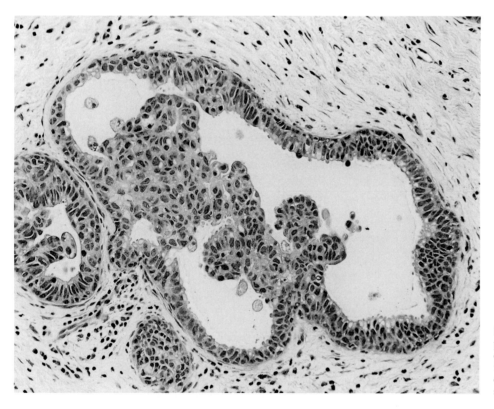

FIGURE 10-35 Typical hyperplasia: papillary and solid proliferation. Note the small size and irregular shapes of hyperplastic cells, with some spindling and swirling.

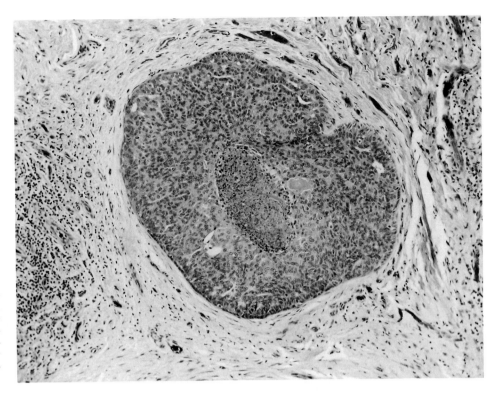

FIGURE 10-36 Typical hyperplasia. The lumina formed in this proliferation vary in size and shape. Central necrosis, although more common in intraductal carcinoma, is occasionally seen in completely benign lesions such as this one.

practicing pathologist, and the reader is referred to our earlier discussion on diagnostic approaches and to pertinent references[23,24] for a discussion of the technical details.

Despite the similarities mentioned above between lobular carcinoma in situ (LCIS) and ductal carcinoma in situ (DCIS), there are significant differences.[100] It is thought that LCIS represents a risk indicator of later invasive carcinoma rather than a fully malignant true precursor lesion, because the eventual invasive cancer may occur anywhere in the ipsilateral or contralateral breast and has an equal likelihood of being lobular or ductal in type. On the other hand, when invasive carcinoma follows DCIS, it appears in the same breast and even in the same quadrant, and is almost invariably of ductal type, indicating that DCIS represents a true precursor of invasive carcinoma.

Ductal Carcinoma In Situ (Intraductal Carcinoma)

Ductal carcinoma in situ (DCIS), which accounted for less than 5% of cases of mammary carcinoma in the pre-mammography era, is reported today to represent 15% to 22% of breast carcinomas.[22,98,100,153] Studies suggest that two forms of DCIS exist. The first is a lesion that does not form a palpable mass, is usually not recognizable macroscopically in excised tissues, and is histologically of non-comedo type. The second form is comedocarcinoma, in which a mass

may be formed and clusters of distended ducts filled with creamy yellow to brown necrotic material may be recognized grossly.[154-158] Either form may be associated with a serosanguineous nipple discharge. Mammography reveals the presence of microcalcifications of granular, linear, or branching type. This finding is not specific, because only 25% of biopsies performed for these calcifications contain carcinoma, and 50% of these carcinomas are invasive.[22,98]

Microscopic Appearance. Intraductal carcinoma is distinguished by proliferation of the lining epithelia of the lactiferous ducts without stromal invasion. These epithelial proliferations occur in three common and two rare architectural patterns. The three common forms are:

Micropapillary, in which papillae (usually lacking connective tissue axes) project into the lumen (Figs. 10-38 and 10-39)

Cribriform, in which the tumor cells form bridges over uniform spaces, producing a uniformly punched-out pattern referred to as "cartwheels" or "Roman bridges" (Figs. 10-40 and 10-41)

Comedocarcinoma, in which the lumina are filled with solid plugs of large, pleomorphic tumor cells, in which central necrosis becomes a prominent feature (Fig. 10-42).

The two less common types are:

Solid, in which solid plugs of tumor cells that are less anaplastic than those of comedocarci-

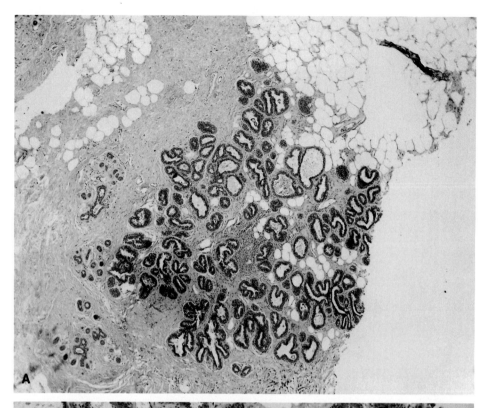

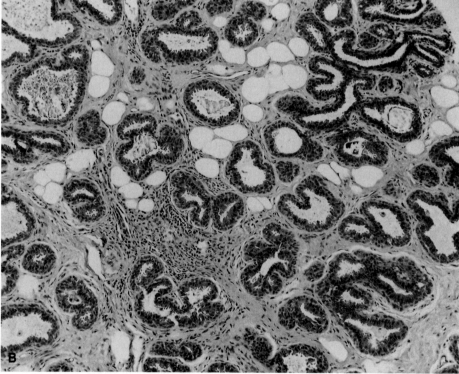

FIGURE 10-37 Unfolded lobules. **(A)** Low-power view showing the crowding of the enlarged and dilated lobules. **(B)** Detail showing double layer of cells without true hyperplasia or atypia.

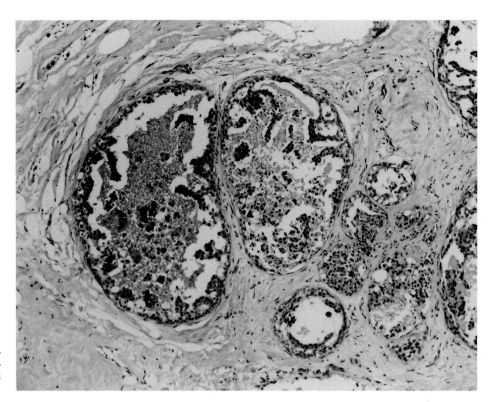

FIGURE 10-38 Intraductal carcinoma, micropapillary type. Low-power view of a group of involved ductal profiles.

noma fill duct lumina (Fig. 10-43) without (or occasionally with) the development of central necrosis (although solid intraductal cellular proliferations without necrosis are more frequently benign)

Papillary stratified spindle cell, in which large papillae with central connective tissue axes are lined by tall columnar cells with their nuclei oriented perpendicular to the basement membrane (Fig. 10-44).

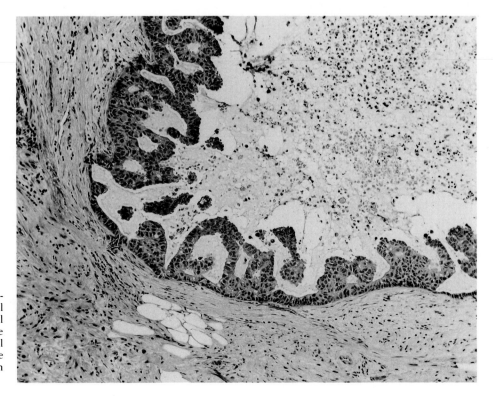

FIGURE 10-39 Intraductal carcinoma, micropapillary type. Detail of an involved duct showing small papillae lacking connective tissue axes and lined by a uniform cell population. Some papillae have fused to form so-called Roman bridges.

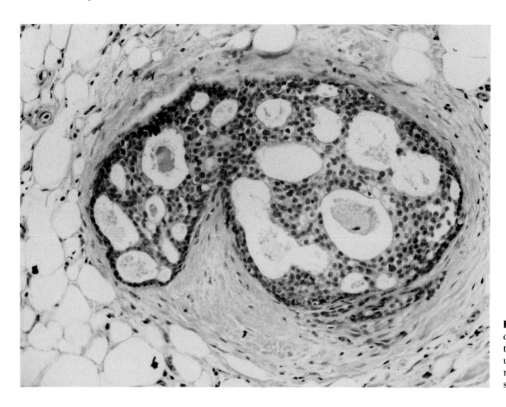

FIGURE 10-40 Intraductal carcinoma, cribriform type. Note the punched-out pattern of regular lumina and the uniform round cells without spindling or swirling.

A sixth type, so-called clinging carcinoma, is more poorly documented as representing carcinoma rather than a form of atypical hyperplasia.[159] In this pattern, a few layers of dyspolaric atypical cells line ducts with minimal architectural abnormalities. Even rarer variants are a mucinous type (Fig. 10-45), which may accompany infiltrating mucinous (colloid) carcinoma; hypersecretory duct carcinoma (Fig. 10-46), in which the malignant ducts are cystically dilated and contain colloid-like material; and intraductal carcinoma showing prominent apocrine differentiation (Fig. 10-47).

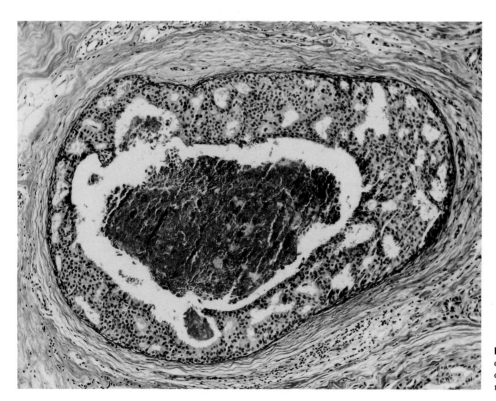

FIGURE 10-41 Intraductal carcinoma, cribriform type. This duct displays prominent central necrosis.

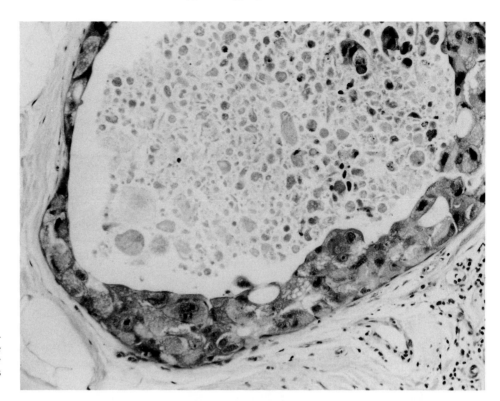

FIGURE 10-42 Intraductal comedocarcinoma. Tumor cells are large and pleomorphic and grow in a solid sheet. Central necrosis is present.

The cells forming the tumor range from small and uniform in the cribriform type to large, pleomorphic, and bizarre in comedocarcinoma, with intermediate differentiation in the other forms. Nevertheless, the prognosis of completely noninvasive intraductal carcinoma is identical in all forms; lymph nodal metastases are extremely rare, as is death resulting from tumor.[154–162]

Diagnosis of a mammary carcinoma as intraductal requires multiple sections to rule out minute foci of stromal invasion. A diagnosis therefore cannot be guaranteed based on a frozen section.[162–164] If

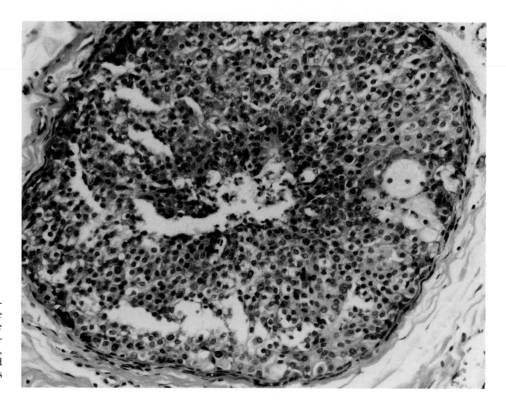

FIGURE 10-43 Intraductal carcinoma, solid type. Despite the solid growth of this tumor, the cells are relatively small and uniform (compare with Fig. 10-42, at the same magnification), and a plug of central necrotic debris is not seen.

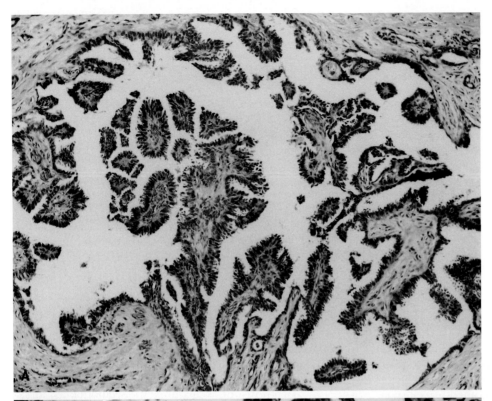

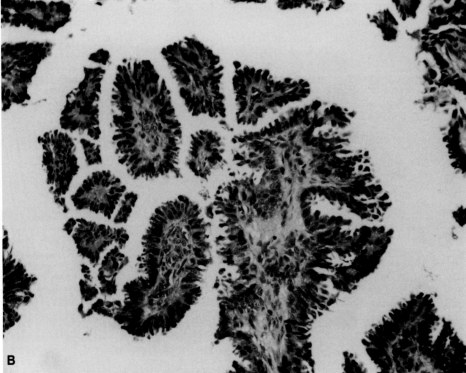

FIGURE 10-44 Intraductal carcinoma, papillary stratified spindle cell type. **(A)** Papillary growth pattern with central connective tissue axes. **(B)** The papillae are lined by tall columnar cells oriented perpendicular to the basement membrane, with no underlying myoepithelial cells.

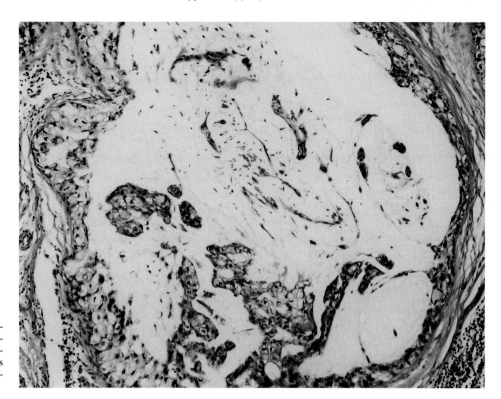

FIGURE 10-45 Intraductal carcinoma, mucinous type. Voluminous intracellular and extracellular mucin is present. This breast was removed for mucinous (colloid) carcinoma.

the diagnostic problem is suspected in advance, frozen sections should not be performed, because freezing artifact renders the interpretation of subsequent permanent sections more difficult. At least eight blocks should be examined to exclude the presence of stromal infiltration. This careful study is important because the incidence of nodal metastases and a lethal course rise sharply when there is even limited invasion of the stroma (Fig. 10-48), although in this situation these eventualities are less likely than with diffusely infiltrative cancer.[163–167] Invasion can be demonstrated ultrastructurally in many instances

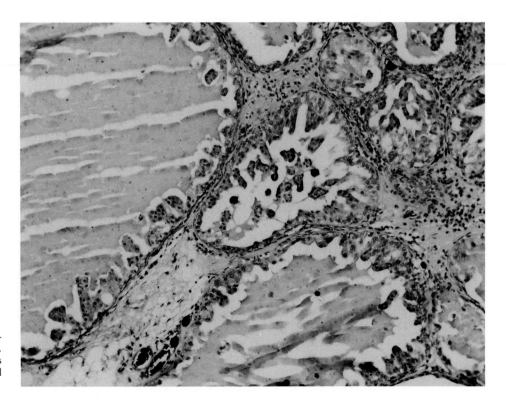

FIGURE 10-46 Intraductal carcinoma, hypersecretory type. This micropapillary tumor has cystically dilated ducts filled with colloid-like material.

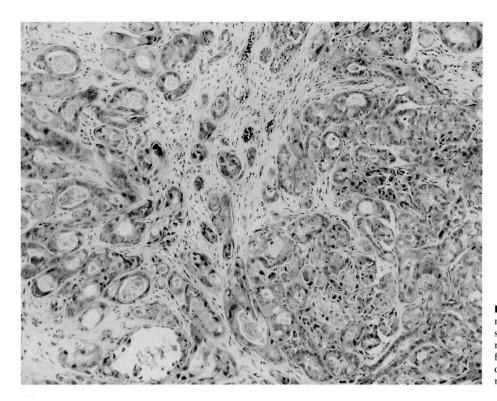

FIGURE 10-47 Intraductal carcinoma, apocrine type, arising in sclerosing adenosis. The sclerosing architecture raises the differential diagnosis of infiltrating carcinoma, but the usual stromal reaction is absent.

when it cannot be seen with the light microscope, but prognostically the light microscopic findings are the important ones. The presence of smooth muscle actin in myoepithelial cells may help in the differential diagnosis, because these cells are said to be lacking in early invasive foci.[168] Immunohistochemical studies for laminin and type IV collagen may be useful.[169] Ultimately, classic light microscopy remains diagnostic.

Differential Diagnosis. The comedo type of DCIS is usually easily diagnosed by virtue of the large

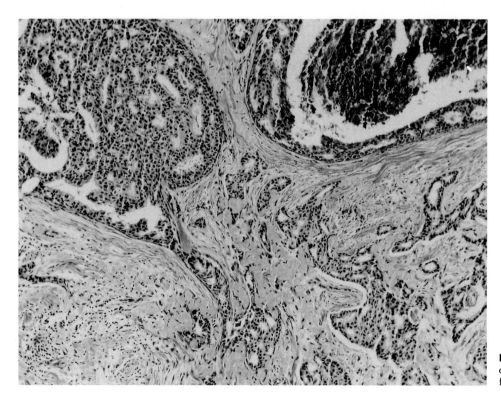

FIGURE 10-48 Intraductal carcinoma, cribriform type, with focal stromal infiltration.

number of ducts involved, the marked atypia and mitotic activity of the tumor cells, and the central necrosis. On the other hand, diagnostic problems are common with the non-comedo forms, which in our experience are more often overdiagnosed than underdiagnosed. If the diagnosis of intraductal carcinoma is being considered, the pathologist should always ask himself or herself into which subtype the lesion fits and be sure that the criteria for that subtype are met. Quantitative criteria are important. Page and colleagues[100] demand that at least two ductal profiles be completely involved by the malignant changes, and Tavassoli and Norris[148] demand that the lesion measure at least 2 mm in diameter. In practice, these criteria usually yield the same results, because two or more adjacent involved ducts usually measure more than 2 mm. Lesser degrees of involvement, or lesions that meet some but not all of the qualitative criteria for the diagnosis of non-comedo DCIS, are diagnosed as atypical ductal hyperplasia (see below).

In theory, ductal hyperplasias without atypia should not enter into the differential diagnosis of DCIS, but in practice they frequently do.[94] The same statement can be made for solitary and multiple intraductal papillomas, juvenile papillomatosis, nipple adenoma, and radial scar, all of which are discussed in more detail in earlier sections. In our experience, the most common reason for diagnostic confusion between these lesions and DCIS is suboptimal histotechnique. This problem is frequently compounded by the fact that frozen sections have been performed on these tissues, and the subsequent artifact in the permanent sections may make the diagnosis difficult if not impossible to render. Therefore, we cannot emphasize too strongly the admonition against performing frozen sections on grossly benign mammographically directed biopsy specimens or in instances in which DCIS is suspected clinically or grossly.

Cytologic Appearance. Because DCIS is only occasionally a palpable lesion, few reports have characterized its FNA cytologic characteristics. One report emphasized that an inadequate specimen was obtained in 44% of the cases, and only 37% were considered diagnostic or suspicious for malignancy.[170] Compared with positive smears from infiltrating duct carcinomas, those from DCIS showed less irregular nuclear spacing and less pronounced nuclear overlapping, and they were more likely to be hypocellular and to contain benign epithelial cells and macrophages. Our experience supports the conclusion of the authors of this study that FNA cannot reliably differentiate DCIS from infiltrating duct carcinoma.

Because the comedo type of DCIS is generally more extensive, often forming a palpable mass, and is cytologically more anaplastic, the likelihood of a positive diagnosis of cancer is greater in FNA cytology of this subtype. The malignant cells are large

and poorly differentiated (Color Figure 10-11) and are arranged largely in relatively cohesive groups, with fewer single tumor cells seen compared with infiltrating carcinomas.[171] Necrotic cellular debris may be prominent. As with non-comedo DCIS, the distinction of this form of DCIS from its microinvasive or more extensively invasive counterpart is difficult and probably should not be attempted.

Treatment. *Treatment,* as for other breast cancers, is still controversial. It should be based on what is clearly known about the lesion:[154-162,165,166,172-174]

When intraductal carcinoma is diagnosed on frozen section, or even on permanent sections of an incisional biopsy, stromal infiltration may be found in 5% to 10% of subsequent material examined.

Axillary lymph node metastases are found in 1% or less of well-documented cases of intraductal carcinoma without stromal infiltration, and distant metastases are even less frequent.

If intraductal carcinoma is untreated after biopsy (usually because of misdiagnosis as a benign lesion), the risk of recurrent carcinoma is about 50% within 10 years, and many of these cancers recur rapidly and are infiltrating.

Although intraductal carcinoma is frequently multifocal and bilateral, the vast majority of clinical recurrences in untreated cases are at the same site in the same breast.

These data may be interpreted to suggest mastectomy as the elected treatment in view of the incidence of multicentric disease, or very wide local excision or quadrantectomy with or without radiation therapy in view of the low risk of recurrence outside the involved quadrant. Probably the best interpretation is that treatment should be individualized, and the patient should be an active participant in the decision and should be aware of the risk involved.

Radiation therapy often is used with conservative surgery in the treatment of DCIS. Some reports suggest that radiation therapy is less active against DCIS than against invasive carcinoma.[174] In any event, local recurrence rates appear to be halved by the addition of radiation therapy, with rates of 10% to 54% reported for excision alone, compared with rates of 4% to 21% for excision with radiation.[173] Even after local recurrence, about 80% of patients can be treated successfully.

The relation of the microscopic findings to results of treatment for DCIS are still being established. Nevertheless, there is a definite indication that intraductal comedocarcinoma is more likely to progress to infiltrating carcinoma if not successfully treated initially. This impression fits with the biologic data that comedocarcinomas are more frequently aneuploid and receptor-negative and more frequently express the protein product of the c-*erb*-B2 oncogene than do non-comedo type intra-ductal carcinomas.[175-177] Large or widespread DCIS lesions would appear to be at greater risk of recurrence after conservative treatment as well.

Atypical Ductal Hyperplasia

Atypical ductal hyperplasia (ADH) is in the middle of the spectrum that includes ductal hyperplasia without atypia at its lower end and in situ ductal carcinoma at its upper end. Although we hope that an acceptable definition for ADH independent of these other entities will be established, at the moment ADH is best defined by what it does not represent—specifically, DCIS. ADH may be thought of as a lesion that possesses some but not all of the characteristics of DCIS.

In ADH, the epithelial cells have a monotonous appearance and display round, often centrally located nuclei with a moderately increased nuclear–cytoplasmic ratio. Hyperchromasia, if present, is discrete. Rosette-like arrangement of the nuclei may be observed. The architectural features may be cribriform, micropapillary, spindle cell papillary, or solid with secondary lumens. There is no central necrosis. Peripheral fenestration is present.

The diagnosis of ADH is usually made because these features, classic for non-comedo DCIS, are present filling only one duct profile or incompletely filling more than one duct profile (Fig. 10-49).[149] In the system of Tavassoli and Norris, the lesion mea-sures less than 2 mm in diameter.[148] An equally compelling reason for making the diagnosis of ADH is that the lesion quantitatively but not qualitatively satisfies the diagnostic criteria for non-comedo DCIS. In such an instance, the lesion is generally well-differentiated and involves only a few ducts, and it is appropriate to choose the less malignant diagnosis and avoid overtreatment.

ADH carries a risk of development of subsequent carcinoma that is intermediate between those of proliferative breast disease without atypia and in situ carcinoma.[98,100,134,148] The relative risk is generally quoted as fourfold, but it should be remembered that a relative risk of four still represents an absolute risk of less than 10% for the development of carcinoma.

Lobular Carcinoma In Situ

Lobular carcinoma in situ (LCIS) is the noninfiltrating form of lobular carcinoma. Despite the fact that it was first described independently in 1941 by Foote and Stewart[178] and Muir,[179] its natural history has been defined only recently. Its mean age of incidence is in the forties, but it may occur at any age; two thirds of the patients are premenopausal. Bilaterality is found at diagnosis in about one third of the cases. The lesion is defined as a proliferation of uniform abnormal cells that distends and fills at least one half of the acini in at least one lobular unit (Figs. 10-50 and 10-51).[149] These cells are definitely larger than normal lobular cells but are not volumi-

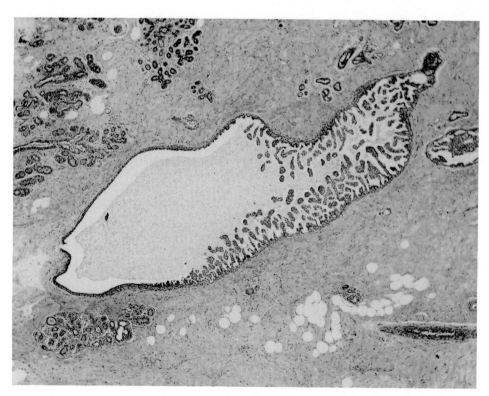

FIGURE 10-49 Atypical ductal hyperplasia. A micropapillary intraductal carcinoma pattern involves less than one complete duct profile.

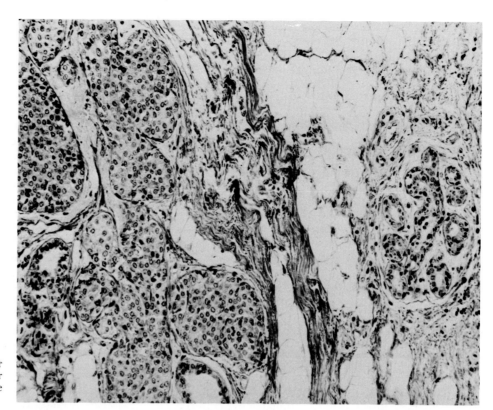

FIGURE 10-50 In situ lobular carcinoma. Contrast the lobular size on left with the normal lobule on right.

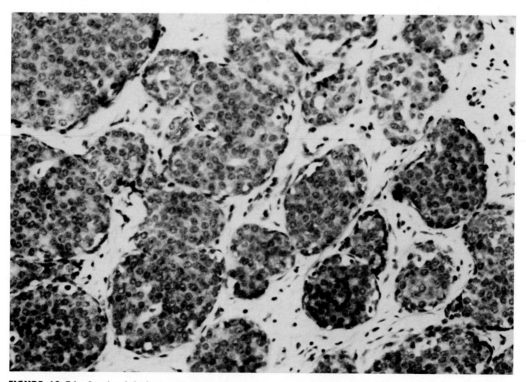

FIGURE 10-51 In situ lobular carcinoma, showing uniformity of neoplastic cells.

nous. They lack cohesion or regular orientation. Their nuclei are round and normochromatic. Nucleoli are small but usually apparent. The cytoplasm is moderately eosinophilic. Intracytoplasmic lumina containing neutral mucosaccharides may be common and represent a characteristic finding (Fig. 10-52). These "bullseye" or "targetoid" structures are a common feature of infiltrating lobular carcinoma as well. Normal or benign hyperplastic lobules are usually found adjacent to the neoplastic lobules, the contrast aiding in the recognition of the lesion. Neoplastic cells may infiltrate adjacent ductules in a pagetoid fashion between the ductal epithelial cells and the myoepithelial elements. The diagnosis, like many others in mammary pathology, is usually made under the scanning lens of the microscope, because the enlarged acini with obliterated lumina are characteristic. On frozen section, pictures of benign but atypical lobular hyperplasia are often confusing, and for this reason we never make a definitive diagnosis of LCIS until we have the opportunity of examining the permanent sections.

The significance of this lesion is that, like intraductal carcinoma, it is a marker of increased risk for the development of infiltrating carcinoma. Unlike intraductal carcinoma, LCIS may not be the lesion from which the infiltrating carcinoma actually develops. The statistics and their translation into therapeutic action are even more vehemently argued than those for intraductal carcinoma.[98,180–186]

The main similarities and differences may be summarized as follows:

LCIS occurs on the average in younger women than DCIS and is even less likely to present as a palpable or otherwise symptomatic lesion, the diagnosis almost invariably being incidental (in a biopsy performed for another lesion, usually fibrocystic change) or mammographic.

Occult stromal infiltration is much less frequently associated with an initial diagnosis of LCIS than of DCIS.

Positive axillary lymph nodes are as rare or rarer with pure LCIS than with DCIS.

LCIS is somewhat less likely than DCIS to progress to infiltrating cancer if untreated (15% to 35% in published series, compared with an average of 50% for DCIS).

When recurrence and progression take place in LCIS, the interval is usually greater than with DCIS (often 20 years or more).

A minimum of one third to a maximum of one half or more of the recurrent cancers occur in the contralateral breast, probably only partially as a result of the greater tendency of LCIS than DCIS to be multifocal (50% or more) and bilateral.

Although a greater proportion of infiltrating carcinomas after LCIS are of infiltrating lobular type than in unselected series of breast cancer, about half are ductal.

The main therapeutic recommendations include lifetime follow-up, in which mammography should

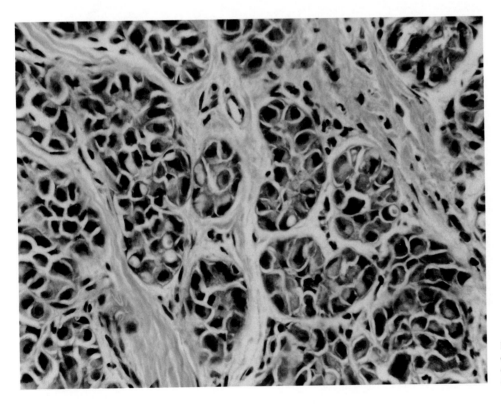

FIGURE 10-52 In situ lobular carcinoma with numerous intracytoplasmic lumina (signet-ring cells).

play an important role, although it is not infallible;[187,188] ipsilateral total mastectomy with contralateral biopsy (mirror image, upper outer quadrant, or mammographically directed); and bilateral total mastectomy. We believe that all of these options should be presented to the patient, although the pendulum has clearly swung toward conservatism in recent years.

Differential Diagnosis. The main differential diagnosis is with atypical lobular hyperplasia and is discussed below. Less commonly, LCIS may be confused with non-comedo DCIS extending into lobules (lobular cancerization; Fig. 10-53). However, the lobular extensions of DCIS often contain some residual cribriform spaces or papillae, whereas LCIS is totally solid. The cells of DCIS are less uniform, usually larger, and may be mitotically active; some central necrosis is frequently present. More typical DCIS involving larger ductal spaces is usually present nearby, although DCIS and LCIS can certainly coexist in the breast, so that the presence of one should not rule out the other.

LCIS in unusual locations may be difficult to diagnose. For example, if the only disease in a section is in small ducts, the differential diagnosis with DCIS and atypical lobular hyperplasia is even more problematic. LCIS within a fibroadenoma usually demonstrates the classic features,[69,70] but LCIS occurring within a focus of sclerosing adenosis is easy to overlook,[141,142] because the usual uniform large round acini are compressed and irregular. Here it is important to recognize the typical LCIS cells filling whatever acini are still recognizable as such.

In sclerosing adenosis, and occasionally without it, the differential diagnosis between LCIS and infiltrating lobular carcinoma (particularly the alveolar variant) may be raised. The latter lesion is usually a palpable or grossly detectable mass that consists of more round nests of tumor cells than would be appropriate to a lobular unit. It invokes the usual stromal reaction to invasive carcinoma.

Atypical Lobular Hyperplasia

Just as ADH is best defined by its relation to DCIS, atypical lobular hyperplasia (ALH) is characterized by its relation to LCIS. Because we have defined LCIS (see previous section) as a proliferation of uniform abnormal cells that distends and fills at least one half of the acini in at least one lobular unit, the definition of ALH is then a qualitatively similar cellular proliferation that differs quantitatively from LCIS in that it does not (1) distend or (2) fill the acini, or (3) it does distend and fill acini, but less than one-half of the acini in one lobular unit (Fig. 10-54). The criterion of LCIS that most often is not met is filling of acini, in that intercellular (not intracellular) lumina are present focally. It also is common for the acini to be filled but not distended. This is best demonstrated by comparing their diameters with those of the acini of the closest uninvolved lobular unit. As with LCIS, ALH is generally detected incidentally or

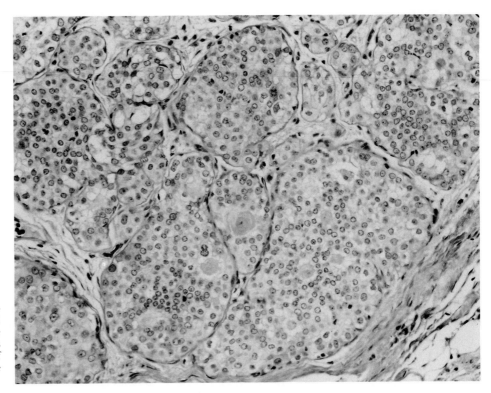

FIGURE 10-53 Lobular cancerization. A cribriform intraductal carcinoma has extended into the lobular unit; note the numerous small lumina. Most cases of lobular cancerization show more pleomorphism and necrosis.

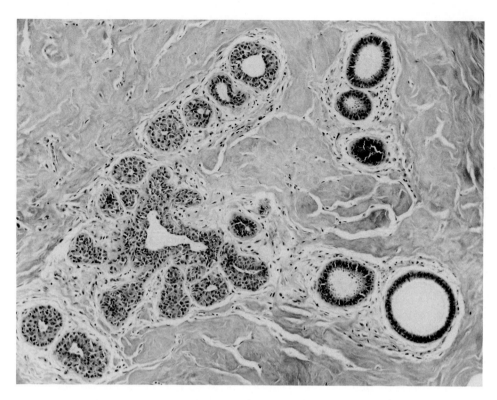

FIGURE 10-54 Atypical lobular hyperplasia. The acini in this lobular unit are slightly distended (as are adjacent uninvolved unfolded lobules) but not filled by the proliferated atypical cells. The terminal duct is also involved by the same process.

mammographically and does not form palpable masses. It also is found predominantly in premenopausal and perimenopausal women.

The term *lobular neoplasia* is sometimes used to include both ALH and LCIS and sometimes is used as a synonym for ALH.[181] Because of this imprecision, we prefer to avoid this term. Nonetheless, ALH and LCIS form a continuous spectrum, perhaps with banal lobular hyperplasia at the lower end.

The *clinical significance* of ALH, again like LCIS, is that it is a marker of increased risk for the development of invasive breast cancer. The relative risk, as with ADH, is about fourfold (absolute risk slightly less than 10%). As with LCIS, subsequent cancers may be of lobular or ductal type and may occur in either breast. The risk of uncomplicated ALH is doubled in the presence of a family history of breast cancer in a first-degree relative (mother, sister, or daughter) and is almost doubled when the ALH extends into ducts beyond the lobular unit (Fig. 10-55).[98,100,189] The usual *management* is careful and lifelong follow-up.

The *differential diagnosis* of ALH is predominantly with LCIS, as discussed above. Although the distinction is basically quantitative, it should be remembered that LCIS may involve only a single lobular unit and ALH may involve many. ALH extending into ducts (see Fig. 10-55) is difficult if not impossible to differentiate from LCIS extending into ducts unless the lobular unit primarily involved can be evaluated by the usual criteria. Lobular hyperplasia without atypia, unfolding lobules, and atypical ductal proliferations extending into lobules may also pose diagnostic problems (see the section on LCIS).

MALIGNANT EPITHELIAL TUMORS

The malignant epithelial tumors of the breast constitute the most important group of cancers in women. More than 5% of all women in the United States develop breast cancer, and some estimates are even higher. In Japan, on the other hand, it is a relatively rare disease (although increasing in frequency), whereas in most European countries the incidence is intermediate between these two extremes but closer to that of America.[190] The incidence curve rises progressively after the age of 35 years and reaches its peak between 50 and 60 years (Fig. 10-56). Mammary cancer is uncommon below the age of 30 years[191] and is very rare below 20 years.[192] It appears with greater frequency and earlier in life in women whose mothers or other primary relatives have also had mammary cancer.[193]

Etiology and Epidemiology

Probably more studies have been done on the epidemiology of breast cancer than of any other human malignant tumor, but the etiology of this neoplasm is still unknown. However, clinical and experimental data point out certain factors that favor its appearance. These generally fall into the major headings of genetic, dietary, and hormonal factors, and there are probably numerous interrelations both within and between these major categories.

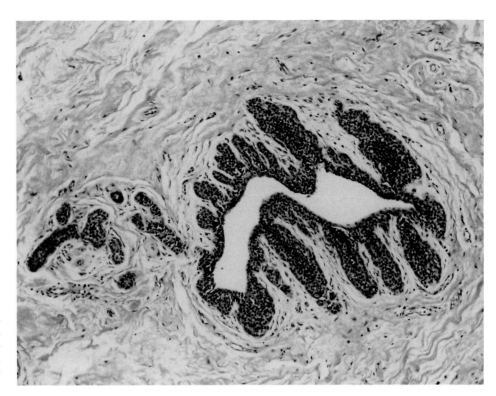

FIGURE 10-55 Atypical lobular hyperplasia with ductal extension. The buds of atypical lobular cells form an architectural pattern easily recognizable at low magnification.

Genetic Factors

Studies related to genetic factors in breast cancer development focus predominantly on populations and families. As mentioned above, breast cancer is much more common in American and European women than in Japanese and Chinese women, but even in America there are differences among such populations as white non-Hispanic, white Hispanic, and Native American.[135] Breast cancer rates in the daughters and granddaughters of Japanese immigrants to the United States show a gradual rise, but not to the level of the Caucasian population.[194] These and other population differences generally have been thought to be related to dietary and hormonal factors more than to genetic ones.

On the other hand, there are certainly strong indications of a genetic basis for the development of breast cancer in families.[193] Two major findings have been known for many years. First, a family history of breast cancer increases a woman's risk twofold to threefold. Second, patients with familial breast cancer are younger when the diagnosis is made and have a higher frequency of bilateral disease than patient with sporadic breast cancer. Studies conducted on families with high frequencies of breast cancer already have identified four distinct inherited patterns of the disease. These include a predisposition to breast cancer only; a predisposition to breast and ovarian cancer; Cowden's disease, which includes breast cancer, thyroid neoplasms, and multiple hamartomas of the skin and oral cavity; and the Li-Fraumeni syndrome, which includes soft-tissue and bone sarcomas, brain tumors, leukemias, and adrenal cortical carcinoma.[193] More such syndromes will probably be reported in the future. The specific chromosomal lesion involved has been identified in some of these situations (see Chap. 12 for further discussion).

Dietary Factors

Numerous dietary factors have been studied in an attempt to determine their relation to breast can-

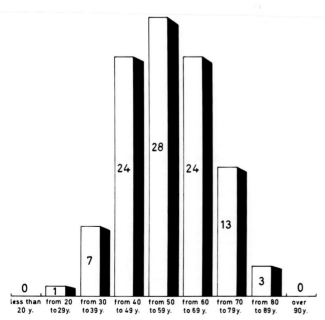

FIGURE 10-56 Frequency of appearance (in percentage) of mammary cancers as a function of age (6590 cases).

cer.[195–198] The long-held opinion has been that a Western diet plays a significant role in increasing the risk of breast cancer in the Western world, but the exact mechanisms involved have been controversial. It has been found recently that a diet high in animal fats elevates plasma levels of sex hormones and decreases the concentration of sex hormone binding globulin, thus increasing the availability of these steroids for peripheral tissues.[195] Obese women, who are at a greater risk for the development of breast cancer, have been found to have lower sex hormone-binding globulin levels.[196] On the other hand, the consumption of soy protein in the Asian diet may be protective, perhaps due to the phytoestrogens in these products.[197] Alcohol consumption has been associated with an increased risk of breast cancer in some studies but not in others, and the mechanism involved is still unknown.[198] These and other dietary factors are still under investigation, but the general assumption is that they ultimately relate to alterations in hormonal levels.

Hormonal Factors

Hormonal factors involved in mammary carcinogenesis are in many ways the most difficult to investigate, because it is postulated that the hormonal events that take place early in life may influence the development of breast cancer many years later. Nevertheless, it has been recognized for many years that, for example, late age at menarche, early artificial or natural menopause, early term pregnancy, and breast feeding are factors that appear to be protective against the development of breast cancer. The exact hormonal mechanisms involved have been searched for in human and animal studies, with considerable differences in the results obtained. There seems to be a definite interplay among genetic, dietary, and hormonal factors, so that, for example, upper body obesity—influenced by inheritance and diet—is a marker for hyperandrogenemia, which is associated with an increased risk of breast cancer.[199]

It is not surprising that, considering the known effect of endogenous hormones on the development of breast cancer, the attention of many epidemiologists has turned to a possible relation with exogenous hormone administration.[200–203] Most studies have not demonstrated a significantly increased risk for estrogen replacement therapy or oral contraception, but several have shown possible risk factors in subsets of women (eg, younger versus older women, long-term versus short-term use, and current users versus former users). Use of these hormones is a matter of informed choice, with individual considerations of the risk-benefit ratio.

Given what is known about breast cancer epidemiology, certain investigators have suggested the possibility of breast cancer prevention by alterations in diet, hormonal milieu, or both.[204–206] It is still far too early to comment on these suggestions, which will require trials involving many thousands of women, careful monitoring of compliance, and analysis of the results only after many years.

Classification

Different classifications of malignant neoplasms of the breast have been proposed, but the most widely used is the one established by the World Health Organization (WHO; Table 10-5).[207] This classification does not include many lesions described or better characterized in recent years, and accordingly the ensuing discussion will use a modification of it.

Malignant epithelial tumors (carcinomas) of the breast classically have been thought to be derived from the lactiferous ducts or from the acinar structures of the breast lobules. More recent studies have suggested that most if not all breast cancers actually originate in the ductules (terminal ducts).[208,209] By far the most common type of carcinoma seen in all populations is infiltrating duct carcinoma of not otherwise specified type, which occurs alone or in combination with other histologic types in about 70% of all cases. The proportion of noninfiltrating ductal and lobular carcinomas has increased in recent years in screened populations, and the remainder of the tumors consist of the specific histologic types of infiltrating carcinoma mentioned in the WHO classification, as well as others that will be discussed. Primary sarcomas and carcinosarcomas of the breast are rare tumors, as are leukemic, lymphomatous, and metastatic lesions.

TABLE 10-5.
World Health Organization Classification of Malignant Epithelial Tumors of the Breast

1. Noninvasive
   a. Intraductal carcinoma
   b. Lobular carcinoma in situ
2. Invasive
   a. Invasive ductal carcinoma
   b. Invasive ductal carcinoma with a predominant intraductal component
   c. Invasive lobular carcinoma
   d. Mucinous carcinoma
   e. Medullary carcinoma
   f. Papillary carcinoma
   g. Tubular carcinoma
   h. Adenoid cystic carcinoma
   i. Secretory (juvenile) carcinoma
   j. Apocrine carcinoma
   k. Carcinoma with metaplasia
      i. Squamous type
      ii. Spindle-cell type
      iii. Cartilaginous and osseous type
      iv. Mixed type
   l. Others
3. Paget's disease of the nipple

Clinical Signs

All the malignant epithelial tumors of the breast present with similar signs and symptoms. In most cases, the patient consults a physician because she has noted the presence of a painless breast mass. With the introduction of mammography, more lesions are detected at a subclinical level.

More rarely, the tumor manifests itself by nipple discharge, retraction or erosion, cutaneous redness or roughening, local pain or tenderness, an axillary mass, or evidence of disseminated metastatic disease, such as bone pain (Fig. 10-57). The median period of time elapsed between the first symptom and the first medical consultation is 6 to 12 months, which underscores the advisability of disseminating to the public more information regarding the technique and necessity of breast self-examination, the necessity of seeking immediate medical consultation on the discovery of a mass, and the value of routine mammography after the age of 40 years or earlier in high-risk groups.

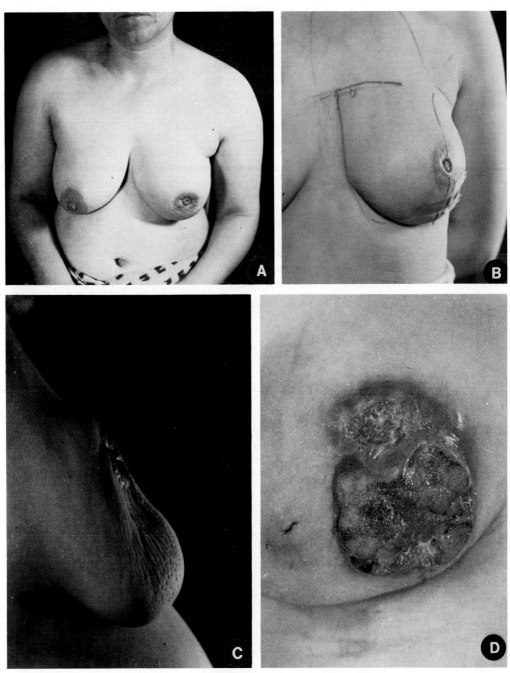

FIGURE 10-57 Mammary duct carcinoma. **(A,B)** Retraction of nipple. **(C)** Retraction of nipple and *peau d'orange*. **(D)** Carcinoma ulcerating through skin.

On the other hand, even the earliest possible diagnosis and treatment does not result in a 100% cure rate. Many authors have noted that, with the exception of asymptomatic tumors and those treated within 1 month of the onset of symptoms, those tumors treated after a long symptomatic period tend to show a more favorable prognosis than those treated with less delay. The reason for this appears to be that slowly growing tumors of low malignant potential will be tolerated by the patient for a longer time before she consults a physician, whereas rapidly growing, highly malignant tumors will alarm their hosts sooner. Some tumors, by their nature and their interaction with the host, can be treated even after considerable delay with good results, whereas others may be fated from their onset to terminate unhappily. This concept of "biologic predeterminism," which is new in the field of oncology and is still not accepted by many authors, has been discussed by MacDonald[209a] and by Gershon-Cohen.[209b] The latter author, by means of serial mammographic studies, has estimated "doubling times" in several breast cancer cases and has indicated that about three fourths of the life histories of these tumors take place in the preclinical phase. Others, using mathematical models, have suggested that tumors can only rarely be detected before metastases have already taken place. Perhaps the key to improving our therapeutic results is held in those techniques, such as mammography or methods yet to be developed, that are capable of detecting breast cancers before they become clinically apparent. It already has been noted that patients with impalpable tumors diagnosed by screening procedures are much more likely to have noninvasive and "minimal" invasive tumors, with less likelihood of metastatic disease.[19–22,210,211]

Invasive Carcinomas

Infiltrating Duct Carcinoma

Infiltrating duct carcinoma (IDC) is also known as *invasive ductal carcinoma, carcinoma of no special type* (not otherwise specified [NOS], *carcinoma with pro-*ductive fibrosis, scirrhous carcinoma, stellate carcinoma,* and *carcinoma simplex.* The WHO classification is one of exclusion: IDC is the most frequently encountered malignant tumor of the breast not falling into any of the other categories of invasive mammary carcinoma.

The tumor arises, in order of decreasing frequency, in the upper outer quadrant, the central region, the upper inner quadrant, the lower outer quadrant, or the lower inner quadrant.[212,213] The diameter of the tumor is most often between 1 and 5 cm.

Macroscopic Appearance. The macroscopic appearance varies, but two main types are encountered. The first and more frequent appearance is that of a round or ovoid hard mass, more or less adherent to adjacent tissues. Section reveals gray-yellow or white tissue with a granular surface, the central region of which is depressed. Attentive examination shows yellow or white streaks disposed in radial fashion around the center of the tumor; these streaks correspond to fibroelastic stroma separating neoplastic cell cords (Fig. 10-58).[214,215] The peripheral fibroadipose tissue adheres to the tumor and emphasizes its radial pattern. When cut, the tumor has a characteristic gritty consistency, which has been likened to that of an unripe pear.

The other appearance, less common, is represented by a spherical yellow-pink mass of softer consistency, which appears better demarcated from adjacent structures. Section in this instance shows white, granular, homogeneous tissue, with only moderate peripheral retraction. This different picture is attributed to more limited fibrosis.

Occasionally, there are several tumor nodules present macroscopically in a breast. Subserial whole organ sections have shown that multiple nodules are actually present in about half of all cases of infiltrating cancer.[216] Although even random sections confirm this in a lower percentage of cases,[217,218,219] clinical recurrences in the breast after partial mastectomy and radiation therapy occur in less than 20% of cases.[220–222]

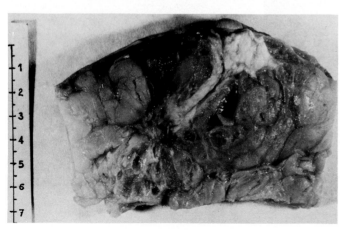

FIGURE 10-58 Mammary duct carcinoma: macroscopic appearance on section.

When the skin is involved, it becomes thickened, indurated, and invaginated over the tumor. Velpeau compared this appearance of the skin to that of a firm hide (carcinoma en cuirasse).[15]

A certain number of breast cancers are bilateral from their onset. These may represent rapid metastatic involvement of the contralateral breast or two independent tumors.[223,224]

Microscopic Appearance. The neoplastic glandular formations are disposed in cords, solid cell nests, tubes, glands, anastomosing bundles, and mixtures of all of these. They are disseminated in a stroma, the prominence of which varies from one tumor to another and from one region to another within a single tumor (Figs. 10-59 through 10-61). There is an abundant framework of collagen, reticulin, and elastic fibers. The epithelial cells present diverse cytologic anomalies. All appearances are encountered, from the small cell with a moderately hyperchromatic regular nucleus to the monstrous cell with a voluminous, lobulated, irregular, and hyperchromatic nucleus. The number of mitoses is variable. Cytoplasm is found in variable abundance.

The stroma may be reduced to a few thin bundles or it may consist of many large homogeneous plaques.[214,215] Hyaline degeneration is uncommon. The neoplastic cell cords rapidly overflow the parenchyma of the breast lobules and infiltrate the adjacent adipose tissue as centrifugal cellular streaks that confer on the tumor its star-shaped gross appearance.

Many tumors express one or more characteristics of the specific tumor types in the classification, but these minor foci do not influence the prognosis, which is more favorable only if the lesions are entirely or mostly composed of the specific patterns.

Histologic Grading. The variable appearance of IDC has led to numerous grading systems, most of which correlate to some extent with biologic tumor behavior. The best validated and most reproducible of these, which has the advantage of using both architectural and cytologic features, is the Nottingham system, a modification of the Bloom and Richardson method as reported by Elston and Ellis.[225] This system is summarized in Table 10-6. Elston and Ellis reported acceptable concurrence (more than 90%) between two pathologists independently using this system, and an excellent correlation with prognosis in a series of almost 2000 cases. They recommend that all invasive breast cancer be graded in this manner, but our preference is to limit its use to IDC not otherwise specified (IDC-NOS), because most histologic subtypes discussed below have unique natural histories and histologic features.

Electron Microscopic Appearance. Electron microscopic studies of mammary carcinomas have contributed interesting morphologic data (Figs. 10-62 and 10-63) but have failed to accomplish the two main tasks in which success might be hoped for: (1) to delineate absolute criteria for differentiating benign from malignant lesions, and (2) to establish a rational

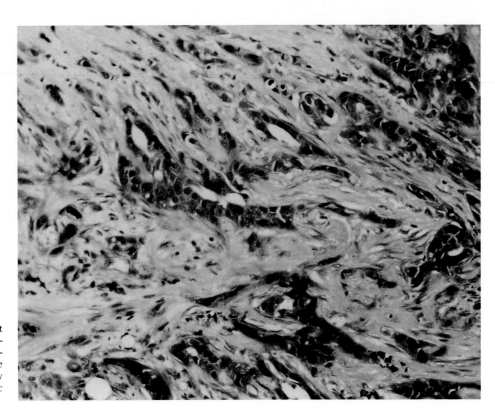

FIGURE 10-59 Infiltrating duct carcinoma, not otherwise specified. The infiltrating ductal formations contain lumina and are lined by cells showing relatively slight pleomorphism and mitotic activity.

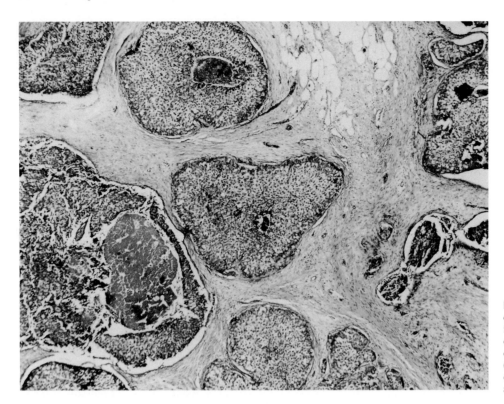

FIGURE 10-60 Infiltrating duct carcinoma, not otherwise specified. In this tumor, large nests of poorly differentiated tumor cells with foci of central necrosis (mimicking intraductal comedocarcinoma) invade through a reactive stroma.

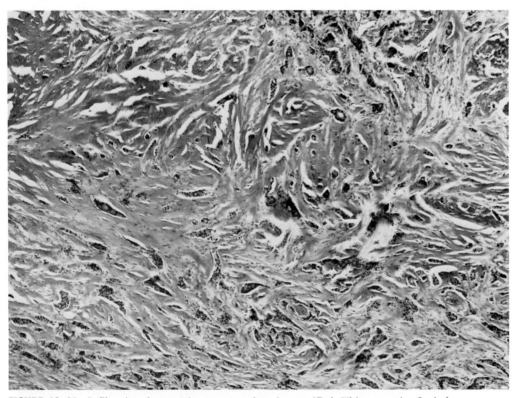

FIGURE 10-61 Infiltrating duct carcinoma, not otherwise specified. This tumor is of scirrhous type, showing a paucicellular pattern and a dense fibroelastotic stroma.

TABLE 10-6.
Combined Architectural and Cytologic Grading System for Infiltrating Duct Carcinoma

Feature	Assessment	Numerical Score*
Tubule formation	In >75% of tumor	1
	10%–75%	2
	<10%	3
Nuclear pleomorphism	Small, regular uniform cells	1
	Moderate increase in size and variability	2
	Marked variation	3
Mitotic counts at tumor periphery	0–9/10 HPF†	1
	10–19	2
	20 or more	3

*The three scores are added together. A final tally of 3 to 5 = grade I (well differentiated); 6 or 7 = grade II (moderately differentiated); and 8 or 9 = grade III (poorly differentiated).

†HPF = high-power fields, defined by use of a Leitz Ortholux microscope with wide-angle eyepieces and 25× objective (field area 0.274 mm²). This must be recalculated for other microscopes.

Adapted from Elston CW, Ellis IO: Pathological prognostic factors in breast cancer. I. The value of histological grade in breast cancer: Experience from a large study with long-term follow-up. Histopathology 19:403–410, 1991

classification of breast cancers based on their exact cell of origin. With regard to the former task, several studies have shown a spectrum from hyperplastic and atypical to malignant lesions.[10,11] The presence of such structures as intracytoplasmic lumina and fibrils and the absence of basal lamina appear to be more frequent in malignant tumors but certainly are not pathognomonic; other features such as nuclear hyperchromatism, increased nuclear–cytoplasmic ratio, and so forth, can be detected as easily (if not more so) with the light microscope.

A histogenetic classification based largely on ultrastructure has been attempted by Murad.[226] He defines a myoepithelial cell (scirrhous), a ductal epithelial cell (medullary), and a ductular (lobular) carcinoma, but he fails to account for other known variants in this rather controversial study. At present, the identification of the various forms of mammary carcinoma still depends on light microscopy.

Cytologic Appearance. The criteria for a diagnosis of carcinoma in an FNA specimen are similar to standard cytologic criteria of malignancy in other organs.[26,28,29] In IDC, the smears generally are highly cellular and are composed of single tumor cells and large clusters, usually in a hemorrhagic background (see Color Figures 10-1 and 10-2). The clusters often show a loss of the tight cellular cohesiveness seen in aspirates from fibroadenomas and other benign conditions that show numerous cell clusters. They lack the bimorphism of most benign breast aspirates, in which the single cells demonstrate bipolar nuclei and little or no cytoplasm. At higher magnification, the

cells are large and exhibit anisonucleosis, high nuclear–cytoplasmic ratios, hyperchromatism, and nuclei that are often eccentrically situated and occasionally bizarre. The degree of atypia in the aspirate generally reflects the differentiation of the tumor, but the correlation is not perfect.

Differential Diagnosis. The most frequent histopathologic differential diagnostic problems associated with IDC-NOS relate to its distinction from other types of infiltrating mammary carcinomas, especially those with a more favorable prognosis. In general terms, the safest statement that can be made is that one of the favorable rarer types (eg, tubular, adenoid cystic, papillary, cribriform, mucinous, and medullary) should not be diagnosed unless the tumor in question is a perfect fit with the classic features of that type. Suggestive but atypical variants are best diagnosed as IDC and graded appropriately. Most of the favorable histologic types must be pure or at least dominant (the rule varies with the type) to maintain their favorable natural history; therefore, when one of these types occurs together with IDC-NOS, the proportion of each should be specified in the surgical pathology report. The diagnostic features of the various subtypes are discussed individually below.

Less common but potentially more serious diagnostic problems concern the distinction of IDC from a noninfiltrating duct carcinoma (DCIS) or a benign lesion. The problem of sclerosing adenosis is probably overemphasized in the literature and usually involves tubular carcinoma more than IDC (see Table 10-2 for the most useful differential diagnostic features). Nipple adenomas, radial scars, and sclerosing papillomas can present problems and are discussed above. They are all cytologically benign lesions and most of them have prominent myoepithelial cells (demonstrable by standard light microscopy or, when necessary, by immunohistochemistry). They all have classic—albeit different—architectural features that are generally lacking in the more haphazardly arranged IDC. The reactive, inflamed, myxoid to fibroelastotic stroma of IDC is in sharp contrast to the totally unreactive stroma of nipple adenoma and the generally hyalinized stroma of a sclerosing papilloma.

DCIS can present a major diagnostic problem, particularly when it occurs within an architecturally abnormal lesion such as sclerosing adenosis or a radial scar (see Figs. 10-32, 10-33, and 10-47). The background lesion, however, is usually apparent, and the diagnosis of IDC should be made only rarely in this situation. Another problem with DCIS involves tangential sectioning through a branch of an involved duct, giving the false appearance of extension of a tongue of tumor out into the stroma. In this situation, additional levels through the block may be helpful if they demonstrate more obvious stromal infiltration. If they do not, we prefer to be conservative and retain the diagnosis of DCIS, because a

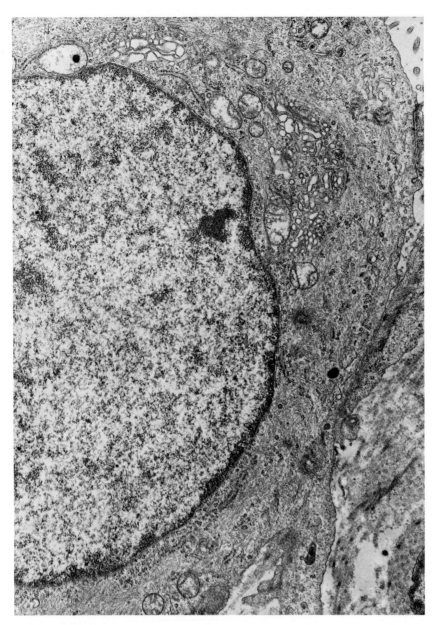

FIGURE 10-62 Infiltrating duct carcinoma: electron micrograph shows tumor cell in intimate contact with collagen fibers at lower right. Myoepithelial cells and basement membrane are absent here. Golgi apparatus, free ribosomes, and microfibrils are prominent.

single microscopic tongue of invasive carcinoma is unlikely to alter the natural history of the tumor. IDC and other mammary carcinomas present differential diagnostic problems when they are detected in a metastatic focus in the absence of a known primary tumor in the breast, or when both a breast primary and a different primary adenocarcinoma have been diagnosed in the past. Despite claims to the contrary, we know of no antibody in immunohistochemical use that is totally specific for breast cancer, so the final estimation—and it often is just that—must still be made on the basis of the basic light microscopic features.

Prognostically Favorable Variants of Infiltrating Carcinoma

Because IDC-NOS makes up about 70% of all primary infiltrating carcinomas of the breast, the less

common variants are defined by virtue of (1) their distinctive histopathologic and (occasionally) gross pathologic features, and (2) their prognostic differences, if any, from IDC-NOS. Most of the variants that have been well characterized are associated with a more favorable prognosis, although in some instances this advantage is present only when the variant is present in its pure form, and in others minor proportions of admixed IDC-NOS apparently do not worsen the prognosis. In some of the prognostically favorable variants, it is difficult to determine whether the clinical behavior is determined by the histologic type alone, or by type in concert with such factors as tumor size and grade. Finally, some of the types that are generally thought to be prognostically favorable by most authors have not had such an excellent prognosis when studied by others, and data derived from the era of treatment by radical mastec-

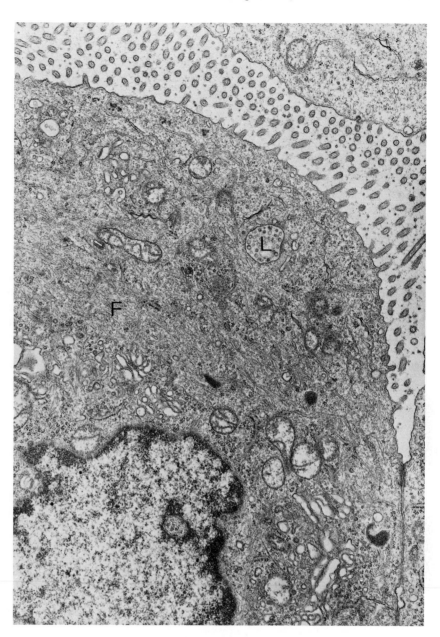

FIGURE 10-63 Infiltrating duct carcinoma: electron micrograph shows considerable similarity to benign mammary ductal epithelial cells, but with numerous microfibrils (*F*) and small intracellular lumen (*L*).

tomy alone are being supplanted by new studies in which the treatment is often conservative surgery with adjuvant radiation therapy, chemotherapy, or both. This is a rapidly changing field, and the reader must keep up with new developments.

A final caveat in this area concerns the tendency for breast cancer tissues to be submitted for numerous prognostic studies in which tumor histopathology is not taken into consideration. Particularly when the cancer is small to begin with—as is often the case today—it becomes more and more difficult to be sure what proportion of a tumor the prognostically favorable variant really represents.

Tubular Carcinoma. When it was first fully characterized in the 1970s, tubular carcinoma was considered to be a rare tumor, representing no more than 1% of all infiltrating carcinomas of the breast. With the advent of mammographic screening, the proportion of tubular carcinomas in most series has increased to close to 10% of all infiltrating cancers.[227-232] A corollary of this observation is the fact that tubular carcinomas tend to be small, usually measuring about 1 cm or less in greatest dimension, and rarely measuring more than 2 cm. It is generally thought that tubular carcinoma represents a stage in the growth phase of IDC, and that if the tumor is allowed to grow to a large size, it will ultimately assume the IDC-NOS morphology.

Clinically, these tumors are often impalpable and are usually discovered by mammography. When a tubular carcinoma is palpable, it generally appears as a small, hard, stellate mass. Skin and nipple retraction are very rare. The age distribution is similar to that of patients with IDC-NOS.

Macroscopically, there is little to differentiate tubular carcinoma from IDC-NOS except its small size. Some tumors are so small (1 to 2 mm) that they even escape detection on examination of the gross biopsy specimen and are initially diagnosed on microscopic examination.

Microscopically, the tumor is characterized by the presence of oval or round tubular structures with open lumina surrounded by a single layer of small, rather uniform cells (Figs. 10-64 through 10-66). The tumor often grows in a stellate pattern but may lack any special form, simply infiltrating around and between benign ducts and into adjacent fat. The ducts may be compressed into an angulated teardrop shape or may grow together to form a focal cribriform pattern (see Fig. 10-66). Stroma between the malignant tubular structures is usually reactive, but it may be hyalinized or even unremarkable. Occasional tubular carcinomas arise within a radial scar, and they share some of the architectural features of that lesion. The tumor cells are, by definition, well differentiated. Mitotic figures are rare, necrosis is absent, and tumor cell stratification is absent or minimal. Myoepithelial cells are not seen.

The above description applies to pure tubular carcinoma, but many cases are admixed with intraductal, in situ lobular, or other infiltrating carcinoma patterns.

Differential Diagnosis. The most important differential diagnosis is with benign sclerosing lesions such as sclerosing adenosis (see Table 10-2) and radial scar. The most useful features of tubular carcinoma in making this distinction are the infiltrative pattern, the uniformity and open appearance of the tubular structures, the presence of a reactive stroma, and the absence of a myoepithelial cell layer. When the presence or absence of myoepithelial cells is in doubt, they can be identified immunohistochemically with antibodies to actin and S-100 protein[233] or ultrastructurally.[139] A more difficult differential diagnosis

is with the rare condition known as *microglandular adenosis* (Fig. 10-67).[234-236] This lesion may present as a palpable mass of several centimeters or may be an incidental microscopic finding. There is a haphazard distribution of small round glands extending through fibrous stroma and fat, without any surrounding stromal reaction. The gland lumina usually contain dense hyaline eosinophilic material that is generally PAS-positive. The cell cytoplasm may be clear and often can be demonstrated to contain glycogen. Nuclear atypia and mitotic figures are absent. Although this condition is benign, it may be associated with simultaneous or subsequent carcinoma.[236] The main differentiating features from tubular carcinoma are the smaller size of the glands, the absence of a reactive stroma, and the hyaline material present within the lumina.

Other differential diagnostic problems for tubular carcinoma involve its distinction from other forms of infiltrating carcinoma, particularly cribriform and infiltrating duct NOS. The former distinction is largely of interest to the histologic purist, because the clinical behavior of tubular and cribriform carcinomas is identical. The distinction from IDC-NOS is more important, because the latter has a poorer prognosis (see below).

Clinical Features and Prognosis. It is universally agreed that pure tubular carcinoma, whether or not admixed with patterns of noninfiltrating carcinoma, has an excellent prognosis, with distant metastases and death recorded only rarely. More controversial is the prognostic significance of admixed infiltrating carcinoma of other histologic types. Most authors allow up to 25% of IDC-NOS within the definition of tubular carcinoma with a favorable prognosis.[227,230,232] However, we believe that if part of the tumor has been submitted for nonhistologic studies, and any IDC-NOS is present in the material examined histologically, the possibility of distant metas-

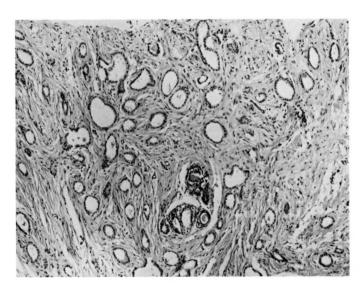

FIGURE 10-64 Tubular carcinoma. Uniform tubular structures in a reactive stroma swirl around benign ducts at bottom center.

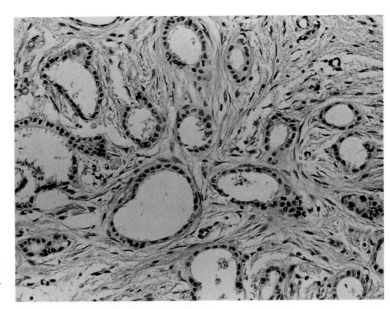

FIGURE 10-65 Tubular carcinoma. Note the stellate pattern, open tubular structures, and single layer of well-differentiated tumor cells.

tases may exist. As mentioned above, the not infrequent coexistence of infiltrating cribriform carcinoma does not worsen the prognosis of tubular carcinoma.

Axillary lymph node metastases are not rare in tubular carcinoma, occurring in about 10% to 15% of cases in most series. Even node-positive cases do not seem to be at much risk for the development of distant metastases, because these occur in 2% or less of all cases. Tubular carcinomas are virtually always estrogen and progesterone receptor-rich and diploid.

Infiltrating Cribriform Carcinoma. Infiltrating cribriform carcinoma is a recently described tumor that comprises slightly more than 3% of infiltrating carcinomas of the breast.[237,238] The size of the tumor is usually between that of tubular carcinoma and that of IDC-NOS, and foci of either or both of these may be present in tumors that are predominantly cribriform. This relation led Venable and colleagues to suggest that infiltrating cribriform carcinoma may represent a transitional form as small tubular carcinomas mature into larger IDCs.[238]

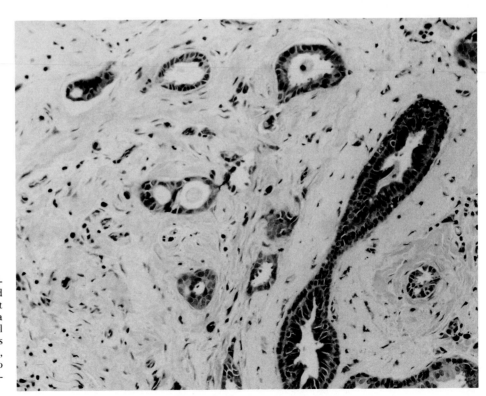

FIGURE 10-66 Tubular carcinoma. Compare the single-layered carcinoma with the benign duct at lower right, which contains a prominent myoepithelial cell layer. Some of the carcinomatous tubules are teardrop-shaped, whereas two others are fused to form the beginning of a cribriform pattern.

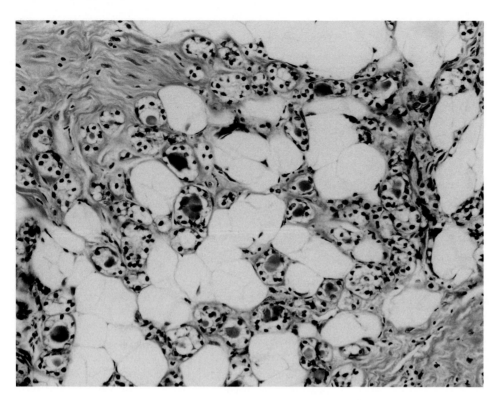

FIGURE 10-67 Microglandular adenosis. Small glandular structures lined by a single cell layer and containing dense eosinophilic material in their lumina infiltrate haphazardly into connective tissue and fat.

Microscopically, the tumor is characterized by irregular infiltrating islands of tumor displaying rather uniform cribriform spaces lined by moderately- to well-differentiated cells (see Fig. 10-68). The word *infiltrating* is part of the name of this tumor to differentiate it from the cribriform pattern of DCIS, which it closely resembles and which forms one of the major differential diagnoses. Important differentiating features are the angular nature of the islands in the infiltrating tumor and the reactive intervening stroma. The other main lesions to be considered in the differential diagnosis are tubular, infiltrating duct, and adenoid cystic carcinomas. The latter entity, which is the most difficult to

differentiate from infiltrating cribriform carcinoma, is discussed below.

Clinical Features and Prognosis. In the reports of Page and colleagues[237] and Venable and colleagues,[238] no patient died of recurrent or metastatic infiltrating cribriform carcinoma, although metastases to axillary lymph nodes were not infrequent. Venable and colleagues emphasized that these always involved three or fewer nodes if IDC-NOS did not comprise more than 50% of the infiltrating component of the primary tumor. Mixed cribriform-tubular carcinomas did well regardless of the respective proportions of these two histologic types. The

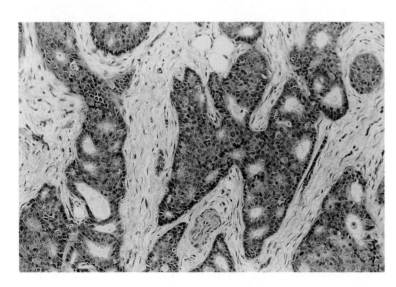

FIGURE 10-68 Infiltrating cribriform carcinoma. Irregularly shaped nests of small, uniform cells form regular cribriform spaces. The intervening stroma is spindled and edematous.

favorable prognosis of these two histologic types was also confirmed in the large study of Ellis and colleagues.[239]

Cytologic Features. The cytologic features of infiltrating cribriform carcinoma and tubular carcinoma are not well established in the literature. We have found that FNA biopsies and intraoperative smears of these two lesions resemble those of very well-differentiated IDCs. In both tumors, lumen formation is occasionally seen and may suggest the specific diagnosis.

Adenoid Cystic Carcinoma. Adenoid cystic carcinoma is a rare primary neoplasm of the breast.[240-242] A recent review suggests that only 140 cases have been reported.[242] It represents far less than 1% of all breast carcinomas.

Macroscopically, the tumors are usually small, well-circumscribed, and white-gray, with a mean diameter ranging from 2 to 3 cm. A significant number occur in the subareolar region, but nipple discharge is not noted.

Microscopically, the tumor is identical to its more common salivary gland counterpart. The tumor cells are arranged in cribriform (Fig. 10-69), trabecular, tubular, or solid patterns, with mixtures of these occurring in many tumors. The tumor cells are small with a round, hyperchromatic nucleus and sparse cytoplasm. The stroma is often myxoid or hyaline and surrounds the epithelial structures. Myoepithelial cells can generally be demonstrated immunohistochemically.

In typical cribriform areas, basement membrane material invaginates into the tumor cell nests to form PAS-positive hyaline cores. As in adenoid cystic carcinoma of salivary glands, perineural infiltration is common.

The *cytologic features* are characteristic and consist of small, uniform neoplastic cells with round, moderately hyperchromatic nuclei grouped in small clusters or large sheets and dispersed in an intercellular matrix that stains pale pink or green with the Papanicolaou stain and intensely red in Giemsa-stained specimens.[243] Frequently, lakes of hyaline stroma are surrounded by a layer of epithelial cells, suggesting the characteristic feature of this tumor at the histopathologic level (Color Figure 10-12).

The *differential diagnosis* of this tumor is predominantly with infiltrating cribriform carcinoma. The main differentiating features characteristic of adenoid cystic carcinoma are the presence of extracellular basement membrane material within pseudocysts; the presence of myoepithelial cells within the tumor; the absence of a noninfiltrating component; the absence of an admixture of tubular or IDC; and the absence of estrogen and progesterone receptors. Infiltrating cribriform carcinoma is virtually always estrogen receptor-positive and usually progesterone receptor-positive.

The *prognosis* of adenoid cystic carcinoma is excellent, with axillary nodal metastases and distant metastases being rare. Few cases with long-term follow-up have been reported in which conservative surgical treatment was undertaken.

Mucinous (Mucoid, Colloid, Gelatinous) Carcinoma. In most mammary carcinomas, there is discrete mucin production in the glandular cells. However, when extracellular mucin comprises 50% or more of tumor volume the tumor is called a *mucinous carcinoma* (Fig. 10-70). This tumor originally was characterized by Saphir[244] in 1941 as having a favorable prognosis, and numerous subsequent studies have confirmed this observation.[212,239,245-247] In its pure form, the tumor comprises about 2% of all mammary carcinomas.

Clinically, the tumor tends to occur in older

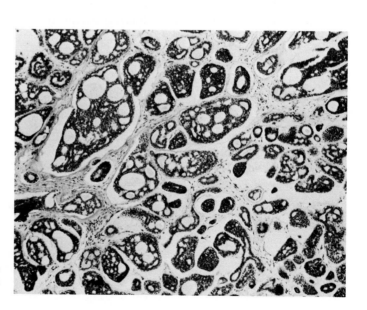

FIGURE 10-69 Adenoid cystic carcinoma: microscopic appearance. Invaginations of basement membrane material into cystic cavities are seen.

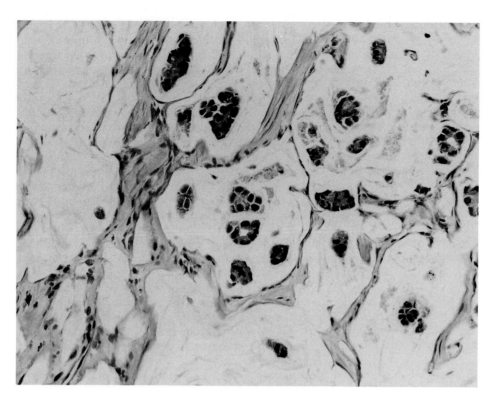

FIGURE 10-70 Mucinous carcinoma. Small glandular structures lined by well-differentiated tumor cells float in lakes of extracellular mucin.

women as a slowly expanding, well-circumscribed, soft mass. It frequently has expanded to a large size by the time that histopathologic diagnosis is made.

The *gross appearance* of the tumor is well circumscribed, soft, and gelatinous. This gross appearance is characteristic (Color Figure 10-13), although it may occasionally be confused with an unusually large and soft fibroadenoma.

Microscopically, the characteristic appearance is one of small solid or glandular nests of well-differentiated tumor cells floating in lakes of extracellular mucin (see Fig. 10-70). For the tumor to display its favorable prognosis, this pattern must be seen uniformly throughout the tumor, because even small amounts of IDC-NOS dilute the clinical behavior. Intraductal carcinoma, on the other hand, does not worsen the prognosis. When it is present, it is usually of non-comedo type and may display voluminous extracellular mucin (Fig. 10-71).

Neuroendocrine differentiation, characterized by the presence of cells showing argyrophilia, immunohistochemical positivity for chromogranin or synaptophysin, or dense-core neurosecretory granules by electron microscopy, is a common feature of mucinous carcinoma but does not seem to alter the prognosis when present.[248,249]

Cytologic examination reveals cellular cohesive groups and isolated cells in a background of abundant mucin (Color Figure 10-14). The nuclei are regular in size and shape, and the chromatin is finely dispersed. In those tumors in which an admixture of IDC-NOS is present, nuclear abnormalities are focally more pronounced. Intracellular (as opposed to extracellular) mucin usually is not prominent.

The *differential diagnosis* is with the rare benign condition known as *mucocele-like tumor of the breast*.[250,251] This lesion is characterized by a palpable mass composed of multiple cysts containing mucinous material, with rupture and discharge of acellular mucin into the surrounding stroma. These tumors may closely resemble mucinous carcinoma at both the cytologic and histologic levels. In the series of Ro and colleagues, all mucocele-like tumors were associated with microscopic foci of either mucinous carcinoma or ADH with abundant intraluminal mucin.[250] These authors caution against considering this tumor an entirely benign lesion.

The *prognosis* of pure mucinous carcinoma is favorable, although not as favorable as that of tubular, cribriform, and adenoid cystic carcinomas. In most series, despite the frequent large size of the tumors, only 10% to 15% of patients have died of metastatic carcinoma. When a minor IDC component is present, the prognosis is intermediate between that of pure mucinous carcinoma and the usual IDC.[239,245–247,252] Early reports suggest that conservative surgery and radiation therapy are effective in the treatment of this tumor type.[253]

Papillary Carcinoma. Although papillary carcinomas generally have been considered to be prognostically favorable mammary carcinomas, it often has been unclear in the literature whether the tumors being analyzed were papillary variants of intraductal carcinoma, papillary intracystic carcino-

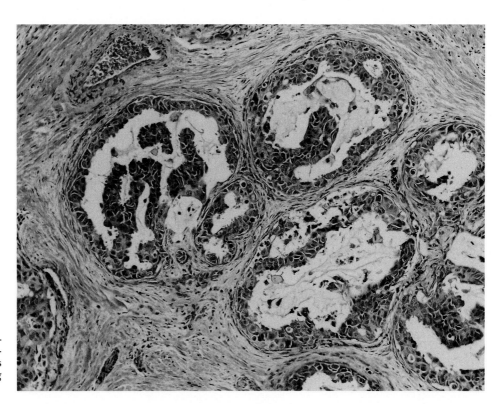

FIGURE 10-71 Intraductal carcinoma with voluminous intraluminal mucin. This lesion was associated with an infiltrating mucinous carcinoma.

mas,[254,255] or invasive papillary carcinomas.[256] Classic intraductal carcinoma has already been discussed in an earlier section, but the other two forms of papillary carcinoma are considered here.

Intracystic papillary carcinoma usually presents as a bulky, soft, well-circumscribed mass in an older woman. Microscopically, the lesion is confined to a large cystic space, but it may extend into adjacent smaller ducts (Fig. 10-72). Stromal infiltration is absent or very focal. These tumors are usually curable by wide local excision alone, and certainly by mastectomy.

Even less common is *invasive papillary carcinoma,* which may actually represent several rare entities but is defined as any infiltrating carcinoma containing papillary formations. Many of the tumors reported by Fisher and colleagues may have represented examples of mucinous carcinoma with some papillary growth, whereas others were histologically similar to serous papillary carcinoma of the ovary.[256] As a group, the 5-year disease-free survival rate was in the range of 90%, although 30% of cases with axillary dissection had nodal metastases.

Secretory Carcinoma. Secretory carcinoma is a rare type of mammary carcinoma that has been known as *juvenile carcinoma,* but several reports have indicated that the tumor also occurs in adults.[257-260] The tumor is usually well circumscribed grossly and is characterized histologically by the presence of vacuolated cells arranged in solid, cystic, or ductal patterns (Fig. 10-73). The secretory material is present in the cytoplasm and in extracellular secretions. The

material is PAS-positive, diastase-resistant, and mucicarmine-negative. Ultrastructural examination reveals the presence of numerous membrane-bound secretory vacuoles. The exact nature of this secretory material remains unknown, but the tumor appears to be different from the *glycogen-rich clear cell carcinomas* recently reported.[261]

The intracytoplasmic vacuoles that are a characteristic feature of secretory carcinoma may also be seen in FNA cytologic material and may result in the correct diagnosis being made preoperatively.[260] When secretory carcinoma occurs in a patient younger than 20 years, it is apparently always curable by surgery alone. In older patients, axillary nodal metastases are not uncommon, and death as a result of distant metastases has been reported in rare cases. Nevertheless, the prognosis is still considerably more favorable than for IDC-NOS.

Medullary Carcinoma. The special tumor variants that have been discussed up to this point all share a well-differentiated nuclear appearance and a favorable prognosis that is acknowledged by virtually all authors. Medullary carcinoma is an exception to both of these rules. One of the characteristic features of the tumor is its high-grade nuclear morphology, and the favorable prognosis initially noted by Moore and Foote[262] has been confirmed by most[263-268] but not all[239,269] authors.

Clinically and mammographically, medullary carcinoma presents as a lobulated circumscribed mass more or less similar to fibroadenoma. Microcalcifiations are rare. The tumor often acquires a large

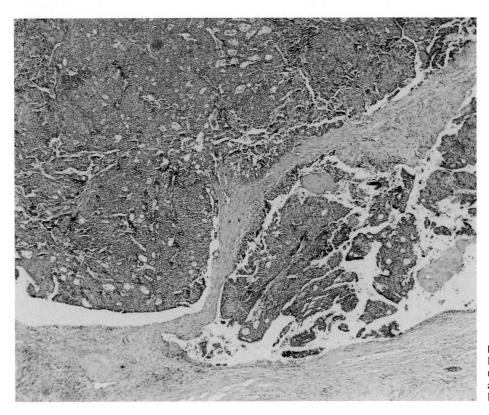

FIGURE 10-72 Intracystic papillary carcinoma. Only a portion of this tumor, which was confined to a large cystic cavity, is shown here.

volume without becoming adherent to the skin or surrounding tissues.

Macroscopically, the tumor is spherical and well demarcated, with a rubbery consistency and yellow-white color (Fig. 10-74). Foci of necrosis and hemorrhage are often prominent.

The classic *microscopic features* of this tumor are shown in Figures 10-75 and 10-76 and are outlined in Table 10-7. These features include the following:

- A predominantly circumscribed border
- A so-called syncytial growth pattern (a solid growth without glandular or papillary features)

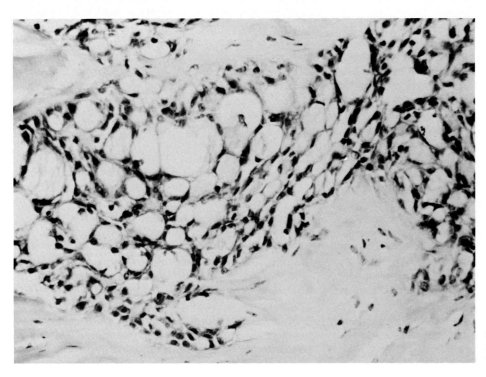

FIGURE 10-73 Secretory carcinoma. Note the feathery secretory material in cells and lumina.

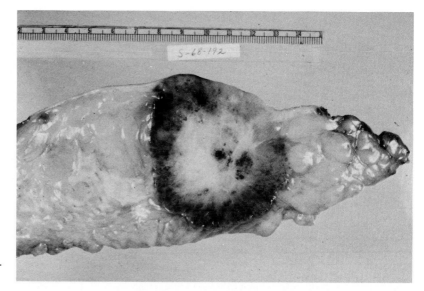

FIGURE 10-74 Medullary carcinoma: macroscopic appearance.

- The presence of a prominent stromal lympho-plasmacytic infiltrate
- Nuclei that are generally poorly differentiated or, at best, moderately differentiated.

Ridolfi and colleagues proposed in 1977 a category of *atypical medullary carcinoma* for tumors that met some but not all of the criteria for classic medullary carcinoma, and they suggested that the prognosis in this group was intermediate between the favorable prognosis of classic medullary carcinoma and the less favorable IDC-NOS.[264] More recently, Wargotz and Silverberg[267] and Pedersen and colleagues[268] have

tried to simplify the diagnostic criteria, because it appears that many breast cancers with inflammatory stroma are overdiagnosed as medullary,[265,266] perhaps leading to the differences in opinion concerning the prognostic significance of this diagnosis. In our system, the term *atypical medullary carcinoma* is not used, and the diagnosis of IDC is mandatory if any of the primary criteria mentioned above are not met, and also if two or more of three secondary criteria (complete microscopic circumscription, moderate to marked mononuclear infiltrate, and absence of surrounding in situ carcinoma) are not met (see Table 10-7).

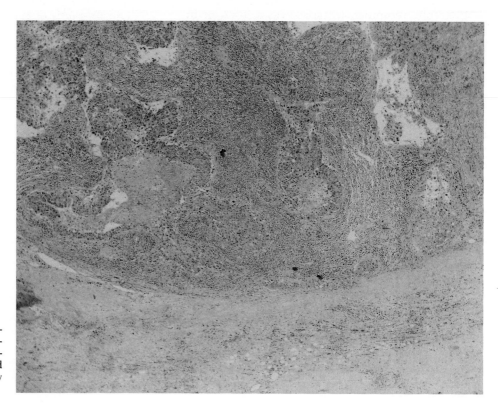

FIGURE 10-75 Medullary carcinoma. Low-power photomicrograph showing tumor circumscription, foci of necrosis, and lack of glandular or papillary differentiation.

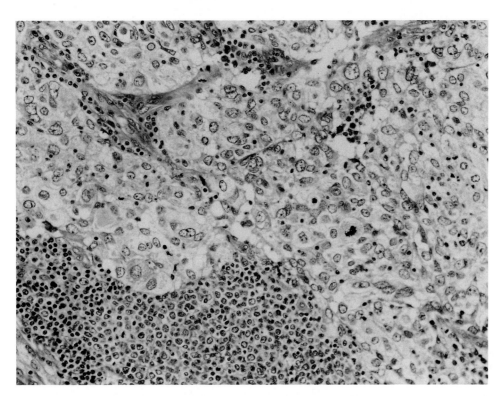

FIGURE 10-76 Medullary carcinoma. Detail of solid sheets of pleomorphic tumor cells and lymphoid infiltrate.

Ultrastructural studies have shown that the tumor cells are characterized by specialization of the cell surfaces into microvilli, formation of ducts and solid islands, and moderately well-developed rough endoplasmic reticulum.[270,271] They resemble the true epithelial cells of the mammary duct.

These tumors rarely, if ever, contain estrogen or progesterone receptors. In typical cases, FNA or intraoperative *cytology* (Color Figure 10-15) shows pleomorphic malignant epithelial cells interspersed with

numerous lymphocytes and plasma cells. Glandular and papillary formations are not seen, and bizarre lobulated nuclei with macronucleoli are common. Unfortunately, medullary-like IDCs (defined by the histologic criteria discussed above) can have identical cytologic features, so the diagnosis is not precise until the entire tumor is studied histopathologically.

The *prognosis* of typical medullary carcinoma is thought to be favorable by most authors. In our series, the 5-year survival rate was greater than 90%.[267] Axillary nodal metastases are fairly common, but the prognosis in most series is better than that of IDC-NOS in node-negative and node-positive cases.

Because the usual prognostic features for breast carcinoma (tumor grade, receptor status, and ploidy) are all unfavorable in medullary carcinoma, an explanation must be sought for the probably favorable prognosis. Most widely studied has been the lymphoid infiltrate that is a characteristic feature of these tumors.[272] It has been suggested that these cells become effector cells capable of killing the tumor cells by mechanisms similar to those of natural killer lymphocytes.

Other Infiltrating Carcinomas

In addition to the prognostically favorable histologic types of mammary carcinoma mentioned above, there are a number of other variants that are prognostically neutral or unfavorable when compared with IDC-NOS. These types are discussed in the following sections.

TABLE 10-7.
Proposed Histologic Criteria for the Diagnosis of Medullary Carcinoma

*Primary**
 1. Predominantly circumscribed border
 2. Syncytial growth ≥ 75%
 3. Presence of admixed stromal mononuclear infiltrate
 4. Grade 2 or 3 nuclei
 5. Absence of glandular features

Secondary†
 1. Microscopically completely circumscribed
 2. 2+ to 3+ mononuclear infiltrate
 3. Absence of in situ carcinoma

---

*Diagnosis of infiltrating duct carcinoma is mandatory if any one of these criteria is not met.

†Diagnosis of infiltrating duct carcinoma is mandatory if two or more of these criteria are not met.

Adapted from Wargotz ES, Silverberg SG: Medullary carcinoma of the breast: A clinicopathologic study with appraisal of current diagnostic criteria. Hum Pathol 19:1340–1346, 1988

Infiltrating Lobular Carcinoma. The most common of the histologic types with no probable prognostic significance is infiltrating lobular carcinoma, which comprises between 5% and 10% of all infiltrating carcinomas of the breast. We emphasize the word "probable" because the prognostic significance of lobular carcinoma is still uncertain. In recent monographs on breast pathology, lobular carcinoma is referred to as a prognostically favorable type of breast cancer by Page and Anderson and an unfavorable type by Carter.[149,151] Furthermore, some authors note prognostic differences between different histologic subtypes of infiltrating lobular carcinoma, whereas others deny this assertion.[239,273–277]

Clinically and *macroscopically,* infiltrating lobular carcinoma is essentially identical to IDC, presenting as a stellate, firm, infiltrative mass of variable size. Several studies have noted a higher frequency of bilaterality in infiltrating lobular carcinoma than in IDC.[273,278]

Microscopically, the so-called classic pattern described initially is still the most common (Fig. 10-77). In this pattern, the neoplastic cells line up in long rows one cell thick, surrounded by fairly abundant stroma, in a single-file pattern. The tumor cells also exhibit a circumferential growth around uninvolved benign ducts. There is no tendency to form glandular or papillary structures, nor are wide sheets of cells noted. The individual cells are small and show little cytologic atypia.

In addition to this classic form, alveolar, solid, mixed, tubulolobular, and pleomorphic variants have been described. In the alveolar pattern, the tumor grows in round aggregates of 20 or more cells, reminiscent of LCIS but with obvious stromal infiltration (Fig. 10-78). In the solid variant, the tumor cells grow in a sheet-like pattern or in irregularly shaped nests (Fig. 10-79). The mixed group shows a combination of classic, alveolar, or solid growth patterns in a single tumor. In all these tumor types, the cytologic appearance of the tumor cells is identical, as it is in tubulolobular carcinoma,[279] in which the cells additionally form small tubules with definite lumina (Fig. 10-80). On the other hand, a group of tumors showing the architectural features of classic infiltrating lobular carcinoma but with a much greater degree of cytologic pleomorphism have been described as the pleomorphic variant of lobular carcinoma.[277] These tumors also are characterized by an eosinophilic, slightly granular cytoplasm and immunohistochemical positivity for the antigen GCDFP-15, suggesting apocrine differentiation.

Ultrastructurally, the most prominent feature of infiltrating lobular carcinoma is the frequency of intracellular lumina (Fig. 10-81). The exact cell of origin is not clear from these studies.[280–282] *Cytologically,* infiltrating lobular carcinoma of classic type differs from IDC by virtue of paucicellular smears or aspirates containing smaller tumor cells arranged singly or in small groups rather than forming larger ductal aggregates (Color Figure 10-16). Because of their low cellularity and lack of marked atypia, these tumors are well-known causes of false-negative cytologic diagnoses.[283] The solid, alveolar, and mixed patterns, on the other hand, may be diagnosed incorrectly as IDC because of the more abundant cellularity of cytologic material from these tumors. A prominent feature in all the variants is intracytoplasmic vacuoles representing the intracellular lumina demonstrated ultrastructurally.

The most difficult *differential diagnosis* of infiltrating lobular carcinoma is with malignant lymphoma or a leukemic infiltrate, and we have seen cases misinterpreted in both directions. If any doubt exists of the correct diagnosis, immunohistochemical stains for keratins and leukocyte common antigen should easily resolve the problem. Lobular carcinomas are also confused histologically with IDCs, especially of the paucicellular scirrhous variety. In this situation, the characteristic small uniform cells of lobular carcinoma should be present before this diagnosis is made.

The *prognosis* is controversial, with some authors claiming better survival than for IDC-NOS and others considering lobular carcinoma to be prognostically unfavorable. Within the histopathologic spectrum of infiltrating lobular carcinoma itself, most authors consider the so-called nonclassic types (alveolar, solid and mixed) of worse prognosis than the classic types,[273–275] whereas others deny this assertion.[276] Nesland and colleagues believe that the alveolar growth pattern signifies neuroendocrine differentiation and is not prognostically unfavorable.[276] Ellis and colleagues find the solid pattern to be unfavorable, but all the others to have a relatively good prognosis.[239] Weidner and Semple state that tumors with the classic architectural features of infiltrating lobular carcinoma but nuclei of grade of 2 or 3 have a poorer prognosis, and label the latter tumors the *pleomorphic variant.*[284] This term is used differently by Eusebi and his colleagues, who also find that their "pleomorphic lobular carcinoma" is an aggressive tumor, with 9 of their 10 cases recurring or proving lethal within short intervals from diagnosis.[277] We have recently noted that the presence of light microscopically detected intracellular lumina (signet-ring cells) in more than 10% of the cells of an infiltrating lobular carcinoma is associated with a poorer prognosis (see the following section).

Several authors believe that infiltrating lobular carcinoma is more likely to be bilateral than IDC. Nevertheless, several studies have demonstrated that conservative surgical therapy and radiation therapy provide as good local control of the primary tumor in cases of lobular carcinoma as in IDC.[285,286]

A recent autopsy study has suggested that metastasis to unusual sites such as peritoneum and retroperitoneum, hollow viscera, internal genital organs, leptomeninges, and myocardium is more common with lobular than ductal carcinoma.[287] The metastases to these and other sites are characterized by a

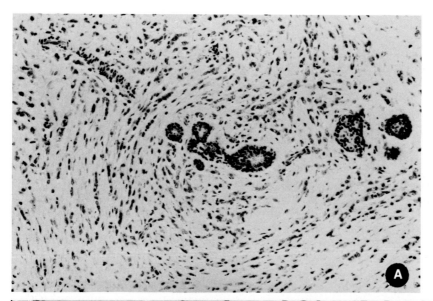

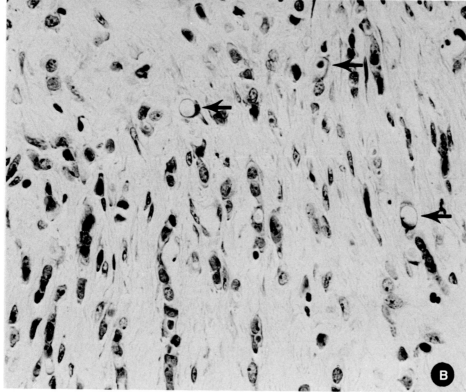

FIGURE 10-77 Infiltrating lobular carcinoma, classical type, with numerous signet-ring cells. **(A)** Low-power view showing single tumor cells swirling around benign ductules. **(B)** Detail of tumor cells with intracellular lumina containing mucin (*arrows*).

diffuse growth that infiltrates in a lymphoma- or leukemia-like manner. As with the primary tumor, immunohistochemistry may be necessary to identify the lesions correctly.

Infiltrating lobular carcinoma has been stated to be more often positive than IDC for estrogen receptors, probably because low nuclear grade is usually part of the definition.[288] The alveolar variant, according to Shousha and colleagues, is the most likely to be receptor-positive.[288]

Signet-Ring Cell Carcinoma. In the late 1970s and early 1980s, a number of studies were published on a variant of breast cancer that usually had the architectural features of classic infiltrating lobular carcinoma but was additionally characterized by the presence of numerous signet-ring cells.[289–291] These cells displayed nuclei that were compressed to the periphery by large globular intracytoplasmic inclusions, many of which showed a "bull's eye" appearance with a central dense mucicarminophilic core surrounded

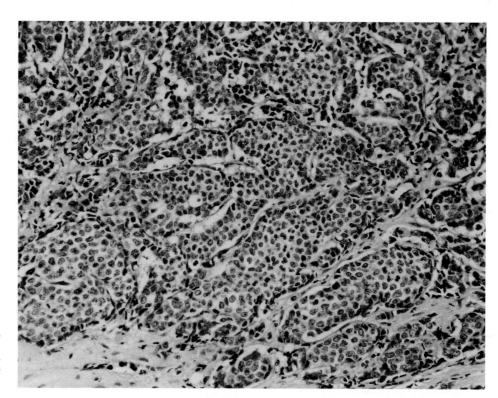

FIGURE 10-78 Infiltrating lobular carcinoma, alveolar type. The rounded nests of small uniform cells suggest in situ lobular carcinoma.

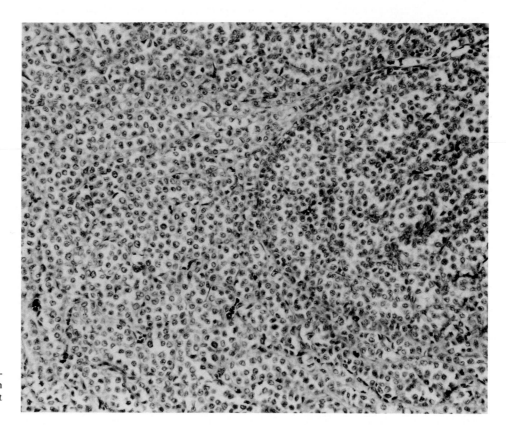

FIGURE 10-79 Infiltrating lobular carcinoma, solid type, with suggestion of alveolar pattern at right.

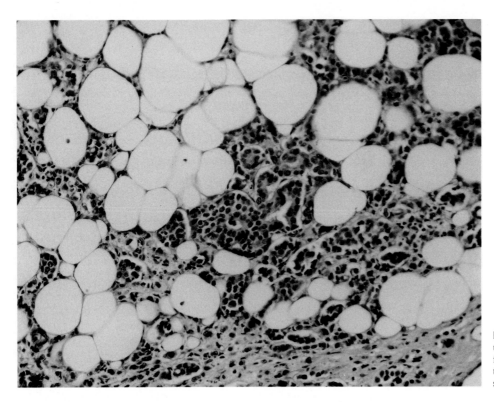

FIGURE 10-80 Infiltrating tubulolobular carcinoma: small cells focally form tubules. Elsewhere this was a mixed classical and solid lobular carcinoma.

by an empty space (see Fig. 10-77). Steinbrecher and Silverberg first suggested that this type of tumor was a mucinous variant of infiltrating lobular carcinoma and that it had a poorer prognosis than other lobular carcinomas,[289] and most other publications on the subject agreed.

At the George Washington University Medical Center and the Hospital of The University of Pennsylvania, we have recently reviewed all our infiltrating lobular carcinomas and have found that the great majority include at least some signet-ring cells. There is a tendency for the prognosis to be poorer as the proportion of these cells increases, with 10% of signet-ring cells appearing to represent a dividing line between favorable and unfavorable cases. Accordingly, we prefer to diagnose these tumors as infiltrating lobular carcinoma, then specifying both the architectural type (eg, classic, alveolar, solid) and the prominence of signet-ring cells if they comprise more than 10% of the tumor cell population.

Apocrine Carcinoma. The term *apocrine carcinoma* is used for an infiltrating carcinoma in which the ductal or glandular structures are lined by large cells with abundant eosinophilic cytoplasm, recalling the apocrine cells of sweat glands (Fig. 10-82). Intraductal carcinomas in which the malignant cells are exclusively apocrine also occur,[292,293] but intraductal proliferations with focal apocrine changes are almost always benign. In a classic publication, Frable and Kay showed that the prognosis of apocrine carcinoma was no different than that for equally differentiated IDCs of non-apocrine type.[292] More recent

studies have expanded on but not changed this impression.[293] On the other hand, the apocrine variant of lobular carcinoma, known as *pleomorphic lobular carcinoma,*[277] does appear to be associated with a particularly unfavorable prognosis.

Neuroendocrine Tumors. In 1977, Cubilla and Woodruff reported 8 cases of a distinctive small cell tumor of the breast containing argyrophilic granules by light microscopy and neurosecretory-type granules on electron microscopic examination, and they designated this tumor *primary carcinoid tumor of the breast.*[294] Subsequent studies have indicated that argyrophilia may be seen in from 5%[72] to 50%[295] of breast carcinomas if appropriate stains are done. Many of these are otherwise typical IDCs and appear to have the usual prognosis for this tumor type. A higher than expected proportion are mucinous carcinomas and appear to share the favorable prognosis of that tumor variant.[248,249] A small proportion of the argyrophilic tumors resemble either the alveolar variant of infiltrating lobular carcinoma[273,276] or the mammary counterpart of small cell or oat cell carcinoma of the lung.[248,296] These *small cell carcinomas* are notable, as are their pulmonary counterparts, for clinical aggressiveness and early metastatic dissemination.

Metaplastic Carcinoma. Metaplastic carcinomas are a heterogeneous group of uncommon neoplasms characterized by foci of squamous, spindle cell, osseous, or chondroid differentiation. Most of these tumors have at least some ductal component, but this

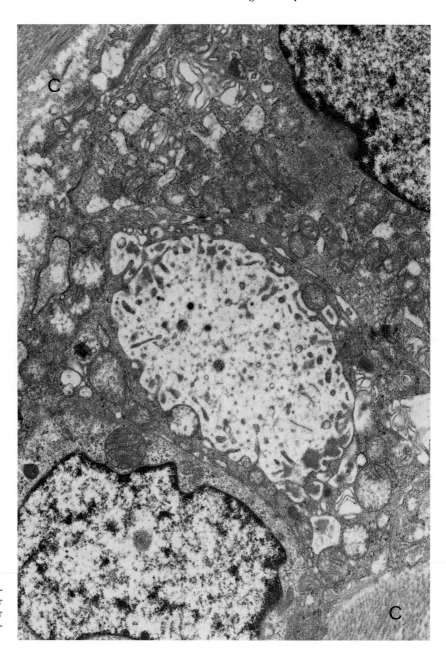

FIGURE 10-81 Infiltrating lobular carcinoma: single-file arrangement of tumor cells surrounded by collagen. Intracellular lumina (*center*) are larger and more numerous than in infiltrating duct carcinoma.

may be difficult or even impossible to find. Confusion about the true nature, classification, and clinical significance of these lesions is exemplified by the fact that even manuscripts from the same department have used different classification systems.[297-302] The largest and most thoroughly studied series of cases has been that of Wargotz and Norris, which we summarize here and in Table 10-8.[298-302]

Basically, Wargotz and Norris divide their metaplastic carcinomas into five separate types. *Matrix-producing carcinoma* is defined as overt carcinoma with direct transition to a cartilaginous or osseous stromal matrix without an intervening spindle cell zone. *Spindle cell carcinoma* is characterized by a dominant spindle cell proliferation composed of bland-appearing bipolar cells with insignificant pleo-

morphism and low mitotic activity, growing in fascicles and producing collagen (Fig. 10-83). To make this diagnosis, either in situ or infiltrating carcinoma must be present merging with the spindle cell component or the epithelial nature of the spindle cells must be proved by immunohistochemistry or electron microscopy.

In *carcinosarcoma* (Fig. 10-84), the neoplasm is biphasic, with both the epithelial and the spindle cell component appearing histologically malignant. Pure *squamous cell carcinoma* of ductal origin is characterized as an infiltrating carcinoma that is exclusively squamous (Fig. 10-85) without involvement of the skin, or as an intraductal carcinoma that is exclusively squamous. Finally, *metaplastic carcinoma with osteoclastic giant cells* consists of an intraductal or in-

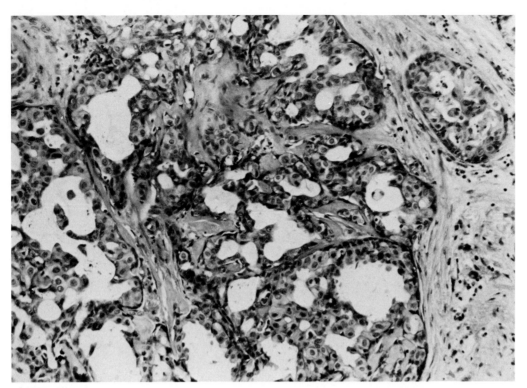

FIGURE 10-82 Apocrine carcinoma.

filtrating carcinoma contiguous to or admixed with a bland-appearing spindle cell stroma or a sarcomatous stroma in which osteoclastic-like giant cells are intermingled.

In the forms dominated by spindle cells—particularly bland-appearing spindle cells—immunohistochemistry may be necessary to demonstrate the epithelial derivation of this cell population.[303] Epithelial antigens may demonstrate somewhat subtle epithelial elements and may mark the apparent mesenchymal elements in many of these cases.

In the material of Wargotz and Norris, spindle cell carcinoma was the most common of the five

types reported, consisting of almost half of the total cases, whereas carcinosarcoma was easily the second most common type. The bland appearance of spindle cell carcinoma must be emphasized, because we have seen cases of this sort misdiagnosed as fibromatosis or reactive scarring. We believe that any infiltrative spindle cell population in the breast that cannot be explained by previous trauma or surgery should be investigated immunohistochemically.

In the publications of Wargotz and Norris, the 5-year survival rates ranged between 63% and 68% for all tumor types except carcinosarcoma, which had a poorer survival of 49%. It is not clear what the survival rate was for IDC-NOS during this time period at the same institution, but in all likelihood only carcinosarcoma had a significantly less favorable prognosis.

The main *differential diagnosis* of most of these lesions is with pure sarcomas of the breast, and the main clinical significance of making the distinction is that metaplastic carcinomas are far more likely to involve axillary lymph nodes.

Lipid-Rich Carcinoma. Lipid-rich carcinoma is another rare mammary tumor, characterized by sheets of epithelial cells containing intracytoplasmic lipid (Fig. 10-86).[304] The histologic pattern, particularly in metastases, may mimic that of a lymphoma. Another significant differential diagnosis is with the signet-ring cell type of infiltrating lobular carcinoma, which can be differentiated by a positive PAS or mucin stain.

TABLE 10-8.
Metaplastic Carcinomas of the Breast

Type	No. of Cases	5-Year Survival(%)
Matrix-producing carcinoma	26	68
Spindle cell carcinoma	100	64
Carcinosarcoma	70	49
Pure squamous cell carcinoma of ductal origin	22	63
Metaplastic carcinoma with osteoclastic giant cells	29	68

Wargotz ES, Norris HJ: Metaplastic carcinomas of the breast. V. Metaplastic carcinoma with osteoclastic giant cells. Hum Pathol 21:1142–1150, 1990

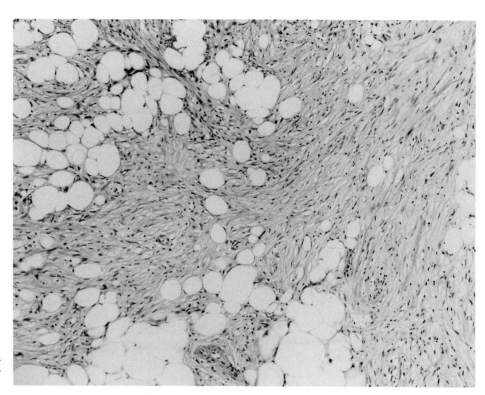

FIGURE 10-83 Spindle cell carcinoma. Fascicles of bland spindle cells infiltrate adipose tissue.

Van Bogaert and Maldague have subdivided the lipid-rich tumors into three types: histiocytoid (the most common), sebaceous, and a type with apocrine-like features.[305] They emphasize a similarity of the first type to the histiocytoid mammary carcinoma reported by Hood and colleagues that frequently metastasized to the eyelid.[306] This latter tumor, however, was said to be negative when stained for lipids. The prognosis in the few lipid-rich carcinomas appropriately analyzed has been poor, but they have tended to be high-grade carcinomas, so that the prognostic significance of the lipid component is not clear.

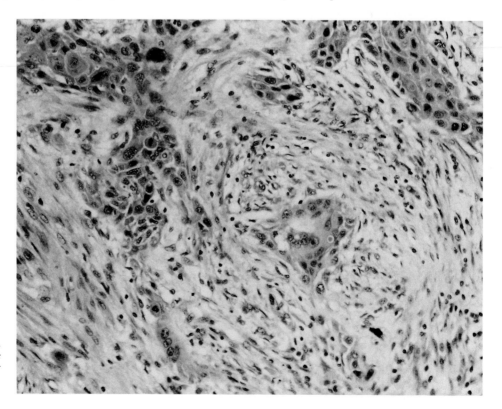

FIGURE 10-84 Carcinosarcoma. Both the epithelial and the stromal components of this tumor appear histologically malignant.

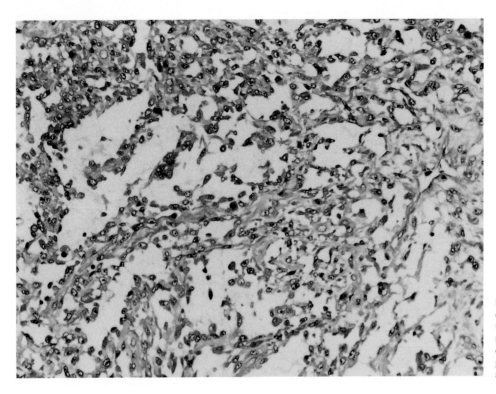

FIGURE 10-85 Squamous cell carcinoma of ductal origin. In this example, the malignant squamous cell nests display a cavitated pattern resembling angiosarcoma (acantholytic squamous cell carcinoma).

Types of Carcinoma Characterized by Their Site of Involvement

In addition to the variants of mammary cancer discussed above, which are characterized by the histologic appearance of the tumor itself, two specific types are characterized by their location within the breast. Paget's disease is a mammary carcinoma involving the epidermis of the nipple, whereas inflammatory carcinoma is a breast cancer that has spread within dermal lymphatics.

Paget's Disease. Paget's disease, described in 1874 by Paget,[307] is a cutaneous alteration of the nipple

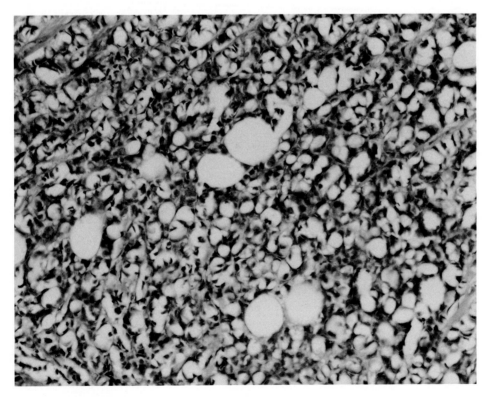

FIGURE 10-86 Lipid-rich carcinoma. Prominent lipid vacuoles distend the tumor cell cytoplasm.

almost always associated with an underlying mammary carcinoma. Paget erroneously thought that the skin lesion was benign but induced the cancer below. It is characterized clinically by a crusted and verrucous lesion of the skin of the nipple (Fig. 10-87). It is encountered especially in women older than 40 years, and is associated with about 5% of mammary carcinomas. The lesion begins as a more or less round, red, pruritic plaque with a granular surface, which eventually ulcerates and bleeds. It is surrounded by a squamous collar, which tends to grow toward the pe-

riphery. The nipple becomes progressively retracted and finally disappears in the neoplastic mass. This evolution may extend over several years, the underlying tumor mass not becoming palpable until the end of this period in some cases. When no tumor is palpable at the time of diagnosis, the underlying carcinoma is usually intraductal, and the prognosis is excellent. When a palpable tumor is present, the tumor is usually infiltrative, axillary and other metastases may have taken place, and the prognosis is that of the infiltrating carcinoma. In the absence of a palpable mass,

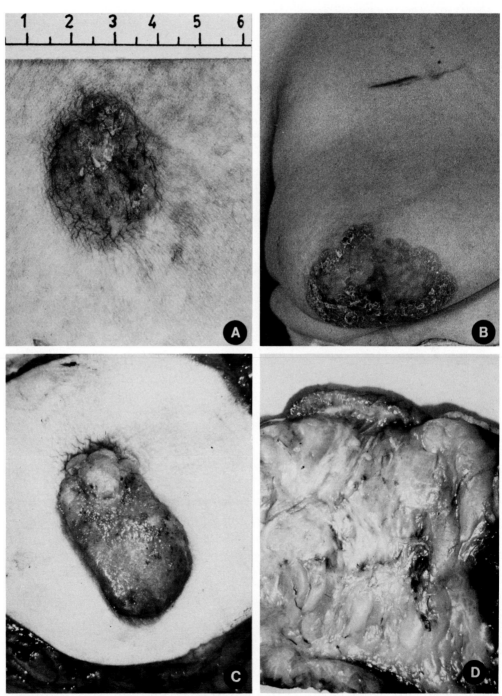

FIGURE 10-87 Paget's disease: macroscopic appearances.

mammography may detect a nodule, microcalcifications, or abnormal architectural changes that may reveal the underlying carcinoma.

Microscopically, Paget's disease is characterized by invasion of the epidermis of the nipple by large, round, neoplastic cells with voluminous clear cell cytoplasm, disposed singly or in small groups (Fig. 10-88). Outlines of gland formation are occasionally distinguishable. The Paget cells are usually located in deep layers of the epidermis, but they also may be found in the superficial layers as dyskaryotic cellular debris. They may also largely replace the nipple epidermis, giving an appearance similar to that of Bowen's disease or in situ squamous carcinoma; the term *anaplastic Paget's disease* has been used in this situation.[308] An inflammatory infiltrate of the underlying dermis or the involved epidermis is occasionally seen.

When the main lactiferous ducts underlying the nipple are examined carefully, the same neoplastic cells usually are found infiltrating the ductal epithelium as isolated cells (Fig. 10-89) or small cords. In the great majority of cases, examination of mastectomy specimens reveals a typical mammary carcinoma of intraductal or infiltrating duct type or both (96% in the series of Dixon and colleagues).[309]

What is the primary site of the tumor? Toker has demonstrated intraepidermal clear cells in about 10% of normal nipples, which may be the cells from which the tumor arises.[310] Similarly, the ultrastructural study of Sagebiel has suggested in situ transformation of epidermal cells to Paget cells.[311] On the other hand, the almost consistent association with an underlying duct carcinoma suggests either a "field cancerization" or invasion of the epidermis by tumor cells growing up the ducts.[309] The origin of the neoplastic cells in the nipple is still controversial.

The *differential diagnosis* of Paget's disease involves other intraepidermal and infiltrating tumors of the nipple, including Bowen's disease (in situ squamous carcinoma), malignant melanoma, and basal cell carcinoma.[308,312,313] All these conditions are far rarer than Paget's disease. A positive stain for mucin is diagnostic, but many cases of Paget's disease stain negatively. Some authors conclude that immunohistochemical staining—specifically for carcinoembryonic antigen (CEA), epithelial membrane antigen (EMA), gross cystic disease fluid protein (GCDFP-15), cytokeratin CAM 5.2, and c-erb-B2—is more reliable.[308,312]

The *prognosis* of Paget's disease depends entirely on the underlying carcinoma, and the treatment should be aimed at that tumor as well.

Inflammatory Carcinoma. Inflammatory carcinoma is characterized clinically by the presence of cutaneous edema (*peau d'orange*), erythema of greater than one third of the breast, and diffuse brawny induration with or without a discrete underlying mass (Fig. 10-90).[314–316] The diagnostic pathologic sign is histologic evidence of carcinomatous invasion of dermal lymphatics (Fig. 10-91). Although histologic confirmation of carcinoma is necessary before treatment can be instituted, numerous studies have indicated that either the clinical or the histopathologic definition may be used to characterize a carcinoma as of inflammatory type. Parenthetically, it should be noted that the name of the tumor does not imply an acute or chronic inflammatory infiltrate seen histologically.

The condition is rare and is encountered in from 1% to 4% of all carcinomas of the breast. It may be associated with any histologic type. Mammography shows a diffuse increased density of the affected parenchyma or a tissue mass and an increase in skin thickness. The tumor mass is often difficult to palpate in the swollen and massively indurated breast. The skin of the breast is red, warm, tender and edematous.

The clinical significance of this type of cancer is that, regardless of the tumor type or grade, the prognosis is extremely poor. For many years, mastec-

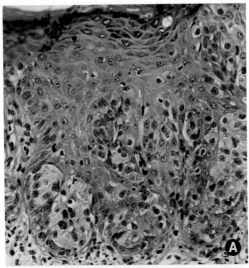

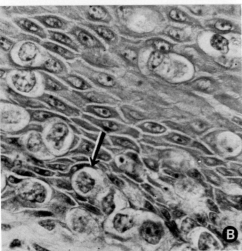

FIGURE 10-88 Paget's disease. **(A)** Nests of Paget cells. **(B)** Detail of Paget cells (*arrow*).

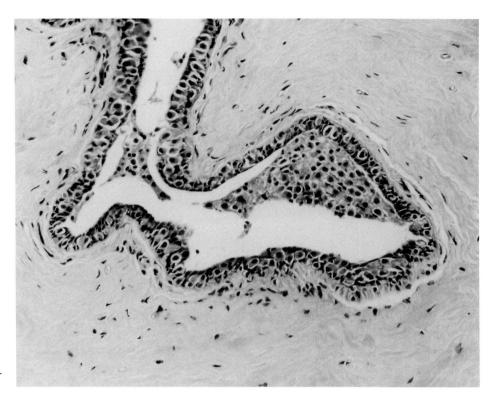

FIGURE 10-89 Pagetoid cancerization of a mammary duct.

tomy was not even attempted, because 5-year survival was almost unknown. Recent investigators have obtained 5-year survival rates in the vicinity of 30% with a combination of irradiation, surgery, and chemotherapy.[315,316]

Prognostic Factors in Breast Carcinoma

The previous discussion in this chapter has emphasized some of the areas of histopathologic typing and grading of carcinomas of the breast that are said to be of prognostic significance. The reader has undoubtedly realized by now that many of the factors

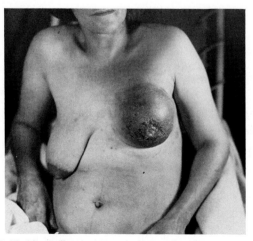

FIGURE 10-90 Inflammatory carcinoma (carcinomatous mastitis) appearing a few weeks after delivery in a 37-year-old woman.

are controversial. The same statement may be applied to other histopathologic, clinical, and laboratory features of breast carcinoma that have been claimed to be of significance in planning therapy and estimating the prognosis.

Some (but by no means all) of the prognostic factors reported in breast carcinoma are listed in Table 10-9. It should be obvious from perusal of this table that we have entered the age of information overload with regard to breast cancer. Furthermore, we have also entered an age in which—thanks to screening programs leading to early detection—the size of the tumor presented to the pathologist has generally become smaller than that seen in past years. Therefore, the pathologist must become more selective about what to do with tumor tissue; the paradox is that, as more tissue is diverted to nonhistologic studies, fewer of the pertinent histologic observations are capable of being made.

The purpose of conveying prognostic information to the clinician treating a patient with breast cancer also has changed. Years ago, all patients underwent radical mastectomy, and prognostic information was used largely to inform the patient or her family what her likelihood of survival was. In unfavorable situations, adjuvant radiation therapy or chemotherapy might be used, but more often these modalities were used only for recurrent carcinoma. In the current era, on the other hand, prognostic factors are used prospectively to determine what type of operative treatment should be undertaken and what type of adjuvant therapy should be given. An often valid assumption is that favorable

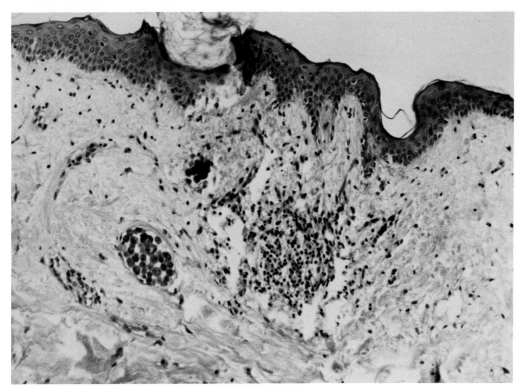

FIGURE 10-91 Inflammatory carcinoma: neoplastic infiltration of subcutaneous lymphatics.

prognostic factors will be used to define that small subset of patients who do not receive adjuvant therapy.[317-319]

Few investigations have compared the entire spectrum of prognostic factors available. Many of the published manuscripts have reported the value of only a single determination, or perhaps the comparison of a single determination with two or three others. Almost never has the cost of the various determinations been taken into account. In this era of cost-conscious medicine, we believe that cost-benefit ratios of performing specific determinations need to be investigated.

Clinical Prognostic Factors

As Table 10-9 indicates, many clinical determinations affect the prognosis of a woman with breast cancer. Older women are believed by many to have a poorer prognosis, and their general physical condition may make them ineligible for certain types of treatment. In the United States, black women with breast cancer do more poorly than white women, partially but not totally on the basis of more extensive disease at the time of diagnosis. The role of pregnancy has been debated for years, with some authorities claiming a poorer outcome for breast cancer in pregnant or lactating women and others denying this assertion.[320,321] Clinical evidence of a large tumor, a locally extensive tumor (see the discussion of inflammatory carcinoma above), or distant metastases will alter the clinical stage, which in turn will usually alter the treatment.

A few words should be included here about staging of breast cancer. Although it would appear that at least clinical staging should be uniform and noncontroversial, in actuality there are four different staging systems—the Columbia, Manchester, International, and American systems—each of which has its proponents. In general terms, both the International Union against Cancer (UICC) and the American Joint Committee for Cancer (AJCC) use a comparable TNM system, with the T stage reflecting the size of the primary tumor, the N stage the extent of regional lymph node metastases, and the M stage the presence or absence of distant metastases.[322-325] This TNM system is presented in Table 10-10. Both primary tumor factors and axillary node factors are indicative of the ability of the tumor to spread to distant sites, because the exact M status may not be known at the time of initial treatment.

"Routine" Gross and Microscopic Pathologic Prognostic Factors

The list of factors included in Table 10-9 is long but by no means comprehensive. It indicates that the final surgical pathology report in a case of breast cancer ought to comment on as many of these factors as is feasible given the specimen examined.[326] Histologic tumor type and tumor grade have been discussed above and will not be covered again here.

TABLE 10-9.
Selected Prognostic Factors in Breast Carcinoma

Clinical
    Age
    Race
    Pregnancy/lactation
    Tumor size estimate
    Locally extensive tumor*
    Distant metastases*
    General physical condition

"Routine" Gross/Microscopic Pathology
    Tumor size*
    Axillary node involvement*
    Histologic tumor type(s)
    Histologic grade
    Lymphatic invasion
    Blood vessel invasion
    Lymphoid host response
    Pushing vs infiltrating border
    Tumor necrosis
    Stromal elastosis
    Mitotic activity
    Nuclear grade
    Proportion of noninvasive carcinoma[†]
    Resection margins[†]
    Multifocality/multicentricity[†]

Other
    Hormone receptors
    Ploidy
    S-phase fraction
    Oncogene overexpression
    Tumor suppressor genes
    Proliferative indices
    Morphometric analyses
    Microvessel quantitation
    Cathepsin D
    P-glycoprotein

*Used in determination of stage and independently.
[†]To evaluate breast conservation surgery.

The tumor size should be measured carefully by the first pathologist to come in contact with the specimen, often in the intraoperative situation. The reporting of axillary node involvement is controversial, because it is not entirely clear how many nodes must be obtained by the surgeon, what techniques are necessary for the pathologist to identify them grossly, how thoroughly lymph nodes submitted for histologic examination should be sectioned, and whether immunohistochemical detection of additional metastases adds information of prognostic value.[327–329] Our general impression is that the more carefully lymph node specimens are examined, the more micrometastases will be found, and the less clinically significant this information will be.

Tumor invasion of blood vessels and lymphatic spaces provides important prognostic information, but in a different manner. Blood vessel invasion appears to be associated with poorer survival regardless of the status of the axillary lymph nodes,[269,330]

whereas peritumoral lymphatic space invasion serves more as a marker of the likelihood of metastases in the axillary lymph nodes.[331,332] Both types of vascular invasion must be distinguished from shrinkage artifact around nests of tumor in stroma—a determination that is sometimes easier to speak or write about than to attempt in practice.

Mitotic activity is included in most grading systems, but it is thought by some authors to be an independent prognostic factor of major significance.[333–335] The best method of expressing mitotic activity is unclear, with both mitotic figures per 10 high-power fields and mitotic figures per 1000 cells proposed as different methods.

The other factors listed in Table 10-9 are probably of less clinical significance with respect to tumor-free survival. In conservative surgical procedures, however, the presence of an extensive intraductal component, multifocal tumor, or positive resection margins may indicate that the patient requires more extensive surgery (perhaps mastectomy) for local tumor control.[220–222,336,337] A similar approach is used to predict the efficacy of primary radiation therapy.[338,339]

Other Prognostic Factors

Table 10-9 again represents only a partial list of nonroutine factors (histologic or otherwise) for which prognostic implications have been claimed. Levels of estrogen and progesterone receptors head the list because, as specific predictors of a tumor's response to hormonal therapy, these determinations

TABLE 10-10.
TNM Clinical Stages for Carcinoma of the Breast, 1988

TNM Stage	Primary Tumor (T) (cm)	Nodal Metastases (N)*	Distant Metastases (M)
0	In situ	No	No
I	≤ 2	No	No
IIA	≤ 2	Yes	No
	> 2 ≤ 5	No	No
IIB	> 2 ≤ 5	Yes	No
	> 5	No	No
IIIA	> 5	Mobile or fixed	No
	> 5	Fixed	No
IIIB	Skin or chest wall	Any	No
	Any	Internal mammary	No
IV	Any	Any	Yes[†]

*Pertains to ipsilateral axillary nodes unless otherwise stated.
[†]Including supraclavicular nodes.
Adapted from Beahrs OH, Henson DE, Hutter RVP, Kennedy BJ, eds: American Joint Committee on Cancer: Manual for staging cancer, 4th ed, pp 149–154. Philadelphia, JB Lippincott, 1992

remain the only ones that provide both prognostic and therapeutic information.[340-344] Fortunately, the biochemical method has been superseded in many laboratories by methods that can determine receptors directly on histologically examined tissue.[342-344]

DNA ploidy and S-phase fraction studies have been reported enthusiastically by many authors, but recent review articles and large studies have suggested that the data should be used with care.[345-348] These studies can be performed both on archival paraffin-embedded tissues and on FNA biopsies. The study of oncogenes and antioncogenes (tumor suppressor genes) has taken on an increased significance in breast cancer in recent years, but reservations have been expressed on the interpretation of these data as well.[349-354] Indices of tumor proliferation other than those that are determined by flow cytometry—such as bromodeoxyuridine and thymidine labeling, argyrophilic nucleolar organizer region counts, Ki67 scores, and similar techniques—are also said to provide useful information.[355-359] Again, it is still not clear whether any of these techniques offer enough additional information beyond routine studies such as tumor grade and mitotic activity to justify the increased labor and cost involved in their performance.

A similar statement might be made of morphometric techniques,[360,361] which, although microscopic pathologic determinations, are hardly routine. They certainly can be said to have less interobserver variability than the routine studies.

Microvessel quantitation is a new prognostic indicator in breast carcinoma.[362] The microvessels are identified by immunohistochemistry using antibodies to endothelial markers. Higher microvessel counts within tumors tend to be associated with a higher frequency of distant metastasis. Again, it remains to be determined whether the additional effort is justified on a cost-benefit basis.

Other markers, such as cathepsin D and P-glycoprotein, have been studied.[363,364] The latter shows some correlation with chemotherapy resistance, but more studies must be done to evaluate its overall clinical significance. Cathepsin D seems to be less important today than it was thought to be several years ago.

In summary, numerous nonroutine prognostic markers are available. With the single exception of estrogen and progesterone receptor determination, further studies are necessary to document the usefulness, reproducibility, and cost-benefit ratio for each of these markers.

The Surgical Pathology Report in Cases of Infiltrating Carcinomas of the Breast

Given the extensive therapeutic menu available to the patient and her physicians, it is more important than ever that the surgical pathology report in a case of breast cancer convey the information necessary for intelligent therapeutic decisions to be made. The compilation of this information begins when the pathologist first encounters the specimen, because at this point a careful measurement of tumor size must be made and recorded, and the decision must be made with regard to how much of the gross tumor tissue (if any) is to be sent for nonhistologic studies, and which studies are to be requested. The complexities of this decision have been discussed above, but for the purposes of the surgical pathology report it should be noted that we always include a statement about which special studies were requested. Ultimately, the results of these studies—receptors, flow cytometry, oncogenes, and so forth—are integrated into the final surgical pathology report, usually in the form of addenda.

A careful and thorough *gross description* continues to be a mainstay of the surgical pathology report in breast cancer, as in other diseases. In addition to the measurement of tumor size, the location of the tumor—relative to margins in a local excision specimen, and to breast quadrant as well in a mastectomy—should be recorded, as should grossly evident multicentricity, skin involvement, and axillary nodal metastases.

Microscopic observations to be recorded are primarily those that have been mentioned above as being of major prognostic significance. The tumor type or types (with the proportion of each if more than one type is found), tumor grade (at least in all cases of IDC-NOS), presence or absence of lymphatic and blood vessel invasion, evaluation of the host lymphoid response, and evaluation of the character of the tumor border, tumor necrosis, and stromal elastosis should be included. In institutions in which protocols call for this information separate from histologic grade, the nuclear grade of the tumor and an estimation of its mitotic activity may be recorded separately. Multicentricity or multifocality should be noted when present. In breast conservation surgical specimens, the proportion of intraductal carcinoma and its localization (within or immediately adjacent to versus distant from the infiltrating component) should be clearly stated, as should the condition of the resection margins.

Beyond these general comments, specific circumstances call for specific observations to be included in the surgical pathology report. Treatment or research protocols at certain institutions may call for information other than that mentioned here, and the pathologist at such institutions must comply with these requests. Because some patients will have had radiation therapy, hormonal therapy, or chemotherapy before the initial operative treatment, or biopsy or excision of a recurrence, it is important for the pathologist to recognize the effects of these treatments on normal and neoplastic breast tissues and to be able to differentiate residual or recurrent carcinoma from therapy-induced changes.[365-367]

Because so many factors require comment in the surgical pathology report, a standard protocol is useful in most institutions, so that errors of omission are not committed. In many departments, this is done by means of a computer-generated list of observations to be made. It is important for the pathologist to be able to add additional comments when they are appropriate.

Evolution

Local tumor extension takes place by infiltration of the lactiferous ducts, the connective tissue network, and the mammary adipose tissue. Infiltration appears to occur after a much shorter noninvasive phase in ductal than in lobular carcinomas.

Lymphatic dissemination within the breast proceeds by two pathways: the centripetal route toward the areolar and retroareolar plexus, and the deep route toward the prepectoral fat (Fig. 10-92). Invasion of local lymphatics is responsible for edema, cutaneous infiltration (*peau d'orange*), and multiple foci of tumor within the breast, especially beneath the nipple. Lymphatic permeation even without lymph node invasion is a local manifestation of histologic aggressiveness, but the accurate histopathologic assessment of lymphatic involvement is difficult.[368,369] The axillary lymph nodes are invaded in most cases in older series, but in a much smaller proportion of cases detected in screening programs.[165,370,371] The clinical estimation of lymph node involvement is often inaccurate; many cases with clinically negative nodes actually have metastases. The converse is also true, in that greatly enlarged clinically positive nodes may merely be the seat of hyperplastic changes or fatty infiltration. The nodes of the internal mammary chain are also frequently involved by metastases. Their involvement appears to be favored by three factors: the presence of axillary metastases, a large (5 cm or more) primary tumor, and a tumor located centrally or medially in the breast. Intramammary lymph nodes may be present in the mammary parenchyma and should be recognized as such.[7] Their involvement by tumor has a prognostic value, particularly in stage I carcinomas. Invasion of the supraclavicular nodes signals the presence of metastases disseminated beyond the possibility of surgical cure and is a grave prognostic sign.[372] More

distant nodes subsequently involved are the cervical, mediastinal, and inguinal nodes.

Hematogenous metastases lead to generalized dissemination of cancer in the bones, lungs, liver, ovaries, adrenals, pleura, peritoneum, and other sites.[373,374] An interesting and unexplained phenomenon is the occasional finding of metastatic mammary cancer massively involving one organ or system (usually liver, bones, or lungs) without significant replacement of other organs.[375–377] The commonly involved bones, in decreasing order of frequency, are the vertebrae, pelvis, femur, humerus, skull, ribs, and clavicle.

Morphologic changes may be present in bone marrow adjacent to foci of metastatic tumor. These consist of medullary fibrosis and increased numbers of erythroblasts, eosinophils, plasma cells, and monocytes. The mechanism of production of this medullary reaction is not known. Micrometastases in bone marrow can be detected immunohistochemically at initial treatment in 25% of cases and are associated with decreased survival.[378]

Breast cancer metastases in bone are, like most other types of cancer, usually osteolytic, but in about 10% of cases the metastases are osteoblastic. Although prostatic carcinomatous metastases are usually blastic, breast cancer is one of the few metastatic lesions in women commonly producing this picture. Hypercalcemia is a frequent finding in mammary cancer with osseous metastases, but it is occasionally encountered in patients without osseous involvement as well; a direct metabolic action by the tumor, probably hormonal in nature, has been postulated in these cases.[373,379] Some data suggest the role of a direct route to bones by retrograde venous seeding. The presence of bone metastases caudad to the lumbosacral junction is said to be predictive of visceral metastases.[375]

Pulmonary involvement in metastatic breast cancer can take many different forms, but diffuse lymphangitic spread[380] is more common, and large solitary metastases rarer, than in other types of cancer. Pulmonary metastases are often accompanied by pleural involvement with recurrent pleural effusions that are difficult to treat successfully.[381]

Local chest wall recurrences after mastectomy arise from neoplastic cells in the deep lymphatics that migrate superficially to constitute multiple subcutaneous nodules of variable size (Fig. 10-93). They usually appear first at or near the mastectomy scar, later extending to involve the entire thoracic region. They may not become evident until several years after initial treatment, but in any event they usually herald widespread metastatic disease.[382]

These and other late recurrences constitute an important clinical and pathologic problem. It is not rare to see recurrences appearing 10 or even 20 years after initial therapy. The reasons for this peculiar behavior in certain cases are not known; exhaustion of immunologic defense mechanisms has been suggested, but this is little more than pure hypothe-

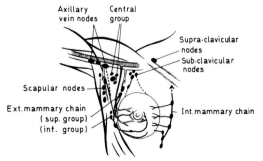

FIGURE 10-92 Diagram of the lymph nodes draining the breast.

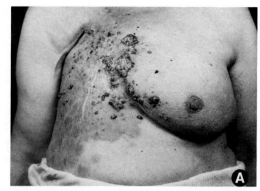

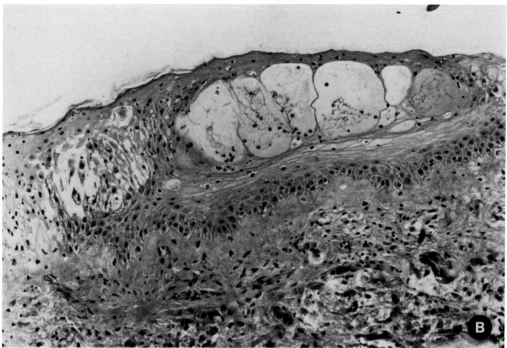

FIGURE 10-93 Infiltrating duct carcinoma. **(A)** Local cutaneous recurrence. **(B)** Dermal neoplastic invasion with bullous degeneration of overlying epidermis (local recurrence).

sis.[383] This phenomenon is much more common in breast cancer than in cancers of most other sites: between 5 and 10 years after treatment, from 14% to 18% of patients apparently cured at 5 years will develop recurrences, and virtually all of these patients will eventually die of their disease. It is meaningless to speak of 5-year "cure" in this disease.

Many of these late recurrences occur in the contralateral breast. For example, in the series of 1458 breast cancer patients followed by Robbins and Berg, 94 developed carcinoma in the opposite breast, representing a fivefold increase over the breast cancer expectancy in a similar population without the first tumor.[384] Stewart underscored this problem when he stated that "the most frequent precancerous lesion of the breast is a cancer of the opposite breast."[385] In these cases, it is not always possible to determine if this represents a metastatic lesion or a new primary cancer (Table 10-11).[386] Subserial whole organ sectioning, however, indi-

cates that the true incidence of bilateral breast cancer may approach 100%.[216,217,219,387]

Primary malignant tumors of other sites develop in breast cancer patients as frequently as contralateral breast cancer (13% of cases in the large series of

TABLE 10-11.
Pathologic Distinction Between Second Primary Mammary Cancer and Metastasis to Contralateral Breast

Second Primary Cancer	*Metastasis*
In mammary tissue	In fat
Usual distribution (UOQ)	Midline or axillary tail
Solitary	Multiple
Infiltrating margins	Pushing margins
Any histologic type	Like primary tumor (high grade)
In situ changes present	In situ changes absent

Rosen and colleagues[388]) and are responsible for many more deaths. Most lethal nonmammary cancers in this series arose in the ovary, stomach, pancreas, and lung.

Therapy

Changes in the primary therapy of breast cancer have progressed so rapidly that it is almost useless to summarize them in great detail in any text that will be published after a hiatus of more than a few months. Nevertheless, we will attempt a brief summary of the state of the art at this time.

First, as discussed above, the primary operative treatment of operable breast cancer has changed dramatically, with few radical mastectomies being performed in the Western world, and a trend toward more and more patients having breast conservation procedures (tylectomy, lumpectomy, local excision) rather than modified radical mastectomy.[389,390] The great majority of these patients will receive postoperative radiation therapy, and some may have received preoperative radiation therapy to convert a large tumor into a smaller one more amenable to breast conservation surgery.[390,391] Preoperative chemotherapy is used in the same manner.[392] The analysis of biopsies, excisions, and fine-needle aspirations of breasts after previous chemotherapy or radiation therapy may pose diagnostic pitfalls for the pathologist.

In addition to its preoperative and postoperative adjuvant roles, radiation therapy may be the only treatment for primary breast cancer in patients deemed to be inoperable because of tumor extent or other medical factors, in patients who refuse surgical treatment, and in certain other instances.[391,393]

Another development in the treatment of breast cancer is that this neoplasm is now considered to be a systemic rather than a localized disease, even in the absence of demonstrable distant metastases. Axillary lymph node dissection is an important part of the primary surgical treatment, because the status of the nodes is a primary factor in determining whether adjuvant hormonal or nonhormonal chemotherapy will be given. Patients with involved lymph nodes are now routinely treated with chemotherapy if they are premenopausal and with tamoxifen (an antiestrogen) if they are postmenopausal, especially if their tumors contain estrogen receptors.[394,395] More controversial is the question of adjuvant therapy in the treatment of node-negative breast cancers, with some studies recommending treatment for all patients and others suggesting that prognostic factors such as tumor size, receptor status, proliferation indices, and others be used to define a subset of node-negative patients who do not need adjuvant therapy.[394-397] Particularly important in making these decisions is expanded information that is accruing concerning the risk of both nonhormonal chemotherapy and tamoxifen.[394,397,398] Tamoxifen has also been suggested as prophylaxis against the development of breast cancer in high-risk women.[204-206]

Treatment of patients with distant metastases is less controversial, although new hormonal and nonhormonal chemotherapeutic regimens are being developed at a rapid rate.[373] The median survival after the development of metastases is about 2 to 3 years in most series,[373,374,377] although the pattern of metastatic spread may result in significantly shorter or longer survival. For example, patients who develop purely osseous metastases[376,377] tend to have much longer survival than patients whose metastases are predominantly visceral. Unlike primary breast cancer, there are studies suggesting that the survival of patients with metastatic breast cancer has not increased significantly over the past 25 years.[374]

MALIGNANT NONEPITHELIAL NEOPLASMS

Malignant Soft-Tissue Tumors (Sarcomas)

Primary sarcomas of the breast are rare (0.6% of mammary malignant tumors at the Institut Bordet and less than 1% in other reported series).[399] In most series, the most common form is malignant phyllodes tumor (periductal fibrosarcoma and liposarcoma). These tumors have been discussed in an earlier section.

Of the remaining primary sarcomas of the breast, the most common in older series is fibrosarcoma[400] and in recent series malignant fibrous histiocytoma.[399] Jones and colleagues have suggested that these two neoplasms be classified together because they have many features in common and a single tumor may contain foci resembling the classic appearance of each.[401]

As a group, the mammary sarcomas share certain clinical features. They tend to present as bulky masses, usually without evidence of metastatic dissemination. Axillary nodal metastases are rare, and dissemination occurs almost exclusively by the hematogenous route.

These tumors often recur locally before they metastasize, and local control is often difficult to obtain with surgical procedures short of mastectomy. Finally, unlike mammary carcinoma, the vast majority of all recurrences occur within the first 5 years after initial treatment.

Fibrosarcoma and Malignant Fibrous Histiocytoma

Although the relative proportions of these two tumors vary in different reported series, they represent together more than 50% of all pure mammary sarcomas.[399-401] As with other sarcomas, they present as large, firm, poorly limited, rapidly growing masses (Fig. 10-94).

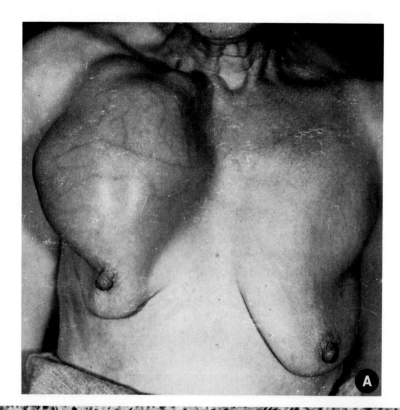

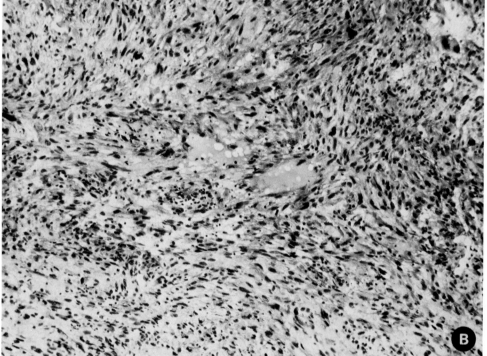

FIGURE 10-94 Fibrosarcoma of breast. **(A)** Clinical appearance. **(B)** Microscopic appearance.

Microscopically, they are composed of fusiform cells with hyperchromatic, often bizarre nuclei, with variable numbers of mitotic figures. The cells are arranged in a herringbone or storiform pattern according to the fibrosarcomatous or malignant fibrous histiocytomatous differentiation. Jones and associates found that the herringbone pattern was associated with a more favorable prognosis, as was low-grade atypia and mitotic activity.[401]

Liposarcoma

Liposarcomas form large, rounded masses of soft to firm yellow tissue. Histologically, they resemble the myxoid or the pleomorphic type of liposarcoma seen elsewhere. Unlike the other mammary sarcomas, they display a tendency to metastasize by the lymphatic as well as the hematogenous route.[402]

Other Nonvascular Sarcomas

Stromal sarcoma of the breast is a term that was popularized by Berg and colleagues in 1962 to unify the diagnosis of all connective tissue sarcomas of the breast other than malignant phyllodes tumor.[403] More recent studies suggest—and we agree—that it is more useful to classify mammary sarcomas as accurately as possible according to histopathologic type.[399,404] In addition to the forms mentioned above, rare examples of leiomyosarcoma,[405] clear cell sarcoma,[399] malignant peripheral nerve sheath tumor,[399] and alveolar soft part sarcoma[399] have been reported. Occasional osteosarcomas and chondrosarcomas have been described, but these may represent matrix-forming metaplastic carcinomas, as recently characterized by Wargotz and Norris.[298]

Differential Diagnosis

The differential diagnosis of the sarcomas mentioned thus far, in addition to each other, is primarily with metaplastic carcinomas and malignant phyllodes tumors, both of which have been described in more detail in earlier sections of this chapter. A careful search of many sections for histologically malignant (in the former case) or benign (in the latter) epithelial elements is essential to the correct diagnosis. Immunostaining for epithelial markers may be necessary to rule out the diagnosis of one of the forms of metaplastic carcinoma.

Other differential diagnostic possibilities, particularly for the low-grade sarcomas, include benign lesions such as fibromatosis, fasciitis, and fat necrosis. These are also discussed earlier in this charter and in standard texts of soft-tissue tumor pathology.

Angiosarcoma

Angiosarcoma of the breast, although rare, is one of the most lethal of all mammary neoplasms.[406] Although it was once taught that all vascular tumors of the breast proper (as opposed to the overlying skin or underlying chest wall) were sarcomatous, it is now known that a variety of benign vascular and pseudo-vascular lesions can be seen in the breast.[116–122] These are discussed in greater detail in an earlier section of this chapter. Unlike these lesions, angiosarcomas almost always present as large palpable masses of firm consistency and pink color, honeycombed with darker red foci. They consist of blood vessels the lining cells of which show varying degrees of differentiation (Figs. 10-95 through 10-97). Several studies have shown a definite relation between tumor

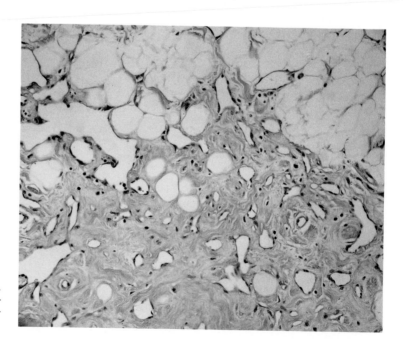

FIGURE 10-95 Well-differentiated angiosarcoma. The blood vessels in this field are infiltrative and irregular in shape, but they lack papillary or solid features and atypia.

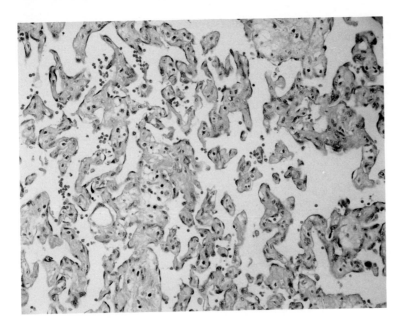

FIGURE 10-96 Moderately differentiated angiosarcoma. Papillary tufting is prominent, but cytologic atypia is still slight.

grade and prognosis, with a poor survival rate (20% or less) for poorly differentiated tumors.[407,408] Well-differentiated angiosarcomas may be difficult to differentiate from benign hemangiomas; the main features favoring a diagnosis of angiosarcoma are a tumor size large enough to form a palpable mass and the presence of communicating vascular channels.

Most patients with mammary angiosarcoma are young, and some have been pregnant at the time of diagnosis, raising the suspicion of hormone dependence. Cases with estrogen receptors have been reported, but it is not clear whether the receptors were actually in the tumor cells or in infiltrated benign mammary tissue.[409]

Angiosarcomas of the breast have been reported after lumpectomy and radiation therapy for breast carcinoma,[410,411] but these appear to be cutaneous rather than true mammary angiosarcomas. Cutaneous angiosarcoma is obviously part of the differential diagnosis of mammary angiosarcoma, as are the benign vascular lesions mentioned above. An additional differential diagnostic possibility is an acantholytic squamous cell carcinoma, such as that illustrated in Figure 10-85. Immunostains for endothelial and epithelial markers are important here.

Postmastectomy Lymphangiosarcoma

Postmastectomy lymphangiosarcoma (Stewart-Treves syndrome)[412] was first described in 1948, and subsequently close to 200 cases have been reported. Although not a breast tumor per se, it merits consider-

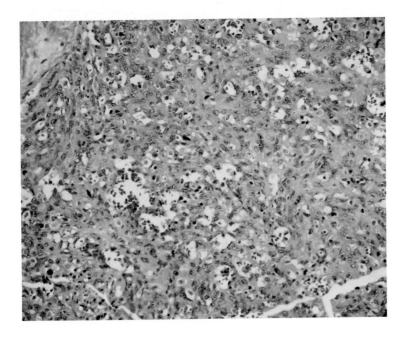

FIGURE 10-97 Poorly differentiated angiosarcoma. Tumor growth is largely in the form of spindled cells with nuclear atypia and mitotic figures. A background of blood-filled vascular channels identifies the tumor as angiosarcoma.

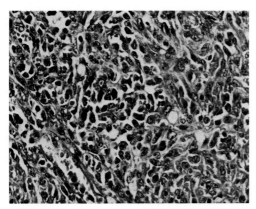

FIGURE 10-98 Postmastectomy lymphangiosarcoma: microscopic appearance.

ation here because of its tendency to develop in lymphedematous arms after mastectomy. Considerably rarer is the appearance of this tumor in lower extremities that are the site of chronic lymphedema of different etiology, but this occurrence supports the concept of the etiologic significance of lymphatic stasis. The lesion first presents as a cutaneous ecchymosis or nodule, rapidly becoming multiple and coalescent; reported cases have appeared an average of almost 10 years after mastectomy. Histologic examination usually easily demonstrates the lymphatic character of the tumor (Fig. 10-98), but a small biopsy specimen may occasionally be confused with metastatic mammary carcinoma. Ultrastructural and immunohistochemical studies may be nec-

essary in such cases to confirm the vascular and nonepithelial nature of the tumor.[413,414] The prognosis is poor.

Lymphoid and Hematopoietic Neoplasms

Mammary localizations of malignant lymphomas[415-417] and leukemic infiltrates[418] are not rare, but they usually are part of the spectrum of disseminated malignant disease. We have seen cases of lymphoma that were difficult to differentiate from lobular, lipid-rich, or medullary carcinoma (Fig. 10-99). Immunostains for leukocyte common antigen and epithelial markers assist in this differential diagnosis. A chloracetate esterase stain identifies the granules of a granulocytic leukemic infiltrate. So-called lymphoid pseudotumors are occasionally encountered in the breast; they are characterized by a pleomorphic but benign cytologic appearance and the frequent formation of follicles with germinal centers.[419] They are benign. More easily differentiated lymphoid lesions are benign intramammary lymph nodes[7] and lymphocytic mastopathy.[46,47]

The *prognosis* of malignant lymphomas depends on the clinical stage and the histologic type, with primary mammary lymphomas of low stage and low histologic grade having a more favorable prognosis. These primary lymphomas are thought to be of B cell type, and may originate in preexisting lymphocytic mastopathy.[415,417]

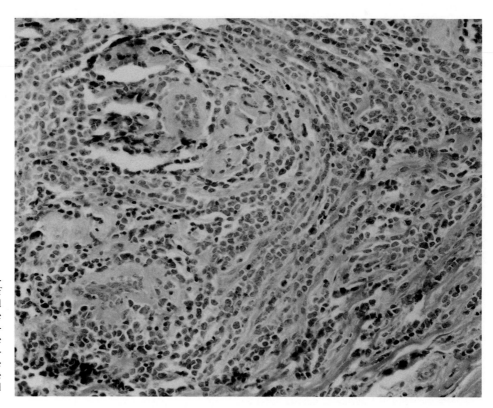

FIGURE 10-99 Malignant lymphoma, small cell type, of breast. Tumor cells swirl around residual benign ducts in the same manner as in classical infiltrating lobular carcinoma. The tumor cells were immunohistochemically positive for leukocyte common antigen and negative for cytokeratins and epithelial membrane antigen.

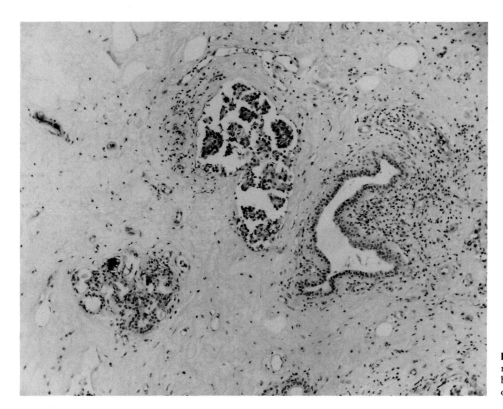

FIGURE 10-100 Metastatic serous carcinoma of ovary in breast tissue. Note involvement of periductal vascular space.

TUMORS METASTATIC TO THE BREAST

Metastatic involvement of the breast is uncommon as an autopsy finding and is a great rarity as a clinical phenomenon; only a few dozen cases of the latter have been reported, whereas the former occurs in about 5% of patients dying of malignant neoplasms other than breast cancer.[420,421] The most common primary tumors seen, other than malignant lymphomas and leukemias, are carcinomas (of the stomach, uterus, ovary, and thyroid) and malignant melanomas. These are generally recognized by the clinical history, the absence of a single dominant mass, and the presence of diffuse lymphatic or vascular infiltration (Fig. 10-100). Primary tumors of the breast—both carcinomas and sarcomas—appear simultaneously or at a later date in the opposite breast with a much greater frequency than do primary tumors of other organs.[386,387]

REFERENCES

1. McCarty KS Jr, Tucker JA: Breast. In Sternberg SS, ed. Histology for pathologists, pp 893–902. New York, Raven Press, 1992
2. Page AL, Anderson TJ: Stages of breast development. In Diagnostic histopathology of the breast, pp 11–29. Edinburgh, Churchill-Livingstone, 1987
3. Smith DM Jr, Peters TG, Donegan WL: Montgomery's areolar tubercle: A light microscopic study. Arch Pathol Lab Med 106:60–63, 1982
4. Halsell JT, Smith JR, Bentlage CR et al: Lymphatic drainage of the breast demonstrated by vital dye staining and radiography. Ann Surg 162:221–226, 1965
5. Turner-Warwick RT: The lymphatics of the breast. Br J Surg 46:574–582, 1959
6. Hultborn KA, Larsson L-G, Ragnhult I: The lymph drainage from the breast to the axillary and parasternal lymph nodes, studied with the aid of colloidal Au[198]. Acta Radiol 43:52–64, 1955
7. Egan RL, McSweeney MB: Intramammary lymph nodes. Cancer 51:1838–1842, 1983
8. Wellings SR, Jensen HM, Marcum RG: An atlas of subgross pathology of the human breast with special reference to possible precancerous lesions. J Natl Cancer Inst 55:231–273, 1975
9. Squartini F, Sarnelli R: Structure, functional changes, and proliferative pathology of the human mammary lobule in cancerous breasts. J Natl Cancer Inst 67:33–46, 1981
10. Ahmed A: Atlas of the ultrastructure of human breast diseases. Edinburgh, Churchill-Livingstone, 1978
11. Ozzello L: Ultrastructure of the human mammary gland. In Sommers SC, ed. Pathology annual, pp 1–60. New York, Appleton-Century-Crofts, 1971
12. Forsyth IA: The mammary gland. Baillieres Clin Endocrinol Metab 5:809–832, 1991
13. Vogel PM, Georgiade NG, Fetter BF et al: The correlation of histologic changes in the human breast with the menstrual cycle. Am J Pathol 104:23–34, 1981
14. Strombeck JO: Macromastia in women and its surgical treatment: A clinical study based on 1,042 cases. Acta Chir Scand (Suppl) 341:1–129, 1964
15. Velpeau A: Traité des maladies du sein et de la région mammaire. Paris, Masson, 1858
16. American College of Radiology: College policy reviews use of thermography. American College of Radiology Bulletin 40:13, 1984
17. Bassett LW, Kimme-Smith C: Breast sonography. Am J Roentgenol 156:449–455, 1991
18. Okazaki A, Okazaki M, Asaishi K, Satoh H et al: Fiberoptic ductoscopy of the breast: A new diagnostic procedure for nipple discharge. Jpn J Clin Oncol 21:188–193, 1991

19. Holland R, Hendriks JHCL, Mravunac M: Mammographically occult breast cancer: A pathologic and radiologic study. Cancer 52:1810–1819, 1983

20. Woolf SH: United States Preventive Services Task Force recommendations on breast cancer screening. Cancer 69:1913–1918, 1992

21. Shapiro S: Periodic breast cancer screening in seven foreign countries. Cancer 69:1919–1924, 1992

22. Stock RJ, Kunschner A, Mazer J, Murphy A: Mammographic localization and biopsy: The experience of a gynecologic oncology group. Gynecol Oncol 33:172–176, 1989

23. Lagios MD, Bennington JL: Protocol for the pathologic examination and tissue processing of the mammographically directed breast biopsy. In Bennington JL, Lagios MD, eds. The mammographically directed biopsy, pp 23–46. Philadelphia, Hanley & Belfus, 1992

24. Schnitt SJ, Connolly JL: Processing and evaluation of breast excision specimens: A clinically oriented approach. Am J Clin Pathol 98:125–137, 1992

25. Stewart FW: The diagnosis of tumors by aspiration. Am J Pathol 9:801–812, 1933

26. Oertel YC, Galblum LI: Fine needle aspiration of the breast: Diagnostic criteria. Pathol Annu 18(1):375–407, 1983

27. Giard RWM, Hermans J: The value of aspiration cytologic examination of the breast: A statistical review of the medical literature. Cancer 69:2104–2110, 1992

28. Oertel YC: Fine needle aspiration of the breast. Boston, Butterworths, 1987

29. Kline TS: Handbook of fine needle aspiration cytology. St. Louis, CV Mosby, 1988

30. Zajdela A, Zillhardt P, Voillemot N: Cytological diagnosis by fine needle sampling without aspiration. Cancer 59:1201–1205, 1987

31. Pestana CB, Donozo N, Pinto AJ et al: Sequential determination of immunocytochemical estrogen receptor and nuclear DNA content in fine needle biopsies from breast carcinoma. Breast Cancer Res Treat 19:39–46, 1991

32. Ciatto S, Cariaggi P, Bulgaresi P: The value of routine cytologic examination of breast cyst fluids. Acta Cytol 31:301–304, 1987

33. Layfield LJ, Parkinson B, Wong J, Giuliano AE, Bassett LW: Mammographically guided fine-needle aspiration biopsy of nonpalpable breast lesions: Can it replace open biopsy? Cancer 68:2007–2011, 1991

34. Millis RR: Needle biopsy of the breast. In McDivitt RW, Oberman HA, Ozzello L, Kaufman N, eds. The breast, pp 186–203. Baltimore, Williams & Wilkins, 1984

35. Takeda T, Suzuki M, Sato Y, Hase T: Cytologic studies of nipple discharges. Acta Cytol 26:35–36, 1982

36. Esteban JM, Zaloudek C, Silverberg SG: Intraoperative diagnosis of breast lesions: Comparison of cytologic with frozen section technics. Am J Clin Pathol 88:681–688, 1987

37. Mair S, Lash RH, Suskin D, Mendelsohn G: Intraoperative surgical specimen evaluation: Frozen section analysis, cytologic examination, or both? A comparative study of 206 cases. Am J Clin Pathol 96:8–14, 1991

38. Oberman HA: A modest proposal. Am J Surg Pathol 16:69–70, 1992

39. Schnitt SJ, Silen W, Sadowsky NL et al: Ductal carcinoma in situ (intraductal carcinoma) of the breast. N Engl J Med 318:898–903, 1988

40. Owings DV, Hann L, Schnitt SJ: How thoroughly should needle localization breast biopsies be sampled for microscopic examination? A prospective mammographic/pathologic correlative study. Am J Surg Pathol 14:578–583, 1990

41. Schnitt SJ, Wang HH: Histologic sampling of grossly benign breast biopsies: How much is enough? Am J Surg Pathol 13:505–512, 1989

42. Thomsen AC, Espersen T, Maigaard S: Course and treatment of milk stasis, noninfectious inflammation of the breast and infectious mastitis in nursing women. Am J Obstet Gynecol 149:492–495, 1984

43. Catania S, Zurrida S, Veronesi P, Galimberti V et al: Mondor's disease and breast cancer. Cancer 69:2267–2270, 1992

44. Winkler JM: Galactocele of the breast. Am J Surg 108:357–360, 1964

45. Kessler E, Wolloch Y: Granulomatous mastitis: A lesion clinically simulating carcinoma. Am J Clin Pathol 58:642–646, 1972

46. Schwartz IS, Strauchen JA: Lymphocytic mastopathy: An autoimmune disease of the breast? Am J Clin Pathol 93:725–730, 1990

47. Tomaszewski JE, Brooks JSJ, Hicks D, LiVolsi VA: Diabetic mastopathy: A distinctive clinicopathologic entity. Hum Pathol 23:780–786, 1992

48. Whitaker HT, Moore RM: Gumma of the breast. Surg Gynecol Obstet 98:473–477, 1954

49. Banik S, Bishop PW, Ormerod LP, O'Brien TE: Sarcoidosis of the breast. J Clin Pathol 39:446–448, 1986

50. Martin BF, Phillips JD: Gangrene of the female breast with anticoagulant therapy: Report of two cases. Am J Clin Pathol 53:622–626, 1970

51. Jordan JM, Rose WT, Allen NB: Wegener's granulomatosis involving the breast: Report of three cases and review of the literature. Am J Med 83:159–164, 1987

52. Dixon JM, Anderson TJ, Lumsden AB et al: Mammary duct ectasia. Br J Surg 70:601–603, 1983

53. Mansel RE, Morgan WP: Duct ectasia in the male. Br J Surg 66:660–662, 1979

54. Wilhelmus JL, Schrodt GR, Mahaffey LM: Cholesterol granuloma of the breast: A lesion which clinically mimics carcinoma. Am J Clin Pathol 77:592–597, 1982

55. Meyer JE, Silverman P, Gandbhir L: Fat necrosis of the breast. Arch Surg 113:801–805, 1978

56. Clarke D, Curtis JL, Martinez A et al: Fat necrosis of the breast simulating recurrent carcinoma after primary radiotherapy in the management of early stage breast carcinoma. Cancer 52:442–445, 1983

57. Silverstein, MJ, Gierson ED, Gamagami P, Handel N, Waisman JR: Breast cancer diagnosis and prognosis in women augmented with silicone gel-filled implants. Cancer 66:97–101, 1990

58. Raven RW: Paraffinoma of the breast. Clin Oncol 7:157–161, 1981

59. Rickert RR, Rajan S: Localized breast infarcts associated with pregnancy. Arch Pathol 97:159–161, 1974

60. Flint A, Oberman HA: Infarction and squamous metaplasia of intraductal papilloma: A benign breast lesion that may simulate carcinoma. Hum Pathol 15:764–767, 1984

61. Robitaille Y, Seemayer TA, Thelmo WL, Cumberlidge MC: Infarction of the mammary region mimicking carcinoma of the breast. Cancer 33:1183–1189, 1974

62. Haggitt RC, Booth JL: Bilateral fibromatosis of the breast in Gardner's syndrome. Cancer 25:161–166, 1970

63. Ward AM: The structure of the breast in mucoviscidosis. J Clin Pathol 25:119–122, 1972

64. Carney JA, Toorkey BC: Myxoid fibroadenoma and allied conditions (myxomatosis) of the breast: A heritable disorder with special associations including cardiac and cutaneous myxomas. Am J Surg Pathol 15:713–721, 1991

65. Carney JA, Toorkey BC: Ductal adenoma of the breast with tubular features: A probable component of the complex of myxomas, spotty pigmentation, endocrine overactivity, and schwannomas. Am J Surg Pathol 15:722–731, 1991

66. O'Hara MF, Page DL: Adenomas of the breast and ectopic breast under lactational influences. Hum Pathol 16:707–712, 1985

67. Fechner RE: Fibroadenomas in patients receiving oral contraceptives: A clinical and pathologic study. Am J Clin Pathol 53:857–864, 1970

68. Hertel BF, Zaloudek C, Kempson RL: Breast adenomas. Cancer 37:2891–2905, 1976

69. Ozzello L, Gump FE: The management of patients with carcinomas in fibroadenomatous tumors of the breast. Surg Gynecol Obstet 160:99–104, 1985

70. Diaz NM, Palmer JO, McDivitt RW: Carcinoma arising within fibroadenomas of the breast. Am J Clin Pathol 95:614–622, 1991

71. Pike AM, Oberman HA: Juvenile (cellular) fibroadenomas: A clinicopathologic study. Am J Surg Pathol 9:730–736, 1985

72. Azzopardi JG, Muretto P, Goddeeris P et al: Carcinoid tumours of the breast: The morphological spectrum of argyrophil carcinomas. Histopathology 6:549–569, 1982

73. Dejmek A, Lindholm K: Frequency of cytologic features in fine needle aspirates from histologically and cytologically diagnosed fibroadenomas. Acta Cytol 35:695–699, 1991

74. Oberman HA: Breast lesions in the adolescent female. Pathol Annu 14(Part 1):175–201, 1979

75. Rao BR, Meyer JS, Fry CG: Most cystosarcoma phyllodes and fibroadenomas have progesterone receptor but lack estrogen receptor. Stromal localization of progesterone receptor. Cancer 47:2016–2021, 1981

76. Müller J: Uber den feinern Bau und die Formen der Krankhaften Geschwülste. Berlin, G. Reimer, 1838

77. Lindqvist KD, Van Heerden JA, Weiland LH, Martin JK Jr: Recurrent and metastatic cystosarcoma phyllodes. Am J Surg 144:341–343, 1982

78. Cohn-Cedermark G, Rutqvist LE, Rosendahl I, Silfverswärd C: Prognostic factors in cystosarcoma phyllodes: A clinicopathologic study of 77 patients. Cancer 68:2017–2022, 1991

79. Hawkins RE, Schofield JB, Fisher C, Wiltshaw E, McKinna JA: The clinical and histologic criteria that predict metastases from cystosarcoma phyllodes. Cancer 69:141–147, 1992

80. Grimes MM: Cystosarcoma phyllodes of the breast: Histologic features, flow cytometric analysis, and clinical correlations. Mod Pathol 5:232–239, 1992

81. Auger M, Hanna W, Kahn HJ: Cystosarcoma phyllodes of the breast and its mimics: An immunohistochemical and ultrastructural study. Arch Pathol Lab Med 113:1231–1235, 1989

82. Reddick RL, Shin TK, Sawhney D, Siegal GP: Stromal proliferations of the breast: An ultrastructural and immunohistochemical evaluation of cystosarcoma phyllodes, juvenile fibroadenoma and fibroadenoma. Hum Pathol 18:45–49, 1987

83. Yeh IT, Francis DJ, Orenstein JM, Silverberg SG: Ultrastructure of cystosarcoma phyllodes and fibroadenoma: A comparative study. Am J Clin Pathol 84:131–136, 1985

84. El-Naggar AK, Ro JY, McLemore D, Garnsy L: DNA content and proliferative activity of cystosarcoma phyllodes of the breast: Potential prognostic significance. Am J Clin Pathol 93:480–485, 1990

85. Layfield LJ, Hart J, Neuwirth H, Bohman R et al: Relation between DNA ploidy and the clinical behavior of phyllodes tumors. Cancer 64:1486–1489, 1989

86. Mottot C, Pouliquen X, Bastien H et al: Fibroadenomes et tumeurs phyllodes: Approche cytopathologique. Ann Anat Pathol 23:233–240, 1978

87. Simi U, Moretti D, Iacconi P et al: Fine needle cytopathology of phyllodes tumor: Differential diagnosis with fibroadenoma. Acta Cytol 32:63–66, 1988

88. West TL, Weiland LH, Clagett OT: Cystosarcoma phyllodes. Ann Surg 173:520–528, 1971

89. Carter D: Intraductal papillary tumors of the breast: A study of 78 cases. Cancer 39:1689–1692, 1977

90. McDivitt RW, Holleb AI, Foote FW: Prior breast disease in patients treated for papillary carcinoma. Arch Pathol 85:117–124, 1968

91. Murad TM, Contesso G, Mouriesse A: Papillary tumors of large lactiferous ducts. Cancer 48:122–133, 1981

92. Kraus FT, Neubecker RD: The differential diagnosis of papillary tumors of the breast. Cancer 15:444–455, 1962

93. Raju UB, Lee MW, Zarbo RJ, Crissman JD: Papillary neoplasia of the breast: Immunohistochemically defined myoepithelial cells in the diagnosis of benign and malignant papillary breast neoplasms. Mod Pathol 2:569–576, 1989

94. Rosai J: Borderline epithelial lesions of the breast. Am J Surg Pathol 15:209–221, 1991

95. Schnitt SJ, Connolly J, Tavassoli F, Fechner R et al: Interobserver reproducibility in the diagnosis of ductal proliferative breast lesions using standarized criteria. Am J Surg Pathol 16:1133–1143, 1992

96. Rosen PP, Kimmel M: Juvenile papillomatosis of the breast: A follow-up study of 41 patients having biopsies before 1979. Am J Clin Pathol 93:599–603, 1990

97. Lammie GA, Millis RR: Ductal adenoma of the breast: A review of fifteen cases. Hum Pathol 20:903–908, 1989

98. Kamel OW, Kempson RL, Hendrickson MR: In situ proliferative lesions of the breast. In Bennington JL, Lagios MD, eds. The mammographically directed biopsy, pp 65–102. Philadelphia, Hanley & Belfus, 1992

99. Ohuchi N, Abe R, Kasai M: Possible cancerous change of intraductal papillomas of the breast: A 3-D reconstruction study of 25 cases. Cancer 54:605–611, 1984

100. Page DL, Dupont WD: Anatomic markers of human premalignancy and risk of breast carcinoma. Cancer 66:1326–1335, 1990

101. Perzin KH, Lattes R: Papillary adenoma of the nipple (florid papillomatosis, adenoma, adenomatosis): A clinicopathologic study. Cancer 29:996–1009, 1972

102. Diaz NM, Palmer JO, Wick MR: Erosive adenomatosis of the nipple: Histology, immunohistology, and differential diagnosis. Mod Pathol 5:179–184, 1992

103. Rosen PP, Caicco JA: Florid papillomatosis of the nipple: A study of 51 patients including nine with mammary carcinoma. Am J Surg Pathol 10:87–101, 1986

104. Mazzara PF, Flint A, Naylor B: Adenoma of the nipple: Cytopathologic features. Acta Cytol 33:188–190, 1989

105. Finck FM, Schwinn CP, Keasbey LE: Clear cell hidradenoma of the breast. Cancer 22:125–135, 1968

106. Moran CA, Suster S, Carter D: Benign mixed tumors (pleomorphic adenomas) of the breast. Am J Surg Pathol 14:913–921, 1990

107. Jones MW, Norris HJ, Snyder RC: Infiltrating syringomatous adenoma of the nipple: A clinical and pathological study of 11 cases. Am J Surg Pathol 13:197–201, 1989

108. Tavassoli FA: Myoepithelial lesions of the breast: Myoepitheliosis, adenomyoepithelioma, and myoepithelial carcinoma. Am J Surg Pathol 15:554–568, 1991

109. Grignon DJ, Ro JY, Mackay BN, Ordoñez NG, Ayala AG: Collagenous spherulosis of the breast: Immunohistochemical and ultrastructural studies. Am J Clin Pathol 91:386–392, 1989

110. Fisher CJ, Hanby AM, Robinson L, Millis RR: Mammary hamartoma: A review of 35 cases. Histopathology 20:99–106, 1992

111. Oberman HA: Hamartomas and hamartoma variants of the breast. Semin Diagn Pathol 6:135–145, 1989

112. Marsh WL Jr, Lucas JG, Olsen J: Chondrolipoma of the breast. Arch Pathol Lab Med 113:369–371, 1989

113. Tavassoli FA, Yeh I: Lactational and clear cell changes of the breast in nonlactating, nonpregnant women. Am J Clin Pathol 87:23–29, 1987

114. DeMay RM, Kay S: Granular cell tumor of the breast. Pathol Annu 19(Part 2):121–148, 1984

115. Lauwers G, de Roux S, Terzakis J: Leiomyoma of the breast. Anat Cytol Pathol 38:108–110, 1990

116. Jozefczyk MA, Rosen PP: Vascular tumors of the breast. II. Perilobular hemangiomas and hemangiomas. Am J Surg Pathol 9:491–503, 1985

117. Lesueur GC, Brown R, Bhathal PS: Incidence of perilobular hemangioma in the female breast. Arch Pathol Lab Med 107:308–310, 1983

118. Rosen PP, Jozefczyk MA, Boram LH: Vascular tumors of the breast. IV. The venous hemangioma. Am J Surg Pathol 9:659–665, 1985

119. Rosen PP: Vascular tumors of the breast. III. Angiomatosis. Am J Surg Pathol 9:652–658, 1985

120. Hoda SA, Cranor ML, Rosen PP: Hemangiomas of the breast with atypical histological features: Further analysis of

histological subtypes confirming their benign character. Am J Surg Pathol 16:553–560, 1992

121. Mittal KR, Gerald W, True LD: Hemangiopericytoma of breast: Report of a case with ultrastructural and immunohistochemical findings. Hum Pathol 17:1181–1183, 1986

122. Ibrahim RE, Sciotto CG, Weidner N: Pseudoangiomatous hyperplasia of mammary stroma: Some observations regarding its clinicopathologic spectrum. Cancer 63:1154–1160, 1989

123. Lefkowitz M, Wear DJ: Cat-scratch disease masquerading as a solitary tumor of the breast. Arch Pathol Lab Med 113:473–475, 1989

124. Pettinato G, Manivel JC, Insabato L, De Chiara A, Petrella G: Plasma cell granuloma (inflammatory pseudotumor) of the breast. Am J Clin Pathol 90:627–632, 1988

125. Rosen PP, Ernsberger D: Mammary fibromatosis: A benign spindle-cell tumor with significant risk for local recurrence. Cancer 63:1363–1369, 1989

126. Bhargava V, Miller TR, Cohen MB: Mucocele-like tumors of the breast: Cytologic findings in two cases. Am J Clin Pathol 95:875–877, 1991

127. Ro JY, Sneige N, Sahin AA, Silva EG et al: Mucocelelike tumor of the breast associated with atypical ductal hyperplasia or mucinous carcinoma: A clinicopathologic study of seven cases. Arch Pathol Lab Med 115:137–140, 1991

128. Reclus P: La maladie kystique des mamelles. Rev Chir 3:761–775, 1883

129. Schimmelbusch C: Das Cystadenom der Mamma. Arch Klin Chir 44:117–134, 1892

130. Love SM, Gelman RS, Sclen W: "Fibrocystic disease" of the breast: A non-disease? N Engl J Med 307:1010–1014, 1982

131. Hutter RVP: Goodbye to "fibrocystic disease." N Engl J Med 312:179–181, 1985

132. Vorheer H: Fibrocystic breast disease: Pathophysiology, pathomorphology, clinical picture and management. Am J Obstet Gynecol 154:161–179, 1986

133. Hutter RVP: Consensus meeting: Is "fibrocystic disease" of the breast precancerous? Arch Pathol Lab Med 110:171–173, 1986

134. Carter CL, Corle DK, Micozzi MS et al: A prospective study of the development of breast cancer in 16,692 women with benign breast disease. Am J Epidemiol 128:467–477, 1988

135. Bartow SA, Pathak DR, Black WC et al: Prevalence of benign, atypical, and malignant breast lesions in populations at different risk for breast cancer: A forensic autopsy study. Cancer 60:2751–2760, 1987

136. Nielsen BD: Adenosis tumor of the breast: A clinicopathological investigation of 27 cases. Histopathology 11:1259–1275, 1987

137. Silverman JF, Dabbs DJ, Gilbert CF: Fine needle aspiration cytology of adenosis tumor of the breast, with immunocytochemical and ultrastructural observations. Acta Cytol 33:181–187, 1989

138. Page DL, Anderson TJ: Cysts and apocrine change. In: Diagnostic histopathology of the breast, pp 43–50. Edinburgh, Churchill-Livingstone, 1987

139. Jao W, Recant W, Swerdlow MA: Comparative ultrastructure of tubular carcinoma and sclerosing adenosis of the breast. Cancer 38:180–186, 1976

140. Davies JD: Neural invasion in benign mammary dysplasia. J Pathol 109:225–231, 1973

141. Eusebi V, Collina G, Bussolati G: Carcinoma in situ in sclerosing adenosis of the breast: An immunocytochemical study. Semin Diagn Pathol 6:146–152, 1989

142. Oberman HA, Markey BA: Noninvasive carcinoma of the breast presenting in adenosis. Mod Pathol 4:31–35, 1991

143. Carter DJ, Rosen PP: Atypical apocrine metaplasia in sclerosing lesions of the breast: A study of 51 patients. Mod Pathol 4:1–5, 1991

144. Jensen RA, Page DL, Dupont WD, Rogers LW: Invasive breast cancer risk in women with sclerosing adenosis. Cancer 64:1977–1983, 1989

145. McDivitt RW, Stevens JA, Lee NC, Wingo PA et al: Histologic types of benign breast disease and the risk for breast cancer. Cancer 69:1408–1414, 1992

146. Andersen JA, Carter D, Linell F: A symposium on sclerosing duct lesions of the breast. Pathol Annu 21(2):145–179, 1986

147. Nielsen M, Christensen L, Andersen JA: Radial scars in women with breast cancer. Cancer 59:1019–1025, 1987

148. Tavassoli FA, Norris HJ: A comparison of the results of long-term follow-up for atypical intraductal hyperplasia and intraductal hyperplasia of the breast. Cancer 65:518–529, 1990

149. Page DL, Anderson TJ, Rogers LW: Epithelial hyperplasia. In Page DL, Anderson TJ, eds. Diagnostic histopathology of the breast, pp 120–156. Edinburgh, Churchill-Livingstone, 1987

150. Fechner RE, Mills SE: Breast pathology: Benign proliferations, atypias and in situ carcinomas, pp 147–171. Chicago, ASCP Press, 1990

151. Carter D: Interpretation of breast biopsies, 2nd ed, pp 116–133. New York, Raven Press, 1990

152. Fechner RE, Mills SE: Breast pathology: Benign proliferations, atypias and in situ carcinomas, pp 89–106. Chicago, ASCP Press, 1990

153. Simon MS, Schwartz AG, Martino S, Swanson GM: Trends in the diagnosis of in situ breast cancer in the Detroit metropolitan area, 1973 to 1987. Cancer 69:466–469, 1992

154. Gump FE, Jicha DL, Ozzello L: Ductal carcinoma in situ (DCIS): A revised concept. Surgery 102:790–795, 1987

155. Holland R, Hendriks JHCL, Verbeek ALM et al: Extent, distribution, and mammographic/histological correlations of breast ductal carcinoma in situ. Lancet 335:519–522, 1990

156. Lagios MD: Duct carcinoma in situ: Pathology and treatment. Surg Clin North Am 70:853–871, 1990

157. Lagios MD, Margolin FR, Westdahl PR et al: Mammographically detected duct carcinoma in situ: Frequency of local recurrence following tylectomy and prognostic effect of nuclear grade on local recurrence. Cancer 63:618–624, 1989

158. Patchefsky AS, Schwartz GF, Finkelstein SD et al: Heterogeneity of intraductal carcinoma of the breast. Cancer 63:731–741, 1989

159. Eusebi V, Foschini MP, Cook MG et al: Long-term follow-up of in situ carcinoma of the breast with special emphasis on clinging carcinoma. Semin Diagn Pathol 6:165–173, 1989

160. Lagios MD, Westdahl PR, Margolin FR, Rose MR: Duct carcinoma in situ: Relationship of extent of noninvasive disease to the frequency of occult invasion, multicentricity, lymph node metastases, and short-term treatment failures. Cancer 50:1309–1314, 1982

161. Page DL, Dupont WD, Rogers LW et al: Intraductal carcinoma of the breast: Follow-up after biopsy only. Cancer 49:751–758, 1982

162. Silverstein MJ, Waisman JR, Gamagami P et al: Intraductal carcinoma of the breast (208 cases): Clinical factors influencing treatment choice. Cancer 66:102–108, 1990

163. Rosner D, Lane WW, Penetrante R: Ductal carcinoma in situ with microinvasion: A curable entity using surgery alone without need for adjuvant therapy. Cancer 67:1498–1503, 1991

164. Carter CL, Allen C, Hensen DE: Relation of tumor size, lymph node status and survival in 24,470 breast cancer cases. Cancer 63:181–187, 1989

165. Rosen PP: Clinical implications of preinvasive and small invasive breast carcinoma. Pathol Annu 16(2):337–356, 1981

166. Rosen PP, Senie R, Schottenfeld D, Ashikari R: Noninvasive breast carcinoma: Frequency of unsuspected invasion and implications for treatment. Ann Surg 189:377–382, 1979

167. Matsukuma A, Enjoji M, Toyoshima S: Ductal carcinoma of the breast: An analysis of proportions of intraductal and invasive carcinoma. Pathol Res Pract 187:62–67, 1991

168. Gillett CE, Bobrow LG, Millis RR: S-100 protein in human

mammary tissue: Immunoreactivity in breast carcinoma, including Paget's disease of the nipple, and value as a marker of myoepithelial cells. J Pathol 160:19–24, 1990

169. Palmer JO, Ghiselli RW, McDivitt RW: Immunohistochemistry in the differential diagnosis of breast diseases. Pathol Annu 25(Part 2):287–316, 1990

170. Wang HH, Ducatman BS, Eick D: Comparative features of ductal carcinoma in situ and infiltrating ductal carcinoma of the breast on fine-needle aspiration biopsy. Am J Clin Pathol 92:736–740, 1989

171. Lilleng R, Hagmar B: The comedo subtype of intraductal carcinoma: Cytologic characteristics. Acta Cytol 36:345–352, 1992

172. Rosen PP: Axillary lymph node metastases in patients with occult non-invasive breast carcinoma. Cancer 46:1298–1306, 1980

173. Bornstein BA, Recht A, Connolly JL, Schnitt SJ et al: Results of treating ductal carcinoma in situ of the breast with conservative surgery and radiation therapy. Cancer 67:7–13, 1991

174. Howard PW, Locker AP, Dowle CS et al: In situ carcinoma of the breast. Eur J Surg Oncol 15:328–332, 1989

175. Bartkova J, Barnes DM, Millis RR, Gullick WJ: Immunohistochemical demonstration of c-erb B-2 protein in mammary ductal carcinoma in situ. Hum Pathol 21:1164–1167, 1990

176. Bur ME, Zimarowski MJ, Schnitt SJ, Baker S, Lew R: Estrogen receptor immunohistochemistry in carcinoma in situ of the breast. Cancer 69:1174–1181, 1992

177. Killeen JL, Namiki H: DNA analysis of ductal carcinoma in situ of the breast. Cancer 68:2602–2607, 1991

178. Foote FW Jr, Stewart FW: Lobular carcinoma in situ: A rare form of mammary cancer. Am J Pathol 17:491–496, 1941

179. Muir R: The evolution of carcinoma of the mamma. J Pathol Bacteriol 52:155–172, 1941

180. Anderson JA: Lobular carcinoma in situ: A long term follow-up in 52 cases. Acta Pathol Microbiol Scand Sect A 82:519–533, 1974

181. Haagensen CD, Lane N, Lattes R, Bodian C: Lobular neoplasia (so-called lobular carcinoma in situ of the breast). Cancer 42:737–769, 1978

182. Hutter RVP, Foote FW Jr: Lobular carcinoma in situ. Long term follow-up. Cancer 24:1081–1085, 1969

183. Newman W: Lobular carcinoma of the female breast: Report of 73 cases. Ann Surg 164:305–314, 1966

184. Rosen PP, Lieberman PH, Braun DW Jr et al: Lobular carcinoma in situ of the breast: Detailed analysis of 99 patients with average follow-up of 24 years. Am J Surg Pathol 2:225–251, 1978

185. Tulusan AH, Egger H, Schneider ML, Willgeroth FA: Contribution to the natural history of breast cancer. IV. Lobular carcinoma in situ and its relation to breast cancer. Arch Gynecol 231:219–226, 1982

186. Wheeler JE, Enterline JT, Roseman JM et al: Lobular carcinoma in situ of the breast: Long-term follow-up. Cancer 34:554–563, 1974

187. Morris DM, Walker AP, Coker DC: Lack of efficacy of xeromammography in preoperatively detecting lobular carcinoma in situ of the breast. Breast Cancer Res Treat 1:365–367, 1982

188. Snyder RE: Mammography and lobular carcinoma in situ. Surg Gynecol Obstet 122:255–260, 1966

189. Page DL, Dupont WD, Rogers LW: Ductal involvement by cells of atypical lobular hyperplasia of the breast: A long-term follow-up study of cancer risk. Hum Pathol 19:201–207, 1988

190. Kelsey JL, Hildreth NG: Breast and gynecologic cancer epidemiology. Boca Raton, CRC Press, 1983

191. Noyes RD, Spanos WJ Jr, Montague ED: Breast cancer in women aged 30 and under. Cancer 49:1302–1307, 1982

192. McDivitt RW, Stewart FW: Breast carcinoma in children. JAMA 195:388–390, 1966

193. Anderson DE: Familial versus sporadic breast cancer. Cancer 70:1740–1746, 1992

194. Goodman MJ: Breast cancer in multi-ethnic populations: The Hawaii perspective. Breast Cancer Res Treat 18(Suppl 1):5–9, 1991

195. Adlercreutz H, Monsavi Y, Hockerstedt K: Diet and breast cancer. Acta Oncol 31:175–181, 1992

196. Schapira DV, Kumar NB, Lyman GH: Obesity, body fat distribution, and sex hormones in breast cancer patients. Cancer 67:2215–2218, 1991

197. Lee HP, Gaurley L, Duffy SW et al: Dietary effects on breast-cancer risk in Singapore. Lancet 337:1197–1200, 1991

198. Howe G, Rohan T, DeCarli A et al: The association between alcohol and breast cancer risk: Evidence from the combined analysis of six dietary case-control studies. Int J Cancer 47:707–710, 1991

199. Stoll BA, Secreto G: New hormone-related markers of high risk to breast cancer. Ann Oncol 3:435–438, 1992

200. Steinberg KK, Thacker SB, Smith SJ et al: A meta-analysis of the effect of estrogen replacement therapy on the risk of breast cancer. JAMA 265:1985–1990, 1991

201. Bernstein L, Ross RK, Henderson BE: Relationship of hormone use to cancer risk. Monogr Natl Cancer Inst 12:137–147, 1992

202. Thomas DB, Noonan EA: Breast cancer and specific types of combined oral contraceptives: The WHO collaborative study of neoplasia and steroid contraceptives. Br J Cancer 65:108–113, 1992

203. Khoo SK, Chick P: Sex steroid hormones and breast cancer: Is there a link with oral contraceptives and hormone replacement therapy? Med J Aust 156:124–132, 1992

204. Women's Health Initiative. Proposed plan. National Institutes of Health, December 1991

205. Nayfield SG, Kapp JE, Ford LG et al: Potential role of tamoxifen in the prevention of breast cancer. J Natl Cancer Inst 83:1450–1459, 1991

206. Baum M, Ziv Y, Colletta AA: Can we prevent breast cancer? (Editorial). Br J Cancer 64:205–207, 1991

207. Azzopardi JG, Chepick OF, Hartmann WH, et al: The World Health Organization: Histological typing of breast tumors, 2nd ed. Am J Clin Pathol 78:806–816, 1982.

208. Wellings SR, Jensen HM, Marcum RG: An atlas of subgross pathology of the human breast with special reference to possible precancerous lesions. J Natl Cancer Inst 55:231–273, 1975

209. Van Bogaert LJ: The proliferative behavior of the human adult mammary epithelium. Acta Cytol 23:252–257, 1979

209a. MacDonald I: The natural history of mammary carcinoma. Am J Surg 111:435–442, 1966

209b. Gershon-Cohen J, Berger SM, Klickstein HS: Roentgenography of breast cancer moderating concept of "biologic predeterminism." Cancer 16:961–964, 1963

210. Duffy SW, Tabar L, Fagerberg G et al: Breast screening prognostic factors and survival: Results from the Swedish two county study. Br J Cancer 64:1333–1338, 1991

211. Frisell J, Eklund G, Hellstrom L et al: Randomized study of mammography screening: Preliminary report on mortality in the Stockholm trial. Breast Cancer Res Treat 18:49–56, 1991

212. Fisher ER, Gregorio RM, Fisher B: The pathology of invasive breast cancer—A syllabus derived from findings of the National Surgical Adjuvant Breast Project (Protocol No. 4). Cancer 36:1–85, 1975

213. Fisher B, Slack NH, Ausman RK, Bross IDJ: Location of breast carcinoma and prognosis. Surg Gynecol Obstet 129:705–716, 1969

214. Robertson AJ, Brown RA, Cree IA et al: Prognostic value of measurement of elastosis in breast carcinoma. J Clin Pathol 34:738–743, 1981

215. Schurch W, Lagace R, Seemayer TA: Myofibroblastic stromal reaction in retracted scirrhous carcinoma of the breast. Surg Gynecol Obstet 154:351–358, 1982

216. Gallager HS, Martin JE: Early phases in the development of breast cancer. Cancer 24:1170–1178, 1969

217. Egan RL: Multicentric breast carcinoma: Clinical-radio-

graphic-pathologic whole organ studies and 10-year survival. Cancer 49:1123–1130, 1982

218. Lagios MD, Westdahl PR, Rose MR: The concept and implications of multicentricity in breast carcinoma. Pathol Annu 18(2):83–102, 1981

219. Westman-Naeser S, Bengtsson E, Eriksson O et al: Multifocal breast carcinoma. Am J Surg 142;255–257, 1981

220. Fisher B, Anderson S, Fisher ER et al: Significance of ipsilateral breast tumor recurrence after lumpectomy. Lancet 338:327–331, 1991

221. Clark RM, McCulloch PB, Levine MN et al: Randomized clinical trial to assess the effectiveness of breast irradiation following lumpectomy and axillary dissection for node negative cancer. J Natl Cancer Inst 84:683–689, 1992

222. Vicini FA, Eberlein TJ, Connolly JL et al: The optimal extent of resection for patients with stages I or II breast cancer treated with conservative surgery and radiotherapy. Ann Surg 214:200–204, 1991

223. Fracchia AA, Borgen PI: Bilateral breast cancer. Semin Surg Oncol 7:300–305, 1992

224. Smith BL, Bertagnolli M, Klein BB et al: Evaluation of the contralateral breast: The role of biopsy at the time of treatment of primary breast cancer. Ann Surg 216:17–21, 1992

225. Elston CW, Ellis IO: Pathological prognostic factors in breast cancer. I. The value of histological grade in breast cancer: Experience from a large study with long-term follow-up. Histopathology 19:403–410, 1991

226. Murad TM: A proposed histochemical and electron microscopic classification of human breast cancer according to cell of origin. Cancer 27:288–299, 1971

227. Carstens PHB, Greenberg RA, Francis D, Lyon H: Tubular carcinoma of the breast: A long term follow-up. Histopathology 9:271–280, 1985

228. Deos PH, Norris HJ: Well-differentiated (tubular) carcinoma of the breast. Am J Clin Pathol 78:1–7, 1982

229. Lagios MD, Rose MR, Margolin FR: Tubular carcinoma of the breast: Association with multicentricity, bilaterality and family history of mammary carcinoma. Am J Clin Pathol 73:25–30, 1980

230. McDivitt RW, Boyce W, Gersell D et al: Tubular carcinoma of the breast: Clinical and pathological observations concerning 135 cases. Am J Surg Pathol 6:401–411, 1982

231. Parl FF, Richardson LD: The histologic and biologic spectrum of tubular carcinoma of the breast. Hum Pathol 14:694–698, 1983

232. Peters GN, Wolff M, Haagensen CD: Tubular carcinoma of the breast. Ann Surg 193:138–149, 1981

233. Hijazi YM, Lessard JL, Weiss MA: Use of anti-actin and S-100 protein antibodies in differentiating benign and malignant sclerosing breast lesions. Surg Pathol 2:125–135, 1989

234. Tavassoli FA, Norris HJ: Microglandular adenosis of the breast: A clinicopathologic study of 11 cases with ultrastructural observations. Am J Surg Pathol 6:731–737, 1983

235. Eusebi V, Foschini MP, Betts CM et al: Microglandular adenosis, apocrine adenosis, and tubular carcinoma of the breast: An immunohistochemical comparison. Am J Surg Pathol 17:99–109, 1993

236. Rosenblum MK. Purrazella R, Rosen PP: Is microglandular adenosis a precancerous disease? A study of carcinoma arising therein. Am J Surg Pathol 10:237–245, 1986

237. Page DL, Dixon JM, Andersen TJ et al: Infiltrating cribriform carcinoma of the breast. Histopathology 7:525–536, 1983

238. Venable JG, Schwartz AM, Silverberg SG: Infiltrating cribriform carcinoma of the breast: A distinctive clinicopathologic entity. Hum Pathol 21:333–338, 1990

239. Ellis IO, Galea M, Broughton N, Locker A et al: Pathological prognostic factors in breast cancer. II. Histological type: Relationship with survival in a large study with long-term follow-up. Histopathology 20:479–490, 1992

240. Sumpio B, Jennings T, Sullivan P et al: Adenoid cystic carcinoma of the breast. Am Surg 205:295–301, 1987

241. Ro JY, Silva EG, Gallager HS: Adenoid cystic carcinoma of the breast. Hum Pathol 18:1276–1281, 1987

242. Leeming R, Jenkins M, Mendelsohn G: Adenoid cystic carcinoma of the breast. Arch Surg 127:233–235, 1992

243. Zaloudek C, Oertel YC, Orenstein JM: Adenoid cystic carcinoma of the breast. Am J Clin Pathol 81:297–307, 1984

244. Saphir O: Mucinous carcinoma of the breast. Surg Gynecol Obstet 72:908–914, 1941

245. Silverberg SG, Kay S, Chitale AR, Levitt SH: Colloid carcinoma of the breast. Am J Clin Pathol 55:355–363, 1971

246. Clayton F: Pure mucinous carcinomas of breast. Hum Pathol 17:34–38, 1986

247. Rasmussen BB, Rose C, Christensen I: Prognostic factors in primary mucinous breast carcinoma. Am J Clin Pathol 87:155–160, 1987

248. Papotti, M, Macri L, Finzi G et al: Neuroendocrine differentiation in carcinomas of the breast: A study of 51 cases. Semin Diagn Pathol 6:174–188, 1989

249. Maluf HM, Zukerberg LR, Dickersin GR, Koerner FC: Spindle-cell argyrophilic mucin-producing carcinoma of the breast: Histological, ultrastructural, and immunohistochemical studies of two cases. Am J Surg Pathol 15:677–686, 1991

250. Ro JY, Sneige N, Sahin AA, Silva EG et al: Mucocelelike tumor of the breast associated with atypical ductal hyperplasia or mucinous carcinoma. Arch Pathol Lab Med. 115:137–140, 1991

251. Bhargava V, Miller TR, Cohen MB: Mucocele-like tumors of the breast: Cytologic findings in two cases. Am J Clin Pathol 95:875–877, 1991

252. Page DL: Prognosis and breast cancer: Recognition of lethal and favorable prognostic types. Am J Surg Pathol 15:334–349, 1991

253. Kurtz JM, Jacquemier J, Torhorst J et al: Conservation therapy for breast cancers other than infiltrating ductal carcinoma. Cancer 63:1630–1635, 1989

254. Squires JE, Betsill WL Jr: Intracystic carcinoma of the breast: A correlation of cytomorphology, gross pathology, microscopic pathology and clinical data. Acta Cytol 25:267–271, 1981

255. Carter D, Orr SL, Merino MJ: Intracystic papillary carcinoma after mastectomy, radiotherapy, or biopsy alone. Cancer 52:14–19, 1983

256. Fisher ER, Palekar AS, Redmond C et al: Pathologic findings from the National Surgical Adjuvant Breast Project (protocol no. 4). VI. Invasive papillary cancer. Am J Clin Pathol 73:313–322, 1980

257. Tavassoli FA, Norris HJ: Secretory carcinoma of the breast. Cancer 45:2404–2413, 1980

258. Krausz T, Jenkins D, Grontoft O et al: Secretory carcinoma of the breast in adults: Emphasis on late recurrence and metastasis. Histopathology 14:25–36, 1989

259. Rosen PP, Cranor ML: Secretory carcinoma of the breast. Arch Pathol Lab Med 115:141–144, 1991

260. Dominguez F, Riera JR, Junco P, Sampedro A: Secretory carcinoma of the breast: Report of a case with diagnosis by fine needle aspiration. Acta Cytol 36:507–510, 1992

261. Fisher, ER, Tavares J, Bulatao IS et al: Glycogen-rich, clear cell breast cancer: With comments concerning other clear cell variants. Hum Pathol 16:1085–1090, 1985

262. Moore OS, Foote FW: The relatively favorable prognosis of medullary carcinoma of the breast. Cancer 2:635–642, 1949

263. Bloom HJG, Richardson WW, Field JR: Host resistance and survival in carcinoma of the breast: A study of 104 cases of medullary carcinoma in a series of 1,411 cases of breast cancer followed for 20 years. Br Med J 3:181–188, 1970

264. Ridolfi RL, Rosen PP, Port A et al: Medullary carcinoma of the breast: A clinicopathologic study with 10 year followup. Cancer 40:1365–1385, 1977

265. Rubens JR, Lewandrowski KB, Kopans DB et al: Medullary carcinoma of the breast: Overdiagnosis of a prognostically favorable neoplasm. Arch Surg 125:601–604, 1990

266. Rapin V, Contesso G, Mouriesse H et al: Medullary breast

carcinoma: A reevaluation of 95 cases of breast cancer with inflammatory stroma. Cancer 61:2503–2510, 1988

267. Wargotz ES, Silverberg SG: Medullary carcinoma of the breast: A clinicopathologic study with appraisal of current diagnostic criteria. Hum Pathol 19:1340–1346, 1988

268. Pedersen L, Zedeler K, Holck S et al: Medullary carcinoma of the breast: Proposal for a new simplified histopathological definition. Br J Cancer 63:591–595, 1991

269. Fisher ER, Sass R, Fisher B et al: Pathologic findings from the National Surgical Adjuvant Project for Breast Cancers (protocol no. 4). X. Discriminants for tenth year treatment failures. Cancer 53:712–723, 1984

270. Gould VE, Miller J, Jao W: Ultrastructure of medullary, intraductal, tubular and adenocystic breast carcinomas: Comparative patterns of myoepithelial differentiation and basal lamina deposition. Am J Pathol 78:401–407, 1975

271. Murad TM, Scarpelli DG: The ultrastructure of medullary and scirrhous mammary duct carcinoma. Am J Pathol 50:335–360, 1967

272. Tanaka H, Hori M, Ohki T: High endothelial venule and immunocompetent cells in typical medullary carcinoma of the breast. Virchows Arch A Pathol Anat Histopathol 420:253–261, 1992

273. Dixon J, Anderson TJ, Page DL et al: Infiltrating lobular carcinoma of the breast. Histopathology 6:149–161, 1982

274. Du Toit RS, Locker AP, Ellis IO et al: Invasive lobular carcinoma of the breast: The prognosis of histopathological types. Br J Cancer 60:605–609, 1989

275. DiConstanzo D, Rosen PP, Gareen I et al: Prognosis in infiltrating lobular carcinoma: An analysis of "classical" and variant tumors. Am J Surg Pathol 14:12–23, 1990

276. Nesland JM, Grude TH, Ottestad L, Johannessen JV: Invasive lobular carcinoma of the breast: The importance of an alveolar growth pattern. Pathol Annu 27(1):233–247, 1992

277. Eusebi V, Magalhaes F, Azzopardi JG: Pleomorphic lobular carcinoma of the breast: An aggressive tumor showing apocrine differentiation. Hum Pathol 23:655–662, 1992

278. Lewis TR, Casey J, Buerk CA, Cammack KV: Incidence of lobular carcinoma in bilateral breast cancer. Am J Surg 144:635–638, 1982

279. Fisher ER, Gregorio RM, Redmond C, Fisher B: Tubulolobular invasive breast cancer: A variant of lobular invasive cancer. Hum Pathol 8:679–683, 1977

280. Carter D, Yardley JH, Shelley WM: Lobular carcinoma of the breast: An ultrastructural comparison with certain duct carcinomas and benign lesions. John Hopkins Med J 125:25–43, 1969

281. Murad TM: Ultrastructure of ductular carcinoma of the breast (in situ and infiltrating lobular carcinoma). Cancer 27:18–28, 1971

282. Schäfer A, Bässler R: Vergleichende elektronen-mikroskopische Untersuchungen am Drüsenepithel und am sog: Lobulären Carcinom der Mamma. Virchows Arch A Pathol Anat Histopathol 346:269–286, 1969

283. Leach C, Howell LP: Cytodiagnosis of classic lobular carcinoma and its variants. Acta Cytol 36:199–202, 1992

284. Weidner N, Semple JP: Pleomorphic variant of invasive lobular carcinoma of the breast. Hum Pathol 23:1167–1171, 1992

285. Schnitt SJ, Connolly JL, Recht A et al: Influence of infiltrating lobular histology on local tumor control in breast cancer patients treated with conservative surgery and radiotherapy. Cancer 64:448–454, 1989

286. Poen JC, Tran L, Juillard G et al: Conservation therapy for invasive lobular carcinoma of the breast. Cancer 69:2789–2795, 1992

287. Lamovec J, Bracko M: Metastatic pattern of infiltrating lobular carcinoma of the breast: An autopsy study. J Surg Oncol 48:28–33, 1991

288. Shousha S, Backhous CM, Alaghband-Zadeh J, Burn I: Alveolar variant of invasive lobular carcinoma of the breast. Am J Clin Pathol 85:1–5, 1986

289. Steinbrecher JS, Silverberg SG: Signet-ring cell carcinoma of the breast: The mucinous variant of infiltrating lobular carcinoma? Cancer 37:828–840, 1976

290. Harris M, Wells S, Vasudev KS: Primary signet ring cell carcinoma of the breast. Histopathology 2:171–176, 1978

291. Merino MJ, LiVolsi VA: Signet ring carcinoma of the female breast: A clinicopathologic analysis of 24 cases. Cancer 48:1830–1837, 1981

292. Frable WJ, Kay S: Carcinoma of the breast: Histologic and clinical features of apocrine tumors. Cancer 21:756–763, 1968

293. Abati AD, Kimmel M, Rosen PP: Apocrine mammary carcinoma: A clinicopathologic study of 72 cases. Am J Clin Pathol 94:371–377, 1990

294. Cubilla AL, Woodruff JM: Primary carcinoid tumor of the breast: A report of eight patients. Am J Surg Pathol 1:283–292, 1977

295. Taxy JB, Tischler AS, Insalaco SJ, Battfora H: "Carcinoid" tumor of the breast: A variant of conventional breast cancer? Hum Pathol 12:170–179, 1981

296. Papotti M, Gherardi G, Eusebi V, Pagani A, Bussolati G: Primary oat cell (neuroendocrine) carcinoma of the breast: Report of four cases. Virch Arch A Pathol Anat Histopathol 290:103–108, 1992

297. Tavassoli FA: Classification of metaplastic carcinomas of the breast. Pathol Annu 27(Part 2):89–120, 1992

298. Wargotz ES, Norris HJ: Metaplastic carcinomas of the breast. I. Matrix-producing carcinoma. Hum Pathol 20:628–635, 1989

299. Wargotz ES, Deos PH, Norris HJ: Metaplastic carcinomas of the breast. II. Spindle cell carcinoma. Hum Pathol 20:732–740, 1989

300. Wargotz ES, Norris HJ: Metaplastic carcinomas of the breast. III. Carcinosarcoma. Cancer 64:1490–1499, 1989

301. Wargotz ES, Norris HJ: Metaplastic carcinomas of the breast. IV. Squamous cell carcinoma of ductal origin. Cancer 65:272–276, 1990

302. Wargotz ES, Norris HJ: Metaplastic carcinomas of the breast. V. Metaplastic carcinoma with osteoclastic giant cells. Hum Pathol 21:1142–1150, 1990

303. Pitts WC, Rojas VA, Gaffey MJ, Rouse RV et al: Carcinomas with metaplasia and sarcomas of the breast. Am J Clin Pathol 95:623–632, 1991

304. Ramos CV, Taylor HB: Lipid-rich carcinoma of the breast: A clinicopathologic analysis of 13 examples. Cancer 33:812–819, 1974

305. Van Bogaert LJ, Maldague P: Histologic variants of lipid-secreting carcinoma of the breast. Virschows Arch A Pathol Anat Histopathol 375:345–353, 1977

306. Hood CI, Font RL, Zimmerman LE: Metastatic mammary carcinoma in the eyelid with histiocytoid appearance. Cancer 31:793–800, 1973

307. Paget J: On disease of the mammary areola preceding cancer of the mammary gland. St. Bartholomew's Hospital Reports 10:87–89, 1874

308. Rayne SC, Santa Cruz DJ: Anaplastic Paget's disease. Am J Surg Pathol 16:1085–1091, 1992

309. Dixon AR, Galea MH, Ellis IO et al: Paget's disease of the nipple. Br J Surg 78:722–723, 1991

310. Toker C: Clear cells of the nipple epidermis. Cancer 25:601–610, 1970

311. Sagebiel RW: Ultrastructural observations on epidermal cells in Paget's disease of the breast. Am J Pathol 57:49–64, 1969

312. Hitchcock A, Topham S, Bell J et al: Routine diagnosis of mammary Paget's disease: A modern approach. Am J Surg Pathol 16:58–61, 1992

313. Shertz WT, Balogh K: Metastasizing basal cell carcinoma of the nipple. Arch Pathol Lab Med 110:761–762, 1986

314. Lucas FV, Perez-Mesa C: Inflammatory carcinoma of the breast. Cancer 41:1595–1605, 1978

315. Fields JN, Kuske RR, Perez CA et al: Prognostic factors in inflammatory breast cancer. Cancer 63:1225–1232, 1989

316. Pisansky TM, Schaid DJ, Loprinzi CL, Donohue JH et al: Inflammatory breast cancer: Integration of irradiation, surgery, and chemotherapy. Am J Clin Oncol 15:376–387, 1992

317. Rosner D, Lane WW: Should all patients with node-negative breast cancer receive adjuvant therapy? Identifying additional subsets of low-risk patients who are highly curable by surgery alone. Cancer 68:1482–1494, 1991

318. Winchester DP: Adjuvant therapy for node-negative breast cancer: The use of prognostic factors in selecting patients. Cancer 67:1741–1743, 1991

319. Ziegler LD, Buzdar AU: Current status of adjuvant therapy of early breast cancer. Am J Clin Oncol 14:101–110, 1991

320. Petrek JA: Pregnancy-associated breast cancer. Semin Surg Oncol 7:306–310, 1991

321. Zemlickis D, Lishner M, Degendorfer P et al: Maternal and fetal outcome after breast cancer in pregnancy. Am J Obstet Gynecol 166:781–787, 1992

322. Nachlas MM: Irrationality in the management of breast cancer. I. The staging system. Cancer 68:681–690, 1991

323. Barr LC, Baum M: Time to abandon TNM staging of breast cancer? Lancet 339:915–917, 1992

324. Carter CL, Allen C, Henson DE: Relation of tumor size, lymph node status, and survival in 24,740 breast cancer cases. Cancer 63:181–187, 1989

325. Henson DE, Ries L, Freedman LS, Carriaga M: Relationship among outcome, stage of disease, and histologic grade for 22,616 cases of breast cancer. Cancer 68:2142–2149, 1991

326. Royal College of Pathologists Working Group: Pathology reporting in breast cancer screening. J Clin Pathol 44:710–725, 1991

327. Noel P, Chauvin F, Michot JP et al: Prognostic value of lymph node micrometastases detected by immunohistochemistry: Study of 168 cases of breast cancer with a 10-year follow-up. Ann Pathol 11:309–315, 1991

328. Galea MH, Athanassiou E, Bell J, Dilks B et al: Occult regional lymph node metastases from breast carcinoma: Immunohistological detection with antibodies CAM 5.2 and NCRC-11. J Pathol 165:221–227, 1991

329. Kiricuta CI, Tausch J: Mathematical model of axillary lymph node involvement based on 1446 complete axillary dissections in patients with breast carcinoma. Cancer 69:2496–2501, 1992

330. Hartveit F, Thorensen S, Thorsen T, Tangen T: Histological grade and efferent vascular invasion in human breast carcinoma. Br J Cancer 44:81–84, 1981

331. Orbo A, Stalsberg H, Kunde D: Topographic criteria in the diagnosis of tumor emboli in intramammary lymphatics. Cancer 66:972–977, 1990

332. Clement CG, Boracchi P, Andreola S, Del Vecchio M et al: Peritumoral lymphatic invasion in patients with node-negative mammary duct carcinoma. Cancer 69:1396–1403, 1992

333. Clayton F: Pathologic correlates of survival in 378 lymph node-negative infiltrating ductal breast carcinomas: Mitotic count is the best single predictor. Cancer 68:1309–1317, 1991

334. Simpson JF, Dutt PL, Page DL: Expression of mitoses per thousand cells and cell density in breast carcinomas: A proposal. Hum Pathol 23:608–611, 1992

335. van Diest PJ, Baak JP, Matze-Cok P et al: Reproducibility of mitosis counting in 2,469 breast cancer specimens: Results from the multicenter morphometric mammary carcinoma project. Hum Pathol 23:603–607, 1992

336. Pezner RD, Terz J, Ben-Ezra J, Hill LR: Now there are two effective conservation approaches for patients with Stage I and II breast cancer: How pathological assessment of inked resection margins can provide valuable information for the radiation oncologist. Am J Clin Oncol 13:175–179, 1990

337. Kurtz JM, Jacquemier J, Amalric R, Brandone H et al: Risk factors for breast recurrence in premenopausal and postmenopausal patients with ductal cancer treated by conservation therapy. Cancer 65:1867–1878, 1990

338. Schnitt SJ, Connolly JL, Harris JR et al: Pathologic predictors of early local recurrence in stage I and II breast cancer treated by primary radiation therapy. Cancer 53:1049–1057, 1984

339. Mate TP, Carter D, Fisher DB et al: A clinical and histopathologic analysis of the results of primary radiation therapy in stage I and II breast carcinomas. Cancer 58:1995–2002, 1986

340. Chevallier B, Heintzmann F, Mosseri V, Dauce JP et al: Prognostic value of estrogen and progesterone receptors in operable breast cancer: Results of a univariate and multivariate analysis. Cancer 62:2517–2524, 1988

341. Nomura Y, Miura S, Koyama H, Enomoto K et al: Relative effect of steroid hormone receptors on the prognosis of patients with operable breast cancer. Cancer 69:153–164, 1992

342. Cudahy TJ, Boeryd BR, Franlund BK, Nordenskjöld BA: A comparison of three different methods for the determination of estrogen receptors in human breast cancer. Am J Clin Pathol 90:583–590, 1988

343. Baddoura FK, Cohen C, Unger ER, DeRose PB, Chenggis M: Image analysis for quantitation of estrogen receptor in formalin-fixed paraffin-embedded sections of breast carcinoma. Mod Pathol 4:91–95, 1991

344. Graham DM, Jin L, Lloyd RV: Detection of estrogen receptor in paraffin-embedded sections of breast carcinoma by immunohistochemistry and in situ hybridization. Am J Surg Pathol 15:475–485, 1991

345. Visscher DW, Zarbo RJ, Greenawald KA, Crissman JD: Prognostic significance of morphological parameters and flow cytometric DNA analysis in carcinoma of the breast. Pathol Annu 25(1):171–210, 1990

346. Frierson HF Jr: Ploidy analysis and S-phase fraction determination by flow cytometry of invasive adenocarcinomas of the breast. Am J Surg Pathol 15:358–367, 1991

347. Fisher B, Gunduz N, Costantino J, Fisher ER et al: DNA flow cytometric analysis of primary operable breast cancer: Relation of ploidy and S-phase fraction to outcome of patients in NSABP B-04. Cancer 68:1465–1475, 1991

348. Robinson RA: Defining the limits of DNA cytometry. Am J Clin Pathol 98:275–277, 1992

349. Yee LD, Kacinski BM, Carter D: Oncogene structure, function, and expression in breast cancer. Semin Diagn Pathol 6:110–125, 1989

350. Naber SP, Tsutsumi Y, Yin S, Zolnay SA et al: Strategies for the analysis of oncogene overexpression: Studies of the neu oncogene in breast carcinoma. Am J Clin Pathol 94:125–136, 1990

351. Leslie KO, Howard P: Oncogenes and antioncogenes in human breast carcinoma. Pathol Annu 27(Part 1): 311–342, 1992

352. Anderson TJ: c-erb B-2 oncogene in breast cancer: The right target or a decoy? Hum Pathol 23:971–973, 1992

353. Battifora H, Gaffey M, Esteban J, Mehta P et al: Immunohistochemical assay of neu/c-erb B-2 oncogene product in paraffin-embedded tissues in early breast cancer: Retrospective follow-up study of 245 stage I and II cases. Mod Pathol 4:466–474, 1991

354. Barbareschi M, Leonardi E, Mauri FA, Serio G, Dalla Palma P: p53 and c-erb B-2 protein expression in breast carcinomas: An immunohistochemical study including correlations with receptor status, proliferation markers, and clinical stage in human breast cancer. Am J Clin Pathol 98:408–418, 1992

355. Dervan PA, Gilmartin LG, Loftus BM, Carney DN: Breast carcinoma kinetics: Argyrophilic nucleolar organizer region counts correlate with Ki67 scores. Am J Clin Pathol 92:401–407, 1989

356. Tham KY, Page DL: AgNor and Ki-67 in breast lesions. Am J Clin Pathol 92:518–520, 1989

357. Sahin AA, Ro J, Ro JY et al: Ki-67 immunostaining in

node-negative stage I/II breast carcinoma: Significant correlation with prognosis. Cancer 68:549–557, 1991

358. Waldman FM, Chew K, Ljung B-M, Goodson W et al: A comparison between bromodeoxyuridine and ³H thymidine labeling in human breast tumors. Mod Pathol 4:718–722, 1991

359. Kennedy JC, El-Badawy N, DeRose PB, Cohen C: Comparison of cell proliferation in breast carcinoma using image analysis (Ki-67) and flow cytometric systems. Anal Quant Cytol Histol 14:304–311, 1992

360. Van Diest PJ, Baak JPA: The morphometric prognostic index is the strongest prognosticator in premenopausal lymph node-negative and lymph node-positive breast cancer patients. Hum Pathol 22:326–330, 1991

361. Pienta KJ, Coffey DS: Correlation of nuclear morphometry with progression of breast cancer. Cancer 68:2012–2016, 1991

362. Weidner N, Folkman J, Pozza F et al: Tumor angiogenesis: A new significant and independent prognostic indicator in early-stage breast carcinoma. J Natl Cancer Inst 84:1875–1887, 1992

363. Rochefort H: Biological and clinical significance of cathepsin D in breast cancer. Acta Oncol 31:125–130, 1992

364. Ro J, Sahin A, Ro JY, Fritsche H et al: Immunohistochemical analysis of P-glycoprotein expression correlated with chemotherapy resistance in locally advanced breast cancer. Hum Pathol 21:787–791, 1990

365. Kennedy S, Merino MJ, Swain SM, Lippman ME: The effects of hormonal and chemotherapy on tumoral and nonneoplastic breast tissue. Hum Pathol 21:192–198, 1990

366. Solin LJ, Fowble BL, Schultz DJ, Rubenstein JR, Goodman RL: The detection of local recurrence after definitive irradiation for early stage carcinoma of the breast. Cancer 65:2497–2502, 1990

367. Dornfeld JM, Thompson SK, Shurbaji MS: Radiation-induced changes in the breast: A potential diagnostic pitfall on fine-needle aspiration. Diagn Cytopathol 8:79–81, 1992

368. Gilchrist KW, Gould VE, Hirschl S et al: Interobserver variation in the identification of breast carcinoma in intramammary lymphatics. Hum Pathol 13:170–172, 1982

369. Lee AKC, DeLellis RA, Silverman ML et al: Lymphatic and blood vessel invasion in breast carcinoma: A useful prognostic indicator? Hum Pathol 17:984–987, 1986

370. Schwartz GF, Feig SA, Rosenberg AL et al: Staging and treatment of clinically occult breast cancer. Cancer 53:1379–1384, 1984

371. Tabar I, Fagerberg G, Day NE, Duffy O, Kitchin R: Breast cancer treatment and natural history: New insights from results of screening. Lancet 339:412–414, 1992

372. Jackson SM: Carcinoma of the breast: The significance of supraclavicular lymph node metastases. Clin Radiol 17:107–114, 1966

373. Rubens RD: Metastatic breast cancer and its complications. Curr Opin Oncol 4:1050–1054, 1992

374. Debonis D, Terz JJ, Eldar S, Hill LR: Survival of patients with metastatic breast cancer diagnosed between 1955 and 1980. J Surg Oncol 48:158–163, 1991

375. Yamashita K, Ueda T, Komatsubara Y et al: Breast cancer with bone-only metastases: Visceral metastases-free rate in relation to anatomic distribution of bone metastases. Cancer 68:634–637, 1991

376. Leone BA, Romero A, Rabinovich MG, Vallejo CT et al: Stage IV breast cancer: Clinical course and survival of patients with osseous versus extraosseous metastases at initial diagnosis. Am J Clin Oncol 11:618–622, 1988

377. Perez JE, Machiavelli M, Leone BA, Romero A et al: Bone-only versus visceral-only metastatic pattern in breast cancer: Analysis of 150 patients. A GOCS study. Am J Clin Oncol 13:294–298, 1990

378. Mansi JL, Easton D, Berger U, Gazet JC et al: Bone marrow micrometastases in primary breast cancer: Prognostic significance after 6 years' follow-up. Eur J Cancer 27:1552–1555, 1991

379. Bundred NJ, Ratcliffe WA, Walker RA et al: Parathyroid hormone related protein and hypercalcaemia in breast cancer. BMJ 303(6816):1506–1509, 1991

380. Goldsmith HS, Bailey HD, Callahan EL, Beattie EJ: Pulmonary lymphangitic metastases from breast carcinoma. Arch Surg 94:483–488, 1967

381. Fentiman IS, Millis R, Sexton S, Hayward JL: Pleural effusion in breast cancer: A review of 105 cases. Cancer 47:2087–2092, 1981

382. Peled IJ, Okon E, Weschler Z, Wexler MR: Distant, late metastases to skin of carcinoma of the breast. J Dermatol Surg Oncol 8:192–195, 1982

383. Dickson R: Regulation of tumor-host interactions in breast cancer. J Steroid Biochem Mol Biol 41:389–400, 1992

384. Robbins GF, Berg JW: Bilateral primary breast cancer. A prospective clinicopathological study. Cancer 17:1501–1527, 1964

385. McDivitt RW, Stewart FW, Berg JW: Tumors of the breast. Atlas of tumor pathology, second series. Fascicle 2. Washington, DC, Armed Forces Institute of Pathology, 1968

386. Dawson PJ, Maloney T, Gimotty P et al: Bilateral breast cancer: One disease or two? Breast Cancer Res Treat 19:233–244, 1991

387. Ringberg A, Palmer B, Linell F: The contralateral breast at reconstructive surgery after breast cancer operation: A histopathological study. Breast Cancer Res Treat 2:151–161, 1982

388. Rosen PP, Groshen S, Kinne DW, Hellman S: Non-mammary malignant neoplasms in patients with stage I ($T_1N_0M_0$) and stage II ($T_1N_1M_0$) breast carcinoma: A long-term follow-up study. Am J Clin Oncol 12:369–374, 1989

389. Forbes J: The surgery of early breast cancer. Curr Opin Oncol 4:1027–1034, 1992

390. Vicini FA, Eberlein TJ, Connolly JL et al: The optimal extent of resection for patients with stages I or II breast cancer treated with conservative surgery and radiotherapy. Ann Surg 214:200–204, 1991

391. McCormick B: Radiation therapy for breast cancer. Curr Opin Oncol 4:1035–1040, 1992

392. Bonadonna G, Veronesi V, Brambilla C et al: Primary chemotherapy to avoid mastectomy in tumours with diameters of three centimeters or more. J Natl Cancer Inst 82:1539–1545, 1990

393. Harris JR, Connolly JL, Schnitt SJ et al: Clinical-pathologic study of early breast cancer treated by primary radiation therapy. J Clin Oncol 3:184–189, 1985

394. Tripathy D, Henderson IC: Systemic adjuvant therapy for breast cancer. Curr Opin Oncol 4:1041–1049, 1992

395. Early Breast Cancer Trialists' Collaborative Group: Systemic treatment of early breast cancer by hormonal, cytotoxic, or immune therapy: 33 randomised trials involving 31,000 recurrences and 24,000 deaths among 75,000 women. Lancet 339:1–15, 71–85, 1992

396. Fisher B, Redmond C: Systemic therapy in node-negative patients: Updated findings from NSABP clinical trials. National Surgical Adjuvant Breast and Bowel Project. Monogr Natl Cancer Inst 11:105–116, 1992

397. McGuire WL, Tandon AK, Allred DC et al: Prognosis and treatment decisions in patients with breast cancer without axillary node involvement. Cancer 70:1775–1781, 1992

398. Jordan VC: Overview from the international conference on long-term tamoxifen therapy for breast cancer. J Natl Cancer Inst 84:231–234, 1992

399. Pollard SG, Marks PV, Temple LN, Thompson HH: Breast sarcoma: A clinicopathologic review of 25 cases. Cancer 66:941–944, 1990

400. Lerner HJ: Fibrosarcoma of the breast: Case report and literature review. Am Surg 31:196–199, 1965

401. Jones MW, Norris HJ, Wargotz ES, Weiss SW: Fibrosarcoma–malignant fibrous histiocytoma of the breast: A clinicopathological study of 32 cases. Am J Surg Pathol 16:667–674, 1992

402. Austin RM, Dupree WB: Liposarcoma of the breast: A clinicopathologic study of 20 cases. Hum Pathol 17:906–913, 1986

403. Berg JW, De Cosse JJ, Fracchia AA, Farrow J: Stromal sarcomas of the breast: A unified approach to connective tissue sarcomas other than cystosarcoma phyllodes. Cancer 15:418–424, 1962

404. Callery CD, Rosen PP, Kinne DW: Sarcoma of the breast: A study of 32 patients with reappraisal of classification and therapy. Ann Surg 201:527–532, 1985

405. Arista-Nasr J, Gonzales-Gomez I, Angeles-Angeles A et al: Primary recurrent leiomyosarcoma of the breast: Case report with ultrastructural and immunohistochemical study and review of the literature. Am J Clin Pathol 92:500–505, 1989

406. Chen TKK, Kirkegaard DD, Bocian JJ: Angiosarcoma of the breast. Cancer 46:368–371, 1980

407. Merino MJ, Carter D, Berman M: Angiosarcoma of the breast. Am J Surg Pathol 7:53–60, 1983

408. Rosen PP, Kimmel M, Ernsberger D: Mammary angiosarcoma: The prognostic significance of tumor differentiation. Cancer 62:2145–2151, 1988

409. Brentani MM, Pacheco MM, Oshima TF et al: Steroid receptors in breast angiosarcoma. Cancer 51:2105–2111, 1983

410. Moskaluk CA, Merino MJ, Danforth DN, Medeiros LJ: Low-grade angiosarcoma of the skin of the breast: A complication of lumpectomy and radiation therapy for breast carcinoma. Hum Pathol 23:710–714, 1992

411. Stokkel MPM, Peterse HL: Angiosarcoma of the breast after lumpectomy and radiation therapy for adenocarcinoma. Cancer 69:2965–2968, 1992

412. Stewart FW, Treves N: Lymphangiosarcoma in postmastectomy lymphedema. Cancer 1:64–81, 1948

413. Miettinen M, Lehto V-P, Virtanen I: Postmastectomy angiosarcoma (Stewart-Treves syndrome): Light-microscopic, immunohistological, and ultrastructural characteristics of two cases. Am J Surg Pathol 7:329–340, 1983

414. Silverberg SG, Kay S, Koss LG: Postmastectomy lymphangiosarcoma: Ultrastructural observations. Cancer 27:100–108, 1971

415. Cohen PL, Brooks JJ: Lymphomas of the breast: A clinicopathologic and immunohistochemical study of primary and secondary cases. Cancer 67:1359–1369, 1991

416. Giardini R, Piccolo C, Rilke F: Primary non-Hodgkin's lymphomas of the female breast. Cancer 69:725–735, 1992

417. Aozasaki K, Ohsawa M, Saeki K et al: Malignant lymphoma of the breast: Immunologic type and association with lymphocytic mastopathy. Am J Clin Pathol 97:699–704, 1992

418. Pascoe HR: Tumors composed of immature granulocytes occurring in the breast in chronic granulocytic leukemia. Cancer 15:697–704, 1970

419. Oberman HA: Primary lymphoreticular neoplasms of the breast. Surg Gynecol Obstet 123:1047–1051, 1966

420. Nielsen M, Andersen JA, Henriksen FW et al: Metastases to the breast from extramammary carcinomas. Acta Pathol Microbiol Scand (A) 89:251–256, 1981

421. Yamasaki H, Saw D, Zdanowitz J, Faltz LL: Ovarian carcinoma metastasis to the breast: Case report and review of the literature. Am J Surg Pathol 17:193–197, 1993

Pathology in Gynecology and Obstetrics, Fourth Edition, edited by Claude Gompel and Steven G. Silverberg. J. B. Lippincott Company, Philadelphia © 1994.

11 Extragenital Pathology in Obstetrics and Gynecology

Hernando Salazar and Richard J. Stock

Most disease processes can occur in women of any age, regardless of their reproductive state. However, there are specific extragenital problems that occur as causes, complications, or secondary effects of gynecologic or obstetric conditions and may alter reproductive function. This chapter discusses the most important extragenital problems related to gynecologic and obstetric practice, focusing on those that may come to the pathologist by way of biopsy or autopsy material. The problems are presented by organ system.

ENDOCRINE SYSTEM

About 30% of patients with amenorrhea-galactorrhea syndrome also have a prolactin-producing adenoma of the pituitary gland.[1-4] Hyperprolactinemia also results from blockage or destruction of the prolactin-producing dopaminergic centers or their hypothalamic-hypophyseal tracts by tumors (eg, craniopharyngioma, meningioma, or pituitary neoplasms other than prolactinomas), inflammatory lesions (eg, sarcoid or tuberculous granulomas), degenerative lesions (eg, amyloidosis), traumatic or surgical stalk transection, or irradiation.[5,6] Hyperprolactinemia may be secondary to hormonal therapy (eg, estrogens, oral contraceptives, or thyrotropin-releasing hormone), anesthesia, dopamine or dopamine-receptor blocking agents (eg, reserpine, methyldopa, MAO inhibitors, phenothiazines, and opiates), hypothyroidism, renal failure, chronic nipple stimulation, or ectopic production of prolactin by neuroendocrine tumors (eg, lung and

kidney).[6] Most of these patients are infertile but regain their fertility and can become pregnant once prolactin levels drop close to normal after surgical (transsphenoidal partial hypophysectomy) or medical (bromocriptine) treatment.[7-9]

In the past, pituitary tumors associated with amenorrhea-galactorrhea syndrome were usually classified as "nonfunctional" or "chromophobic" adenomas because they were formed by degranulated cells that did not stain with the standard methods.[10] It was not until 1971, when the identification of prolactin-producing cells of "lactotrophs" by immunoassay was standardized, that prolactinomas were recognized as functional neoplasms capable of causing hyperprolactinemia.[11-14]

Prolactin-producing adenomas are the most common tumors of the human pituitary gland.[15,16] Most are microadenomas measuring less than 1 cm in diameter, but they may be larger (macroadenomas) and capable of causing deformation of the sella or compression of the hypothalamus, optic chiasm, and other neighboring structures. Macroadenomas may be diagnosed clinically and radiologically by standard radiographic techniques. The diagnosis of microadenomas requires computed tomography (CT) scans because they usually do not produce deformities of the sella.

Before the introduction of bromoergocriptine (bromocriptine), a potent antiprolactin agent that is now the preferred method of treatment of prolactinomas, the only therapeutic approaches were surgery and radiation.[17] Surgical removal of the tumor by partial transsphenoidal hypophysectomy has been the source of specimens suitable for biochemical and morphologic studies. Prolactin-secreting pituitary adenomas are usually "chromophobic" with standard stains because they contain scant secretory granules (Fig. 11-1). The prolactin content of the neoplastic cells is high, although it does not take the form of granules.[18,19]

Ultrastructurally, the cells are large and oval with irregular nuclei and abundant cytoplasm rich in mitochondria and rough endoplasmic reticulum. There is a prominent Golgi system. The secretory granules usually are scant and small (<100 nm in diameter), in sharp contrast to the characteristic large and irregular granules of the normal lactotrophs (600 to 800 nm in diameter). The neoplastic lactotrophs apparently are incapable of forming normal granules. The high prolactin content is present as particulate or homogeneous, medium-dense material within the endoplasmic reticulum cisternae and Golgi apparatus or as discrete droplets with abnormal granular organization (Fig. 11-2). The secretory granules are frequently released ectopically into the intercellular spaces rather than through the vascular pole of the cells into the capillaries.[18,19]

The content of prolactin in the tumor can be assessed qualitatively by immunocytochemical labeling with specific antiprolactin antibodies.[20] It can be assessed quantitatively by incubation of tumor fragments and measurement of hormone levels in the effluent, expressed as nanograms per milligram of tissue.[18]

There is moderate hyperplasia of the nonsecretory stellate cells surrounding the microadenomas, the significance of which is not clear.[21] Significant hyperplasia of lactotrophs within the parenchyma surrounding the adenoma may account for the resid-ual elevated serum prolactin levels observed after "complete" removal of the tumors.[22,23]

The pituitary gland normally increases in size during pregnancy. The size increase is probably due to a physiologic hyperplasia of lactotrophs and somatotrophs, with corresponding increases in the levels of prolactin and growth hormone secondary to the normal increase of placental estrogen during pregnancy.[6] Estrogen seems to exert direct and indirect (antidopaminergic) stimulating actions on lactotrophs. This may explain the chronic hyperprolactinemia observed in patients receiving hormone contraceptives. However, galactorrhea is absent in these cases, probably due to the inhibitory effect of estrogen and progesterone on the breast's lactogenic functions. Contrary to previous indications that oral contraceptives or estrogen therapy would result in the development of prolactinomas,[24–28] multicenter studies with large numbers of patients have failed to prove such a cause-effect relation.[29,30]

Postpartum Pituitary Necrosis (Sheehan's Syndrome)

Although pituitary necrosis resulting in hypopituitarism had been known as part of the so-called Simmonds' syndrome (panhypopituitarism with cachexia), it was Sheehan who first recognized the problem of an ischemic necrosis or infarction of the pituitary gland during the postpartum period (Sheehan's syndrome).[31] The mechanism by which hypophyseal infarction sometimes occurs in these patients seems to be part of a general circulatory deficit secondary to postpartum uterine bleeding. Systemic

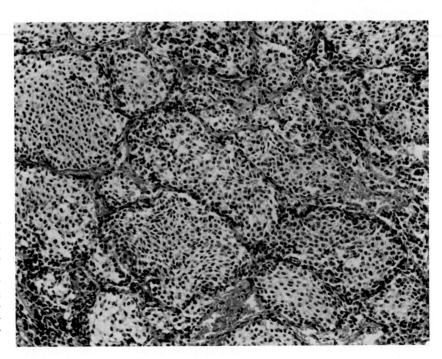

FIGURE 11-1 Panoramic view of a pituitary adenoma removed by transsphenoidal partial hypophysectomy from a 25-year-old patient with hyperprolactinemia, galactorrhea, and history of oral contraception. The tumor is lobulated and formed by cords and masses of monotonous, uniform cells with clear unstained (degranulated) cytoplasm. High prolactin content was demonstrated by a prolactin-specific peroxidase-antiperoxidase (PAP) method.

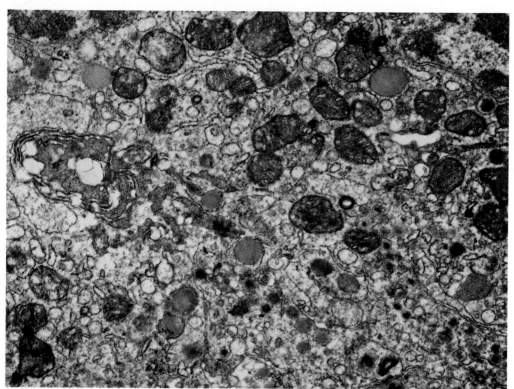

FIGURE 11-2 Portion of lactotroph in a prolactin-producing microadenoma removed from a 22-year-old woman with galactorrhea-amenorrhea. Serum prolactin levels were 490 ng/mL (normal < 25 ng/mL) and tumor levels were 1.24 µg/mg of tissue (normal <0.37 µg/mg). Note well-developed organelles, small membrane-bound secretory granules, and poorly formed granules with decreased density and amorphous material of similar density in Golgi structures. These suggest abundant hormonal content but abnormal packing of secretory granules (×47,000).

vascular collapse and shock are, in turn, probably related to hypofibrinogenemia and disseminated intravascular coagulation. The acute infarction of the hypertrophied gland at the end of gestation results in rapid loss of most or all of the hypophyseal trophic hormones. Often, the entire gland is involved, although the neurohypophysis is sometimes preserved.

The magnitude of the clinical picture depends on the extent of the infarct. If more than 75% of the gland is necrotic, the result is severe panhypopituitarism with morphologic changes and functional deficits of the target organs.[32–35] Lactation is terminated, and the thyroid, adrenals, and gonads atrophy. This is followed by amenorrhea, loss of libido, loss of pubic and axillary hair, trophic and pigmentary changes of the skin, general muscle weakness, decreased tolerance to cold temperature, and other conditions of endocrine deficit. If the posterior lobe is compromised, the problem is complicated by diabetes insipidus.

Grossly, the pituitary gland appears enlarged and congested and has a burgundy-red discoloration. It is friable in the necrotic areas if the infarction is recent. After some time, healing by fibrosis occurs, and the gland appears small, firm, gray-brown, and irregular due to scarring. Microscopically, the necrotic areas are replaced by dense, poorly vascular-ized fibroconnective tissue with islands of preserved parenchyma usually containing largely degranulated cells (Fig. 11-3). The noninfarcted areas may show compensatory hyperplasia and hypergranulation. Recovery is highly variable.

Diabetes Mellitus and Pregnancy

The advances of the past decades in the understanding of diabetes and abnormal glucose metabolism have resulted in great improvements in the management of the pregnant diabetic patient. These improvements have translated into decreased fetal and neonatal morbidity and mortality. Before 1922, no infant of a diabetic mother survived.[36] With the availability of insulin, the infant survival rate improved to about 70% in 1960 and to more than 90% in the 1980s, reaching the neonatal mortality rate of the general population.[37] Likewise, the recognition and adequate management of patients with so-called diabetes of pregnancy (transient abnormal glucose metabolism of gestation), which occurs in about 2.5% of all pregnancies, have prevented maternal and fetal morbidity and death.

Adult-onset (type II) diabetes differs etiologically and pathogenetically from juvenile, insulin-depen-

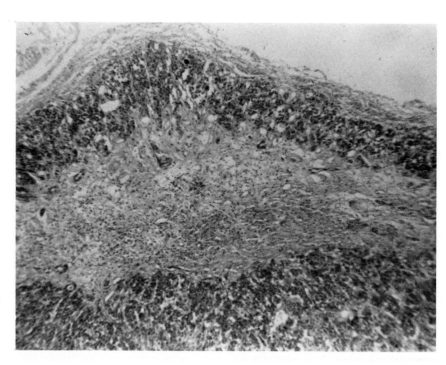

FIGURE 11-3 Adenohypophysis with a large central infarct in the process of healing. Note the density of cells in the preserved areas and fibroblastic proliferation in the infarcted area.

dent (type I) diabetes. In adult-onset diabetic pregnancies, decreased insulin secretion and markedly reduced insulin sensitivity are pathophysiologically important, independent of the effect of obesity.[38,39] The main pathogenetic mechanism in juvenile diabetes, on the other hand, is an absolute deficiency of insulin.

During pregnancy, whether normal or diabetic, metabolic changes occur in a biphasic fashion, with significant changes at about the 27th week of gestation (the beginning of the third trimester). These changes are related to factors of maternal fuel utilization, such as storage of adipose tissue, insulin secretion and resistance, glucose utilization, and concentrations of high-density lipoprotein cholesterol.[40,41] At about the 27th week, the diabetic mother switches from a glucose-based to a lipid-based source of energy from stored reserves and insulating fats. This saves glucose and other nutrients for fetal nutrition and growth, with a significant increase in transplacental transport to the fetus. This may explain the fetal macrosomia of diabetic pregnancies, with uncontrolled glucose assimilated by the fetus. Infant survival is directly related to the degree of control of maternal glucose.[42] At the time of metabolic transition in the mother, gestational diabetes usually becomes apparent or ketoacidosis occurs in the pregnant diabetic. The management of the diabetic pregnancy, therefore, is geared to the regulation of concentrations of plasma glucose and other circulating fuels.

Microvascular disease or diabetic microangiopathy is the most significant complication, resulting in renal, retinal, cardiac, cutaneous, and soft-tissue chronic ischemia.[43]

Diabetic Nephropathy

Diabetic nephropathy is a progressive disease of the microvasculature of the glomerulus that results in increased permeability to protein, glomerular scarring, and, finally, irreversible peripheral edema and chronic progressive renal failure.[44–46] The risk of developing nephropathy varies from 30% to 50% in type I and type II diabetes. The incidence of nephropathy among pregnant diabetic women is about 5% in the general population and 10% to 25% in obstetric referral centers.

Histologic changes in the kidney precede the clinical diagnosis of nephropathy by several years. These changes consist primarily of basement membrane thickening of afferent and efferent glomerular arterioles. Nodular or diffuse intercapillary sclerosis of the glomerular tuft results from increased accumulation of plasma proteins on the capillary basement membranes and the mesangium (Fig. 11-4). Progression of these abnormalities leads to gradual glomerular sclerosis, secondary tubular atrophy, and chronic renal failure. By the time azotemia appears and creatinine clearance drops to less than 25 mL/min, hypertension occurs and accelerates the progression of the vascular disease, contributing to mortality.

Diabetic nephropathy has implications for pregnancy mainly because it is complicated by hypertension and results in a high incidence of preeclampsia, accelerated hypertension, fetal distress, fetal growth retardation, and perinatal mortality. Pregnancy in itself apparently does not accelerate or worsen the progression of nephropathy in the diabetic patient. The main objective in the management of these

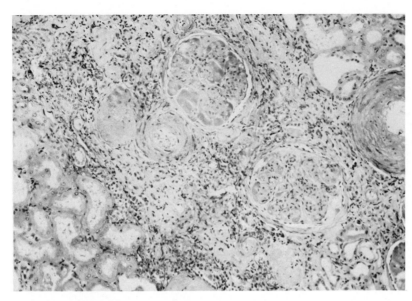

FIGURE 11-4 Diabetic nephropathy, showing both nodular glomerulosclerosis (Kimmelstiel-Wilson lesion) and severe arterial and arteriolar sclerosis. (Courtesy of Dr. A. Andrew Abraham, George Washington University, Washington, DC)

pregnancies is to save the fetus and the mother, and preterm delivery is frequently required. Improvements in perinatal and neonatal intensive care facilities have greatly reduced the perinatal morbidity and mortality associated with the preterm delivery of infants of diabetic mothers. The incidence of spontaneous abortions and congenital malformations is much higher in diabetic mothers with poor glycemic control.[47]

Diabetic Retinopathy

Retinopathy is the most prevalent form of microvascular lesion in diabetics.[48,49] It is generally divided into three main types according to the kind and magnitude of the lesions:

1. Nonproliferative or background retinopathy is characterized by microaneurysms, microhemorrhages, hard exudates, and edema. Unless these lesions occur in the perimacular area, vision is not affected.
2. Preproliferative retinopathy is characterized by intraretinal microvascular abnormalities, microhemorrhages, and soft or "cotton-wool" exudates. This lesion may progress to neovascularization.
3. Proliferative retinopathy is the final stage, with extensive neovascularization at the disc and elsewhere. Fibrosis, preretinal and massive vitreal hemorrhages, and retinal detachment result in permanent loss of vision.

The pathogenesis of diabetic retinopathy is not clear. It does not seem to be based, as is the case elsewhere, on thickening of the capillary basement membranes. Instead, it is based on a breakdown of the blood-retinal barrier with vascular damage, leakage of blood and plasma proteins, hyperglycemia-in-

duced hypercoagulation, and decreased fibrinolysis, with endothelial deposits, microthrombosis, and proliferation of pericytes and fibroblasts.[50]

The role of pregnancy as a complicating factor in diabetic retinopathy is not clear. Apparently, it depends on the magnitude of the problem. Background nonproliferative retinopathy progresses in severity during pregnancy, with a maximum peak in the third trimester, and regresses postpartum. Problems occur in pregnant patients with active proliferative retinopathy, mainly due to intraocular hemorrhage, and blindness may occur during pregnancy. The proliferating neovascularization of the disc and other areas progresses through pregnancy if untreated. Laser-beam pararetinal photocoagulation and therapeutic abortion are indicated in cases of florid discal neovascularization in early pregnancy. Cases in therapeutic or spontaneous remission at the onset of pregnancy do not seem to progress to catastrophic stages.

Because excessive elevation of blood glucose levels for prolonged periods is the most important factor in the origin and development of diabetic retinopathy, strict glycemic control is the most crucial therapeutic measure for the prevention and control of retinal sequelae in diabetic patients. The following risk factors have been identified in diabetic pregnant subjects:[48]

Pregnancy per se accelerates the natural progression of retinopathies.

Hyperglycemia and hypertension potentiate this acceleration.

The rate of acceleration depends on the duration of diabetes and the state of the retina at the onset of pregnancy.

Rapid normalization of blood glucose may be counterproductive, requiring intensive surveillance and aggressive retinal therapy.

VASCULAR SYSTEM

Thromboembolism Associated With Pregnancy and Contraception

Virchow first described clots in the lungs that had arisen elsewhere in the body, excluding the pulmonary arteries, and termed this process *embolia*.[51] He postulated that the intravascular clots were the result of vascular trauma, vascular stasis, and a state of hypercoagulability (Virchow's triad). Although our knowledge of the clotting mechanism has grown by leaps and bounds in the last few decades, our concepts of the actual causes of thrombosis and embolization still remain fairly nonspecific and within the boundaries of Virchow's triad.

There are several possible risk factors for thrombosis and embolization in the obstetric or gynecologic patient. In general, pregnancy has been viewed as a high-risk state.[52,53] However, it appears that the period of highest relative risk is the postpartum period; the antepartum period does not appear to be associated with excess risk. In contrast to popular belief, there is no evidence that varicose veins constitute a positive risk factor. Prolonged immobilization, pelvic surgery, obesity, increasing age, and malignancy do constitute increased risks. It has been postulated that oral contraceptives and estrogens, when used for lactation suppression, are associated with increased risks for thromboembolic phenomena.[54–57] Peculiar to pregnancy and the use of oral contraceptives are the rare occurrences of highly localized vascular intimal proliferation, sometimes with thrombosis, that may involve the pulmonary, renal, hepatic, ovarian, and intracranial vessels, including the sagittal sinuses (Fig. 11-5). Pulmonary embolization, on the other hand, is a problem of major clinical significance in obstetric practice, particularly in the postpartum period. Although the incidence of death secondary to pulmonary embolism is decreasing, it is still the second leading cause of death in the post-cesarean section patient.[58]

Of Virchow's triad, vascular trauma has predominated as the focal point in thrombosis research. Major steps in the initiation of localized coagulation are localized platelet aggregation, subsequent release of adenosine diphosphate, and availability of platelet factor 3. There is little evidence that this chain of events is actually responsible for localized thrombosis in humans. Rather, it is believed that vascular stasis and altered coagulability play major roles because they occur in the area of the venous valves. In the postpartum state, significant alterations occur in the diameters and pressures of the ovarian veins, which are important sites of thrombosis. Principles other than changes in procoagulant and anticoagulant factors must be considered. Rheologic aspects may play a significant role, especially when considering the changing vessel diameters and flow patterns.[59] Hypercoagulability in pregnancy is thought to exist and may be related to the increases in all the plasma factors involved in the coagulation mechanism, except for factors XI and XIII.

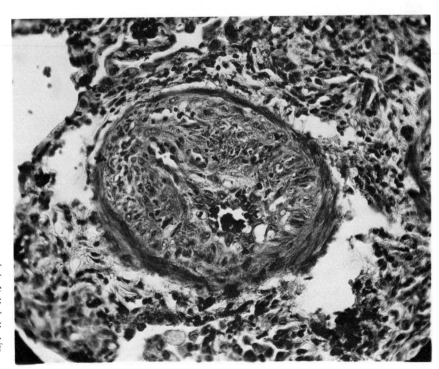

FIGURE 11-5 Branch of a pulmonary artery in a pregnant woman: marked cellular intimal proliferation with almost complete luminal obliteration. (Irey NS, Norris HJ: Intimal vascular lesions associated with female reproductive steroids. Arch Pathol 96: 227–234, 1973. (Courtesy of Dr. Henry J. Norris and the Armed Forces Institute of Pathology, Washington, DC)

Oral Contraception and Cardiovascular Disease

Initial studies of oral contraceptive use focused on the alterations in coagulation activation factors and fibrinolytic systems. Changes were identified that affected both systems, but whether the overall effect clinically resulted in increased risk for thrombosis generally was not clear.[60] Many epidemiologic studies have suggested an increased risk of cardiovascular disease with oral contraceptive use. Unfortunately, these studies have been hampered by the many oral contraceptives available and their changing formulation with time, by the fact that women use different contraceptives for varying periods, by the generally unreliable information regarding the use of a product, and by variable familial, work, and medical conditions or habits that might contribute to cardiovascular events.[61,62] In general, there appears to be an increased risk of venous thrombosis with the use of preparations with high estrogen doses (most of which are no longer on the market).[63]

More recent studies have focused on changes in serum cholesterol, triglycerides, and lipoproteins. The progestins, especially formulations containing levonorgestrel, tend to affect adversely the markers for coronary heart disease.[64] Epidemiologic studies do not suggest a increased risk after discontinuation of oral contraceptives.[65]

Lower-Extremity Thrombophlebitis in Pregnancy

Deep vein thrombosis is difficult to diagnose accurately. Depending on the criteria used, the incidence in pregnancy ranges from 1.9 in 1000 to 30 in 100. This problem is rare antepartum but is 10 times more frequent in the postpartum period. It is correlated with increased age, traumatic and operative deliveries, preeclampsia, dehydration, anemia, prolonged bed rest, infection, and nutritional deficiencies. Often these major problems arise in the postpartum state, in which pulmonary embolization constitutes a major threat. In the event of a death secondary to pulmonary embolism and suspected deep vein thrombosis of the lower extremities, it is imperative to evaluate these vessels at autopsy. This is done in routine autopsies by "milking" the veins of the leg while observing the free flow of blood from the transected pelvic vessels. If there is a high degree of suspicion, the vascular spaces of the legs should be opened and examined thoroughly.

Ovarian Vein Thrombosis and Thrombophlebitis

In the third trimester of pregnancy, the ovarian veins increase in diameter as much as 60-fold to about 26 mm.[66] Although venous pressure does not appear to rise in pregnancy, there is a precipitous fall in the ovarian vein pressure immediately postpartum and a shift in the pattern in venous drainage from the uterus. These changes are probably the major factors associated with the occurrence of ovarian vein thrombosis in the immediate postpartum period.[67] The clinical picture of this condition is characterized by fever, abdominal pain, and, at times, a palpable mass. The differential diagnosis often includes appendicitis, because ovarian vein thrombosis more often occurs on the right side. Diagnosis frequently is made at the time of exploratory laparotomy. Cultures from the vessels usually are negative. This is in contrast to a frequent occurrence of positive cultures from ovarian vein thrombosis associated with septic abortion or pelvic inflammatory disease. Ovarian vein thrombi are probably the major source of postpartum pulmonary emboli; therefore, examination of these vessels at autopsy is imperative.

Renal Vein Thrombosis

Renal vein thrombosis appears to be a rare complication of pregnancy and has been said to be secondary to uterine compression of the inferior vena cava.[68] The main symptoms often consist of lumbar or abdominal pain, which is associated with proteinuria if the process is acute. The process may be gradual and first identified by the discovery of a mass on abdominal postpartum examination. Besides the occlusion of vessels, the histologic changes noted in the kidneys are similar to those of membranous glomerulonephritis. Interstitial edema occurs, and there may be mild to moderate atrophy of the convoluted tubules. In more chronic cases, interstitial fibrosis and severe tubular atrophy may be seen.

Hepatic Vein Thrombosis (Budd-Chiari Syndrome)

Occlusion of the hepatic venous outflow tract is a rare condition that was described by Budd in 1845 and Chiari in 1898. The cause may be tumor or localized venous thrombosis. The latter has been associated with conditions in which there is an underlying predisposition to thrombosis, such as polycythemia rubra vera or paroxysmal nocturnal hemoglobinuria. The occurrence of this syndrome in pregnancy and with the use of oral contraceptives has been attributed to induced changes in the coagulation factors, but the possibility of estrogen- or progesterone-induced intimal vascular changes cannot be excluded.[69,70] In pregnancy and with oral contraceptives, the onset of symptoms is sudden, developing over a period of 1 to 3 months.

Clinically, patients present with abdominal pain and distention, hepatomegaly, and ascites. Jaundice usually is not present at the time of diagnosis, and liver enzyme studies are not helpful. The hepatic scintiscan may be useful in diagnosis; however, hepatic vein catheterization is the most important diagnostic technique.

Liver biopsy generally shows intense vascular congestion, localized necrosis, and cell atrophy. Demonstration of thrombi in the small hepatic sinusoids or antral veins is unusual. The histologic findings in general reflect localized ischemia and, although nonspecific, may be useful in suggesting the appropriate diagnosis.

The Budd-Chiari syndrome in association with pregnancy has a poor prognosis, with a mortality of about 50%.[71] The prognosis does not appear to be as grave when the syndrome occurs in association with the use of oral contraceptives, and remission has occurred with discontinuation of the medication. Death, if it occurs, is usually within a period of 6 to 12 months. At autopsy, the hepatic veins are found to be occluded by thrombi. The inferior vena cava is patent. In rare cases, associated portal, mesenteric, and splenic vein thrombi have been seen. Liver changes, in addition to thrombosis of central and suprahepatic veins, vary from marked dilatation and congestion of sinusoids to focal necrosis resulting from ischemia. Extravasation of blood into Disse's spaces and progressive atrophy of hepatocytes in the less congested areas are characteristic. Coalescing fibrosis of centrilobular regions is the form of healing in surviving cases.

Intracranial Thrombosis

Cerebral venous and dural sinus thrombi occur in several conditions, including pregnancy.[72,73] Intracranial thrombosis most commonly occurs in the latter part of pregnancy but has been reported in the first trimester. The hypercoagulable state of pregnancy has been implicated, as has the predisposition of the cortical venous system to thrombotic episodes by virtue of the lack of valves, low pressure, fibrous septa, and transient changes in pressure during pregnancy.

Intracranial thrombosis has been associated with the use of oral contraceptives.[72,73] These hormones may cause arterial changes including eccentric intimal thickening with clumping of the internal elastic membrane and the occurrence of plaques. These findings are most often noted in strokes associated with the use of oral contraceptives. Although it is frequently stated that cerebral venous thrombosis in pregnancy and the puerperium is not uncommon, occurring in about 1 in 10,000 pregnancies, few cases have been reported.

Clinical manifestations frequently include headache with or without convulsions. When accompanied by convulsions, cerebral venous thrombosis may be confused with eclampsia; however, hypertension is absent. Focal neurologic signs or coma may be presenting features. Definite antemortem diagnosis is made by cerebral angiography. CT scans can reliably and noninvasively suggest the diagnosis. The mortality is high, and the autopsy findings include cerebral edema, basilar herniation, multiple petechial hemorrhages, and organizing venous thrombosis. In pregnancy-associated intracranial venous thrombosis, the sinus endothelial proliferation described in cases associated with oral contraceptive use is not observed as frequently.

Pulmonary Thromboembolism

Pulmonary thromboembolism in patients receiving oral contraceptives usually is believed to be secondary to alterations in the coagulation process similar to those seen in pregnancy.[74] Some reports suggest that the pathogenesis of pulmonary thromboembolism in oral contraceptive users may be different from that in pregnancy, in that the pulmonary vascular obstruction usually is secondary to local vascular changes and subsequent thrombosis rather than to an embolic phenomenon (see Fig. 11-5).

Pulmonary embolism is the second leading cause of death in pregnancy.[74,75] It is the leading cause of death in cesarean section patients. The major clinical signs of pulmonary embolism are dyspnea and tachypnea. The classic signs of hemoptysis—pleural friction rub, gallop rhythm, cyanosis, and sharp chest pain—are present in less than 25% of these patients. The most helpful auxiliary studies include arterial PO_2, electrocardiogram, chest x-ray films, lung scans, and pulmonary arteriography. The latter constitutes a definitive diagnostic tool but usually is reserved for those patients in whom surgery is contemplated. Massive pulmonary embolism occurs suddenly, usually from the second postpartum day to several weeks postpartum. The risk increases with age, parity, restricted activity, traumatic or operative deliveries, dehydration, anemia, and the use of estrogens to suppress lactation.

One of the major problems in delineating the probable causes and origins of pulmonary embolism has been the incomplete reporting of the investigation of deaths secondary to suspected pulmonary embolism. In cases in which a careful search was conducted, about one half of the thrombi originated in the pelvic veins. In cases of death occurring soon after delivery, the emboli may be unorganized and therefore difficult to differentiate from postmortem clotting. In autopsies of sudden death shortly after delivery, opening the pulmonary veins in situ might reveal folds in the obstructing clot that would be diagnostic of embolization (Fig. 11-6).

To define risk factors that may be associated with anesthesia or surgical techniques used during cesarean section, every effort should be made to identify the sources of the emboli. This type of information may allow modification of techniques or procedures to lessen the risk of pulmonary embolism after cesarean section.

Chorionic Embolism

Chorionic tissue can be identified in the maternal circulation throughout pregnancy. Chorionic tissue has been found sequestered in the pulmonary vasculature postpartum and is considered a normal event.

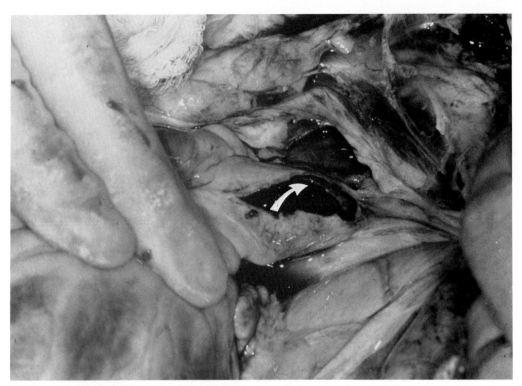

FIGURE 11-6 Pulmonary embolism. This patient died within 4 hours of a cesarean section. At the time of surgery, marked broad ligament and ovarian vein varicosities had been noticed without evidence of thrombosis. The fresh, folded embolus (*arrow*) that can be seen obstructing the main pulmonary artery originated from the right ovarian vein.

Acute pulmonary embolism with chorionic tissue has been identified in association with hydatidiform mole and choriocarcinoma. In hydatidiform mole, it is usually associated with uterine evacuation, occurring in about 10% of cases, and is self-limited and rarely fatal.[76]

Fat Embolism

Fat embolism appears to be encountered more frequently when the pregnant patient sustains bone and extensive soft-tissue injuries.[77] The predominant symptoms are tachypnea, hypotension, altered consciousness, petechial rash about the neck and shoulders, and pyrexia. Hypoxemia, leukocytosis, and hypocalcemia are frequently present. Demonstration of fat globules in sputum, circulating blood, and spinal fluid may be of help in the diagnosis, but they are not specific. At autopsy, neutral fat should be looked for in frozen section material from the lungs and choroid plexus. Fat embolism may play some role in amniotic fluid embolism and may be a component of air embolism.

Air Embolism

Air embolism is associated with many different types of operative procedures and circumstances, but it appears to be most common in association with pregnancy.[78] After Leonet reported the first death

associated with pregnancy in 1845, most of the reported gynecologic fatalities of air embolism were associated with pregnancy, except those in which the precipitating events were diagnostic pneumoperitoneum, tubal insufflation, or, rarely, hysterectomy.[79] In 1960, Nelson reviewed all the cases reported to be associated with pregnancy and the puerperium and estimated that the incidence of air embolism was about 1 in 100,000 live births.[79] Of the 199 proved fatal cases of embolism, 40% were associated with attempted illegal abortion, most of them by douching with various substances.

Two factors are necessary for venous air embolization. First, there must be a partially open venous space. Second, the air pressure must exceed the venous pressure. The mechanism suggested for air entry before labor is the forcing of air through the cervix, with displacement of the membranes in the lower uterine segment and entry into the exposed rich vascular bed. A douche bulb can provide 200 to 300 mL of air with a fluid mixture in this fashion. The rich, open vascular spaces associated with delivery provide easy access to the vascular system. The hemodynamic changes associated with delivery, along with decompression of the abdomen and Trendelenburg's position, are believed to create negative venous pressure that potentiates air embolism.

The effect of the bolus of air in the venous system is almost immediate. Clinically, there is marked apprehension, tachycardia with loss of peripheral pulse, dyspnea, cyanosis, and vascular collapse. In arterial air embolism, the lethal dose is considerably less, and the mechanism of death is secondary to cerebral embolism, which produces neurologic manifestations, including blindness. Ophthalmologic examination may reveal air in the retinal vessels.

Gynecologic laparoscopy is a common procedure in which large volumes of gas are injected into the peritoneal cavity. The most commonly used gases are carbon dioxide and nitrous dioxide, both of which have high solubility constants. Usually, large intravascular volumes are required to cause a symptomatic embolism. Fatal gas embolism secondary to laparoscopy has been reported.[80] Laser ablation of the endometrium has been associated with at least 2 deaths from gas embolization; the use of air and nitrogen were involved.[81] In operative hysteroscopy, the uterine cavity is distended by a fluid medium. With operative trauma to the wall, intravasation of fluid easily occurs, and acute fluid overload with pulmonary edema is a common complication. With the advent of laser ablation using artificial sapphire tips, an additional cooling mechanism must be used to keep the sapphire tip from overheating. This has been accomplished by use of a gas flow around the fiber, usually air, nitrogen, or carbon dioxide, which is the source of the gas embolization in fatal cases. Air embolism can be associated with forced infusion of blood, insertion of subclavian catheters or central venous lines, and the placement of the needle for epidural anesthesia.[82]

The autopsy findings in venous air embolism are usually evident, with air frequently found in the uterine vessels, the veins of the broad ligament, the inferior vena cava, and the right heart. Pulmonary congestion and right heart dilatation are dominant findings. In performing the autopsy, no major veins should be transected until the inferior vena cava is adequately exposed and examined for air and the right heart opened under water. This may be achieved by filling the chest cavity with water or carefully clamping all the major heart vessels and transferring the heart to a water-filled basin. The gas found within the heart and great vessels can be trapped and analyzed by such devices as the Erben and Nadvornik apparatus.

Antemortem air embolism must be differentiated from septic death associated with a gas-forming organism and from postmortem gas formation secondary to gas-forming bacilli. In the former, the clinical course is different; blood culture should identify the problem in both cases. In both situations, gas is found in arteries and veins. In the rare case of arterial gas embolism, gas may be found in the coronary arteries and the brain, particularly the choroid plexus. The main central nervous system finding is that of disseminated foci of ischemic necrosis.

Most cases of air embolism are seen in pregnancy and associated with the use of a vaginal douche, cunnilingus, or aberrant sexual activity. These histories may not be readily available and must be carefully ferreted out. A detailed description of the external and internal genitalia should be made. When the event is associated with delivery, the uterus should be examined carefully for lacerations or rupture.

Amniotic Fluid Embolism

Amniotic fluid embolism is one of the most dangerous and untreatable conditions in obstetrics.[58,82,83] Although previously recognized, the clinical entity was not widely appreciated until the publication by Steiner and Lushbaugh in 1941.[84] It is characterized by hypotension, hypoxia, and coagulopathy, with an incidence of anywhere from 1 in 3,400 to 1 in 80,000 deliveries.[85,86] Amniotic fluid embolism accounts for 5% to 10% of maternal deaths, and when combined with pulmonary thromboembolism represents the leading group of causes of maternal mortality in the United States.[85] The syndrome usually occurs in the term patient in labor or immediately postpartum, but it has been described in the first and second trimesters and, in rare cases, hours to days after delivery. The dramatically acute symptoms are sometimes heralded by chills, apprehension, emesis, and a need for micturition, followed by sudden respiratory distress, cyanosis, cardiovascular collapse, and coma. Eighty percent of patients die within 6 hours of onset of symptoms, with 25% to 50% of those dying in the first hour. For those surviving the first hour, coagulation problems develop in 30% to 45% and are manifested by a range of changes from minor drops in the platelet counts to full-blown disseminated intravascular coagulation. Coagulation problems constitute the presenting symptom in about 12% of cases.[86,87]

Because the respiratory symptoms are so acute and the main autopsy finding consists of intravascular amniotic debris in the pulmonary vasculature, it has long been postulated that the symptom complex is precipitated by a sudden and massive intravasation of amniotic fluid. For this reason, particular attention was directed at the clinical notations of tumultuous labor patterns and the use of oxytocin with chlorobutanol (Pitocin). Because of the acuteness of the onset of symptoms, the differential diagnosis includes ruptured uterus, eclampsia, pulmonary embolism, air embolism, abruptio placentae with shock, supine hypotension syndrome, myocardial infarction, cerebrovascular accident, Gram-negative sepsis, bilateral pneumothorax, aspiration syndrome, and anaphylactic reaction to an administered drug.

Amniotic fluid embolism is rare. Only slightly more than 300 cases are recorded in the literature, many of them single case reports, often with incomplete clinical and pathologic data.[86] The single major diagnostic feature is the autopsy finding of amniotic fluid debris in the pulmonary vasculature, which usually is described as consisting of squamous epithelial cells, mucin, fat, and fetal hair.[87] These findings, combined with the acute nature of the pulmonary symptoms, has been viewed in the past as evidence for an acute obstructive or possible anaphylactoid reaction to a massive intravasation of fluid with subsequent cor pulmonale. There have been only a limited number of animal studies, and their results have yielded conflicting data regarding the effects of intravenous infusion of amniotic fluid with and without meconium.[86] The only two studies carried out in primates have shown that amniotic fluid infusion is clinically innocuous.[86] In more recent years, careful clinical documentation of hemodynamic events in affected patients has tended to refute the earlier view that the clinical symptoms are a result of mechanical obstruction or anaphylactoid reaction.[87] The findings in larger series of carefully compiled autopsies and in cytologic analyses of right heart blood in affected and unaffected patients have altered past suggestions about the sequence of events and mechanisms of response in patients with amniotic fluid embolism.[87,88]

The patient suffering from amniotic fluid embolism tends to be older (average age of 32) and is more often parous (88%). Most cases occur at term and during the course of labor. Sudden dyspnea accompanied by hypotension and cardiorespiratory arrest occur in nearly 80% of the cases, with subsequent convulsions in 10%. It has been postulated that the acute symptoms are secondary to pulmonary hypertension, transient right ventricular dysfunction, and interpulmonary vascular shunting with arterial hypoxia and acidosis. Of those patients surviving the first hour, hemodynamic observations fail to identify evidence of pulmonary hypertension, and it is presumed that there was resolution of any acute changes. Left ventricular dysfunction or failure is identified with resultant pulmonary edema. The myocardial dysfunction is believed to be due to the initial hypoxia and acidosis, which may in part account for the subsequent findings of renal failure, hepatic injury, and cerebral edema.

The autopsy findings usually are not dramatic. Right heart dilatation is sometimes identified in sudden death, which tends to refute the mechanical obstruction theory of the presumed initial right heart failure. The more usual macroscopic findings include the following: pulmonary edema (consistent with left heart failure); pulmonary, subendocardial, subepicardial, and subcapsular hepatic hemorrhages; multiple organ vascular congestion; and cerebral edema. The pulmonary vasculature often appears to be bloodless, but on microscopic examination contains squames, mucin, lanugo, fat, and leukostasis.[87] The quantity of intravascular material identified does not completely correlate with the duration of symptoms before death and, in fact, may be sparse.[87]

Squames, mucin, fat, and lanugo may not be readily appreciated in slides stained with hematoxylin and eosin (Fig. 11-7). Squames must be differentiated from detached endothelial cells, especially when the interval between death and autopsy is prolonged. Multiple frozen sections of lung should be obtained and stained for fat, which is good evidence for the diagnosis of amniotic fluid embolism without

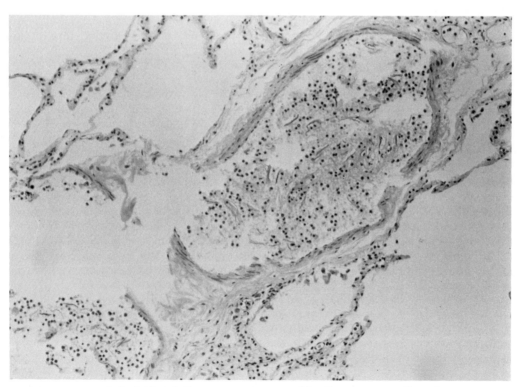

FIGURE 11-7 Amniotic fluid embolism. Numerous neutrophils, flat squamous cells, and amorphous material fill the pulmonary vascular spaces.

the risk of contamination or misdiagnosis that exists with the identification of squames. Multiple pulmonary sections should be stained for mucin, using Mowry's colloidal iron stain, and for squames, using Alcian green-phloxine. Lanugo is best seen with polarized light and is rarely identified. Mucin positivity is the most common finding. Unlike the presence of trophoblastic tissue in the lungs of pregnant patients, the finding of amniotic debris in the maternal circulation has always been considered abnormal and pathognomonic of amniotic fluid embolism. Amniotic debris has been found in the systemic circulation. It has been reported in the vessels of the myocardium, cerebrum, kidneys, pancreas, gallbladder, pituitary, adrenals, small bowel, and spleen. Apparently, no clinical significance is attached to these latter findings.[87]

In recent years, it has been thought possible to diagnose amniotic fluid embolism by examining right heart blood.[88,89] On centrifugation, three distinct zones have been noted in right heart blood of patients with the clinical syndrome of amniotic fluid embolization. The topmost layer is usually positive for mucin, the presence of which may be confirmed by cytologic preparations. Squames are usually identified in cell block material taken from the uppermost layer. However, the presence of squames alone may be an artifact, because squames may be identified in right heart blood recovered from non-pregnant women.[90,91] Because the initial reports suggested that a positive diagnosis could be made on the basis of squames in the blood from the right heart circulation, amniotic fluid embolism has a tendency to be overdiagnosed.

The idea that a massive intravasation occurs abruptly is partially supported by the frequent autopsy finding of uterine lacerations.[87] Vascular access for the amniotic fluid has been postulated to occur by one of the following three mechanisms:

1. Via the endocervical veins, in that as the fetal head descends, it blocks the birth canal, and the transmitted pressure of the contractions drives the trapped fluid into the traumatized and opened cervical veins[92]
2. Via the placental site secondary to premature placental separation, which allows access to large maternal veins (premature separation was clinically evident in 45% of the cases in one series)[83]
3. By way of the uterine wall.

Careful examination of the uteri of women who died of amniotic fluid embolism has disclosed partial rupture or localized tears with venous sinuses filled with amniotic debris.[87] Trauma to the endometrial surface has been implicated. Amniotic fluid embolism occurs in a disproportionate number of women in association with an intrauterine device and has been associated with intrauterine catheters, cesarean sections, and intrauterine manipulations. The observation of uterine intravascular amniotic debris and blood clot is not necessarily correlated with the occurrence of amniotic fluid embolization.

When death occurs early after the onset of symptoms, large numbers of neutrophils and histiocytes with phagocytized meconium-like debris have been observed to obstruct the pulmonary vessels. This suggests that amniotic fluid containment may be a mediator for the clinical response. Meconium and prostaglandins have been implicated; the latter, especially prostaglandin F_2, are found in the amniotic fluid in patients in labor. This theory would not explain amniotic fluid embolism occurring in the first and second trimesters.

The bleeding diathesis that may occur is not readily explained. The picture is that of disseminated intravascular coagulation, with an increase in serum fibrinolytic activity, thrombocytopenia, hypofibrinogenemia, and fibrin split products. Amniotic fluid has been shown to contain an activator of factor X; however, the amount present in amniotic fluid is not sufficient to precipitate a systemic effect.

Disseminated Intravascular Coagulopathy

Disseminated intravascular coagulopathy (DIC) is a clinical syndrome that occurs during the course of several different disease states. The manifestations probably can best be regarded as a consequence of the formation of thrombin. The thrombin catalyzes the activation and consumption of certain coagulant proteins and the production of fibrin thrombi. The consumption of fibrin leads to hypofibrinogenemia, which in pregnancy may be associated with any of the conditions associated with DIC listed below:

Abruptio placentae
Intrauterine fetal death with retention
Intra-amniotic injection of saline
Amniotic fluid embolism
Septic abortion
Retained placenta
Toxemia
Transfusion reaction
Septicemia

The laboratory diagnosis is made in patients with evidence of hemorrhage or thrombosis by the findings of a decreased platelet count, hypofibrinogenemia, prolonged prothrombin time, and fibrin degradation products. The histologic findings are those of multiple, small-vessel fibrin thrombi in different organ systems (Fig. 11-8).

LIVER

Toxemia of Pregnancy

Acute toxemia of pregnancy, a complex disorder of the third trimester of pregnancy (after the 24th week), is characterized by edema, hypertension, and

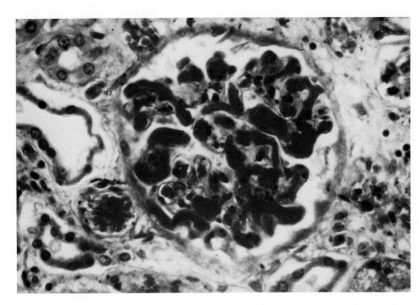

FIGURE 11-8 Renal glomerulus in a case of disseminated intravascular coagulation (DIC). Multiple fibrin thrombi are demonstrated well in this periodic acid-Schiff stain. (Courtesy of Dr. A. Andrew Abraham, George Washington University, Washington, DC)

proteinuria. It usually is classified into two groups: preeclampsia, which may be mild or severe, and eclampsia.[93-97] In mild preeclampsia, patients have edema of the face and hands, hypertension of at least 140/90 mm Hg, and persistent proteinuria (1+ to 2+). In severe preeclampsia, these signs are increased and there is marked edema, including anasarca and pulmonary edema. The blood pressure rises to at least 166/110 mm Hg, and the proteinuria is of the order of 5 g or more per 24 hours (3+ to 4+). Oliguria of less than 500 mL per 24 hours, visual and cerebral disturbances, headaches, and epigastric pain are common in severe preeclampsia. If the patient develops convulsions, becomes comatose, or both, the diagnosis of eclampsia is made.

In recent years, the HELLP syndrome (hemolysis, elevated liver enzymes, and low platelets) has been characterized as a form of severe preeclampsia.[98] The syndrome is related to a marked increase in maternal and perinatal morbidity and mortality. The hematologic and serologic changes can be identified before the appearance of proteinuria and hypertension and are identified in 23% of proteinuric hypertensive patients.[99] It is particularly in association with this syndrome that hepatic necrosis, subcapsular hemorrhage, and renal dysfunction are encountered.

In the United States, preeclampsia occurs in about 5% to 10% of all pregnancies. Eclampsia represents only 0.1% to 0.2% of all pregnancies, or 2% of all cases of preeclampsia.[100] Although these conditions may occur in multiparous women, they are more prevalent in primigravidas. Progress in prenatal care during the past decades has notably reduced the incidence of severe preeclampsia and eclampsia, and therefore of fetal and maternal morbidity and mortality.

The systemic complications of severe preeclampsia and eclampsia include abruptio placentae, hypofibrinogenemia, hemolysis, cerebral hemorrhage (a common cause of death), retinal hemorrhage, pulmonary edema, glomeruloendotheliosis with secondary oliguria, and liver necrosis and hemorrhage.[94,101] In this section, only the hepatic alterations in preeclampsia and eclampsia are discussed.[97,102-105]

The liver changes in toxemia of pregnancy are just part of the systemic vascular disorder resulting, presumably, from renin activation (the trigger mechanism is unknown). This is followed by retention of sodium in the vascular walls, which in turn induces a generalized vascular hyperreactivity to pressor substances (catecholamines and angiotensin) with development of an insidious vasospastic state characteristic of toxemia.[97,99,104-106] The vasospasm is considered the basic cause for the hypertensive state and the changes seen in different organs in preeclampsia and eclampsia.

Less than 50% of toxemic patients present with liver function changes, which usually consist of elevated alkaline phosphatase levels, moderate elevations in transaminase levels, and decreased platelet levels (HELLP syndrome). Markedly elevated lactate dehydrogenase levels are associated with liver necrosis, whereas alkaline phosphatase and γ-glutamyltransferase levels apparently are not related to the occurrence or extent of liver necrosis.[99] Hepatic injury may be detected before clinical signs by ultrasonography.[107] Elevation in bilirubin levels is rare, and only 10% of patients with eclampsia develop jaundice.[108]

Only in severe cases are the functional changes complicated by hepatic necrosis and hemorrhage and, eventually, spontaneous rupture.[101,109] These lesions may be fatal. A sudden complaint of right upper quadrant pain, accompanied by hepatomegaly, elevated serum levels of hepatic enzymes, fever, and leukocytosis, should suggest the presence of liver necrosis and hemorrhage. At times oliguria and shock complete the clinical picture.

The main histologic findings consist of fibrinous thrombosis of sinusoids with panlobar, multifocal periportal hemorrhage. In severe cases, multiple areas of intraparenchymal and subcapsular hemorrhage may occur, as well as centrilobular ischemic necrosis with inflammatory exudate (Fig. 11-9). Liver rupture, a potentially fatal complication, may occur in rare severe cases.[110–114]

Liver biopsy is a hazardous procedure usually not attempted in the eclamptic patient. Most of the morphologic changes have been described from autopsy material.

Liver Tumors and Steroid Therapy

Since the introduction of oral contraceptive drugs in 1960, contraceptive steroids have been implicated in liver function alterations resulting in intrahepatic cholestasis, abnormal bromsalphthalein (BSP) excretion, jaundice, and neoplastic and nonneoplastic mass lesions. Other nonspecific alterations of the hepatocyte can be seen in pregnancy and with estrogen replacement therapy, chiefly the presence of megamitochondria with crystalline inclusions (Fig. 11-10), intracellular bile inclusions, and cholestasis.[115]

During the past decades, there have been numerous reports of liver tumors associated with a history of steroid contraception.[116–127] Although the lesions have been diagnosed using a variety of terms, they can be grouped into three main categories: focal nodular hyperplasia, hepatocellular adenoma, and hepatocellular carcinoma.[118,121,122,125,128,129]

Focal Nodular Hyperplasia

Focal nodular hyperplasia is a nonneoplastic, tumorous lesion of the liver that affects women more often than men, is most frequent in the third and fourth decades of life, and is frequently associated with hormonal contraception.[125,128,130–132] Most patients with this association are symptomatic and are more likely than focal nodular hyperplasia patients not using oral contraception to develop spontaneous rupture of the liver with hemoperitoneum, a potentially fatal complication.[133]

In asymptomatic patients, the lesion may be found incidentally at the time of surgery for other conditions. When symptomatic, patients commonly present with acute or chronic abdominal pain and a palpable mass. Liver function tests are negative, but a CT scan is usually diagnostic. The lesion is usually single (in rare cases it is multiple) and less than 5 cm in diameter. It is frequently located at the surface of the liver and may be pedunculated. Although not encapsulated, it is well circumscribed, firm, fibrous, and distinct from the adjacent hepatic tissue. It characteristically contains a central stellate scar.

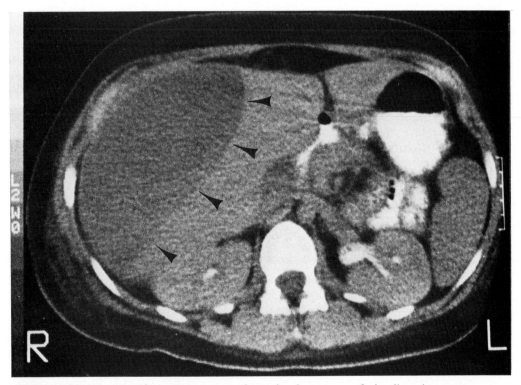

FIGURE 11-9 CT scan of a spontaneous subcapsular hematoma of the liver in severe preeclampsia. This patient presented with severe epigastric pain immediately postpartum associated with marked elevation of liver enzymes. Both ultrasound and CT scan revealed a large subcapsular lesion (*arrows*). Fine-needle aspiration confirmed the lesion to be an encapsulated hematoma. Resolution occurred without surgery over a period of 7 months.

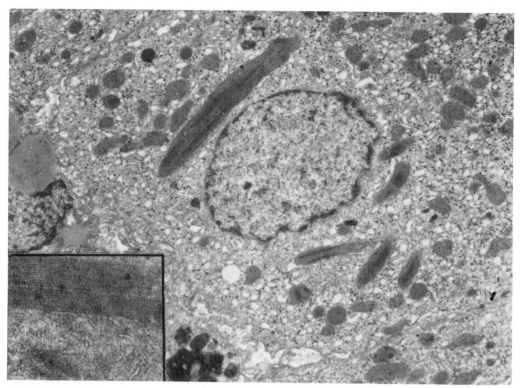

FIGURE 11-10 Hepatocyte with abundant mitochondria, some of them gigantic and containing crystalline structures (*detail in inset*). Note the dispersed glycogen granules and well-developed endoplasmic reticulum. The specimen is from the liver biopsy of a 28-year-old woman who took oral contraceptives for 5 years (×9800; inset, ×69,200).

Histologically, the lesion is composed of multiple small, confluent nodules of normal-appearing hepatocytes arranged in compact plates and cords around irregular foci of hyperplastic bile ducts and small blood vessels, within a fibrous collagenous stroma with lymphocytic infiltration (Figs. 11-11 and 11-12). Hemorrhage may occur within the tumor or may progress to rupture of the liver and hemoperitoneum, a catastrophic complication that requires immediate surgical treatment and occurs particularly in cases associated with steroid contraception.[132] The lesions of focal nodular hyperplasia may regress spontaneously after discontinuance of the steroid medication.

Hepatocellular Adenoma

Hepatocellular adenoma is the benign liver lesion most commonly associated with oral steroid contraception.[118,119,128,134–136] This lesion was rare until the 1970s, ten years after the introduction of hormonal contraception. Since then, an increasing number of reports have confirmed this association, supporting a causal relation. Adenomas also occur in female and male patients receiving androgens for therapeutic reasons.

Clinically, most patients are symptomatic, presenting with chronic right upper quadrant or epigastric pain or pressure and usually with a palpable

mass. If intratumorous or subcapsular hemorrhage has occurred, the complaint is of acute upper abdominal pain. If rupture of the liver and hemoperitoneum complicate the problem, the picture is that of an acute abdomen. Liver function tests are within normal limits. Hepatic angiography and CT scan are diagnostic of the tumor mass. Needle biopsies may be considered with caution due to the high risk of hemorrhage. Like focal nodular hyperplasia, adenomas may regress after discontinuance of the steroid medication.[137,138]

Macroscopically, these tumors are usually single, although about 25% are multiple. They are well-circumscribed and partially encapsulated masses of lobulated, firm, gray-tan tissue that contrast with the surrounding darker and homogeneous liver parenchyma. These adenomas are usually larger than focal nodular hyperplasias, but most measure less than 10 cm in diameter. They are usually located in the right lobe of the liver. Some may be very large and can be located in the left lobe (Fig. 11-13). These tumors may become hemorrhagic and may result in liver rupture and hemorrhage. Greatly dilated veins are characteristically present within and around these hepatocellular adenomas, a factor that plays an important role in hemorrhagic complications.

Histologically, these tumors are composed of closely packed cords and masses of slightly pleomorphic hepatocytes with clear granular cytoplasm, sepa-

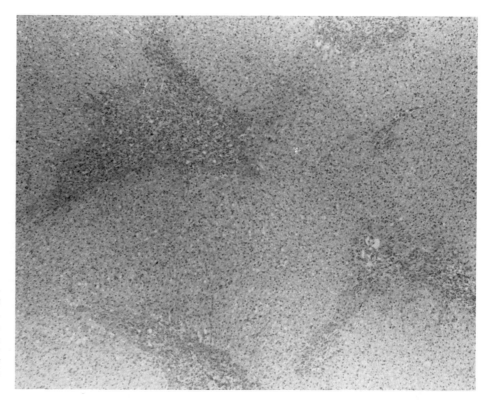

FIGURE 11-11 Panoramic view of focal nodular hyperplasia of the liver in a patient with a history of oral contraception. The irregular dark areas correspond to foci of fibrosis containing vascular proliferation and hyperplasia of bile ducts. They are separated by normal-appearing parenchyma.

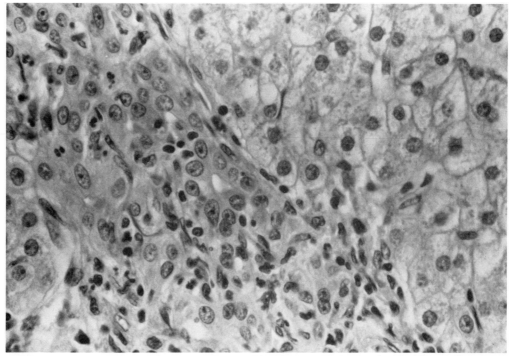

FIGURE 11-12 High-power view of an area of focal nodular hyperplasia, showing abundant, well-preserved cords of hepatocytes surrounding a triangular zone of fibrosis with bile duct hyperplasia, proliferation of small blood vessels, and predominantly mononuclear inflammatory infiltrate.

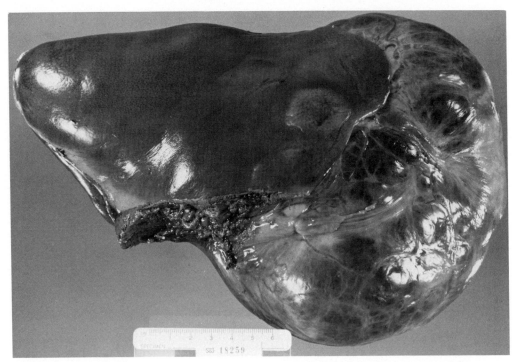

FIGURE 11-13 Large hepatocellular adenoma (18 × 16 × 12 cm) occupying most of the left lobe of the liver. A partial lobectomy was performed in this patient, who had a long history of oral contraception before conception. The tumor was found at 12 weeks of gestation. Therapeutic abortion failed to induce regression of the tumor. Its cut surface was lobulated, focally necrotic, and hemorrhagic, thus confirming a CT scan impression. The tumor was negative for estrogen and progesterone receptors, but the adjacent normal liver was positive.

rated by irregular sinusoids, with obliteration of the lobular hepatic architecture and absence of portal spaces and central veins (Fig. 11-14). Dilated veins are present randomly throughout the tumors. Bile ducts are absent. Fatty metamorphosis may be present focally. Areas of ischemic necrosis and hemorrhage are frequently seen. Resection is the treatment of choice (see Fig. 11-13).

Hepatocellular Carcinoma

Hepatocellular carcinoma is a distinctive malignant neoplasm. It is epidemiologically associated with environmental factors, mainly chemical exposure, and is related to viral hepatitis, cirrhosis, irradiation, and steroid therapy.[120,129,139–144] In geographic areas of high prevalence, these tumors affect young and middle-aged adults, mainly men (5:1). In areas of low frequency, such as Europe and North America, they usually occur in elderly men.

A possible etiologic relation between hepatic malignant tumors and long-term use of steroid hormones (contraceptive steroids and anabolic androgens) has been evolving in recent years on the basis of strong circumstantial evidence.[120,127,139–141,145] This evidence for a relation is strongly suggested by a marked increase in the relative risk with continuous use of oral contraceptives for more than 5 years. The risk is postulated to be secondary to es-

trogen; however, a recent study did not show an increased risk with long-term use of replacement estrogen.[146] More than 100 cases of oral contraceptive-associated hepatocellular carcinoma have been reported since 1977, and although there is no proof of a causal relation, the epidemiologic evidence suggests a strong correlation that must be considered seriously and evaluated.[127,146] This becomes especially evident when the common risk factors of alcoholism and hepatitis B virus are absent.[127]

Most of these contraceptive-associated malignant hepatic tumors have been hepatocellular carcinomas occurring in young women, a population at minimal risk for this type of lesion in the past. The tumors appear de novo, with the exception of a few alleged to have resulted from malignant transformation of an adenoma. In addition to their ability to metastasize, these tumors had spontaneous rupture with severe hemorrhage in about 10% of cases.

Histologically, hepatocellular carcinomas are differentiated from focal nodular hyperplasia by the absence of central scarring and vascular and bile duct proliferation and by the presence of architectural and cytologic criteria of malignancy. These latter criteria (irregular cell nests, trabeculae, and acini; infiltrating tumor borders; cellular atypia and pleomorphism; presence of numerous mitotic figures) are even more important in the differential diagnosis of hepatocellular adenoma, because both lesions are

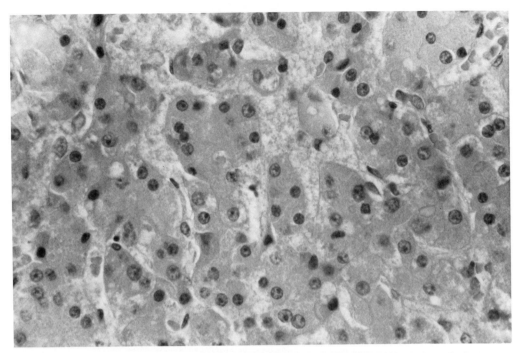

FIGURE 11-14 Needle biopsy of the hepatocellular adenoma shown in Figure 11-13. Note the irregular cords and sheets of slightly pleomorphic hepatocytes with focal necrosis and hemorrhage.

monomorphous proliferations of hepatocytes only, but adenomas lack the malignant phenotype. In young women, many of the carcinomas are of the *fibrolamellar oncocytic* type, a recently characterized and prognostically favorable variant in which cords and nests of large eosinophilic cells that show ultrastructural features of oncoctyes (packed with large and pleomorphic mitochondria) are separated by prominent bands of dense collagen (Figs. 11-15 and 11-16).[147,148]

Spontaneous Rupture of the Liver

Spontaneous rupture of the liver is not a common occurrence. Usually the patients are older, multiparous, in the third trimester of pregnancy, and hypertensive.[110–113] Eclampsia is diagnosed in only about 25% of the cases. Usually, the patient presents with epigastric pain, right upper quadrant pain, or both. The pain may have been present for several weeks. Usually, there is marked elevation of all liver enzymes. Spontaneous rupture of a subcapsular hematoma usually occurs in association with delivery. Hemoperitoneum, shock, and death occur in 60% of cases. The subcapsular hematoma is usually seen in association with histologic findings of fibrin emboli in the sinusoids and hepatic arterioles, with periportal hemorrhagic necrosis. Unlike the diffuse subcapsular hematomas noted in eclamptic patients, the hematomas in spontaneous hepatic rupture usually are confined to the anterior and superior aspects of the liver. In pregnant patients presenting with epi-

gastric or right upper quadrant pain, it has been recommended that hepatic scans or ultrasound be performed to detect the subcapsular hematoma before rupture. This may be achieved by CT scan. Most of these instances are associated with the HELLP syndrome. Hemangiomas, amebic abscesses,

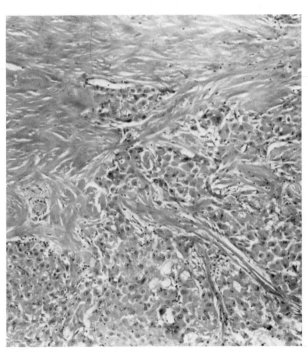

FIGURE 11-15 Fibrolamellar oncocytic hepatocellular carcinoma in a 23-year-old woman. Dense, laminated collagen separates solid nests of tumor cells.

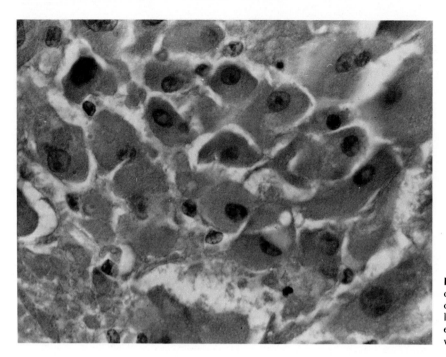

FIGURE 11-16 The tumor cells (oncocytes) in fibrolamellar oncocytic hepatocellular carcinoma are characterized by large size, pleomorphism, and voluminous eosinophilic granular cytoplasm packed with mitochondria.

and hepatic adenomas and carcinomas have been noted as rare causes of hepatic rupture in pregnancy. Fine-needle aspiration may be useful in confirming the nature of the observed hepatic defect. Large-bore needle biopsies should be avoided because they are more likely to precipitate a surgical emergency.

SEXUAL, CONTRACEPTIVE, AND SANITARY PRACTICES

Death Related to Sexual Activity

Unlike men, women almost never suffer an acute myocardial infarct during sexual activity. However, air embolism secondary to cunnilingus or air injection for eroticism does occur (see the section on air embolism). Although death due to airway obstruction secondary to an aspirated condom is evident, asphyxiation secondary to aspiration of semen or the impaction of the penis in the hypopharynx may not be readily evident. Diagnosis may be established by tracheobronchial cytology for the identification of sperm.

Complications of Intrauterine Contraception

Although intrauterine contraceptive devices (IUDs) were first introduced early in this century, not until the advent of inert plastic materials did a multitude of devices appear on the medical scene. The main problems with the devices included intrauterine retention, uterine cramping, bleeding, and myometrial embedding of the devices. Critical illness and deaths associated with intrauterine devices were first reported in 1968 by Scott.[149] The deaths attributed to the IUD were secondary to septicemia occurring shortly after insertion. Two deaths occurred secondary to amniotic fluid embolism, with devices that were found to be partially protruding through the myometrium. Subsequent problems with septicemia occurred mostly with the Dalkon Shield. With this device, the element responsible for infection was the multifilament string that protruded through the cervix (Fig. 11-17). This string allowed bacteria to migrate through its protected interstices and into the endometrial cavity. Intrauterine infection became an especially important problem when pregnancy occurred in the patient wearing the Dalkon Shield. More recent evaluation of IUDs has revealed little in the way of an increased risk for pelvic inflammatory disease.[150]

Beyond these immediate problems was the question of the fate of the IUD that perforated through the myometrium into the peritoneal cavity. Originally, some IUDs such as the Bromberg Bow were of a "closed" loop construction. In the peritoneal cavity, a loop of bowel could become entrapped within the closed loop of this device, resulting in intestinal obstruction.[151] IUDs are now made of relatively inert polyethylene plastic impregnated with barium salts. The salts enable the device to be seen by radiographic procedures. Some devices are "medicated," containing elemental copper or a progestin (Cu7, Tatum T, Dalkon Shield, Progestasert). The devices containing copper tend to invoke an intense fibrous reaction when located in the endometrial cavity. Perforation of the uterus is usually thought to be a consequence of insertion. If the uterus is perforated, the device may simultaneously perforate adjacent structures such as the bladder or colon. The nonmedicated devices usually provoke little peritoneal reaction and therefore can be located and removed by means of laparoscopy, but the copper-wrapped (Cu7, Tatum T) and copper-impregnated (Dalkon Shield) devices tend to be encapsulated by fibrous tissue.

Under experimental conditions, the copper devices are immobilized by fibrous tissue, and visceral perforation is not seen. Clinically, there have been well-documented cases of perforation of the appendix, jejunum, and colon by copper-wrapped devices that do not appear to be secondary to perforation at the time of insertion.

Other complications of intrauterine contraception are discussed in the chapters on the uterine corpus (Chap. 4), the fallopian tube (Chap. 5), and ectopic pregnancy (Chap. 9).

LAPAROSCOPIC AND PELVISCOPIC INJURIES

Laparoscopy is achieved with a trocar that is sharply and blindly introduced transcutaneously into the peritoneal cavity. Pelviscopy involves operative manipulation, usually via additional abdominal wall puncture sites. Peritoneal insufflation with carbon dioxide (CO_2) is usually achieved via a Verres needle, which is 2 mm in diameter, followed by a primary trocar of 10 to 12 mm diameter, and by secondary trocars ranging from 5 to 10 mm in diameter. The most frequently used primary trocars have sharp pyramidal tips that cut through the anterior abdominal wall fascia when the instrument is thrust against the tented lower abdominal wall. Trocars with conical tips are available but are much less frequently used; the conical tip is somewhat blunted and has no cut-

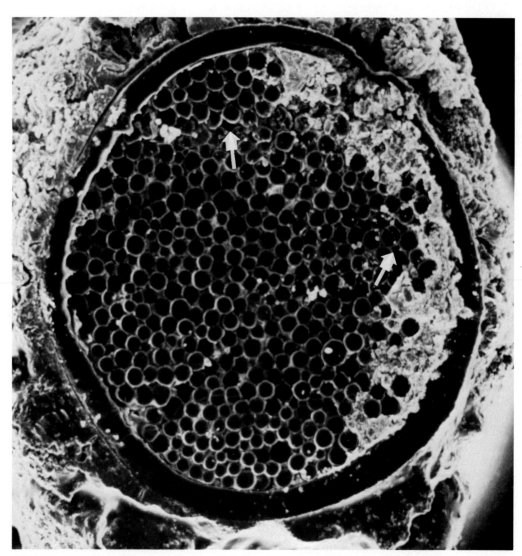

FIGURE 11-17 Scanning electron photomicrograph of a cross section of the tail of an intrauterine contraceptive device (Dalkon Shield) that had been in place for 12 years. Note the multifilament structure with internal spaces (*arrow*) that permit safe movement of bacteria.

ting edge. The Verres needle and primary trocar are inserted around or within the umbilicus and directed in the midline toward the hollow of the pelvis. Secondary trocars are usually inserted off the midline, through the rectus muscle, and the internal puncture site is usually viewed from the primary trocar site through a laparoscope. Recently, disposable pyramidal trocars have become available and are widely used because they are exceedingly sharp. This characteristic tends to reduce the force necessary to penetrate the anterior abdominal wall and hence may reduce uncontrolled thrust injuries to the peritoneal contents and the retroperitoneal structures.[152] The disposable pyramidal-tipped trocars have a retractable plastic shield that is supposed to advance over the sharp pyramidal point once anterior wall penetration is achieved. Gynecologic operative procedures by laparoscopy (pelviscopy) include the use of scissors, scalpels, clips, thermocoagulation, monopolar and bipolar electrical coagulation, and lasers.

The single most common use of laparoscopy is for female sterilization. The most serious direct complication has arisen from the use of intraperitoneal electrofulguration by monopolar techniques.[153] During the 1970s, unrecognized bowel injury with delayed perforation, sepsis, and death related to these techniques led to significant modifications of the electrosurgical generators and to a trend away from the use of monopolar electrical current to bipolar current and to the development of mechanical devices designed to obstruct the fallopian tubes. Another associated injury is intravasation of the insufflating gas with gas embolization.[153] The medium used most often is CO_2, which because of its solubility constant requires large volumes before symptoms are precipitated. The clinical and pathologic changes are discussed under the topic of gas embolization.

Other significant injuries that occur secondary to laparoscopic and pelviscopic procedures include penetration and laceration injuries occurring with the Verres needle or trocar and electrical burns and laser injuries to structures near the operative sites.[154] Complications necessitating laparotomy are reported in about 3 of 1,000 cases, and deaths are reported in 1 in 11,000 procedures.[154] Lethal vascular injuries have occurred secondary to Verres needle and trocar injuries to the aorta, vena cava, or the common iliac vessels. Most often, deaths follow obvious trocar injuries to the major vessels.[155] Verres needle vascular injuries can be detected by careful dissection of the major vessels. In these cases, there usually is extensive retroperitoneal hemorrhage.

Unrecognized gastrointestinal injuries of a significant nature are common and often become medicolegal issues. The nature of these injuries is important in ascertaining causation and instituting or designing preventive techniques or equipment. The main question has been whether there are distinctive histologic changes attributable to a thermally induced injury versus a perforation-type injury.[156,157] From the clinical perspective, surgically induced perforations manifest within a day or so after the injury, whereas perforations induced by thermal injury occur some days later. With sterilization by unipolar electrofulguration, death most commonly followed sepsis that developed after presumed electrical bowel injury with subsequent perforation. The exact mechanism for the injury is unknown, although it was attributed to spark gapping, inadvertent touching of adjacent bowel with an active electrode or hot instrument, or even by the heat retained within the fulgurated tissue itself. In 1981, this led to an admonition by the American Association of Gynecologic Laparoscopists that methods other than unipolar sterilization should be used for female sterilization.

Levy and colleagues studied the effects of four types of intestinal injuries in rabbits at 24, 28, 72, and 96 hours.[156] They felt that there were distinct differences between electrical injuries (unipolar and monopolar) and puncture injuries. As in a previous report by Thompson and Wheeless in a small series of human cases with presumed unipolar electrical injury, it was noted that, in contrast to a puncture injury, electrically induced injuries had coagulative necrosis with a relative absence of white cell infiltrates within the lesion site.[157] In contrast to the observations of Thompson and Wheeless, Levy and colleagues did not correlate more extensive necrosis of the outer muscular bundle of the bowel with an electrical injury. From our own observations of 3 known electrical injuries and 3 puncture injuries, the former injury to the outer muscle layer was notably more extensive and somewhat characteristic, as Thompson and Wheeless reported.[157] We have noted similar patterns of injury to the muscularis of the fallopian tube after unipolar and bipolar electrofulguration procedures (Figs. 11-18 and 11-19). Puncture injuries tend to tear or cut muscle bundles, with muscular retraction being somewhat greater in the outer muscle bundle. The sharp nature of the injury is usually apparent, even in injuries to the bladder, where the muscle pattern is not as distinct as in the bowel (Figs. 11-20 and 11-21). The excised bowel segment at the perforation site should be sectioned carefully to exclude a surgically independent cause of perforation, such as a ruptured diverticulum.

Large and small bowel puncture injuries occur most often because of adhesions and frequently are unrecognized by the surgeon because the segment of involved bowel adheres to the anterior abdominal wall at the peritoneal trocar site. The surgeon, therefore, is unable to recognize the possibility at the time of surgery unless a 360° scan of the anterior peritoneum is carried out and the bowel is visualized coming up to the trocar site. For an accurate assessment of the cause of injury, careful observations at the time of corrective surgery should be recorded.

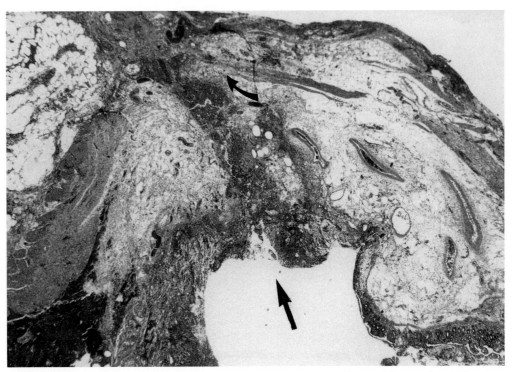

FIGURE 11-18 Exit trocar injury to the small bowel (*straight arrow*) with stretching, tearing, and acute inflammatory infiltrate involving the muscularis (*curved arrow*). The injury occurred during a laparoscopic sterilization procedure 8 hours before this specimen was taken and was identified by bowel contents leaking through the umbilical trocar site.

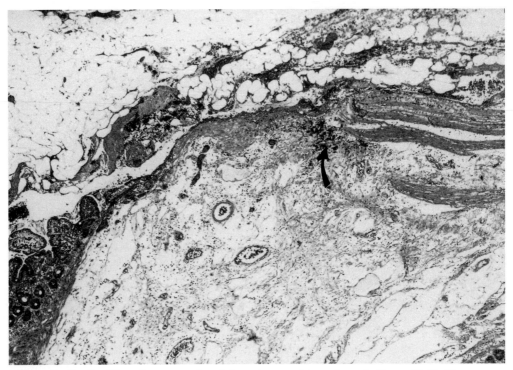

FIGURE 11-19 Small bowel puncture site of the exit trocar injury shown in Figure 11-18. Note the retracted but severed ends of the muscularis and the acute inflammatory infiltrate (*arrow*).

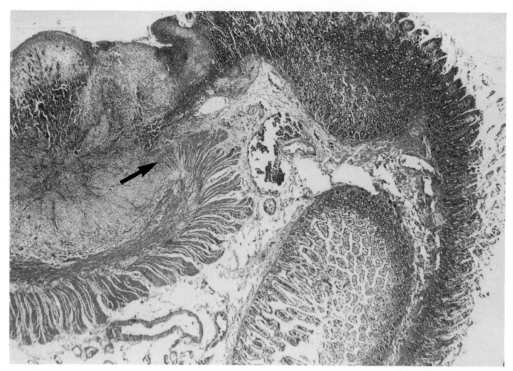

FIGURE 11-20 Site of a perforation 6 days after lysis of bowel adhesions using monopolar electrosurigcal devices. Note the contracted muscularis with more marked loss of the outer muscle layer (*arrow*).

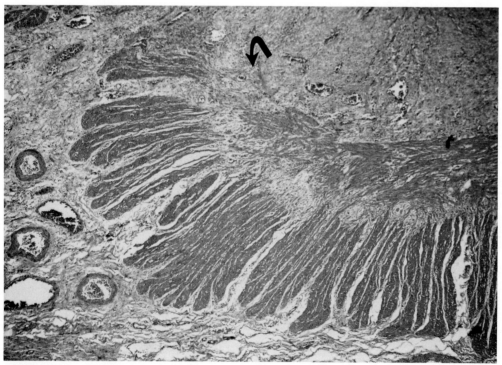

FIGURE 11-21 Detail of Figure 11-20, showing the differential loss of outer muscle mass (*arrow*) with contraction pattern and little local acute inflammatory infiltrate.

VAGINAL DOUCHING

Air embolism is a potential hazard of vaginal douching during pregnancy (see the section on air embolism). Air and fluids injected intravaginally may pass through the endometrial cavity and fallopian tubes to enter the peritoneal cavity, much in the same fashion as in diagnostic tests such as hysterosalpingography. Two problems may be seen secondary to such an event. First, the patient may present with abdominal discomfort and, if in the process of medical evaluation an upright x-ray film of the abdomen is obtained, free air may be visualized beneath the diaphragm. This could lead to an unnecessary laparotomy with a preoperative diagnosis of ruptured viscus. The second problem is the intraperitoneal instillation of nonsterile fluid, irritating chemicals, or both. Acute bacterial salpingitis or peritonitis or chemical peritonitis may ensue. Some researchers believe that talc powders are implicated in the pathogenesis of malignant epithelial tumors of the ovary.

TOXIC SHOCK SYNDROME

Toxic shock syndrome was originally described in 1978 by Todd and associates.[158] They showed a relation between the syndrome and the finding of *Staphylococcus aureus,* phage group 1, in mucosal or sequestered sites. The systemic syndrome is a multisystem illness with a wide range of signs and symptoms. The Centers for Disease Control definition for the syndrome includes the following:

Fever of 38.9°C (102°F) or higher
Diffuse macular erythroderma
Hypotension
Systemic symptoms involving three or more of the following organ systems: gastrointestinal, muscular, mucosal membranes, renal, hepatic, hematologic, or central nervous system
Desquamation 1 to 2 weeks after the onset of the illness
Negative serologic tests (Rocky Mountain spotted fever, leptospirosis, or measles)
No evidence of another cause for the illness.

The toxic shock cases rapidly gained national attention because they were reported in large numbers among young, previously healthy women who were menstruating.[159] By October 1981, 1330 cases were reported to the Centers for Disease Control, with a case fatality rate of 5.9%.[160] Although toxic shock syndrome has been reported in males and is associated with a multitude of surgically and nonsurgically caused focal infections, about 90% of cases occur in women at or near the time of menstruation, most of whom have been using tampons. Early in the 1980s, epidemiologic data suggested that the syndrome had a direct relation with the chemical composition and absorbency capacity of newer tampons introduced in the late 1970s.[161] Although the chemical composition of these tampons has been modified, toxic shock syndrome remains a risk for tampon users, especially those in their late teens. The mechanism for initial mucosal injury was thought to be secondary to vaginal mucosal drying with point ulceration, allowing staphylococcal colonization.[160] There has been some question regarding the association of toxic shock syndrome with features other than menstruation and the use of tampons. Lanes and colleagues noted a positive association with a recent history of vaginitis and a negative association with oral contraceptive use.[162] After high absorbency tampons were withdrawn from the market in 1981 and the absorbency of other tampons was lowered through 1985, the incidence of menstrual-associated toxic shock syndrome has markedly decreased. The fatality rate has declined to about 2%.

Recently, cases of toxic shock syndrome have been reported in association with the use of vaginal contraceptive sponges made of polyurethane. The symptoms and signs are not related to menstruation. Toxic shock syndrome also has been reported in association with genital laser procedures, and there have been similar clinical presentations secondary to group A streptococcal infections involving spontaneous abortion.[163,164]

The major cause for the syndrome complex is almost always an infection with a strain of *S. aureus* that produces exoprotein toxins. Most of the menstrual-associated toxic shock cases are related to *S. aureus* strains producing toxic shock syndrome toxins.[165] Other toxins, particularly enterotoxins B and C, can produce identical symptoms, as can some of the streptococcal toxins.

The histopathologic changes noted in fatal cases are similar to the changes previously reported in scarlet fever.[166] The predominant pathologic lesion appears to be that of vascular injury. The main findings have been in the skin, vaginal mucosa, lung, liver, and kidney. Mucosal edema, ulceration, and perivasculitis are seen in the vagina. In the lung, pulmonary congestion, alveolar hemorrhage, edema, and hyaline membrane formation are frequently noted. Periportal inflammation and microvesicular fatty change are seen in the liver. The renal changes are most consistent with acute tubular necrosis. In addition, occasional cases of adrenal hemorrhage have been recorded.

References

1. Boyar R, Kapen S, Weitzman ED et al: Pituitary microadenoma and hyperprolactinemia. N Engl J Med 294:263–265, 1976
2. Chang RJ: Hyperprolactinemia and menstrual dysfunction. Clin Obstet Gynecol 26:736–748, 1983
3. Child DF, Nader S, Mashiter K et al: Prolactin studies in "functionless" pituitary tumors. Br Med J 1:604–611, 1975

4. Schlechte J, Sherman B, Halins H et al: Prolactin secreting pituitary tumors. Endocr Rev 1:295, 1980

5. Doody KM, Carr BR: Amenorrhea. Obstet Gynecol Clin North Am 17:361–387, 1990

6. Yen SSC, Jaffe RG: Reproductive endocrinology: Physiology, pathophysiology and clinical management, 2nd ed. Philadelphia, WB Saunders, 1986

7. Archer DF, Lattanzi DR, Moore EE et al: Bromocriptine treatment of women with suspected pituitary prolactin secreting microadenomas. Am J Obstet Gynecol 143:620, 1982

8. Post K, Biller B et al: Selective transsphenoidal adenomectomy in women with galactorrhea-amenorrhea. JAMA 242:158, 1979

9. Thorner MD, Martin WH, Rogol AD et al: Rapid regression of pituitary prolactinoma during bromocriptine treatment. J Clin Endocr Metab 51:438, 1980

10. Horvath E, Kovacs K: Misplaced exocytosis, distinct ultrastructural feature in some pituitary adenomas. Arch Pathol Lab Med 97:221–224, 1974

11. Hwang P, Guyda H, Friesen H: A radioimmunoassay for human prolactin. Proc Natl Acad Sci USA 68:1902–1906, 1971

12. Kovacs K: Morphology of prolactin-producing adenomas. Clin Endocrinol (Oxf): 6:715–795, 1977

13. Kovacs K, Corenblum B, Sirek AMT et al: Localization of prolactin in chromophobe pituitary adenomas: Study in human necropsy material by immunoperoxidase technique. J Clin Pathol 29:250–258, 1976

14. Lloyd RV, Gikas PW, Chandler WF: Prolactin and growth hormone-producing pituitary adenomas: An immunohistochemical and ultrastructural study. Am J Surg Pathol 7:251–260, 1983

15. Keye WR Jr, Chang RJ, Monroe SE et al: Prolactin-secreting pituitary adenomas in women. Am J Obstet Gynecol 134:360–367, 1979

16. Kovacs K, Horvath E: Hypothalmic-pituitary abnormalities in ovulatory disorders. In Gondos B, Riddick DH, eds. Pathology of infertility, p 189. New York, Thieme, 1987

17. Friesen H, Tolis G: The use of bromocriptine in the galactorrhea-amenorrhea syndromes: The Canadian Cooperative Study. Clin Endocrinol (Oxf) 6(Suppl):915–995, 1977

18. Archer DF, Salazar H, Maroon JC et al: Prolactin-secreting pituitary adenomas: Serum and tissue prolactin levels with ultrastructural correlation. Am J Obstet Gynecol 137:646–652, 1980

19. Dingemans KP, Assies J, Jansen N et al: Sparsely granulated prolactin cell adenomas of the pituitary gland. Virchows Arch A Pathol Anat Histopathol 396:167–186, 1982

20. Kameya T, Tsumuraya M, Adachi I et al: Ultrastructure, immunohistochemistry and hormone release of pituitary adenomas in relation to prolactin production. Virchows Arch A Pathol Anat Histopathol 387:31–46, 1980

21. Salazar H: Ultrastructural evidence for the existence of a non-secretory sustentacular cell in the human adenohypophysis. Anat Rec 160:419–420, 1968

22. Kovacs K, Ryan N, Horvath E, Ezrin C, Penz G: Prolactin cell adenomas of the human pituitary: Morphological features of prolactin cells in the nontumorous portions of the anterior lobe. Horm Metab Res 10:409–412, 1978

23. Landolt AM, Yasargil MG: Possible causes of failure in prolactinoma surgery. Proceedings of the Annual Meeting of the American Association of Neurological Surgery, Los Angeles, April 1979

24. Badawi SZ, Rebscher F, Kohn L et al: The relationship between oral contraceptive use and subsequent development of hyperprolactinemia. Fertil Steril 36:464, 1981

25. Frantz A: Prolactin secretion in physiologic and pathologic human conditions measured by bioassay and radioimmunoassay. In Josimovich JB, Reynolds M, Cobo E, eds: Lactogenic hormones, fetal nutrition and lactation, pp 379–412. New York, John Wiley & Sons, 1974

26. March CM, Kletzky OA, Israel R, Davajan V, Mishell DR: Amenorrhea, galactorrhea and pituitary tumors: Postpill and non-postpill. Fertil Steril 28:346–352, 1977

27. March CM, Mishell DR Jr, Kletzky OA et al: Galactorrhea and pituitary tumors in post-pill and non-postpill secondary amenorrhea. Am J Obstet Gynecol 134:45–50, 1979

28. Shy KK, McTiernan AM, Daling JR, Weiss NS: Oral contraceptive use and the occurrence of pituitary prolactinoma. JAMA 249:2204–2207, 1983

29. Caulam CB, Anagers JF, Abboud CF et al: Pituitary adenoma and oral contraceptives: A cast-control study. Fertil Steril 31:25, 1979

30. Coulom CB, Annegers JF, Abbond CF et al: Pituitary adenomas and oral contraceptives: A multicenter case control study. Fertil Steril 39:753, 1983

31. Sheehan HL: Post-partum necrosis of the anterior pituitary. Journal of Pathology and Bacteriology 45:189–214, 1937

32. Aono T, Minagawa J, Kinugasa T et al: Response of pituitary LH and FSH to synthetic LH-releasing hormone in normal subjects and patients with Sheehan's syndrome. Am J Obstet Gynecol 117:1046, 1973

33. Drury MI, Keelan DM: Sheehan's syndrome. Br J Obstet Gynaecol 73:802–809, 1966

34. Kovacs K: Necrosis of anterior pituitary in humans. Neuroendocrinology 4:170–241, 1969

35. Sheehan HL: The frequency of postpartum hypopituitarism. Br J Obstet Gynecol 72:103–107, 1965

36. Jovanovic L, Peterson CM: Optimal insulin delivery for pregnant diabetic patient. Diabetes Care 5(Suppl 1):24, 1982

37. Coustan DR: Management of the pregnant diabetic. In Olefky JM, Sherwin RS, eds. Diabetes mellitus: Management and complications, p 311. New York, Churchill-Livingstone, 1985

38. National Diabetes Data Group: Classification and diagnosis of diabetes mellitus and other categories of glucose intolerance. Diabetes 28:1039–1057, 1979

39. Spellacy WN: Diabetes and pregnancy. In Sciarra JJ, ed. Gynecology and obstetrics, rev ed, vol 2, pp 1–10. Philadelphia, Harper & Row, 1983

40. Knopp RH, Montes A, Childs M et al: Metabolic adjustments in normal and diabetic pregnancy. Clin Obstet Gynecol 24:21–49, 1981

41. Seeds AE, Knowles HC Jr: Metabolic control of diabetic pregnancy. Clin Obstet Gynecol 24:51–64, 1981

42. Karlsson K, Kjellmer I: The outcome of diabetic pregnancies in relation to the mother's glucose level. Am J Obstet Gynecol 112:213, 1972

43. Kitzmiller JL, Aiello LM, Kaldany A et al: Diabetic vascular disease complicating pregnancy. Clin Obstet Gynecol 24:107–123, 1981

44. Bertoli S, Botteli R, Confalonieri R, et al: Diabetic nephropathy: Clinical and histological study in 22 patients. Acta Diabetol 20:125–133, 1983

45. Dachs S, Churg J, Mautner W et al: Diabetic nephropathy. Am J Pathol 44:155–161, 1964

46. Selby JV, Fitzsimmons SC, Newman JM et al: The natural history and epidemiology of diabetic nephropathy: Implications for prevention and control. JAMA 263:1954, 1990

47. Combs CA, Kitzmiller JL: Diabetic nephropathy and pregnancy. Clin Obstet Gynecol 34:505–515, 1991

48. Javanovic-Peterson L, Peterson CM: Diabetic retinopathy. Clin Obstet Gynecol 34:516–525, 1991

49. Moloney JB, Drury MI: The effect of pregnancy on the natural course of diabetic retinopathy. Am J Ophthalmol 93:745–756, 1982

50. Bresnick GH, Davis MD, Myers FL et al: Clinicopathologic correlations in diabetic retinopathy II. Arch Ophthalmol 95:1215, 1977

51. Virchow R: Phlogose und Thrombose in Gefas-system. In Virchow R. Gesammelte Abhandlugen Zur Wissenschaftlichen Medicin, pp 458–636. Frankfurt, Von Meidinger Sohn, 1856

52. Laros RK, Alger LS: Thromboembolism and pregnancy. Clin Obstet Gynecol 22:871–888, 1979

53. Ullery JC: Thromboembolic disease complicating pregnancy and the puerperium. Am J Obstet Gynecol 68:1243–1250, 1954

54. Bergqvist A, Bergqvist D, Hedner U: Oral contraceptives and venous thromboembolism. Br J Obstet Gynaecol 89:381–386, 1982

55. Huppert LC: Vascular effects of hormonal contraception. Clin Obstet Gynecol 24:951–963, 1981

56. Irey NS, Norris HJ: Intimal vascular lesions associated with female reproductive steroids. Arch Pathol 96:227–234, 1973

57. Meade TW: Oral contraceptives, clotting factors and thrombosis. Am J Obstet Gynecol 142:758–761, 1982

58. Laos O, Schoultz BV: Amniotic fluid embolism: A review of the literature and 2 case reports. Int J Gynaecol Obstet 15:48–55, 1977

59. Goldsmith HL, Turitto V: Rheological aspects of thrombosis and haemostasis: Basic principles and applications. Thromb Haemost 55(3):415–435, 1986

60. Farag AM, Bottoms SF, Mammen EF et al: Oral contraceptives and the hemostatic system. Obstet Gynecol 71:584–588, 1988

61. Realini JP, Goldzieher JW: Oral contraceptives and cardiovascular disease: A critique of the epidemiologic studies. Am J Obstet Gynecol 152:729–798, 1985

62. Stolley PD, Strom BL, Startwell PE: Oral contraceptives and vascular disease. Epidemiol Rev 11:241–243, 1989

63. Gerstman BB, Piper JM, Freiman JP et al: Oral contraceptive oestrogen and progestin potencies and the incidence of deep venous thromboembolism. Int J Epidemiol 19:931–6, 1990

64. Godsland IF, Crook D, Wynn V: Coronary heart disease risk markers in users of low-dose oral contraceptives. J Reprod Med 36:226–37, 1991

65. Rosenberg L, Palmer JR, Lesko SM, Shapiro S: Oral contraceptive use and the risk of myocardial infarction. Am J Epidemiol 131:1009–1106, 1990

66. Hodgkinson CP: Physiology of the ovarian veins during pregnancy. Obstet Gynecol 1:26–37, 1953

67. Lotze EC, Kaufmann RH, Kaplan AL: Postpartum ovarian vein thrombophlebitis. Obstet Gynecol Surv 21:853–859, 1966

68. Baum NH, Moriel E, Carlton E: Renal vein thrombosis: Review. J Urol 119:443–454, 1978

69. Hoyumpa AM, Schiff L, Helfman EL: Budd-Chiari syndrome in women taking oral contraceptives. Am J Med 50:137–140, 1971

70. Mitchell MC, Boitnott JK, Kaufman S, Cameron JL, Maddrey WC: Budd-Chiari syndrome: Etiology, diagnosis, and management. Medicine 61:199–207, 1982

71. Khuroo MS, Daha DU: Budd-Chiari syndrome following pregnancy. Am J Med 68:113–117, 1980

72. Auerback P: Primary cerebral venous thrombosis of young adults: The disease manifestations of an under recognized disease. Ann Neurol 3:81–90, 1978

73. Polterz AA: The pathology of intracranial venous thrombosis in oral contraceptives. J Pathol 106:209–214, 1972

74. Sabiston DC: Pathophysiology, diagnosis and management of pulmonary embolism. Am J Surg 138:384–394, 1978

75. Arthure H: Maternal deaths from pulmonary embolism. Br J Obstet Gynaecol 75:1309–1313, 1968

76. Twiggs LB, Morrow CP, Schlaertl JB: Acute pulmonary complications of molar pregnancy. Am J Obstet Gynecol 135:189–198, 1979

77. Moore P, Janes O, Saltos N: Fat embolism syndrome: Incidence, significance and early features. Aust N Z J Surg 51:546–551, 1981

78. Ragan WD: Antepartum air embolism. Indiana Med 74:30–32, 1981

79. Nelson PH: Pulmonary gas embolism in pregnancy and the puerperium. Obstet Gynecol Surv 15:449–459, 1960

80. Yacoub OF, Cardona I, Coveler LA, Dodson MG: Carbon dioxide embolism during laparoscopy. Anesthesiology 57:533–535, 1982

81. Baggish MS, Daniell JF: Catastrophic injury secondary to the use of coaxial gas-cooled fibers and artificial sapphire tips for intrauterine surgery: A report of five cases. Lasers Surg Med 9:581–84, 1989

82. Morgan M: Amniotic fluid embolism. Anesthesia 34:20–32, 1979

82. Naulty JS, Ostheimer GW, Datta S, Knapp B, Weiss JB: Incidence of venous air embolism during epidural catheter insertion. Anesthesiology 57:410–413, 1982

83. Peterson EP, Taylor HB: Amniotic fluid embolism: An analysis of 40 cases. Obstet Gynecol 35:787–795, 1970

84. Steiner PE, Lushbaugh CC: Maternal pulmonary embolism by amniotic fluid. JAMA 117:1245–1254, 1340–1345, 1941

85. Clark SL: New concepts of amniotic fluid embolism: A review. Obstet Gynecol Surv 45:360–368, 1990

86. Gabel HD: Maternal mortality in South Carolina from 1970 to 1984: An analysis. Obstet Gynecol 69:307–311, 1987

87. Liban E, Raz S: A clinicopathologic study of fourteen cases of amniotic fluid embolism. Am J Clin Pathol 51:477–486, 1969

88. Clark SL, Cotton DB, Gonik B, Greenspoon J, Phelan JP: Central hemodynamic alterations in amniotic fluid embolism. Am J Obstet Gynecol 158:1124–1126, 1988

89. Masson RG, Ruggieri J, Siddiqui MM: Amniotic fluid embolism: Definitive diagnosis in a survivor. Am Rev Resp Dis 120:187–192, 1979

90. Clark SL, Pavlova Z, Greenspoon J, Horenstein J, Phelan JP: Squamous cells in the maternal pulmonary circulation. Am J Obstet Gynecol 154:104–106, 1986

91. Giampaolo C, Schneider V, Kowalski BH, Bellaver LA: The cytologic diagnosis of amniotic fluid embolism: A critical reappraisal. Diagn Cytopathol 3:126–8, 1987

92. Attwood HD: Fatal pulmonary embolism by amniotic fluid. J Clin Pathol 9:38–46, 1956

93. Chesley LC: Vascular reactivity in normal and toxemic pregnancy. Clin Obstet Gynecol 9:871–881, 1966

94. Ferris TF: Toxemia and hypertension. In Burrow GN, Ferris TF, eds. Medical complications during pregnancy, pp 53–104. Philadelphia, WB Saunders, 1975

95. Finnerty FA Jr: Hypertension and pregnancy. J Cardiovasc Med 5:559–565, 1980

96. Gallery EDM: Hypertension in pregnancy. Aust Fam Physician 9:250–254, 1980

97. Zuspan FP: Toxemia of pregnancy. In Sciarra JJ, ed. Gynecology and obstetrics, rev ed, vol 2, pp 1–20. Philadelphia, Harper & Row, 1983

98. Weinstein L: Syndrome of hemolysis, elevated liver enzymes and low platelet count: A severe consequence of hypertension in pregnancy. Am J Obstet Gynecol 142:159–167, 1982

99. Verhaeghe J, Anthony J, Davey DA: Platelet count and liver function tests in proteinuric and chronic hypertension in pregnancy. South Afr Med J 79:590–594, 1991

100. Davies AM: Epidemiology of the hypertensive disorders of pregnancy. Bull World Health Organ 57:373–386, 1979

101. Miller FG: Hepatic hemorrhage due to eclampsia. Can Med Assoc J 106:964–968, 1972

102. Douvas SG, Meeks O, Phillips JC et al: Liver disease in pregnancy. Obstet Gynecol Surv 38:531–536, 1983

103. Fallon HJ: Liver diseases. In Burrow GN, Ferris TF, eds. Medical complications during pregnancy, pp 351–381. Philadelphia, WB Saunders, 1975

104. Sheehan HL, Lynch JB: Pathology of toxemia of pregnancy. Baltimore, Williams & Wilkins, 1973

105. Steven MM: Pregnancy and liver disease. Gut 22:592–614, 1981

106. Page EW: On the pathogenesis of pre-eclampsia and eclampsia. Br J Obstet Gynaecol 79:883–894, 1972

107. Strauss S, Walden R, Mashiach S, Graif M: Sonographic liver changes prior to clinical signs of preeclampsia. Gynecol Obstet Invest 31:114–115, 1991

108. Hurwitz MB: Jaundice in pregnancy: A 10-year study and review. S Afr Med J 44:219–226, 1972

109. Castaneda H, Garcia-Romera H, Canto M: Hepatic hemorrhage in toxemia of pregnancy. Am J Obstet Gynecol 107:578–584, 1970

110. Bis KA, Wayman B: Rupture of the liver associated with

pregnancy: A review of the literature and report of two cases. Obstet Gynecol Surv 31:763–767, 1976

111. Herbert WN, Brenner WE: Improving survival with liver rupture complicating pregnancy. Am J Obstet Gynecol 142:530–534, 1982

112. Mokotoff R, Weiss LS, Brandon LH et al: Liver rupture complicating toxemia of pregnancy: An example of thrombo-hemorrhagic disease. Arch Intern Med 119:375–380, 1967

113. Portnuff J, Ballon S: Hepatic rupture in pregnancy. Am J Obstet Gynecol 114:1102–1104, 1972

114. Roopnarinesingh S, Jankey N, Gopeesingh T: Rupture of the liver as a complication of pre-eclampsia: Case report and review of the literature. Int Surg 66:169–170, 1981

115. Gonzalez-Angulo A, Salazar H: Pathology of the reproductive system, breast and liver in women during hormonal contraception. In Josimovich JB, ed. Uterine contraction-hormonal contraception, pp 343–380. New York, John Wiley & Sons, 1973

116. Barrows GH, Christopherson WM, Mays ET: Human liver tumors in relation to steroidal usage. Environ Health Perspect 50:201–208, 1983

117. Baum IK, Bookstein JJ, Holtz F et al: Possible association between hepatomas and oral contraceptives. Lancet 2:926–929, 1973

118. Christopherson WM, Mays ET: Liver tumors and contraceptive steroids: Experience with the first one hundred registry patients. J Natl Cancer Inst 58:167–172, 1977

119. Christopherson WM, Mays ET, Barrows G: A clinicopathologic study of steroid-related liver tumors. Am J Surg Pathol 1:31–36, 1977

120. Christopherson WM, Mays ET, Barrows G: Hepatocellular carcinoma in young women on oral contraceptives. Lancet 2:38–39, 1978

121. Fechner RE: Benign hepatic lesions and orally administered contraceptives. Hum Pathol 8:255–268, 1977

122. Ishak KG, Rabin L: Benign tumors of the liver. Med Clin North Am 59:995–1010, 1975

123. Klatskin G: Hepatic tumors: Possible relationship to use of oral contraceptives. Gastroenterology 73:386–394, 1977

124. Knowles DM II, Casavella WJ, Johnson PM, Wolff M: The clinical, radiologic, and pathologic characterization of benign hepatic neoplasms. Medicine 57:223–237, 1978

125. Mays ET, Christopherson WM, Barrows GH: Focal nodular hyperplasia of the liver: Possible relationship to oral contraceptives. Am J Clin Pathol 61:735–746, 1974

126. Mays ET, Christopherson WM, Mahr MM et al: Hepatic changes in young women ingesting contraceptive steroids. JAMA 235:730–732, 1976

127. Rosenberg L: The risk of liver neoplasia in relation to combined oral contraceptive use. Contraception 43:643–662, 1991

128. Kerlin P, Davis GL, McGill DB et al: Hepatic adenoma and focal nodular hyperplasia: Clinical, pathologic and radiologic features. Gastroenterology 84:994–1002, 1983

129. Neuberger J, Nunnerly HB, Davis M et al: Oral-contraceptive-associated liver tumours: Occurrence of malignancy and difficulties in diagnosis. Lancet 1:273–276, 1980

130. Grabowski GM, Stenram U, Berqvist Z: Focal nodular hyperplasia of the liver, benign hepatomas, oral contraceptives and other drugs affecting the liver. Acta Pathol Microbiol Scand (A) 83:615–622, 1975

131. Knowles DM II, Wolff M: Focal nodular hyperplasia of the liver: A clinicopathologic study and review of the literature. Hum Pathol 7:533–545, 1976

132. Staufer JQ, Lapinski MW, Honold DJ et al: Focal nodular hyperplasia of the liver and intrahepatic hemorrhage in young women on oral contraceptives. Ann Intern Med 83:301–306, 1975

133. Kent DR, Nissen ED, Nissen SE et al: Maternal death resulting from rupture of liver adenoma associated with oral contraceptives. Obstet Gynecol 50(Suppl):5–6, 1977

134. Albritton DR, Tompkins RK, Longmire WP Jr: Hepatic cell adenoma: A report of four cases. Ann Surg 180:14–24, 1974

135. Ameriks JA, Thompson NW, Norman W et al: Hepatic cell adenomas, spontaneous liver rupture and oral contraceptives. Arch Surg 110:548–557, 1975

136. Edmondson HA, Henderson B, Benton A: Liver cell adenomas associated with the use of oral contraceptives. N Engl J Med 294:470–472, 1976

137. Buhler H, Pirovino M, Akovbiantz A et al: Regression of liver cell adenoma. Gastroenterology 82:775–782, 1982

138. Edmondson HA, Reynolds TB, Henderson B et al: Regression of liver cell adenomas associated with oral contraceptives. Ann Intern Med 86:180–184, 1977

139. Davis M, Portmann B, Searle M et al: Histological evidence of carcinoma in a hepatic tumor associated with oral contraceptives. Br Med J 4:496–498, 1975

140. Dudley AG et al: Hepatocellular carcinoma associated with oral contraceptive use and pregnancy. Diagn Gynecol Obstet 4:301–304, 1982

141. Glassberg AB, Rosenbaum EH: Oral contraceptives and malignant hepatoma. Lancet 1:479, 1976

142. Menzies-Gow N: Hepatocellular carcinoma associated with oral contraceptives. Br J Surg 65:316–324, 1978

143. O'Sullivan JP, Rosswick RP: Oral contraceptives and malignant hepatic tumours. Lancet 1:1124–1130, 1976

144. Shar SR, Kew MC: Oral contraceptives and hepatocellular carcinoma. Cancer 49:407–410, 1982

145. Thalassinos NC, Lymberatos C, Hadjionnou J et al: Liver cell carcinoma after long term use of estrogen-like drugs. Lancet 1:270, 1974

146. Adami HO, Persson I, Hoover R, Schairer C, Bergkvist L: Risk of cancer in women receiving hormone replacement therapy. Int J Cancer 44:833–839, 1989

147. Farhi DC, Shikes RH, Murari PJ, Silverberg SG: Hepatocellular carcinoma in young people. Cancer 52:1516–1525, 1983

148. Farhi DC, Shikes RH, Silverberg SG: Ultrastructure of fibrolamellar oncocytic hepatoma. Cancer 50:702–709, 1982

149. Scott RB: Critical illness and deaths associated with intrauterine devices. Obstet Gynecol 31:322–328, 1968

150. Lee NC, Rubin GL, Borucki R: The intrauterine device and pelvic inflammatory disease revisited: New results from the Women's Health Study. Obstet Gynecol 72:1–6, 1988

151. Key TC, Kreutner AK: Gastrointestinal complications of modern intrauterine devices. Obstet Gynecol 55:239–243, 1980

152. Yuzpe AA: Pneumoperitoneum needle and trocar injuries in laparoscopy: A survey on possible contributing factors and prevention. J Reprod Med 35:485–490, 1990

153. Peterson HB, DeStefano F, Rubin GL et al: Deaths attributable to tubal sterilization in the United States, 1977 to 1981. Am J Obstet Gynecol 146:131–136, 1983

154. Riedel HH, Lehmann-Willenbrock E, Conrad P, Semm K: German pelviscopic statistics for the years 1978–1982. Endoscopy 18:219–222, 1986

155. Peterson HB, Greenspan JR, Ory HW: Deaths following puncture of the aorta during laparoscopic sterilization. Obstet Gynecol 59:133–134, 1982

156. Levy BS, Soderstrom RM, Dail DH: Bowel injuries during laparoscopy: Gross anatomy and histology. J Reprod Med 30:168–172, 1985

157. Thompson BH, Wheeless CR Jr: Gastrointestinal complications of laparoscopy sterilization. Obstet Gynecol 41:669–676, 1973

158. Todd J, Fishaut M, Kapral F et al: Toxic shock syndrome associated with phage group I staphylococci. Lancet 2:1116–1118, 1978

159. Wager GP: Toxic shock syndrome: A review. Am J Obstet Gynecol 146:93–99, 1983

160. Crowder WE, Shannon FL: Colposcopic diagnosis of vaginal ulcerations in toxic shock syndrome. Obstet Gynecol 61:50S–53S, 1983

161. Reingold AI: Toxic shock syndrome: An update. Am J Obstet Gynecol 165:1236–1239, 1991

162. Lanes SF, Poole C, Dreyer NA, Lanza LL: Toxic shock syndrome, contraceptive methods, and vaginitis. Am J Obstet Gynecol 154:989–91, 1986

163. Bowe LW, Sand PK, Ostergard DR: Toxic shock syndrome following carbon dioxide laser treatment of genital tract condyloma accuminatum. Am J Obstet Gynecol 154:145–146, 1986

164. Dotters DJ, Katz VL: Streptococcal toxic shock associated with septic abortion. Obstet Gynecol 78:549–551, 1991

165. Schlievert PM: TSST-1: Structure, function, purification, and detection. Role of toxic shock syndrome toxin 1 in toxic shock syndrome: Overview. Rev Infect Dis 2:107S–109S, 1989

166. Paris AL, Loreen AH, Blum D et al: Pathologic findings in twelve fatal cases of toxic shock syndrome. Ann Intern Med 96:852–857, 1982

Pathology in Gynecology and Obstetrics, Fourth Edition, edited by Claude Gompel and Steven G. Silverberg. J. B. Lippincott Company, Philadelphia © 1994.

12 | *New Technologies in Gynecologic Pathology*

Alain Verhest, Hironobu Sasano, Shinji Sato, and Akira Yajima

CYTOMETRY

Measurement of DNA content has been a valuable technique in the study of gynecologic tumors for many years.[1] The clinical relevance of DNA content is based on the linkage between extensive chromosome aberrations and shifts from euploidy with loss of modal value. The goal is to better assess prognostic indicators by supplementing subjective histologic type and grading with more objective measurements.

Methodology

There are basic differences between flow cytometry (FCM) and static DNA analyzers. FCM favors the measurement of a huge number of signals, supposed to be single unaltered cells, so that the information on the quantity of "events" is valuable. In static devices, the technique is based on the stoichiometric character of the Feulgen stain, which is directly proportional to the amount of DNA in the nucleus. Individual cells are submitted interactively to a skilled observer, and each single cell is taken into consideration. Superpositions, fragments, and benign accompanying cells are discarded, making the total number of measured cells much lower (200 to 300 nuclei). This interactive morphonuclear analysis allows a stepwise multiparametric discriminant analysis, selecting for each pathologic entity between the most significant morphometric (nuclear area) and densitometric (DNA index) parameters and ana-

lyzing the spatial distribution and condensation of the chromatin.[2]

Both FCM and ICM (interactive computerized cytometry) can be applied to fine-needle aspiration material if adequately sampled. A cell suspension at a minimal concentration of 2×10^6 cells/mL in buffer solution is needed for FCM; full details of the procedure are explained elsewhere.[3,4] For ICM, smears can be obtained from aspirates, surgical specimens, or resuspension of paraffin-embedded blocks.[5] Small aneuploid stem lines and intratumoral heterogeneity are detected more easily in aspirates than in tumor pieces.[6] The smears are immediately fixed in EFA (96% ethanol, 75 vol; 40% neutral formol, 20 vol; 5% acetic acid, 5 vol). They can be stored at 4°C.

Comparison of FCM with ICM shows 80% agreement in ploidy assessment. However, some cases judged as diploid by FCM were reclassified as aneuploid by ICM. It is therefore recommended that FCM diploid cases be confirmed by an ICM analysis.[7] The major pitfalls in the accuracy of interactive computerized cytometry arise in the reproducibility of the sampling and staining procedures and in the standardization of the digital analyses.[8]

Ovary

Abnormal karyotypes and DNA values in ovarian cancer have been found in some reports to be independent adverse prognostic indicators of patient survival.[9] The DNA index combined with the number of aneuploid clones and the S-phase fraction is prognostically significant.[10] The DNA content in both primary tumors and metastatic ascites is predominantly hypodiploid and paratriploid.[11-15] Aneuploid tumor cells are more often identified in advanced cases than in earlier stages of the disease.[3] Paratriploid tumors also are more disseminated at the time of diagnosis, which could be due to an early loss of chromosomes followed by duplication of the hypodiploid clones leading to near triploidy.[16] Near-diploid tumors have a more favorable prognosis.[17]

Tumors of low malignant potential (borderline tumors) should perhaps be reassessed in the light of their DNA analysis. Five of 35 of these ovarian borderline tumors studied by our group (unpublished data) were hyperdiploid and aneuploid, suggesting that they should be considered early carcinomas.

Corpus Uteri

In endometrial carcinoma, diploid tumors have a better prognosis than aneuploid tumors,[17] and the ploidy group is related to the degree of differentiation. Attempts to differentiate between atypical hyperplasia and carcinoma give inconclusive results by DNA analysis, because diploidy with occasional peridiploidy is present in atypical hyperplasia and in early carcinoma.[9] Morphometry sometimes helps in the differential diagnosis of papillary carcinoma with or without a background of atypical hyperplasia.[18]

Cervix

Premalignant lesions show two groups of modal values, one at the diploid level and one at the hypertriploid-tetraploid level, with in situ carcinoma having undergone less change than invasive carcinoma. Histograms obtained from severe dysplasia and carcinoma in situ were found sufficiently different compared with those from mild lesions to be proposed as an automatic prescreening procedure for cancer diagnosis.[19]

Changes in nuclear shape and chromatin structure observed in cervical intraepithelial neoplasia (CIN) have been compared with normal cells on reference smears. Not surprisingly, significant deviations were also detected close to the intraepithelial lesion in histologically normal-appearing cells, auguring possible recurrence after surgical excision or ablation of the visible lesion.[20] The risk is highlighted by the demonstration of human papillomavirus in the nuclei of "normal" epithelium adjacent to lesions and persisting in the residual tissue after local treatment.[21]

A comparative study between a group of pure CIN III cases and selected CIN areas adjacent to the invasive component of cervical cancers revealed significant differences in a panel of photometric features. The CIN lesions associated with invasive cancer all showed features consistent with potentially progressive lesions, whereas the pure CIN cases could be divided into a similar cluster (62% of patients younger than 45 years, and 27% of those older than 45 years) and a separate cluster suggesting the possibility of regression.[22]

Cervical squamous cell carcinomas are near diploid or hypertriploid.[23] DNA analyses tend to suggest that tumors with large nuclei and a triploid to tetraploid range have a better survival rate and late distant metastases. Those peridiploid tumors with a worse prognosis can be identified histologically as of the small cell type.[17]

Breast

Many prognostic indicators have already proved to be relevant in breast cancer, and every new machine-generated parameter or combination of parameters must provide nonredundant information. They can be used to quantify objectively the subjective appraisal of the shape, size, and hyperchromatism used in the scoring of Bloom and Richardson.[24] They are equally informative with fresh imprints or with smears from fine-needle aspiration.[25,26]

DNA content and its derivatives (DNA index, DNA malignancy grade) have been correlated more or less successfully with histologic grading, receptor status, and lymph node status.[27,28] Involvement of the axillary lymph nodes is most important in the prediction of disease-free interval.[29] By DNA measurements, both node-negative and node-positive cases can be split into separate prognostic subgroups.[30]

Correlation of aneuploidy with tumor size is biased by the frequency of diploid, small, nonpalpable tumors easily detected by mammography during their indolent course. Aneuploidy often precedes the invasive stage; aneuploid tumors grow more rapidly, and their aggressive behavior is correlated with absent estrogen receptors and poorly differentiated histologic type.[30-33]

Measurements of the nuclear area in invasive cancers are in agreement with the concept that less aggressive tumors contain cells with smaller nuclei.[25,34] These measurements have been used to differentiate between atypical ductal hyperplasia and in situ carcinoma.[35]

Nuclear DNA distribution is supposed to predict the outcome of the disease, but results from different groups remain contradictory. Clinical application to the care of individual patients should be considered questionable. In this regard, study of the S-phase fraction in combination with ploidy[27] or the combined use of DNA content and histologic characterization[9] seem better than either method alone. For some authors, there is no clear relation between histogram distribution of DNA and 5-bromodeoxyuridine (BrdU) labeling index. There may be tumors with hyperdiploid or frankly aneuploid cells but with low S-phase fraction, raising the question of the biological significance of these aneuploid cells.[36]

Another promising application is the study of morphometric and textural modifications of breast tumor cells related to their response during chemotherapy.[37] These studies promise to be useful in the identification of chemosensitive stem lines and may help to develop new therapeutic strategies.

Conclusion

The ability of DNA ploidy to predict recurrence and survival is more reliable in early stages of cancer, but ploidy and other cytometric determinations do not facilitate the early diagnosis of malignancy. Moreover, no single parameter threshold has a specific meaning. When assessing the information that a single parameter provides, it is necessary to consider whether that factor has a direct impact on other relevant prognostic factors.

DNA content is a stable, easily measured marker of tumor cells. It gives valuable information about the biology of the cell, which must not be confused with the clinical behavior of the clone. How these measurements may be applied to the management of individual patients with cancer remains controversial. The measurements should not be used for individual therapeutic decisions.

IMMUNOHISTOCHEMICAL ANALYSIS OF CELL CYCLE-RELATED ANTIGENS

Cell kinetic information is becoming a valuable adjunct to histopathologically based tumor classification. It is well known that the identification of proliferating compartments in human tumor tissues is important in predicting biological behavior. Among the various methods used to assess cell proliferation or cell kinetics in human surgical specimens submitted to pathology laboratories, immunohistochemical analysis of cell cycle-related antigens has several advantages over other reported methods, including thymidine labeling index, BrdU, and FCM: cellular and tissue architectures are maintained (especially compared with FCM), the method is relatively simple and rapid, and the use of radioactivity is avoided. Therefore, immunohistochemical detection of cell cycle-related antigens has the potential to become important in assessment of tumor cell kinetics in pathologic material routinely submitted to the laboratory. This section reviews the three cell cycle-related nuclear antigens most extensively studied in human tumors by immunohistochemical methods.

DNA Polymerase α

DNA polymerase α is an enzyme that plays a central role in DNA replication in mammalian cells.[38] The production of a monoclonal antibody against DNA polymerase α provided a new method for detecting proliferative activity of both tumor cells and normal cells with high proliferative activity.[39] The enzyme is localized in the nucleus at the G_1/S or G_2 phase and in the cytoplasm at the M phase of cultured human cells; it is not detected in resting cells.[40] DNA polymerase α was extensively studied immunohistochemically in various human neoplasms by Tsutsumi and colleagues.[41] In human gynecologic tumors, Mushika and associates reported that the proportion of cells positive for DNA polymerase α increased progressively in dysplasia, carcinoma in situ, and invasive squamous carcinoma of the cervix.[42] However, immunostaining of DNA polymerase α requires frozen sections, and in our experience the results are easily affected by fixation. Therefore, analysis of DNA polymerase α is not widely used in diagnostic laboratories.

Ki67

Ki67 is a mouse monoclonal antibody that was produced by Gerdes and colleagues in 1983.[43] The precise nature and composition of the antigen are unknown, but it is considered to be a nuclear antigen present in all phases of the cell cycle except for the G_0 phase.[44] It has been postulated that the number of cells with positive immunoreactivity of Ki67 per total number of tumor cells represents the number of cells cycling at any one time (ie, the growth fraction). However, Ki67 labeling obtained by immunohistochemistry in various tumors has not necessarily been consistent with flow cytometric studies and the usual clinical and histologic parameters used to predict clinical outcome.[45] Ki67 labeling also requires frozen sections, as in the case of DNA polymerase α, but can be demonstrated on cytologic smears if appropriately processed.[46] Ki67 labeling eventually may be worth incorporating into a routine diagnostic service, but it awaits further investigations to be established as an independent prognostic indicator.

Proliferating Cell Nuclear Antigen

Proliferating cell nuclear antigen (PCNA) was discovered initially by Miyachi and associates as a nuclear antigen that reacts with an autoantibody in the sera of some patients with systemic lupus erythematosus.[47] Subsequent studies have revealed that the expression of this 36-kd nuclear antigen correlates with the late G_1 and S-phase of the cell cycle.[48] PCNA later turned out to be an auxiliary protein of DNA polymerase δ and is considered to play an important role in the initiation of cell proliferation.[49] Recently, Hall and colleagues employed monoclonal antibody PC-10, which recognizes a fixation- and processing-resistant epitope of PCNA and thus is appropriate for immunohistochemistry in routinely processed surgical pathology specimens.[50] With the introduction of this antibody, immunolocalization of PCNA has a practical advantage over that of Ki67 and DNA polymerase α for assessing cell kinetics on tissue sections: PCNA can be detected to some extent in formalin-fixed and paraffin-embedded specimens. This makes retrospective studies of cell kinetics possible. However, PCNA immunoreactivity is considerably influenced by tissue preparation, especially choice of fixatives and duration of fixation. In addition, intra- and interobserver errors in interpretation are still prominent. The PCNA labeling index has been demonstrated to be consistent with the Ki67 labeling index,[50,51] BrdU incorporation,[50] and flow-cytometric S-phase analysis,[52] although conflicting data have been reported. Contradictory results have been reported in correlation of the PCNA labeling index with the clinical outcome of various malignant tumors.

The variability of PCNA data obtained in previous investigations may be due to lack of sensitivity in the immunohistochemical detection system, lack of uniformity in preparing the tissue specimens, the choice of antibodies, or differences in scoring methods (eg, how to interpret weakly stained PCNA immunoreactivity). At this juncture, PCNA labeling is best assessed by (1) using immediately and briefly fixed (10% formalin or 4% paraformaldehyde) and paraffin-embedded specimens; (2) employing a monoclonal antibody against a tissue-processing-resistant epitope of PCNA; and (3) counting all PCNA-reactive nuclei as positive regardless of intensity of immunostain. Under these conditions, PCNA was successfully and reproducibly localized in our laboratory in surgical pathology materials including gynecologic specimens (Figs. 12-1 and 12-2). We recommend incorporating PCNA immunohistochemistry into the techniques available in pathology laboratories.

AgNORS

Nucleolar organizer regions (NORs) are loops of ribosomal DNA (rDNA) present in the nuclei of cells that possess ribosomal RNA (rRNA) genes.[53] These rRNA are transcribed by RNA polymerase I and ultimately direct the synthesis of protein. Therefore, NOR numbers appear to reflect cellular and nuclear activity. NORs can be easily visualized by a silver impregnation technique originally described on metaphase chromosome spreads and then applied to histologic sections. Since Crocker and Nar reported a one-step silver staining technique for nucleolar organizer regions applicable to routinely processed formalin-fixed and paraffin-embedded tissues,[54] the method has been widely used in the study of human neoplasms. The argyrophilic structures obtained by a one-step silver stain (AgNORs) are NOR-associated nonhistone nucleoproteins.

AgNORs appear as multiple granular, well-defined, black, silver-stained intranuclear structures, sometimes in aggregates within the nucleolus (Color Figure 12-1). In human ovarian epithelial tumors (Sasano and associates, unpublished observations), the mean number of AgNORs per nucleus is correlated with histologic nuclear grade (Fig. 12-3) and histologic type of the neoplasms (Fig. 12-4). However, Wilkinson and colleagues studied AgNORs in human endometrial lesions and found no significant differences of the mean number of AgNORs per nucleus among intraendometrial neoplasia, hyperplastic mucosa, and normal proliferative mucosa, with a slight increase in invasive adenocarcinoma.[55]

AgNOR staining and counting is a relatively easy and simple method, and only a darkroom facility is required when performing this stain in diagnostic pathology laboratories. AgNORs are, however, associ-

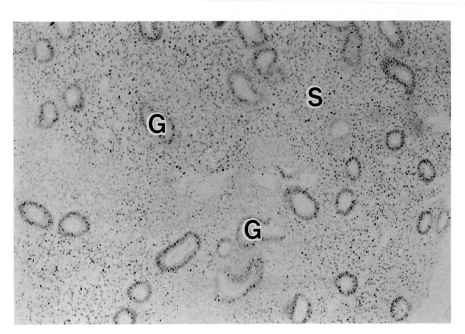

FIGURE 12-1 Immunolocalization of proliferating cell nuclear antigen in proliferative human endometrium. Immunoreactivity is observed in stroma (*S*) and glands (*G*).

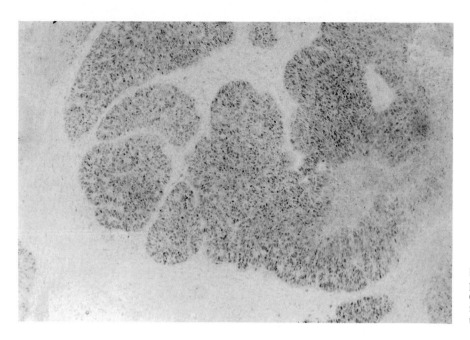

FIGURE 12-2 Immunolocalization of proliferating cell nuclear antigen (PCNA) in poorly differentiated endometrial adenocarcinoma. Almost all the tumor cells are positive for PCNA.

ated with several major technical problems, including intra- and interobserver errors in counting the silver grains, and the effects of fixation (increasing fixation time resulting in a tendency for the smaller intranucleolar dots to coalesce).[56] In addition, increasing numbers of reports have demonstrated no relation between AgNORs and prognosis, clinical course, cell proliferation indices, and DNA ploidy.[57] Therefore, the practical value of AgNORs remains to be evaluated at this juncture.

KARYOTYPING

At the beginning of the century, Boveri expressed the theory that mitotic anomalies lead to malignant transformations.[58] The results of cytogenetic studies conducted on animal and human tumors over the subsequent three quarters of a century have favored this hypothesis, and chromosome anomalies are today considered a major event in carcinogenesis.[59] The current karyotype nomenclature is based on the banding techniques of the 1970s,[60] which individualized 500 to 600 chromatin segments and was crucial in proving that almost all tumor metaphases are actually abnormal.[61]

For a couple of decades, cytogenetic studies have been more rewarding in human leukemia than in solid tumors, because the higher mitotic rate and natural suspension state of bone marrow aspirates fa-

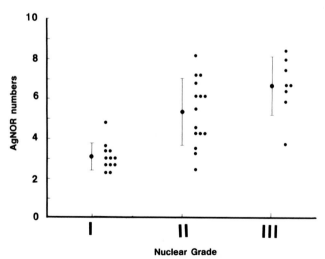

FIGURE 12-3 Correlation between nuclear grade and mean number of AgNORs per nucleus in serous and mucinous carcinoma of the ovary.

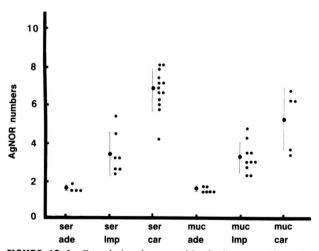

FIGURE 12-4 Correlation between histologic types of ovarian serous and mucinous neoplasms and pooled mean AgNOR numbers per nucleus. *ser ade,* serous cystadenoma; *ser lmp,* serous adenocarcinoma of low malignant potential; *ser car,* serous adenocarcinoma; *muc ade,* mucinous cystadenoma; *muc lmp,* mucinous adenocarcinoma of low malignant potential; *muc car,* mucinous carcinoma.

vored cytogenetic analyses in the leukemias. Although appropriate studies of chromosomes in solid tumors are still few (less than 20% of more than 14,000 cancer cases in one major analysis[62]), they prove that nonrandom specific changes occur in solid tumors the same way they do in leukemias and lymphomas, hallmarked by an abnormal clone with markers and consistent chromosome breakpoints in the whole cell population.

It is now well established that chromosome rearrangements are nonrandom and often specific for the histologic pattern of the neoplastic proliferation.[63] Some cytogenetic findings are pathognomonic of tumor subtypes, such as t(X;18) in synovial sarcoma, t(12;16) in myxoid liposarcoma, and t(11;22) in Ewing's sarcoma, or of their embryologic origin (iso12p in testicular germ cell tumors).[64,65] This morphology-associated profile may be helpful in cases of uncertain differentiation or origin and is becoming accepted as an aid in the diagnosis of soft-tissue tumors. Despite the fact that epithelial tumors are much more common than sarcomas, sarcomas still constitute the bulk of the reports. This is because their chromosome rearrangements are unique and simple, as they are in hematologic neoplasms, and because they may retain a relative karyotypic stability through clinical progression and metastasis.

The recurrent chromosome breakpoints of benign tumors are not the same as those of their malignant counterparts. There may be specific regions preferentially affected in certain benign neoplasms.[66] It is, however, possible that the underlying cause is the same, although the biological effects depend on the affected breakpoints distinguishing benign neoplasms from their malignant counterparts.[67] Probably at its very beginning, a tumor is still polyclonal and occasionally multicentric. One or a small number of cells initiate the process of neoplasia by monoclonal selection, with the genetic alteration itself allowing the outgrowth of the dominant cell by clonal expansion. The tumors remain monoclonal but heterogeneous, composed of different subclones with subsequent (secondary) chromosome changes selected by their growth advantage, their drug resistance, and the more aggressive biological behavior they can offer.

At the time of surgery and sampling for cytogenetic studies, carcinomas are already fully developed. Their karyotype at that stage is far more complex and is blurred by many secondary changes often not related to a specific disease. Significant primary changes tend to be obscured, and their analysis is puzzling; interpretation is time-consuming and sometimes meaningless. Nevertheless, detection of minor DNA changes remains beyond the resolution of "metaphase cytogenetics" and needs more sophisticated methods, such as molecular genetics or in situ hybridization. This promising new approach uses fluorescent DNA probes specific to known regions of the genome to measure numerical heterogeneity in tumors and even in normal tissues and to demon-

strate structural rearrangements.[68,69] Combining in situ hybridization on nuclei isolated from fresh tissue and metaphase cytogenetics will certainly improve the interpretation of complex karyotypes.[70] The major advantage of interphase cytogenetics is that it requires only a small number of cells, its sensitivity allowing the detection of minimal residual disease.[68]

Karyotyping is the first step of recognition of the chromosome profiles of the tumors. Once the profile is characterized, interphase cytogenetics becomes relevant to the study of a larger series, including archival material, allowing an assessment of the prognostic significance of every deviation from normal.

Malignant Tumors

Ovary

The first karyotypic studies in the ovary were conducted on metastatic fluids or cell lines and yielded confusing results. Throughout the bulk of this complex information, chromosomes 1 and 6 and, to a lesser degree, chromosome 11 remain the more consistently involved in structural rearrangements (Fig. 12-5).[14,71-73]

Published studies deal mostly with the common epithelial adenocarcinomas, which represent more than 80% of all ovarian cancers. A t(6;14) translocation was described in 12 papillary cystadenocarcinomas,[74] but it could not be confirmed as specifically and systematically involved in ovarian carcinomas.[72,75-77] However, aberrations of 6q could be an important constituent of ovarian cancer, having been recognized in various histologic types and cell lines.[72,78,79] Chromosome 7 has also been reported in structural or numerical rearrangements.[76,80-82]

In a recent survey, structural rearrangement breakpoints in 53 ovarian carcinomas appeared nonrandomly clustered in certain chromosome regions and could be related to tumor-specific allele loss.[16] The potential existence of a tumor suppressor gene has been suggested in deletions of 6q and 17p, whose loss favors transformation.[83] In the survey, 7 of the 53 carcinomas of the ovary displayed simple karyotypic changes: 5 had numerical changes only (2 of these being trisomic 12) and 2 had a single translocation as the sole anomaly.[16] Such simple karyotypic changes appear to be preferentially demonstrated in well-differentiated carcinomas or in borderline tumors.[84,85] These changes might precede complex aneuploidies acquired during the progressive dedifferentiation of the tumor, according to the theory of clonal evolution as a cause of more aggressive phenotype.[84,86]

Complex karyotypes are more frequent in serous papillary tumors than in mucinous and clear cell carcinomas.[16] Among 46 cases with complex aberrations, chromosomes 1, 3, and 6 were commonly altered, as already mentioned in previous studies; chromosome 19p arms were affected 26 times, and q arms 14 times. Twelve tumors had a breakpoint in

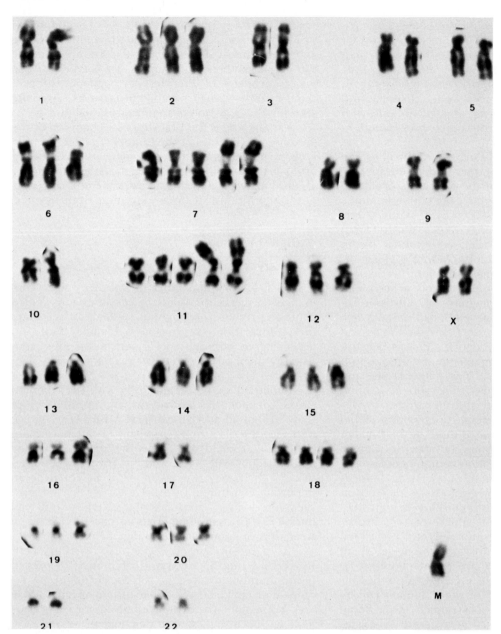

FIGURE 12-5 Karyotype from an ovarian metastatic ascites. Tetraploidization with subsequent losses and structural anomalies affects almost all pairs. Short arms of chromosome 6 are deleted; p arms of derivative chromosome 7 contain a homogeneous staining region; and abnormal chromosomes in pair 11 are der (1;11). (Verhest A, Van Schoubroek F, Lambot M: Identification of abnormal chromosomes in a metastic ovarian tumor. Abstract from the 5th European Congress of Cytology. European Federation of Cytology Societies, Milano, 1975)

11p13. Nevertheless, a common cytogenetic event in the development of ovarian carcinoma has not been detected. A study by Atkin and associates suggested an inverse correlation between the presence of chromosome 1 and survival rate,[75] but this correlation was not significant in another series.[81]

Carcinosarcoma (malignant mixed mesodermal tumor) has been reported only twice: isochromosome for the short arms of nb 5 was noted, and both cases were also triploid.[75,87] Nonepithelial tumors are still poorly documented: two studies of immature teratomas suggest a possible link between poor prognosis and deviations in karyotype.[88,89] Cytogenetic studies of sex cord-stromal tumors deal mainly with the fibroma-thecoma group, in which trisomy 12 was found as a nonrandom change. The same anomaly is shared by some granulosa cell tumors[85,90,91] and uterine leiomyomas.[92] Two reported cases of granulosa cell tumor are comparable, with a structural rearrangement of 6q leading to loss of genetic material.[93,94]

Once again, these simple numerical or structural

anomalies may reflect a low-grade malignant potential,[84] as they do in epithelial tumors. It is premature to draw any prognostic conclusion, however, because 6q breakpoints are found in a broad spectrum of carcinomas, including those of ovarian origin.[62]

Breast

Breast cancer is the most frequently occurring cancer in women living in Europe and North America. It displays a variable and somewhat unpredictable outcome, even in small tumors, and therefore is in need of accurate predictors of behavior. Technical difficulties encountered in solid tumor cytogenetic studies are conspicuous in breast cancer; therefore, specificity of primary changes remains to be confirmed. A recent large study claims a rate of success of 18% (banded karyotypes available), with a final tally of 26 meaningful cases.[95] The results show the great instability of the population, often without clearly defined modal values. Two ductal carcinomas with early invasion had a diploid karyotype; most tumors were in the triploid range, sometimes with a hypodiploid sideline. One or more sites were involved in almost 80% of the published observations on chromosome 1, and chromosomes 3 and 11 were affected in 45% of the cases.[62,95] In other series, rearrangements of chromosomes 6, 7, 11, 16, and 17 were noted;[96–99] they are not considered as primary but rather as secondary (acquired during tumor progression), and they may confer a selective advantage in cell proliferation. In another study, trisomic cells for chromosomes 1 and 18 were detected by in situ hybridization in an otherwise diploid DNA pattern.[100]

Several regions on chromosome 1 are the targets of rearrangements that result in genic imbalance between alleles,[96,97,99,101] implicated in breast cancer development.[102] Loss of chromosome 16 is another interesting feature.[98,99] This loss is sometimes preceded in a first evolutionary step by long-arm rearrangements leading to homozygosity of the 16q21-24 segment in early carcinomas. This segment thus has been proposed as a site of a putative breast cancer suppressor gene relevant to cancer initiation.[95] This chromosome could be discarded in later stages by further multiple abnormalities related to tumor progression. Allelic defect is not limited to chromosome 16 in breast cancer.[98,103] A 17p deletion has been identified,[104,105] including the locus of the p53 gene.[106] The protein product of this gene plays a role in the regulation of the cell cycle and is considered a potential antioncogene (see below).

As expected, loss of heterozygosity (LOH) and oncogene amplification are not limited to breast cancer; 1q, 3p, 11p, 13q, and 17p sites of mutation are shared with other epithelial tumors of the lung, gastrointestinal tract, and kidney and urinary tract, and with some sarcomas.[107]

Somatic mutations have been related to other prognostic factors, such as hormone receptors and histologic grade.[108] However, no significant association with disease-free interval and overall survival can be accurately drawn due to the lack of reproducibility of the results among different authors. Lack of uniformity in the statistical management of the data is another pitfall.[107,109] Quantitative DNA analysis appears more relevant to prognostic assessment.

Corpus Uteri

In a recent comprehensive survey, only 25 cases of cytogenetically analyzed endometrial carcinoma could be collected from the literature.[15] More recently, 24 new observations have been reported in detail.[110] Trisomy and tetrasomy 1q appear the most consistent anomaly in these series, with a mean frequency of 75%. Breakpoints on chromosome 1 are common in human neoplasia but are generally considered nonspecific.[111] Trisomy as a sole anomaly would suggest a real primary change, possibly related to the early stage of development of carcinoma. Although trisomy 10 is the second most frequent anomaly,[110,112] about 30% of stage I carcinomas remain diploid or beyond the resolution of current banding techniques. Whether those "normal" mitoses originate from cancer cells or from stromal benign cells is still controversial.

No correlation could be found between chromosome patterns and prognostic parameters such as age, hormonal status, histologic grade, and TNM stage.[110] There thus seems to be little chance to get any relevant information relating to progression to carcinoma from karyotypic rearrangements in borderline endometrial lesions.

Carcinosarcomas (malignant mixed mesodermal tumors) are reported to present complex abnormalities with no identical rearrangements.[110]

Cervix

Invasive Carcinoma. Cytogenetic mapping of genes involved in the initiation, development, and progression of cancer provides some clues to which regions are more susceptible to mutagenicity. It appears that cytogenetic changes related to cervical cancer are variable, some directly related to the neoplastic transformation itself, others to the viral integration process or to the step of progression to invasive cancer. These nonrandomly distributed structural rearrangements affect highly significantly both arms of chromosomes 1 and 11, but also 3p, 6q, 17p, 18p, and 21q in deletions, duplications or translocations.[113] Duplication resulted in iso17q in one case, with anomalies emerging early in the microinvasive phase.[78] No correlation could be drawn with the histologic type,[113] but chromosome 1 rearrangement is suggested to be linked with a proliferation advantage for the cell.

Cervical Intraepithelial Neoplasia (CIN). Cytogeneticists have been attracted from the beginning to this model of human carcinogenesis. The continuous slow evolution through the dysplastic changes fluctuating from regression to relapse has shown precocious minimal structural anomalies and modal deviations.[114] Multiple preinvasive lesions with different karyotypes in the same cone biopsy raised the question of the multiclonality of such lesions before their clonal expansion.[115]

The high rate of failure in obtaining a sufficient number of suitable mitoses (about 1 per 1000 cells) has led and still leads to the wide use of morphometric and densitometric analyses of the interphase nuclei. For the same reasons, no relevant information is available for carcinomas of the vagina and the vulva.

Benign Tumors

Diploidy remains the rule in benign conditions. However, clonal evolution in the ovary was reported more than 20 years ago,[116,117] and in a recent survey trisomy 12 was detected in 3 cases of mucinous and serous cystadenomas.[118]

The recent recognition of nonrandom, clonal chromosome abnormalities in benign tumors rests largely on the study of *leiomyomas* of the corpus uteri. Series are numerous from different groups of investigators.[119,120] Recurrent findings point out that breakpoints affect specific regions such as 7q21 in deletions or 12q14 in translocation. This last band is also involved in benign lipomas, which suggests that the same growth-controlling genes might affect mesenchymal cells in different types of benign soft-tissue tumors but are different from those of their malignant counterparts.[121] Trisomy 12,[92] ring chromosomes, and monosomy 22 are other nonrandom abnormalities described in leiomyomas.[119] Specific regions on chromosomes 1, 7, and 13 and t(12;14) could be important at the molecular level in the control of muscle cell proliferation.[120,122] A normal chromosome complement is retained in about 50% of benign uterine leiomyomas, but 80% of cellular and atypical leiomyomas show clonal abnormalities.[122] The possibility of clonal evolution with additional anomalies is worth keeping in mind because of a relation with increased cellularity and mitotic activity; such cases could be of some unexplained clinical significance.[123]

Fibroadenoma is to the breast what leiomyoma is to the corpus uteri: the most frequent benign tumor, generally considered as an innocuous lesion without risk of malignant transformation. Few studies deal with this tumor. Clonal structural rearrangement was present in one fourth of the cases in a recent series,[124] focusing on 12p anomaly as already noted in a previous report.[125] It is suggested that in the "co-proliferation" of epithelial and mesenchymal cells, cytogenetic aberrations are limited to vimentin-positive metaphases.[126]

Borderline epithelial breast lesions remain to be clearly defined before being compared cytogenetically, because they still generate many controversies.[127] Malignant but preinvasive epithelial proliferations do not yield reproducible or convincing results.[128] Because of their focal and widely dispersed nature, they will probably be investigated more satisfactorily by techniques such as in situ hybridization or immunohistochemistry, which can preserve their architecture.

Technical Addendum

The technical difficulties in obtaining a sufficient number of suitable mitoses are beginning to be overcome by the use of collagenase for disaggregation and methotrexate for synchronization.[129,130] A 5-cm³ specimen in sterile growth medium is enough for transportation to the laboratory. The initiation of the procedure should be as fast as possible and requires a perfect collaboration with the surgeon and the pathologist, who will ensure both good clinical information and a representative, viable sample of the tumor.

ONCOGENES AND TUMOR SUPPRESSOR GENES

Understanding the fundamental nature of human malignancy has been the central theme of a large body of molecular biological research performed during the last two decades. This work has led to the identification of dominantly acting DNA sequences whose expression appears to be associated with conversion of normal cells to cancer cells. These DNA sequences are known as *oncogenes* and were first identified in the genomes of acutely transforming rodent and avian retroviruses, which efficiently transform cells and induce tumors in vivo within 2 to 3 weeks. During the retroviral life cycle, retroviruses incorporate certain genes from their infected hosts in a process known as *transduction*. These transduced DNA sequences have turned out to be so-called viral oncogenes. These findings demonstrated that the genetic sequences responsible for neoplastic transformation by the retroviruses are actually of mammalian or avian DNA origin. There generally are genetic differences between retroviral oncogenes and cellular progenitors because transduction is frequently associated with genetic mutations, including point mutations, deletions, and genetic substitutions. The homologous genes present in mammalian or avian DNA generally are referred to as *cellular oncogenes* or *proto-oncogenes*.

Occasionally, retroviral oncogenes are fused products of more than one cellular oncogene, and oncogenes in some human retroviruses are not homologous to any genes present in eukaryotes but are still responsible for oncogenic activity by the virus.[131] Increasing numbers of cellular and viral transforming genes are continuing to be detected, characterized, and reported in many scientific journals. Many readers may have noticed the prefixes "v-" or "c-" preceding the names of these genes in various articles. The term v-*onc* denotes an actual retroviral oncogene (ie, the gene of an acutely transforming retrovirus that causes malignant transformation in target cells). On the other hand, c-*onc* denotes a cellular oncogene or proto-oncogene as described above, derived from normal cells, which usually requires activation to cause cellular transformation.

Structure and Function of Oncogenes

The fact that cellular oncogenes are conserved in DNA sequences in mammals led to the postulation that oncogene products might play important roles in normal cell growth and differentiation. Experimental studies have revealed that oncogenes appear to be regulated in a specific manner during fetal development, and that transcription levels for different cellular oncogenes vary in the same tissues at different stages of development. Oncogene products have been investigated and placed into a number of functional categories based on their location in the cell or on knowledge of their action at the cellular level.

Classification

Proto-oncogenes are classified into five major categories.[132,133] The first and largest class of proto-oncogenes encodes protein kinases. This group of proto-oncogenes can be further subclassified into two functional groups: those encoding tyrosine-specific kinases (including *src, abl, fes, fgr, ros, rel, yes,* and *syn*) and those that encode proteins that have a kinase-like domain but do not possess detectable tyrosine kinase activity in vitro (which include *raf, pks, kit, mos,* and *sea*).[133]

The second class of proto-oncogenes is the so-called *ras* family and consists of H-*ras*, K-*ras* and N-*ras*. The *ras* family has different degrees of homology in their effector regions. Each of the genes in the *ras* family is composed of four coding exons with identical intron spacing, and each encodes a 21,000-d polypeptide (p21)[134] that binds GTP and GDP and has a GTPase and autokinase activity. It is located on the plasma membrane when active. The p21 of the different members of the *ras* oncogene family differ slightly in their carboxyl terminus. Members of the *ras* oncogene family containing activating point mutations are generally capable of transforming cell lines.

The third class of proto-oncogenes encodes growth factors themselves. This group includes the *int* and *sis* genes. The *int*-1 gene was identified in mammary neoplasms and encodes a protein in the fibroblast growth factor family. The proto-oncogene v-*sis* is derived from genes encoding a platelet-derived growth factor (PDGF), with 92% homology with the nonglycosylated β-chain of PDGF.

The fourth class encodes polypeptide growth factor receptors or proteins with the characteristic transmembrane structure of a growth factor receptor. This group of proto-oncogenes includes *erb*-A, *erb*-B, *fms,* and *kit*. Characteristically, these proteins span the cell membrane and possess an intracellular cytoplasmic domain and an extracellular domain. Binding of ligands to the extracellular domain of these growth factor receptors generally leads to the activation of the intrinsic tyrosine kinase activity of the intracellular cytoplasmic domain of the receptor molecule, which subsequently results in the induction of cell proliferation.

The last class of proto-oncogenes are those located in the nucleus. They are considered to regulate gene expression with possible DNA binding. This class of proto-oncogenes includes the *myc* group (c-*myc*, N-*myc* and L-*myc*), *myb, fos, ets*-1, *ets*-2, and *ski*. Some of these genes have been demonstrated to encode nuclear proteins that bind regulatory regions in DNA, which subsequently regulate transcription of cellular genes. Gene products of these proto-oncogenes are also considered to play major roles in the transition from quiescence to proliferation in the cell cycle.

Oncogene Activation

Proto-oncogenes or cellular oncogenes derived from normal cells usually do not cause cellular transformation. Therefore, many studies have attempted to explain how cellular oncogenes become involved in the biology of malignant tumors. The data indicate that for proto-oncogenes to play any role in neoplastic transformation and progression, they must go through the process called *activation*. Activation of proto-oncogenes occurs as a result of structural changes that create qualitative changes in their genes and expression levels or quantitative changes in their genes and encoded proteins. The types of structural changes that can cause activation include point mutations, chromosomal rearrangements, and DNA amplification. These changes in the DNA can lead to increased expression of the protein, enhanced activity of the protein, or deregulation of protein expression. The best characterized system demonstrating activation of oncogenes by point mutations occurs in the *ras* gene family, in which point mutations interfere with the binding of *ras* protein to the GAP protein.

DNA amplification of various oncogenes has been documented in numerous human tumors. Gene amplification may be associated with readily recognizable chromosomal abnormalities but, in most cases, DNA amplification of proto-oncogenes occurs without significant quantitative change of the entire DNA content of the cells. Some amplification genes are also rearranged or mutated. Amplification of proto-oncogene can lead to overexpression, by increasing the amount of DNA template available for mRNA production. An increased level of oncogene expression is believed to be a prerequisite for the selective growth advantage exhibited by cells containing additional gene copies. It could also be the principal contribution of gene amplification to tumorigenesis.[135]

Despite these features of proto-oncogene activation, in most naturally occurring human tumors, activation of a single proto-oncogene probably does not lead to immediate malignant transformation. Experiments have indicated that naturally occurring human cancers result from multiple events that may involve activation of more than one proto-oncogene, as well as loss of other cellular genes that suppress the development of the tumor cell type (tumor suppressor genes).

Laboratory Methods to Detect Oncogene Abnormalities in Clinical Laboratories

The initial step in studying whether a proto-oncogene may be involved in the biological or clinical behavior of a human neoplasm is to determine whether it has been activated through one of the processes previously described (point mutation, gene rearrangement, overexpression, or amplification) or through other processes. From the practical standpoint, methods to detect changes of cellular oncogenes in clinical laboratories are classified based on the level of oncogene abnormality the pathologist attempts to study (ie, at the DNA, mRNA, or protein level). The major methods classified by this schema are summarized in Table 12-1. The remainder of this section briefly describes the characteristics of these respective methods, with particular emphasis on advantages and disadvantages from the standpoint of diagnostic laboratories.

TABLE 12-1.
Major Methods to Detect Changes of Cellular Oncogenes in the Clinical Laboratory

  I. DNA levels
      1. Dot/slot blot hybridization
      2. Southern blot hybridization and restriction fragment length polymorphism
      3. Polymerase chain reaction–dot/slot blot hybridization and nuclear sequencing
      4. Others

 II. mRNA levels
      1. Northern blot hybridization
      2. In situ hybridization

III. Protein levels
      1. Immunoblotting
      2. Immunohistochemistry

DNA Levels

DNA transfection techniques have led to the isolation of genes that cause transformation of NIH3T3 cells, but transfection assays are still tools of basic science laboratories, as is insertional mutagenesis assay. Therefore, DNA abnormalities are generally examined on immobilized DNA sequences, with the possible exception of nucleotide sequencing in the clinical laboratory setting.

Dot/Slot Blotting. This technique is the most simple of the DNA hybridization methods and has been used in various clinical laboratories. The technique itself is based on hybridization of a single-stranded radiolabeled probe on immobilized target sequences on a membrane. After washing the membrane, autoradiographs or colorimetric reactions can reveal binding of the DNA probe employed. After stripping the membrane and reprobing with a control probe, one can examine the presence or absence of DNA amplification by comparing the intensity of hybridization between the proto-oncogene DNA probes and the control probes. This technique is simple and straightforward and can examine DNA extracted from formalin-fixed and paraffin-embedded materials to some extent. A major disadvantage is that it is impossible to determine what sizes of DNA fragment one is analyzing (ie, whether increased hybridization signals really represent DNA amplification). This disadvantage is augmented by the fact that results are occasionally in conflict with the data obtained by Southern blotting. Therefore, dot/slot hybridization may remain a method of studying the degree of DNA amplification in cases known to have oncogene DNA amplification, but the technique is being largely replaced by Southern blot hybridization.

Southern Blot Hybridization and Restriction Fragment Length Polymorphism. The principle of Southern blot hybridization is summarized in Figure 12-6. Southern blot analysis can provide information on (1) gene structure, including gene rearrangement or chromosomal alteration; (2) the copy number of a particular gene, including the presence or absence of DNA amplification (Fig. 12-7) and the degree of amplification by dilution of the applied DNA (Fig. 12-8); and (3) the presence of polymorphism in the DNA sequences. Southern blot hybridization is still the best method for the study of oncogene abnormalities, especially with regard to the first two sets of information. Diagnostic pathologists must have at least basic knowledge about this method.

Restriction fragment length polymorphism (RFLP), which can demonstrate the presence of point mutations, is also studied by Southern blot analysis by digestion of DNA with appropriate restriction endonuclease. This method is based on the fact that, without DNA mutations, all the restriction sites are present in the stretch of DNA that hybri-

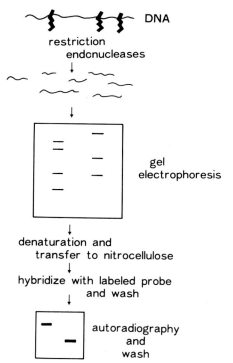

FIGURE 12-6 The principle of Southern blot hybridization analysis.

dizes to the probe when an appropriate restriction enzyme is employed. The recent use of allele-specific oligonucleotide probes has contributed to the detection of point mutations of oncogenes.

Polymerase Chain Reaction–Dot/Slot Hybridization. Since its introduction in 1985, the polymerase chain reaction (PCR) has transformed the way DNA analysis is carried out in clinical and research laboratories.[136] The PCR reaction is based on the annealing and extension of two oligonucleotide primers that flank the target region in duplex DNA.[136] Thus, PCR technique overcomes the problem of detecting DNA abnormalities that occur at low frequency in the target population as well as the problem of too little DNA for analysis. Amplified DNA fragments may be run on a gel and visualized with ethidium bromide staining, but generally the DNA is analyzed by hybridization, direct sequencing, or the RNase A mismatch cleavage method. Because of the extreme

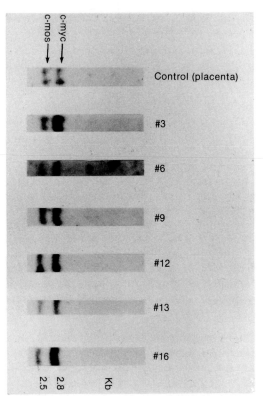

FIGURE 12-7 Amplification of c-*myc* in 6 cases of ovarian carcinoma. Lanes are from an autoradiograph of a Southern blot of Hind III-digested DNA from normal placenta and 6 ovarian carcinomas. The intensity of signal of c-*myc* relative to that for the placental control DNA indicates amplification of the c-*myc* oncogene in the tumors. (Sasano H, Garrett CT, Wilkinson DS et al: Proto-oncogene amplification and tumor ploidy in human ovarian neoplasms. Hum Pathol 21:382–391, 1990)

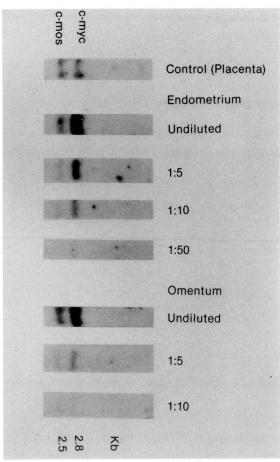

FIGURE 12-8 Dilution study of c-*myc* amplification in DNA extracted from endometrial and omental tumors analyzed by Southern blot hybridization. DNA from the endometrial tumor exhibited about 10-fold c-*myc* amplification. DNA from the omental lesion showed about 5-fold c-*myc* amplification. (Sasano H, Comerford J, Wilkinson DS et al: Serous papillary adenocarcinoma of the endometrium: Proto-oncogene amplification, flow cytometry, estrogen and progesterone receptors and immunohistochemical analysis. Cancer 65:1545–1551, 1990)

sensitivity of PCR, DNA contamination can become a serious problem.

The major application of PCR to oncogene analysis is the detection of point mutations. PCR is able to detect minor structural changes, rearrangements, or both in single-copy genes. PCR has been used effectively to test tumors (including human gynecologic neoplasms) for single nucleotide mutations with the H-, K-, and N-*ras* cellular genes (Fig. 12-9). The presence of the mutation may not be diagnostic of malignancy but does provide information concerning one of the abnormal growth-controlling mechanisms within the neoplastic cells.

It is true that determination of the specific sites of point mutation can be achieved only by nucleotide sequencing of PCR products. However, DNA sequencing is time-consuming, labor-intensive, and expensive to perform, despite advances in automation. Therefore, to determine the presence of point mutations, it is more feasible to analyze PCR products by selective oligonucleotide probe hybridization, RNAase A cleavage, or the single-strand conformation polymorphism method. These methods can provide information comparable to DNA sequencing in most diagnostic laboratories.

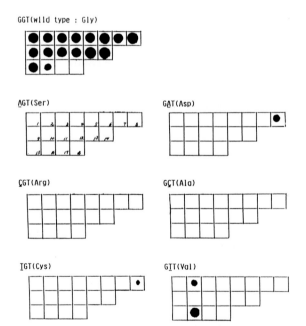

FIGURE 12-9 Detection of K-*ras* codon 12 mutation. Polymerase chain reaction and dot blot hybridization were done three times in each case. Point mutations were recognized in three cases in this figure: No. 6, GGT → GAT (endometrial carcinoma); No. 15, GGT, GAT, and GCT (cervical adenocarcinoma); No. 16, GGT → GTT (cervical adenocarcinoma). Control cases are shown from No. 18 to No. 21: No. 18, human placenta as negative control; No. 19, SW 480 (100%) as positive control (GGT → GTT); No. 20, SW 480 (10%); No. 21, SW 480 (5%). (Sato S, Ito K, Ozawa N, et al: Analysis of point mutations at codon 12 of k-ras in human endometrial carcinoma and cervical adenocarcinoma by dot blot hybridization and polymerase chain reaction. Tohoku J Exp Med 165:131–136, 1991.)

Other Methods. Other methods to study abnormalities of proto-oncogenes of human tumors at the DNA level are pulse field gel electrophoresis[137] and fluorescent in situ hybridization. They may be less cumbersome and labor-intensive than the transfection method or insertional mutagenesis, as described above, but they are not used routinely in diagnostic laboratories.

mRNA Levels

The first step in analyzing gene expression of proto-oncogenes in human tumors is to determine whether their mRNA is present in the specimen obtained. Techniques for the analysis of gene expression include one that examines immobilized mRNA on membranes (Northern blot analysis) and one that studies the localization of mRNA in tissue sections (in situ hybridization) by the use of radioactively labelled or nonisotopic probes.

Northern Blot. Total RNA obtained from fresh or quick-frozen tissue is fractionated and separated in a denaturing gel during electrophoresis, as was described in the section on Southern blot analysis. RNA is then transferred after electrophoresis to a nylon or nitrocellulose membrane, followed by hybridization with a specific radiolabeled or nonisotopic probe, washing, and development of a colorimetric reaction. Northern blot can demonstrate the molecular size of mRNA transcripts and the degrees of expression of a particular transcript. Overexpression of proto-oncogenes can be observed by this technique after reprobing with such control probes as β-actin. Northern blot analysis is thus considered a standard method of analyzing proto-oncogene expression in human neoplasms.

From the practical standpoint, it is difficult to install this technique in diagnostic laboratories because the technique is time-consuming and labor-intensive. Great care must be taken during the procedure, including sampling of the specimen, to avoid degrading the fragile RNA by RNase contamination. Thus, in the study of proto-oncogenes, Northern blot is a powerful tool in basic science laboratories but may not play such an important role in diagnostic laboratories dealing with surgical pathology specimens.

In Situ Hybridization. Northern blot analysis, like Southern blot analysis, treats the specimen as a mass and cannot provide information on the localization of mRNA expression, which is a serious disadvantage when studying human specimens. Human solid tumors, including almost all gynecologic tumors, are composed of stroma and cancer cells, and Northern blot analysis cannot demonstrate cancer cell-specific mRNA expression of proto-oncogenes. In situ hybridization is a technique that visualizes RNA molecules in a tissue section through hybridization with a radiolabeled or nonisotopic probe of the specimen affixed to a glass slide. As an example, in situ hybridization analysis of the *c-myc* oncogene in human ovarian carcinoma is shown in Figure 12-10. The results of in situ hybridization are easily influenced by tissue preparation, choice of probes, and conditions of hybridization and washing.

A method by which we have consistently demonstrated good and reproducible hybridization signals is summarized in Figure 12-11. Fixation of tissues in 4% paraformaldehyde and subsequent paraffin embedding have provided reliable retention of the mRNA targets as well as excellent preservation of cell and tissue architecture compared with frozen sections.[138,139] Oligonucleotide probes generally permit greater specificity than cDNA or cRNA probes because redundant or conserved nucleotide sequences can be avoided during probe design and synthesis. In our experience, radiolabeled probes have a much higher sensitivity than the nonisotopic probes available, including digoxigenin. Therefore, the combination of 4% paraformaldehyde-fixed, wax-embedded specimens with radiolabeled oligonucleotide DNA probes is probably the ideal method for in situ hybridization. In addition, one can perform immunohistochemistry and in situ hybridization on the same tissue sections with the appropriate choice of chromogens. This simultaneous immunohistochemistry and in situ hybridization on the same section allows study of the expression of proto-oncogenes in the same carcinoma cells (Color Figure 12-2).

Thus, mRNA in situ hybridization can provide information regarding both the localization of mRNA expression and, to some extent, the level of expression. This technique has a potential wide appeal to surgical pathologists because the analysis is performed on tissue sections, making it possible to correlate mRNA expression with histopathologic findings. In situ hybridization cannot provide qualitative information regarding the size or structure of the mRNA, and the technique itself is still time-consuming and labor-intensive. Therefore, further improvements—especially introduction of much better colorimetric agents—are required for this technique to be widely used in diagnostic laboratories.

Protein Levels

Analysis of proto-oncogene expression in human cancers by determining protein levels is in most cases performed by employing specific antibodies against the oncogene products. Technically, analysis is classified into two groups: Western (or immunoblotting) and immunohistochemistry. For practicing pathologists, the latter method is probably the easiest of all of the techniques discussed thus far for the study of oncogene abnormalities. However, as in the case of in situ hybridization, results are easily influenced by tissue preparation—especially fixation—and the choice of antibodies. Many of the oncogene products are transmembrane or nuclear proteins, and extra care should be taken not to disrupt their intracellular localization and antigenicity when performing immunostains. A large number of antibodies are commercially available, including antibodies against *ras*-p21, *c-myc*, N-*myc*, *c-erb*-B2, EGFR, and *c-fos*. Pathologists or technologists in charge of histopathology laboratories should check the following points before ordering these antibodies:

1. The antibodies should be usable for immunostaining of routinely processed surgical pathology specimens.
2. The antibodies should have been generated against processing-resistant epitopes of the molecule.
3. The specificity of the antibodies must have been checked by immunoblotting.

Some commercially available antibodies against oncogene products are not suitable for immunostaining of surgical pathology material. Even if immunostains can be performed successfully on tissue sections, it is still difficult to interpret the immunoreactivity obtained, for two main reasons. First, immunohistochemistry cannot provide information on the quantity of the products. Second, the oncogene products examined by immunohistochemistry are also present in nonneoplastic cells, with the possible exception of *c-erb*-B2.

In summary, immunohistochemistry of oncogene products can be easily done in most diagnostic pathology laboratories if one chooses appropriate methods of tissue preparation and suitable antibodies, but great care should be taken in interpreting the findings.

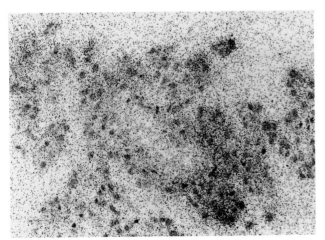

FIGURE 12-10 In situ hybridization of *c-myc* in a case of serous papillary adenocarcinoma of the ovary. Hybridization signals are observed as black dots on autoradiography. Intense hybridization signals were observed in the tumor cells.

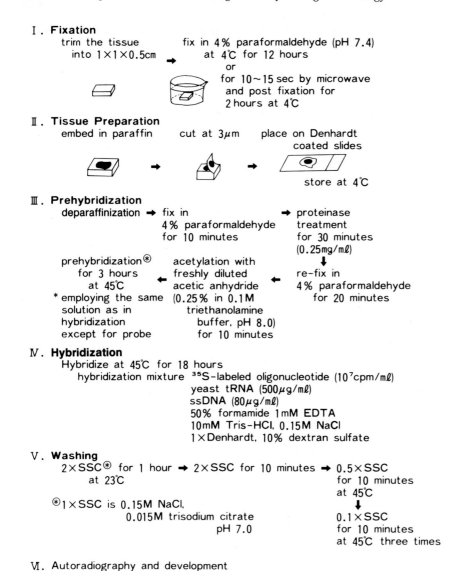

I. Fixation

trim the tissue into 1×1×0.5cm → fix in 4% paraformaldehyde (pH 7.4) at 4°C for 12 hours
or
for 10~15 sec by microwave and post fixation for 2 hours at 4°C

II. Tissue Preparation

embed in paraffin → cut at 3μm → place on Denhardt coated slides

store at 4°C

III. Prehybridization

deparaffinization → fix in 4% paraformaldehyde for 10 minutes → proteinase treatment for 30 minutes (0.25mg/ml)

prehybridization⊛ for 3 hours at 45°C ← acetylation with freshly diluted acetic anhydride (0.25% in 0.1M triethanolamine buffer, pH 8.0) for 10 minutes ← re-fix in 4% paraformaldehyde for 20 minutes

* employing the same solution as in hybridization except for probe

IV. Hybridization

Hybridize at 45°C for 18 hours
hybridization mixture ^{35}S-labeled oligonucleotide (10^7cpm/ml)
yeast tRNA (500μg/ml)
ssDNA (80μg/ml)
50% formamide 1mM EDTA
10mM Tris-HCl, 0.15M NaCl
1×Denhardt, 10% dextran sulfate

V. Washing

2×SSC⊛ for 1 hour at 23°C → 2×SSC for 10 minutes → 0.5×SSC for 10 minutes at 45°C

⊛1×SSC is 0.15M NaCl, 0.015M trisodium citrate pH 7.0

0.1×SSC for 10 minutes at 45°C three times

VI. Autoradiography and development

immersed in Kodak NTB-2 emulsion for 72 hours at 4°C

FIGURE 12-11 In situ hybridization methods routinely used in our laboratory. (Courtesy of the Department of Pathology, Tohoku University School of Medicine)

Oncogenes in Human Gynecologic Tumors

At this point, no definitive correlation has been established between abnormalities of cellular oncogenes and the biological behavior or clinical outcome of any gynecologic cancers. However, considerable evidence suggests that activation of cellular oncogenes is involved in the pathogenesis or development of at least some of these tumors. This section reviews the frequency with which cellular oncogene abnormalities have been found in ovarian, cervical, and endometrial cancers.

Ovarian Cancer

Ovarian cancer remains a common and lethal disease. It is the most common cause of death from gynecologic cancer and the fourth most common cause of female cancer death in the United States.[140] There is now a greater understanding of the numerous prognostic factors that are predictive for outcome of patients with ovarian cancer. These prognostic variables provide not only a framework for appropriate selection of therapy, but also a valid comparison between treatment options. In this regard, there have been an increasing number of studies that indicate that activated oncogenes should be among the factors considered.

Results of major published studies are summarized in Table 12-2.[141-164] This table shows the conflicting results obtained regarding the involvement of the *ras* oncogene group and c-*erb*-B2. The proto-oncogene c-*erb*-B2 probably has associated tyrosine kinase activity similar to that of EGFR, and the immunohistochemistry of c-*erb*-B2 is well established in human ovarian cancer (Fig. 12-12). Slamon and colleagues reported a high prevalence of c-*erb*-B2 amplification in human ovarian cancer.[141] They claimed that both amplification and overexpression were associated with decreased survival of the patients.[141] Press and associates subsequently reported similar findings.[142] Other reports have observed neither the

TABLE 12-2.
Summary of Major Studies on Abnormalities of Proto-oncogenes in Ovarian Cancer

Investigators	Oncogenes Examined	Type of Abnormality	Summary of Results
Sasano et al[145]	c-erb-B2	Amplification	0/12
	int 2	Amplification	1/12
	c-myc	Amplification	6/12
Zang et al[151]	c-erb-B1	Amplification	0/15
	c-erb-B2	Amplification	3/15
Berchuck et al[152]	c-erb-B2	Overexpression (immunohistochemistry)	Intense staining is associated with poor survival.
Slamon et al[141]	c-erb-B2	Amplification	20/31*
Zhou et al[153]	c-K-ras	Amplification	3/7
	c-H-ras	Amplification	1/12
	c-myc	Amplification	3/12
	c-erb-B-2	Amplification	1/12
Masuda et al[154]	c-myc	Amplification	3/11
	c-erb-B-2	Amplification	1/11
	c-erb-B-1	Amplification	0/5
	c-K-ras	Amplification	2/5
	c-H-ras	Amplification	1/11
	myb	Amplification	0/8
	N-myc	Amplification	0/4
	sis	Amplification	0/6
Van't Veer et al[155]	c-K-ras	Amplification	3/37
		Point mutation	0/30
Fukumoto et al[156]	c-K-ras	Amplification	2/8
		Point mutation	None
Boltz et al[157]	c-K-ras	Amplification	2/81†
Enomoto et al[158]	K-ras	Transfection	0/7
		Point mutation	2/13
Press et al[142]	c-erb-B2	Amplification	31/120
		Overexpression (Northern blot)	23/67
		Overexpression (immunohistochemistry)	69/72
Garuti et al[143]	c-erb-B2	Amplification (Northern blot)	0/20
Chien et al[159]	K-ras	Amplification	4/12
		Overexpression (Northern blot)	4/12
Schreiber et al[148]	c-myc	Amplification	5/30
Sasano et al[160]	c-myc	Overexpression (immunohistochemistry)	No significant difference of immunostain between invasive carcinoma and carcinoma of LMP
Ito et al[144]	EGFR	Overexpression (immunohistochemistry)	
	c-erb-B2	Overexpression (immunohistochemistry)	
Haas et al[161]	ras group	Transfection	1/18 active in serous papillary carcinoma
Watson et al[162]	c-myc	Overexpression (flow cytometry)	Overexpression in serous papillary carcinoma
Polacarz et al[163]	c-myc	Overexpression (immunohistochemistry)	Difference of staining pattern among mucinous neoplasms

(continued)

TABLE 12-2. *(continued)*

Investigators	Oncogenes Examined	Type of Abnormality	Summary of Results
Rodenburg et al[147]	*ras* group	Overexpression (immunohistochemistry)	More intense staining in carcinoma than in normal ovary‡
Slamon et al[149]	*abl*	Overexpression (mRNA)	0/6
	fes	Overexpression	0/6
	fos	Overexpression	6/6
	fms	Overexpression	4/6
	c-myc	Overexpression	6/6
	myb	Overexpression	0/6
	c-H-*ras*	Overexpression	6/6
	c-K-*ras*	Overexpression	4/6
Lee et al[164]	c-H-*ras*	Rearrangement	1/17
		Allele loss	5/17

*Overexpression generally correlated with amplification.

†Specimen consisted of 26 patients and seven xenografted ovarian cancer cell lines.

‡No correlation of *ras* expression with histologic type of ovarian cancer, tumor ploidy, or clinical outcome.

frequency nor the correlation with clinical outcome reported by Slamon.[143-145] Therefore, it is premature to assign any role to the *c-erb*-B2 oncogene in the development or progression of human ovarian carcinoma.

The *ras* oncogenes are the most frequently identified transformation-associated genes found in human solid tumors. The frequency of mutation or amplification of *ras,* especially K-*ras,* in ovarian cancer is in the range of 10% to 25% (see Table 12-2), which is consistent with the reported prevalence of activated *ras* in other human solid cancers.[146] However, Rodenburg and colleagues reported no correlation of *ras* expression with histo-

logic type of ovarian cancer, tumor ploidy, or clinical outcome.[147] Therefore, the biological significance of *ras* oncogenes in human ovarian carcinoma requires further evaluation.

Expression of the *c-myc* proto-oncogene is highly regulatable and usually is correlated with cell proliferation; *c-myc* activation, overexpression, or both have been demonstrated in from 17%[148] to 100%[149] of ovarian cancers. Adequate information regarding the clinical characteristics and outcomes of patients with ovarian cancers that overexpress the *c-myc* oncogene is not available in all reports. However, the presence of *c-myc* amplification (see Fig. 12-7) was reported to be associated with a higher degree of nu-

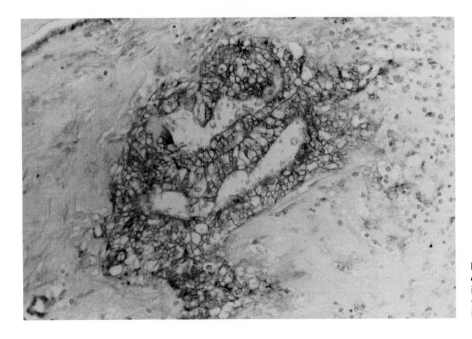

FIGURE 12-12 Mucinous adenocarcinoma of the ovary showing *c-erb*-B2 immunolocalization. Immunoreactivity was present at the cell membrane and in the cytoplasm.

clear atypia and high mitotic rate,[145] which are established as prognostic factors in human ovarian cancer.[150] Direct correlation of c-*myc* activation with clinical outcome in patients with ovarian cancer awaits further investigation.

Uterine Cervical Cancer

Results of major studies on proto-oncogene abnormalities in uterine cervical cancer are summarized in Table 12-3. Invasive carcinoma of the uterine cervix is the second most frequent cancer in women worldwide. The biological behavior of cervical cancer is complicated by the possible involvement of human papillomavirus (HPV) in carcinogenesis. Therefore, many studies of proto-oncogenes have been performed in cervical invasive carcinoma and its precursors to clarify the correlation with HPV and with malignant transformation of HPV-related lesions.[165–182] Numerous reports (summarized in Table 12-3) suggest that certain proto-oncogenes are involved in the development and progression of uterine cervical cancers.

Most studies have focused on c-*myc*. The data from both amplification and overexpression are not necessarily consistent, but it appears that activation of c-*myc* occurs in advanced stages of carcinoma, suggesting its possible role in tumor progression.[165–167] Bourhis and colleagues recently reported that overexpression of c-*myc* is a strong and independent indicator of the risk of overall relapse and distant metastases, even in early-stage carcinoma.[168] Durst and associates suggested that one mechanism by which HPV might induce neoplasia was through integration into cellular DNA in the proximity of c-*myc* and induction of c-*myc* expression.[169] This finding may be reevaluated in light of recent findings that suggest that the tumor-inducing properties of HPV may be related more to inhibition of tumor suppressor genes than to activation of proto-oncogenes.[170]

Results of c-*erb*-B2 studies in uterine cervical squamous carcinoma are consistent with the overall low frequency of c-*erb*-B2 abnormalities in squamous cell carcinomas in general. In addition, even in cervical squamous cancer cells with c-*erb*-B2 abnormalities, the results may merely reflect the conserved potential of glandular differentiation in exocervical squamous epithelia and their malignant counterparts.[171] Most of the proto-oncogene studies were performed on uterine cervical squamous cell carcinoma, with the exception of that of Sato and colleagues, who studied the immunohistochemical localization of c-*myc*, c-*erb*-B2, and EGFR in 7 cases of cervical adenocarcinoma.[172] These were positive in 5, 2, and 7 of the cases, respectively. Because cervical adenocarcinoma is known to be an aggressive tumor, further investigations are needed to clarify which proto-oncogenes play roles in the pathogenesis and development of this tumor.

Endometrial Carcinoma

The results of major studies on oncogene abnormalities in human endometrial carcinoma are summarized in Table 12-4. When analyzing abnormalities of proto-oncogenes in clinical samples of human endometrial carcinoma, it is important to note that many of these tumors are intimately associated with hyperplasia. Therefore, proto-oncogene studies should be performed by a morphology-based technique such as in situ hybridization or immunohistochemistry; otherwise, the carcinoma itself may not be the lesion studied. Enomoto and colleagues proposed that point mutations in codon 12 of K-*ras* are significant events in the etiology of adenocarcinoma of the endometrium,[158] but other reports have shown a lower frequency of c-K-*ras* point mutation.[182,183] This discrepancy may be due to the degree of contamination of nontumor cells, but further studies are required.

Other studies have indicated a possible correlation of clinical outcome in human breast carcinoma with abnormalities of c-*erb*-B2[141,184] and c-*myc*.[184] Some endometrial carcinomas may depend on sex steroid hormones, as in breast cancer, and both human breast and endometrial cancers share common clinical risk factors. Therefore, it is reasonable to postulate possible roles of these two proto-oncogenes in the biological behavior of human endometrial carcinoma. Abnormalities of these two oncogenes have been reported recently in human endometrial carcinoma (see Table 12-4).[185–189]

A high degree of c-*myc* amplification was reported in endometrial serous papillary adenocarcinoma (see Fig. 12-8), which is known to be associated with aggressive biological behavior and poor prognosis.[185] Borst and associates reported that amplification of the c-*erb*-B2 or c-*myc* oncogene was correlated with clinically advanced-stage disease and poorly differentiated lesions, indicating that oncogene amplification may predict biologically aggressive endometrial cancers.[187] Berchuck and colleagues demonstrated a correlation of high expression of c-*erb*-B2 with increased mortality in patients with endometrial cancer.[188] Further studies are needed, but c-*myc* and c-*erb*-B2 appear to play important roles in the biological behavior of human endometrial carcinoma.

Tumor Suppressor Genes

The molecular biology of cancer encompasses far more than the simple activation of oncogenes. Cancer has been recognized as a genomic disease, which progresses stochastically through a series of steps to ultimately produce malignant neoplasia. In most human cancers, neoplastic transformation involves activation of oncogenes (as described earlier) and simultaneous escape from the control of counterbalancing suppressor genes.[190]

TABLE 12-3.
Summary of Major Studies on Abnormalities of Proto-oncogenes in Uterine Cervical Cancer

Investigators	Oncogenes Examined	Type of Abnormality	Summary of Results
Riou et al[166]	c-H-*ras*	Locus analysis Point mutation	Loss of one allele in 36% 24%*
DiLuca et al[173]	c-*myc*	Amplification	0/14
Ocadiz et al[174]	c-*myc*	Amplification	17/35
Baker et al[175]	c-*myc*	Amplification	14/44
Hendy-Ibbs et al[176]	c-*myc*	Overexpression (flow cytometry)	Normal cervix higher than carcinoma
Riou et al[165]	c-*myc*	Overexpression (Northern and slot blot)	25/72
Hughes et al[177]	c-*myc*	Overexpression (immunohistochemistry)	Normal cervix more positive than carcinoma
Sagae et al[178]	*ras*(p21)	Overexpression (immunohistochemistry)	57.1%† 54.2%‡ 38.7%§
Berchuck et al[179]	c-*erb*-B2 EGFR	Overexpression (immunohistochemistry) Overexpression (immunohistochemistry)	1/26 22/26
Hayashi et al[180]	*ras*(p21) EGFR	Overexpression (immunohistochemistry) Overexpression (immunohistochemistry)	6/52‖ 3/52
Riviere et al[181]	c-*erb*-B2 c-*myc*	Overexpression (Northern blot) Overexpression (Northern blot)	3/27 5/18
Riou et al[167]	c-*myc*	Amplification Overexpression (Northern blot)	35/182 70/151#
Bourhis et al[168]	c-*myc*	Amplification Overexpression (Northern blot)	8/93 31/93
Brumm et al[171]	c-*erb*-B2	Overexpression (Northern blot) Overexpression (immunohistochemistry)	3/8 2/8
Sato et al[172]	c-*erb*-B2 c-*myc* EGFR	Overexpression (immunohistochemistry) Overexpression (immunohistochemistry) Overexpression (immunohistochemistry)	2/7** 5/7** 7/7**
Sato et al[182]	K-*ras*	Point mutation	2/7**

*Mutation at codon 12.
†Keratinizing type of squamous cell carcinoma.
‡Large cell nonkeratinizing type.
§Small cell type.
‖Positive cases have higher incidence of lymph node metastasis.
#Overexpression associated with aggressive biological behavior.
**Cervical adenocarcinoma.

TABLE 12-4.
Summary of Major Studies on Abnormalities of Proto-oncogenes in Endometrial Cancer

Investigators	Oncogenes Examined	Type of Abnormality	Summary of Results
Sasano et al[185]	c-*myc* *int*-2 c-*erb* B-2	Amplification Amplification Amplification	1/4 0/4 0/4*
Kacinski et al[186]	*fms* *fos* c-*erb* B-2 c-K-*ras*	Overexpression (in situ hybridization)	High levels of expression
Long et al[183]	*ras* group (p21)	Overexpression (immunohistochemistry)	Higher rate of positivity in high grade carcinoma[†]
Brumm et al[171]	c-*erb*-B2	Overexpression (Northern)	4/11
Enomoto et al[158]	c-K-*ras*	Point mutation	4/10
Borst et al[187]	c-*erb*-B2 c-*myc*	Amplification Amplification	11/16 10/15
Berchuck et al[188]	c-*erb*-B2	Overexpression (immunohistochemistry)	9/95
Nasim et al.[220]	c-K-*ras*	Point mutation	2/12
Sato et al[182]	c-K-*ras*	Point mutation	3/21
Sato et al[172]	c-*erb*-B2 EFGR	Overexpression (immunohistochemistry) Overexpression (immunohistochemistry)	7/23 21/23
Sato et al[189]	c-*myc*	Overexpression (in situ hybridization)	Intense hybridization in high grade carcinoma

*Amplification was seen only in serous papillary carcinoma, not in classical endometrioid carcinoma.
[†]Positivity of p21 was also seen in stromal cells.

The genetic predisposition to certain malignant neoplasms was first postulated because certain forms of cancer cluster in families that demonstrated certain chromosomal abnormalities inherited as an autosomal dominant Mendelian trait. From this observation, the presence of genes that predispose individuals to the development of cancer by loss of their function has been postulated. The putative genes have been called *tumor suppressor genes, recessive oncogenes, antioncogenes,* and *cancer predisposition genes.* Laboratory studies have indicated that loss of function may occur through mutation or deletion of these genes in a variety of malignant neoplasms.[191–193]

Two types of experimental evidence have pointed to the identification of tumor suppressor genes. The first type of evidence is provided by somatic cell hybridization: malignant cells fused to nonmalignant cells of the same species remain nonmalignant as long as these cells retain certain chromosomes donated by the parents. The loss of these sets of chromosomes results in the malignant phenotype in the hybrid cells.[194] In addition, cancer cell proliferation and the transformed phenotype can be suppressed by contact with normal cells[195] or by the introduction of individual chromosomes into the tumor cells of interest.[196] Mapping of putative tumor suppressor genes to specific chromosomes derived from normal cells has been attempted by analyzing the loss of chromosomes in the hybrid cells that re-express tumorigenicity.

The second type of evidence has come from the study of familial hereditary predisposition to cancers such as retinoblastoma. Cytogenetic and molecular studies have indicated that loss of genes on specific chromosomal loci occurs frequently in certain types of tumors. This may be explained by the so-called genetic instability associated with malignant transformation, but it is also true that recurrent and nonrandom chromosomal abnormalities are present in a variety of tumors, although all these chromosomal deletions may not necessarily indicate the presence of tumor suppressor genes.[191]

Tumor suppressor genes have been postulated to encode proteins that regulate normal growth and to suppress neoplastic development indirectly. These genes may act recessively so that both maternal and paternal copies of the gene product must be inactivated for the involvement of tumor suppressor genes in the development of malignant phenotypes. Numerous chromosome abnormalities have been proposed as putative tumor suppressor genes, but at this juncture there are only three well-established and widely accepted tumor suppressor genes in human cancer. These are the retinoblastoma (*RB*) gene on chromosome 13q, the p53 gene on chromosome 17p,[196] and the DCC gene on chromosome 18q.[197] The retinoblastoma gene is located on the long arm of chromosome 13 (13q 14), and the expression of this gene is altered in virtually all cases of retinoblastoma[198–200] and in some other tumors.[198] Retinoblastoma cells lack a functional Rb protein and their tumor-forming propensity is suppressed by introducing the wild-type *Rb*-1 gene into the cells. Increasing evidence suggests that retinoblastoma protein plays a critical role in control of the cell cycle.[201]

The p53 protein was first identified as a host cell protein bound to T antigen, the dominant transforming oncogene of the DNA tumor virus SV-40.[202] This gene, which is located on the short arm of chromosome 17, was at first considered a proto-oncogene rather than a tumor suppressor gene because transfection of mutant variants into cells along with *ras* oncogene leads to malignant transformation.[203] It was subsequently shown that the study above actually employed mutated p53 genes and that the wild-type gene is incapable of the transformation described.[194]

The gene DCC, which is located on the long arm of chromosome 18, was originally described by Fearon and colleagues in 1990.[197] This gene is considered to play a role in the pathogenesis of human colorectal neoplasia through alteration of the normal cell-cell interactions controlling growth.[197]

Tumor Suppressor Genes in Human Gynecologic Tumors

Studies on involvement of tumor suppressor genes, mostly the retinoblastoma gene and p53, and on chromosomal deletion in human gynecologic cancers are summarized in this section. Emphasis is placed on their clinical significance and on clinical methods of laboratory detection.

Chromosomal Allelic Deletion. Certain genetic predispositions to develop gynecologic cancers have been known for years. In these cases, it has been postulated that the patient inherits one defective tumor suppressor gene from one parent and then inactivates the other gene through spontaneous mutation

or deletion in cells that give rise to the tumor.[193] Therefore, tumors that arise in individuals without such a genetic predisposition must be associated with inactivation or loss of both normal alleles.[193] This is generally detected by observing that a tumor contains only one of the two alleles for a given gene that is present in the corresponding normal tissue. Therefore, allelic deletion in tumor cells generally represents the loss of a functioning tumor suppressor gene on the deleted allele and retention of a mutated nonfunctional cancer suppressor gene on the remaining allele.[193] Studies on allelic loss or loss of heterozygosity (LOH) in human gynecologic tumors are summarized in Table 12-5.[204–211]

Retinoblastoma (RB) Gene. Analysis of the retinoblastoma gene is usually done by detecting DNA abnormalities in the specimen, because immunohistochemical study of the *RB* product is not well established. *RB* gene abnormalities have not been

TABLE 12-5.
Summary of Loss of Heterozygosity in Human Gynecologic Tumors

Investigators	Tumor Site	Chromosome	Frequency
Yokota et al[204]	Uterine cervix	3p	9/9
Lee et al[164]	Ovary	11p (c-H-*ras*)	5/10
Sato et al[205]	Ovary	3p	6/33
		7p	3/7
		11p	7/29
		17p	13/28
		17q	12/31
		19p	11/32
		19q	4/16
		20	4/32
		21	0/12
		22	2/10
Okamoto et al[206]	Endometrium	Loss of heterozygosity at 27 loci in 10 chromosomes	
Ehlen et al[207]	Ovary	High frequency in 3p, 6q, 11p	
Eccles et al[208]	Ovary	17p	69%
		17q	77%
Russell et al[209]	Ovary	17q	10/13
Viel et al[210]	Ovary	11p (c-H-*ras*)	4/7
Lee et al[211]	Ovary	6q	9/14
		17p	6/8(D17S28)
			9/14(DI7S30)
		11p	5/11
Riou et al[166]	Uterine cervix	11p	10/28

studied extensively in human gynecologic tumors. Sasano and colleagues recently demonstrated a possible involvement of the *RB* gene in an ovarian carcinoma of low malignant potential with aggressive behavior.[212] One of 16 cases of ovarian carcinoma demonstrated evidence of homozygous deletion of the gene (Fig. 12-13). This tumor was classified histologically as being of low malignant potential but behaved in an aggressive fashion, suggesting that the structural alteration of the *RB* gene was involved in the behavior of this tumor. Recently Li and associates demonstrated allelic loss at the *RB* locus in 6 of 20 cases of human ovarian cancer.[213] What is becoming of great interest in the story of involvement of the *RB* gene in human gynecologic cancer is the fact that the oncogenic HPV types encode transformation proteins (E7) that form complexes with the protein product of the *RB* gene.[170] Further study should clarify the possible role of the *RB* gene and its gene products in the clinical behavior of human gynecologic cancers, especially HPV-associated lesions.

p53. Increasing numbers of studies of p53 have been reported in a variety of human neoplasms, and gynecologic cancers are no exception. The major studies of p53 abnormalities in human gynecologic cancer are summarized in Table 12-6.[214–216]

The major methods of detecting p53 abnormalities (ie, the presence of mutated p53) in human surgical pathology specimens are the nucleic acid-based approach and immunohistochemical methods. The nucleic acid-based approach was initially the detection of DNA abnormalities by direct sequencing of PCR products (Fig. 12-14). In human cancers, most activating mutations seem to be present in a portion of the gene spanning codons 132 to 281 (corresponding to exons 5, 6, 7, 8, and 9), which is known to include the SV-40 large T-binding domain as well as four highly conserved sequence blocks.[196] The patterns of DNA mutations vary from DNA point mutation to deletions of variable length. Although activating mutations are not necessarily confined to these areas, most studies have used PCR-amplified DNA fragments of these regions. Direct nucleotide sequencing of these fragments is a well established conventional method of detecting p53 abnormalities. However, the method is not used in diagnostic laboratories because of its time-consuming, expensive, and cumbersome nature. Recently, a relatively simple and sensitive method for detection of structural alterations of DNA fragments, known as the SSCP (single-strand conformation polymorphism) technique, was developed.[217] This technique employs radiolabeled PCR fragments, which allow the mutated molecule to be separated before sequencing (Fig. 12-15). This method is much simpler and less time-consuming then conventional DNA direct sequencing but is still cumbersome and labor-intensive, and the use of radioactivity prevents its widespread use in diagnostic laboratories.

It has been demonstrated that p53 mutations, which cause amino acid substitutions, appear to change the structure of the protein, resulting in a

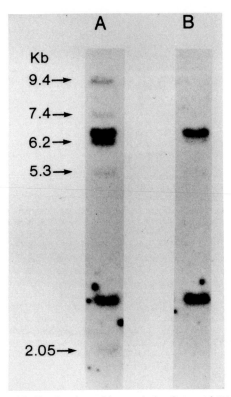

FIGURE 12-13 Southern blot analysis of control DNA (*lane A*) and endometrioid carcinoma of low malignant potential (*lane B*) using a probe to the *RB* gene and a probe to monitor DNA transfer. The intensity of the band monitoring the amount of DNA on the filter (two intense bands in this figure) was nearly identical in the control and tumor tissues. Compared with the control tissue in lane A, the 9.4-kb and 7.4-kb bands detected by the probe to the *RB* gene were deleted in lane B. (Sasano H, Comerford J, Silverberg SG, Garrett CT: Analysis of abnormalities of the retinoblastoma gene in human ovarian and endometrial carcinoma. Cancer 66:2150–2154, 1990)

TABLE 12-6.
Analysis of p53 Abnormalities in Gynecologic Tumors

Investigators	Tumor Site	Methods	Results (Mutations)
Okamoto et al[206]	Endometrium	PCR-SSCP DNA sequencing	3/24
Mazars et al[214]	Ovary	PCR-SSCP	11/30
Marks et al[215]	Ovary	Immunohisto-chemistry	54/107
Kihana et al[216]	Ovary	PCR-SSCP DNA sequencing	11/22

PCR, polymerase chain reaction; *SSCP,* single-strand conformation polymorphism.

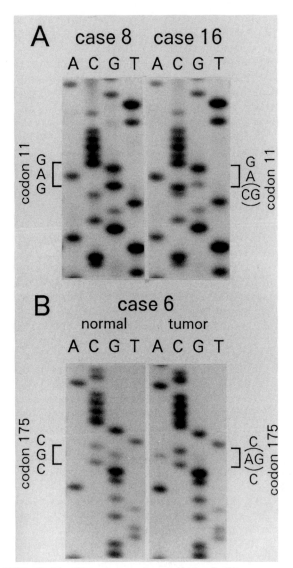

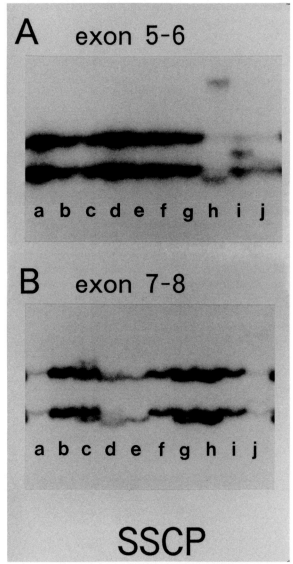

FIGURE 12-14 Direct sequencing analysis of p53 gene mutations in human ovarian carcinoma. **(A)** Sequencing of DNA of tumor tissues from cases 8 and 16 (serous papillary adenocarcinoma) around codon 11. **(B)** Sequencing of DNA from tumor and normal tissue from case 6 (serous papillary adenocarcinoma) around codon 175. Point mutational alterations were detected at codon 11 (sense, CAG from GAG) in case 16 and at codon 175 (sense, CAC from CGC) in case 6 tumor. Case 8 and normal tissue from case 6 demonstrated the wild-type sequence. (Kihana T, Tsuda H, Okada S et al: Analysis of abnormalities of p53 tumor suppressor gene in ovarian cancer. Jpn J Cancer Res 50:107, 1991; Courtesy of Dr. Kihana, Ehime University School of Medicine, Ehime, Japan)

FIGURE 12-15 Single-strand conformation polymorphic (SSCP) analysis of PCR-amplified DNA fragments of p53 in human ovarian cancer. **(A)** Analysis of exon 5–6 of the p53 gene using a gel with glycerol at room temperature. Lanes A and B show fragments of normal and tumor DNA from the same case. Lanes C through J show tumor tissue DNA from carcinoma cases. Mobility shift of single-stranded fragments, differing from normal control DNA in lane A, was detected in lanes H, I, and J. **(B)** Analysis of exon 7–8 of the p53 gene on gel without glycerol at room temperature. Lane A represents normal tissue, and lanes B through J show fragments of tumor DNA. By SSCP analysis of the PCR product encompassing exons 7 and 8, two or four constitutional bands were observed for each case because of DNA polymorphism within the intron between exons 7 and 8 of the p53 gene. Mobility shift was detected in lanes C, D, and J. (Kihana T, Tsuda H, Okada S et al: Analysis of abnormalities of p53 tumor suppressor gene in ovarian cancer. Jpn J Cancer Res 50:107, 1991; Courtesy of Dr. Kihana, Ehime University School of Medicine, Ehime, Japan)

longer half-life, which can be detected as overexpression of p53.[218] In various human neoplasms, overexpression of the p53 protein as determined by immunohistochemistry is closely correlated with the presence of a DNA mutation in the p53 gene. Therefore, simple immunohistologic methods can provide strong evidence of such a p53 DNA mutation. Immunolocalization of p53 has two other advantages over a conventional nucleic acid-based approach to detecting p53 abnormalities. First, immunostaining is a rapid, inexpensive, and straightfor-

ward method of identifying p53 mutations. The second and more important advantage is that the expression of p53 can be localized and correlated with other histopathologic parameters (Fig. 12-16).

A nucleic acid-based approach usually involves contamination by nonmalignant and nonviable

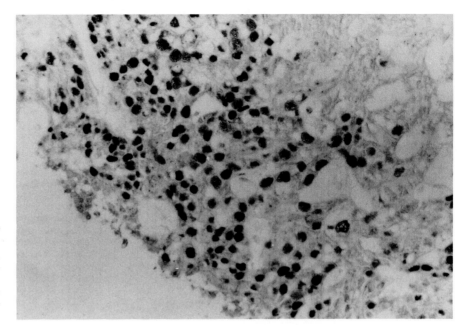

FIGURE 12-16 Immunolocalization of p53 in human ovarian carcinoma. Immunoreactivity, which represents overexpression of p53, is seen exclusively in the nuclei of carcinoma cells. The specimen was fixed in 4% paraformaldehyde for 18 hours and then embedded in paraffin.

cancer cells, because the tissue is processed as a mass. Therefore, the results are strongly influenced by the percentage of viable cancer cells present in the specimen examined. An immunohistochemical approach has a number of drawbacks, including the difficulty of demonstrating immunoreactivity in routinely processed specimens and of detecting all mutated forms of the p53 gene. These difficulties may be overcome by future technical advances. Despite these potential drawbacks, the immunohistochemical approach to p53 is considered to be of potential value in the study of human cancers including gynecologic tumors, especially for surgical pathologists.

Abnormalities of p53 appear to be correlated strongly with malignant phenotypes, but no significant correlation has been reported between p53 abnormalities and prognosis or clinical outcome in a variety of human tumors, including ovarian carcinoma. The practical value of detecting p53 abnormalities is thus limited both by technical difficulties and by the lack of immediate prognostic and therapeutic application of the results. However, the strong relation between p53 and malignant transformation is of potential value in differentiating premalignant conditions, and the possible involvement of p53 with the behavior of HPV-associated gynecologic lesions may be important in the near future.[219]

Conclusion

Increasing evidence suggests that proto-oncogenes and tumor suppressor genes are involved in the development or progression of human gynecologic cancer, or both. Although conventional morphologic approaches will no doubt remain an indispensable tool of the surgical pathologist in the diagnosis and evaluation of these tumors, the development of novel technologies and new knowledge of the molecular features of neoplastic transformation will provide an opportunity to improve our understanding of their behavior. It is important for those engaged in the care of patients with gynecologic tumors to follow and understand the developments in this field.

References

1. Atkin NB, Richards BM: Deoxyribonucleic acid in human tumors as measured by microspectrophotometry of Feulgen stain: A comparison of tumors arising at different sites. Br J Cancer 10:769–786, 1956
2. Brugal G, Garbay C, Giroud F, Adhel D: A double scanning microphotometer for image analysis: Hardware, software and biomedical applications. J Histochem Cytochem 27:144–152, 1979
3. Dressler LG, Bartow SA: DNA flow cytometry in solid tumors: Practical aspects and clinical applications. Semin Diagn Pathol 6:55–82, 1989
4. Mellin W: Cytophotometry in tumor pathology; A clinical review of methods and applications, and some results of DNA analysis. Pathol Res Pract 186:37–62, 1990
5. Van Driel-Kulker A, Mesker W, Van Den Burg N, Ploem J: Preparation of cells from paraffin-embedded tumor for cytometry and cytomorphologic evaluation. Anal Quant Cytol Histol 9:225–231, 1987
6. Spyratos F, Briffod M, Gentile A et al: Flow cytometric study of DNA distribution in cytopunctures of benign and malignant breast lesions. Anal Quant Cytol Histol 9:485–494, 1987
7. Kaern J, Wetteland J, Tropé CG et al: Comparison between flow cytometry and image cytometry in ploidy distribution assessments in gynecologic cancer. Cytometry 13:314–321, 1992
8. Kiss R, Gasperin P, Verhest A, Pasteels JL: Modification of tumor ploidy level by the choice of the tissue taken as diploid reference in digital cell image analysis of Feulgen-stained nuclei. Mod Pathol 1993
9. Ellis CN, Burnette JJ, Sedlak R et al: Prognostic applica-

tions of DNA analysis in solid malignant lesions in humans. Surg Gynecol Obstet 173:329–342, 1991

10. Kallioniemi OP, Punnonen R, Mattila J et al: Prognostic significance of DNA index, multiploidy and S-phase fraction in ovarian cancer. Cancer 61:334–339, 1988

11. Atkin NB: Modal DNA value and chromosome number in ovarian neoplasia. Cancer 27:1064–1073, 1971

12. Atkin NB, Baker MC, Robinson R, Gaze SE: Chromosome studies on 14 near-diploid carcinomas of the ovary. Eur J Cancer 10:141–146, 1974

13. Kusyk CF, Turpening EL, Edwards CL: Karyotype analysis of four solid gynecologic tumors. Gynecol Oncol 14:324–338, 1982

14. Mackillop WJ, Trent JM, Stewart SS: Tumor progression studied by analysis of cellular features of serial ascitic ovarian carcinoma tumors. Cancer Res 43:874–878, 1983

15. Sandberg AA: The chromosomes in human cancer and leukemia, 2nd ed. New York, Elsevier, 1990

16. Pejovic T: Cytogenetic analysis of ovarian tumors. Doctoral Thesis, Lund University, 1991

17. Atkin NB: Prognostic value of cytogenetic studies in tumors of the female genital tract. In LG Koss, DV Coleman, eds. Advances in clinical cytology II, pp 103–121. New York, Masson, 1984

18. Deligdisch L, Gil J, Heller D, Cohen CJ: Two types of endometrial papillary neoplasm: A morphometric study. Pathol Res Pract 188:473–477, 1992

19. Nishiya I, Kikushi T, Moriya S: Cytophotometric study of premalignant and malignant cells of the cervix in an approach toward automatic cytology. Acta Cytol 21:271–275, 1977

20. Montag AG, Bartels PH, Lerma-Puertas E et al: Karyometric marker features in tissue adjacent to in situ cervical carcinomas. Anal Quant Cytol Histol 11:275–280, 1989

21. Colgan TJ, Percy ME, Suri M et al: Human papillomavirus infection of morphologically normal cervical epithelium adjacent to squamous dysplasia and invasive carcinoma. Hum Pathol 20:316–319, 1989

22. Hanselaar AGJM, Vooijs GP, Van't Hof-Grootenboer AE, Pahlplatz MMM: Cytophotometric analysis of cervical intraepithelial neoplasia grade III, with and without synchronous invasive squamous cell carcinoma. Cytometry 11:901–906, 1990

23. Teyssier JR: The chromosomal analysis of human solid tumors: A triple challenge. Cancer Genet Cytogenet 37:103–125, 1989

24. Bloom HJG, Richardson WW: Histological grading and prognosis in breast cancer. Br J Cancer 11:369–377, 1957

25. Larsimont D, Kiss R, d'Olne D et al: Relationship between computerized morphonuclear image analysis and histopathologic grading of breast cancer. Anal Quant Cytol Histol 11:433–439, 1989

26. Salmon I, Coibion M, Larsimont D et al: Comparison of fine needle aspirates of breast cancers to imprint smears by means of digital cell image analysis. Anal Quant Cytol Histol 13:193–200, 1991

27. Frierson HF Jr: Ploidy analysis and S-phase fraction determination by flow cytometry of invasive adenocarcinomas of the breast. Am J Surg Pathol 15:358–367, 1991

28. Longin A, Fontainière B, Pinzani V et al: An image cytometric DNA-analysis in breast neoplasms—parameters of DNA—aneuploidy and their relationship with conventional prognostic factors. Pathol Res Pract 188:466–472, 1992

29. McGuire WL: Prognostic factors for recurrence and survival in human breast cancer. Breast Cancer Res Treat 10:5–9, 1987

30. Fallenius AG, Franzén SA, Auer GU: Predictive value of nuclear DNA content in breast cancer in relation to clinical and morphologic factors. Cancer 62:521–530, 1988

31. Auer GU, Caspersson TO, Gustafsson SA et al: Relationship between nuclear DNA distribution and estrogen receptors in human mammary carcinomas. Anal Quant Cytol Histol 2:280–284, 1980

32. Bichel P, Poulsen S, Andersen J. Estrogen receptor content and ploidy of human mammary carcinoma. Cancer 50:1771–1774, 1982

33. Larsimont D, Kiss R, d'Olne D et al: Correlation between nuclear cytomorphometric parameters and estrogen receptor levels in breast cancer. Cancer 63:2162–2168, 1989

34. Wittekind C, Schulte E: Computerized morphometric image analysis of cytologic nuclear parameters in breast cancer. Anal Quant Cytol Histol 9:480–484, 1987

35. Bhattacharjee DK, Harris M, Faragher EB: Nuclear morphometry of epitheliosis and intraduct carcinoma of the breast. Histopathology 9:511–516, 1985

36. Mayall B, Waldman F, Chew K et al: Does DNA cytometry have a place in the clinical laboratory? In Burger G, Oberholzer M, Vooijs GP, eds. Advances in analytical cellular pathology, pp 181–182. New York, Elsevier, 1990

37. Briffod M, Spyratos F, Hacène K et al: Evaluation of breast carcinoma chemosensitivity by flow cytometric DNA analysis and computer assisted image analysis. Cytometry 13:250–258, 1992

38. Hubscher H: DNA polymerases in prokaryotes and eukaryotes: Mode of action and biological implications. Experientia 39:1–25, 1983

39. Tanaka S, Hu S-Z, Wang TS-F, Korn D: Preparation and preliminary characterization of monoclonal antibodies against human polymerase α. J Biol Chem 257:8386–8390, 1982

40. Matsukage A, Yamamoto S, Yamaguchi M et al: Immunocytochemical localization of chick DNA polymerase α and β. J Cell Physiol 117:266–271, 1983

41. Tsutsumi Y, Hori S, Onoda N: DNA polymerase α: An immunohistochemical marker for proliferating cells in normal and neoplastic human tissues. Am J Pathol 93:643–650, 1991

42. Mushika M, Miwa T, Suzuoki Y et al: Detection of positive cells in dysplasia, carcinoma in situ and invasive carcinoma of the uterine cervix by monoclonal antibody against DNA polymerase alpha. Cancer 61:1182–1186, 1988

43. Gerdes J, Schwab U, Lemke H, Stein H: Production of a mouse monoclonal antibody reactive with a human nuclear antigen associated with cell proliferation. Int J Cancer 31:13–20, 1983

44. Baisch H, Gerdes J: Simultaneous staining of exponentially growing versus plateau phase cells with the proliferation associated antibody Ki67 and propidium iodide: Analysis by flow cytometry. Cell Tissue Kinet 20:387–391, 1987

45. Quinn CM, Wright NA: The clinical assessment of proliferation and growth in human tumors: Evaluation of methods and applications as prognostic variables. J Pathol 160:93–102, 1990

46. Sasano H, Miyazaki S, Nishihara T et al: The proliferative cell fraction in cytology specimens: A study in human esophageal carcinoma. Am J Clin Pathol 98:161–166, 1992

47. Miyachi K, Fritzler MJ, Tan EM: Autoantibody to a nuclear antigen in proliferating cells. J Immunol 121:2228–2234, 1978

48. Celis JE, Celis A: Cell cycle dependent variations in the distribution of the nuclear protein cyclin, proliferating cell nuclear antigen in cultured cells: Subdivision of S phase. Proc Natl Acad Sci U S A 82:3262–3266, 1985

49. Bravo R, Frank R, Blundell PA, MacDonald-Bravo H: Cyclin/PCNA is the auxiliary protein of DNA polymerase delta. Nature 326:515–517, 1987

50. Hall PA, Levison DA, Woods AL et al: Proliferating cell nuclear antigen (PCNA) immunolocalization in paraffin sections: An index of cell proliferation with evidence of deregulated expression in some neoplasms. J Pathol 162:285–294, 1990

51. Kamel OW, LeBrun DP, Davis RE et al: Growth fraction estimation of malignant lymphomas in formalin-fixed paraffin-embedded tissue using anti-PCNA/cyclin 19A2. Am J Pathol 138:1471–1477, 1991

52. Garcia RL, Coltrera MD, Gown AM: Analysis of proliferative grade using anti-PCNA/cyclin monoclonal antibodies in fixed, embedded tissues: Comparison with flow cytometric analysis. Am J Pathol 134:733–739, 1989

53. Gall JG, Pardue ML: Formation of RNA-DNA hybrid molecules in cytological preparations. Proc Natl Acad Sci U S A 63:378–383, 1969

54. Crocker J, Nar P: Nucleolar organizer regions in lymphomas. J Pathol 151:111–118, 1987

55. Wilkinson N, Buckley CH, Chawner L, Fox H: Nucleolar organizer regions in normal, hyperplastic and neoplastic endometria. Int J Gynecol Pathol 9:55–59, 1990

56. Griffiths AP, Butler CW, Roberts P et al: Silver-stained structures (AgNORs), their dependence on tissue fixation and absence of prognostic relevance in rectal adenocarcinoma. J Pathol 159:121–129, 1989

57. Sasano H, Saito Y, Sato I et al: Nucleolar organizer regions in human adrenocortical disorders. Mod Pathol 3:591–595, 1990

58. Boveri T: Zur Frage der Entstehung malinger Tumoren. Jena, Gustav Fischer Verlag, 1914

59. Sasaki M: Current status of cytogenetic studies in animal tumors with special reference to nonrandom chromosome changes. Cancer Genet Cytogenet 5:153–172, 1982

60. Harnden DG, Klinger HP, eds: ISCN: An international system for human cytogenetic nomenclature: Published in collaboration with Cytogenet Cell Genet. Basel, Karger, 1985

61. Yunis JJ: The chromosomal basis of human neoplasia. Science 221:227–236, 1983

62. Mitelman F: Catalog of chromosome aberrations in cancer, 4th ed. New York, Wiley Liss, 1991

63. Sandberg AA, Turc-Carel C: The cytogenetics of solid tumors: Relation to diagnosis, classification and pathology. Cancer 59:387–395, 1987

64. Heim S, Mitelman F: Cancer cytogenetics. New York, Alan R Liss, 1987

65. Sandberg AA, Turc-Carel C, Gemmill R: Chromosomes in solid tumors and beyond. Cancer Res 46:6019–6023, 1988

66. Turc-Carel C, Dal Cin P, Limon J et al: Cytogenetic and molecular studies of adipose tissue tumors. Cancer Genet Cytogenet 28:33, 1987

67. Sandberg AA: Editorial: The cytogenetic route of benign tumors. Cancer Genet Cytogenet 32:11–12, 1988

68. Arnoldus EPJ, Wiegant J, Noordermeer IA et al: Detection of the Philadelphia chromosome in interphase nuclei. Cytogenet Cell Genet 54:108–111, 1990

69. Hopman AHN, Ramaekers FCS, Raap AK et al: In situ hybridization as a tool to study numerical chromosome aberrations in solid bladder tumors. Histochemistry 89:307–316, 1988

70. Smit VTHBM, Wessels JW, Mollevanger P et al: Combined GTG-banding and nonradioactive in situ hybridization improves characterization of complex karyotypes. Cytogenet Cell Genet 54:20–23, 1990

71. Atkin NB, Pickthall VJ: Chromosome 1 in 14 ovarian cancers: Heterochromatin variants and structural changes. Hum Genet 38:25–33, 1977

72. Trent JM, Salmon SE: Karyotypic analysis of human ovarian carcinoma cells cloned in short term agar culture. Cancer Genet Cytogenet 3:279–291, 1981

73. Verhest A, Van Schoubroeck F, Lambot M: Identification of abnormal chromosomes in a metastatic ovarian tumor. Abstract from the 5th European Congress of Cytology. Milano, European Federation of Cytology Societies, 1975

74. Wake N, Hreshchyshyn MM, Piver SM et al: Specific cytogenetic changes in ovarian cancer involving chromosomes 6 and 14. Cancer Res 40:4512–4518, 1980

75. Panani AD, Ferti-Passantonopoulou AD: Common marker chromosomes in ovarian cancer. Cancer Genet Cytogenet 16:65–71, 1985

76. Atkin NB, Baker MC: Abnormal chromosomes including small metacentrics in 14 ovarian cancers. Cancer Genet Cytogenet 26:355–361, 1987

77. Whang-Peng J, Knutsen T, Douglass EC et al: Cytogenetic studies in ovarian cancer. Cancer Genet Cytogenet 11:91–106, 1984

78. Atkin N, Baker MC, Ferti-Passantonopoulou A: Chromosome changes in early gynecologic malignancies. Acta Cytol 27:450–453, 1983

79. Sheer D, Sheppard DM, Gorman PA et al: Cytogenetic analysis of four ovarian cell lines. Cancer Genet Cytogenet 26:339–349, 1987

80. Atkin NB, Baker MC: Specific chromosome change in ovarian cancer. Cancer Genet Cytogenet 3:275–276, 1981

81. Roberts CG, Tattersall MHN: Cytogenetic study of solid ovarian tumors. Cancer Genet Cytogenet 48:243–253, 1990

82. Tharapel SA, Qumsiyeh MB, Photopulos G: Numerical chromosome abnormalities associated with early clinical stages of gynecologic tumors. Cancer Genet Cytogenet 55:89–96, 1991

83. Lee JH, Kavanagh JJ, Wildrick DM et al: Frequent loss of heterozygosity on chromosomes 6q, 11 and 17 in human ovarian carcinomas. Cancer Res 50:2724–2728, 1990

84. Pejovic T, Heim S, Örndal C et al: Simple numerical chromosome aberrations in well-differentiated malignant epithelial tumors. Cancer Genet Cytogenet 49:95–101, 1990

85. Samuelson J, Leung WY, Schwartz PE et al: Trisomy 12 in various ovarian tumors of benign to low malignancy. Am J Hum Genet 47[Suppl]:A16, 1990

86. Samuelson J, Katz S, Schwartz PE, Yang-Feng TI: Chromosomal evolution through tumor progression in ovarian cancers. Am J Hum Genet 43[Suppl]:A33, 1988

87. Pejovic T, Heim S. Mandahl N et al: Complex karyotypic anomalies, including an i(5p) marker chromosome, in malignant mixed mesodermal tumor of the ovary. Cancer Genet Cytogenet 46:65–69, 1990

88. Ohama K, Nomura K, Okamoto E et al: Origin of immature teratoma of the ovary. Am J Obstet Gynecol 152:896–900, 1985

89. Ihara T, Ohama K, Satoh H et al: Histologic grade and karyotype of immature teratoma of the ovary. Cancer 54:2988–2994, 1984

90. Fletcher JA, Bibas Z, Donovan K et al: Ovarian granulosa-stromal cell tumors are characterized by trisomy 12. Am J Pathol 138:515–520, 1991

91. Leung WY, Schwartz PE, Ng HT, Yang-Feng TL: Trisomy 12 in benign fibroma and granulosa cell tumor of the ovary. Gynecol Oncol 38:28–31, 1990

92. Nilbert M, Heim S, Mandahl N et al: Trisomy 12 in uterine leiomyomas: A new cytogenetic subgroup. Cancer Genet Cytogenet 45:85–92, 1990

93. Teyssier JR, Adnet JJ, Pigeon B, Barjolle F: Chromosomal changes in an ovarian granulosa cell tumor: Similarity with carcinoma. Cancer Genet Cytogenet 14:147–152, 1985

94. Verhest A, Nedoszytko B, Noël JC et al: Translocation (6;16) in a case of granulosa cell tumor of the ovary. Cancer Genet Cytogenet 60:41–44, 1992

95. Hainsworth PJ, Raphael KL, Stillwell R et al: Cytogenetic features of twenty-six primary breast cancers. Cancer Genet Cytogenet 52:205–218, 1991

96. Dutrillaux B, Gerbault-Seureau M, Zafrani B: Characterization of chromosomal anomalies in human breast cancer: A comparison of 30 paradiploid cases with few chromosome changes. Cancer Genet Cytogenet 49:203–217, 1990

97. Ferti-Passantonopoulou AD, Panani AD: Common cytogenetic findings in primary breast cancer. Cancer Genet Cytogenet 27:289–298, 1987

98. Geleick D, Müller H, Matter A et al: Cytogenetics of breast cancer. Cancer Genet Cytogenet 46:217–229, 1990

99. Gerbault-Seureau M, Vielh P, Zafrani B et al: Cytogenetic study of twelve human near-diploid breast cancers with chromosomal changes. Ann Genet 30:138–145, 1987

100. Devilee P, Thierry RF, Kievits T et al: Detection of chromosome aneuploidy in interphase nuclei from human primary breast tumors using chromosome-specific repetitive DNA probes. Cancer Res 48:5825–5830, 1988

101. Genuardi M, Tsihira H, Anderson DE, Saunders GF: Distal deletion of chromosome 1p in ductal carcinoma of the breast. Am J Hum Genet 45:73–82, 1989

102. Devilee P, van Vliet M, Bardoel A et al: Frequent somatic

imbalance of marker alleles for chromosome 1 in human primary breast carcinoma. Cancer Res 51:1020–1025, 1991

103. Scott D, Heighway J: Meeting report: Human breast cancer genetics. Br J Cancer 59:654–656, 1989

104. Devilee P, Cornelisse CJ, Kuipers-Dijkshoorn N et al: Loss of heterozygosity on 17p in human breast carcinomas: Defining the smallest common region of deletion. Cytogenet Cell Genet 53:52–54, 1990

105. Mackay J, Steel CM, Elder PA et al: Allele loss on short arm of chromosome 17 in breast cancers. Lancet 2:1384–1385, 1988

106. Miller C, Mohandas T, Wolf D et al: Human p53 gene localized to short arm of chromosome 17. Nature 319:783–784, 1986

107. Callahan R, Campbell G: Mutations in human breast cancer: An overview. J Natl Cancer Inst 81:1780–1786, 1989

108. Ali IU, Lidereau R, Theillet C, Callahan R: Reduction to homozygosity of genes on chromosome 11 in human breast neoplasia. Science 238:185–188, 1987

109. Van der Meulen EA, Boon ME, Böcking A et al: Sense and nonsense of cytomorphometry and cytophotometry in predicting survival. In Goerttler K, Feichter GE, Wittle S, eds: New frontiers in cytology. Berlin, Springer-Verlag, 1988:116–129

110. Milatovich A, Heerema NA, Palmer CG: Cytogenetic studies of endometrial malignancies. Cancer Genet Cytogenet 46:41–54, 1990

111. Brito-Babapulle V, Atkin NB: Break points in chromosome 1 abnormalities of 218 human neoplasms. Cancer Genet Cytogenet 4:215–225, 1981

112. Couturier J, Vielh P, Salmon RJ et al: Chromosome imbalance in endometrial adenocarcinoma. Cancer Genet Cytogenet 33:67–76, 1988

113. Sreekantaiah CH, De Braekeleer M, Haas O: Cytogenetic findings in cervical carcinoma: A statistical approach. Cancer Genet Cytogenet 53:75–81, 1991

114. Wakonig-Vaartaja T, Kirkland JA: A correlated chromosomal and histopathologic study of preinvasive lesions of the cervix. Cancer 18:1101–1112, 1965

115. Granberg I: Chromosomes in preinvasive, microinvasive and invasive carcinoma. Hereditas 68:165–218, 1971

116. Atkin NB, Baker MC: Chromosome and DNA abnormalities in ovarian cystadenomas. Lancet 1:470, 1970

117. Fraccaro M, Mannini A, Tiepolo L: Karyotypic clonal evolution in a cystic adenoma of the ovary. Lancet 1:613–614, 1968

118. Pejovic T, Heim S, Mandahl N et al: Trisomy 12 is a consistent chromosomal aberration in benign ovarian tumors. Genes Chromosom Cancer 2:48–52, 1990

119. Kiechle-Schwarz M, Sreekantaiah C, Berger CS et al: Nonrandom cytogenetic changes in leiomyomas of the female genitourinary tract: A report of 35 cases. Cancer Genet Cytogenet 53:125–136, 1991

120. Vanni R, Lecca U, Faa G: Uterine leiomyoma cytogenetics. II. Report of forty cases. Cancer Genet Cytogenet 53:247–256, 1991

121. Dal Cin P, Sandberg AA: Chromosome changes in soft tissue tumors: Benign and malignant. Cancer Invest 7:63–76, 1989

122. Meloni AM, Surti U, Contento AM et al: Uterine leiomyomas: Cytogenetic and histologic profile. Obstet Gynecol 80:209–217, 1992

123. Pandis N, Heim S, Bardi G et al: Chromosome analysis of 96 uterine leiomyomas. Cancer Genet Cytogenet 55:11–18, 1991

124. Calabrese G, DiVirgilio C, Cianchetti E et al: Chromosome abnormalities in breast fibroadenomas. Genes Chromosomes Cancer 3:202–204, 1991

125. Nielsen KV, Briand P: Cytogenetic analysis of in vitro karyotype evolution in a cell line established from nonmalignant human mammary epithelium. Cancer Genet Cytogenet 39:103–118, 1989

126. Fletcher JA, Pinkus GS, Morton CC: Combined immunohistochemical/cytogenetic (IH/C) approach reveals lineage

127. Rosai J: Borderline epithelial lesions of the breast. Am J Surg Pathol 15:209–221, 1991

128. Nielsen KW, Blichert-Toft M, Andersen JA: Chromosome analysis of in situ breast cancer. Acta Oncol 28:919–922, 1989

129. Limon J, Dal Cin P, Sandberg AA: Applications of long-term collagenase disaggregation for the cytogenetic analysis of human solid tumors. Cancer Genet Cytogenet 23:305–313, 1986

130. Pandis N, Heim S, Bardi G et al: Improved technique for short-term culture and cytogenetics analysis of human breast cancer. Genes Chromosom Cancer 5:14–20, 1992

131. Haseltine WA, Sodroski J, Patarca R et al: Structure of 3′ terminal region of type II human lymphotrophic virus: Evidence for a new coding region. Science 225:419–421, 1984

132. Garrett CT: Oncogenes. Clin Chim Acta 156:1–40, 1986

133. Brodeur GM: The involvement of oncogenes and suppressor genes in human neoplasia. Adv Pediatr 34:1–44, 1987

134. Taparowsky E, Suara Y, Fasano O et al: Activation of the T-24 bladder carcinoma transforming gene is linked to a single amino acid change. Nature 300:762–765, 1982

135. Schimke RT: Gene amplification in cultured animal cells. Cell 37:705–713, 1984

136. Erlich HA, Gelfand D, Sninsky JJ: Recent advances in the polymerase chain reaction. Science 252:1643–1650, 1991

137. Lai E, Birren BW, Clark SM, Simon SI, Hood L: Pulse field electrophoresis. Biotechniques 7:1–9, 1989

138. Couwenhoven RI, Luo W, Snead ML: Colocalization of EGF transcripts and peptides by combined immunohistochemistry and in situ hybridization. J Histochem Cytochem 38:1853–1860, 1990

139. Hayashi M, Ninomiya Y, Parsons J et al: Differential localization of mRNAs of collagen types I and II in chick fibroblasts, chondrocytes and corneal cells by in situ hybridization using cDNA probes. J Cell Biol 102:2302–2307, 1986

140. Piver MS, Baker TR, Piedmonte M, Sandecki AM: Epidemiology and etiology of ovarian cancer. Semin Oncol 18:177–185, 1991

141. Slamon DJ, Godolphin W, Jones LA et al: Studies of the HER-2/neu proto-oncogene in human breast and ovarian cancer. Science 244:707–712, 1989

142. Press MF, Jones LA, Godolphin W et al: HER-2/neu oncogene amplification and expression in breast and ovarian cancers. Prog Clin Biol Res 354:209–221, 1990

143. Garuti G, Genazzani AR: Human neu oncogene is expressed in endometrial but not in ovarian adenocarcinoma. Cancer 67:1713, 1991

144. Ito K, Sasano H, Ozawa N, Sato S, Silverberg SG, Yajima A: Immunolocalization of EGFR and c-erb-B2 oncogene products in human ovarian cancer. Int J Gynecol Pathol 11:253–257, 1992

145. Sasano H, Garrett CT, Wilkinson DS et al: Proto-oncogene amplification and tumor ploidy in human ovarian neoplasms. Hum Pathol 21:382–391, 1990

146. Perez RP, Godwin AK, Hamilton TC, Ozols RF: Ovarian cancer biology. Semin Oncol 18:186–204, 1991

147. Rodenburg CJ, Koelma IA, Nap M, Fleuren GJ: Immunohistochemical detection of the ras oncogene product p21 in advanced ovarian cancer: Lack of correlation with clinical outcome. Arch Pathol Lab Med 112:151–154, 1988

148. Shreiber G, Dubeau L: C-myc proto-oncogene amplification detected by polymerase chain reaction in archival human ovarian carcinomas. Am J Pathol 137:653–658, 1990

149. Slamon DJ, de Kernion JB, Verma IM, Cline MJ: Expression of cellular oncogenes in human malignancy. Science 224:256–262, 1984

150. Silverberg SG: Prognostic significance of pathologic features in ovarian carcinoma. Curr Top Pathol 78:85–109, 1989

151. Zang X, Silva E, Gershenson D, Hung M-C: Amplification and rearrangement of c-erb-proto-oncogene in cancer of human female genital tract. Oncogene 4:985–989, 1989

152. Berchuck A, Kamel A, Whitaker R et al: Overexpression of HER-2/neu is associated with poor survival in advanced epithelial ovarian cancer. Cancer Res 50:4087–4091, 1990

153. Zhou DJ, Gonzales-Cadavid N, Ahuva H et al: A unique pattern of proto-oncogene abnormalities in ovarian adenocarcinoma. Cancer 62:1573–1576, 1988

154. Masuda H, Battifora H, Yokota J et al: Specificity of proto-oncogene amplification in human malignant diseases. Mol Biol Med 4:213–227, 1987

155. Van't Veer LJ, Hermens R, van der Bakker LAM et al: Ras oncogene activation in human ovarian carcinoma. Oncogene 2:157–165, 1988

156. Fukumoto M, Estensen RD, Sha L et al: Association of ki-ras with amplified DNA sequences detected in human ovarian carcinomas by a modified in-gel renaturation assay. Cancer Res 49:1693–1697, 1989

157. Boltz EM, Kefford RF, Leary JA et al: Amplification of c-ras-ki oncogene in human ovarian tumors. Int J Cancer 43:423–430, 1989

158. Enomoto T, Inoue M, Perantoni AO et al: K-ras activation in neoplasms of the human female reproductive tract. Cancer Res 50:6139–6145, 1990

159. Chien C-H, Chang K-T, Chow S-N: Amplification and expression of c-ki-ras oncogene in human ovarian cancer. Proc Natl Sci Counc Repub China [B] 14:27–32, 1990

160. Sasano H, Nagura H, Silverberg SG: Immunolocalization of c-myc oncoprotein in mucinous and serous adenocarcinomas of the ovary. Hum Pathol 23:491–495, 1992

161. Haas M, Isakov J, Howell SB: Evidence against ras activation in human ovarian carcinomas. Mol Biol Med 4:265–275, 1987

162. Watson JV, Curling OM, Munn CF, Hudson CN: Oncogene expression in ovarian cancer: A pilot study of c-myc oncoprotein in serous papillary ovarian cancer. Gynecol Oncol 28:137–150, 1987

163. Polacarz SV, Hey NA, Stephenson TJ, Hill AS: C-myc oncogene product p62$^{c\text{-}myc}$ in ovarian mucinous neoplasms: Immunohistochemical study correlated with malignancy. J Clin Pathol 42:148–152, 1989

164. Lee JH, Kavanagh JJ, Wharton JT et al: Allele loss at the c-Ha-ras1 locus in human ovarian cancer. Cancer Res 49:1220–1222, 1989

165. Riou G, Barrois M, Le MG et al: C-myc proto-oncogene expression and prognosis in early carcinoma of the uterine cervix. Lancet 1(8536):761–763, 1987

166. Riou G, Barrois M, Sheng ZM et al: Somatic deletion and mutations of c-Ha-ras gene in human cervical cancers. Oncogene 3:329–333, 1988

167. Riou G, Bourhis J, Le MG: The c-myc proto-oncogene in invasive carcinomas of the uterine cervix: Clinical relevance of overexpression in early stages of the cancer. Anticancer Res 10:1225–1232, 1990

168. Bourhis J, Le MG, Barrois M et al: Prognostic value of c-myc proto-oncogene overexpression in early invasive carcinoma of the cervix. J Clin Oncol 8:1789–1796, 1990

169. Durst M, Crose CM, Grissman L et al: Papilloma virus sequences integrate near cellular oncogenes in some cervical carcinomas. Proc Natl Acad Sci U S A 84:1070–1074, 1987

170. Dyson N, Howley PM, Munger K, Harlow E: The human papilloma virus-16E7 oncoprotein is able to bind to the retinoblastoma gene product. Science 243:934–940, 1989

171. Brumm C, Riviere A, Wilckens C, Loning T: Immunohistochemical investigation and northern blot analysis of c-erb-B2 expression in normal, premalignant and malignant tissues of the corpus and cervix uteri. Virchows Arch A Pathol Anat Histopathol 417:477–484, 1990

172. Sato S, Ito K, Ozawa N, Yajima A, Sasano H: Expression of c-myc, epidermal growth factor receptor and c-erb-B2 in human endometrial carcinoma and cervical adenocarcinoma. Tohoku J Exp Med 165:137–145, 1991

173. DiLuca D, Costa S, Monini P et al: Search for human papillomavirus, herpes simplex virus and c-myc oncogene in human genital tumors. Int J Cancer 43:570–577, 1989

174. Ocadiz R, Sauceda R, Cruz M et al: High correlation between alterations of c-myc oncogene and carcinoma of the uterine cervix. Cancer Res 47:4173–4177, 1987

175. Baker VV, Hatch KD, Shingleton HM: Amplification of c-myc proto-oncogene in cervical carcinoma. J Surg Oncol 39:225–228, 1988

176. Hendy-Ibbs P, Cox H, Evan GI, Watson JV: Flow cytometric quantitation of DNA and c-myc oncoprotein in archival biopsies of uterine cervix neoplasia. Br J Cancer 55:275–282, 1987

177. Hughes RA, Neill WA, Norval M: Papilloma virus and c-myc antigen expression in normal and neoplastic cervical epithelium. J Clin Pathol 42:46–51, 1989

178. Sagae S, Kuzumaki N, Hisada T et al: Ras oncogene expression and prognosis of invasive squamous carcinoma of the uterine cervix. Cancer 63:1577–1582, 1989

179. Berchuck A, Rodriguez G, Kamel A et al: Expression of epidermal growth factor receptor and HER-21 neu in normal and neoplastic cervix, vulva and vagina. Obstet Gynecol 76:381–387, 1990

180. Hayashi Y, Hachisuga T, Iwasaka T et al: Expression of ras oncogene product and EGF receptor in cervical squamous cell carcinoma and its relationship to lymph node involvement. Gynecol Oncol 40:147–151, 1991

181. Riviere A, Wilckens C, Loning T: Expression of c-erb-B2 and c-myc in squamous cell carcinomas of the head and neck and the lower female genital tract. J Oral Pathol Med 19:408–413, 1990

182. Sato S, Ito K, Ozawa N et al: Analysis of point mutations at codon 12 of k-ras in human endometrial carcinoma and cervical adenocarcinoma by dot blot hybridization and polymerase chain reaction. Tohoku J Exp Med 165:131–136, 1991

183. Long CA, O'Brien TJ, Sanders MM et al: A ras oncogene is expressed in adenocarcinoma of the endometrium. Am J Obstet Gynecol 159:1512–1515, 1988

184. Machotka SV, Garrett CT, Schwartz AM, Callahan R: Amplification of the proto-oncogenes int-2, c-erbB-2 and c-myc in human breast cancer. Clin Chim Acta 184:207–218, 1989

185. Sasano H, Comerford J, Wilkinson DS et al: Serous papillary adenocarcinoma of the endometrium: Proto-oncogene amplification, flow cytometry, estrogen and progesterone receptors and immunohistochemical analysis. Cancer 65:1545–1551, 1990

186. Kacinski BM, Carter D, Mittal K et al: High level expression of fms proto-oncogene mRNA is observed in clinically aggressive human endometrial adenocarcinoma. Int J Radiat Oncol Biol Phys 15:823–829, 1988

187. Borst MP, Baker VV, Dixon D et al: Oncogene alterations in endometrial carcinoma. Gynecol Oncol 38:364–366, 1990

188. Berchuck A, Rodriguez G, Kinney RB et al: Overexpression of HER-2/neu in endometrial cancer is associated with advanced stage disease. Am J Obstet Gynecol 164:15–21, 1991

189. Sato S, Jiko K, Ito K et al: Expression of c-myc RNA and protein in human endometrial carcinoma: Simultaneous study of in situ hybridization and immunohistochemistry. Tohoku J Exp Med 1993

190. Anderson G, Mihich E, Nishimura S et al: Molecular aspects of growth control. Cancer Res 49:6852–6866, 1989

191. Klein G: The approaching era of the tumor suppressor genes. Science 238:1539–1550, 1987

192. Sager R: Genetic suppression of tumor formation: A new frontier in cancer research. Cancer Res 46:1573–1580, 1986

193. Sager R: Tumor suppressor genes: The puzzle and the promise. Science 246:1406–1412, 1989

194. Hinds P, Finlay C, Levine AJ: Mutation is required to acti-

vate the p53 gene for cooperation with the ras oncogene and transformation. J Virol 63:739–746, 1989

195. Stoker M: Regulation of growth and orientation in hamster cells transformed by polyoma virus. Virology 24:165–174, 1964

196. Soussi T, Caron de Fromentel C, May P: Structural aspects of the p53 protein in relation to gene evolution. Oncogene 5:945–952, 1990

197. Fearon ER, Cho KR, Nigro JM et al: Identification of a chromosome 18q gene that is altered in colorectal cancer. Science 247:49–56, 1990

198. Friend SH, Bernard SR, Rogelj S et al: A human DNA segment with properties of the gene that predisposes to retinoblastoma and osteosarcoma. Nature 323:643–646, 1986

199. Fung Y-KT, Murphree AL, T'Ang A et al: Structural evidence for the authenticity of the human retinoblastoma gene. Science 244:217–221, 1987

200. Lee EY-HP, To H, Shew J-Y et al: Inactivation of the retinoblastoma susceptibility gene in human breast cancers. Science 241:218–221, 1988

201. Xu H-J, Hu S-X, Benedict WF: Lack of nuclear RB protein staining in GO/ middle G1 cells: Correlation to changes in total RB protein levels. Oncogene 6:1139–1146, 1991

202. Lane DP, Crawford LV: T antigen is bound to a host protein in SV40 transformed cells. Nature 278:261–263, 1979

203. Eliyahu D, Raz A, Gruss P et al: Participation of p53 cellular tumor antigen in transformation of normal embryonic cells. Nature 312:646–649, 1984

204. Yokota J, Tsukada Y, Nakajima T et al: Loss of heterozygosity on the short arm of chromosome 3 in carcinoma of the uterine cervix. Cancer Res 49:3598–3601, 1989

205. Sato T, Saito H, Morita R et al: Allelotype type of human ovarian cancer. Cancer Res 51:5118–5122, 1991

206. Okamoto A, Sameshima Y, Yamada Y et al: Allelic loss of chromosome 17p and p53 mutations in human endometrial carcinoma of the uterus. Cancer Res 51:5632–5635, 1991

207. Ehlen T, Dubeau L: Loss of heterozygosity on chromosomal segments 3p, 6q, and 11p in human ovarian carcinomas. Oncogene 5:219–224, 1990

208. Eccles DM, Cranston G, Steel CM et al: Allele losses on chromosome 17 in human epithelial ovarian carcinoma. Oncogene 5:1599–1601, 1990

209. Russell SEH, Hickey GI, Lowry WS et al: Allele loss from chromosome 17 in ovarian cancer. Oncogene 5:1581–1583, 1990

210. Viel A, De Pascale L, Toffoli G et al: Frequent occurrence of Ha-ras1 allelic deletion in human ovarian adenocarcinomas. Tumori 77:16–20, 1991

211. Lee JH, Kavanagh JJ, Wildrick DM et al: Frequent loss of heterozygosity on chromosomes 6q, 11 and 17 in human ovarian carcinomas. Cancer Res 50:2724–2728, 1990

212. Sasano H, Comerford J, Silverberg SG, Garrett CT: Analysis of abnormalities of the retinoblastoma gene in human ovarian and endometrial carcinoma. Cancer 66:2150–2154, 1990

213. Li SB, Schwartz PE, Lee W-H, Yang-Feng TL: Allele loss at the retinoblastoma locus in human ovarian cancer. J Natl Cancer Inst 83:637–640, 1991

214. Mazars R, Pujol P, Maudelonde T et al: p53 mutations in ovarian cancer: A late event? Oncogene 6:1685–1690, 1991

215. Marks JR, Davidoff AM, Kerns BJ et al: Overexpression and mutation of p53 in epithelial ovarian cancer. Cancer Res 51:2979–2984, 1991

216. Kihana T, Tsuda H, Okada S et al: Analysis of abnormalities of p53 tumor suppressor gene in ovarian cancer. Jpn J Cancer Res 50:107, 1991

217. Mashiyama S, Murakami Y, Yoshimoto T et al: Detection of p53 gene mutations in human brain tumors by single strand conformation polymorphism analysis of polymerase chain reaction products. Oncogene 6:1313–1318, 1991

218. Levine AJ, Moman J, Finlay CA: The p53 tumor suppressor gene. Nature 351:453–456, 1991

219. Crook T, Wrede D, Tidy J et al: Status of c-myc, p53 and retinoblastoma genes in human papillomavirus positive and negative squamous cell carcinoma of the anus. Oncogene 6:1251–1257, 1991

220. Nasim S, Mizuuchi H, Garrett CT: Direct DNA sequencing of polymerase chain reaction amplified fragments in evaluation of neoplastic disease. Proc Ann Am Assoc Cancer 31:328, 1990

Index

Page numbers followed by f *indicate figures; page numbers followed by* t *indicate tables;* CF *indicates color figures.*